AF731616

REVIEW OF SURGERY FOR NEET SS/INI SS

Reference: Sabiston's Textbook of Surgery, 21st Edition

Authors

Alhad Naragude
MBBS, MS

Sourabh Ghewade
MBBS, MS

Peepee Publishers and Distributors (P) Ltd.®

REVIEW OF SURGERY FOR NEET SS/INI SS

Published by
Pawaninder P. Vij and Anupam Vij

Peepee Publishers and Distributors (P) Ltd.
Head Office: 160, Shakti Vihar, Pitam Pura, Delhi-110 034 (India)

Correspondence Address:
7/31, First Floor, Ansari Road, Daryaganj
New Delhi-110 002 (India)
Ph: 011-41512412, 011-23246245, 9811156083
e-mail: peepee160@yahoo.co.in
e-mail: peepee160@gmail.com
www.peepeepub.com
join us on facebook.com/pp.publishers

© 2023 Peepee Publishers and Distributors (P) Ltd.

All rights reserved

No part of this publication may be reproduced or transmitted in any form or by any means, electronic, mechanical, photocopy, recording, translated, or any information storage and retrieval system, without permission in writing from the editor and the publisher.

This book has been published in good faith that the material provided by authors/contributors is original. Every effort is made to ensure accuracy of material, but publisher and printer will not be held responsible for any inadvertent errors. In case of any dispute, all legal matters to be settled under Delhi jurisdiction only.

First Edition: 2023

ISBN: 978-81-9523-445-5

FOREWORD

Review of Surgery for NEET SS/INI SS is an excellent compilation of multiple choice questions from Sabiston's Textbook of Surgery. It covers the entire gamut of general surgery topics which is essential for a surgical postgraduate student who wishes to superspecialise. This book is a comprehensive and yet concise source of information. Reading a chapter from Sabiston's Textbook of Surgery and then reviewing the MCQs from this book should help the learner grasp and recollect important facts and concepts needed to clear the entrance exam with flying colors.

Dr Alhad Naragude and Dr Sourabh Ghewade, both being students of LTMM College, have co-authored this book. Dr Naragude and Dr Ghewade are well mannered, knowledgeable, sincere and hard-working surgeons who have always evinced a keen interest in teaching undergraduate and postgraduate students. It gives me immense pleasure to write a foreword to this book which, I am sure, will benefit and guide young surgeons to clear the NEET super specialty entrance examinations successfully. I wish both the authors the very best in all their future endeavors.

Dr Sandhya P Iyer
Professor of Surgery
LTMM College and LTMGH
Mumbai, India

PREFACE

The idea to write this book came to us when we were preparing for our exam. It brings us immense pleasure while presenting this book to our fellow NEET SS aspirants. In our maiden attempt to author a book, we have compiled over **7000 MCQs** from **Sabiston Textbook of Surgery, 21st Edition**.

It took a significant period of time to ensure that all essential facts and concepts from the book were covered in detail. Efforts have been made to cross refer and arrange every MCQ and check its authenticity with **Sabiston Textbook of Surgery, 21st Edition**.

We sincerely thank all our friends and colleagues who have supported us during our residency and preparations for the entrance exam. We thank our teachers and parents for being there for us at all times.

We express our gratitude to Mr Pawaninder Paul Vij and the whole team of Peepee Publishers and Distributors (P) Ltd for supporting us through this process of authoring our first book. It was an amazing experience working with them. Their constant support and follow-up was essential during the entire process of MCQ compilation with guidance when needed.

Finally, we have faith that this book will definitely help future NEET SS General Surgery aspirants **(150 Qs)** and INI-SS aspirants **(40 Qs)** get through this tough phase of something every medical student never fancies but has to go through, to enter the field of his/her choice. During this process of solving the MCQs, if the reader comes across any errata, they can mail the corrections to ***sushrutasamhitasurgery@gmail.com*** or our Instagram page ***sushrutasamhita_sx*** or our Facebook page ***sushrutasamhita_sx***.

Dr Alhad Naragude
MBBS, MS
Dr Sourabh Ghewade
MBBS, MS

HOW TO USE THIS BOOK?

- Read a chapter from Sabiston Textbook of Surgery.
- Solve the MCQs and check the knowledge retained.
- Mark and revise important missed points while reviewing the book.
- Follow us on Instagram and Facebook for errata and daily free MCQs ***sushrutasamhita_sx***.

CONTENTS

1

The Rise of Modern Surgery: An Overview

KNOWLEDGE OF ANATOMY

1. **De Humani Corporis Fabrica Libri Septem was written by:**

   A. William Cowper   B. Andreas Vesalius
   C. Ambroise Paré   D. Harvey Cushing

2. **Who showed that the heart acts as a pump and forces blood along the arteries and back via veins, forming a closed loop?**

   A. William Cowper   B. Andreas Vesalius
   C. Ambroise Paré   D. William Harvey

CONTROL OF BLEEDING

3. **Who proposed a method to control hemorrhage during a surgical operation?**

   A. William Cowper   B. Andreas Vesalius
   C. Ambroise Paré   D. William Harvey

4. **Combination of concoction of egg yolk, rose oil (a combination of ground-up rose petals and olive oil) and turpentine, was used for haemostasis by:**

   A. William Cowper   B. Andreas Vesalius
   C. Ambroise Paré   D. William Harvey

5. **Instrument named crow's beak which is used to control bleeding was introduced by:**

   A. William Cowper   B. Andreas Vesalius
   C. Ambroise Paré   D. William Harvey

6. **Screw compressor tourniquet was invented by:**

   A. William Cowper   B. Jean-Louis Petit
   C. Ambroise Paré   D. William Harvey

7. **Electrocautery was developed by:**

   A. Ambroise Paré   B. Jean-Louis Petit
   C. Ambroise Paré   D. William Bovie

CONTROL OF PAIN

8. **Who used sulfuric ether for inhalational anaesthesia?**

   A. Charles T. Jackson   B. Horace Wells
   C. Morton   D. James Corning

9. **Who used nitrous oxide for inhalational anaesthesia?**

   A. Charles T. Jackson   B. Horace Wells
   C. Morton   D. James Corning

10. **Who used cocaine and infiltration anaesthesia with great success?**

    A. Morton   B. Horace Wells
    C. William Halsted   D. James Corning

11. **Who carried out the earliest experiments on spinal anaesthesia?**

    A. Morton   B. Horace Wells
    C. William Halsted   D. James Corning

CONTROL OF INFECTION

12. **Who popularized use of gloves during surgery?**

    A. Halsted   B. Lister
    C. Carrel   D. Nussbaum

13. **Who hypothesized that these invisible "germs", or, as they became known, bacteria, were the cause of wound healing difficulties in surgical patients?**

    A. Halsted   B. Lister
    C. Carrel   D. Nussbaum

14. **Who used chemical antisepsis with carbolic acid (phenol)?**

    A. Halsted   B. Lister
    C. Louis Pasteur   D. Nussbaum

15. **Who developed sterile absorbable sutures?**

    A. Halsted   B. Lister
    C. Louis Pasteur   D. Bergmann

16. Who recommended steam sterilisation?

A. Nussbaum B. Lister
C. Louis Pasteur D. Bergmann

17. The principle of wound treatment by means of surgical debridement and mechanical irrigation with an antiseptic solution was developed by:

A. Nussbaum B. Lister
C. Alexis Carrel D. Volkmann

18. Who devised a single-layer gauze mask to be worn during a surgical operation?

A. Alexis Carrel
B. Jan Mikulicz Radecki
C. Lister
D. Volkmann

OTHER ADVANCES THAT FURTHERED THE RISE OF MODERN SURGERY

19. Who discovered X-rays?

A. Karl Landsteiner B. Louis Harold Gray
C. Wilhelm Roentgen D. George Crile

20. Who discovered human major blood groups?

A. Karl Landsteiner B. Louis Harold Gray
C. Wilhelm Roentgen D. George Crile

21. Who performed the first surgical operation during which a blood transfusion was used?

A. Karl Landsteiner B. Louis Harold Gray
C. Wilhelm Roentgen D. George Crile

22. Who showed how blood could be separated into two main components, red blood cells and plasma, and that the plasma could be frozen for long-term storage leading to the creation of large-scale blood banking?

A. Karl Landsteiner B. Louis Harold Gray
C. Charles Drew D. George Crile

23. Who recommended "freezing microtome" to be used as an aid in diagnosis during a surgical operation?

A. Thomas Cullen B. Joseph Bloodgood
C. Charles Drew D. Nicholas Senn

ASCENT OF SCIENTIFIC SURGERY

24. Who is regarded as "Adam" in American surgery?

A. Halsted B. Harvey
C. Hunter D. Hippocrates

25. Halsted's triad of educational principles?

A. Knowledge of the basic sciences
B. Experimental research
C. Graduated patient responsibility
D. All of the above

26. Who found that antiandrogenic treatment, consisting of orchiectomy or the administration of estrogens, could produce long-term regression in patients with advanced prostatic cancer?

A. Huggins B. Harvey
C. Hunter D. Hippocrates

27. Who won the 1990 Nobel Prize in Physiology or Medicine for his work on organ and cell transplantation in the treatment of human disease, specifically kidney transplant?

A. Joseph Murray B. Helen Taussig
C. Charles Huggins D. Vivien Thomas

THE MODERN ERA

28. Who did the first successful aortic valve homograft?

A. Donald Murray B. Charles Hufnagel
C. Hale Williams D. Luther Hill

29. Who designed and inserted the first workable prosthetic heart valve in a man?

A. Donald Murray B. Charles Hufnagel
C. Hale Williams D. Luther Hill

30. Who devised heart lung bypass machine?

A. Michael DeBakey B. René Favaloro
C. Hale Williams D. John H. Gibbon

31. Who pioneered the use of Dacron grafts?

A. Michael DeBakey B. René Favaloro
C. Hale Williams D. John H. Gibbon

32. Who did the first successful human heart transplant successfully?

A. Michael DeBakey B. Christiaan Barnard
C. Hale Williams D. John H. Gibbon

33. Decompression of mechanical bowel obstruction by a suction apparatus was first demonstrated by:

A. Joseph Murray
B. Charles Huggins
C. Theodor Kocher
D. Owen H. Wangensteen

34. Subclavian artery–pulmonary artery shunt for increasing blood flow to the lungs of a "blue baby" was developed by:

A. Alfred Blalock

B. Helen Taussig

C. Vivien Thomas

D. All of the above

35. DeBakey is probably the best-known American surgeon of the modern era. His contributions include all except:

A. Invented the roller pump

B. Developed ventricular assist devices

C. Created an early version of what became the Mobile Army Saving Hospital (MASH) unit

D. Pioneered the use of Dacron grafts to replace or repair blood vessels

ANSWERS

1. **Ans: B. Andreas Vesalius**
Ref: Chapter No.1, Page No.3-4
2. **Ans: D. William Harvey**
Ref: Chapter No.1, Page No.4
3. **Ans: C. Ambroise Paré**
Ref: Chapter No.1, Page No.4
4. **Ans: C. Ambroise Paré**
Ref: Chapter No.1, Page No.5
5. **Ans: C. Ambroise Paré**
Ref: Chapter No.1, Page No.5
6. **Ans: B. Jean-Louis Petit**
Ref: Chapter No.1, Page No.5
7. **Ans: B. Jean-Louis Petit**
Ref: Chapter No.1, Page No.5
8. **Ans: C. Morton**
Ref: Chapter No.1, Page No.5-6
9. **Ans: B. Horace Wells**
Ref: Chapter No.1, Page No. 5-6
10. **Ans: C. William Halsted**
Ref: Chapter No.1, Page No.5-6
11. **Ans: D. James Corning**
Ref: Chapter No.1, Page No.5-6
12. **Ans: A. Halsted**
Ref: Chapter No.1, Page No.7
13. **Ans: B. Lister**
Ref: Chapter No.1, Page No.6
14. **Ans: B. Lister**
Ref: Chapter No.1, Page No.7
15. **Ans: B. Lister**
Ref: Chapter No.1, Page No.7
16. **Ans: D. Bergmann**
Ref: Chapter No.1, Page No.7
17. **Ans: C. Alexis Carrel**
Ref: Chapter No.1, Page No.7
18. **Ans: B. Jan Mikulicz Radecki**
Ref: Chapter No.1, Page No.7
19. **Ans: C. Wilhelm Roentgen**
Ref: Chapter No.1, Page No.8
20. **Ans: A. Karl Landsteiner**
Ref: Chapter No.1, Page No.8
21. **Ans: D. George Crile**
Ref: Chapter No.1, Page No.8
22. **Ans: C. Charles Drew**
Ref: Chapter No.1, Page No.8
23. **Ans: D. Nicholas Senn**
Ref: Chapter No.1, Page No.8
24. **Ans: A. Halsted**
Ref: Chapter No.1, Page No.10
25. **Ans: D. All of the above**
Ref: Chapter No.1, Page No.10
26. **Ans: A. Huggins**
Ref: Chapter No.1, Page No.11
27. **Ans: A Joseph Murray**
Ref: Chapter No.1, Page No.11
28. **Ans: A. Donald Murray**
Ref: Chapter No.1, Page No.15
29. **Ans: B. Charles Hufnagel**
Ref: Chapter No.1, Page No.15
30. **Ans: D. John H. Gibbon**
Ref: Chapter No.1, Page No.16
31. **Ans: A. Michael DeBakey**
Ref: Chapter No.1, Page No.16
32. **Ans: B. Christiaan Barnard**
Ref: Chapter No.1, Page No.16
33. **Ans: D. Owen H. Wangensteen**
Ref: Chapter No.1, Page No.14
34. **Ans: D. All of the above**
Ref: Chapter No.1, Page No.15
35. **Ans: C. Created an early version of what became the Mobile Army Saving Hospital (MASH) unit**
Ref: Chapter No.1, Page No.16

2

Ethics and Professionalism in Surgery

1. **Foundational elements by which we view ethical issues includes all except:**
   A. Autonomy B. Beneficence
   C. Maleficence D. Justice

2. **Edmond Pellegrino, indicated that essential virtues of medical practice include all except:**
   A. Fidelity to trust
   B. Suppression of self-interest
   C. Speciality training
   D. Compassion, courage and prudence

3. **The method in which, one would attempt to derive principles from previously resolved cases and apply them to the issues or conflicts at hand is called as:**
   A. Consequentialism
   B. Nonconsequentialism
   C. Casuistry
   D. Feminism

4. **Topics commonly used to analyse ethical dilemmas in health care are all except:**
   A. Medical Indications B. Doctor's Preferences
   C. Quality of Life D. Contextual Features

5. **Principles used in the topic of Quality-of-Life includes all except:**
   A. Beneficence
   B. Nonmaleficence
   C. Respect for Autonomy
   D. Justice

6. **Principle used in the topic of patient preference includes:**
   A. Beneficence
   B. Nonmaleficence
   C. Respect for Autonomy
   D. Justice

7. **Justice (Fairness) as a principle, is used in which topic to analyse ethical dilemmas in health care?**
   A. Medical Indications B. Doctor's Preferences
   C. Quality of Life D. Contextual Features

8. **The "Informed consent" honours which of the following principle of ethical practice?**
   A. Beneficence
   B. Nonmaleficence
   C. Respect for Autonomy
   D. Justice

9. **The Hippocratic notion of *"primum non nocere"* is often invoked as a maxim to convey our commitment to the care and healing of the patient. Which of the following ethical principles are followed by this notion?**
   a. Beneficence b. Nonmaleficence
   c. Respect for Autonomy d. Justice
   A. a,b,c B. a,b,c,d
   C. a,c,d D. a,b

10. **All of the following are true about casuistry except:**
    A. Advantage of a casuistic approach is that it is steeped in clinical reality, which may offer concrete, pragmatic solutions to ethical dilemmas
    B. In this method, one would attempt to derive principles from previously resolved cases and apply them to the issues or conflicts at hand
    C. Single case is usually enough to abstract grand notions for ethical analysis
    D. Casuistry is one of the mechanisms for ethical enquiry, which refers to case-based analysis

11. **Collecting significant facts and understanding the perspectives of relevant stakeholders is important step in ethical issue resolution. Which of the following is the most commonly used tool to**

collect relevant information to analyse an ethical dilemma?

A. Four Topics Method

B. Three Topics Method

C. Sequence analysis collection

D. Two Topics Method

12. Mrs Geeta is an 80-year-old woman with advanced breast cancer who presents with a fungating malodorous lesion. The cancer is treatment-refractory and her current goals of care, in coordination with the palliative care team, include a focus on quality of life and comfort. She was referred to surgery for lesion resection. She is currently not receiving therapeutic interventions and has an Out-of-Hospital Do Not Resuscitate (DNR) order. Ms. Smith informs the team that someone told her the DNR order must be rescinded or she cannot have the procedure. What should be the next best plan of action for this patient?

A. Do not offer surgery unless Ms. Smith agrees to full resuscitation

B. Offer surgery with the explicit agreement and Ms. Smith's consent that no attempts at resuscitation will be made during the procedure

C. Reach an agreement with Ms. Smith that limited attempts at resuscitation can be made, if appropriate

D. Explain all the possibilities with possible consequences (good or bad) to the patient and relatives and finally reach a shared decision

ANSWERS

1. **Ans: C. Maleficence**

   Ref: Chapter No.2, Page No.20

2. **Ans: C. Speciality training**

   Ref: Chapter No.2, Page No.21

3. **Ans: C. Casuistry**

   Ref: Chapter No.2, Page No.21

4. **Ans: B. Doctor's Preferences**

   Ref: Chapter No.2, Page No.22

5. **Ans: D. Justice**

   Ref: Chapter No.2, Page No.22

6. **Ans: C. Respect for Autonomy**

   Ref: Chapter No.2, Page No.22

7. **Ans: D. Contextual Features**

   Ref: Chapter No.2, Page No.22

8. **Ans: C. Respect for Autonomy**

   Ref: Chapter No.2, Page No.20

9. **Ans: D. a,b**

   Ref: Chapter No.2, Page No.20

10. **Ans: C. Single case is usually enough to abstract grand notions for ethical analysis**

    Ref: Chapter No.2, Page No.21

11. **Ans: A. Four Topics Method**

    Ref: Chapter No.2, Page No.21

12. **Ans: D. Explain all the possibilities with possible consequences (good or bad) to the patient and relatives and finally reach a shared decision**

    Ref: Chapter No.2, Page No.23

3

The Inflammatory Response

COMPONENTS OF THE INFLAMMATORY RESPONSE

1. **About Neutrophils, all statements are true except:**
   A. A potent mediator of acute inflammation
   B. Last cell type recruited in response to injury and infection
   C. The neutrophil granules contain a number of proteases that are essential for tissue remodeling and wound healing
   D. They directly stimulate angiogenesis via release of vascular endothelial growth factors (VEGFs)

2. **Production of Neutrophils is regulated by __ from T-cells.**
   A. IL 5 B. IL 17
   C. IL 23 D. IL 4

3. **Production of Neutrophils is regulated by __ from macrophages.**
   A. IL 5 B. IL 17
   C. IL 23 D. IL 4

4. **Neutrophils have a half-life of approximately __ hours.**
   A. 24 hrs B. 6 hrs
   C. 12 hrs D. 8 hrs

5. **About Neutrophils, all statements are true except:**
   A. Neutrophils contain three types of proinflammatory granules
   B. Extracellular pathogens are trapped within the NET to prevent spread of the pathogen and aid phagocytosis
   C. Neutrophils also release fiber meshwork to which histones, proteins, and enzymes adhere; this is the neutrophil extracellular trap (NET)
   D. All of the above are true

6. **Wrong about neutrophil recruitment and migration from blood to peripheral tissue:**
   A. Tethering–E-Selectin
   B. Adhesion–ICAM
   C. Transmigration–PECAM
   D. Adhesion–Cadherin

7. **About Macrophages, all statements are true except:**
   A. Monocytes, the precursor to the macrophage, differentiate into macrophages in response to infection and tissue injury
   B. Macrophages also process antigenic substances and present them on their surface to help stimulate the differentiation of helper T cells
   C. Kupffer cells of the liver and microglia of the central nervous system are macrophages
   D. High concentrations of M2-type cytokines correlate with mortality in sepsis models

8. **About M1 macrophages, all statements are true except:**
   A. High concentrations of M1-type cytokines correlate with mortality in sepsis models
   B. M1 are predominant in viral and bacterial infection
   C. High concentrations of M1-type cytokines correlate with mortality in sepsis models
   D. M1 macrophages are essential for tissue remodelling and wound healing; they express a variety of anti-inflammatory markers, including IL-10

9. **About Dendritic cells, all statements are true except:**
   A. Dendritic cells bridge the innate and adaptive immune response as the major professional APC

B. These antigenic proteins are loaded onto a major histocompatibility (MHC) complex class I or class II molecule
C. Intracellular proteins are processed within the cytosol by the proteasome, and they are presented via the MHC class I molecule to CD8+ cytotoxic T cells
D. Extracellular proteins are processed within the dendritic cell lysosome, and they are presented in conjunction with the MHC class I molecule to activate CD8+ cytotoxic T cells

10. Which of the following match is wrong?

A. Interferon (IFN) type 1 - antiviral predominant response and drives activation of CD8+ cytotoxic T cells
B. IL-17 - differentiation of helper T cell type 1 (Th1) cells
C. IL-4 - differentiation to Th2 cells
D. IL-6 and transforming growth factor-β (TGF-β) - differentiation of Th17 cells

11. About T cells, all statements are true except:

A. Th1 cells primarily fight intracellular pathogens and do so via upregulation of IFN-γ
B. Th2 cells function to clear extracellular pathogens and mediate the allergic response through production of IL-4, IL-5 and IL-13
C. Th17 cells differentiate in response to extracellular pathogens and fungi
D. Th17 cells can acquire the characteristic of Th2 cells in chronic inflammatory states

12. About T cells, all statements are true except:

A. T cells play a role in the destruction of circulating tumor cells and the prevention of micro metastasis
B. The regulatory T cells increase at 72 hours postoperatively correlated with a larger tumor size, human epidermal growth factor receptor-2 (HER2) positivity, and decrease in the length of disease-free survival
C. A lower burden of Th1 cells was correlated with a greater tumor burden and HER2 positivity
D. All of the above

13. Studies have shown that the adaptive T cell–dependent inflammatory response is dampened after all of the following except:

A. General anaesthesia B. Blood transfusion
C. Hyperthermia D. Hyperglycaemia

14. About B cells, all statements are true except:

A. B cells undergo a process termed V(D)J recombination
B. Immunoglobulins have the capacity to recognize more than 5×10^{13} different antibodies
C. Marginal zone B cells function in the spleen as the first line of defense against blood borne invaders
D. Dependent of T cells, marginal zone B cells can rapidly produce soluble IgM during the early stages of infection

15. CD80 is also called as:

A. B7-1 B. B7-2
C. PD-L1 D. PD-L2

16. CD86 is also called as:

A. B7-1 B. B7-2
C. PD-L1 D. PD-L2

17. CD274 is also called as:

A. B7-1 B. B7-2
C. PD-L1 D. PD-L2

18. Major function of CTLA-4 is:

A. Activation of naive T cells
B. Inhibition of T cell
C. Generation of Tfh cells
D. Induction of immune responses

19. Generation of Tfh cells is by:

A. CTLA-4 B. CD28
C. ICOS D. PD-1

20. About TLRs', true statement is:

A. TLR4 plays a key role in recognition of bacterial LPS
B. TLR1, TLR2 and TLR6 recognize other common bacterial lipoproteins
C. TLR4 plays a role in recognition of high-mobility group box protein 1 (HMGB1) and heat shock protein 70
D. All of the above

21. Key cytokines involved in the acute proinflammatory response include:

A. TNF-α B. IL-2
C. L-8 D. IFN-γ

22. False statement about TNF-α is:

A. TNF-α is a protein secreted by both innate and adaptive immune cells, as well as nonimmune cells, such as fibroblasts

B. Along with IL-1, it is released rapidly in response to foreign invaders and tissue injury
C. TNF-α prompts cell signalling by binding to TNF receptor 1 (TNFR1) or TNFR2 – two transmembrane receptors found on a large variety of cells
D. All of the above are true statements

23. False statement about IL 1 is:

A. IL-1 is a hyperacute proinflammatory cytokine with a half-life of approximately 10 minutes
B. Increased platelet count
C. Hepatocellular injury
D. All of the above are true

24. True statement about IL 6 is:

A. Induces hepatic synthesis of acute-phase proteins
B. In trauma patients with SIRS, sepsis, or multiorgan dysfunction syndrome (MODS), IL-6 is currently considered the most accurate prognosticator of outcome with increased and sustained levels of IL-6 directly correlating with a poorer prognosis
C. IL-6 also has anti-inflammatory effects
D. All of the above are true

25. Physiologic effects are induced by infusing IL 1 or TNF into human subjects. Effect that is seen only by IL 1 and not by TNF is:

A. Pulmonary edema
B. Hepatocellular injury
C. Increased platelet count
D. Hypozincemia

26. False statement about TGF-β is:

A. TGF-β1 is found within the bone, cartilage and skin
B. TGF-β2 is expressed in neurons and astroglial cells
C. TGF-β3 is localized to the palate and lung tissue
D. All of the above are true

27. False statement about TGF-β is:

A. In late malignancy, TGF-β functions as a tumor suppressor
B. In healthy cells, TGF-β arrests the cell in the G1 phase of mitosis and thus limits cell division
C. Malignant cells can turn TGF-β to their advantage and use it to promote tumor cell proliferation, invasion and metastasis
D. Malignant cells can use TGF-β to proliferate, metastasize, and evade phagocytic and chemotoxic cells of the immune response

28. Food and Drug Administration (FDA) approved drug in the treatment of paroxysmal nocturnal hemoglobinuria and atypical hemolytic uremic syndrome (aHUS) is:

A. Nivolumab
B. Pembrolizumab
C. Eculizumab
D. Vedozulimab

29. True statement about complement system is:

A. First in its class, the therapeutic agent eculizumab is an anti-C5 antibody
B. It is approved by the U.S. Food and Drug Administration (FDA) in the treatment of paroxysmal nocturnal hemoglobinuria and atypical hemolytic uremic syndrome (aHUS)
C. Eculizumab has off-label uses in many processes, ranging from nephropathies to transplant medicine
D. All of the above are true

30. False statement about Neural regulation of the innate immune system is:

A. The vagus participates in the cholinergic anti-inflammatory pathway
B. This pathway has been demonstrated in the liver, heart, pancreas, and gastrointestinal tract to suppress excess inflammation
C. Many efferent motor vagal nerve fibres travel to the spleen via the vagus nerve
D. Both A and B

31. True statement about Neural regulation of the adaptive immune system is:

A. The inflammatory reflex arc has been linked to antibody production in B cells following exposure to blood borne antigens
B. In response to Streptococcus pneumoniae infection, vagus nerve signalling has been shown to promote retention of B cells within the marginal zone of the spleen
C. Daily treatment of the α7 nicotinic receptor with an agonist result in a 50% reduction of antibody production within the spleen during times of infection
D. All of the above

32. Proinflammatory cytokines that exert effects at all three levels of the HPA axis are all except:

A. TNF-α
B. IL 1
C. IL 2
D. IL-6

INFLAMMATION AND THE CRITICALLY ILL

33. Mortality of multiorgan failure is:

A. 20% to 40% B. 40% to 80%
C. 60% to 90% D. 80% to 90%

34. Late mortality in Multiorgan failure was attributed to:

A. Secondary nosocomial infections
B. Single Severe insult
C. Genetic Causes
D. Trauma

35. False statement among the following is:

A. Early mortality in MOF can occur following a single severe insult or a series of amplifying insults
B. Late mortality in MOF was attributed to secondary nosocomial infections
C. As overall deaths from MOF decline, more patients are moving into a state of chronic critical illness
D. All of the above are true

36. Therapies to counter SIRS includes all except:

A. Anti-TNF antibody
B. Recombinant IL-1Ra
C. Recombinant activated protein C
D. Interferons

37. True regarding Compensatory Anti-inflammatory Response 9 (CARS) is all except:

A. CARS can be described as suppression of the adaptive immune system
B. CARS has been tied to an increase in anti-inflammatory IL-10 and IL-6 and a downregulation of the human leukocyte antigen DR
C. HLA-DR is one of several molecules that can make up the MHC class I surface complex
D. In both CD4+ and CD8+ populations, memory T cells fail to develop

38. True regarding diagnosis and immunotherapy in sepsis is/are all except:

A. The loss of HLA-DR in the acute postoperative period has been linked to increased postoperative infection
B. Granulocyte-macrophage colony-stimulating factor (GM-CSF) may also improve expression of HLA-DR among critically ill patients
C. Treatment in vitro with IFN-γ, however, improved antigen presentation among monocytes postoperatively
D. All of the above are true

39. Which of the following is not a diagnostic gene expression microarray?

A. Sepsis MetaScore B. FAIM3:PLAC8 ratio
C. Septicyte Lab D. Denver Score

40. What remains one of the strongest MOF risk factors?

A. Abdominal Compartment Syndrome
B. Early transfusion requirement
C. Infection
D. Advanced Age

41. Those patients who develop MOF exhibit a profound neutropenia within __ hours postinjury.

A. 2 to 4 B. 4 to 6
C. 6 to 12 D. 12 to 24

42. Risk factors for Multiorgan Failure includes all except:

A. Advanced age
B. Increased body mass index (BMI)
C. Female sex
D. Injury severity score

43. True Statement in the following is/are all except:

A. Male sex confers a greater risk of death
B. Early transfusion requirement remains one of the strongest MOF risk factors
C. Blood products contain numerous immunoactive substances, including proinflammatory lipids and cytokines within the red blood cells that remain despite leukodepletion of blood products
D. All of the above true

44. The most widely accepted scoring systems of MOF includes:

A. Denver Postinjury Multiple Organ Failure Score
B. The Sequential Organ Failure Assessment (SOFA)
C. The Marshall Multiple Organ Dysfunction Score (MODS)
D. All of the above

45. The Denver scoring system uses laboratory values representing all except:

A. Respiratory system

B. Renal system
C. Central Nervous system
D. Cardiac systems

46. Denver scoring system uses laboratory values in patients with:

A. With an injury severity score >15 who have survived more than 24 hours from injury to predict various outcomes
B. With an injury severity score >25 who have survived more than 48 hours from injury to predict various outcomes
C. With an injury severity score >15 who have survived more than 48 hours from injury to predict various outcomes
D. With an injury severity score >25 who have survived more than 24 hours from injury to predict various outcomes

47. False statement about Persistent Inflammation, Immunosuppression and Catabolism Syndrome:

A. Severe cellular stress creates a state of "emergency myelopoiesis" at the expense of lymphopoiesis and erythropoiesis
B. The mechanism of this – (PICS) – is based on a pathophysiologic maintenance of low-grade inflammation with increased serum levels of IL-6 and neutrophils in conjunction with immunosuppression through lymphocyte depletion and dysfunction
C. The expansion of MDSCs (myeloid-derived suppressor cells) after sepsis correlates with good clinical outcomes
D. There is a strong correlation between acute kidney injury and the development of sepsis

48. Within skeletal muscle, sepsis and severe cellular stress induces all except:

A. Dysfunction in the mitochondria
B. Increase in protein synthesis
C. Breakdown of myofibrillar proteins
D. Severe muscle wasting and cachexia

49. The recommended daily protein supplementation for critically ill patients is:

A. >0.5 g/kg/day
B. >1.0 g/kg/day
C. >1.5 g/kg/day
D. >2.5 g/kg/day

50. False statement among the following is/are:

A. Administration of propranolol and oxandrolone, with the intent to decrease catabolic requirements, has shown poor outcomes in the paediatric burns population
B. Chronic critical illness confers an increased risk of death following hospital discharge
C. Discharge to a skilled nursing facility remains one of the strongest predictors of mortality in patients with chronic critical illness
D. The recommended daily protein supplementation for critically ill patients has recently been increased to >1.5 g/kg/day

ANSWERS

1. **Ans: B. Last cell type recruited in response to injury and infection**
Ref: Chapter No.3, Page No.26

2. **Ans: B. IL 17**
Ref: Chapter No.3, Page No.26

3. **Ans: C. IL 23**
Ref: Chapter No.3, Page No.26

4. **Ans: D 8 hrs**
Ref: Chapter No.3, Page No.26

5. **Ans: D. All of the above are true**
Ref: Chapter No.3, Page No.26

6. **Ans: D. Adhesion-Cadherin**
Ref: Chapter No.3, Page No.27

7. **Ans: D. High concentrations of M2-type cytokines correlate with mortality in sepsis models**
Ref: Chapter No.3, Page No.27

8. **Ans: D. M1 macrophages are essential for tissue remodelling and wound healing; they express a variety of anti-inflammatory markers, including IL-10**
Ref: Chapter No.3, Page No.27

9. **Ans: D. Extracellular proteins are processed within the dendritic cell lysosome, and they are presented in conjunction with the MHC class I molecule to activate CD8+ cytotoxic T cells**
Ref: Chapter No.3, Page No.27

10. **Ans: B. IL-17 - differentiation of helper T cell type 1 (Th1) cells**
Ref: Chapter No.3, Page No.28

11. **Ans: D. Th17 cells can acquire the characteristic of Th2 cells in chronic inflammatory states**
Ref: Chapter No.3, Page No.28

12. **Ans: D. All of the above**
Ref: Chapter No.3, Page No.28

13. **Ans: C. Hyperthermia**

Ref: Chapter No.3, Page No.28

14. **Ans: D. Dependent of T cells, marginal zone B cells can rapidly produce soluble IgM during the early stages of infection.**

Ref: Chapter No.3, Page No.28

15. **Ans: A. B7-1**

Ref: Chapter No.3, Page No.29

16. **Ans: B. B7-2**

Ref: Chapter No.3, Page No.29

17. **Ans: C. PD-L1**

Ref: Chapter No.3, Page No.29

18. **Ans: B. Inhibition of T cell**

Ref: Chapter No.3, Page No.29

19. **Ans: C. ICOS**

Ref: Chapter No.3, Page No.29

20. **Ans: D. All of the above**

Ref: Chapter No.3, Page No.30

21. **Ans: B. IL-2**

Ref: Chapter No.3, Page No.31

22. **Ans: D. All of the above are true statements**

Ref: Chapter No.3, Page No.31

23. **Ans: C. Hepatocellular injury**

Ref: Chapter No.3, Page No.32-33

24. **Ans: D. All of the above are true**

Ref: Chapter No.3, Page No.32-33

25. **Ans: C. Increased platelet count**

Ref: Chapter No.3, Page No.33

26. **Ans: D. All of the above are true**

Ref: Chapter No.3, Page No.33

27. **Ans: A. In Late malignancy, TGF-β functions as a tumor suppressor**

Ref: Chapter No.3, Page No.33-34

28. **Ans: C. Eculizumab**

Ref: Chapter No.3, Page No.35

29. **Ans: D. All of the above are true**

Ref: Chapter No.3, Page No.35

30. **Ans: C. Many efferent motor vagal nerve fibres travel to the spleen via the vagus nerve**

Ref: Chapter No.3, Page No.36

31. **Ans: D. All of the above**

Ref: Chapter No.3, Page No.36

32. **Ans: C. IL 2**

Ref: Chapter No.3, Page No.36

33. **Ans: B. 40% to 80%**

Ref: Chapter No.3, Page No.37

34. **Ans: A. Secondary nosocomial infections**

Ref: Chapter No.3, Page No.37

35. **Ans: D. All of the above are true**

Ref: Chapter No.3, Page No.37

36. **Ans: D. Interferons**

Ref: Chapter No.3, Page No.38

37. **Ans: C. HLA-DR is one of several molecules that can make up the MHC class I surface complex**

Ref: Chapter No.3, Page No.38

38. **Ans: D. All of the above are true**

Ref: Chapter No.3, Page No.39

39. **Ans: D. Denver Score**

Ref: Chapter No.3, Page No.39

40. **Ans: B. Early transfusion requirement**

Ref: Chapter No.3, Page No.40

41. **Ans: C. 6 to 12**

Ref: Chapter No.3, Page No.39

42. **Ans: C. Female sex**

Ref: Chapter No.3, Page No.40

43. **Ans: A. Male sex confers a greater risk of death**

Ref: Chapter No.3, Page No.40

44. **Ans: D. All of the above**

Ref: Chapter No.3, Page No.40

45. **Ans: C. Central Nervous system**

Ref: Chapter No.3, Page No.40

46. **Ans: C. With an injury severity score >15 who have survived more than 48 hours from injury to predict various outcomes**

Ref: Chapter No.3, Page No.40

47. **Ans: C. The expansion of MDSCs (myeloid-derived suppressor cells) after sepsis correlates with good clinical outcomes**

Ref: Chapter No.3, Page No.40

48. **Ans: B. Increase in protein synthesis**

Ref: Chapter No.3, Page No.40

49. **Ans: C. >1.5 g/kg/day**

Ref: Chapter No.3, Page No.41

50. **Ans: A. Administration of propranolol and oxandrolone, with the intent to decrease catabolic requirements, has shown poor outcomes in the paediatric burn population**

Ref: Chapter No.3, Page No.41

4

Shock, Electrolytes and Fluid

HISTORY

1. Who provided one of the first clear descriptions of intravenous (IV) fluid therapy?

A. Ambroise Pare B. Herman
C. O'Shaughnessy D. Gross

2. Who defined shock as "a manifestation of the rude unhinging of the machinery of life"?

A. Ambroise Pare B. Herman
C. O'Shaughnessy D. Gross

3. Who concluded that the lowering of the central venous pressure in the shock state in animal experiments was due to a failure of the autonomic nervous system?

A. Crile C. O'Shaughnessy
C. Herman D. Gross

4. Who proposed the kinetic system theory?

A. Crile C. O'Shaughnessy
C. Herman D. Gross

5. Who found that epinephrine was released in response to pain or emotion, shifting blood from the intestines to the brain and extremities?

A. Crile B. Henderson
C. Herman D. Walter B. Cannon

6. Who recognized the importance of decreased venous return and its effect on cardiac output and arterial pressure?

A. Crile B. Henderson
C. Herman D. Walter B. Cannon

7. Who first described the concept of "irreversible shock"?

A. Blalock B. Henderson
C. Wiggers D. Walter B. Cannon

8. The concept of IV fluids was first introduced in the treatment of which disease?

A. Cholera
B. Typhoid
C. Plague
D. Inflammatory Bowel Disease

9. Regarding *Wiggers Prep*, which of the following is false?

A. It is a controlled Hemorrhage
B. It is a Pressure controlled Hemorrhage
C. It is a Volume controlled Hemorrhage
D. None of the above

10. Causes of shock according to Blalock includes:

A. Hematogenic B. Neurogenic
C. Vasogenic D. All of the above

11. Normal Saline was first described by:

A. Robert Lewins B. Sydney Ringer
C. Wiggers D. Jakob Hamburger

12. Lewins described Latta's saline solution. Latta's solution was found to equate to having:

A. 134 mmol per liter of Na+
B. 118 mmol per liter of Cl–
C. 16 mmol per liter of bicarbonate (HCO_3–)
D. All of the above

13. Who is regarded as the originator of modern fluid treatment? Also introduced the concept of the continued IV drip but also warned of potential dangers of saline infusions:

A. Rudolph Matas B. Sydney Ringer
C. Wiggers D. Jakob Hamburger

14. Few hours after infusion of 1 litre of NS, how much fluid is retained in intravascular space?

A. 50 ml B. 200 ml
C. 750 ml D. 500 ml

15. Who showed that blood was interchangeable?

A. Crile B. Sydney Ringer
C. Wiggers D. Alexis Carrel

16. Who was able to sew blood vessels together with his triangulation technique, using it to connect blood vessels from one person to another for the purpose of transfusions?

A. Crile B. Sydney Ringer
C. Wiggers D. Alexis Carrel

17. Who developed a short cannula to facilitate transfusions?

A. Crile B. Sydney Ringer
C. Wiggers D. Alexis Carrel

PHYSIOLOGY OF SHOCK

18. According to ATLS Classes of Hemorrhagic Shock, blood loss of 25% is classified as:

A. Class I B. Class II
C. Class III D. Class IV

19. According to ATLS Classes of Hemorrhagic Shock, decreased blood pressure is seen in which class?

A. Class I B. Class II
C. Class III D. All of the above

20. According to ATLS Classes of Hemorrhagic Shock, decreased pulse pressure is not seen in which class?

A. Class I B. Class II
C. Class III D. Class IV

21. In class III hemorrhagic shock as per ATLS Hemorrhagic shock classification, urine output is:

A. 20-30 ml/hr B. 5-15 ml/hr
C. Negligible D. <5 ml/hr

22. False statement regarding hemorrhagic shock is:

A. The change in pulse pressure is thought to be caused by an epinephrine response constricting vessels, resulting in higher diastolic pressures
B. Pain and mere nervousness doesn't increase heart rate
C. Not until patients are in class III shock does BP theoretically decrease
D. Important key when a patient is in shock due to hemorrhage is recognizing that blood loss is the cause of their shock and identify the source of bleeding and treat it

23. Relative bradycardia is defined as a heart rate less than:

A. 90 beats/min while simultaneously having a systolic BP below 90 mm Hg
B. 100 beats/min while simultaneously having a systolic BP below 100 mm Hg
C. 100 beats/min while simultaneously having a systolic BP below 90 mm Hg
D. 90 beats/min while simultaneously having a systolic BP below 100 mm Hg

24. Heart rate of bleeding patient who have the highest survival rate:

A. < 60 beats/min B. 60 to 90 beats/min
C. 90 to 120 beats/min D. > 120 beats/min

25. False statement among the following statements is:

A. Venous blood loss can be massive before hypotension occurs
B. A lacerated artery bleeds more than a transected artery
C. In Arterial bleeding patients, measurements of lactate or base deficit can yield normal results
D. Venous bleeding is typically faster, allowing the human body no time to compensate

26. False statement regarding venous bleeding is:

A. Venous bleeding is typically slower, allowing the human body time to compensate
B. Slower progression provides the time necessary for recruitment of water from the intracellular and interstitial spaces
C. Large volumes of blood that can be lost before hypotension ensues
D. Lactate and base deficit levels are normal

27. Shock Index is defined as:

A. Heart rate divided by pulse pressure
B. Heart rate divided by diastolic BP
C. Heart rate divided by systolic BP
D. Heart rate divided by MAP (Mean arterial pressure)

28. Modified Shock Index is defined as:

A. Heart rate divided by pulse pressure
B. Heart rate divided by diastolic BP
C. Heart rate divided by systolic BP
D. Heart rate divided by MAP (Mean arterial pressure)

29. Regarding Modified shock index, false statement is:

A. MSI considers Diastolic BP also
B. Low MSI indicates Hyperdynamic state

C. MSI is a better marker than SI for mortality prediction
D. Low MSI Hypodynamic Circulatory State

30. Preferred fuel in brain during rest is:

A. Lactate
B. Glucose
C. Ketones
D. Amino Acids

31. False regarding lactate:

A. It's the preferred fuel in brain during rest and exercise
B. Can be protective in TBI
C. It has glucose sparing effect
D. Stress causes decrease in lactate

32. Base deficit is defined as:

A. Number of millimoles of base required to correct the pH of ½ liter of whole blood to 7.4
B. Number of millimoles of base required to correct the pH of 1 liter of whole blood to 7.2
C. Number of millimoles of base required to correct the pH of ½ liter of whole blood to 7.2
D. Number of millimoles of base required to correct the pH of 1 litre of whole blood to 7.4

33. In the acute stage of renal failure, a base deficit of less than _________ mmol/L is associated with poor outcome.

A. 2 mmol/L
B. 4 mmol/L
C. 6 mmol/L
D. 8 mmol/L

34. False statement about base deficit is:

A. Base deficit, a measure of the number of millimoles of base required to correct the pH of a liter of whole blood to 7.4
B. Problem with base deficit is that it is commonly influenced by the chloride in various resuscitation fluids, resulting in a hyperchloremic non anion gap acidosis
C. Problem with base deficit is that it is commonly influenced by the chloride in various resuscitation fluids, resulting in a hyperchloremic anion gap acidosis
D. In the acute stage of renal failure, a base deficit of less than 6 mmol/L is associated with poor outcome

35. Lethal triad of death includes all except:

A. Hypothermia
B. Acidosis
C. Coagulopathy
D. Hyperthermia

36. True statement regarding compensatory mechanisms in shock is:

A. Antidiuretic hormone (ADH) is released from the adrenal gland, causing retention of free water at the level of the kidney
B. Although the role of glucose elevation in hemorrhagic shock is not fully understood, it does seem to affect outcome
C. Angiotensin II causes the reabsorption of sodium through a direct action on the renal tubules
D. The earliest compensatory mechanism in response to a decrease in intravascular volume is an increase in parasympathetic activity

37. False statement among the following is:

A. Hypothermia and acidosis affect the efficiency of enzymes, which work best at 37°C and a pH of 7.4
B. The optimal method to break the "vicious circle of death" is to stop the bleeding and the causes of hypothermia
C. In most typical scenarios, hypothermia is spontaneous from ischemia
D. If ATP production is inadequate to maintain body temperature, the body will trend toward the ambient temperature

38. Regarding THAM, which is used as alternate to bicarbonate to correct acidosis; Which of the following is not true?

A. Biologically inert amino alcohol of low toxicity
B. It's sodium free but generates more CO_2
C. More effective than Sodium bicarbonate
D. THAM is effective in a closed or semi closed system, and it maintains its buffering ability during hypothermia

39. True statement regarding THAM is:

A. Not suitable for closed systems
B. Less effective than soda bicarb
C. May cause hyperglycaemia
D. May cause respiratory depression

40. The initial loading dose of THAM is calculated by using the formula:

A. Lean Body Weight × Base deficit
B. Lean Body Weight / Base deficit
C. Lean Body Weight × Serum Lactate
D. Lean Body Weight / Serum Lactate

41. True Statement regarding hypothermia is:

A. Cold water near-drowning victims have higher death rates

B. The average temperature drop is to about 34°C
C. Trauma patients with a postoperative core temperature below 35°C have a four-fold increase in death
D. Even a drop in core temperature of just a few degrees results in 100% inefficiency in some of the enzymes

42. In Hypothermia due to trauma, severe is considered as below:

A. < 30°C B. < 32°C
C. < 26°C D. < 28°C

43. In accidental Hypothermia, severe hypothermia is considered as below:

A. < 30°C B. < 32°C
C. < 26°C D. < 28°C

44. Loss of ________ Kcal of energy would lead to 1°C decrease of body temperature.

A. 52 B. 62
C. 72 D. 82

45. True Statement regarding hypothermia is all except:

A. The normal basal metabolic heat generation is about 70 kcal/ hr; Shivering can increase this to 250 kcal/hr
B. Convection is an extremely inefficient way to transfer heat as the air molecules are so far apart compared with liquids and solids
C. Conduction and radiation are the most efficient ways to transfer heat
D. Although IV fluids can be warmed, the U.S. Food and Drug Administration (FDA) allows fluid warmers to be set at a maximum of 44°C

46. IV fluids can be warmed; the U.S. Food and Drug Administration (FDA) allows fluid warmers to be set at a maximum of __°C.

A. 36 B. 40
C. 44 D. 42

47. 1 L of warmed fluids can transfer only ____ Kcal to the patient.

A. 2 B. 4
C. 6 D. 8

48. Max calories delivered by active warming is by:

A. Cardiopulmonary Bypass
B. Heating Blankets
C. Airway from ventilator
D. Continuous arteriovenous rewarming

49. Clinitron bed is a ________ method of rewarming technique.

A. Passive warming technique
B. Active External Rewarming
C. Active Internal warming technique
D. None of these

50. Which of the following is not an Active External Warming device:

A. Bair Hugger B. Clinitron Bed
C. Radiant warmers D. Warm the room

51. Amount of energy delivered by Cardiopulmonary bypass:

A. 200 KCal/Hr B. 400 KCal/Hr
C. 600 KCal/Hr D. 700 KCal/Hr

52. False statement among the following is:

A. A method that can actively rewarm a patient and also assist in the treatment of shock is extracorporeal membrane oxygenation (ECMO)
B. With ECMO, the patient's blood is pumped through an artificial lung and then back into the bloodstream, which can support either a failing pulmonary or cardiac system
C. If gastric lavage is desired, one method is continuous lavage by infusion of warmed fluids through the sump port while the fluid is sucked out of the main tube
D. All the above statements are true

53. Identify what the letter R denotes in this thromboelastography:

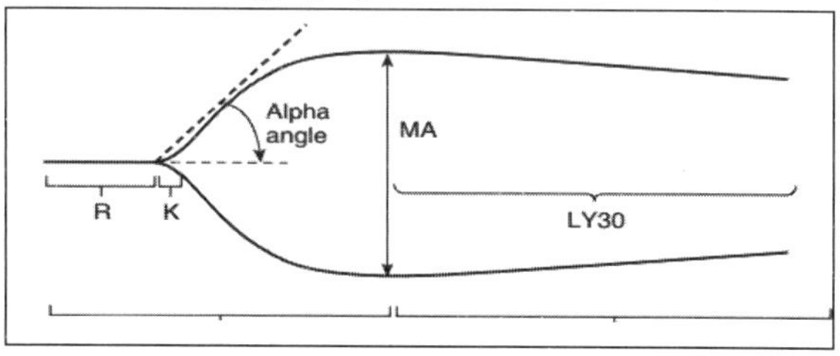

A. Reaction Time
B. Clot Elasticity
C. Rate of fibrin formation
D. Measure of clot strength

54. Identify what does alpha angle denote in the thromboelastography (Question No. 53):

A. Reaction Time
B. Clot Elasticity
C. Rate of fibrin formation
D. Measure of clot strength

55. Identify what does MA denote in the thrombo-elastography (Question No. 53):

A. Reaction Time
B. Clot Elasticity
C. Rate of fibrin formation
D. Measure of clot strength

56. True statements about Tranexamic acid is all except:

A. Tranexamic acid (TXA) is a synthetic analogue of the amino acid lysine and is an antifibrinolytic medication that competitively inhibits the activation of plasminogen to plasmin
B. TXA has about eight times the antifibrinolytic activity of an older analogue, ε aminocaproic acid
C. (CRASH-2) trial, a multicentre randomized controlled civilian trial, showed that TXA reduced all-cause mortality versus placebo and risk of death caused by bleeding was also reduced
D. All the above are true

57. CRASH-2 also suggested that TXA was less effective and could even be harmful if treatment was delayed more than __ hours after admission.

A. 1 hr B. 3 hrs
C. 8 hrs D. 12 hrs

58. False statement among the following is:

A. The most conventional method of sampling the venous oxygen content is by drawing blood from the most proximal port of a pulmonary artery catheter
B. The sample is taken from the pulmonary artery because venous blood is mixed there from all parts of the body
C. Oxygen content in the inferior vena cava is typically higher than in the superior vena cava, which is higher than in the coronary sinus
D. The average mixed venous sample is 75% saturated, so the oxygen consumption is thought to be, on average, 25% of the oxygen delivered

59. Following is not a trail not related to Tranexamic acid:

A. CRASH-4 study B. CRASH-2 study
C. MATTERS study D. PED-TRAX study

60. Pulse Oximeter uses which technology:

A. NIR technology
B. Tonometry technology
C. Microwave technology
D. Ultraviolet technology

61. Gastric tonometry measures the adequacy of blood flow in the GI tract through placement of a CO_2-permeable balloon filled with saline in the stomach of a patient after gastric acid suppression. The balloon is left in contact with the mucosa of the stomach for _____ mins.

A. 10 mins B. 20 mins
C. 30 mins D. 40 mins

62. NIR spectroscopy uses the NIR region of the electromagnetic spectrum from about:

A. 300 nm to 800 nm B. 800 nm to 2500 nm
C. 2500 nm to 5500 nm D. 5500 nm to 8000 nm

63. False about NIR spectroscopy is:

A. NIR spectroscopy uses the NIR region of the electromagnetic spectrum from about 800 nm to 2500 nm
B. Optical devices that use NIR wavelengths can determine the redox potential of copper atoms on cytochrome aa3 and have been used to study intracellular oxidative processes noninvasively
C. The NIR probe was found to be as sensitive as base deficit in predicting death and MODS in hypotensive trauma patients
D. The superiority of NIR results over conventional measurements of shock has not been proven

64. Which is not included in SIRS criteria?

A. Body temperature >38°C
B. >90 beats per min
C. Respiratory rate >30/min
D. WBC >12,000/mm^3 or 10% immature neutrophils

65. qSOFA includes all except:

A. Respiratory rate ≥22
B. Altered mental status
C. Systolic blood pressure ≤100 mm Hg
D. Pulse rate >100

66. According to Surviving Sepsis campaign, which statement is false?

A. Surviving Sepsis campaign clinical guidelines published in 2016
B. Instead of using SIRS criteria, sepsis was now defined as an increase in a patient's sequential organ failure assessment (SOFA) score by 2 points from baseline
C. The qSOFA can be calculated at a patient bedside by identifying tachypnea, altered mental status and hypotension

D. If the patient meets 2 of the 4 criterias in qSOFA and they are at risk for sepsis, further workup for an infectious source should be conducted

PROBLEMS WITH RESUSCITATION

67. Da Nung lung refers to:

A. Pneumonitis
B. ARDS
C. ALI
D. Streptococcal Lung infection

68. Mattox study refers to:

A. Administering of prehospital IV fluids affected outcomes in hypotensive patients after a blunt torso injury
B. Administering of prehospital IV fluids affected outcomes in hypotensive patients after a penetrating torso injury
C. With holding of prehospital IV fluids affected outcomes in hypotensive patients after a blunt torso injury
D. With holding of prehospital IV fluids affected outcomes in hypotensive patients after a penetrating torso injury

69. Which organ suffers the most ischemia during shock and is the most susceptible to reperfusion injury?

A. Brain
B. Heart
C. Gut
D. Lung

70. To avoid muscle cells from undergoing ischemia and reperfusion in which the cells will start to swell, which can then result in compartment syndrome in the lower leg; Femoral artery injury's circulation should be restored by:

A. 2-4 hrs
B. 4-6 hrs
C. 6-8 hrs
D. 8-12 hrs

EVOLUTION OF MODERN RESUSCITATION

71. Neutrophils are activated after a __% blood volume hemorrhage when followed by resuscitation with LR solution.

A. 20%
B. 30%
C. 40%
D. 50%

72. All the following statements are true except:

A. Lactic acid occurs in two stereoisomeric forms as well as in a true racemic mixture of the isomers
B. l(+)- lactate is a normal intermediary of mammalian metabolism
C. l(+)- lactate has low toxicity
D. d(–)- lactate has low toxic potential

73. Among the resuscitation fluids of choice for casualties in hemorrhagic shock, most preferred is:

A. Plasma or RBCs alone
B. Plasma, RBCs and platelets in a 1:1:1 ratio
C. Plasma and RBCs in a 1:1 ratio
D. Whole blood

74. Among the resuscitation fluids of choice for casualties in hemorrhagic shock, least preferred is:

A. Plasma or RBCs alone
B. Plasma, RBCs and platelets in a 1:1:1 ratio
C. Plasma and RBCs in a 1:1 ratio
D. Whole blood

75. Following statements are true except:

A. The use of Hextend was limited to 1 L, given its potential for exacerbating coagulopathy
B. With the rapid sequence induction of anaesthesia, aspiration is a minimal risk
C. As per fluid resuscitation from the U.S. military by the Committee on Tactical Combat Casualty Care; If Vital signs and mental status is normal IV access should be taken and encourage oral fluids
D. As per fluid resuscitation from the U.S. military by the Committee on Tactical Combat Casualty Care; If Vital signs and mental status is normal IV access should be taken and IV fluid should be administered

76. Components of Damage Control Surgery are all except:

A. Permissive hypotension until definitive surgical control
B. Minimize crystalloid use and Initial use of 5% hypertonic saline
C. Delayed use of blood products (PRBCs, FFP, platelets, cryoprecipitates)
D. Consider drugs to treat coagulopathy (rFVIIa, prothrombin complex concentrate, TXA)

77. The whole blood is stored at ___°C.

A. 0°C
B. 4°C
C. -20°C
D. 25°C

78. Citrate-phosphate-dextrose (CPD) with whole blood allows storage up to ____days.

A. 21 Days
B. 14 Days
C. 35 Days
D. 42 Days

79. Most hospitals use apheresis platelets, which are pooled platelets; 1 unit is equivalent to:

A. 2 pack of platelets
B. 4 pack of platelets
C. 6 pack of platelets
D. 8 pack of platelets

80. Debate about transfusing patients with a blood product ratio of 1:1:1 was settled by which trial?

A. PROMMTT trial
B. PROPPR trial
C. Mattox trial
D. CRASH trial

81. Endotheliopathy of trauma; true statements are all except:

A. The delivery of increased clotting factors to exsanguinating patients may explain part of the benefit of a high-ratio approach in massive transfusion
B. Trauma and shock result in degradation of the vascular glycocalyx and increased endothelial permeability
C. Phenomenon likely explains the development of ARDS and abdominal compartment syndrome
D. All of the above are true

CURRENT STATUS OF FLUID TYPES

82. Which of the following has highest osmolarity?

A. Ringer's Lactate
B. Normal Saline
C. Plasma
D. Normosol

83. Which of the following has max sodium and chloride?

A. Ringer's Lactate
B. Normal Saline
C. Plasma
D. Normosol

84. pH of Ringer's lactate is:

A. 5.5
B. 6.5
C. 7.4
D. 8.5

85. Which of the following is not a content of Ringer's lactate?

A. Sodium
B. Calcium
C. Magnesium
D. Lactate

86. Amount of lactate present in Ringer's Lactate:

A. 25 mOsm/L
B. 28 mOsm/L
C. 5 mOsm/L
D. 30 mOsm/L

87. Osmolarity of Ringer's lactate is __ mOsm/L.

A. 273
B. 294
C. 308
D. 295

88. Which of the following is absent in PLASMA-LYTE A?

A. Sodium
B. Calcium
C. Magnesium
D Gluconate

89. Which of the following is absent in NORMOSOL?

A. Sodium
B. Bicarbonate
C. Potassium
D. Gluconate

90. The result of massive normal saline infusion is a:

A. Hyperchloremic metabolic alkalosis
B. Hyperchloremic anion gap metabolic acidosis
C. Hyperchloremic non anion gap metabolic acidosis
D. None of the above

91. Regarding Hypertonic Saline, false statement is:

A. It has consistently been shown to reduce the inflammatory response
B. HTS infusion is highly effective in decreasing ICP and can do this while increasing blood volume, BP and blood flow to the brain
C. Compared with mannitol, which is customarily used for lowering ICP, HTS might do this with dehydrating patients
D. The method used in trauma patients is to give 5% HTS in 250-mL infusions and, if more than 500 mL is needed, to check sodium levels

92. True statements about Human albumin are all except:

A. Other than its dilutional effect, albumin is associated with coagulopathy
B. SAFE study in Australia has shown 4% albumin to be safe, compared with normal saline, in ICU patients
C. Albumin has a proven immunologic anti-inflammatory effect and five times less volume than current artificial colloids
D. It is considered to be the reference colloidal solution

93. False statement regarding colloids is:

A. Because of the potential for accumulation in tissues, the recommended maximal daily dose of hetastarch is 33 to 55 mL/kg/day
B. Colloids such as hetastarch can have proinflammatory effects similar to those of crystalloids
C. Hetastarch solutions are produced from amylopectin obtained from sorghum, maize or potatoes

D. Despite extensive randomized controlled trials, the safety and efficacy of 5% albumin, 6% hetastarch, and 6% dextran has not been examined

FUTURE RESUSCITATION RESEARCH

94. The ideal blood substitute would do all of the following except:

A. Deliver oxygen
B. Have few side effects
C. Not persist in the circulation
D. Be cost-effective

95. Problems with free hemoglobin includes all except:

A. Osmotic diuretic effects
B. Renal toxicity
C. Coagulation abnormalities
D. Long half-life

96. All of the following statements about Blood substitutes are true except:

A. Referred to as hemoglobin oxygen carriers (HBOCs)
B. Current second-generation HBOCs are pasteurized and thus free of communicable pathogens; they also have no ABO/Rh or other blood antigens
C. The hemoglobin for blood substitutes comes from a variety of sources, such as outdated donated human blood, bovine or swine blood, and transgenic E. coli
D. About 4 units of discarded blood are required to make 1 unit of the HBOC

97. Number of units of discarded blood that are required to make 1 unit of the HBOC:

A. 2 B. 4
C. 6 D. 8

98. Troublesome side effects of blood substitutes that are still present includes all except:

A. Free radical generation and exacerbation of reperfusion injury
B. Methaemoglobin production
C. Renal toxicity
D. Immunologic effects

99. True statements about Recombinant hemoglobin is/are:

A. Volumes of bacterial culture and the stringent processing methods are costly
B. It is estimated that only 0.1 g of hemoglobin can be generated from 1 L of E. coli culture
C. Production of 3 million units would require more than 1.125 billion litres of culture
D. All of the above

100. True statements about HBOC-201 are all except:

A. Also called Hemopure
B. It is universally compatible and is stable at room temperature for up to 3 years
C. The vasoconstrictive properties of Hemopure may have caused myocardial infarction in susceptible patients
D. FDA has approved Hemopure

101. Regarding Perfluorocarbons, all statements are true except:

A. Perfluorocarbons (PFCs) are completely inert biologically
B. Altering the molecule (by fluoridating the ring structure) lowers the melting point and thus makes it a liquid at room temperature
C. The liquid form is mixable in water
D. PFCs has a linear relationship to the PO_2

102. Regarding Second-generation PFCs, false statement is:

A. Compounds can also be stored at 4°C, whereas previous solutions had to be frozen
B. Oxygent is a 60% perflubron emulsion with a median particle diameter of less than 0.2 μm
C. The use of lecithin as an emulsifier eliminated the adverse effects of complement activation observed in earlier studies of PFCs
D. Oxygent possibly decreased the incidence of strokes

103. Which of the following is a PFCs?

A. OxyFluor B. Oxygent
C. Oxycyte D. All of the above

104. Advantage of dried plasma are all except:

A. Long shelf life
B. It does not need refrigeration
C. It does not transmit viruses
D. It does not need tight temperature control

105. Freeze dried and secured plasma needs __ ml of water and for use in less than __ mins.

A. It is easily rehydrated with 400 mL of water for use in less than 5 minutes
B. It is easily rehydrated with 200 mL of water for use in less than 5 minutes

C. It is easily rehydrated with 400 mL of water for use in less than 3 minutes

D. It is easily rehydrated with 200 mL of water for use in less than 3 minutes

106. FDSP is shelf stable in ambient temperatures for _____ years.

A. 1 year B. 2 years
C. 3 years D. 4 years

107. Regarding Freeze-dried platelets, all are true except:

A. Frozen platelets are cryopreserved in 6% dimethyl sulfoxide and can be stored for up to 10 years at –80°C

B. Modern preparations, which are treated with 1.8% paraformaldehyde, frozen in 5% albumin, and then lyophilized

C. Once rehydrated, they seem structurally intact, contain most of the glycoproteins, and are capable of supporting thrombin generation and fibrin deposition

D. In vivo testing shows that the duration of haemostatic activity is brief, approximately 4 to 6 hours, and sometimes limited to 2 hrs

108. False statements about histone deacetylases (HDACs) and histone acetyltransferases is/are:

A. Animal experiments showed that hemorrhagic shock and resuscitation were associated with HDAC/histone acetyltransferase activity misbalance and that the acetylation status of cardiac histones is influenced by the choice of resuscitation strategy

B. Shock-induced changes can be reversed through the infusion of a pharmacologic HDAC inhibitor, even when it is administered for only a limited period after the insult

C. The role of HDAC inhibitors, such as valproic acid (VPA, an anticonvulsant) and suberoylanilide hydroxamic acid

D. All statements are true

109. The current length of time that flow to the brain can be halted is only about _____ minutes.

A. 30 B. 45
C. 60 D. 90

110. Who is the father of modern-day cardiopulmonary resuscitation?

A. DeBakey B. Gibbons
C. Peter Safar D. Crile

PERIOPERATIVE FLUID MANAGEMENT

111. Best used to calculate body fat is:

A. MRI
B. Body Weight
C. Bioimpedance Spectroscopy
D. Triceps thickness

112. Principal anion intracellularly is:

A. Phosphates B. Chloride
C. Oxygen D. Iron

113. Major electrolyte responsible for the osmotic pressure is:

A. Potassium B. Calcium
C. Chloride D. Sodium

114. Which of the following statements is false?

A. In surgical patients, assessing the intravascular status is a pivotal task but also one of the most difficult.

B. The main daily task of perioperative patient care is assessing the intravascular status

C. Patients about to undergo major surgery requiring inpatient hospitalization after surgery, IV fluids the night before are necessary

D. The current standard for maintenance fluid is to use 5% dextrose in half-normal saline with 20 mEq per liter of potassium

115. A 50-year-old patient has been admitted in your ward. The patient is NPO and the sister asks you to write orders for maintenance fluid to be started. The weight is 50 kgs; calculate the amount of fluid needed:

A. 75 ml/hr B. 80 ml/hr
C. 85 ml/hr D. 90 ml/hr

116. A 10-year-old patient has been admitted in your ward. The patient is NPO and the sister asks you to write orders for maintenance fluid to be started. The weight is 30 kgs; calculate the amount of fluid needed:

A. 60 ml/hr B. 65 ml/hr
C. 70 ml/hr D. 75 ml/hr

117. A 4-year-old patient has been admitted in your ward. The patient is NPO and the sister asks you to write orders for maintenance fluid to be started. The weight is 11 kgs; calculate the amount of fluid needed:

A. 40 ml/hr B. 42 ml/hr
C. 52 ml/hr D. 50 ml/hr

118. A 7-year-old patient has been admitted in your ward. The patient is NPO and the sister asks you to write orders for maintenance fluid to be started. The weight is 23 kgs; calculate the amount of fluid needed:

A. 50 ml/hr
B. 53 ml/hr
C. 60 ml/hr
D. 63 ml/hr

119. A 32-year-old patient has been admitted in your ward. The patient is NPO and the sister asks you to write orders for maintenance fluid to be started. The weight is 77 kgs; calculate the amount of fluid needed:

A. 107 ml/hr
B. 117 ml/hr
C. 127 ml/hr
D. 100 ml/hr

120. Normal sodium needs for a 70-kg man per day is:

A. 4-5 g
B. 2-4 g
C. 1-2 g
D. 10-12 g

121. Patients undergoing brain herniation have:

A. Tachycardic hypertensive state to a profoundly bradycardic and hypotensive state
B. Tachycardic hypotensive state to a profoundly bradycardic and hypertensive state
C. Bradycardic hypertensive state to a profoundly tachycardic and hypotensive state
D. Bradycardic hypotensive state to a profoundly tachycardic and hypertensive state

122. Laboratory findings suggesting adrenal insufficiency are all except:

A. Hyperkalemia
B. Acidemia
C. Hyponatremia
D. Decreased serum creatinine levels

123. False regarding adrenal glucocorticoid insufficiency among the following is:

A. The chief complaint may be vague cramping abdominal pain, nausea, and a change in bowel habits
B. Patients with a complete loss of circulating glucocorticoids can die within hours after irreversible hypotension
C. Treatment of glucocorticoid deficiency in adults consists of an IV infusion of dexamethasone, methylprednisolone, or hydrocortisone
D. Using dexamethasone is avoided if sending simultaneous laboratory tests to confirm the diagnosis of acute hypercortisolism as this medication interferes with the cosyntropin test

124. All of the following statements are true except:

A. ADH causes water to be reabsorbed and thus reduces urine output
B. Excess production or release of ADH causes overhydration; water is retained and thus sodium levels are lowered
C. In SIADH urine osmolality will be low (<300 mmol/kg) even though serum osmolality is high
D. Treatment of patients with DI should include desmopressin; and of patients with SIADH, water restriction

ELECTROLYTES

125. Normal range of serum sodium concentration is:

A. 125 to 135 mEq/L
B. 135 to 145 mEq/L
C. 145 to 155 mEq/L
D. 115 to 125 mEq/L

126. All of the following statements are true except:

A. Hyponatremia and hypernatremia, heavily controlled by ADH, are common problems in surgical patients
B. Mild forms of hyponatremia and hypernatremia are not a problem
C. Hypernatremia is more concerning than hyponatremia
D. None of the signs or symptoms alone would lead a clinician to diagnose a sodium abnormality, a blood test is always required

127. Severe hyponatremia is sodium levels:

A. <130 mEq/liter
B. <120 mEq/liter
C. <115 mEq/liter
D. 120-130 mEq/liter

128. True statement among the following is:

A. The measured sodium level is lowered by 1.8 mEq/L for every 100 mg/dL of glucose above 100
B. The measured sodium level is lowered by 1.6 mEq/L for every 100 mg/dL of glucose above 100
C. The measured sodium level is lowered by 1.6 mEq/L for every 100 mg/dL of glucose above 200
D. The measured sodium level is lowered by 1.8 mEq/L for every 100 mg/dL of glucose above 200

129. The correct equation for clinical use:

A. Sodium deficit (mEq) = ([Na] goal + [Na] plasma) × TBW
B. Sodium deficit (mEq) = ([Na] goal – [Na] plasma) × TBW

C. Sodium deficit (mEq) = ([Na] goal – [K] plasma) × TBW
D. Sodium deficit (mEq) = ([Na] goal – [Cl] plasma) × TBW

130. The correct equation for clinical use:
A. Corrected sodium = [Na] + 0.018 × (Glucose – 100)
B. Corrected sodium = [Na] + 0.016 × (Glucose – 100)
C. Corrected sodium = [Na] + 0.018 × (Glucose + 100)
D. Corrected sodium = [Na] + 0.016 × (Glucose + 100)

131. The correct equation for clinical use:
A. Free water deficit = (([Na]/140) + 1) × TBW
B. Free water deficit = (([Na]/100) – 1) × TBW
C. Free water deficit = (([Na]/140) – 1) × TBW
D. Free water deficit = (([Na]/100) + 1) × TBW

132. The correct equation for clinical use:
A. Serum osmolality = 2 × [Na] + BUN/2.8 + Glucose/18
B. Serum osmolality = 2 × [Na] + BUN/1.8 + Glucose/28
C. Serum osmolality = 2 × [K] + BUN/2.8 + Glucose/18
D. Serum osmolality = 2 × [Cl] + BUN/2.8 + Glucose/18

133. All of the following statements are true about hyponatremia except:
A. Patients with hyponatremia are usually hypotonic
B. No specific therapy is required other than treating the hyperglycaemia; artificially lowered sodium concentrations will return to normal once the plasma glucose level is normalized
C. In hypovolemic patients, baroreceptors also stimulate the hypothalamus to retain water through ADH release since the homeostatic mechanism for maintaining intravascular volume is stronger than maintaining proper sodium concentration
D. If urologic or gynecologic surgery is performed with hypoosmotic irrigation, acute hypernatremia can occur

134. Severe hypernatremia is:
A. >150 mEq/L B. >160 mEq/L
C. >165 mEq/L D. >170 mEq/L

135. Patients with Diabetes Insipidus have:
A. Euvolemic hypernatremia
B. Hypovolemic hypernatremia
C. Hypervolemic hypernatremia
D. Euvolemic hyponatremia

136. Drugs which can induce Diabetes Insipidus include all except:
A. Lithium B. Amiloride
C. Demeclocycline D. Amphotericin B

137. The treatment of patients with lithium-induced nephrogenic DI is:
A. Glyburide B. Amiloride
C. Demeclocycline D. Amphotericin B

138. False regarding Hypernatremia is:
A. Hypernatremia is usually defined as serum sodium concentration above 145 mEq/L
B. Nephrogenic DI is defined as an impaired capacity of the renal tubules to respond to ADH and to concentrate urine
C. Hypocalcaemia or severe hyperkalaemia also impairs the capacity of renal tubular cells to absorb sodium
D. Hypervolemic hypernatremia is usually iatrogenic caused by resuscitation with hypertonic solutions or a result of excess mineralocorticoids in Conn or Cushing syndrome

139. False regarding Hypernatremia is:
A. In patients with acute hypernatremia, the rate is usually no more than 1 to 2 mEq/hr
B. In patients with chronic hypernatremia, the rate is usually no more than 0.5 mEq/hr
C. Sodium levels should not be corrected at a rate of more than 8 mEq/day
D. All of the above are true

140. False statement among Diabetes Insipidus among the following is:
A. Patients with DI are producing dilute urine at rates of hundreds of milliliters per hour
B. They should be treated with desmopressin (DDAVP)
C. DDAVP increases water movement out of the collecting duct, and also has vasoconstrictive properties like ADH
D. DDAVP can be administered orally, intranasally, subcutaneously, or intravenously. The intranasal dose is 10 μg once or twice daily

141. Symptoms of hypokalaemia includes:
A. Generalized fatigue and weakness
B. Acute renal insufficiency
C. Atrial arrhythmia
D. All of the above

142. Flaccid paralysis with respiratory compromise can occur as [K+] decreases to less than:
A. 2.5 mmol/L B. 2 mmol/L
C. 1.5 mmol/L D. 1 mmol/L

143. Rhabdomyolysis occurs in patients whose [K+] drops below:
A. 2.5 mmol/L B. 2 mmol/L
C. 1.5 mmol/L D. 1 mmol/L

144. The electrocardiogram of patients with hypokalemia will show:
A. Peaked T waves
B. Development of U waves
C. T waves higher than R waves
D. None of the above

145. False regarding Hypokalemia is:
A. Patients with hypokalemia have a [K+] lower than 3.5 mmol/L
B. Hypokalemia is a common problem in patients with congestive heart failure who are receiving multiple drugs
C. Patients with a chronic potassium deficiency can develop a cardiac rhythm disturbance
D. Hypokalemia is also frequently associated with hypermagnesemia and alkalosis

146. Potassium infusion at rates of more than __ mEq/hr, cardiac monitoring is required.
A. 10 mEq/hr B. 15 mEq/hr
C. 20 mEq/hr D. 25 mEq/hr

147. In the treatment of acute hypokalaemia, following statements are true except:
A. Oral supplementation is generally 40 to 100 mEq/day, in two to four doses
B. The IV rate is 10 to 20 mEq/hr
C. In emergency situations, the rate can be as high as 40 mEq/hr
D. All of the above are true

148. All of the following statements are true except:
A. Hypomagnesemia can produce refractory hypokalaemia
B. Supplemental magnesium increases the risk of arrhythmia
C. Hypokalaemia patients with concurrent acidemia are treated with potassium replacement before their pH is corrected by bicarbonate administration
D. Spironolactone blocks the effect of aldosterone and reduces potassium loss in urine

149. All of the following statements are true except:
A. Hyperkalemia is defined as [K+] of more than 5.0 mmol/L
B. The primary clinical problem with hyperkalemia is cardiac arrhythmia
C. Dangerous hyperkalemia (6–7 mmol/L) is indicated by T waves higher than R waves
D. The most common cause of hyperkalemia is heart failure in hospitalized patients

150. All of the following statements are true except:
A. The most common cause of hyperkalemia is acute onset of renal dysfunction or failure
B. At least 50% of normal renal function is required to respond to aldosterone and to maintain normal potassium levels
C. Succinylcholine, a depolarizing paralytic agent, can cause severe hyperkalemia
D. Revascularization after an ischemic injury may cause severe hyperkalemia; it is usually recommended to administer bicarbonate before reperfusion

151. In the treatment of acute hyperkalaemia, following statements are true except:
A. Calcium administered via IV can immediately reduce the risk of arrhythmia
B. Bicarbonate therapy is most effective in hyperkalemic patients with metabolic acidemia
C. Insulin and glucose infusions prompt an increase in Na+, K+-ATPase activity and a decline in extracellular water potassium concentration as the extracellular water potassium is driven into the cell
D. All of the above are true

152. As per guidelines for treatment of adult patients with hyperkalemia, with electrocardiographic evidence of pending arrest following is true except:
A. Stop all infusion of potassium
B. Intravenous (IV) infusion of calcium salts 10 mL of 10% calcium chloride during a 10-minute period
C. IV infusion of sodium bicarbonate 50-100 mEq during a 10- to 20-minute period
D. Immediate hemodialysis

153. In patients at risk for development of cardiac arrhythmia from hyperkalemia; first therapy administered is:

A. IV Calcium
B. Insulin and glucose infusions
C. Bicarbonate therapy
D. Haemodialysis

154. Most effective in hyperkalemic patients with metabolic acidemia is:

A. IV Calcium
B. Insulin and glucose infusions
C. Bicarbonate therapy
D. Haemodialysis

155. In patients with acute renal failure, the most reliable method to control hyperkalemia is:

A. IV Calcium
B. Insulin and glucose infusions
C. Bicarbonate therapy
D. Haemodialysis

156. The correct equation for corrected calcium levels is:

A. Corrected [iCa+2] = Total [Ca] + [(0.8 × [4.0 - Albumin level])]
B. Corrected [iCa+2] = Total [Ca] + [(0.8 × [4.5 - Albumin level])]
C. Corrected [iCa+2] = Total [Ca] + [(0.6 × [4.0 - Albumin level])]
D. Corrected [iCa+2] = Total [Ca] + [(0.6 × [4.5 - Albumin level])]

157. All of the following statements are true except:

A. Hypocalcemia is defined as total serum concentration below 8.4 mg/dL or ionized calcium concentration below 4.5 mg/dL
B. Hypocalcemic patients can have paresthesias, muscle spasms (including tetany), and seizures
C. Hypocalcemic patients have a prolonged QT interval on electrocardiograms that may progress to complete heart block or ventricular fibrillation
D. All of the above are true

158. The most common cause of hypocalcemia:

A. Hypoparathyroidism
B. Acute Pancreatitis
C. Tumor lysis syndrome
D. Malignancy

159. False statement regarding Pseudohypoparathyroidism is:

A. Pseudohypoparathyroidism is a group of disorders characterized by postreceptor resistance to PTH
B. Classic variant is Albright hereditary osteodystrophy
C. Albright hereditary osteodystrophy, associated with low stature, round facies, short digits and mental retardation
D. Hypermagnesemia induces PTH resistance

160. False statement regarding treatment of hypocalcemia:

A. Calcium gluconate is preferred to calcium chloride as it causes less tissue necrosis if it extravasates
B. Calcium chloride is preferred to calcium gluconate as it causes less tissue necrosis if it extravasates
C. Coexisting hypomagnesemia should be corrected in every patient
D. Magnesium is given by infusion, initiated with 2 g of magnesium sulfate during 10 to 15 minutes, followed by 1 g/hr

161. False statement regarding treatment of hypocalcemia:

A. During pregnancy, vitamin D requirements gradually increase, up to three times as high as the pre pregnancy requirements
B. If the baby is to be nursed, the dose of calcitriol should be decreased to 50% of the pre pregnancy dose
C. If the phosphorus level is higher than 6.0 mg/dL when the calcium level is satisfactory, an unabsorbable phosphate binder should be added
D. All of the above are true

162. The most common cause of hypercalcemia is:

A. Primary hyperparathyroidism
B. Secondary hyperparathyroidism
C. Malignancy
D. Milk Alkali syndrome

163. Hypercalcemic crisis is a syndrome in which total serum calcium levels exceeds:

A. 10 mg/dL
B. 13 mg/dL
C. 17 mg/dL
D. 15 mg/dL

164. Patients have severe hypercalcemia when serum calcium levels exceeds:

A. 10 mg/dL
B. 13 mg/dL
C. 17 mg/dL
D. 15 mg/dL

165. The most common malignant cause of hypercalcemia:

A. Prostate cancer B. Breast cancer
C. Pancreatic cancer D. Renal cancer

166. True regarding Humoral hypercalcemia of malignancy (HHM) is all except:

A. It is a clinical syndrome in which elevated calcium levels are caused by synthesis of the humoral factor by the tumoral process
B. Applied to patients with excessive tumoral production of PTHrP
C. Patients with HHM constitute about 20% of all patients with hypercalcemia associated with malignant disease
D. HHM patients usually have a clinically obvious malignant disease and a poor prognosis

167. False statement regarding treatment of hypercalcemia:

A. Administration of exogenous calcitonin is often initially effective in patients with hypercalcemia
B. Chelating agents (EDTA or phosphate salts) that bind and neutralize [iCa2+] are always indicated
C. Patients with a malignant neoplasm and hypercalcemia may respond to surgical excision, radiation therapy, or chemotherapy
D. All of the above are true

168. Humoral hypercalcemia of malignancy (HHM) is most commonly seen with:

A. Squamous cell carcinomas
B. Prostate cancer
C. Breast cancer
D. Pancrcatic cancer

169. The normal concentration of magnesium [Mg2+] in plasma ranges between:

A. 1.0 and 1.5 mEq/L B. 1.5 and 2.0 mEq/L
C. 2.0 and 2.5 mEq/L D. 2.5 and 3.0 mEq/L

170. Magnesium is protein bound; Most commonly it is bound with:

A. Prealbumin B. Albumin
C. Transferrin D. Globulin

171. False statement among the following:

A. Magnesium is primarily intracellular, with less than 1% of body stores in the ECF
B. Clinical sequelae of altered magnesium content depends on blood magnesium concentration
C. Patients who retain more than 30% of an 800 mg load of magnesium via IV are thought to be magnesium depleted, whereas those who retain less than 20% are said to be magnesium replete
D. In response to magnesium depletion or decreased intake, the fractional resorption of magnesium can rise to 99.5% to minimize urinary losses

172. Symptoms of hypomagnesemia become more common as the serum magnesium level falls below:

A. 1.8 mg/dL B. 1.2 mg/dL
C. 1.0 mg/dL D. 1.5 mg/dL

173. False statement regarding treatment of hypomagnesemia:

A. Symptomatic hypomagnesemia should be treated with an IV magnesium infusion
B. 1 g of magnesium sulfate contains 1 g of elemental magnesium
C. Optimal regimen for magnesium replacement is 8 to 12 g of magnesium sulfate in the first 24 hours followed by 4 to 6 g/day for 3 or 4 days to replete body stores
D. The American College of Cardiology and the American Heart Association recommend 1 to 2 g of magnesium sulfate as an IV bolus during 5 minutes for torsade de pointes therapy

174. False statement regarding treatment of hypomagnesemia:

A. Magnesium replacement should be done cautiously in patients with renal insufficiency, and recommendations call for dose reductions of 50% to 75% of baseline
B. Severe hypomagnesemia requires intermittent therapy because of the slow equilibration of extracellular magnesium with intracellular stores
C. The magnitude of magnesium deficiency frequently parallels the magnitude of hypocalcemia
D. Hypocalcemia in patients with magnesium deficiency is resistant to calcium replacement alone, so such patients should receive magnesium concurrently

175. Higher magnesium level leads to all except:

A. Prolonged PR interval
B. Increased QRS duration

C. Prolonged QT interval
D. Elevated ST segment

176. False statement regarding treatment of hypermagnesemia:

A. Severe hypermagnesemia is treated calcium gluconate 10% (10–20 mL for 10 minutes) administered via IV
B. Patients are typically given 100 to 200 mg IV of elemental calcium during 5 to 10 minutes
C. Unlike magnesium depletion, hypermagnesemia is a rare but frequently iatrogenic and fatal problem
D. Peritoneal dialysis or continuous renal replacement therapy corrects hypermagnesemia more rapidly than intermittent hemodialysis

ANSWERS

1. **Ans: B. Herman**
Ref: Chapter No.4, Page No.45

2. **Ans: D. Gross**
Ref: Chapter No.4, Page No.45

3. **Ans: A. Crile**
Ref: Chapter No.4, Page No.46

4. **Ans: A. Crile**
Ref: Chapter No.4, Page No.46

5. **Ans: D. Walter B. Cannon**
Ref: Chapter No.4, Page No.46

6. **Ans: B. Henderson**
Ref: Chapter No.4, Page No.46

7. **Ans: C. Wiggers**
Ref: Chapter No.4, Page No.46

8. **Ans: A. Cholera**
Ref: Chapter No.4, Page No.45

9. **Ans: C. It is a Volume controlled Hemorrhage**
Ref: Chapter No.4, Page No.47

10. **Ans: D. All of the above**
Ref: Chapter No.4, Page No.47

11. **Ans: D. Jakob Hamburger**
Ref: Chapter No.4, Page No.47

12. **Ans: D. All of the above**
Ref: Chapter No.4, Page No.48

13. **Ans: A. Rudolph Matas**
Ref: Chapter No.4, Page No.48

14. **Ans: B. 200 ml**
Ref: Chapter No.4, Page No.48-49

15. **Ans: A. Crile**
Ref: Chapter No.4, Page No.49

16. **Ans: D. Alexis Carrel**
Ref: Chapter No.4, Page No.49

17. **Ans: A. Crile**
Ref: Chapter No.4, Page No.49

18. **Ans: B. Class II**
Ref: Chapter No.4, Page No.49

19. **Ans: C. Class III**
Ref: Chapter No.4, Page No.49

20. **Ans: A. Class I**
Ref: Chapter No.4, Page No.49

21. **Ans: B. 5-15 ml/hr**
Ref: Chapter No.4, Page No.49

22. **Ans: B. Pain and mere nervousness don't increase heart rate.**
Ref: Chapter No.4, Page No.50-51

23. **Ans: C. 100 beats/min while simultaneously having a systolic BP below 90 mm Hg**
Ref: Chapter No.4, Page No.51

24. **Ans: B. 60 to 90 beats/min**
Ref: Chapter No.4, Page No.51

25. **Ans: D. Venous bleeding is typically faster, allowing the human body no time to compensate.**
Ref: Chapter No.4, Page No.51

26. **Ans: D. Lactate and base deficit levels are normal**
Ref: Chapter No.4, Page No.51

27. **Ans: C. Heart rate divided by systolic BP**
Ref: Chapter No.4, Page No.51

28. **Ans: D. Heart rate divided by MAP (Mean arterial pressure)**
Ref: Chapter No.4, Page No.51

29. **Ans: D. Low MSI Hypodynamic Circulatory State**
Ref: Chapter No.4, Page No.51-52

30. **Ans: A. Lactate**
Ref: Chapter No.4, Page No.51-52

31. **Ans: D. Stress causes decrease of Lactate**
Ref: Chapter No.4, Page No.51-52

32. **Ans: D. Number of millimoles of base required to correct the pH of 1 litre of whole blood to 7.4**
Ref: Chapter No.4, Page No.52

33. **Ans: C. 6 mmol/L**
Ref: Chapter No.4, Page No.52

34. **Ans: C. Problem with base deficit is that it is commonly influenced by the chloride in various resuscitation fluids, resulting in a hyperchloremic anion gap acidosis.**
Ref: Chapter No.4, Page No.52

35. **Ans: D. Hyperthermia**
Ref: Chapter No.4, Page No.52

36. **Ans: C. Angiotensin II causes the reabsorption of sodium through a direct action on the renal tubules.**
Ref: Chapter No.4, Page No.52-53

37. **Ans: C. In most typical scenarios, hypothermia is spontaneous from ischemia**
Ref: Chapter No.4, Page No.53

38. **Ans: B. It's sodium free but generates more CO_2**
Ref: Chapter No.4, Page No.53

39. **Ans: D. May cause respiratory depression**
Ref: Chapter No.4, Page No.53-54

40. **Ans: A. Lean Body Weight × Base deficit**
Ref: Chapter No.4, Page No.54

41. **Ans: C. Trauma patients with a postoperative core temperature below 35°C have a fourfold increase in death**
Ref: Chapter No.4, Page No.54

42. **Ans: B. < 32°C**
Ref: Chapter No.4, Page No.54

43. **Ans: D. < 28°C**
Ref: Chapter No.4, Page No.54

44. **Ans: B. 62**
Ref: Chapter No.4, Page No.54

45. **Ans: D. Although IV fluids can be warmed, the U.S. Food and Drug Administration (FDA) allows fluid warmers to be set at a maximum of 44°C**
Ref: Chapter No.4, Page No.54-55

46. **Ans: B. 40**
Ref: Chapter No.4, Page No.55

47. **Ans: C. 6**
Ref: Chapter No.4, Page No.55

48. **Ans: A. Cardiopulmonary Bypass**
Ref: Chapter No.4, Page No.55

49. **Ans: B. Active External Rewarming**
Ref: Chapter No.4, Page No.55

50. **Ans: D. Warm the room**
Ref: Chapter No.4, Page No.55

51. **Ans: D. 700 KCal/Hr**
Ref: Chapter No.4, Page No.55

52. **Ans: D. All the above statements are true**
Ref: Chapter No.4, Page No.55-56

53. **Ans: A. Reaction Time**
Ref: Chapter No.4, Page No.56

54. **Ans: C. Rate of fibrin formation**
Ref: Chapter No.4, Page No.56

55. **Ans: B. Clot Elasticity**
Ref: Chapter No.4, Page No.56

56. **Ans: D. All the above are true**
Ref: Chapter No.4, Page No.57

57. **Ans: B. 3 hrs**
Ref: Chapter No.4, Page No.57

58. **Ans: A. The most conventional method of sampling the venous oxygen content is by drawing blood from the most proximal port of a pulmonary artery catheter.**
Ref: Chapter No.4, Page No.58

59. **Ans: A. CRASH-4 study**
Ref: Chapter No.4, Page No.58

60. **Ans: A. NIR technology**
Ref: Chapter No.4, Page No.58

61. **Ans: C. 30 mins**
Ref: Chapter No.4, Page No.60

62. **Ans: B. 800 nm to 2500 nm**
Ref: Chapter No.4, Page No.60

63. **Ans: D. The superiority of NIR results over conventional measurements of shock has not been proven**
Ref: Chapter No.4, Page No.60-61

64. **Ans: C. Respiratory rate >30/min**
Ref: Chapter No.4, Page No.62

65. **Ans: D. Pulse rate >100**
Ref: Chapter No.4, Page No.62-63

66. **Ans: D. If the patient meets 2 of the 4 criteria's in qSOFA and they are at risk for sepsis, further workup for an infectious source should be conducted.**
Ref: Chapter No.4, Page No.62

67. **Ans: B. ARDS**
Ref: Chapter No.4, Page No.63

68. **Ans: D. With holding of prehospital IV fluids affected outcomes in hypotensive patients after a penetrating torso injury**
Ref: Chapter No.4, Page No.64

69. **Ans: C. Gut**
Ref: Chapter No.4, Page No.66

70. **Ans: B. 4-6 hrs**
Ref: Chapter No.4, Page No.66

71. **Ans: C. 40%**
Ref: Chapter No.4, Page No.66

72. **Ans: D. d(–)- lactate has low toxic potential**
Ref: Chapter No.4, Page No.67

73. **Ans: D. Whole blood**
Ref: Chapter No.4, Page No.68

74. **Ans: A. Plasma or RBCs alone**
Ref: Chapter No.4, Page No.68

75. **Ans: D. As per fluid resuscitation from the U.S. military by the Committee on Tactical Combat Casualty Care; If Vital signs and mental status is normal IV access should be taken and IV fluid should be administered**
Ref: Chapter No.4, Page No.69

76. **Ans: C. Delayed use of blood products (PRBCs, FFP, platelets, cryoprecipitates)**
Ref: Chapter No.4, Page No.69

77. **Ans: B. 4°C**
Ref: Chapter No.4, Page No.70

78. **Ans: A. 21 Days**
Ref: Chapter No.4, Page No.70

79. **Ans: C. 6 pack of platelets**
Ref: Chapter No.4, Page No.70

80. **Ans: B. PROPPR trial**
Ref: Chapter No.4, Page No.70

81. **Ans: D. All of the above true**
Ref: Chapter No.4, Page No.71

82. **Ans: B. Normal Saline**
Ref: Chapter No.4, Page No.72

83. **Ans: B. Normal Saline**
Ref: Chapter No.4, Page No.72

84. **Ans: B. 6.5**
Ref: Chapter No.4, Page No.72

85. **Ans: C. Magnesium**
Ref: Chapter No.4, Page No.72

86. **Ans: B. 28 mOsm/L**
Ref: Chapter No.4, Page No.72

87. **Ans: A. 273**
Ref: Chapter No.4, Page No.72

88. **Ans: B. Calcium**
Ref: Chapter No.4, Page No.72

89. **Ans: B. Bicarbonate**
Ref: Chapter No.4, Page No.72

90. **Ans: C. Hyperchloremic non anion gap metabolic acidosis**
Ref: Chapter No.4, Page No.72

91. **Ans: C. Compared with mannitol, which is customarily used for lowering ICP, HTS might do this with dehydrating patients**
Ref: Chapter No.4, Page No.73

92. **Ans: A. Other than its dilutional effect, albumin is associated with coagulopathy**
Ref: Chapter No.4, Page No.74

93. **Ans: D. Despite extensive randomized controlled trials, the safety and efficacy of 5% albumin, 6% hetastarch, and 6% dextran has not been examined**
Ref: Chapter No.4, Page No.74-75

94. **Ans: C. Not persist in the circulation**
Ref: Chapter No.4, Page No.75

95. **Ans: D. Long half-life**
Ref: Chapter No.4, Page No.75

96. **Ans: D. About 4 units of discarded blood are required to make 1 unit of the HBOC**
Ref: Chapter No.4, Page No.75

97. **Ans: A. 2**
Ref: Chapter No.4, Page No.75

98. **Ans: C. Renal toxicity**
Ref: Chapter No.4, Page No.75

99. **Ans: D. All of the above**
Ref: Chapter No.4, Page No.75

100. **Ans: D. FDA has approved Hemopure**
Ref: Chapter No.4, Page No.76

101. **Ans: C. The liquid form is mixable in water**
Ref: Chapter No.4, Page No.76

102. **Ans: D. Oxygent possibly decreased the incidence of strokes**
Ref: Chapter No.4, Page No.77

103. **Ans: D. All of the above**
Ref: Chapter No.4, Page No.77

104. **Ans: C. It does not transmit viruses**
Ref: Chapter No.4, Page No.77

105. **Ans: C. It is easily rehydrated with 400 mL of water for use in less than 3 minutes**
Ref: Chapter No.4, Page No.78

106. **Ans: B. 2 years**
Ref: Chapter No.4, Page No.78

107. **Ans: D. In vivo testing shows that the duration of haemostatic activity is brief, approximately 4 to 6 hours, and sometimes limited to 2 hrs**
Ref: Chapter No.4, Page No.78

108. **Ans: D. All statements are true**
Ref: Chapter No.4, Page No.78

109. **Ans: B. 45**
Ref: Chapter No.4, Page No.78

110. **Ans: C. Peter Safar**
Ref: Chapter No.4, Page No.79

111. **Ans: C. Bioimpedance Spectroscopy**
Ref: Chapter No.4, Page No.80

112. **Ans: A. Phosphates**
Ref: Chapter No.4, Page No.80

113. **Ans: D. Sodium**
Ref: Chapter No.4, Page No.80

114. **Ans: C. Patients about to undergo major surgery requiring inpatient hospitalization after surgery, IV fluids the night before are necessary**
Ref: Chapter No.4, Page No.81

115. **Ans: D. 90 ml/hr**
Ref: Chapter No.4, Page No.81

116. **Ans: C. 70 ml/hr**
Ref: Chapter No.4, Page No.81

117. **Ans: B. 42 ml/hr**
Ref: Chapter No.4, Page No.81

118. **Ans: D. 63 ml/hr**
Ref: Chapter No.4, Page No.81

119. **Ans: B. 117 ml/hr**
Ref: Chapter No.4, Page No.81

120. Ans: B. 2-4 g

Ref: Chapter No.4, Page No.81

121. Ans: C. Bradycardic hypertensive state to a profoundly tachycardic and hypotensive state

Ref: Chapter No.4, Page No.83

122. Ans: D. Decreased serum creatinine levels

Ref: Chapter No.4, Page No.83

123. Ans: D. Using dexamethasone is avoided if sending simultaneous laboratory tests to confirm the diagnosis of acute hypercortisolism as this medication interferes with the cosyntropin test

Ref: Chapter No.4, Page No.83

124. Ans: C. In SIADH urine osmolality will be low (<300 mmol/kg) even though serum osmolality is high

Ref: Chapter No.4, Page No.83

125. Ans: B. 135 to 145 mEq/L.

Ref: Chapter No.4, Page No.83

126. Ans: C. Hypernatremia is more concerning than hyponatremia

Ref: Chapter No.4, Page No.83-84

127. Ans: B. <120 mEq/liter

Ref: Chapter No.4, Page No.84

128. Ans: B. The measured sodium level is lowered by 1.6 mEq/L for every 100 mg/dL of glucose above 100

Ref: Chapter No.4, Page No.84

129. Ans: B. Sodium deficit (mEq) = ([Na] goal – [Na] plasma) × TBW

Ref: Chapter No.4, Page No.84

130. Ans: B. Corrected sodium = [Na] + 0.016 × (Glucose – 100)

Ref: Chapter No.4, Page No.84

131. Ans: C. Free water deficit = (([Na]/140) – 1) × TBW

Ref: Chapter No.4, Page No.84

132. Ans: A. Serum osmolality = 2 × [Na] + BUN/2.8 + Glucose/18

Ref: Chapter No.4, Page No.84

133. Ans: D. If urologic or gynecologic surgery is performed with hypoosmotic irrigation, acute hypernatremia can occur

Ref: Chapter No.4, Page No.84

134. Ans: B. >160 mEq/L

Ref: Chapter No.4, Page No.85

135. Ans: A. Euvolemic hypernatremia

Ref: Chapter No.4, Page No.85

136. Ans: B. Amiloride

Ref: Chapter No.4, Page No.85

137. Ans: B. Amiloride

Ref: Chapter No.4, Page No.85

138. Ans: C. Hypocalcaemia or severe hyperkalaemia also impairs the capacity of renal tubular cells to absorb sodium

Ref: Chapter No.4, Page No.85

139. Ans: D. All of the above are true

Ref: Chapter No.4, Page No.85

140. Ans: C. DDAVP increases water movement out of the collecting duct, and also has vasoconstrictive properties like ADH

Ref: Chapter No.4, Page No.85

141. Ans: D. All of the above

Ref: Chapter No.4, Page No.85

142. Ans: B. 2 mmol/L

Ref: Chapter No.4, Page No.85

143. Ans: A. 2.5 mmol/L

Ref: Chapter No.4, Page No.85

144. Ans: B. Development of U waves

Ref: Chapter No.4, Page No.86

145. Ans: D. Hypokalemia is also frequently associated with hypermagnesemia and alkalosis

Ref: Chapter No.4, Page No.86

146. Ans: A. 10 mEq/hr

Ref: Chapter No.4, Page No.86

147. Ans: D. All of the above are true

Ref: Chapter No.4, Page No.86

148. Ans: B. Supplemental magnesium increases the risk of arrhythmia

Ref: Chapter No.4, Page No.86

149. Ans: D. The most common cause of hyperkalemia is heart failure in hospitalized patients

Ref: Chapter No.4, Page No.86

150. Ans: B. At least 50% of normal renal function is required to respond to aldosterone and to maintain normal potassium levels

Ref: Chapter No.4, Page No.86-87

151. Ans: D. All of the above are true

Ref: Chapter No.4, Page No.87

152. Ans: D. Immediate hemodialysis

Ref: Chapter No.4, Page No.87

153. Ans: A. IV Calcium

Ref: Chapter No.4, Page No.87

154. Ans: C. Bicarbonate therapy

Ref: Chapter No.4, Page No.87

155. Ans: D. Haemodialysis

Ref: Chapter No.4, Page No.87

156. Ans: B. Corrected [iCa+2] = Total [Ca] + [(0.8 × [4.5 - Albumin level])]

Ref: Chapter No.4, Page No.87

157. Ans: D. All of the above are true

Ref: Chapter No.4, Page No.88

158. Ans: A. Hypoparathyroidism

Ref: Chapter No.4, Page No.88

159. Ans: D. Hypermagnesemia induces PTH resistance

Ref: Chapter No.4, Page No.88

160. Ans: B. Calcium chloride is preferred to calcium gluconate as it causes less tissue necrosis if it extravasates

Ref: Chapter No.4, Page No.88

161. Ans: D. All of the above are true

Ref: Chapter No.4, Page No.88

162. Ans: A. Primary hyperparathyroidism

Ref: Chapter No.4, Page No.88-89

163. Ans: C. 17 mg/dL

Ref: Chapter No.4, Page No.89

164. Ans: D. 15 mg/dL

Ref: Chapter No.4, Page No.89

165. Ans: B. Breast cancer

Ref: Chapter No.4, Page No.89

166. Ans: C. Patients with HHM constitute about 20% of all patients with hypercalcemia associated with malignant disease

Ref: Chapter No.4, Page No.89-90

167. Ans: B. Chelating agents (EDTA or phosphate salts) that bind and neutralize [iCa2+] are always indicated

Ref: Chapter No.4, Page No.90

168. Ans: A. Squamous cell carcinomas

Ref: Chapter No.4, Page No.90

169. Ans: B. 1.5 and 2.0 mEq/L

Ref: Chapter No.4, Page No.90

170. Ans: B. Albumin

Ref: Chapter No.4, Page No.90

171. Ans: B. Clinical sequelae of altered magnesium content depends on blood magnesium concentration

Ref: Chapter No.4, Page No. 90-91

172. Ans: B. 1.2 mg/dL

Ref: Chapter No.4, Page No.91

173. Ans: B. 1 g of magnesium sulfate contains 1 g of elemental magnesium

Ref: Chapter No.4, Page No. 91

174. Ans: B. Severe hypomagnesemia requires intermittent therapy because of the slow equilibration of extracellular magnesium with intracellular stores

Ref: Chapter No.4, Page No. 91

175. Ans: D. Elevated ST segment

Ref: Chapter No.4, Page No. 91

176. Ans: D. Peritoneal dialysis or continuous renal replacement therapy corrects hypermagnesemia more rapidly than intermittent hemodialysis

Ref: Chapter No.4, Page No. 91

5

Metabolism in Surgical Patients

METABOLIC SCIENCE

1. **Who pioneered the use of carbolic acid to prevent infection, and surgical mortality predictably began to decline?**
   A. Joseph Priestly
   B. Joseph Lister
   C. David Cuthbertson
   D. Antone-Laurent de Lavoisier

2. **Who had described the phenomenon of negative nitrogen balance after tissue trauma and argued that the losses were mostly due to muscle wasting?**
   A. Joseph Priestly
   B. Joseph Lister
   C. David Cuthbertson
   D. Antone-Laurent de Lavoisier

3. **Who had previously demonstrated that a mouse could not survive in a sealed flask if a flame had first burned in it; likewise, a flame could not burn in a flask in which a mouse had first breathed?**
   A. Joseph Priestly
   B. Joseph Lister
   C. David Cuthbertson
   D. Antone-Laurent de Lavoisier

4. **Who discovered the fundamental overlap between chemistry and biology that sits at the core of bioenergetics: oxidation?**
   A. Joseph Priestly
   B. Joseph Lister
   C. David Cuthbertson
   D. Antone-Laurent de Lavoisier

5. **True statement among the following is:**
   A. Adenosine triphosphate (ATP) is the most common currency of cellular bioenergetics by virtue of the chemical energy stored within the terminal phosphate bond
   B. ATP is synthesized from adenosine diphosphate (ADP) and phosphate via a reaction known as phosphorylation
   C. Multiple enzymes are capable of phosphorylating ADP to create ATP, with the most relevant to bioenergetics being ATP synthase, phosphoglycerate kinase and pyruvate kinase
   D. All of the above

6. **False about Kreb's cycle is:**
   A. Occur almost exclusively in the mitochondrial matrix
   B. TCA cycle only proceeds when oxygen delivery is high
   C. Baseline concentration of lactate production is not present at all times in the human body
   D. The citric acid (TCA/tricarboxylic acid/Krebs) cycle harnesses high energy electrons via the oxidation of pyruvate to power the electron transport chain

7. **No. of ATP molecules generated per glucose molecule via TCA cycle is:**
   A. 24 ATP B. 32 ATP
   C. 36 ATP D. 40 ATP

8. **False statement about Oxidative Phosphorylation:**
   A. The electron transport chain involves the transfer of electrons from NADH and FADH2 to ubiquinone through a series of 4 large protein complexes that reside in the mitochondrial inner membrane
   B. Without oxygen, the electrons in the electron transport chain cannot continue to fall down their potential energy gradient, and progression of electrons through the transport chain stops

C. The accumulation of electrons at Complex I and Complex III that occurs when substrate delivery is high and ADP concentrations are low contributes most to superoxide creation
D. All of the above are true

9. **No. of ATP molecules generated per glucose molecule via glycolysis is:**
A. 2 ATP B. 4 ATP
C. 6 ATP D. 8 ATP

10. **The most important of the starting substrates for gluconeogenesis are all except:**
A. Lactate B. Pyruvate
C. Fatty acids D. Amino acids

11. **The term ketone body generally refers to all except:**
A. β hydroxybutyrate
B. Acetoacetate
C. Acetone
D. Beta-hydroxypentanoate

12. **By the fourth day of fasting, the brain obtains ____ of its energy from ketone bodies.**
A. 30% B. 50%
C. 70% D. 90%

13. **True statement about brown adipose tissue (BAT) is:**
A. Adult humans have very small depots of BAT, generally located above the clavicle, near the vertebrae, in the mediastinum, and around the kidney
B. BAT is characterized by abundant uncoupling protein expression, leading to mitochondria that are highly thermogenic due to elevated expression of uncoupling protein-1
C. BAT cells are thought to be derived from cells positive for the myogenic factor 5 surface marker
D. All of the above

14. **No of amino acids that appear in human proteins:**
A. 18 B. 19
C. 22 D. 21

15. **Essential amino acids include all except:**
A. Leucine B. Threonine
C. Tyrosine D. Tryptophan

16. **Essential amino acids among the following is:**
A. Cysteine B. Phenylalanine
C. Asparagine D. Serine

17. **No. of essential amino acids are:**
A. 8 B. 9
C. 12 D. 6

18. **Non-essential amino acids includes all except:**
A. Alanine B. Glutamine
C. Selenocysteine D. Glutamate

19. **BCCA includes all except:**
A. Isoleucine B. Leucine
C. Valine D. Phenylalanine

20. **Which of the following amino acid cannot be oxidized into glucose?**
A. Asparagine B. Glutamine
C. Leucine D. Methionine

21. **Among the following amino acids, which can't be converted to either ketones or glucose?**
A. Isoleucine B. Lysine
C. Tryptophan D. Phenylalanine

22. **Tyrosine is converted to all of the catecholamine neurotransmitters, including all except:**
A. Dopamine B. Epinephrine
C. Norepinephrine D. Serotonin

23. **Regarding Cholesterol false statement among the following is:**
A. Cholesterol is a steroid alcohol that consists of three cyclohexanes and a single cyclopentane
B. The first reaction to synthesize all steroid hormones is the conversion of cholesterol to pregnenolone by a cholesterol side chain cleavage enzyme
C. The starting substrate of the cholesterol biosynthesis pathway is acetyl-CoA and the key rate-limiting enzyme, β-hydroxy β methylglutaryl-CoA reductase
D. Cholesterol can't be fully synthesized by the human body, is a dietary essential requirement

24. **Regarding fatty acids false statement is:**
A. Omega-3 and omega-6 fatty acids can be synthesized in the human body, making them non-essential nutrients
B. When the first saturated bond occurs at the third carbon-carbon bond when counted from the tail of the aliphatic chain, the fatty acid is called an "omega-3" fatty acid
C. When the bond is at the sixth carbon-carbon bond when counted from the tail, the fatty acid is called an "omega-6" fatty acid

D. Omega-3 and omega-6 fatty acids are converted into eicosanoids, powerful but short-lived 20-carbon molecules that are synthesized in response to tissue injury and stress

25. Regarding nucleotide synthesis and degradation all statements are true except:

A. Aspartate, glycine and glutamine are required to synthesize the pyrimidine nucleotides
B. Adenine and guanine are purine nucleotides, while cytosine, uracil and thymine are pyrimidine nucleotides
C. Nucleotides are small organic molecules composed of a five-carbon sugar, a nitrogenous base, and a phosphate group
D. In pyrimidine nucleotides, the nitrogenous base is a pyrimidine ring, while purine nucleotides contain a purine ring

26. Half-life of endogenous Insulin is between:

A. 1-2 mins B. 2-5 mins
C. 5-15 mins D. 15-45 mins

SURGICAL METABOLISM

27. Regarding Nutritional Assessment Scores all statements are true except:

A. Malnutrition Universal Screening Tool, the Mini Nutritional Assessment, and the newer Perioperative Nutrition Screen only take into account current nutritional status
B. Nutrition Risk Screening (NRS 2002) and the Nutrition Assessment in Critically Ill (NUTRIC) scores are currently the only two scores that take into account the severity of disease as well as nutritional factors
C. If malnutrition is considered, a nutrition risk score should also be utilized
D. Serum markers have been found to be effective for stratifying risk of malnutrition postoperatively

28. NUTRIC score includes all of the following variables except:

A. Sex B. Age
C. APACHE II D. SOFA

29. IL-6 concentrations of ___ adds 1 point to NUTRIC score.

A. $\geq$200 B. $\geq$300
C. $\geq$400 D. $\geq$500

30. High malnutrition risk means NUTRIC scores of more than:

A. 4 B. 5
C. 6 D. 7

31. If IL-6 concentrations are obtained, high malnutrition risk means NUTRIC scores of more than:

A. 4 B. 5
C. 6 D. 7

32. 30-day mortality rate if serum albumin levels of <2.1 g/dl is:

A. 5 B. 9
C. 15 D. 30

33. 30-day mortality rate if serum albumin levels of 3 g/dl is:

A. 5 B. 9
C. 15 D. 30

34. Gold standard, capable of providing highly accurate measures of bone and soft tissues is:

A. Ultrasound
B. DEXA
C. Computed tomography
D. MRI

35. Which of the following is a rapid and reliable bedside method to assess muscle mass, especially when the age and sex of the patient are incorporated into the assessment?

A. Ultrasound
B. DEXA
C. Computed tomography
D. MRI

36. Ideal body weight for males is:

A. 40 kg +2.3 kg for every 2.54 cm over 152.4 cm
B. 45 kg +2.3 kg for every 2.54 cm over 152.4 cm
C. 50 kg +2.3 kg for every 2.54 cm over 152.4 cm
D. 55 kg +2.3 kg for every 2.54 cm over 152.4 cm

37. Ideal body weight for females is:

A. 40 kg +2.3 kg for every 2.54 cm over 152.4 cm
B. 45 kg +2.3 kg for every 2.54 cm over 152.4 cm
C. 50 kg +2.3 kg for every 2.54 cm over 152.4 cm
D. 55 kg +2.3 kg for every 2.54 cm over 152.4 cm

38. Adjusted body weight is often used by nutritionists for energy calculations in bariatric surgery. It can be calculated as:

A. Adjusted body weight = Ideal body weight + 0.4 Current body weight–Ideal Body Weight
B. Adjusted body weight = Ideal body weight + 0.4 Current body weight+Ideal Body Weight
C. Adjusted body weight = Ideal body weight + 0.6 Current body weight–Ideal Body Weight

D. Adjusted body weight = Ideal body weight + 0.6 Current body weight+Ideal Body Weight

39. Harris-Benedict equation includes all except:

A. Weight
B. Age
C. Sex
D. BMI

40. Harris-Benedict energy expenditure multiplier for the scenario of major sepsis:

A. 1.2
B. 1.35
C. 1.6
D. 2.1

41. Harris-Benedict energy expenditure multiplier for the scenario of severe thermal injury:

A. 1.2
B. 1.35
C. 1.6
D. 2.1

42. Harris-Benedict energy expenditure multiplier for the scenario of skeletal trauma:

A. 1.2
B. 1.35
C. 1.6
D. 2.1

43. Harris-Benedict energy expenditure multiplier for the scenario of patient being febrile:

A. 1 + 0.09 per 0.5°C >38.5
B. 1 + 0.06 per 0.8°C >38.5
C. 1 + 0.09 per 0.8°C >38.5
D. 1 + 0.06 per 0.5°C >38.5

44. Underfeeding below ___ of the true REE can increase mortality.

A. 30%
B. 50%
C. 70%
D. 80%

45. A patient with 40% total body surface area burn; how much extra protein is needed in order to compensate for protein losses?

A. 10 to 20 g of extra protein per liter of intraperitoneal fluid lost
B. 15 to 30 g of extra protein per liter of intraperitoneal fluid lost
C. 25 to 40 g of extra protein per liter of intraperitoneal fluid lost
D. 5 to 10 g of extra protein per liter of intraperitoneal fluid lost

46. Baseline daily caloric intake at normal BMI is:

A. 30–40 kcal/kg actual body weight
B. 25–30 kcal/kg actual body weight
C. 11–14 kcal/kg actual body weight
D. 22–25 kcal/kg ideal body weight

47. Baseline daily caloric intake at BMI <18.5:

A. 30–40 kcal/kg actual body weight
B. 25–30 kcal/kg actual body weight
C. 11–14 kcal/kg actual body weight
D. 22–25 kcal/kg ideal body weight

48. Baseline daily caloric intake at BMI >50:

A. 30–40 kcal/kg actual body weight
B. 25–30 kcal/kg actual body weight
C. 11–14 kcal/kg actual body weight
D. 22–25 kcal/kg ideal body weight

49. Baseline daily caloric intake at BMI of 25.0–29.9:

A. 30–40 kcal/kg actual body weight
B. 25–30 kcal/kg actual body weight
C. 11–14 kcal/kg actual body weight
D. 22–25 kcal/kg ideal body weight

50. In the absence of hard contraindications for enteral feeding, such as intestinal discontinuity, enteral nutrition (EN) can safely begin within:

A. 6 hours postoperatively
B. 12 hours postoperatively
C. 24 hours postoperatively
D. 48 hours postoperatively

51. After gastrointestinal anastomosis parenteral nutrition is indicated after ____ for low-risk patients.

A. 1-2 days
B. 2-4 days
C. 5-7 days
D. >7 days

52. ASPEN recommended intensive care unit (ICU) nutrition bundle includes all except:

A. Initiate enteral nutrition (EN) within 24–48 hours following the onset of critical illness and admission to the ICU, and increase to goals over the first week of ICU stay
B. Use gastric residual volumes as part of routine care to monitor ICU patients receiving EN
C. Initiate enteral nutrition (EN) within 24–48 hours following the onset of critical illness and admission to the ICU, and increase to goals over the first week of ICU stay
D. Start parenteral nutrition early when EN is not feasible or sufficient in high risk or poorly nourished patients

53. False statement among the following is:

A. ASPEN guidelines currently recommend enteral feeding over parenteral nutrition based on best available evidence

B. Current evidence suggests that gastric feeding is unsafe as there is a high risk for aspiration
C. Lack of enteral feeding can lead to dysbiosis of the gut microbiome, allowing bacteria to traverse the intestinal wall, leading to sepsis and multisystem organ failure
D. EN has been shown to improve intestinal blood flow, cause release of bile salts and gastrin, and assist in tight junction maintenance in the gut

54. Recommendations of soluble fiber are usually:

A. 20 to 30 g/day B. 10 to 20 g/day
C. 30 to 40 g/day D. 25 to 35 g/day

55. The initial "ebb" phase occurs approximately after how long, after trauma or surgical stress?

A. 12 hours B. 24 hours
C. 72 hours D. 1 week

56. For an average adult, even early in starvation, the body degrades approximately:

A. 25 g of muscle protein per day
B. 50 g of muscle protein per day
C. 75 g of muscle protein per day
D. 100 g of muscle protein per day

57. False regarding Vit A deficiency is all except:

A. Deficiency causes impaired gut epithelial integrity
B. Cofactor in collagen synthesis and cross linking
C. Deficiency can result in diminished activity of helper T cells
D. Essential for coagulation

58. Which vitamin deficiency leading to poor wound healing and skin graft take?

A. Vitamin B1 B. Vitamin B5
C. Vitamin A D. Vitamin C

59. Which vitamin deficiency leading to prolonged steatorrhea and neuronal degeneration?

A. Vitamin B1 B. Vitamin E
C. Vitamin K D. Vitamin D

60. Which micronutrient losses can cause significant wound exudate?

A. Copper B. Selenium
C. Magnesium D. Calcium

61. False statement about Zinc is:

A. Deficiency can cause impaired wound healing
B. Reduces intracellular hydroperoxides
C. Deficiency can cause hair loss, dermatitis
D. None

62. Which micronutrient deficiency causes delayed sexual maturation, testicular atrophy?

A. Zinc B. Selenium
C. Copper D. Magnesium

63. Which micronutrient deficiency causes myopathy, cardiomyopathy?

A. Zinc B. Selenium
C. Copper D. Magnesium

64. Which vitamin deficiency leading to Wernicke-Korsakoff syndrome?

A. Vitamin B1 B. Vitamin B5
C. Vitamin B2 D. Vitamin C

65. The amount of protein needed to overcome anabolic resistance in severe illness is estimated to be at least:

A. 1.2 to 2.0 g/kg/day
B. 1.5 to 2.5 g/kg/day
C. 1.0 to 1.5 g/kg/day
D. 0.7 to 1.2 g/kg/day

66. Which of the following is not seen refeeding syndrome?

A. Hypophosphatemia B. Hypomagnesemia
C. Hypokalaemia D. Hypocalcaemia

67. The hallmark feature of refeeding syndrome is:

A. Hypophosphatemia B. Hypomagnesemia
C. Hypokalaemia D. Hypocalcaemia

68. False statement about refeeding syndrome is:

A. Refeeding syndrome is a potentially fatal condition that occurs in patients who have experienced prolonged periods of starvation
B. As phosphate is shifted to the intracellular compartment for the production of ATP for energy, there are profound decreases in extracellular phosphate concentrations
C. If refeeding syndrome is anticipated, high-potency B vitamins and daily vitamin supplementation is recommended prior to starting EN
D. Feedings should commence at 25 kcal/kg/day with slow increases over 4 to 7 days.

69. In aggregate, transplant patients have been noted to have elevated REEs for up to:

A. 6 months B. 1 year
C. 2 years D. 5 years

70. Current recommendations for caloric and protein intake in post-transplant patients is:
A. 30 to 35 kcal/kg and 1.5 to 2.0 g/kg/day, respectively
B. 35 to 40 kcal/kg and 1.3 to 1.5 g/kg/day, respectively
C. 35 to 40 kcal/kg and 1.5 to 2.0 g/kg/day, respectively
D. 30 to 35 kcal/kg and 1.3 to 1.5 g/kg/day, respectively

71. True about nutritional recommendations in case of inflammatory bowel disease is/are:
A. These dietary modifications can lead to significant improvement in symptoms over the long term
B. Diets high in meat and alcohol increase the likelihood of ulcerative colitis relapse
C. Diets high in sucrose, refined carbohydrates, and omega-6 fatty acids and diets low in fruit and vegetables increase the risk of inflammatory bowel disease, especially Crohn's disease
D. All of the above

72. The most successful regimens to improve oral food intake in inflammatory bowel disease patients include:
A. Low-protein, low-fat, high-carbohydrate diets
B. High-protein, high-fat, low-carbohydrate diets
C. High-protein, low-fat, low-carbohydrate diets
D. High-protein, low-fat, high-carbohydrate diets

73. False regarding short bowel syndrome is:
A. After resection of the small bowel, the endothelial lining of remaining bowel hypertrophies within 48 hours
B. The most common causes of short bowel syndrome in adults is necrotising enterocolitis
C. Treatment recommendations for SBS revolve around aggressive enteral support to stimulate hypertrophy of the villi
D. As a last resort, the treatment is home TPN, which has been shown to increase life expectancy between 10 and 20 years and promote survival

74. In cases of acute pancreatitis enteral nutrition should be started within:
A. 24 hrs B. 48 hrs
C. 72 hrs D. 12 hrs

75. The symptoms of exocrine pancreatic failure, such as steatorrhea, are only apparent after loss of exocrine tissue of about:
A. 20% to 30% B. 30% to 50%
C. 50% to 80% D. 80% to 90%

76. False among the following is:
A. Nasogastric route causes erosive esophagitis
B. Gastrostomy has risks include bleeding, perforation
C. Nasojejunal tube can be easily clogged or displaced
D. Jejunostomy is used for short term feeding

77. Regarding nutrition in burns patient all are true except:
A. The metabolic dysregulation associated with massive thermal injury directly contributes to clinical complications, delayed recovery and increased mortality
B. Even in the context of aggressive delivery of nutrition, significant lean-body mass loss over the course of acute burn treatment is inevitable with the current standard of care
C. Propranolol is a selective β-AR antagonist that has been shown to reduce thermogenesis, tachycardia, and REE in burn patients
D. Negative nitrogen balance, insulin resistance, lipolysis, and protein wasting may persist for as long as 2 years following severe injuries, leading to a significant delay in rehabilitation

78. The recommended amount of protein for septic patients during acute resuscitation is approximately:
A. 0.8 g/kg/day B. 1.0 g/kg/day
C. 1.2 g/kg/day D. 1.5 g/kg/day

79. The recommended amount of nonprotein calories is approximately:
A. 15 kcal/kg/day B. 20 kcal/kg/day
C. 25 kcal/kg/day D. 30 kcal/kg/day

80. During severe sepsis, oxygen consumption may:
A. Rise 40% to 50% above baseline
B. Rise 50% to 60% above baseline
C. Rise 60% to 70% above baseline
D. Rise 70% to 80% above baseline

81. Pure carbohydrate consumption results in an RQ of:
A. 0.7 B. 0.9
C. 1.0 D. 1.2

82. Supplement that improve cancer cachexia in bile duct and pancreatic cancer:

A. High-dose vitamin D
B. Increasing dietary fibre
C. Omega-3 fatty acid
D. Coffee

83. False statement about Nutrition Support in Hepatic Insufficiency:

A. Up to 70% hepatocyte destruction is required for clinical features of cirrhosis
B. While partial thromboplastin is almost always normal in hepatic insufficiency, bleeding time can either be prolonged or normal
C. A catabolic condition closely resembling burn hypermetabolism or sepsis develops during hepatic insufficiency
D. The treatment of patients with hepatic insufficiency centres around meeting the caloric intake required to maintain lean body mass while maintaining low fluid intake

84. Because encephalopathy is likely a result of the accumulation of ammonia, protein restriction to:

A. <20 g/day
B. <25 g/day
C. <40 g/day
D. <30 g/day

85. The most common nutrient deficiency after the adjustable gastric band procedure is:

A. Iron deficiency anemia
B. B12 deficiency
C. Vit D deficiency
D. Protein malnutrition

86. The most common nutrient deficiency after sleeve gastrectomy procedure is:

A. Iron deficiency anemia
B. B12 deficiency
C. Vit D deficiency
D. Protein malnutrition

87. The most common nutrient deficiency associated with RYGB is:

A. Iron deficiency anemia
B. B12 deficiency
C. Vit D deficiency
D. Protein malnutrition

88. The most common nutrient deficiency in BPD and BPD-DS is:

A. Iron deficiency anemia
B. B12 deficiency
C. Vit D deficiency
D. Protein malnutrition

ANSWERS

1. **Ans: B. Joseph Lister**
Ref: Chapter No.5, Page No.95

2. **Ans: C. David Cuthbertson**
Ref: Chapter No.5, Page No.95

3. **Ans: A. Joseph Priestly**
Ref: Chapter No.5, Page No.95

4. **Ans: D. Antone-Laurent de Lavoisier**
Ref: Chapter No.5, Page No.95

5. **Ans: D. All of the above**
Ref: Chapter No.5, Page No.95

6. **Ans: C. Baseline concentration of lactate production is not present at all times in the human body**
Ref: Chapter No.5, Page No.95-97

7. **Ans: C. 36 ATP molecules**
Ref: Chapter No.5, Page No.97

8. **Ans: D. All of the above are true**
Ref: Chapter No.5, Page No.97-98

9. **Ans: A. 2 ATP**
Ref: Chapter No.5, Page No.98

10. **Ans: B. Pyruvate**
Ref: Chapter No.5, Page No.99

11. **Ans: D. Beta-hydroxypentanoate**
Ref: Chapter No.5, Page No.99

12. **Ans: C. 70%**
Ref: Chapter No.5, Page No.99

13. **Ans: D. All of the above**
Ref: Chapter No.5, Page No.100

14. **Ans: D. 21**
Ref: Chapter No.5, Page No.100

15. **Ans: C. Tyrosine**
Ref: Chapter No.5, Page No.100

16. **Ans: B. Phenylalanine**
Ref: Chapter No.5, Page No.100

17. **Ans: B. 9**

Ref: Chapter No.5, Page No.100

18. **Ans: B. Glutamine**

Ref: Chapter No.5, Page No.100

19. **Ans: D. Phenylalanine**

Ref: Chapter No.5, Page No.100

20. **Ans: C. Leucine**

Ref: Chapter No.5, Page No.100

21. **Ans: B. Lysine**

Ref: Chapter No.5, Page No.100

22. **Ans: D. Serotonin**

Ref: Chapter No.5, Page No.100

23. **Ans: D. Cholesterol can't be fully synthesized by the human body, is a dietary essential requirement**

Ref: Chapter No.5, Page No.101

24. **Ans: A. Omega-3 and omega-6 fatty acids can be synthesized in the human body, making them non-essential nutrients**

Ref: Chapter No.5, Page No.101

25. **Ans: A. Aspartate, glycine and glutamine are required to synthesize the pyrimidine nucleotides**

Ref: Chapter No.5, Page No.101-102

26. **Ans: C. 5-15 mins**

Ref: Chapter No.5, Page No.102

27. **Ans: D. Serum markers have been found to be effective for stratifying risk of malnutrition postoperatively**

Ref: Chapter No.5, Page No.103

28. **Ans: A. Sex**

Ref: Chapter No.5, Page No.104

29. **Ans: C. ≥400**

Ref: Chapter No.5, Page No.104

30. **Ans: B. 5**

Ref: Chapter No.5, Page No.104

31. **Ans: C. 6**

Ref: Chapter No.5, Page No.104

32. **Ans: D. 30**

Ref: Chapter No.5, Page No.104

33. **Ans: B. 9**

Ref: Chapter No.5, Page No.104

34. **Ans: B. DEXA**

Ref: Chapter No.5, Page No.104

35. **Ans: A. Ultrasound**

Ref: Chapter No.5, Page No.104

36. **Ans: C. 50 kg +2.3 kg for every 2.54 cm over 152.4 cm**

Ref: Chapter No.5, Page No.105

37. **Ans: B. 45 kg +2.3 kg for every 2.54 cm over 152.4 cm**

Ref: Chapter No.5, Page No.105

38. **Ans: A. Adjusted body weight = Ideal body weight + 0.4 Current body weight–Ideal Body Weight**

Ref: Chapter No.5, Page No.105

39. **Ans: D. BMI**

Ref: Chapter No.5, Page No.105

40. **Ans: C. 1.6**

Ref: Chapter No.5, Page No.106

41. **Ans: D. 2.1**

Ref: Chapter No.5, Page No.106

42. **Ans: B. 1.35**

Ref: Chapter No.5, Page No.106

43. **Ans: A. 1 + 0.09 per 0.5°C >38.5**

Ref: Chapter No.5, Page No.106

44. **Ans: C. 70%**

Ref: Chapter No.5, Page No.106

45. **Ans: B. 15 to 30 g of extra protein per liter of intraperitoneal fluid lost**

Ref: Chapter No.5, Page No.106

46. **Ans: B. 25–30 kcal/kg actual body weight**

Ref: Chapter No.5, Page No.106

47. **Ans: A. 30–40 kcal/kg actual body weight**

Ref: Chapter No.5, Page No.106

48. **Ans: D. 22–25 kcal/kg ideal body weight**

Ref: Chapter No.5, Page No.106

49. **Ans: C. 11–14 kcal/kg actual body weight**

Ref: Chapter No.5, Page No.106

50. **Ans: C. 24 hours postoperatively**

Ref: Chapter No.5, Page No.107

51. **Ans: C. 5-7 days**

Ref: Chapter No.5, Page No.107

52. **Ans: B. Use gastric residual volumes as part of routine care to monitor ICU patients receiving EN**

Ref: Chapter No.5, Page No.107

53. **Ans: B. Current evidence suggests that gastric feeding is unsafe as there is a high risk for aspiration**

Ref: Chapter No.5, Page No.107

54. **Ans: B. 10 to 20 g/day**

Ref: Chapter No.5, Page No.108

55. **Ans: B. 24 hours**

Ref: Chapter No.5, Page No.108

56. **Ans: C. 75 g of muscle protein per day**

Ref: Chapter No.5, Page No.109

57. **Ans: D. Essential for coagulation**

Ref: Chapter No.5, Page No.110

58. **Ans: B. Vitamin B5**

Ref: Chapter No.5, Page No.110

59. **Ans: B. Vitamin E**

Ref: Chapter No.5, Page No.110

60. **Ans: A. Copper**

Ref: Chapter No.5, Page No.110

61. **Ans: D. None**

Ref: Chapter No.5, Page No.110

62. **Ans: A. Zinc**

Ref: Chapter No.5, Page No.110

63. **Ans: B. Selenium**

Ref: Chapter No.5, Page No.110

64. **Ans: A. Vitamin B1**

Ref: Chapter No.5, Page No.110

65. **Ans: A. 1.2 to 2.0 g/kg/day**

Ref: Chapter No.5, Page No.109

66. **Ans: D. Hypocalcaemia**

Ref: Chapter No.5, Page No.109

67. **Ans: A. Hypophosphatemia**

Ref: Chapter No.5, Page No.109

68. **Ans: D. Feedings should commence at 25 kcal/kg/day with slow increases over 4 to 7 days**

Ref: Chapter No.5, Page No.109

69. **Ans: B. 1 year**

Ref: Chapter No.5, Page No.109

70. **Ans: D. 30 to 35 kcal/kg and 1.3 to 1.5 g/kg/day, respectively**

Ref: Chapter No.5, Page No.111

71. **Ans: D. All of the above**

Ref: Chapter No.5, Page No.111

72. **Ans: C. High-protein, low-fat, low-carbohydrate diets**

Ref: Chapter No.5, Page No.111

73. **Ans: B. The most common causes of short bowel syndrome in adults is necrotising enterocolitis**

Ref: Chapter No.5, Page No.111

74. **Ans: B. 48 hrs**

Ref: Chapter No.5, Page No.112

75. **Ans: D. 80% to 90%**

Ref: Chapter No.5, Page No.112

76. **Ans: D. Jejunostomy is used for short term feeding**

Ref: Chapter No.5, Page No.113

77. **Ans: C. Propranolol is a selective β-AR antagonist that has been shown to reduce thermogenesis, tachycardia and REE in burn patients**

Ref: Chapter No.5, Page No.113-114

78. **Ans: B. 1.0 g/kg/day**

Ref: Chapter No.5, Page No.114

79. **Ans: A. 15 kcal/kg/day**

Ref: Chapter No.5, Page No.114

80. **Ans: B. Rise 50% to 60% above baseline**

Ref: Chapter No.5, Page No.114

81. **Ans: C. 1.0**

Ref: Chapter No.5, Page No.114

82. **Ans: C. Omega-3 fatty acid**

Ref: Chapter No.5, Page No.115

83. **Ans: A. Up to 70% hepatocyte destruction is required for clinical features of cirrhosis**

Ref: Chapter No.5, Page No.115

84. **Ans: C. <40 g/day**

Ref: Chapter No.5, Page No.115

85. **Ans: A. Iron deficiency anemia**

Ref: Chapter No.5, Page No.116

86. **Ans: B. B12 deficiency**

Ref: Chapter No.5, Page No.116

87. **Ans: A. Iron deficiency anemia**

Ref: Chapter No.5, Page No.116

88. **Ans: D. Protein malnutrition**

Ref: Chapter No.5, Page No.116

6

Wound Healing

TISSUE INJURY AND RESPONSE

1. **False statement among the following is:**
   A. During wound repair, flawless reconstruction is sacrificed in order to speed up the return to function
   B. Attempts to restore mechanical integrity, to repair barriers to fluid loss and infection, and to re-establish normal blood and lymphatic flow patterns are termed wound repair.
   C. A chronic wound stalls during a sustained proliferative phase and fails to heal
   D. Regeneration, which is the goal of wound healing, is the perfect restoration of the pre-existing tissue architecture without scar formation

2. **Regeneration is achievable in all except:**
   A. Embryonic development
   B. Liver
   C. Bone
   D. Brain

WOUND-HEALING PHASES

3. **Platelet activation occurs by binding to exposed ___ from the damaged endothelium.**
   A. Type V and type VI collagen
   B. Type IV and type V collagen
   C. Type IV and type VI collagen
   D. Type IV and type VII collagen

4. **Initial contact between platelets and collagen requires:**
   A. Type IV collagen
   B. Von Willebrand factor
   C. Megakaryocytes
   D. Integrins

5. **Platelet alpha granules are storage organelles that contains all except:**
   A. Platelet-derived growth factor (PDGF)
   B. Fibrinogen
   C. Insulin-like growth factor 1 (IGF-1)
   D. Histamine

6. **The dense bodies contain vasoactive amines like:**
   A. Histamine B. Serotonin
   C. Dopamine D. Noradrenaline

7. **Which of the following statement is false?**
   A. MCP-1 is elevated in chronic wounds
   B. CXCL1 (GRO-α) is increased in acute wounds
   C. Interleukin-8 is increased in acute and chronic wounds
   D. High levels of IL-8 are found in fetal wounds

8. **Stromal cell–derived factor-1 (SDF-1, also known as CXCL12) is expressed by all except:**
   A. Endothelial cells B. Myofibroblasts
   C. Megakaryocytes D. Keratinocytes

9. **Peak levels of T lymphocytes in wound are seen on:**
   A. 2nd day B. 3rd day
   C. 7th day D. 5th day

10. **Peak levels of Neutrophils in wound are seen on:**
    A. 2nd day B. 3rd day
    C. 7th day D. 5th day

11. **Integrins are crucial for:**
    A. Cell motility
    B. Normal wound healing
    C. Tumor metastases
    D. All of the above

12. **False statement among the following statements is:**
    A. Spreading is characterized by the development of lamellipodia and filopodia
    B. Retraction at the leading edge of the cell develops through binding of integrin followed by translocation of the cell over the adherent segment of the plasma membrane
    C. Within the assembled framework of the ECM, binding sites for integrins have been identified on collagen, laminin and fibronectin
    D. Four phases of integrin-mediated cell motility have been described: adhesion, spreading, contractility or traction and retraction

13. **Peak levels of Macrophages in wound are seen on:**
    A. 2nd day B. 3rd day
    C. 7th day D. 5th day

14. **False statement among the following statements is:**
    A. Superoxide dismutase catalyzes the formation of hydrogen peroxide (H_2O_2), which is then degraded by myeloperoxidase in the azurophilic granules of neutrophils
    B. The iron-catalyzed reaction between H_2O_2 and O_2 – forms hydroxyl radicals (OH·)
    C. Individual PMNs survive no longer than 72 hours and are replaced predominantly by mononuclear cells
    D. PMNs are not essential for wound healing because their phagocytosis and antimicrobial role can be taken over by macrophages

15. **Monocyte chemotactic factors include all except:**
    A. Thrombin B. TGF-β
    C. Fibrinogen D. Collagen

16. **The activity of the free radicals is potentiated by:**
    A. IL-6 B. IL-2
    C. IL-10 D. IL-12

17. **Macrophages have specific receptors for all except:**
    A. IgG B. C3b
    C. Thrombin D. Fibronectin

18. **ECM turnover is blocked by:**
    (a) Nonsteroidal anti-inflammatory
    (b) Glucocorticoids
    (c) Colchicine
    (d) Retinoic acid
    A. a,b,c B. a,b
    C. b,d D. b,c,d

19. **Collagenase production decreased by:**
    (a) Nonsteroidal anti-inflammatory
    (b) Glucocorticoids
    (c) Colchicine
    (d) Retinoic acid
    A. b,c,d B. a,b,c
    C. b,d D. c,d

20. **Interleukin responsible for febrile response:**
    A. IL-1 B. IL-2
    C. IL-8 D. IL-10

21. **TNF-α is detected in a wound peak after:**
    A. 24 hrs B. 48 hrs
    C. 72 hrs D. 96 hrs

22. **Cytokine responsible for hepatic acute phase protein synthesis:**
    A. TNF-α B. IL-2
    C. IL-6 D. IFN-γ

23. **IL-8 in the acute wound has peak expression within the first:**
    A. 24 hours B. 48 hours
    C. 72 hours D. 96 hours

24. **False statement about IFN-γ is:**
    A. Is secreted by T lymphocytes and macrophages
    B. IFN-γ has been used in the treatment of hypertrophic and keloid scars
    C. Decreases collagenase activity
    D. IFN-γ may improve scar hypertrophy by decreasing the strength of the wound

25. **The only growth factor preparation approved by the U.S. Food and Drug Administration and is the most widely studied clinically:**
    A. PDGF-AA B. PDGF-BB
    C. PDGF-AB D. All of the above

26. **The most potent stimulant of fibroplasia:**
    A. TGF-β B. PDGF
    C. TGF-α D. IGF-1

27. **False statement among the following is:**
    A. Lipopolysaccharide and IFN-γ stimulate the differentiation into M1 macrophages that release TNF-α, NO and IL-6
    B. M2 macrophages are activated by IL-4 and IL-13

C. M2 macrophages can also be involved in different diseases, such as allergy, asthma and fibrosis, which is the result of a helper T-cell (Th2) response predominated by IL-4 or IL-10
D. In the proliferative phase, M1 macrophages predominate

28. T lymphocytes appear by __ after injury.

A. Day 3 B. Day 5
C. Day 7 D. Day 14

29. T lymphocytes peak on __ after injury.

A. Day 3 B. Day 5
C. Day 7 D. Day 14

30. False statement among the following is:

A. T lymphocytes appear to be principally involved in downregulating healing as the wound closes
B. Significant numbers of T lymphocytes appear by day 5 after injury and peak on day 7
C. IFN-γ appears to be an important mediator of chronic nonhealing wounds
D. IFN-γ decreases prostaglandin synthesis, enhancing the effect of inflammatory mediators

31. Which cytokine orchestrates angiogenesis during the inflammatory phase?

A. TNF-α B. VEGF
C. Flt-1 D. FGF

32. Factor required for blood vessel organization:

A. TNF-α B. VEGF
C. Flt-1 D. FGF

33. FGF-2 provides the initial angiogenic stimulus within the first ______ days of wound repair.

A. 2 days B. 3 days
C. 7 days D. 14 days

34. Prolonged stimulus for angiogenesis is mediated by VEGF from:

A. Day 1-3 B. Day 4-7
C. Day 7-14 D. Day 14-21

35. HIF-1α mRNA is prominently present in wound inflammatory cells during the initial:

A. 6 hours B. 12 hours
C. 24 hours D. 48 hours

36. Which factor stimulates fibroblast proliferation?

A. TNF-α B. TGF-α
C. VEGF D. TGF-β

37. The rate of collagen synthesis declines after:

A. 3 weeks B. 4 weeks
C. 6 weeks D. 12 weeks

38. False statement among the following is:

A. The basal layer of the epidermis attaches to the basement membrane zone by desmosomes
B. The migrating cells dissect the wound by separating the desiccated eschar from viable tissue
C. The epithelial cells move in a leapfrog and tumbling fashion until the edges establish contact
D. Topical application of keratinocyte growth factor-2 (KGF-2) in young and aged animals accelerates reepithelialisation

39. Resilience to matrix is given by:

A. Collagen Fibres B. Elastin Fibres
C. Glycosaminoglycans D. Proteoglycans

40. Strength to matrix is given by:

A. Collagen Fibres B. Elastin Fibres
C. Glycosaminoglycans D. Proteoglycans

41. False statement about collagen among the following is:

A. Proline-rich and glycine-rich collagen molecule is a long, stiff, triple-stranded helical structure
B. Proline provides stability to the helical conformation in each α chain
C. In newborns, the content of type I collagen is greater than that found in adults
D. Type I collagens are the fibrillar, or fibril-forming collagens

42. Principal collagen of skin and bone and the most common type of collagen is:

A. Type I B. Type II
C. Type III D. Type IV

43. False statement about collagen among the following is:

A. Hydroxylation results in the stable triple-stranded helix through the formation of interchain hydrogen bonds
B. In conditions such as vitamin C deficiency (scurvy), proline hydroxylation is prevented
C. Vitamin C deficiency is characterized by the gradual loss of pre-existing normal collagen, which leads to fragile blood vessels and loose teeth

D. Covalent cross-linking of the glycine residues provides tensile strength.

44. False statement about collagen among the following is:

A. Covalent cross-linking of the lysine residues provides tensile strength
B. In mammalian skin, the fibrils are organized in a basketweave pattern
C. In tendons, fibrils are in parallel bundles aligned along the major axis of tension
D. None

45. Ehlers-Danlos syndrome is a result of mutations affecting:

A. Type I collagen B. Type II collagen
C. Type III collagen D. Type IV collagen

46. False statement about elastic fibres among the following is:

A. Elastin is composed of hydrophobic and alanine-rich and lysine-rich α-helical segments that alternate along the polypeptide chain
B. Elastin-binding fibrillin is essential for the integrity of the elastic fibers
C. Elastin is produced early in life, stabilizes, and undergo much further synthesis or degradation
D. IGF-1 and TGF-β stimulate the production of elastin

47. Gene mutations in fibrillin result in:

A. Edwards syndrome
B. Marfan syndrome
C. Ehlers-Danlos syndrome
D. Osteogenesis Imperfecta

48. Glycosaminoglycans in matrix provides:

A. Strength B. Turgor
C. Resilience D. All of the above

49. Simplest Glycosaminoglycan is:

A. Keratan sulfate B. Dermatan sulfate
C. Chondroitin sulfate D. Hyaluronan

50. Which GAG is present in abundance in fetal wounds which is a factor in the scarless wound healing seen in fetal tissues?

A. Keratan sulfate B. Dermatan sulfate
C. Chondroitin sulfate D. Hyaluronan

51. Stress fibres in wound healing process are made by:

A. Beta smooth muscle actin
B. Alpha skeletal muscle actin
C. Alpha smooth muscle actin
D. Beta skeletal muscle actin

52. The actin after wounding persists at high levels for:

A. 7 days B. 14 days
C. 15 days D. 30 days

53. Which of the following is not done by proteoglycans after binding to proteins?

A. Immobilizing the protein and restricting its range of action
B. Providing a reservoir of the protein for delayed release
C. Altering the protein to allow more effective presentation to cell surface receptors
D. Shortening the action of the protein by promoting degradation

54. False statement about basal lamina is:

A. Basal laminae are flexible, thin (40–120 nm) mats of specialized ECM that separate cells and epithelia from the underlying or surrounding connective tissue.
B. Composite of basal lamina and collagen is the basement membrane
C. Type IV collagen has a less flexible structure than the fibrillar collagens
D. Laminins generally consist of three long polypeptide chains (α, β and γ)

55. The actin after wounding is gone by:

A. 4 weeks B. 6 weeks
C. 2 weeks D. 8 weeks

56. False statement about wound contraction is:

A. Contractures occur when excessive scar exceeds normal wound contraction
B. Fibroblasts in a contracting wound undergo change to stimulated cells, termed myofibroblasts
C. Wound contraction occurs by centripetal movement of the partial thickness of the surrounding skin
D. Fibroblasts develop a linear arrangement in the line of tension that, when removed, causes the cells to round up

57. The actin after wounding, appears at:

A. Day 3 B. Day 6
C. Day 7 D. Day 14

58. Tensile strength is ___% in the scar.

A. 20% B. 30%
C. 50% D. 70%

59. Breaking strength increases after approximately:

A. 7 days B. 14 days
C. 21 days D. 28 days

60. False statement about remodeling among the following is:

A. In contrast to normal skin, the epidermodermal interface in a healed wound is devoid of rete pegs
B. Wound strength increases rapidly within 1 to 6 weeks and then appears to plateau up to 1 year after the injury
C. Although collagen cross-linking causes further wound contraction and an increase in strength, it also results in a scar that is less brittle and more elastic than normal skin
D. Loss of this anchorage results in increased fragility and predisposes the neoepidermis to avulsion after minor trauma.

ABNORMAL WOUND HEALING

61. All of the following statements about keloids are true except:

A. Proposed pathways include apoptosis, endocytosis, cytokine-cytokine receptor interaction, mitogen-activated protein kinase signaling pathway, tenascin C, jun proto-oncogene, and growth factors such as TGF-β and VEGF
B. They are more prevalent in darkly pigmented skin
C. There are known effective prevention method for keloid formation
D. Keloids, by definition, grow beyond the borders of the original wounds and rarely regress with time

62. Factors that inhibit wound healing includes all except:

A. Adriamycin B. Diabetes mellitus
C. Ionizing radiation D. Young age

63. False statement about hypertrophied scar among the following is:

A. Hypertrophic scars are often preventable
B. Hypertrophic scars primarily contain disorganised-organized type III collagen
C. Hypertrophic scars represent a reversible hyperproliferative scar phenotype that tends to regress when the original stimuli are removed.
D. All of the above

64. True statement among the following is:

A. Keloids, contain islands composed of aggregates of fibroblasts, small vessels, and collagen fibers throughout the dermis
B. Keloids and hypertrophic scars have stretched collagen bundles aligned in the same plane as the epidermis, whereas collagen bundles are randomly arrayed and relaxed in normal scars
C. Keloids primarily contain well-organized type III collagen
D. Hypertrophic scars contain disorganized type I and type III collagen bundles

65. False statement among the following is:

A. Scars parallel to the underlying muscle fibers tend to be flatter and narrower, with less collagen formation than when they are perpendicular to the underlying muscle fibers
B. As muscle fibers contract, the wound edges become reapproximated when they are perpendicular to the underlying muscle and tend to gape if placed parallel to it, leading to greater wound tension and scar formation
C. Hypertrophic scars are often preventable
D. Hypertrophic scars represent a reversible hyperproliferative scar phenotype that tends to regress when the original stimuli are removed.

66. False statement among the following is:

A. Blocking TGF-β activity with antibodies increases scar fibrosis
B. Keloids appear to be genetically predisposed and switched on irreversibly by factors such as TGF-β
C. MMP-1 (collagenase) and MMP-9 (gelatinase, early tissue repair) are decreased, whereas MMP-2 (gelatinase, late tissue remodelling) is significantly elevated
D. All of the above are true

67. False statement about prevention of keloids/ hypertrophic scar among the following is:

A. Avoidance of sun exposure and use of SPF 50+ sunscreens for 1 month postoperatively reduce scar hyperpigmentation and improve clinical appearance
B. Scarring can be reduced by postsurgical taping of the wound for 3 months

C. Pressure garments should be used prophylactically in wounds that are wide
D. Strategies that reduce adverse scarring immediately after wound closure are tension relief, hydration/occlusion, and use of taping/pressure garments

68. Early linear scar hypertrophy (e.g., after trauma or surgery) at 6 weeks to 3 months should be treated with:

A. Intralesional corticosteroids
B. Pressure therapy
C. Silicone therapy
D. Surgical scar revision

69. Intralesional corticosteroids (triamcinolone acetonide, 10–40 mg/mL) is injected into:

A. Epidermis
B. Subcutaneous fat
C. Reticular Dermis
D. Papillary Dermis

70. False statement about Intralesional corticosteroids among the following is:

A. Approximately 50% to 100% of patients respond, and up to 50% experience recurrence
B. Injections should be limited to the scar itself to minimize adjacent fat atrophy
C. Adverse steroid effects include skin atrophy, hypopigmentation, telangiectasias, and excessive pain during injections
D. Intralesional corticosteroids (triamcinolone acetonide, 10–40 mg/mL) injected into the papillary dermis every 2 to 4 months until flat

71. Surgical scar revision may be considered for permanent linear hypertrophic scars present after:

A. 6 months
B. 1 year
C. 2 years
D. 3 years

72. False statement about widespread hypertrophic scars among the following is:

A. Bleomycin, 5-fluorouracil (5-FU), and verapamil have been used as adjuncts to corticosteroid therapy
B. Pressure therapy is believed to act on cellular mechanoreceptors that are involved in cellular apoptosis and linked to the ECM
C. Losartan ointment (5%) was found to significantly decrease vascularity and pliability and improve scar quality after 3 months of treatment, with no recurrences in a 6-month follow-up
D. All of the above are true

73. False statement about keloids among the following is:

A. Excision alone results in a high recurrence rate of 50% to 100% and potential enlargement of the keloid
B. First-line treatments include intralesional corticosteroid injections in combination with silicone dressings and pressure therapy
C. Refractory cases after 12 weeks of therapy should be considered for surgical excision in combination with adjuvant therapy
D. Immediate postoperative electron beam irradiation or brachytherapy reduces recurrence rates by 50% to 95%

74. Chronic wounds are wounds that have failed to proceed through an orderly and timely reparative process to produce anatomic and functional integrity over a period of:

A. 6 months
B. 1 month
C. 3 months
D. 12 months

75. Chronic wound fluid, in contrast to acute wound fluid, has been shown to have greater levels of all except:

A. IL-1
B. IL-6
C. TGF-α
D. TNF-α

76. Triple Keloid therapy includes all except:

A. Surgery
B. Pressure dressing
C. Corticosteroids
D. Silicone sheeting

77. False statement about the mechanisms involved in the development and persistence of chronic wounds is:

A. Reactive oxygen species and proteases, such as matrix metalloproteinases (MMP-1, -2, -3, -9, -13), are the most significant deleterious influences
B. Chronic wounds do not adequately complete the "normal" phases of wound healing
C. Inflammatory cells, particularly neutrophils and macrophages (M1 phenotype > M2 phenotype), persist in the wound, creating a highly pro-oxidant, protease-rich environment with an abundance of proinflammatory cytokines such as interleukin-1
D. All of the above are true

78. False statement about chronic wound is:

A. Cutaneous wound may first exhibit pseudoepitheliomatous hyperplasia a premalignant condition

B. The CD4/CD8 cell ratio is significantly higher in chronic wounds
C. Chronically inflamed wounds are susceptible to neoplastic transformation
D. Squamous cell carcinoma was originally reported in chronic burn scars by Marjolin

79. Hypoxia affects wound healing; collagen assembly proceeds poorly when partial pressure of oxygen (PO_2) becomes less than:

A. 25 mm Hg
B. 30 mm Hg
C. 40 mm Hg
D. 50 mm Hg

80. Presence of molecular oxygen in wound healing is critical for:

A. Pretranslational hydroxylation of the prolyl and lysyl residues
B. Posttranslational hydroxylation of the prolyl and glycine residues
C. Posttranslational hydroxylation of the prolyl and lysyl residues
D. Pretranslational hydroxylation of the prolyl and glycine residues

81. Tobacco product consumption affects wound healing; all are true except:

A. 70% to 80% reduction in wound blood flow
B. Tobacco smoking and consumption of tobacco products causes peripheral vasoconstriction
C. Nicotine also inhibits platelet prostacyclin, promoting platelet adhesiveness, thrombotic microvascular occlusion, and tissue ischemia
D. Most clinicians recommend complete smoking cessation in human patients for 4 to 6 weeks before elective procedures

82. Diabetes affects wound healing; all are true except:

A. Hypoxia is normally a potent upregulator of VEGF, but cells from patients with diabetes do not upregulate VEGF expression in response to hypoxia
B. Lymphocyte and leukocyte function are impaired
C. Diabetic sensory neuropathy leads to repeated trauma and unrelieved wound pressure
D. Collagen degradation is decreased, whereas collagen deposition is improved

83. Diabetes affects wound healing; false statement is:

A. Collagen is brittle secondary to glycosylation in the ECM
B. High glucose exposure also results in changes in cellular morphology, decreased proliferation, and abnormal differentiation of keratinocytes
C. Insulin degrading enzyme activity in wound fluid is not correlated with hemoglobin A1c levels
D. Growth factors are abnormally expressed and degraded rapidly in wound fluids as a result of increased insulin degrading enzyme activity

84. Ionizing radiation has its greatest effect on rapidly dividing cells in phases:

A. G1 to S phase
B. G2 to M phase
C. M to G2 phase
D. All of the above

85. Early side effects of ionising radiation includes all except:

A. Erythema
B. Dry desquamation
C. Telangiectasia
D. Skin hyperpigmentation

86. Late side effects of ionising radiation includes all except:

A. Local hair loss
B. Skin atrophy
C. Telangiectasia
D. Dyschromia

87. Ionising radiation affects wound healing; false statement is:

A. Keratinocytes, which are crucial for wound epithelialization, demonstrate a shift in expression from the high molecular keratins 1 and 10 to the low molecular keratins 5 and 14 after radiation injury
B. NO, is increased in irradiated wounds
C. Expression of MMP-2, MMP-12 and MMP-13 has been shown to be elevated in irradiated human keratinocytes and fibroblasts
D. Hyperbaric oxygen (HBO) therapy may improve tissue oxygen partial pressure in the treatment of osteoradionecrosis via increased capillary density and more complete neovascularization

88. Which of the following is false regarding aging and wound healing?

A. The dermis has fewer fibroblasts, macrophages and mast cells; reduced vascularity; and less collagen and GAGs
B. Skin elasticity is increased because of altered elastin morphology
C. There is reduced sebum secretion and vitamin D3 production

D. Keratinocyte proliferation is reduced, and the turnover time is increased by 50%

89. Delayed wound healing and wound dehiscence is seen when serum albumin levels are less than:

A. 3.0 g/dL B. 2.5 g/dL
C. 2.0 g/dL D. 1.5 g/dL

90. After how long, vitamin C deprivation can cause delayed healing?

A. 3 months B. 6 months
C. 12 months D. 24 months

91. False statement about vitamin deficiency and wound healing among the following is:

A. Vitamin K deficiency limits the synthesis of prothrombin and factors VII, IX and X
B. Delayed healing can occur 3 months after vitamin C deprivation and can be reversed by supplements of 10 mg/day and no more than 2000 mg/day
C. Vitamin D contributes to lysosomal membrane destabilization and directly counteracts the effect of glucocorticoids
D. Vitamin K metabolism is impeded by antibiotics

92. False statement about drug use and wound healing is:

A. Glucocorticosteroids impair fibroblast proliferation and collagen synthesis
B. Steroids inhibit keratinocyte migration and proper wound healing
C. Tamoxifen decreases cellular proliferation, with a decrease in wound-breaking strength that is dose dependent and may be secondary to decreased TGF-β production.
D. Administration of vitamin D can reverse steroid induced effects on wound effects

93. Characteristics of ideal dressing includes all except:

A. Impermeable to microorganisms
B. Prevents desiccation
C. Nontoxic to beneficial host cells
D. Need not provide mechanical protection

94. Occlusive wound dressing like films; false statement is:

A. Waterproof
B. Wound contraction is fastened
C. Clear polyurethane membranes with acrylic adhesive on one side
D. Nonabsorptive, can leak

95. Which of the following is not an occlusive wound dressing?

A. Hydrogels B. Films
C. Skin substitutes D. Foams

96. Which of the following is not an absorptive wound dressing?

A. Foams B. Gauze
C. Hydrocolloids D. All of the above

97. Biologic dressing composed of neonatal dermal fibroblasts on collagen matrix is:

A. Integra B. AlloDerm
C. Apligraf D. Biobrane

98. Epithelialization is slowed by:

A. Mafenide acetate
B. Iodine-containing solutions
C. Silver nitrate
D. Silver sulfadiazine

99. Acceleration of epithelialization of partial-thickness burns is by:

A. Mafenide acetate
B. Iodine-containing solutions
C. Silver nitrate
D. Silver sulfadiazine

100. Hyponatremia is caused by:

A. Mafenide acetate
B. Iodine-containing solutions
C. Silver nitrate
D. Silver sulfadiazine

101. Which of the following penetrates eschar?

A. Mafenide acetate
B. Iodine-containing solutions
C. Silver nitrate
D. Silver sulfadiazine

102. Which of the following stains the clothes black?

A. Mafenide acetate
B. Iodine-containing solutions
C. Silver nitrate
D. Silver sulfadiazine

103. Which of the following causes transient neutropenia?

A. Mafenide acetate
B. Iodine-containing solutions
C. Silver nitrate
D. Silver sulfadiazine

104. Sulfamylon is:

A. Mafenide acetate
B. Iodine-containing solutions
C. Silver nitrate
D. Silver sulfadiazine

105. Silvadene is:

A. Mafenide acetate
B. Iodine-containing solutions
C. Silver nitrate
D. Silver sulfadiazine

106. Neosporin increased reepithelialisation in experimental wounds by __ % compared with wounds with no dressing.

A. 10% B. 25%
C. 40% D. 50%

107. Triple antibiotic ointment includes all except:

A. Polysporin B. Polymyxin B
C. Neomycin D. Bacitracin

108. Antibacterial ointments have all of the following function except:

A. Lubricates wound surface
B. Antibacterial activity lasts 12 hours
C. Absorptive
D. Soothing to apply

109. Leg ulcers can produce _____ of exudate.

A. 6 g/10 cm²/24 hours
B. 12 g/10 cm²/24 hours
C. 24 g/10 cm²/24 hours
D. 36 g/10 cm²/24 hours

110. Dressings with antibacterial properties are indicated when clinical signs of infection are present or if quantitative culture demonstrates more than:

A. 10^3 organisms per gram of tissue
B. 10^4 organisms per gram of tissue
C. 10^5 organisms per gram of tissue
D. 10^6 organisms per gram of tissue

111. Addition of urea increases enzymatic action of papain by:

A. 2X B. 3X
C. 4X D. 5X

OTHER THERAPIES

112. The most common cause of wound-healing failure is:

A. Infection B. Malnutrition
C. Trauma D. Wound ischemia

113. Partial oxygen pressure of less than __ significantly impairs normal metabolic activity.

A. <30 mm Hg B. <40 mm Hg
C. <50 mm Hg D. <60 mm Hg

114. HBO therapy involves inhalation of 100% oxygen at:

A. 1.0 to 1.9 atm B. 1.9 to 2.5 atm
C. 2.9 to 3.5 atm D. 2.5 to 3.5 atm

115. HBO therapy involves inhalation of 100% oxygen at 1.9 to 2.5 atm, which can increase tissue pO_2:

A. 5 times higher than usual
B. 10 times higher than usual
C. 20 times higher than usual
D. 100 times higher than usual

116. False statement about HBO therapy is:

A. Elevated levels of O_2 lasts for 2 to 4 hours after termination of HBO therapy and induces synthesis of endothelial cell NO synthase as well as angiogenesis
B. A higher PaO_2 is sufficient to supply the tissue with all its metabolic requirements, even in the absence of hemoglobin
C. An in-chamber tcp O_2 of 200 mm Hg or more suggests potential benefit from HBO therapy
D. HBO treatments for hypoxic wounds are usually delivered at 1.9 to 2.5 atm for sessions of 30 to 45 minutes each

117. Clinical evidence of wound improvement should be noted after:

A. 15 to 20 treatments B. 10 to 15 treatments
C. 5 to 10 treatments D. 3 to 5 treatments

118. Complications of HBO therapy is:

A. Brain oxygen toxicity B. Pneumothorax
C. Oxygen lung toxicity D. All of the above

119. Absolute contraindications to HBO therapy are all except:

A. Uncontrolled pneumothorax
B. Current or recent treatment with Bleomycin
C. Treatment with Disulfiram
D. All of the above are contraindications

120. The most common complication of HBO therapy:

A. Pneumothorax
B. Barotrauma

C. Intracranial bleeding
D. Intestinal Obstruction

121. Life-threatening common complication of HBO therapy:

A. Pneumothorax
B. Barotrauma
C. Intracranial bleeding
D. Intestinal Obstruction

122. Negative pressure assisted wound therapy (NPWT) includes all except:

A. This technique may be used on acute, subacute and chronic wounds
B. There have been reports of a 78% decrease in hospital stay and a 76% decrease in cost with NPWT
C. With NPWT, there is a tenfold increase in blood flow to cutaneous tissues
D. The reason for increased wound healing is the removal of wound exudates while keeping the wound moist

FETAL WOUND HEALING

123. The transition from scarless to scarring repair occurs at the beginning of the:

A. Infant age
B. Second trimester
C. Third trimester
D. Early neonatal period

124. False statement about fetal wound healing is:

A. Wounds created early in gestation heal without scarring and with dermal appendages
B. Fetal skin retains a reticular pattern
C. Wounds heal faster in a neonate than in a fetus
D. Fetal repair depends on gestational age and wound size

125. False statement about fetal wound healing is:

A. Early-gestation fetal human fibroblasts have increased prolyl hydroxylase activity
B. Collagen types I, III, V and VI appear earlier, and the ratio of type III to type I is greater in fetal wounds
C. Early-gestation fetal human fibroblasts have increased prolyl hydroxylase activity
D. Fetal fibroblasts in vitro have lower collagen production than their adult counterparts

126. False statement about fetal wound healing is:

A. Hyaluronic acid is persistently elevated in fetal wounds
B. Fetal wounds have increased levels of TGF-β and FGF-2
C. Tenascin, an inhibitor of fibronectin, increases earlier and returns to normal more rapidly in the fetus
D. IL-10 levels are higher

127. Which of the following is not seen in fetal wound healing?

A. Higher levels of TGF-β3
B. Higher levels of IL-6, IL-8
C. Higher levels of type III collagen
D. Dot cells are present

128. Which of the following is seen in fetal wound healing?

A. Higher levels of VEGF`
B. Lower levels of HA receptors (fibroblast)
C. Myofibroblast are present
D. Higher levels of PDGF

TISSUE ENGINEERING

129. About Integra™; false statement is:

A. Bilayer substitute containing a silicone outer layer and a deeper layer consisting of bovine cartilage and GAGs
B. Outer layer can be removed after 2 to 3 weeks of application
C. Split-thickness skin graft can be applied over the dermal component.
D. Can't be directly applied to tendon and bone

GENE AND STEM CELL THERAPY

130. Roles of MSCs in Remodelling includes all except:

A. Blocking of T-cell proliferation
B. Production of TGF-3, KGF
C. Regulation of MMPs/TIMP
D. Regulation of collagen deposition

131. Primary function of α2-Macroglobulin in human mesenchymal stem cell containing skin substitutes:

A. Inhibit protease activity, coordinate growth factor bioavailability

B. Antibacterial
C. Stimulate growth and migration
D. Recruit cells to site of tissue damage

132. Primary function of Acrp-30 in human mesenchymal stem cell containing skin substitutes:

A. Inhibit activity of MMPs, angiogenic
B. Recruit cells to site of tissue damage
C. Regulate growth and activity of keratinocytes
D. Regulate IGF and its proliferative effect

133. Primary function of TIMP-1 and TIMP-2 in human mesenchymal stem cell containing skin substitutes:

A. Prevent fibrosis by decreasing TGF-β1 and TGF-β2
B. Inhibit activity of MMPs, angiogenic
C. Matrix and growth factor degradation, facilitate cell migration
D. Inhibit protease activity, coordinate growth factor bioavailability

134. Primary function of TGF-β3, HGF in human mesenchymal stem cell containing skin substitutes:

A. Prevent fibrosis by decreasing TGF-β1 and TGF-β2
B. Stimulate growth and migration
C. Support of angiogenic growth factors
D. Inhibit scar and contracture formation

135. Primary function of IL-1Ra in human mesenchymal stem cell containing skin substitutes:

A. Anti-inflammatory
B. Antibacterial
C. Recruit cells to site of tissue damage
D. Stimulate growth and migration

NEW HORIZONS

136. False statement among the following is:

A. Low-frequency ultrasound has been shown to decrease venous leg ulcer size in 8 weeks
B. Noncontact low-frequency ultrasound has been used in the treatment of venous, diabetic, and pressure wounds.
C. Wounds carry a direct current electrical gradient that can be utilized to hasten the healing process
D. Transcutaneous electrical nerve stimulation treatment plus standard wound care had significant improvements in pain and wound size

137. Regarding Vibration therapy all statements are true except:

A. Low-magnitude, high-frequency vibration therapy was also found to recruit mesenchymal cells to fracture sites in rats with osteoporosis
B. Whole-body vibration may play a role in reducing pain of extremity burn patients
C. Vibration therapy is another modality that may improve wound healing
D. All of the above are true

ANSWERS

1. **Ans: C. A chronic wound stalls during a sustained proliferative Phase and fails to heal**
Ref: Chapter No.6, Page No.119
2. **Ans: D. Brain**
Ref: Chapter No.6, Page No.119
3. **Ans: B. Type IV and type V collagen**
Ref: Chapter No.6, Page No.119
4. **Ans: B. Von Willebrand factor**
Ref: Chapter No.6, Page No.119
5. **Ans: D. Histamine**
Ref: Chapter No.6, Page No.120
6. **Ans: B. Serotonin**
Ref: Chapter No.6, Page No.120
7. **Ans: D. High levels of IL-8 are found in fetal wounds**
Ref: Chapter No.6, Page No.120
8. **Ans: C. Megakaryocytes**
Ref: Chapter No.6, Page No.121
9. **Ans: C. 7th day**
Ref: Chapter No.6, Page No.120
10. **Ans: A. 2nd day**
Ref: Chapter No.6, Page No.120
11. **Ans: D. All of the above**
Ref: Chapter No.6, Page No.121
12. **Ans: B. Retraction at the leading edge of the cell develops through binding of integrin followed by translocation of the cell over the adherent segment of the plasma membrane**
Ref: Chapter No.6, Page No.121
13. **Ans: B. 3rd day**
Ref: Chapter No.6, Page No.120
14. **Ans: C. Individual PMNs survive no longer than 72 hours and are replaced predominantly by mononuclear cells**
Ref: Chapter No.6, Page No.121
15. **Ans: C. Fibrinogen**
Ref: Chapter No.6, Page No.121
16. **Ans: B. IL-2**
Ref: Chapter No.6, Page No.121
17. **Ans: C. Thrombin**
Ref: Chapter No.6, Page No.121
18. **Ans: B. a,b**
Ref: Chapter No.6, Page No.122
19. **Ans: D. c,d**
Ref: Chapter No.6, Page No.122
20. **Ans: A. IL-1**
Ref: Chapter No.6, Page No.122
21. **Ans: C. 72 hrs**
Ref: Chapter No.6, Page No.123
22. **Ans: C. IL-6**
Ref: Chapter No.6, Page No.123
23. **Ans: A. 24 hours**
Ref: Chapter No.6, Page No.123
24. **Ans: C. Decreases collagenase activity**
Ref: Chapter No.6, Page No.123
25. **Ans: B. PDGF-BB**
Ref: Chapter No.6, Page No.123-124
26. **Ans: A. TGF-β**
Ref: Chapter No.6, Page No.124
27. **Ans: D. In the proliferative phase, M1 macrophages predominate**
Ref: Chapter No.6, Page No.124-125
28. **Ans: B. Day 5**
Ref: Chapter No.6, Page No.125
29. **Ans: C. Day 7**
Ref: Chapter No.6, Page No.125
30. **Ans: A. T lymphocytes appear to be principally involved in downregulating healing as the wound closes**
Ref: Chapter No.6, Page No.125
31. **Ans: A. TNF-α**
Ref: Chapter No.6, Page No.125
32. **Ans: C. Flt-1**
Ref: Chapter No.6, Page No.125
33. **Ans: B. 3 days**
Ref: Chapter No.6, Page No.126
34. **Ans: B. Day 4-7**
Ref: Chapter No.6, Page No.126

35. **Ans: C. 24 hours**

Ref: Chapter No.6, Page No.126

36. **Ans: D. TGF-β**

Ref: Chapter No.6, Page No.126

37. **Ans: B. 4 weeks**

Ref: Chapter No.6, Page No.126

38. **Ans: A. The basal layer of the epidermis attaches to the basement membrane zone by desmosomes**

Ref: Chapter No.6, Page No.126

39. **Ans: B. Elastin Fibres**

Ref: Chapter No.6, Page No.127

40. **Ans: A. Collagen Fibres**

Ref: Chapter No.6, Page No.127

41. **Ans: C. In newborns, the content of type I collagen is greater than that found in adults**

Ref: Chapter No.6, Page No.127

42. **Ans: A. Type I**

Ref: Chapter No.6, Page No.127

43. **Ans: D. Covalent cross-linking of the glycine residues provides tensile strength.**

Ref: Chapter No.6, Page No.128

44. **Ans: D. None**

Ref: Chapter No.6, Page No.128

45. **Ans: C. Type III collagen**

Ref: Chapter No.6, Page No.128

46. **Ans: C. Elastin is produced early in life, stabilizes and undergo much further synthesis or degradation**

Ref: Chapter No.6, Page No.128-129

47. **Ans: B. Marfan syndrome**

Ref: Chapter No.6, Page No.129

48. **Ans: B. Turgor**

Ref: Chapter No.6, Page No.129

49. **Ans: D. Hyaluronan**

Ref: Chapter No.6, Page No.129

50. **Ans: D. Hyaluronan**

Ref: Chapter No.6, Page No.129

51. **Ans: C. Alpha smooth muscle actin**

Ref: Chapter No.6, Page No.130

52. **Ans: C. 15 days**

Ref: Chapter No.6, Page No.130

53. **Ans: D. Shortening the action of the protein by promoting degradation**

Ref: Chapter No.6, Page No.129

54. **Ans: C. Type IV collagen has a less flexible structure than the fibrillar collagens**

Ref: Chapter No.6, Page No.129-130

55. **Ans: A. 4 weeks**

Ref: Chapter No.6, Page No.130

56. **Ans: C. Wound contraction occurs by centripetal movement of the partial thickness of the surrounding skin**

Ref: Chapter No.6, Page No.130

57. **Ans: B. Day 6**

Ref: Chapter No.6, Page No.130

58. **Ans: B. 30%**

Ref: Chapter No.6, Page No.130

59. **Ans: C. 21 days**

Ref: Chapter No.6, Page No.130

60. **Ans: C. Although collagen cross-linking causes further wound contraction and an increase in strength, it also results in a scar that is less brittle and more elastic than normal skin**

Ref: Chapter No.6, Page No.130

61. **Ans: C. There are known effective prevention method for keloid formation**

Ref: Chapter No.6, Page No.130-131

62. **Ans: D. Young age**

Ref: Chapter No.6, Page No.131

63. **Ans: B. Hypertrophic scars primarily contain disorganised-organized type III collagen**

Ref: Chapter No.6, Page No.131

64. **Ans: B. Keloids and hypertrophic scars have stretched collagen bundles aligned in the same plane as the epidermis, whereas collagen bundles are randomly arrayed and relaxed in normal scars**

Ref: Chapter No.6, Page No.131

65. **Ans: A. Scars parallel to the underlying muscle fibers tend to be flatter and narrower, with less collagen formation than when they are perpendicular to the underlying muscle fibers**

Ref: Chapter No.6, Page No.131

66. **Ans: A. Blocking TGF-β activity with antibodies increases scar fibrosis**

Ref: Chapter No.6, Page No.131

67. **Ans: A. Avoidance of sun exposure and use of SPF 50+ sunscreens for 1 month postoperatively reduce scar hyperpigmentation and improve clinical appearance**

Ref: Chapter No.6, Page No.131

68. **Ans: B. Pressure therapy**

Ref: Chapter No.6, Page No.131

69. **Ans: D. Papillary Dermis**

Ref: Chapter No.6, Page No.131-132

70. **Ans: D. Intralesional corticosteroids (triamcinolone acetonide, 10–40 mg/mL) injected into the papillary dermis every 2 to 4 months until flat**

Ref: Chapter No.6, Page No.131-132

71. **Ans: B. 1 year**

Ref: Chapter No.6, Page No.132

72. **Ans: D. All of the above are true**

Ref: Chapter No.6, Page No.132

73. **Ans: C. Refractory cases after 12 weeks of therapy should be considered for surgical excision in combination with adjuvant therapy.**

Ref: Chapter No.6, Page No.132

74. **Ans: C. 3 months**

Ref: Chapter No.6, Page No.132

75. **Ans: C. TGF-α**

Ref: Chapter No.6, Page No.132

76. **Ans: B. Pressure dressing**

Ref: Chapter No.6, Page No.132

77. **Ans: D. All of the above are true**

Ref: Chapter No.6, Page No.134

78. **Ans: B. The CD4/CD8 cell ratio is significantly higher in chronic wounds**

Ref: Chapter No.6, Page No.135

79. **Ans: C. 40 mm Hg**

Ref: Chapter No.6, Page No.135

80. **Ans: C. Posttranslational hydroxylation of the prolyl and lysyl residues**

Ref: Chapter No.6, Page No.135

81. **Ans: A. 70% to 80% reduction in wound blood flow**

Ref: Chapter No.6, Page No.135

82. **Ans: D. Collagen degradation is decreased, whereas collagen deposition is improved**

Ref: Chapter No.6, Page No.135

83. **Ans: C. Insulin degrading enzyme activity in wound fluid is not correlated with hemoglobin A1c levels**

Ref: Chapter No.6, Page No.135

84. **Ans: B. G2 to M phase**

Ref: Chapter No.6, Page No.135

85. **Ans: C. Telangiectasia**

Ref: Chapter No.6, Page No.136

86. **Ans: A. Local hair loss**

Ref: Chapter No.6, Page No.136

87. **Ans: B. NO, is increased in irradiated wounds**

Ref: Chapter No.6, Page No.136

88. **Ans: B. Skin elasticity is increased because of altered elastin morphology**

Ref: Chapter No.6, Page No.136

89. **Ans: C. 2.0 g/dL**

Ref: Chapter No.6, Page No.136

90. **Ans: A. 3 months**

Ref: Chapter No.6, Page No.136

91. **Ans: C. Vitamin D contributes to lysosomal membrane destabilization and directly counteracts the effect of glucocorticoids**

Ref: Chapter No.6, Page No.136

92. **Ans: D. Administration of vitamin D can reverse steroid induced effects on wound effects**

Ref: Chapter No.6, Page No.136-137

93. **Ans: D. Need not provide mechanical protection**

Ref: Chapter No.6, Page No.137

94. **Ans: B. Wound contraction is fastened**

Ref: Chapter No.6, Page No.138

95. **Ans: D. Foams**

Ref: Chapter No.6, Page No.138

96. **Ans: C. Hydrocolloids**

Ref: Chapter No.6, Page No.138

97. **Ans: C. Apligraf**

Ref: Chapter No.6, Page No.138

98. **Ans: C. Silver nitrate**

Ref: Chapter No.6, Page No.139

99. **Ans: D. Silver sulfadiazine**

Ref: Chapter No.6, Page No.139

100. **Ans: C. Silver nitrate**

Ref: Chapter No.6, Page No.139

101. **Ans: A. Mafenide acetate**

Ref: Chapter No.6, Page No.139

102. **Ans: C. Silver nitrate**

Ref: Chapter No.6, Page No.139

103. **Ans: D. Silver sulfadiazine**

Ref: Chapter No.6, Page No.139

104. **Ans: A. Mafenide acetate**

Ref: Chapter No.6, Page No.139

105. **Ans: D. Silver sulfadiazine**

Ref: Chapter No.6, Page No.139

106. **Ans: B. 25%**

Ref: Chapter No.6, Page No.139

107. Ans: A. Polysporin

Ref: Chapter No.6, Page No.139

108. Ans: C. Absorptive

Ref: Chapter No.6, Page No.139

109. Ans: B. 12 g/10 cm²/24 hours

Ref: Chapter No.6, Page No.139

110. Ans: C. 10^5 organisms per gram of tissue

Ref: Chapter No.6, Page No.139

111. Ans: A. 2X

Ref: Chapter No.6, Page No.139

112. Ans: D. Wound ischemia

Ref: Chapter No.6, Page No.139

113. Ans: A. <30 mm Hg

Ref: Chapter No.6, Page No.140

114. Ans: B. 1.9 to 2.5 atm

Ref: Chapter No.6, Page No.140

115. Ans: B. 10 times higher than usual

Ref: Chapter No.6, Page No.140

116. Ans: D. HBO treatments for hypoxic wounds are usually delivered at 1.9 to 2.5 atm for sessions of 30 to 45 minutes each

Ref: Chapter No.6, Page No.140

117. Ans: A. 15 to 20 treatments

Ref: Chapter No.6, Page No.140

118. Ans: D. All of the above

Ref: Chapter No.6, Page No.140

119. Ans: D. All of the above are contraindications

Ref: Chapter No.6, Page No.140

120. Ans: B. Barotrauma

Ref: Chapter No.6, Page No.140

121. Ans: A. Pneumothorax

Ref: Chapter No.6, Page No.140

122. Ans: C. With NPWT, there is a tenfold increase in blood flow to cutaneous tissues

Ref: Chapter No.6, Page No.141

123. Ans: C. Third trimester

Ref: Chapter No.6, Page No.141-142

124. Ans: C. Wounds heal faster in a neonate than in a fetus

Ref: Chapter No.6, Page No.141-142

125. Ans: D. Fetal fibroblasts in vitro have lower collagen production than their adult counterparts

Ref: Chapter No.6, Page No.142

126. Ans: B. Fetal wounds have increased levels of TGF-β and FGF-2

Ref: Chapter No.6, Page No.142-143

127. Ans: B. Higher levels of IL-6, IL-8

Ref: Chapter No.6, Page No.143

128. Ans: A Higher levels of VEGF

Ref: Chapter No.6, Page No.143

129. Ans: D. Can't be directly applied to tendon and bone

Ref: Chapter No.6, Page No.143

130. Ans: A. Blocking of T-cell proliferation

Ref: Chapter No.6, Page No.145

131. Ans: A. Inhibit protease activity, coordinate growth factor bioavailability

Ref: Chapter No.6, Page No.145

132. Ans: C. Regulate growth and activity of keratinocytes

Ref: Chapter No.6, Page No.145

133. Ans: B. Inhibit activity of MMPs, angiogenic

Ref: Chapter No.6, Page No.145

134. Ans: D. Inhibit scar and contracture formation

Ref: Chapter No.6, Page No.145

135. Ans: A. Anti-inflammatory

Ref: Chapter No.6, Page No.145

136. Ans: A. Low-frequency ultrasound has been shown to decrease venous leg ulcer size in 8 weeks

Ref: Chapter No.6, Page No.146

137. Ans: D. All of the above are true

Ref: Chapter No.6, Page No.147

7

Regenerative Medicine

STEM CELL SOURCES

1. **Embryonic stem cells (ESCs) are cells derived from the:**
   A. Zona pellucida of the blastocyst
   B. Inner cell mass of the blastocyst
   C. Trophoblast of the blastocyst
   D. Blastocoel of the blastocyst

2. **Ability to form all differentiated cells in the embryo and extraembryonic tissue is seen by:**
   A. Totipotent B. Pluripotent
   C. Unipotent D. Multipotent

3. **Adult stem cells that can form multiple cells in a particular cell lineage is seen by:**
   A. Totipotent B. Pluripotent
   C. Unipotent D. Multipotent

4. **Ability to form all lineages of the body but not extraembryonic tissue is seen by:**
   A. Totipotent B. Pluripotent
   C. Unipotent D. Multipotent

5. **Zygote is an example of:**
   A. Totipotent cell B. Pluripotent cell
   C. Unipotent cell D. Multipotent cell

6. **Embryonic stem cells (ESCs) are:**
   A. Totipotent cell B. Pluripotent cell
   C. Unipotent cell D. Multipotent cell

7. **False statement about somatic cell nuclear transfer is:**
   A. Dolly the sheep was the first mammal to be cloned from a somatic cell in 1997
   B. Somatic cell nuclear transfer (SCNT) involves the transfer of a nucleus from a differentiated somatic cell containing a desired genetic profile into an enucleated ovum
   C. The resultant hybrid cells are perfect copies of the donor cell nucleus
   D. Cloning efficiency remains extremely low in all species

8. **Yamanaka factors include all except:**
   A. Oct4 B. Sox2
   C. Nanong D. cMyc

9. **True statement about Induced Pluripotent Stem Cells is:**
   A. Autologous iPSCs can theoretically reduce the need for immunosuppression post transplantation
   B. The risk of tumorigenicity is a major concern, and genetic mutations in iPSCs in the first human iPSC-mandated trial suspension
   C. CRISPR-Cas9 technology has helped advance iPSC-based disease modelling by introducing disease-causing mutations to wild-type iPSCs and eliminating the same mutations in patient iPSCs
   D. All of the above

10. **Adult stem cells are:**
    A. Totipotent B. Pluripotent
    C. Unipotent D. Multipotent

11. **Which cells were first adult stem cells to be described?**
    A. Mesenchymal stem/stromal cells (MSCs)
    B. Adipose-derived stem/stromal cells (ASCs)
    C. Skeletal stem cells (SSCs)
    D. Hematopoietic stem cells (HSCs)

12. **Which cells are most studied and best characterized adult multipotent stem cell?**
    A. Mesenchymal stem/stromal cells (MSCs)
    B. Adipose-derived stem/stromal cells (ASCs)
    C. Skeletal stem cells (SSCs)
    D. Hematopoietic stem cells (HSCs)

13. The most widely used stem cell therapy to date is:

A. Transplantation of MSCs for joint diseases and malignancies
B. Transplantation of HSCs for hematologic diseases and malignancies
C. Transplantation of SSCs for skeletal diseases and malignancies
D. Transplantation of ASCs for vascular diseases and malignancies

14. Skin follicular bulge cells are:

A. Totipotent cell B. Pluripotent cell
C. Unipotent cell D. Multipotent cell

15. True statement about Mesenchymal Stem/Stromal Cells is/are:

A. MSCs represent the collection of nonhematopoietic progenitor cells of mesodermal origin that have characteristic spindle shapes and can derive colonies from single cells
B. MSCs are thought to mediate their regenerative effects primarily through paracrine signalling
C. MSCs are considered immune-privileged
D. All of the above

16. Human skeletal stem cell (hSSC) are identified by the presence of surface antigens; among the following, all are surface antigens except:

A. CD164 B. CD93
C. PDPN D. CD73

17. In the skin epidermal stem cells are reported to reside in:

A. Outer hair sheath
B. Hair follicles in the bulge region deep to the sebaceous glands
C. Inner hair sheath
D. Base of the crypts

18. In the skin epidermal stem cells are reported to reside in:

A. Deep interfollicular epidermis
B. Superficial dermal layer
C. Inner hair sheath
D. Deep dermal layer

19. In the small intestine, a group of proliferative cells has been identified:

A. Muscularis propria
B. At the isthmus of the crypts
C. At the base of the crypts
D. At the neck of the crypts

BIOENGINEERING FOR REGENERATIVE MEDICINE

20. Commonly used biomaterials as Constructs for Cell Delivery and Cell Differentiation include:

A. Polyethylene glycol hydrogel
B. Polyglycolic acid hydrogel
C. Polylactic-co-glycolic acid
D. All of the above

CLINICAL APPLICATIONS OF STEM CELLS

21. Which of the following is correctly matched?

A. HSC transplantation provides the best chance for cure for a range of malignant and non-malignant diseases
B. ESC tested for their ability to generate insulin-producing pancreatic cells to help correct type 1 diabetes
C. Human ESC–derived retinal pigment epithelium (RPE) cells and found them to improve visual acuity
D. All of the above

ANSWERS

1. **Ans: B. Inner cell mass of the blastocyst**

   Ref: Chapter No.7, Page No.150

2. **Ans: A. Totipotent**

   Ref: Chapter No.7, Page No.151

3. **Ans: D. Multipotent**

   Ref: Chapter No.7, Page No.151

4. **Ans: B. Pluripotent**

   Ref: Chapter No.7, Page No.151

5. **Ans: A. Totipotent cell**

   Ref: Chapter No.7, Page No.151

6. **Ans: B. Pluripotent cell**

   Ref: Chapter No.7, Page No.151

7. **Ans: C. The resultant hybrid cells are perfect copies of the donor cell nucleus**

   Ref: Chapter No.7, Page No.152

8. **Ans: C. Nanong**

   Ref: Chapter No.7, Page No.152

9. **Ans: D. All of the above**

   Ref: Chapter No.7, Page No.152

10. **Ans: D. Multipotent**

    Ref: Chapter No.7, Page No.152

11. **Ans: D. Hematopoietic stem cells (HSCs)**

    Ref: Chapter No.7, Page No.152

12. **Ans: D. Hematopoietic stem cells (HSCs)**

    Ref: Chapter No.7, Page No.152

13. **Ans: B. Transplantation of HSCs for hematologic diseases and malignancies**

    Ref: Chapter No.7, Page No.152

14. **Ans: C. Unipotent cell**

    Ref: Chapter No.7, Page No.151, Fig. 7.1

15. **Ans: D. All of the above**

    Ref: Chapter No.7, Page No.153

16. **Ans: B. CD93**

    Ref: Chapter No.7, Page No.154, Fig. 7.3

17. **Ans: B. Hair follicles in the bulge region deep to the sebaceous glands**

    Ref: Chapter No.7, Page No.154

18. **Ans: A. Deep interfollicular epidermis**

    Ref: Chapter No.7, Page No.154

19. **Ans: C. At the base of the crypts**

    Ref: Chapter No.7, Page No.154

20. **Ans: D. All of the above**

    Ref: Chapter No.7, Page No.155

21. **Ans: D. All of the above**

    Ref: Chapter No.7, Page No.155-156

8

Critical Assessment of Surgical Outcomes and Health Services Research

EVIDENCE-BASED APPROACH TO SURGERY

1. **Evidence-based approach to clinical practice can also be remembered by the five A's; which of the following is not a part of it?**

   A. Acquire
   B. Appeal
   C. Ask
   D. Apply

2. **FINER provides a framework that prompts the reader to ask several important questions when considering a research study; the letter N in FINER means:**

   A. Novel
   B. New
   C. Nice
   D. Neat

3. **FINER means:**

   A. Feasible, intervention, novel, exclusive and repeat
   B. Feasible, innovative, novel, ethical and relevant
   C. Feasible, interesting, novel, ethical and relevant
   D. Feasible, innovative, novel, exclusive and repeat

4. **PICOT framework for evaluating research questions means:**

   A. Population, Intervention, Comparator, Outscore, Time frame
   B. Problem, Intervention, Comparator, Outcome, Time frame
   C. Population, Interesting, Comparator, Outscore, Time frame
   D. Problem, Interesting, Comparator, Outcome, Time frame

5. **Exposure and outcomes measures at same point in time in:**

   A. Randomized controlled trial
   B. Cohort study
   C. Case control study
   D. Cross-sectional study

6. **Which of the following is not used for Hypothesis generating?**

   A. Case series and report
   B. Cohort study
   C. Case control study
   D. Cross-sectional study

7. **Used for describing disease prevalence:**

   A. Randomized controlled trial
   B. Cohort study
   C. Case control study
   D. Cross-sectional study

8. **Which study is used for rare outcomes and multiple exposures?**

   A. Randomized controlled trial
   B. Cohort study
   C. Case control study
   D. Cross-sectional study

9. **Allocation of subjects to experimental or control group by chance is done in:**

   A. Randomized controlled trial
   B. Cohort study
   C. Case control study
   D. Cross-sectional study

10. **Which study is used for rare exposures and multiple outcomes?**

    A. Randomized controlled trial
    B. Cohort study
    C. Case control study
    D. Cross-sectional study

11. **Which of the following is not a weakness of Cohort study?**

A. Selection bias
B. Can be expensive
C. Some potential to establish causal effects
D. Not generalizable

12. False statement about Cohort studies is:

A. STROBE provides guidance on how to report critical components of research studies from all types of observational study designs, including cohort, case-control, and cross-sectional study designs
B. This study design can be conducted from either a forward-looking (i.e., prospective) or backward-looking (i.e., retrospective) viewpoint
C. For both types of cohort studies, a higher incidence of outcomes in the exposed group suggests an association between that factor and the outcome
D. The disadvantages of cohort studies are that they are harder and more expensive to conduct than RCTs

APPRAISING SURGICAL EVIDENCE

13. Strong recommendation means:

A. Our confidence in the effect estimate is limited
B. We are very confident that the true effect lies close to that of the estimate of the effect
C. We are moderately confident in the effect estimate
D. We have very little confidence in the effect estimate

14. Low quality of evidence means:

A. Our confidence in the effect estimate is limited
B. We are very confident that the true effect lies close to that of the estimate of the effect
C. We are moderately confident in the effect estimate
D. We have very little confidence in the effect estimate

15. Factors that increase evidence quality includes all except:

A. Indirectness of evidence
B. Representative patient populations studied
C. Consistency of findings across multiple studies
D. Dose-response gradient

16. Factors that reduce evidence quality includes all except:

A. Lack of information on important health outcomes
B. Dose-response gradient
C. Representative patient populations studied
D. Publication bias

17. All of the following statements are true except:

A. When assessing the validity of scientific evidence, surgeons need not carefully consider the characteristics of the subjects selected for study
B. Selection bias refers to any imperfection in the selection process that results in either the wrong types of subjects
C. Efforts to control measurement bias include blinding (not telling the subject or assessor what intervention was performed) and prospective study design
D. Retrospective studies, in particular, are prone to a variety of types of measurement bias

18. True about confounding is/are:

A. When randomization is not practical, restriction or matching can be used to prevent confounding
B. Confounding refers to differences in outcomes that occur because of differences in the baseline risks of the comparison groups
C. Analytic techniques used to address confounding include stratification and propensity score risk adjustment
D. All of the above

19. When researchers erroneously confirm the null hypothesis it is called:

A. Type I error
B. Type II error
C. Beta Error
D. Both B and C

20. When researchers erroneously reject the null hypothesis, that is, infer that there is a difference in outcomes when there is no difference it is called:

A. Type I error
B. Type II error
C. Beta Error
D. Both B and C

ANSWERS

1. **Ans: B. Appeal**

Ref: Chapter No.8, Page No.159

2. **Ans: A. Novel**

Ref: Chapter No.8, Page No.159

3. **Ans: C. Feasible, interesting, novel, ethical and relevant**

Ref: Chapter No.8, Page No.159

4. **Ans: B. Problem, Intervention, Comparator, Outcome, Time frame**

Ref: Chapter No.8, Page No.160

5. **Ans: D. Cross-sectional study**

Ref: Chapter No.8, Page No.161

6. **Ans: B. Cohort study**

Ref: Chapter No.8, Page No.161

7. **Ans: D. Cross-sectional study**

Ref: Chapter No.8, Page No.161

8. **Ans: C. Case control study**

Ref: Chapter No.8, Page No.161

9. **Ans: A. Randomized controlled trial**

Ref: Chapter No.8, Page No.161

10. **Ans: B. Cohort study**

Ref: Chapter No.8, Page No.161

11. **Ans: D. Not generalizable**

Ref: Chapter No.8, Page No.161

12. **Ans: D. The disadvantages of cohort studies are that they are harder and more expensive to conduct than RCTs**

Ref: Chapter No.8, Page No.162

13. **Ans: B. We are very confident that the true effect lies close to that of the estimate of the effect**

Ref: Chapter No.8, Page No.164

14. **Ans: A. Our confidence in the effect estimate is limited**

Ref: Chapter No.8, Page No.164

15. **Ans: A. Indirectness of evidence**

Ref: Chapter No.8, Page No.165

16. **Ans: B. Dose-response gradient**

Ref: Chapter No.8, Page No.165

17. **Ans: A. When assessing the validity of scientific evidence, surgeons need not carefully consider the characteristics of the subjects selected for study**

Ref: Chapter No.8, Page No.165

18. **Ans: D. All of the above**

Ref: Chapter No.8, Page No.165-166

19. **Ans: D. Both B and C**

Ref: Chapter No.8, Page No.166

20. **Ans: A. Type I error**

Ref: Chapter No.8, Page No.166

9

Safety in the Surgical Environment

1. **Leape and colleagues proposed five transforming concepts for adoption by health care organizations seeking such transformative change, these include all except:**
   A. Transparency must be a practiced value in everything we do
   B. Health care workers need to find their passion and follow it
   C. Care must be delivered by multidisciplinary teams working in integrated care platforms
   D. Patients must become full partners in all aspects of health care
2. **The most common causes of attributable mortality as per NSQIP database is:**
   A. Respiratory failure B. Bleeding
   C. Septic shock D. Renal failure
3. **False statement about National Surgical Quality Improvement Program (NSQIP) database is:**
   A. Probably the most reliable prospectively collected data come from large multi-institutional registries
   B. The most common causes of attributable mortality were bleeding, respiratory failure, septic shock and renal failure
   C. Surgical interventions for traumatic injuries are included in the NSQIP data
   D. Unplanned intubation, bleeding, and septic shock were associated with the greatest number of years of life lost
4. **According to African Surgical Outcomes Study most common post operative complication is:**
   A. Infection B. Bleeding
   C. Respiratory failure D. Renal failure
5. **When trying to estimate a rate for perioperative mortality, which type of study appears to be the most trustworthy?**
   A. Prospective studies
   B. Retrospective studies
   C. Experimental studies
   D. All of the above
6. **As per NSQIP database, most common surgical complication associated with maximum years of life lost per million patients is:**
   A. Bleeding
   B. Unplanned intubation
   C. Septic shock
   D. Superficial infection
7. **What is considered as a potential driver of many of the system-level performance domains in the area of quality improvement?**
   A. Type of surgery
   B. Educational level of surgeon
   C. Technical skill of the surgeon
   D. Duration of surgery

FOSTERING A CULTURE OF SAFETY THROUGH LEADERSHIP

8. **The leadership of the perioperative enterprise is tripartite, which includes all of the following except:**
   A. Chair of surgery
   B. Chair of anaesthesiology
   C. Chair of medicine
   D. Associate chief nursing officer

LOCAL ORGANIZATIONAL STRUCTURES TO PROMOTE PERIOPERATIVE SAFETY

9. **Who serves as the primary input point and clearing house for safety considerations?**
   A. MMI conference
   B. Joint QMMI conference

C. Departmental PSO
D. Division chief

10. The original ERAS protocol was developed for:

A. Thoracic surgery
B. Colorectal surgery
C. Radical Nephrectomy
D. Radical Cystectomy

NATIONAL AND HEALTH CARE SYSTEM–LEVEL SAFETY INITIATIVES

11. Key features of a well-designed ongoing professional practice evaluation process includes all except:

A. Objective criteria for identifying clinicians whose practice falls outside of normative expectations
B. Direct mapping to the clinician's unique medical practice
C. Frequent review
D. Continued medical education

12. Colorectal ERAS perioperative components includes all except:

A. No food after mid night
B. Opioid maximodal analgesia
C. PONV prophylaxis
D. Clear PO up to 2h before surgery

13. According to ERAS Clear fluids PO are allowed up to:

A. 1h before surgery
B. 2h before surgery
C. 4h before surgery
D. 6h before surgery

14. According to ERAS to avoid SSI all of the following is done except:

A. Oxygenation ($FiO_2 > 0.8$)
B. Normothermia: $T > 36°C$
C. Skin prep (CHG)/no Shaving
D. Glycemic control (Glc < 150 mg/dL)

15. Implementing the checklist reduced complication rates from 11% to:

A. 7%
B. 5%
C. 3%
D. 9%

16. Implementing the checklist reduced postoperative death rate from 1.5% to 0.8%:

A. 0.2%
B. 0.4%
C. 0.6%
D. 0.8%

17. Estimates of wrong surgery incidence range from:

A. 1:112,994 to 1:50000
B. 1:112,994 to 1:5000
C. 1:112,994 to 1:500
D. 1:112,994 to 1:50

18. Major initiatives as per Surgical Care Improvement Project are all except:

A. Reduce incidence and impact of SSIs through timely administration and discontinuation of appropriate antibiotics
B. Reduce incidence and impact of SSIs through appropriate glucose control in selected patient populations
C. Reduce incidence and impact of SSIs through hair removal by shaving
D. Reduce incidence and impact of SSIs through maintenance of normothermia

19. Major initiatives as per Surgical Care Improvement Project are:

A. Reduce incidence of perioperative major cardiac events by continuing beta blockade in patients with previous beta blockade
B. Reduce venous thromboembolism and pulmonary embolism by use of thromboprophylaxis when indicated
C. Appropriate removal of urinary catheters
D. All of the above

20. Most common cause of "never" surgical events is:

A. Wrong surgeries
B. Wrong techniques
C. Poor perioperative care
D. Poor infrastructure

21. Universal Protocol is used for the prevention of wrong-site, wrong-patient and wrong-procedure surgery. This protocol includes all of the following elements except:

A. Site marking
B. Pre procedural verification
C. Post procedural verification
D. Final verification during the pre-procedural time-out

22. Surgical safety checklist includes all except:

A. Time in
B. Sign in
C. Time out
D. Sign out

23. The Time-Out phase of surgical safety checklist begins:

A. Before induction of anaesthesia

B. Before skin incision
C. Before the patient leaves the operating room
D. Before administration of prophylactic antibiotic

24. Which of the following is not a component of "Sign in" in surgical safety checklist?

A. All members of the team are aware of whether the patient has a known allergy
B. The surgical site is marked or site marking is not applicable.
C. The patient has verified his or her identity, surgical site and procedure and consent
D. Team confirms that all essential imaging results for correct patient are displayed in operating room

25. The pulse oximeter is on the patient and functioning is checked during which component of surgical safety checklist?

A. Time in
B. Sign in
C. Time out
D. Sign out

26. Which of the following is not a component of "Time out" in surgical safety checklist?

A. That needle, sponge and instrument counts are complete
B. Name of procedure, as recorded
C. Whether there are any issues with equipment that need to be addressed
D. Only anesthesia professional review aloud the key concerns for the recovery and care of the patient

27. The Sign-Out phase of surgical safety checklist begins:

A. Before induction of anaesthesia
B. Before skin incision
C. Before the patient leaves the operating room
D. Before administration of prophylactic antibiotic

28. The Sign-In phase of surgical safety checklist begins:

A. Before induction of anaesthesia
B. Before skin incision
C. Before the patient leaves the operating room
D. Before administration of prophylactic antibiotic

29. All of the following are checked in Sign-In phase of surgical safety checklist except:

A. The patient has verified his or her identity, surgical site and procedure and consent
B. The surgical site is marked
C. Confirmation that prophylactic antibiotics have been administered
D. The patient's airway and risk of aspiration have been evaluated, and appropriate equipment and assistance are available

ANSWERS

1. **Ans: B. Health care workers need to find their passion and follow it**

   Ref: Chapter No.9, Page No.170

2. **Ans: B. Bleeding**

   Ref: Chapter No.9, Page No.170

3. **Ans: C. Surgical interventions for traumatic injuries are included in the NSQIP data**

   Ref: Chapter No.9, Page No.170

4. **Ans: A. Infection**

   Ref: Chapter No.9, Page No.170

5. **Ans: B. Retrospective studies**

   Ref: Chapter No.9, Page No.171

6. **Ans: B. Unplanned intubation**

   Ref: Chapter No.9, Page No.170

7. **Ans: C. Technical skill of the surgeon**

   Ref: Chapter No.9, Page No.171

8. **Ans: C. Chair of medicine**

   Ref: Chapter No.9, Page No.172

9. **Ans: C. Departmental PSO**

   Ref: Chapter No.9, Page No.173-174

10. **Ans: B. Colorectal surgery**

    Ref: Chapter No.9, Page No.174

11. **Ans: D. Continued medical education**

    Ref: Chapter No.9, Page No.174

12. **Ans: B. Opioid maximodal analgesia**

    Ref: Chapter No.9, Page No.175

13. **Ans: B. 2h before surgery**

    Ref: Chapter No.9, Page No.175

14. **Ans: D. Glycemic control (Glc < 150 mg/dL)**

    Ref: Chapter No.9, Page No.175

15. **Ans: A. 7%**

    Ref: Chapter No.9, Page No.175

16. **Ans: D. 0.8%**

    Ref: Chapter No.9, Page No.175

17. **Ans: B. 1:112,994 to 1:5000**

    Ref: Chapter No.9, Page No.176

18. **Ans: C. Reduce incidence and impact of SSIs through hair removal by shaving**

    Ref: Chapter No.9, Page No.177

19. **Ans: D. All of the above**

    Ref: Chapter No.9, Page No.177

20. **Ans: A. Wrong surgeries**

    Ref: Chapter No.9, Page No.176

21. **Ans: C. Post procedural verification**

    Ref: Chapter No.9, Page No.176

22. **Ans: A. Time in**

    Ref: Chapter No.9, Page No.179

23. **Ans: B. Before skin incision**

    Ref: Chapter No.9, Page No.179

24. **Ans: D. Team confirms that all essential imaging results for correct patient are displayed in operating room**

    Ref: Chapter No.9, Page No.179

25. **Ans: B. Sign in**

    Ref: Chapter No.9, Page No.179

26. **Ans: D. Only anesthesia professional review aloud the key concerns for the recovery and care of the patient**

    Ref: Chapter No.9, Page No.179

27. **Ans: C. Before the patient leaves the operating room**

    Ref: Chapter No.9, Page No.179

28. **Ans: A. Before induction of anaesthesia**

    Ref: Chapter No.9, Page No.179

29. **Ans: C. Confirmation that prophylactic antibiotics have been administered**

    Ref: Chapter No.9, Page No.179

10

Principles of Preoperative and Operative Surgery

PRINCIPLES OF SURGICAL EVALUATION

1. **False statement among the following is:**
   A. Within ACS NSQIP, emergency surgery is characterized by an ongoing acute process that can result in rapid deterioration in a patient's condition for which unnecessary delay can potentially threaten the clinical outcome
   B. Within ACS NSQIP, elective operations generally involve a patient who has completed preoperative surgical evaluation during a separate patient surgeon encounter and is subsequently scheduled for operation
   C. Urgent operations are a relatively ill-defined category and have an acuity level in between those of elective and emergent cases
   D. Inpatients, referrals from the emergency department, and direct transfers from clinic are included in elective patient categorization

2. **As per American Society of Anesthesiologists physical status (ASA PS), a patient with severe systemic disease that is a constant threat to life is in:**
   A. ASA PS V B. ASA PS II
   C. ASA PS III D. ASA PS IV

3. **As per American Society of Anesthesiologists physical status (ASA PS), a patient with severe systemic disease is in:**
   A. ASA PS I B. ASA PS II
   C. ASA PS III D. ASA PS IV

4. **False statements among the following is:**
   A. The American Society of Anesthesiologists (ASA) physical status categorization has frequently served as a simple, initial rubric to summarize baseline patient comorbidity
   B. Increasing ASA class was not shown to be associated with early postoperative mortality
   C. The addition of an "E" designation signifies emergent operation, hence indicating a higher risk
   D. Patient categorization into ASA 1 to 5, helps stratify patients as low risk (1–2), intermediate risk (3), and high risk (4–5)

5. **Early postoperative mortality in ASA class 5E is nearly:**
   A. 5% B. 10%
   C. 20% D. 40%

6. **Which of the following surgery doesn't have an intermediate risk of mortality?**
   A. Adrenal resection
   B. Peripheral arterial angioplasty
   C. Renal transplant
   D. Endovascular aneurysm repair

7. **Which of the following surgery doesn't have a high risk of mortality?**
   A. Total cystectomy
   B. Pulmonary or liver transplant
   C. Renal transplant
   D. Aortic and major vascular surgery

8. **Which of the following surgery doesn't have a low risk of mortality?**
   A. Endocrine: thyroid
   B. Intrathoracic: nonmajor
   C. Orthopedic: minor (meniscectomy)
   D. Gynecology: minor

9. **Mortality risk in intermediate risk of mortality is:**
   A. 0.5%–1% B. 1%–5%
   C. 5%–10% D. 10%–20%

10. Number of patient characteristics used in ACS NSQIP Surgical Risk Calculator (SRC) is:

A. 10
B. 15
C. 20
D. 25

11. False statement among the following is:

A. ACS NSQIP universal SRC predicts adverse postoperative outcomes based on 20 preoperative patient-level characteristics, including demographics and comorbidities
B. The ACS NSQIP SRC is specifically designed to facilitate patient counselling and consent prior to surgery; as such, it takes into account intraoperative findings
C. Within the last 5 years, the SRC model has also been adapted for the pediatric population as well
D. The most commonly used and cited example of a surgical risk score is the ACS NSQIP Surgical Risk Calculator (SRC)

12. The common components of a consent discussion should include:

A. Procedure-related risks
B. The proposed procedure
C. Mental capacity of the patient
D. All of the above

13. ACS NSQIP variables used in the universal Surgical Risk Calculator includes all except:

A. History of asthma
B. Hypertension requiring medication
C. Sex
D. Disseminated cancer

14. ACS NSQIP variables used in the universal Surgical Risk Calculator includes all except:

A. System sepsis within 24 hours preoperatively
B. Ventilator dependent
C. Congestive heart failure in 30 days preoperatively
D. BMI class

15. ACS NSQIP variables used in the universal Surgical Risk Calculator includes all except:

A. Dyspnea
B. Current smoker within 1 month
C. Acute renal failure
D. Sex

16. ACS NSQIP universal Surgical Risk Calculator reported outcome measures:

A. Renal failure
B. Any complication (surgical site infections [SSIs], pulmonary embolus, ventilator >48 hours, etc.)
C. Venous thromboembolism
D. All of the above

ASSESSMENT OF GERIATRIC SURGICAL PATIENTS

17. ACS NSQIP/AGS collaborative checklist for preoperative assessment of geriatric surgical patients includes:

A. Assess the patient's cognitive ability and capacity to understand the anticipated surgery
B. Determine the patient's treatment goals and expectations in the context of the possible treatment outcomes
C. Determine the patient's treatment goals and expectations in the context of the possible treatment outcomes
D. All of the above

18. False about interpretation of the Mini-Cog: 3-Item Recall and Clock Draw is:

A. 3-item recall (0 to 3 points): 1 point for each correct word
B. Total score of 3, 4, or 5 suggests no impairment
C. 3 points for normal clock
D. Max score is 5

19. The Mini-Cog's advantages include:

A. Focus on attention and executive function
B. A large body of evidence supporting its usefulness
C. Ease of implementation (3 minutes to complete)
D. All of the above

20. Among geriatric patients, in the postoperative setting, cognitive impairment strongly predicts delirium, which has an incidence of nearly:

A. 10%
B. 30%
C. 50%
D. 70%

21. Risk factors for postoperative delirium includes all except:

A. Alcohol use
B. Age > 55 years
C. Anemia
D. Hypoxia or hypercarbia

22. Risk factors for postoperative delirium includes all except:

A. Adequately controlled pain
B. Electrolyte abnormalities
C. Renal insufficiency
D. Hearing or vision impairment

23. As a pragmatic preoperative screening tool for elderly patients, the ACS NSQIP/AGS guidelines recommend the:

A. The Generalized Anxiety Disorder (GAD-7) questionnaire
B. Patient Health Questionnaire-2
C. The Beck Depression Inventory (BDI)
D. The Hamilton Depression Rating Scale (HAM-D or HDRS)

24. False statement among the following is:

A. Adverse effects of beta blocker initiation too close to the time of surgery include risk of stroke, hypotension and death
B. The American College of Cardiology (ACC) and American Heart Association (AHA) guidelines for perioperative beta blockade supports continued administration of beta blockers for patients already on this medication
C. Patients undergoing intermediate-risk surgery with known coronary artery disease or risk factors for ischemic heart disease may be candidates for perioperative beta blockade
D. If initiation of beta blockers is indicated in the preoperative setting, treatment ideally should start weeks before elective surgery and should be titrated to a target heart rate of 80 to 100 beats/minute

25. The AGS Beers criteria for potentially inappropriate medication use includes all except:

A. Avoid: Cilostazol - potential to increase mortality
B. Parkinson disease: Avoid - dopamine-receptor antagonists with potential to worsen parkinsonian symptoms
C. Urinary incontinence in women: Avoid in women; oral estrogen: lack of efficacy
D. Anticholinergic and anticholinergic: Avoid - decreased risk of cognitive decline

26. False about functional status and frailty is:

A. Frailty can be measured using exhaustive, multidimensional scales such as the CGA or more pragmatic tests such as the Timed Up and Go (TUG) tool, which measures functional mobility
B. Preoperative frailty index was more strongly associated with postoperative cardiac arrest and death than ASA class or history of myocardial infarction (MI)
C. Frailty is associated with major complications and early postoperative mortality for cardiothoracic, orthopedic, otolaryngologic, and elective cancer operations
D. All of the above

27. As the most pervasive gait speed measure, TUG time is calculated by:

A. Measuring the time it takes for a patient to rise from a chair, walk 1 meter, turn, and return to a sitting position in the same chair
B. Measuring the time it takes for a patient to rise from a chair, walk 3 meters, turn, and return to a sitting position in the same chair
C. Measuring the time it takes for a patient to rise from a chair, walk 5 meters, turn, and return to a sitting position in the same chair
D. Measuring the time it takes for a patient to rise from a chair, walk 10 meters, turn, and return to a sitting position in the same chair

28. In a multi-institutional study of patients undergoing minor and major elective operations for solid malignancies, if TUG time >20 seconds, the risk of major complications among patients >70 years is:

A. 10% B. 30%
C. 50% D. 70%

29. The total distance to walk in the (TUG) timed up and go test is:

A. 3 m B. 6 m
C. 9 m D. 12 m

SYSTEMS APPROACH TO PREOPERATIVE EVALUATION

30. As per the ACC and AHA collaborative guidelines regarding perioperative cardiac risk, example of intermediate-risk surgery is:

A. Ambulatory operations
B. Thoracic procedures
C. Peripheral vascular surgery
D. Endovascular surgery

31. Revised cardiac risk index includes all except:

A. History of congestive heart failure
B. Preoperative serum creatinine >2.0 mg/dL
C. High-risk type of surgery
D. Hypertension

32. The most pervasive ACC/AHA guideline on perioperative cardiovascular evaluation and management of patients undergoing noncardiac surgery is:

A. ESTS guidelines
B. Revised Cardiac Risk Index (RCRI)
C. EBCP guidelines
D. STS Clinical Practice Guidelines

33. Class IV of RCRI is:

A. >2 B. >3
C. >4 D. >5

34. ACC/ACH guidelines recommend that patients without symptoms of cardiac disease proceed with elective or urgent operation, when the METS are:

A. ≥3 B. ≥4
C. ≥5 D. ≥8

35. Severe aortic stenosis is aortic valve area of:

A. <0.75 cm^2 B. <1.0 cm^2
C. <1.5 cm^2 D. <2 cm^2

36. For patients considering elective noncardiac surgery after recent coronary revascularization (after balloon angioplasty), surgery should be delayed a minimum of:

A. 7 days B. 14 days
C. 28 days D. 30 days

37. For patients considering elective noncardiac surgery after recent coronary revascularization (after bare-metal stent implantation), surgery should be delayed a minimum of:

A. 7 days B. 14 days
C. 28 days D. 30 days

38. Following DES placement if risk of further surgical delay exceeds the risk of stent thrombosis and ischemia, an operation with interruption of dual antiplatelet therapy can be considered after:

A. 30 days B. 90 days
C. 180 days D. 365 days

39. False about use of perioperative cardiovascular medications is:

A. ACC/AHA guidelines recommend that beta blockers should be continued in the perioperative setting for patients for whom it is an established preoperative medication
B. Perioperative use of aspirin monotherapy is safe in the vast majority of patients who require general and cardiovascular operations
C. Patients taking statins at baseline should stop therapy in the perioperative setting
D. If discontinuation of $P2Y_{12}$-inhibitor (clopidogrel, prasugrel, ticagrelor) is necessary to prevent surgical bleeding, it is recommended that aspirin be continued if possible and that the $P2Y_{12}$-inhibitor be restarted as soon as possible after the operation

40. Perioperative beta blockers can be initiated preoperatively if the RCRI is:

A. ≥2 B. ≥3
C. ≥4 D. ≥1

41. A 68-year-old male with known case of coronary heart disease is to be posted for elective surgery. He has low risk of major adverse coronary events after surgery and doesn't have ACS. What should be the next step of management?

A. Pharmacologic stress testing will be needed
B. No further testing and proceed to surgery
C. Coronary revascularization followed by surgery
D. Cancel surgery and keep on conservative management

42. A 54-year-old male with known case of coronary heart disease is to be posted for elective surgery. He has high risk of major adverse coronary events after surgery and doesn't have ACS. His functional capacity is <4 METs. What should be the next step of management?

A. Pharmacologic stress testing will be needed
B. No further testing and proceed to surgery
C. Coronary revascularization followed by surgery
D. Cancel surgery and keep on conservative management

43. A 56-year-old male with known case of coronary heart disease is to be posted for elective surgery. He has high risk of major adverse coronary events after surgery and does not have ACS. His functional capacity is unknown. What should be the next step of management?

A. Pharmacologic stress testing will be needed
B. No further testing and proceed to surgery
C. Coronary revascularization followed by surgery
D. Cancel surgery and keep on conservative management

44. A 62-year-old male with known case of coronary heart disease is to be posted for elective surgery. He has high risk of major adverse coronary events after surgery and does not have ACS. His functional capacity is unknown. He underwent pharmacologic stress testing which was abnormal. What should be the next step of management?

A. Pharmacologic stress testing will be needed
B. No further testing and proceed to surgery
C. Coronary revascularization
D. Cancel surgery and keep on conservative management

45. After major abdominal operations, postoperative pulmonary complications occur in approximately:

A. 1%   B. 6%
C. 15%   D. 25%

46. ACP guidelines indicate that patient-related risk factors for postoperative pulmonary complications includes all except:

A. Hypoalbuminemia (<2.5 g/dL)
B. Age >50 years
C. Heart failure
D. COPD

47. ACP guidelines indicate that patient-related risk factors for postoperative pulmonary complications if the ASA class is:

A. 1 or above   B. 2 or above
C. 3 or above   D. 4 or above

48. False about postoperative pulmonary complications is:

A. Active smoking is associated with a moderate increase in risk of postoperative complications
B. Congestive heart failure especially when associated with pulmonary hypertension is a considerably stronger predictor of postoperative pulmonary complications than severe COPD
C. Obstructive sleep apnea (OSA) and obesity hypoventilation syndrome, which often complement overweight, metabolic syndrome, and morbid obesity, are associated with pulmonary complications and death
D. Smoking cessation at least 1 week prior to the operation reduces the risk of complications

49. Procedure-related risk factors that increase the risk of pulmonary complications include all except:

A. Emergency surgery
B. Procedure duration (>2 hours)
C. Vascular surgery
D. General anesthesia

50. False about postoperative pulmonary complications is:

A. Routine chest radiography may be indicated in patients >50 years of age who are undergoing high-risk surgery
B. Spirometry and chest radiography should be considered in patients with a preexisting diagnosis of COPD or asthma if history and physical exam cannot determine if the patient is at their optimal baseline physiology
C. Pulse oxygen saturation is a risk factor within the ARISCAT index, and its low resource utilization allows for routine screening
D. There is a prohibitive spirometric threshold below which nonthoracic surgery is strictly contraindicated

51. The most frequently cited predictive indices for pulmonary complications includes:

A. Arozullah index
B. Gupta respiratory failure calculators
C. ARISCAT index
D. All of the above

52. False among the following is:

A. ARISCAT index is the simplest to use, featuring 10 readily available preoperative predictors in a simple score system
B. The Arozullah index, derived from a veteran population, specifically targets postoperative respiratory failure
C. Gupta and colleagues developed risk calculators using the ACS NSQIP dataset with primary outcomes of postoperative respiratory failure and pneumonia
D. The disadvantage of the ARISCAT index is that it may overestimate postoperative complication rate as its complication definition includes minor morbidities such as small radiographic effusions and bronchospasm/wheezing

53. Following is not the component of ARISCAT index:

A. Age
B. Preoperative SpO_2
C. Preoperative anemia (≤7 g/dL)
D. Surgical incision

54. High risk for pulmonary complications after surgery is if the ARISCAT index score is:

A. ≥25 points B. ≥35 points
C. ≥45 points D. ≥50 points

55. Low risk for pulmonary complications after surgery is if the ARISCAT index score is:

A. <16 points B. <10 points
C. <26 points D. <36 points

56. Higher prevalence of OSA is with:

A. Obesity B. Female sex
C. Older age D. Male sex

57. Questionnaire used for OSA is all except:

A. Berlin questionnaire
B. STOP-BANG questionnaire
C. Osaka questionnaire
D. Epworth questionnaire

58. STOP-BANG questionnaire has been developed to screen patients for OSA and to stratify patients into risk categories based on presence of symptoms; All of the following are components of the questionnaire except:

A. Daytime tiredness
B. Snoring
C. Body mass index (BMI) >30
D. Neck diameter >40 cm

59. False about STOP-BANG questionnaire in the following is:

A. Patients with 5 or more risk factors are considered at high risk for moderate to severe OSA
B. If an elective operation is planned, patients with scores of 3 or more should be considered for a sleep study
C. Consideration for postoperative capnography and adherence to OSA screening and postoperative CPAP use can decrease the risk of respiratory failure and death
D. Patients requiring urgent or emergent operations are managed for OSA in the postoperative setting

60. Obesity hypoventilation syndrome is defined as a combination of:

A. BMI >30 with awake $PaCO_2$ >55 mm Hg indicative of hypercapnia
B. BMI >35 with awake $PaCO_2$ >55 mm Hg indicative of hypercapnia
C. BMI >30 with awake $PaCO_2$ >45 mm Hg indicative of hypercapnia
D. BMI >35 with awake $PaCO_2$ >45 mm Hg indicative of hypercapnia

61. False among the following is:

A. Chronic renal disease is a consistent predictor of death and cardiac arrest in the perioperative patient
B. A normal potassium level is a not a prerequisite for patients with chronic renal disease being considered for an elective or urgent operation
C. Patients with stage 1 to 2 chronic renal insufficiency and functional capacity >4 METs who are undergoing low- or intermediate-risk surgery do not require additional preoperative studies
D. Echocardiography should be done in patients with volume overload despite optimal chronic renal disease management to evaluate for concomitant cardiac dysfunction

62. The ideal timing of preoperative dialysis is:

A. The day prior to the operation or the day of surgery
B. The day after operation or the day of surgery
C. The 2 days prior or the 2 days after surgery
D. The 1 week prior or the 1 week after surgery

63. Experts recommend increasing the amount of peritoneal dialysis for:

A. 1 day prior to surgery
B. 1 week prior to surgery
C. 10 days prior to surgery
D. 1 month prior to surgery

64. False statement among the following is:

A. Chronic renal insufficiency impacts platelet count
B. In patients with CKD, after addressing the various etiologies for chronic anemia, erythropoietin or darbepoetin may be started for preoperative optimization
C. Cryoprecipitate and platelet transfusion can be used if necessary
D. Desmopressin (DDAVP) should be readily available and administered if medical bleeding from platelet dysfunction is encountered

65. Which of the following is not a Modified Child-Turcotte-Pugh scoring system variable?

A. Serum Albumin B. Direct bilirubin
C. INR D. Ascitis

66. Modified Child-Turcotte-Pugh score of 7 is:

A. Class A
B. Class B
C. Class C
D. Class D

67. Modified Child-Turcotte-Pugh score of 9 is:

A. Class A
B. Class B
C. Class C
D. Class D

68. Modified Child-Turcotte-Pugh score of a 43 years old male with primary biliary sclerosis with serum albumin 3.0 g/dl, total bilirubin 3.4 mg/dl, INR 2.0, moderate ascites and no encephalopathy is:

A. 8
B. 9
C. 10
D. 11

69. Modified Child-Turcotte-Pugh score of a 33 years old male with primary sclerosing cholangitis with serum albumin 2.7 g/dl, total bilirubin 4.4 mg/dl, INR 1.5, no ascites and no encephalopathy is:

A. 8
B. 9
C. 7
D. 10

70. Modified Child-Turcotte-Pugh score of a 53 years old male with alcoholic liver disease with serum albumin 2.7 g/dl, total bilirubin 4.4 mg/dl, INR 2.5, no ascites and grade 2 encephalopathy is:

A. 10
B. 11
C. 12
D. 13

71. False about patients with hepatic disease is:

A. Contraindications to elective surgery include acute or fulminant hepatitis and alcoholic hepatitis
B. Patients with fibrosis with cirrhosis can usually tolerate elective surgery
C. Common anesthetics, such as propofol, ketamine, etomidate, benzodiazepines, and opioids undergo hepatic metabolism and are modified for use
D. Cirrhosis is associated with increased mortality across all types of major elective surgery, with odds ratios ranging from 3.4 for cholecystectomy to 8.0 for coronary artery bypass graft

72. Common objective measures of surgical risk in cirrhotic patients is/are:

A. MELD score
B. Child-Turcotte-Pugh (CTP) score
C. Residual liver volume
D. All of the above

73. False about CTP classification is:

A. Originally proposed by Child and Turcotte, this score estimated the procedural risk for portosystemic shunting for variceal bleeding
B. The score was modified by Pugh and colleagues to include prothrombin time (PT) and include nutritional status
C. Broad estimates of mortality for abdominal operations are 10%, 20%, and 60% for CTP A, B and C, respectively
D. A CTP score of 5 to 6 is considered class A (well-compensated), 7 to 9 is considered class B (significant compromise), and 10 to 15 is considered class C (decompensated)

74. False statement about MELD score is:

A. The predictive utility of both MELD score may be greater for urgent than for elective operations
B. MELD score is predictive of survival in patients with cirrhosis and was originally developed primarily for transplant selection
C. Unlike MELD score, which includes subjective components such as encephalopathy and ascites, the CTP score is comprised only of objective measures
D. The MELD score has gradually supplanted CTP classification for both liver-directed operations and non-hepatic surgical risk stratification

75. MELD score includes all except:

A. Total bilirubin
B. INR
C. Creatinine
D. Albumin

76. 30-day mortality associated with MELD >20 is:

A. >10%
B. >30%
C. >50%
D. >70%

77. As per 50-50 criteria: post hepatectomy liver failure is associated with mortality rate up to:

A. 10%
B. 30%
C. 50%
D. 70%

78. 50-50 criteria is defined as:

A. PT >50% of normal and serum albumin >2.9 g/dL (50 μmol/L) on postoperative day 7
B. Bleeding time >50% of normal and serum albumin >2.9 g/dL (50 μmol/L) on postoperative day 7
C. PT >50% of normal and serum bilirubin >2.9 mg/dL (50 μmol/L) on postoperative day 5
D. Bleeding time >50% of normal and serum bilirubin >2.9 mg/dL (50 μmol/L) on postoperative day 5

79. For patients without cirrhosis undergoing hepatic resection, a residual liver volume generally considered adequate is:

A. 20% B. 25%
C. 30% D. 40%

80. For patients with compensated cirrhosis undergoing hepatic resection, a residual liver volume generally considered adequate is:

A. 20% B. 35%
C. 30% D. 40%

81. Synthetic function of liver should be evaluated through assessment of:

A. Albumin B. Fibrinogen
C. PT D. All of the above

82. Approximate risk of Febrile reaction per unit transfusion of RBCs is:

A. 1:60 B. 1:100
C. 1:250 D. 1:12,000

83. Approximate risk of Allergic reaction per unit transfusion of RBCs is:

A. 1:1,149,000 B. 1:100
C. 1:250 D. 1:12,000

84. Approximate risk of Fatal hemolysis per unit transfusion of RBCs is:

A. 1:1,150,000 B. 1:1,200,000
C. 1:1,400,000 D. 1:1,972,000

85. Approximate risk of Transfusion-related acute lung injury per unit transfusion of RBCs is:

A. 1:600 B. 1:1000
C. 1:2500 D. 1:12,000

86. For most hemodynamically stable, asymptomatic hospitalized patients, transfusion is not indicated until hemoglobin level is:

A. ≤6 g/dL B. ≤7 g/dL
C. ≤8 g/dL D. ≤9 g/dL

87. For patients with cardiovascular disease and undergoing cardiac surgery, transfusion threshold is of:

A. 6 g/dL B. 7 g/dL
C. 8 g/dL D. 9 g/dL

88. False statement among the following is:

A. Patients with signs of hereditary bleeding disorders should be referred for preoperative hematologic consultation
B. Hemophilia A and B are both are autosomal recessive disorders
C. Perioperative analgesia should not include medications with antiplatelet effects such as aspirin and NSAIDs
D. All of the above are true

89. Spontaneous bleeding generally does not occur unless the platelet count is below:

A. 5,000/µL B. 10,000/µL
C. 30,000/µL D. 50,000/µL

90. The most common inherited disorders in platelet function or storage is:

A. Bernard-Soulier disease
B. von Willebrand disease (vWD)
C. Glanzmann thrombasthenia
D. Myelodysplastic syndromes

91. Acquired causes of platelet dysfunction includes:

A. NSAIDs B. Uremia
C. Cirrhosis D. All of the above

92. Hemophilia A is deficiency of:

A. Factor VII B. Factor VIII
C. Factor IX D. Factor XI

93. Hemophilia B is deficiency of:

A. Factor VII B. Factor VIII
C. Factor IX D. Factor XI

94. Abnormal results on both PT and aPTT usually indicate a defect in all except:

A. Factor V B. Prothrombin
C. Fibrinogen D. Factor VII

95. PTT is only prolonged in deficiency of all except:

A. Factor VII B. Factor XI
C. Factor VIII D. Factor IX

96. DDAVP given the day of surgery for hemophilia A patients, will raise factor VIII levels up to:

A. 3-fold within 30 minutes
B. 5-fold within 90 minutes
C. 7-fold within 60 minutes
D. 10-fold within 120 minutes

97. False statement among the following is:

A. Mild forms of hemophilia B require factor replacement both before and after major surgery to maintain appropriate levels
B. Hyponatremia can be a serious complication of DDAVP
C. Up to 50% of patients with severe hemophilia

A will ultimately develop inhibiting antibodies to factor VIII

D. For hemophilia A & B disorders, severe phenotypes should be treated with administration of factor concentrates in the immediate preoperative setting, within 10 to 20 minutes of incision

98. False about von Willebrand factor (vWF) is:

A. Type 2 vWD comprises a variety of qualitative defects in vWF that can result in decreased binding of factor VIII and disorders in platelet function (2A, 2B and 2M)

B. Type 1 is a partial deficiency of vWF and the most common version of vWD

C. Type 3 vWD is a complete or near-complete deficiency in vWF and universally does not respond to DDAVP

D. DDAVP is contraindicated in type 2A vWD

99. Recommended levels of vWF in patients with vWD for minor surgeries is:

A. 100% vWF preoperatively and trough daily levels of 50% until wound healing (5–10 days)

B. 60% vWF level preoperatively and trough daily levels of 30% until wound healing (2–4 days)

C. 60% vWF level preoperatively (single dose)

D. 80%–100% vWF level predelivery and trough levels of 30% (3–4 days)

100. Recommended levels of vWF in patients with vWD for major surgeries is:

A. 100% vWF preoperatively and trough daily levels of 50% until wound healing (5–10 days)

B. 60% vWF level preoperatively and trough daily levels of 30% until wound healing (2–4 days)

C. 60% vWF level preoperatively (single dose)

D. 80%–100% vWF level predelivery and trough levels of 30% (3–4 days)

101. Recommended levels of vWF in patients with vWD for delivery and puerperium is:

A. 100% vWF preoperatively and trough daily levels of 50% until wound healing (5–10 days)

B. 60% vWF level preoperatively and trough daily levels of 30% until wound healing (2–4 days)

C. 60% vWF level preoperatively (single dose)

D. 80%–100% vWF level predelivery and trough levels of 30% (3–4 days)

102. Landmark trial which concluded that administration of aspirin in the perioperative setting has no impact on death or MI and increases the risk of major bleeding is:

A. ASCEND trial B. ARRIVE trial
C. POISE-2 trial D. ASPIRE trial

103. How many days before elective operations, Warfarin should be discontinued?

A. 2 days B. 3 days
C. 5 days D. 7 days

104. False among the following is:

A. Results from the double-blind, placebo-controlled BRIDGE trial concluded that forgoing bridging with low-molecular–weight heparin for high-risk atrial fibrillation decreases risk for arterial thromboembolism and increases the risk of major bleeding

B. When used in the setting of bridging treatment, unfractionated heparin should be stopped 4 to 6 hours before surgery

C. When used in the setting of bridging treatment, low–molecular-weight heparin should be stopped 24 hours before surgery

D. For operations with high bleeding risk, therapeutic-dose low-molecular–weight heparin should be resumed 48 to 72 hours postoperatively

105. Direct factor Xa inhibitor includes all except:

A. Edoxaban B. Dabigatran
C. Rivaroxaban D. Apixaban

106. False about Dabigatran is:

A. Dabigatran was approved by the US Food and Drug Administration (FDA) for stroke prevention in atrial fibrillation in 2010

B. For patients with normal renal function who are anticipating major surgery, dabigatran should be held for 48 hours prior to surgery and resumed 2 to 3 days after surgery

C. Its clearance is renal with a half-life of 24 - 48 hours

D. Dabigatran can be monitored using dilute thrombin time or liquid chromatography-mass spectrometry (LC-MS/MS) drug level

107. Specific reversal agent for dabigatran is:

A. Adalimumab B. Andexanet alpha
C. Idarucizumab D. Alirocumab

108. Specific reversal agent for Rivaroxaban is:

A. Adalimumab B. Andexanet alpha
C. Idarucizumab D. Alirocumab

109. False about Rivaroxaban is:

A. Rivaroxaban can be monitored using a chromogenic anti-Xa assay or LC-MS/MS

B. Direct factor IXa inhibitors
C. Factor Xa inhibitors are substrates of P-glycoprotein efflux transporters
D. Oral Xa inhibitors have rapid onset (2–4 hours) and relatively short half-lives, allowing for short periods of interruption perioperatively

110. False statement among the following is:

A. DPP-4 inhibitors (gliptins) typically are withheld the day of surgery
B. Hemoglobin A_{1c} helps evaluate the efficacy of glycemic control
C. Administration of metformin the morning of surgery is controversial
D. Sulfonylureas (e.g., glyburide, glipizide, glimepiride, and other single-agent or combination sulfonylureas) are withheld the day of surgery

111. Perioperative supplemental glucocorticoid regimens in patient with no HPAA suppression is:

A. 50 mg hydrocortisone IV before induction of anesthesia, 25 mg hydrocortisone every 8 hours thereafter for 24–48 hours, then resume usual dose
B. Give usual daily glucocorticoid dose during perioperative period
C. 100 mg hydrocortisone IV before induction of anesthesia, 50 mg hydrocortisone every 8 hours thereafter for 48–72 hours, then resume usual dose
D. Give supplemental glucocorticoids as though suppressed

112. Perioperative supplemental glucocorticoid regimen in patient when HPAA suppression is documented for moderate surgical stress is:

A. 50 mg hydrocortisone IV before induction of anesthesia, 25 mg hydrocortisone every 8 hours thereafter for 24–48 hours, then resume usual dose
B. Give usual daily glucocorticoid dose during perioperative period
C. 100 mg hydrocortisone IV before induction of anesthesia, 50 mg hydrocortisone every 8 hours thereafter for 48–72 hours, then resume usual dose
D. Give supplemental glucocorticoids as though suppressed

113. The most commonly cited serum indicators of protein status is/are:

A. Transferrin B. Prealbumin
C. Albumin D. All of the above

114. Transferrin has a half-life of:

A. 4 to 5 days B. 8 to 9 days
C. 11 to 13 days D. 20 to 25 days

115. False about Nutritional Risk Screen (NRS-2002) tool is:

A. Score ≥3: the patient is nutritionally at-risk and a nutritional care plan is initiated
B. Score <3: weekly rescreening of the patient
C. Nutritional risk is defined by the present nutritional status and risk of impairment of present status due to increased requirements caused by stress metabolism of the clinical condition
D. All of the above are true

116. Parenteral nutrition be considered in the postoperative setting when there is an expectation for non-functional gastrointestinal tract of:

A. > 2 days B. > 7 days
C. > 14 days D. > 21 days

117. AHA recommends a preoperative ECG and chest radiography for all patients with BMI:

A. >30 B. >35
C. >40 D. >50

PREOPERATIVE CONSIDERATIONS AND CARE PROTOCOLS

118. Operative wounds in which the respiratory, alimentary, genital, or urinary tracts are entered under controlled conditions and without unusual contamination are:

A. Clean
B. Clean-Contaminated
C. Contaminated
D. Dirty-Infected

119. Open, fresh, accidental wounds and operations with major breaks in sterile technique or gross spillage from the gastrointestinal tract are:

A. Clean
B. Clean-Contaminated
C. Contaminated
D. Dirty-Infected

120. Current data support administration of the first dose of prophylactic antibiotics, before surgical incision within:

A. 30 minutes B. 45 minutes
C. 60 minutes D. 120 minutes

121. Current data support administration of the first dose of vancomycin, before surgical incision within:

A. 30 minutes B. 45 minutes
C. 60 minutes D. 120 minutes

122. Redosing of antibiotics should be performed to maintain therapeutic serum levels, generally after every 2 half-lives or if there is blood loss:

A. >500 mL B. >1000 mL
C. >1500 mL D. >2000 mL

123. After cardiothoracic surgery, the Surgical Infection Society and the Society of Thoracic Surgeons both recommend consideration of antimicrobial prophylaxis for up to:

A. 12 hours B. 24 hours
C. 48 hours D. 72 hours

124. Due to thromboembolic risk, preoperatively Estrogen and tamoxifen should be held for:

A. 1 week B. 2 weeks
C. 4 weeks D. 8 weeks

125. Garlic should be stopped preoperatively for at least:

A. 1 day B. 5 days
C. 7 days D. 14 days

126. Recommended minimum fasting periods between oral intake of breast milk and general anesthesia for elective operations is:

A. 2 hours B. 4 hours
C. 6 hours D. 8 hours

127. Recommended minimum fasting periods between oral intake of Infant formula and general anesthesia for elective operations is:

A. 2 hours B. 4 hours
C. 6 hours D. 8 hours

128. Recommended minimum fasting periods between oral intake of Clear liquids and general anesthesia for elective operations is:

A. 2 hours B. 4 hours
C. 6 hours D. 8 hours

129. Recommended minimum fasting periods between oral intake of Nonhuman milk and general anesthesia for elective operations is:

A. 2 hours B. 4 hours
C. 6 hours D. 8 hours

130. False statement among the following is:

A. Under normal conditions, autonomic control regulates core temperature consistently to between 36°C and 38°C
B. Neuraxial anesthesia (epidural and spinal) further blunts thermoregulatory control by reducing thermal discomfort and blocking efferent nervous control of vasoconstriction and shivering
C. Intraoperative hypothermia causes platelet aggregation and the coagulation cascade are impaired, resulting in an association between hypothermia and nearly a 50% increased operative blood loss
D. Hypothermia is most drastic within the first hour after induction due to the rapid effect of anesthesia-induced vasodilatation

131. Passive insulation (blankets, sheets) can reduce cutaneous heat loss by roughly:

A. 10% B. 30%
C. 50% D. 70%

132. False among the following is:

A. Patients can be cooled by infusion of ambient-temperature fluids, thereby exacerbating anesthesia-induced hypothermia
B. Any intraoperative infusion of >1 L/h should be prewarmed
C. Increasing ambient room temperature can passively mitigate heat loss and is practical for raising core body temperature
D. Active warming with forced air is frequently effective during induction and throughout the operation to compensate for rapid thermal dysregulation

133. The CDC guidelines recommend the following techniques for application of skin preparation except:

A. Wide area to include any potential incision sites
B. Vertical motion
C. Use of a dedicated application instrument
D. Adequate time to allow the solution to dry

134. Common solutions used for skin preparation is:

A. Iodine povacrylex with isopropyl alcohol
B. Chlorhexidine-alcohol scrub

C. Povidone-iodine scrub and paint
D. All of the above

135. Following image shows DuraPrep, what is the composition?

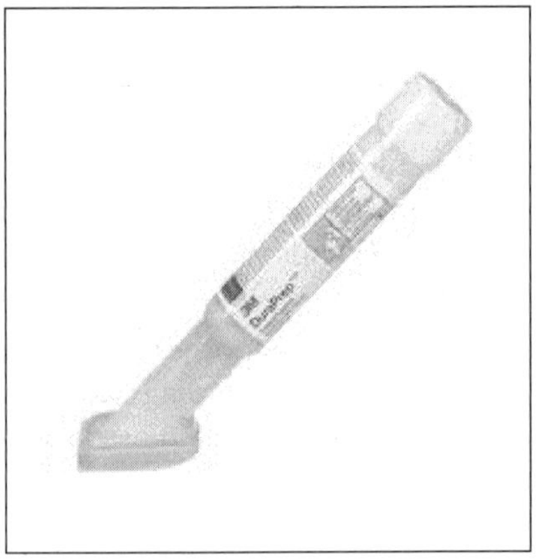

A. Iodine povacrylex with isopropyl alcohol
B. Chlorhexidine-alcohol scrub
C. Povidone-iodine scrub and paint
D. All of the above

136. Following image shows ChloraPrep, what is the composition?

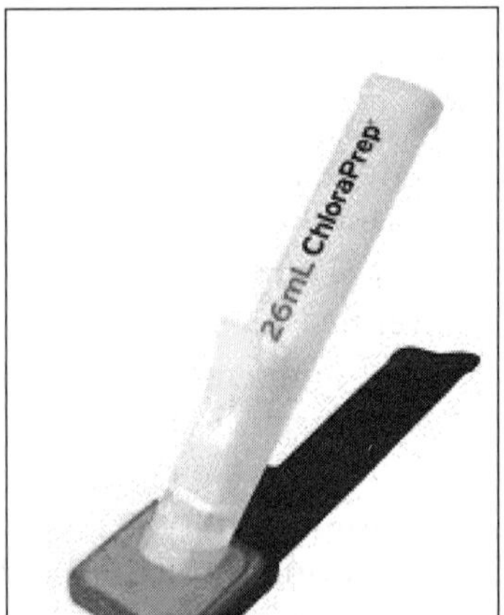

A. Iodine povacrylex with isopropyl alcohol
B. Chlorhexidine-isopropyl alcohol scrub
C. Povidone-iodine scrub and paint
D. All of the above

137. In the surgical safety checklist, steps included before induction of anaesthesia are all except:

A. Is the site marked?
B. Is the pulse oximeter on the patient and functioning?
C. Is essential imaging displayed?
D. Has the patient confirmed his/her identity, site, procedure and consent?

138. In the surgical safety checklist, steps included before skin incision are all except:

A. Is essential imaging displayed?
B. Has antibiotic prophylaxis been given within the last 60 minutes?
C. Difficult airway or aspiration risk
D. Anticipated Critical Events

139. True statement among the following is/are:

A. Dedicated vacuum-assisted closure devices such as the V.A.C. Abdominal Dressing System and the ABThera System have gained popularity due to ease of application
B. Serial closure can be initiated using devices such as a Wittmann patch, which may be serially tightened every 24 to 48 hours
C. Bioprosthetic dermal matrices have gained favor as an alternative material for fascial bridging and is derived from cadaveric dermis (porcine, human, or bovine), acellular dermal matrix is devoid of all cellular components while retaining the extracellular matrix and basement membrane
D. All of the above

140. Dermabond is composed of:

A. Nanocyanoacrylate
B. Octylcyanoacrylate
C. Ethylcyanoacrylate
D. Butylcyanoacrylate

141. Histoacryl is composed of:

A. Nanocyanoacrylate
B. Octylcyanoacrylate
C. Ethylcyanoacrylate
D. Butylcyanoacrylate

142. True about Fibrin sealant is:

A. Fibrin sealant confers both adhesive and hemostatic functions
B. For perianal fistulae, fibrin glue avoids an adverse impact on continence; however, it exhibits inferior durability compared to conventional surgical treatment
C. Fibrin glue has been used to treat bronchopleural fistulae, either as a direct injection of fibrinogen followed by topical thrombin or as a diluted pleurodesis agent
D. All of the above

SURGICAL DEVICES, ENERGY SOURCES AND STAPLERS

143. Diathermy was first described by:

A. Oliver Bernard B. Harvey Cushing
C. William T. Bovie D. Karl Franz

144. Modern electrosurgery was introduced by:

A. Oliver Bernard B. Harvey Cushing
C. William T Bovie D. Karl Franz

145. Following image shows:

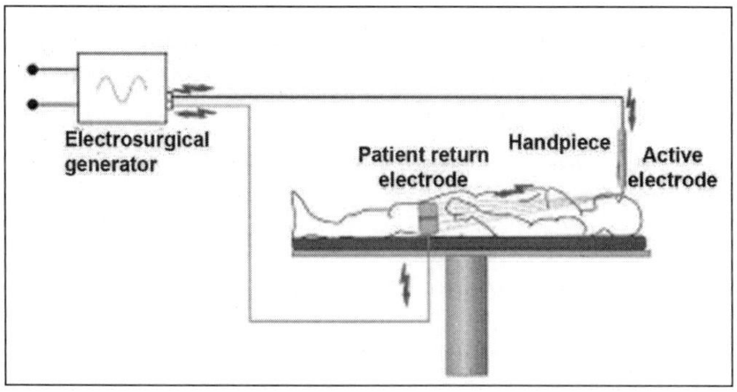

A. Bipolar cautery B. Monopolar cautery
C. Tripolar cautery D. None of the above

146. Following image shows:

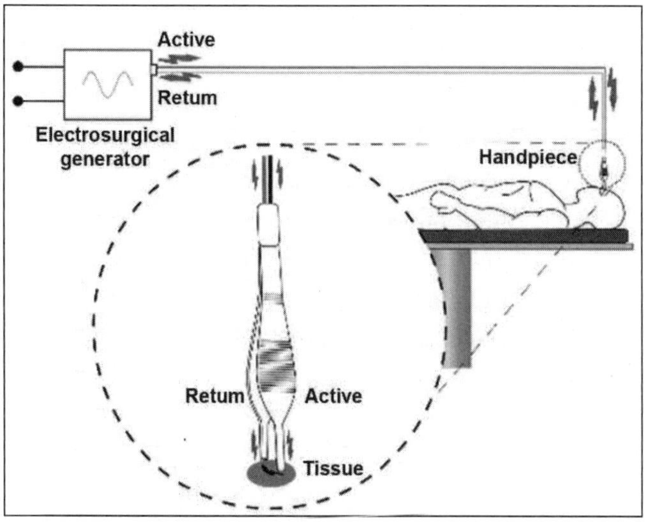

A. Bipolar cautery
B. Monopolar cautery
C. Tripolar cautery
D. None of the above

147. LigaSure and Enseal can seal vessels upto:

A. 3 mm B. 5 mm
C. 7 mm D. 10 mm

148. Which of the following is saline-cooled radio-frequency dissector?

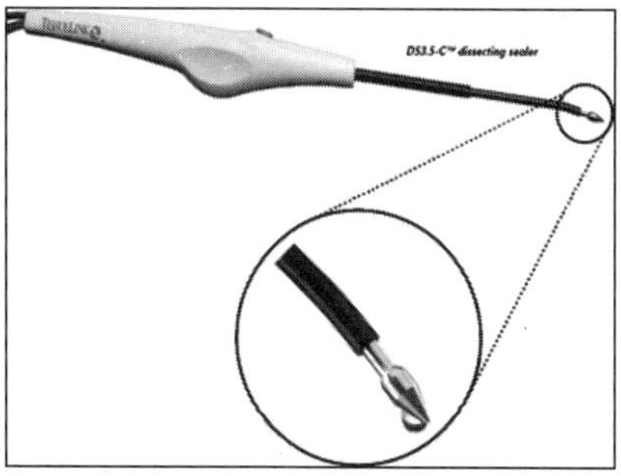

A. Harmonic Scalpel B. TissueLink
C. LigaSure D. Enseal

149. Following image shows:

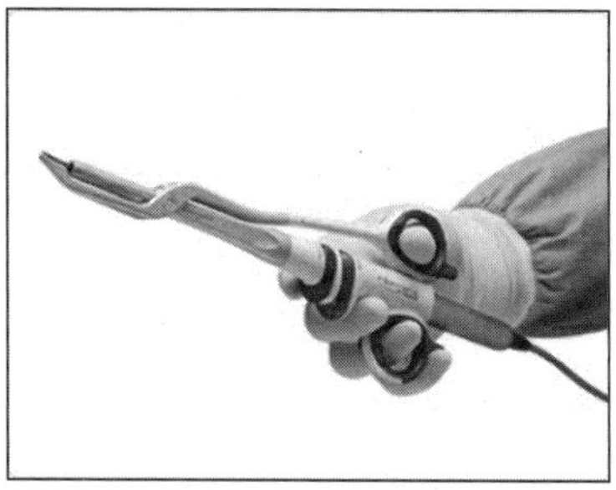

A. Harmonic Scalpel
B. Cavitron ultrasound surgical aspirator (CUSA)
C. LigaSure
D. Enseal

150. Following image shows:

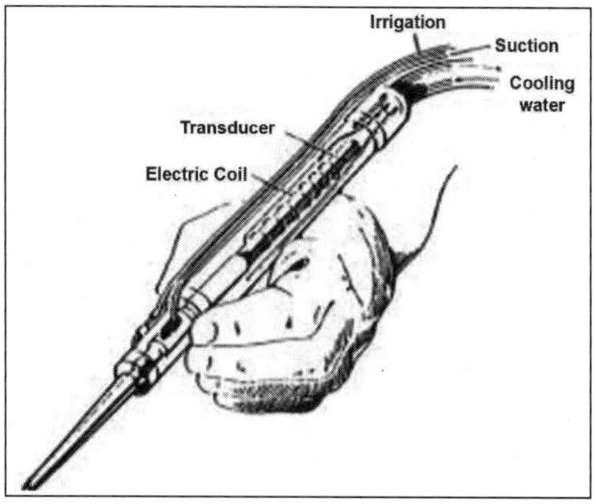

A. Harmonic Scalpel
B. Cavitron ultrasound surgical aspirator (CUSA)
C. LigaSure
D. Enseal

151. False about RFA is:

A. Typically, tumors up to 5 cm can be effectively ablated by RFA; an additional margin of 0.5 cm of healthy parenchyma beyond the target lesion should be ablated to ensure complete ablation of the tumor

B. Applications include esophageal dysplasia, atrial fibrillation, and tumors found within solid organ parenchyma
C. When performed near a blood vessel, thermal energy is dispersed rapidly from the target tissue, creating a "heat sink" and limiting efficacy
D. The electrode at the probe tip transmits high-frequency alternating current to the surrounding tissue, which is converted to kinetic and thermal energy and results in denaturation and coagulation

152. False about Microwave Ablation is:

A. Microwave energy lies between infrared and radio waves in frequency
B. The impact between microwave energy radiation and polar molecules such as water result in oscillation and frictional heat
C. A grounding pad is necessary and use in the presence of metallic clips and implants is unsafe
D. The impact between microwave energy radiation and polar molecules such as water result in oscillation and frictional heat

153. False about Argon beam coagulation (ABC) is:

A. ABC is a laser device
B. Advantages of ABC over conventional electrosurgery include more rapid activity, shallower penetration, and faster heat dispersion
C. Radiofrequency current is transported from a monopolar electrode to the tissue across this pathway of argon gas
D. ABC is most suitable for achieving hemostasis over surfaces of solid organ parenchyma, such as the spleen, liver, kidney, lung and peritoneum

154. Following image shows:

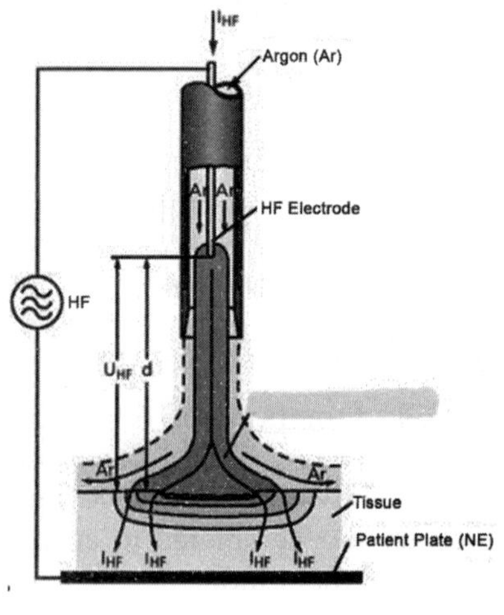

A. Radiofrequency Ablation
B. Microwave Ablation
C. Harmonic Scalpel
D. Argon beam coagulation (ABC)

155. Surgical staples best suited for vascular closure and/or transection is/are:

A. Open - 5.5 mm; Closed - 1 mm
B. Open - 2 mm; Closed - 1 mm
C. Open - 5.5 mm; Closed - 2 mm
D. Open - 2 mm; Closed - 0.5 mm

156. Surgical staples well suited for closure and/or transection of thicker tissues such as the stomach or pancreas is/are:

A. Open - 5.5 mm; Closed - 1 mm
B. Open - 2 mm; Closed - 1 mm
C. Open - 5.5 mm; Closed - 2 mm
D. Open - 2 mm; Closed - 0.5 mm

157. Following image shows:

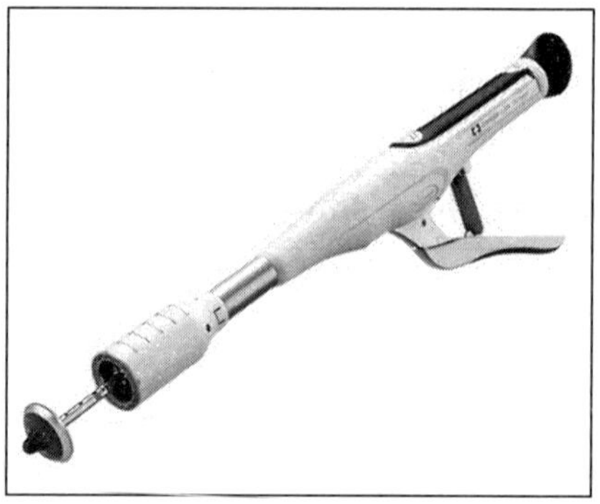

A. Open staplers
B. Circular Stapler
C. Single Use Skin Stapler
D. Signia™ Small Diameter Reload

158. Following image shows:

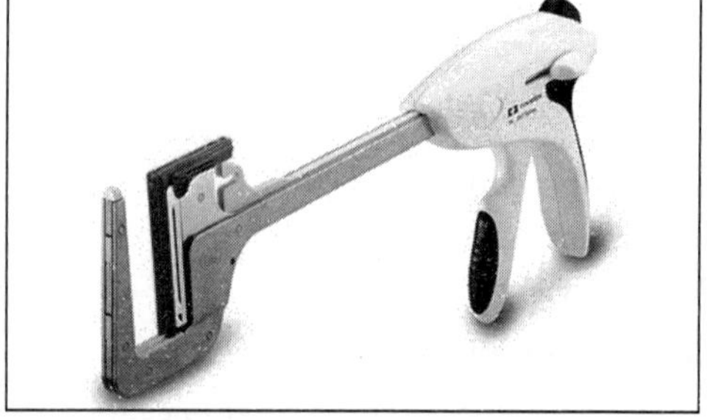

A. Circular Stapler
B. Open staplers
C. Single Use Skin Stapler
D. Signia™ Small Diameter Reload

159. Following image shows:

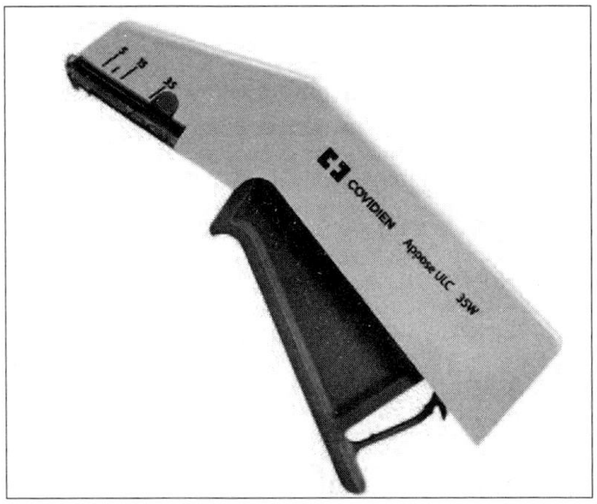

A. Circular Stapler
B. Open staplers
C. Single Use Skin Stapler
D. Signia™ Small Diameter Reload

160. Following image shows:

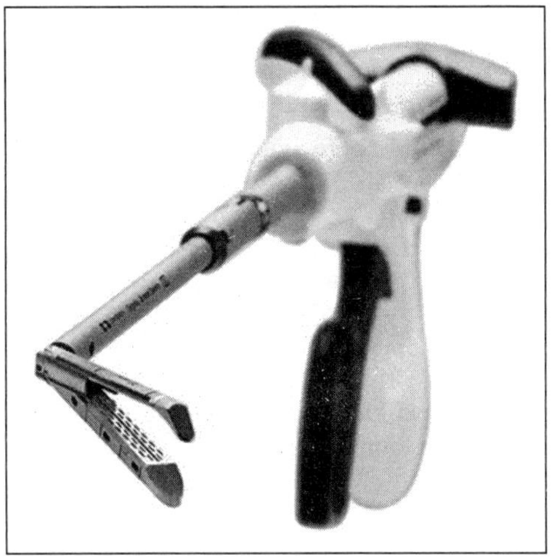

A. Circular Stapler
B. Open staplers
C. Single Use Skin Stapler
D. Signia™ Small Diameter Reload

161. Following image shows:

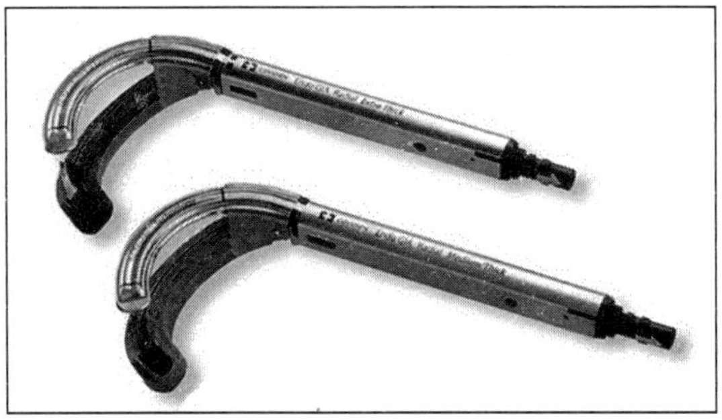

A. Single Use Skin Stapler
B. Endo GIA™ Radial Reload with Tri-Staple™ Technology
C. Signia™ Small Diameter Reload
D. Circular Stapler

POTENTIAL CAUSES OF INTRAOPERATIVE INSTABILITY

162. False about Malignant hyperthermia (MH) is:

A. Malignant hyperthermia (MH) is an acute episode of hypermetabolism as a response to volatile halogenated anesthetic gases (e.g., sevoflurane, isoflurane, and others) and the depolarizing paralytic succinylcholine
B. Most commonly described mutation is in the RYR1 gene
C. Symptoms of MH can occur at any time during general anesthesia or up to 120 minutes after cessation of anesthesia
D. An increase in end tidal CO_2 despite an increase in minute ventilation is one of the earliest intraoperative harbingers of MH

163. False about the management of Malignant hyperthermia (MH) is:

A. MH is treated by immediate discontinuation of volatile gases, IV administration of dantrolene in doses of 5 mg/kg
B. Dantrolene can be re-dosed every 10 to 15 minutes for ongoing fever, acidosis and muscle rigidity
C. Other supportive measures include therapy for arrhythmias, hyperkalemia and acidosis
D. With current advances, mortality with MH has decreased from 60% to 80% a few decades ago to less than 5%

164. False about Gas Embolus is:

A. Intraoperative transoesophageal echocardiography can help confirm the diagnosis and measure the amount of gas trapped within the right heart
B. CO_2 embolus can be a fatal complication of minimally invasive laparoscopic or robotic operations
C. Mortality in patients with gas embolus is approximately 50%
D. Both are a result of air or CO_2 entering the systemic, most often venous, circulation

ANSWERS

1. **Ans: D. Inpatients, referrals from the emergency department, and direct transfers from clinic are included in elective patient categorization**
Ref: Chapter No.10, Page No.188

2. **Ans: D. ASA PS IV**
Ref: Chapter No.10, Page No.188

3. **Ans: C. ASA PS III**
Ref: Chapter No.10, Page No.188

4. **Ans: B. Increasing ASA class was not shown to be associated with early postoperative mortality**
Ref: Chapter No.10, Page No.188

5. **Ans: C. 20%**
Ref: Chapter No.10, Page No.188

6. **Ans: A. Adrenal resection**
Ref: Chapter No.10, Page No.189

7. **Ans: C. Renal transplant**
Ref: Chapter No.10, Page No.189

8. **Ans: B. Intrathoracic: nonmajor**
Ref: Chapter No.10, Page No.189

9. **Ans: B. 1%–5%**
Ref: Chapter No.10, Page No.189

10. **Ans: C. 20**
Ref: Chapter No.10, Page No.189

11. **Ans: B. The ACS NSQIP SRC is specifically designed to facilitate patient counseling and consent prior to surgery; as such, it takes into account intraoperative findings**
Ref: Chapter No.10, Page No.188-189

12. **Ans: D. All of the above**
Ref: Chapter No.10, Page No.189

13. **Ans: A. History of asthma**
Ref: Chapter No.10, Page No.190

14. **Ans: A. System sepsis within 24 hrs preoperatively**
Ref: Chapter No.10, Page No.190

15. **Ans: B. Current smoker within 1 month**
Ref: Chapter No.10, Page No.190

16. **Ans: D. All of the above**
Ref: Chapter No.10, Page No.190

17. **Ans: D. All of the above**
Ref: Chapter No.10, Page No.191

18. **Ans: C. 3 points for normal clock**
Ref: Chapter No.10, Page No.191

19. **Ans: D. All of the above**
Ref: Chapter No.10, Page No.191

20. **Ans: C. 50%**
Ref: Chapter No.10, Page No.191

21. **Ans: B. Age > 55 years**
Ref: Chapter No.10, Page No.192

22. **Ans: A. Adequately controlled pain**
Ref: Chapter No.10, Page No.192

23. **Ans: B. Patient Health Questionnaire-2**
Ref: Chapter No.10, Page No.192

24. **Ans: D. If initiation of beta blockers is indicated in the preoperative setting, treatment ideally should start weeks before elective surgery and should be titrated to a target heart rate of 80 to 100 beats/minute.**
Ref: Chapter No.10, Page No.192

25. **Ans: D. Anticholinergic and anticholinergic: Avoid - decreased risk of cognitive decline**
Ref: http://files.hgsitebuilder.com/hostgator257222/file/ags_2019_beers_pocket_printable_rh.pd

26. **Ans: D. All of the above**
Ref: Chapter No.10, Page No.192-193

27. **Ans: B. Measuring the time it takes for a patient to rise from a chair, walk 3 meters, turn, and return to a sitting position in the same chair**
Ref: Chapter No.10, Page No.193

28. **Ans: C. 50%**
Ref: Chapter No.10, Page No.193

29. **Ans: B. 6 m**
Ref: Chapter No.10, Page No.193

30. **Ans: B. Thoracic procedures**
Ref: Chapter No.10, Page No.193

31. **Ans: D. Hypertension**
Ref: Chapter No.10, Page No.194

32. **Ans: B. Revised Cardiac Risk Index (RCRI)**
Ref: Chapter No.10, Page No.194

33. **Ans: A. >2**
Ref: Chapter No.10, Page No.194

34. **Ans: B. ≥4**
Ref: Chapter No.10, Page No.194

35. Ans: B. <1.0 cm²

Ref: Chapter No.10, Page No.194

36. Ans: B. 14 days

Ref: Chapter No.10, Page No.194

37. Ans: D. 30 days

Ref: Chapter No.10, Page No.194

38. Ans: C. 180 days

Ref: Chapter No.10, Page No.194

39. Ans: C. Patients taking statins at baseline should stop therapy in the perioperative setting

Ref: Chapter No.10, Page No.194-196

40. Ans: B. ≥3 (OR class IV RCRI)

Ref: Chapter No.10, Page No.194-196

41. Ans: B. No further testing and proceed to surgery

Ref: Chapter No.10, Page No.195

42. Ans: A. Pharmacologic stress testing will be needed

Ref: Chapter No.10, Page No.195

43. Ans: A. Pharmacologic stress testing will be needed

Ref: Chapter No.10, Page No.195

44. Ans: C. Coronary revascularization

Ref: Chapter No.10, Page No.195

45. Ans: B. 6%

Ref: Chapter No.10, Page No.196

46. Ans: A. Hypoalbuminemia (<2.5 g/dL)

Ref: Chapter No.10, Page No.196

47. Ans: B. 2 or above

Ref: Chapter No.10, Page No.196

48. Ans: D. Smoking cessation at least 1 week prior to the operation reduces the risk of complications

Ref: Chapter No.10, Page No.196

49. Ans: B. Procedure duration (>2 hours)

Ref: Chapter No.10, Page No.196

50. Ans: D. There is a prohibitive spirometric threshold below which nonthoracic surgery is strictly contraindicated

Ref: Chapter No.10, Page No.196

51. Ans: D. All of the above

Ref: Chapter No.10, Page No.196-197

52. Ans: A. ARISCAT index is the simplest to use, featuring 10 readily available preoperative predictors in a simple score system

Ref: Chapter No.10, Page No.197

53. Ans: C. Preoperative anemia (≤7 g/dL)

Ref: Chapter No.10, Page No.197

54. Ans: C. ≥45 points

Ref: Chapter No.10, Page No.197

55. Ans: C. <26 points

Ref: Chapter No.10, Page No.197

56. Ans: B. Female sex

Ref: Chapter No.10, Page No.197

57. Ans: A. Berlin questionnaire

The **Berlin Criteria** is for ARDS

Epworth questionnaire

- The **Epworth Sleepiness Scale** is widely used in the field of sleep medicine as a subjective measure of a patient's sleepiness
- The test is a list of ***8 situations*** in which you rate your tendency to become sleepy on a scale of 0, no chance of dozing, to 3, high chance of dozing. When you finish the test, add up the values of your responses
- Your total score is based on a scale of ***0 to 24***
- The scale estimates whether you are experiencing excessive sleepiness that possibly requires medical attention

The **Obstructive Sleep Apnea Knowledge and Attitudes (OSAKA)** questionnaire

- OSAKA questionnaire containing sections regarding knowledge about OSA (18 items), attitudes about OSA (five items)

Ref: Chapter No.10, Page No.197-198

https://epworthsleepinessscale.com/about-the-ess/

https://pubmed.ncbi.nlm.nih.gov/14592286/

58. Ans: C. Body mass index (BMI) >30

STOP-Bang questionnaire
Please answer the following questions by checking "Yes" or "No" for earch one.

	Yes	No
Snoring (Do you snore loudly?)	☐	☐
Tiredness (Do you often feel tired, fatigued, or sleepy during the daytime?)	☐	☐
Observed Apnea (Has anyone observed that you stop breathing, or choke or gasp during your sleep?)	☐	☐
High Blood Pressure (Do you have or are you being treated for high blood pressure?)	☐	☐
BMI (Is your body mass index more than 35 kg per m²?	☐	☐
Age (Are you older than 50 years?)	☐	☐
Neck Circumference (Is your neck circumference greater than 40 cm [15.75 inches]?)	☐	☐
Gender (Are you male?)	☐	☐

Score 1 point for each positive response.
Scoring interpretation:0 to 2 = low risk, 3 or 4 = intermediate risk, ≥ 5 = high risk.

STOP BANG

- The STOP-BANG questionnaire is ***not well-validated in the obstetrical population***, a subgroup with increased risk of OSA

- The STOP-BANG questionnaire is ***one of the most widely accepted screening tools*** for OSA.
- Perioperative risks associated with OSA may be modifiable through increased monitoring and treatments (i.e., ***perioperative CPAP***).

Ref: Chapter No.10, Page No.197-198

https://www.mdcalc.com/calc/3992/stop-bang-score-obstructive-sleep-apnea#pearls-pitfalls

59. **Ans: B. If an elective operation is planned, patients with scores of 3 or more should be considered for a sleep study**

Ref: Chapter No.10, Page No.198

60. **Ans: C. BMI >30 with awake $PaCO_2$ >45 mm Hg indicative of hypercapnia**

Ref: Chapter No.10, Page No.198

61. **Ans: B. A normal potassium level is a not a prerequisite for patients with chronic renal disease being considered for an elective or urgent operation**

Ref: Chapter No.10, Page No.198

62. **Ans: A. The day prior to the operation or the day of surgery**

Ref: Chapter No.10, Page No.198

63. **Ans: B. 1 week prior to surgery**

Ref: Chapter No.10, Page No.198

64. **Ans: A. Chronic renal insufficiency impacts platelet count**

Ref: Chapter No.10, Page No.198

65. **Ans: B. Direct bilirubin**

(ABCDE: Albumin, **B**ilirubin-total, **C**oagulation-INR, **D**istension-Ascitis, **E**ncephalopathy**)**

Ref: Chapter No.10, Page No.198

66. **Ans: B. Class B**

Ref: Chapter No.10, Page No.198

67. **Ans: B. Class B**

Ref: Chapter No.10, Page No.198

68. **Ans: B. 9**

Ref: Chapter No.10, Page No.198

69. **Ans: A. 8**

Ref: Chapter No.10, Page No.198

70. **Ans: C. 12**

Ref: Chapter No.10, Page No.198

71. **Ans: B. Patients with fibrosis with cirrhosis can usually tolerate elective surgery**

Ref: Chapter No.10, Page No.199

72. **Ans: D. All of the above**

Ref: Chapter No.10, Page No.199

73. **Ans: B. The score was modified by Pugh and colleagues to include prothrombin time (PT) and include nutritional status**

Ref: Chapter No.10, Page No.199

74. **Ans: C. Unlike MELD score, which includes subjective components such as encephalopathy and ascites, the CTP score is comprised only of objective measures**

Ref: Chapter No.10, Page No.199

75. **Ans: D. Albumin**

Ref: Chapter No.10, Page No.199

76. **Ans: C. >50%**

Ref: Chapter No.10, Page No.199

77. **Ans: C. 50%**

Ref: Chapter No.10, Page No.199

78. **Ans: C. PT >50% of normal and serum bilirubin >2.9 mg/dL (50 µmol/L) on postoperative day 5**

Ref: Chapter No.10, Page No.199

79. **Ans: A. 20%**

Ref: Chapter No.10, Page No.199

80. **Ans: D. 40%**

Ref: Chapter No.10, Page No.199

81. **Ans: D. All of the above**

Ref: Chapter No.10, Page No.199

82. **Ans: A. 1:60**

Ref: Chapter No.10, Page No.200

83. **Ans: C. 1:250**

Ref: Chapter No.10, Page No.200

84. **Ans: D. 1:1,972,000**

Ref: Chapter No.10, Page No.200

85. **Ans: D. 1:12,000**

Ref: Chapter No.10, Page No.200

86. **Ans: B. ≤7 g/dL**

- **These recommendations are supported by the *Transfusion Requirements in Critical Care* (TRICC) *trial***
- **Findings from the TRICC *trial* were recently corroborated by the *Transfusion Requirements in Septic Shock* (TRISS) *trial***
- **The recent *Transfusion Requirements in Cardiac Surgery III* (TRICS III) trial found** *no difference in death, MI, stroke, or renal failure* **between transfusion thresholds of 7.5 g/dL and 8.5 to 9.5 g/dL in cardiac surgery patients**
- **For asymptomatic patients with baseline cardiovascular disease, the *Functional Outcomes in Cardiovascular Patients Undergoing Surgical Hip Fracture* (FOCUS) trial suggests that a transfusion** *threshold of 8 g/dL is not associated with worse postoperative outcomes when compared to a threshold of 10 g/dL*

Ref: Chapter No.10, Page No.200

87. **Ans: C. 8 g/dL**

Ref: Chapter No.10, Page No.200

88. **Ans: B. Hemophilia A and B are both are autosomal recessive disorders**

Ref: Chapter No.10, Page No.201

89. **Ans: C. 30,000/μL**

Ref: Chapter No.10, Page No.201

90. **Ans: B. von Willebrand disease (vWD)**

Ref: Chapter No.10, Page No.201

91. **Ans: D. All of the above**

Ref: Chapter No.10, Page No.201

92. **Ans: B. Factor VIII**

Ref: Chapter No.10, Page No.201

93. **Ans: C. Factor IX**

Ref: Chapter No.10, Page No.201

94. **Ans: D. Factor VII**

Ref: Chapter No.10, Page No.201

95. **Ans: A. Factor VII**

Ref: Chapter No.10, Page No.201

96. **Ans: B. 5-fold within 90 minutes**

Ref: Chapter No.10, Page No.201

97. **Ans: C. Up to 50% of patients with severe hemophilia A will ultimately develop inhibiting antibodies to factor VIII**

Ref: Chapter No.10, Page No.201-202

98. **Ans: D. DDAVP is contraindicated in type 2A vWD**

Ref: Chapter No.10, Page No.202

99. **Ans: B. 60% vWF level preoperatively and trough daily levels of 30% until wound healing (2–4 days)**

Ref: Chapter No.10, Page No.202

100. **Ans: A. 100% vWF preoperatively and trough daily levels of 50% until wound healing (5–10 days)**

Ref: Chapter No.10, Page No.202

101. **Ans: D. 80%–100% vWF level predelivery and trough levels of 30% (3–4 days)**

Ref: Chapter No.10, Page No.202

102. **Ans: C. POISE-2 trial**

1. **POISE-2 trial** showed that among unselected patients undergoing noncardiac surgical procedures, ***neither the perioperative use of aspirin, nor clonidine, was beneficial*** in reducing the incidence of death or myocardial infarction. However, benefit was observed with aspirin among patients with prior stenting
2. **POISE-3 trial (2022):** The goals of the trial were to compare the effects of ***intraoperative tranexamic acid vs. placebo on bleeding, as well as perioperative hypotension-avoidance strategy vs. hypertension-avoidance strategy on major adverse complications***
   - Among patients undergoing noncardiac surgery at risk of vascular events in the POISE-3 trial, ***tranexamic acid resulted in lower bleeding compared with placebo*** but ***did not meet criteria for noninferiority for cardiovascular safety***. Further, a perioperative hypotension-avoidance strategy did not differ from hypertension-avoidance strategy with regard to 30-day major vascular complications
3. **ASCEND** (**A** **S**tudy of **C**ardiovascular **E**vents i**N** **D**iabetes) is a randomised trial looking at the effects of ***aspirin and of omega-3 fatty acids*** (fish oils) in people with diabetes
4. Use of aspirin to reduce risk of ***initial vascular events in patients at moderate risk*** of cardiovascular disease **(ARRIVE)**
5. The Aspirin to ***Prevent Recurrent Venous Thrombo-embolism (ASPIRE) study***

Ref: Chapter No.10, Page No.202

https://www.acc.org/latest-in-cardiology/clinical-trials/2014/05/03/19/28/poise-2

https://www.acc.org/latest-in-cardiology/clinical-trials/2022/04/01/03/11/poise-3

https://pubmed.ncbi.nlm.nih.gov/30158069/

https://www.acc.org/latest-in-cardiology/articles/2019/04/26/09/46/the-ascend-trial-who-benefits-with-aspirin

https://pubmed.ncbi.nlm.nih.gov/28741785/

103. **Ans: C. 5 days**

Ref: Chapter No.10, Page No.202

104. **Ans: A. Results from the double-blind, placebo-controlled BRIDGE trial concluded that forgoing bridging with low-molecular–weight heparin for high-risk atrial fibrillation decreases risk for arterial thromboembolism and increases the risk of major bleeding**

Ref: Chapter No.10, Page No.202

105. **Ans: B. Dabigatran**

Ref: Chapter No.10, Page No.202

106. **Ans: C. Its clearance is renal with a half-life of 24 - 48 hours**

Ref: Chapter No.10, Page No.203

107. **Ans: C. Idarucizumab (Rapid reversal is achieved with a *single 5 g IV dose*)**

Ref: Chapter No.10, Page No.203

108. **Ans: B. Andexanet alpha (Administration involves an *initial bolus of 400 to 800 mg followed by a continuous infusion*)**

Ref: Chapter No.10, Page No.204

109. **Ans: B. Direct factor IXa inhibitors**

Ref: Chapter No.10, Page No.203-204

110. Ans: A. DPP-4 inhibitors (gliptins) typically are withheld the day of surgery

Ref: Chapter No.10, Page No.204

111. Ans: B. Give usual daily glucocorticoid dose during perioperative period

Ref: Chapter No.10, Page No.205

112. Ans: A. 50 mg hydrocortisone IV before induction of anesthesia, 25 mg hydrocortisone every 8 hours thereafter for 24–48 hours, then resume usual dose

Ref: Chapter No.10, Page No.205

113. Ans: D. All of the above

Ref: Chapter No.10, Page No.206

114. Ans: B. 8 to 9 days

Ref: Chapter No.10, Page No.206

115. Ans: D. All of the above are true

Ref: Chapter No.10, Page No.206

116. Ans: B. > 7 days

Ref: Chapter No.10, Page No.206-207

117. Ans: C. >40

Ref: Chapter No.10, Page No.207

118. Ans: B. Clean-Contaminated

Ref: Chapter No.10, Page No.207

119. Ans: C. Contaminated

Ref: Chapter No.10, Page No.207

120. Ans: C. 60 minutes

Ref: Chapter No.10, Page No.207

121. Ans: D. 120 minutes

Ref: Chapter No.10, Page No.207

122. Ans: C. >1500 mL

Ref: Chapter No.10, Page No.207

123. Ans: C. 48 hours

Ref: Chapter No.10, Page No.207

124. Ans: C. 4 weeks

Ref: Chapter No.10, Page No.207

125. Ans: C. 7 days

Ref: Chapter No.10, Page No.213

126. Ans: B. 4 hours

Ref: Chapter No.10, Page No.213

127. Ans: C. 6 hours

Ref: Chapter No.10, Page No.213

128. Ans: A. 2 hours

Ref: Chapter No.10, Page No.213

129. Ans: C. 6 hours

Ref: Chapter No.10, Page No.213

130. Ans: C. Intraoperative hypothermia causes platelet aggregation and the coagulation cascade are impaired, resulting in an association between hypothermia and nearly a 50% increased operative blood loss

Ref: Chapter No.10, Page No.211-213

131. Ans: B. 30%

Ref: Chapter No.10, Page No.213

132. Ans: C. Increasing ambient room temperature can passively mitigate heat loss and is practical for raising core body temperature

Ref: Chapter No.10, Page No.213

133. Ans: B. Vertical motion

Ref: Chapter No.10, Page No.213

134. Ans: D. All of the above (Skin preparation that contains an alcohol-based agent as part of the preparation appears optimal)

Ref: Chapter No.10, Page No.214

135. Ans: A. Iodine povacrylex with isopropyl alcohol

Ref: Chapter No.10, Page No.214

136. Ans: B. Chlorhexidine-isopropyl alcohol scrub

Ref: Chapter No.10, Page No.214

137. Ans: C. Is essential imaging displayed?

Ref: Chapter No.10, Page No.214

138. Ans: C. Difficult airway or aspiration risk?

Ref: Chapter No.10, Page No.214

139. Ans: D. All of the above

Ref: Chapter No.10, Page No.215

140. Ans: B. Octylcyanoacrylate

Ref: Chapter No.10, Page No.215

141. Ans: D. Butylcyanoacrylate

Ref: Chapter No.10, Page No.215

142. Ans: D. All of the above

Ref: Chapter No.10, Page No.215-216

143. Ans: D. Karl Franz

Ref: Chapter No.10, Page No.216

144. Ans: C. William T Bovie

Ref: Chapter No.10, Page No.216

145. Ans: B. Monopolar cautery

Ref: Chapter No.10, Page No.216

146. Ans: A. Bipolar cautery

Ref: Chapter No.10, Page No.216

147. Ans: C. 7 mm

Ref: Chapter No.10, Page No.216

148. Ans: B. TissueLink

Ref: Chapter No.10, Page No.216

149. Ans: A. Harmonic Scalpel

Ref: Chapter No.10, Page No.216

150. Ans: B. Cavitron ultrasound surgical aspirator (CUSA)

Cavitron ultrasound surgical aspirator (CUSA)

- **CUSA probe** consists of 3 distinct components
  1. **Transducer:** A device that converts electromagnetic energy into mechanical vibrations. The transducer is composed of a stack of **nickel alloy plates.** A magnetic field is produced by a coil placed around the plates and causes mechanical motion of approximately ***300 microns***
  2. **Connecting body:** Mechanically conveys the motion of the transducer to the surgical ap. It also ***amplifies the vibration motion*** of the transducer
  3. **Surgical tip:** Completes the amplifications of the motion and also contacts the tissue. Hence tip is relatively long compared to its diameter and this provides adequate motion amplification
- **The CUSA has a *self-contained suction capability*** to remove fragmented tissue and irrigation fluid.

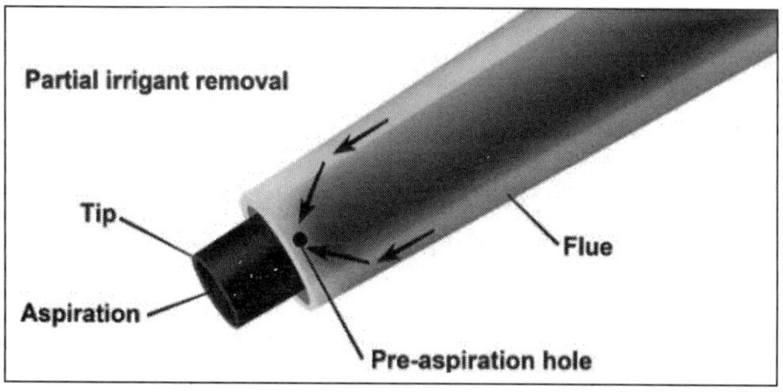

The Suction and Irrigation performs 3 functions in CUSA operation:

1. It draws tissue toward the vibrating tip, and creates a tip/tissue coupling effect
2. It keeps the surgical site clear of irrigation and fragmentation debris
3. Irrigation fluid ***flows coaxially around the outside of the vibrating tip*** to keep the tip cool

- The **CUSA console** provides ***alternating current (24 or 35 kHz)*** to the hand piece.

  In the hand piece, the current passes through ***a coil, which induces a magnetic field***

  The magnetic field in turn excites a transducer of ***nickel alloy laminations,*** resulting in oscillating motion in the transducer laminated structure—vibration—along its long axis

  The transducer transmits vibrations through a metal connecting body to an attached surgical tip

  When the vibrating tip contacts tissue, it breaks cells apart (fragmentation)

  The CUSA system supports different magnetostrictive hand pieces based on frequencies, and each supports multiple tip designs

Ref: Chapter No.10, Page No.217

https://wiins.org/technology-at-glance/cavitron-ultrasonic-surgical-aspirator-cusa/

151. Ans: A. Typically, tumors up to 5 cm can be effectively ablated by RFA; an additional margin of 0.5 cm of healthy parenchyma beyond the target lesion should be ablated to ensure complete ablation of the tumor

Ref: Chapter No.10, Page No.217

152. Ans: C. A grounding pad is necessary and use in the presence of metallic clips and implants is unsafe

Ref: Chapter No.10, Page No.217

153. Ans: A. ABC is a laser device

Ref: Chapter No.10, Page No.217

154. Ans: D. Argon beam coagulation (ABC)

Ref: Chapter No.10, Page No.217

155. Ans: B. Open - 2 mm; Closed - 1 mm

Ref: Chapter No.10, Page No.217

156. Ans: C. Open – 5.5 mm; Closed - 2 mm

Ref: Chapter No.10, Page No.217

157. Ans: B. Circular Stapler

- The EEA™ hemorrhoid and prolapse stapler set with DST Series™ technology is designed for use as a stapler instrument for control of rectal prolapse and hemorrhoid disease
- The instrument places a circular, double-staggered row of titanium DST™ staples and removes a circular tissue specimen

Ref: https://www.medtronic.com/covidien/en-us/products/surgical-stapling/circular-staplers.html

158. Ans: B. Open staplers

Ref: https://www.medtronic.com/covidien/en-us/products/surgical-stapling/

159. Ans: C. Single Use Skin Stapler

Ref: https://www.medtronic.com/covidien/en-us/products/surgical-stapling/

160. Ans: D. Signia™ Small Diameter Reload

Ref: https://www.medtronic.com/covidien/en-us/products/surgical-stapling/

161. Ans: B. Endo GIA™ Radial Reload with Tri-Staple™ Technology

Ref: https://www.medtronic.com/covidien/en-us/products/surgical-stapling/

162. Ans: C. Symptoms of MH can occur at any time during general anesthesia or up to 120 minutes after cessation of anesthesia

Ref: Chapter No.10, Page No.217-218

163. Ans: A. MH is treated by immediate discontinuation of volatile gases, IV administration of dantrolene in doses of 5 mg/kg

Ref: Chapter No.10, Page No.218

164. Ans: C. Mortality in patients with gas embolus is approximately 50%

Ref: Chapter No.10, Page No.218

11

Surgical Infections and Antibiotic Use

1. **Of all hospital infections, SSIs are the most common and costly of all hospital-acquired infections, accounting for:**
   A. 5% B. 10%
   C. 20% D. 40%

2. **With evidence-based guidelines, SSIs are preventable in about:**
   A. 20% B. 40%
   C. 60% D. 80%

3. **False about surgical site infection prevention is:**
   A. In clean and clean-contaminated procedures, additional prophylactic antimicrobial agents should be administered
   B. Preventive measures for SSI include a full-body bath or shower with soap (antimicrobial or nonantimicrobial) or an antiseptic agent the night before or the morning of the operation, appropriate antimicrobial prophylaxis before incision, and skin preparation with an alcohol-based agent unless contraindicated
   C. Maintenance of normothermia, glycemic control with targets less than 200 mg/dL, and the provision of supplemental oxygen are other adjunct measures proposed to reduce SSI in the perioperative bundle
   D. A randomized study showed that prophylactic use of negative pressure dressings for closed laparotomy wounds significantly reduces the incidence of SSI at 30 days postoperatively

4. **A 24-year-old female with complaints of pain in right iliac fossa came to emergency department. She was diagnosed as to have an appendicitis and was taken up for emergency appendicectomy. Intraoperative findings were suggestive of necrotic appendix without evidence of purulent drainage. According to CDC wound classification, this wound is:**
   A. Dirty-Infected
   B. Contaminated
   C. Clean-contaminated
   D. Clean

5. **According to CDC wound classification, an uninfected operative wound in which no inflammation is encountered and the respiratory, alimentary, genital, or uninfected urinary tract is not entered is:**
   A. Dirty-infected
   B. Contaminated
   C. Clean-contaminated
   D. Clean

6. **A 30-year-old female with complaints of pain in right iliac fossa came to emergency department. She was diagnosed as to have an appendicitis and was taken up for emergency appendicectomy. Intraoperative findings were suggestive of appendicitis without evidence of purulent drainage. According to CDC wound classification, this wound is:**
   A. Dirty-infected
   B. Contaminated
   C. Clean-contaminated
   D. Clean

7. **A 55-year-old male with complaints of pain in epigastric region, came to emergency department. He was diagnosed as to have perforative peritonitis and was taken up for emergency exploratory laparotomy. Intraoperative findings were suggestive of gastric antral perforation with evidence of purulent drainage. According to CDC wound classification, this wound is:**
   A. Dirty-infected
   B. Contaminated

C. Clean-contaminated
D. Clean

8. According to CDC wound classification, the procedure of open cardiac massage is:

A. Dirty-infected
B. Contaminated
C. Clean-contaminated
D. Clean

9. According to CDC wound classification, operations with major breaks in sterile technique is:

A. Dirty-infected
B. Contaminated
C. Clean-contaminated
D. Clean

10. Risk factors for the development of surgical site infection includes all except:

A. Alcoholism
B. Hyperbilirubinemia >3 mg/dL
C. Ascites
D. Hypoalbuminemia

11. Risk factors for the development of surgical site infection includes all except:

A. Hypocholesterolaemia
B. Recent radiotherapy
C. Smoking
D. Steroid therapy

12. Risk factors for the development of surgical site infection includes all except:

A. Inadequate antisepsis
B. Inadequate disinfection
C. Inadequate ventilation
D. Decreased operating room traffic

13. Risk factors for the development of surgical site infection includes all except:

A. Blood transfusion
B. Drains
C. Hyperthermia
D. Prolonged operation

14. Treatment strategies for surgical site infection includes:

A. Immediate empiric antibiotic coverage
B. Timely antibiotic de-escalation
C. Local wound care
D. All of the above

NECROTIZING SOFT TISSUE INFECTIONS (NSTI)

15. False about necrotizing soft tissue infections (NSTIs):

A. NSTIs are rapidly progressing skin and soft tissue infections associated with necrosis of the dermis, subcutaneous tissue, superficial fascia, deep fascia, or muscle
B. Mortality rates between 30% and 45%
C. NSTI caused by streptococci and clostridia often have a fulminant course with rapid onset of symptoms and worsening over days or even hours and may be rapidly progressing to death if untreated
D. Increased prevalence of obesity, type 2 diabetes mellitus, and people living with chronic immunosuppression, all of which may predispose an individual to NSTI

16. Laboratory risk indicator for necrotizing fasciitis (LRINEC) includes all except:

A. Hemoglobin
B. Serum albumin
C. Serum creatinine
D. C-reactive protein

17. In laboratory risk indicator for necrotizing fasciitis (LRINEC), 4 points are for:

A. C-reactive protein ≥150 mg/L
B. White blood cell count (per mm) >25
C. Hemoglobin <11 g/dL
D. Serum creatinine >1.6 mg/dL

18. With LRINEC score of 7, the probability of NSTI is:

A. <25%
B. 25–50%
C. 50–75%
D. >75%

19. Risk category of NSTI when LINREC score is 5 is:

A. Very low
B. Low risk
C. Intermediate risk
D. High risk

20. False about diagnosis of NSTI is:

A. The most common clinical features of NSTIs present in 90% of cases are erythema, warmth, and pain—unfortunately, common symptoms and signs that are also present in mild infections such as cellulitis and in almost every case of inflammation from any cause
B. While fever may be present in nearly every infection, hypotension should not be and should serve as a warning sign if present
C. Crepitus, skin necrosis, and bullae are much more specific to NSTI but unfortunately are present >40% of the time

D. Signs of skin and tissue necrosis are pathognomonic and should provoke urgent resuscitation and surgery

21. Features suggestive of NSTI on CT includes:

A. Multiple fluid collections
B. Gas in the soft tissues and significant inflammatory changes under the fascia
C. Absence or heterogeneity of tissue enhancement by intravenous (IV) contrast
D. All of the above

22. The sensitivity of CT in identifying NSTI was:

A. 70%
B. 80%
C. 90%
D. 100%

23. False about Surgical debridement in NSTI is:

A. Surgical debridement is the mainstay of NSTI treatment
B. All affected tissue should be sharply excised with at least 1 cm rim of normal tissue
C. Bleeding is an indication of tissue viability
D. All questionable tissue should be resected at the initial operation; the need for multiple operations and the spread of infection both increase the risk of mortality

24. False about management of NSTI is:

A. Recent studies using 16S ribonucleic acid (RNA) sequencing have demonstrated that anaerobes are likely a significant contributor to mortality in NSTIs
B. There is specific evidence for the use of antioxidants or steroids in NSTIs
C. Once the infection is resolved, the wound is placed in a negative pressure vacuum dressing and reconstructive procedures, usually a skin graft, is planned in 2 to 4 weeks
D. The large soft tissue defects that result from appropriate debridement of NSTI will require extensive reconstructive procedures once the patient has recovered from the acute episode

SPECIFIC INFECTIONS

25. False about Intraabdominal infections is:

A. Intraabdominal abscess refers to a localized walled-off collection of infected fluid within the confines of the abdomen (peritoneal cavity, retroperitoneum and pelvic cavity)
B. Patients with intraabdominal abscess usually present with acute abdominal pain associated with signs and symptoms of infection/inflammation as well as gastrointestinal symptoms
C. CT scan of the abdomen and pelvis with IV contrast is the imaging modality of choice and is the gold standard in high resource countries to assess all these features as well as determine the likely source of the abscess
D. US in the diagnosis of intraabdominal abscess is especially useful for loop of bowel abscesses

26. Ruptured acute appendicitis abscess is a:

A. Primary intraabdominal abscess
B. Delayed primary intraabdominal
C. Secondary intraabdominal abscess
D. Tertiary intraabdominal abscess

27. Intraabdominal fluid secondarily infected by external instrumentation is:

A. Primary intraabdominal abscess
B. Delayed primary intraabdominal
C. Secondary intraabdominal abscess
D. Tertiary intraabdominal abscess

28. Acute diverticulitis with abscess is a:

A. Primary intraabdominal abscess
B. Delayed primary intraabdominal
C. Secondary intraabdominal abscess
D. Tertiary intraabdominal abscess

29. Subhepatic abscess developing later from infected fluid around after cholecystectomy for acute cholecystitis is:

A. Primary intraabdominal abscess
B. Delayed primary intraabdominal
C. Secondary intraabdominal abscess
D. Tertiary intraabdominal abscess

30. Post pancreatitis sterile pseudocyst with secondarily infection from systemic bacteremia is:

A. Primary intraabdominal abscess
B. Delayed primary intraabdominal
C. Secondary intraabdominal abscess
D. Tertiary intraabdominal abscess

31. True about management of intraabdominal abscess is:

A. For the hemodynamically stable patient, source control via percutaneous drainage should be performed as soon as possible, however, this may be delayed up to 24 hours as long as the patient is covered with appropriate spectrum IV antibiotics and monitored closely

B. An intraabdominal abscess requires some form of drainage (percutaneous or operative) in addition to antibiotic treatment to ensure complete resolution
C. Nonsurgical source control is often performed by percutaneous drainage, which is preferably the first-choice approach to source control for the contained walled-off abscess
D. All of the above

32. Key treatment measures according to the "Surviving Sepsis Campaign: International Guidelines for Management of Sepsis and Septic Shock: 2016" is all except:

A. Early clinical endpoint-directed fluid therapy (30 mL/kg of crystalloid fluid within the first 3 to 6 hours)
B. Restore mean arterial pressure to >65 mm Hg with hemodynamic reassessments and additional fluid therapy guided by serum lactate levels as a marker of tissue perfusion
C. No inotropic support for low cardiac output if fluid and vasopressor therapy is given
D. Use of vasopressors in septic shock to maintain mean arterial pressure of 65 mm Hg if not fluid responsive

33. In intraabdominal abscess, can be adequately managed to full resolution by antibiotics and percutaneous aspiration of the abscess contents alone, without leaving a drain in the abscess cavity if the abscess size is:

A. <2 cm B. <5 cm
C. <7 cm D. <10 cm

34. As per surviving sepsis 2021 guidelines, for adults with sepsis or septic shock requiring ICU admission, the patient should be admitted to ICU within:

A. 3 hours B. 6 hours
C. 10 hours D. 12 hours

35. As per surviving sepsis 2021 guidelines, for adults with sepsis or septic shock the first line agent for hemodynamic management is:

A. Norepinephrine B. Dopamine
C. Vasopressin D. Epinephrine

36. As per surviving sepsis 2021 guidelines, for adults with sepsis or septic shock the first line of fluid for resuscitation is:

A. Albumin B. Crystalloids
C. Blood products D. Colloids

37. As per surviving sepsis 2021 guidelines, for adults with septic shock on vasopressors, it is recommendation for MAP is:

A. 60 mm Hg or higher
B. 65 mm Hg or higher
C. 70 mm Hg or higher
D. 75 mm Hg or higher

38. False about Intrathoracic abscess is:

A. Pleural empyema refers to accumulation of purulent fluid between the parietal and visceral pleura, which may be loculated
B. Pleural empyema (abscess) often occurs in patients with poor physical and nutritional status and is often associated with prolonged treatment course
C. Postpneumonectomy empyema is especially feared due to associated high mortality
D. Acute pleural infection that is a few days old consists of thin infected pleural effusion and requires drainage and debridement/decortication to facilitate healing

39. Chronic empyema may develop in:

A. Post thoracic trauma with hemothorax
B. Transdiaphragmatic translocation from an intraabdominal infection
C. A poorly drained post pneumonic infected pleural effusion
D. All of the above

40. True about the management of acute empyema is:

A. In the majority of cases, acute empyema can be treated fully with antibiotics and closed tube thoracostomy drainage of the infected pleural effusion
B. A smaller caliber chest tube may be adequate early on in the course of disease of acute empyema
C. Instillation of fibrinolytic agents may be necessary to facilitate complete drainage by lysing of the fibrinous adhesions that may result in loculations
D. All of the above

41. Treatment of Chronic Empyema includes:

A. Closed pleural drainage (tube thoracostomy, thoracoscopy and thoracotomy)
B. Clagett window (open window thoracostomy with partial rib resection)
C. Eloesser flap thoracostomy window
D. All of the above

42. Surgical treatment of chronic empyema shown in the following image is:

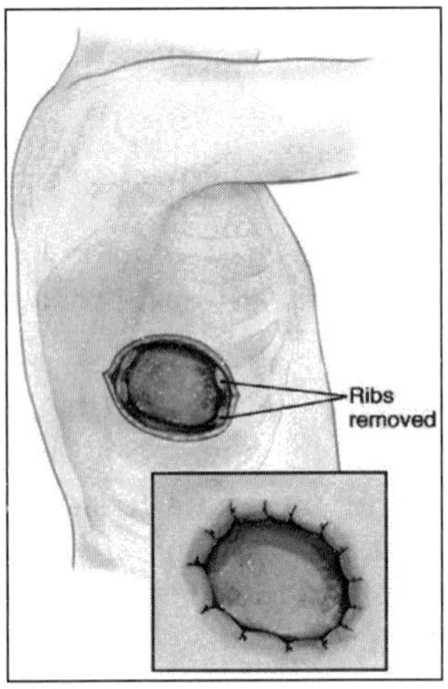

A. Eloesser flap thoracostomy window
B. Clagett window
C. Closed vacuum-assisted closure with open window thoracostomy
D. Closed pleural drainage

43. Surgical treatment of chronic empyema shown in the following image is:

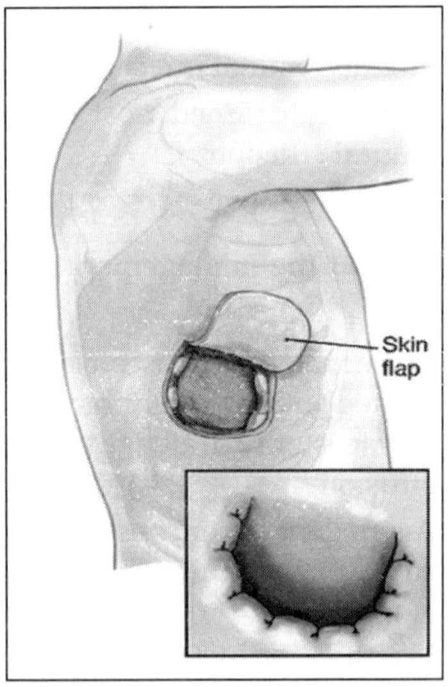

A. Eloesser flap thoracostomy window
B. Clagett window
C. Closed vacuum-assisted closure with open window thoracostomy
D. Closed pleural drainage

44. True about The Eloesser flap thoracostomy window (EFTW) is:

A. It as an operative treatment option for tuberculous the pleural space infection associated with bronchopleural fistula to allow passive drainage of the pleural empyema and to act as a one-way valve to drain pleural space fluid without allowing entry of air into the pleural space
B. The original description of the flap included a 5-cm-wide and two-rib spaces long U-shaped flap of skin and subcutaneous tissue between the posterior axillary line and the caudal portion of the scapula
C. The rib and intercostal muscle deep to the flap are resected, and the flap is placed in the pleural space and sutured to the pleural so that, as the lung re-expands and cavity collapses, the flap acts as a one-way valve
D. All of the above

45. Surgical treatment of chronic empyema shown in the following image is:

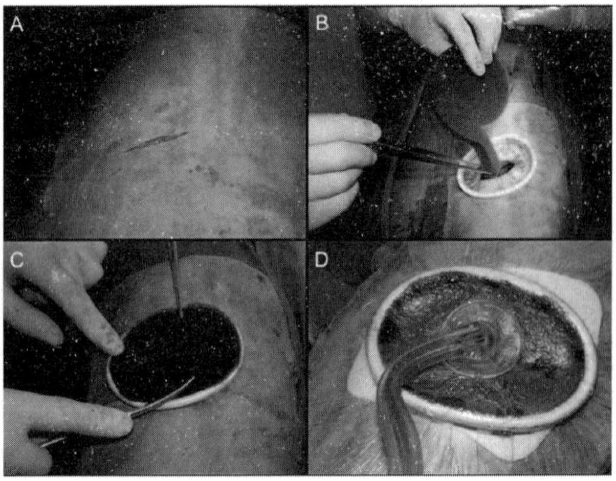

A. Eloesser flap thoracostomy window
B. Clagett window
C. Closed vacuum-assisted closure with open window thoracostomy
D. Closed pleural drainage

46. False about Clostridium difficile infection (CDI) is:

A. Patients with unexplained and new-onset passage of 3 or more unformed stools in 24 hours should be tested for CDI
B. Oral (PO) vancomycin, 125 mg every 6 hours, or fidaxomicin, 200 mg PO twice daily for 10 days is the recommended treatment for the initial episode of CDI
C. Fulminant CDI, defined as presence of hypotension, shock, ileus, or toxic megacolon, the recommended treatment is oral vancomycin 500 mg 3 times daily

D. In the presence of ileus, vancomycin 500 mg in 100 cc normal saline per rectum every 24 hours as a retention enema should be considered

47. Common risk factors for Clostridium difficile infection (CDI) is include:

A. Inflammatory bowel disease
B. Age over 65
C. Use of proton pump inhibitors
D. All of the above

48. False about the treatment of Clostridium difficile infection (CDI) for first recurrence is:

A. Fidaxomicin 200 mg BID for 10 days if Vancomycin was used for the initial episode
B. Vancomycin 500 mg QID for 10 days if metronidazole was used for the initial episode
C. Use a prolonged tapered and pulsed Vancomycin regimen
D. All of the above are true

49. False about the treatment of Clostridium difficile infection (CDI) for second recurrence is:

A. Fidaxomicin 200 mg PO BID for 21 days
B. Vancomycin, 125 mg QID PO for 10 days followed by Rifaximin 400 mg TID for 20 days
C. Vancomycin in a tapered and pulsed regimen
D. Fecal microbiota transplantation

50. A recent systematic review with meta regression analysis showed that administering probiotics at the time of first dose of antibiotic reduces the risk of CDI by:

A. >10% B. >30%
C. >50% D. >70%

HEALTH CARE–ASSOCIATED INFECTIONS

51. While catheter-associated bloodstream infections are uncommon, when they do occur they carry a mortality rate of:

A. 15% B. 25%
C. 40% D. 50%

52. Each day the indwelling urinary catheter remains, it increases the risk of the patient acquiring catheter-associated urinary tract infections by approximately:

A. 2% B. 5%
C. 10% D. 15%

53. The definition of catheter-associated urinary tract infection requires that a patient has an indwelling catheter for:

A. 2 or more days B. 3 or more days
C. 5 or more days D. 7 or more days

54. The definition of catheter-associated urinary tract infection requires:

A. Clinical symptoms of a urinary infection such as suprapubic tenderness, urgency, frequency or fever
B. Urine culture showing >10^5 growth of a pathogenic organism
C. Has an indwelling catheter for 2 or more days
D. All of the above

55. There is agreement on broad principles for the prevention of ventilator-associated pneumonia, which includes:

A. Elevation of the head of the bed above 30 degrees
B. Attempting invasive ventilation where feasible
C. Subglottic suctioning
D. Minimization of interruptions to sterility of the ventilator circuit

ANTIBIOTIC RESISTANCE

56. True statement among the following is:

A. Inappropriate antimicrobial use was defined as use of antimicrobial agents to which the pathogen is resistant or that are not recommended in the treatment guidelines in the setting of established infection
B. Suboptimal antimicrobial use was defined as the use of an inappropriate antimicrobial drug choice, drug route, or drug dose in the setting of established infection
C. Unnecessary antimicrobial use was defined as use of antimicrobials for non-infectious syndromes, antibiotics for nonbacterial infections, antimicrobial duration of use beyond the indicated period without clinical indication
D. All of the above

CLINICALLY IMPORTANT PATHOGENS

57. False about carbapenem-resistant Enterobacteriaceae (CRE) is:

A. CREs are resistant to nearly all antibiotics, including the antibiotics of last resort (i.e., carbapenems)
B. Due to the resultant limited treatment options, CRE infections are associated with a high mortality, with up to 90% of all CRE bloodstream infections leading to death

C. The common mode of transmission for CRE is by direct contact from patient to patient, usually through the hands of the health care personnel
D. Colonized and infected patients are the main reservoirs for CRE organisms

58. Antimicrobials that may be considered for treatment of CRE infections includes all except:

A. Tetracyclines
B. Fosfomycin
C. Tigecycline
D. Polymyxin B

59. False about Vancomycin-Resistant Enterococcus (VRE) is:

A. E. faecalis accounts for the majority of the vancomycin-resistant Enterococcus (VRE)
B. Enterococcus infections are cause by drug-resistant bacteria, resulting in significant morbidity and a mortality rate of 6.5%
C. Patients at high risk for VRE infection include patients who are immunosuppressed, critically ill, on hemodialysis, on broad-spectrum antibiotic therapy
D. The current treatment for invasive VRE infection primarily involves use of daptomycin or linezolid

60. Risk factors for Invasive fungal infections (IFIs) are all except:

A. Immunosuppression therapy for organ transplantation
B. Hypertensive patients
C. Critically ill patients in the ICU
D. Patients with chronic indwelling urinary and central venous catheters

61. True about the diagnosis of invasive fungal infections is/are:

A. Beta D-glycan test for Candida and Aspergillus
B. Galactomannan test for Aspergillus
C. Mannan antigen/antimannan antibody test for Candida spp
D. All of the above

62. False about treatment of invasive fungal infections is:

A. Amphotericin B is the recommended treatment in cases of azole- and echinocandin-resistant invasive Candida infections
B. Echinocandins are still recommended as the initial therapy of candidemia in neutropenic patient
C. A 4-week treatment duration is recommended for candidemia without metastatic complications after documented clearance of candidemia and with appropriate fungal susceptibilities
D. For invasive aspergillosis, the IDSA recommendation for primary treatment is early initiation of voriconazole therapy for 6 to 12 weeks

ANSWERS

1. **Ans: C. 20%**

   Ref: Chapter No.11, Page No.223

2. **Ans: C. 60%**

   Ref: Chapter No.11, Page No.223

3. **Ans: A. In clean and clean-contaminated procedures, additional prophylactic antimicrobial agents should be administered**

   Ref: Chapter No.11, Page No.224

4. **Ans: B. Contaminated**

   Ref: Chapter No.10, Page No.207

5. **Ans: D. Clean**

   Ref: Chapter No.11, Page No.225

6. **Ans: C. Clean-contaminated**

   Ref: Chapter No.11, Page No.225

7. **Ans: A. Dirty-Infected**

   Ref: Chapter No.11, Page No.225

8. **Ans: B. Contaminated**

   Ref: Chapter No.11, Page No.225

9. **Ans: B. Contaminated**

   Ref: Chapter No.11, Page No.225

10. **Ans: B. Hyperbilirubinemia >3 mg/dL**

    Ref: Chapter No.11, Page No.225

11. **Ans: A. Hypocholesterolaemia**

    Ref: Chapter No.11, Page No.225

12. **Ans: D. Decreased operating room traffic**

    Ref: Chapter No.11, Page No.225

13. **Ans: C. Hyperthermia**

    Ref: Chapter No.11, Page No.225

14. **Ans: D. All of the above**

    Ref: Chapter No.11, Page No.225

15. **Ans: B. Mortality rates between 30% and 45%**

    Ref: Chapter No.11, Page No.225

16. **Ans: B. Serum albumin**

    Ref: Chapter No.11, Page No.226

17. **Ans: A. C-reactive protein ≥150 mg/L**

    Ref: Chapter No.11, Page No.226

18. **Ans: C. 50–75%**

    Ref: Chapter No.11, Page No.226

19. **Ans: B. Low risk**

    Ref: Chapter No.11, Page No.226

20. **Ans: C. Crepitus, skin necrosis and bullae are much more specific to NSTI but unfortunately are present >40% of the time**

    Ref: Chapter No.11, Page No.226

21. **Ans: D. All of the above**

    Ref: Chapter No.11, Page No.226

22. **Ans: D. 100%**

    Ref: Chapter No.11, Page No.226

23. **Ans: C. Bleeding is an indication of tissue viability**

    Ref: Chapter No.11, Page No.226

24. **Ans: B. There is specific evidence for the use of antioxidants or steroids in NSTIs**

    Ref: Chapter No.11, Page No.227

25. **Ans: D. US in the diagnosis of intraabdominal abscess is especially useful for loop of bowel abscesses**

    Ref: Chapter No.11, Page No.227-228

26. **Ans: A. Primary intraabdominal abscess**

    Ref: Chapter No.11, Page No.229

27. **Ans: C. Secondary intraabdominal abscess**

    Ref: Chapter No.11, Page No.229

28. **Ans: A. Primary intraabdominal abscess**

    Ref: Chapter No.11, Page No.229

29. **Ans: B. Delayed primary intraabdominal**

    Ref: Chapter No.11, Page No.229

30. **Ans: C. Secondary intraabdominal abscess**

    Ref: Chapter No.11, Page No.229

31. **Ans: D. All of the above**

    Ref: Chapter No.11, Page No.228-229

32. **Ans: C. No inotropic support for low cardiac output if fluid and vasopressor therapy is given**

    Ref: Chapter No.11, Page No.229

33. **Ans: B. <5 cm**

    Ref: Chapter No.11, Page No.229

34. **Ans: B. 6 hours**

    Ref: https://www.esicm.org/resources/sepsis-resources/

35. **Ans: A. Norepinephrine**

    Ref: https://www.esicm.org/resources/sepsis-resources/

36. **Ans: B. Crystalloids**

    Ref: https://www.esicm.org/resources/sepsis-resources/

37. **Ans: B. 65 mm Hg or higher**

Ref: https://www.esicm.org/resources/sepsis-resources/

38. **Ans: D. Acute pleural infection that is a few days old consists of thin infected pleural effusion and requires drainage and debridement/decortication to facilitate healing**

Ref: Chapter No.11, Page No.230

39. **Ans: D. All of the above**

Ref: Chapter No.11, Page No.230

40. **Ans: D. All of the above**

Ref: Chapter No.11, Page No.230

41. **Ans: D. All of the above**

Ref: Chapter No.11, Page No.230-231

42. **Ans: B. Clagett window**

Ref: Chapter No.11, Page No.231

43. **Ans: A. Eloesser flap thoracostomy window**

Ref: Chapter No.11, Page No.231

44. **Ans: D. All of the above**

Ref: Chapter No.11, Page No.231

45. **Ans: C. Closed vacuum-assisted closure with open window thoracostomy**

Ref: Chapter No.11, Page No.231

46. **Ans: D. In the presence of ileus, vancomycin 500 mg in 100 cc normal saline per rectum every 24 hours as a retention enema should be considered**

Ref: Chapter No.11, Page No.231

47. **Ans: D. All of the above**

Ref: Chapter No.11, Page No.231

48. **Ans: B. Vancomycin 500 mg QID for 10 days if metronidazole was used for the initial episode**

Ref: Chapter No.11, Page No.232

49. **Ans: A. Fidaxomicin 200 mg PO BID for 21 days**

Ref: Chapter No.11, Page No.232

50. **Ans: C. >50%**

Ref: Chapter No.11, Page No.232

51. **Ans: B. 25%**

Ref: Chapter No.11, Page No.233

52. **Ans: B. 5% (3 to 7%)**

Ref: Chapter No.11, Page No.233

53. **Ans: A. 2 or more days**

Ref: Chapter No.11, Page No.233

54. **Ans: D. All of the above**

Ref: Chapter No.11, Page No.233

55. **Ans: B. Attempting invasive ventilation where feasible**

Ref: Chapter No.11, Page No.233

56. **Ans: D. All of the above**

Ref: Chapter No.11, Page No.233

57. **Ans: B. Due to the resultant limited treatment options, CRE infections are associated with a high mortality, with up to 90% of all CRE bloodstream infections leading to death**

Ref: Chapter No.11, Page No.234

58. **Ans: A. Tetracyclines**

Ref: Chapter No.11, Page No.234

59. **Ans: A. E. faecalis accounts for the majority of the vancomycin-resistant Enterococcus (VRE)**

Ref: Chapter No.11, Page No.234-235

60. **Ans: B. Hypertensive patients**

Ref: Chapter No.11, Page No.235

61. **Ans: D. All of the above**

Ref: Chapter No.11, Page No.235

62. **Ans: C. A 4-week treatment duration is recommended for candidemia without metastatic complications after documented clearance of candidemia and with appropriate fungal susceptibilities**

Ref: Chapter No.11, Page No.235

12

Surgical Complications

WOUND COMPLICATIONS

1. **False statement about seroma formation is:**
   A. The use of prosthetic mesh in hernia surgery doesn't increase the risk of seroma formation
   B. A seroma is the collection of fluid containing fat, serum and lymph that develops at surgical wound or dead space from surgery
   C. The diagnosis of seroma can be made clinically based on physical examination or radiologically by ultrasound or computed tomography (CT)
   D. Techniques to decrease the risk of seroma include minimization of dead space (e.g., excision of excess skin) and surgical drainage of dead space

2. **False statement about seroma formation is:**
   A. Prosthetic implants that are exposed should be removed in the setting of severe infection
   B. Symptomatic seromas should be aspirated under sterile conditions and have a pressure dressing applied
   C. Several techniques are used to reduce dead space, including the use of fibrin sealant, quilting sutures, and medical talc with consistent results
   D. In refractory seromas, a drain can be placed or the surgical site can be opened and packed to heal by secondary intention or treated with negative pressure therapy

3. **How many days before elective surgery, clopidogrel should be discontinued?**
   A. 1 day B. 3 days
   C. 5 days D. 7 days

4. **A 60-year-old male will undergo elective hernia repair. He has creatinine clearance of <50 ml/min and is on dabigatran. How many days before elective surgery, dabigatran should be discontinued?**
   A. 2–3 days B. 3–5 days
   C. 5–7 days D. 7–10 days

5. **A 50-year-old female will undergo elective hydrocele repair. He is on warfarin for his DVT. How many days before elective surgery, warfarin should be discontinued?**
   A. 1 day B. 3 days
   C. 5 days D. 7 days

6. **False statement about hematoma formation is:**
   A. Hematomas may be caused by incomplete surgical hemostasis or medical conditions that impair clotting, including coagulation disorders, platelet disorders, or other conditions that impair hemostasis
   B. Superficial hematomas may present with skin discoloration, SQ swelling, and pain of the affected area due to pressure
   C. A hematoma is collection of blood clot and blood at the surgical site and occurs only in the subcutaneous tissue plane
   D. Infected hematomas may cause fever, leukocytosis, or sepsis

7. **As per HAS-BLED score, risk of bleeding in a patient 70 years old with history of stroke and normal lab values is:**
   A. Low risk B. Intermediate risk
   C. High risk D. Very high risk

8. **A 42 years old male with H/O alcohol consumption and a recent episode of variceal bleeding that needed hospitalisation, came with yellowish discolouration of skin. His bilirubin levels were 3.2 mg/dl. What is his HAS-BLED score and the risk of bleeding?**
   A. 4 and high risk of bleeding
   B. 3 and high risk of bleeding
   C. 2 and intermediate risk of bleeding
   D. 5 and high risk of bleeding

9. **False about wound dehiscence is:**
   A. Abdominal wound dehiscence describes partial or total disruption of the surgical wound, which can be superficial (skin and SQ fat) or deep (fascial), with or without extrusion of abdominal viscera (evisceration)
   B. After an incision, the aponeurosis will never completely regain its original strength and requires relatively longer time to heal
   C. Wound dehiscence occurs in 10% - 15% of all surgical procedures
   D. Factors contributing to wound failure include inadequate closure (technical failure), increased intraabdominal pressure and local factors like infection or radiation

10. **False about wound dehiscence is:**
   A. Wound dehiscence is more common during the 2nd postoperative week
   B. The fascial layer provides most of the strength and anchor for abdominal incisions
   C. Dehiscence can be caused by technical failure if the suture material breaks, knots become undone, or if the suture material cuts through the suture holding tissues
   D. Infection decreases collagen formation by reducing collagen synthesis and increasing collagen breakdown

11. **In wound dehiscence, infection contributes to aponeurotic breakdown and failure in:**
   A. > 5% cases B. > 30% cases
   C. > 50% cases D. > 80% cases

12. **False about wound dehiscence is:**
   A. Wound dehiscence is associated with a mortality rate as high as 35%
   B. STITCH trial compared large (1 cm every 1 cm) with small (0.5 cm every 0.5 cm) bite techniques for midline fascial closure
   C. Concepts for fascial closure include accurate approximation of anatomic layers, avoiding excessive tension on the suture line, and avoiding the use of prophylactic mesh or retention sutures in "high-risk" patients
   D. Wound dehiscence may be an early manifestation of an intraabdominal process (e.g., abscess or anastomotic leak) presenting with serosanguineous fluid drainage from the wound or in some cases sudden evisceration with no warning

13. **False about management of wound dehiscence is:**
   A. When wound dehiscence presents early after surgery without evisceration, prompt recloser of the fascia is recommended
   B. When wound dehiscence occurs due to local soft tissue infection, the fascial edges should be debrided back to healthy tissue and the wound reclosed without tension
   C. The use of permanent mesh (polypropylene or polytetrafluoroethylene) is recommended in most cases due to the presence of associated infection or bowel injury
   D. Open wounds can be treated with wet-to-dry dressing changes and delayed primary closure in some cases

14. **For proper fascial closure, recommended suture: wound length ratio is:**
   A. > 2:1 B. > 4:1
   C. > 5:1 D. > 6:1

15. **True about negative pressure wound therapy (NPWT) is:**
   A. The application of negative pressure to open wounds reduces tissue edema
   B. NPWT also regulates the inflammatory process by recruiting fibroblasts (through mechanical micro deformation) and induces cell migration, directly reducing bacterial populations through impairment of bacterial enzymatic processes
   C. NPWT increases tissue perfusion and facilitates healing by secondary intention
   D. All of the above

16. **Negative pressure wound therapy is not recommended in all except:**
   A. Necrotic tissue with eschar
   B. Treated osteomyelitis
   C. Contact with exposed blood vessels
   D. Contact with anastomotic sites

17. **Criteria for superficial incisional surgical site infection includes all except:**
   A. Infection that involves only skin and subcutaneous tissue of the incision
   B. Infection occurs within 7 days after the operation
   C. Purulent drainage, with or without laboratory confirmation, from the superficial incision
   D. At least one of the following signs or symptoms of infection: pain or tenderness, localized swelling, redness, or heat and superficial incision is deliberately opened by a surgeon, unless incision is culture-negative

18. Criteria for deep incisional surgical site infection is:

A. Infection involves deep soft tissue (e.g., fascia, muscle) of the incision

B. An abscess or other evidence of infection involving the deep incision found on direct examination, during reoperation, or by histopathologic or radiographic examination

C. Purulent drainage from the deep incision but not from the organ/space component of the surgical site

D. Infection occurs within 30 days after the operation if implant is left in place

19. Patient factors of surgical site infections includes all except:

A. Anemia B. Hypothermia
C. Ascites D. Malnutrition

20. Patient factors of surgical site infections includes all except:

A. High ASA score
B. Diabetic mellitus
C. Decreased BMI
D. Staphylococcal colonization

21. Rate of infection in a contaminated surgical wound is:

A. 5–10% B. 10–15%
C. 20–25% D. 30–35%

22. A 48-year-old male underwent surgery. A drain was left in the abdomen. The rate of surgical site infection is:

A. 1–3% B. 5–8%
C. 10–20% D. 30–40%

23. A 50-year-old female underwent bowel preparation. The category of the surgical wound is:

A. Clean B. Clean contaminated
C. Contaminated D. Dirty

24. While performing a procedure, a resident doctor did a major break in aseptic technique. The category of the surgical wound is:

A. Clean B. Clean contaminated
C. Contaminated D. Dirty

25. While performing a procedure, a resident doctor did a minor break in aseptic technique. The category of the surgical wound is:

A. Clean B. Clean contaminated
C. Contaminated D. Dirty

26. The rate of surgical site infection in a dirty wound is:

A. 20–25% B. 30–40%
C. 40–50% D. 50–66%

27. False about the prevention of surgical site infection is:

A. Use of increased FiO_2 is recommended during general anesthesia and for 2 to 6 hours postoperatively, especially after colon surgery, to ensure adequate tissue oxygen levels which are associated with reduced risk of SSI

B. Decolonizing staphylococcal carriers with 10% mupirocin nasal ointment can reduce the risk of postoperative S. aureus infection in cardiac and orthopedic surgery

C. Preoperative antibiotics should be administered within 60 minutes of the skin incision to reach therapeutic concentration in serum and tissue during the surgical procedure

D. Perioperative glycemic control has been shown to reduce SSIs with a glucose threshold of <200 mg/dL

28. False about the management of surgical site infection is:

A. IV or oral antibiotics should be given when there are signs of systemic infection

B. Empiric antibiotics for operations involving axillae, groin, perineum, genital tract, and gastrointestinal (GI) tract should cover gram-positive and aerobic bacteria

C. Infected surgical wounds should be opened to allow the infection to drain, and debridement should be considered if devitalized or infected tissue is present

D. The wound should be wet dressed with normal saline damped sterile gauze at least daily

THERMAL REGULATION

29. Hypothermia is defined as core body temperature:

A. < 37°C B. < 36°C
C. < 35°C D. < 34°C

30. Severe hypothermia is:

A. < 34°C B. < 32°C
C. < 30°C D. < 28°C

31. False about hypothermia is:

A. Vasoconstriction and shivering are the body's major thermoregulatory protective mechanisms

B. Hypothermia is not associated with increased risk of SSI
C. Preoperatively, the use of muscle relaxants impairs shivering
D. Hypothermia is common after traumatic injury due to shock, alcohol intoxication, environmental exposure, fluid resuscitation, and loss of shivering

32. Risk factors for heat loss and perioperative hypothermia includes all except:

A. Open surgical procedures
B. Burn injuries
C. Prolonged surgeries (>2 hours)
D. Infusion of room-temperature fluids

33. Hypothermia after surgery contributes to organ injury through various mechanisms including all except:

A. Reduced platelet function
B. Ventilation-perfusion (V/Q) mismatch
C. Shift of oxyhemoglobin-dissociation curve to the right
D. Decreases myocardial contractility and peripheral vasoconstriction

34. Pathognomonic of hypothermia on ECG is:

A. Osborn wave
B. ST segment elevation
C. J point depression
D. Tall T waves

35. False about hypothermia is:

A. Hypotension due to shock is the most important impediment to wound oxygenation
B. Severe hypothermia impairs cough reflex and increases the risk of a comatose surgical patient to postoperative pneumonia
C. When the core temperature falls < 32°C., significant reductions in blood pressure and cardiac output occur
D. With mild and moderate hypothermia, renal perfusion and glomerular filtration are decreased, resulting in "cold-induced diuresis"

36. True about the management of hypothermia is:

A. In patients with asystole, defibrillation and drugs have unpredictable efficacy, and cardiopulmonary bypass is essential for rewarming and maintaining perfusion
B. Increasing the ambient room temperature, administering warmed IV fluids, covering patients with blankets, and using forced-air warming devices are commonly used techniques to prevent intraoperative hypothermia
C. When rapid warming is needed, continuous arteriovenous rewarming is more effective
D. All of the above

37. False about Malignant hyperthermia is:

A. Seen most commonly ryanodine receptor mutations
B. It is an autosomal recessive pharmacogenetic disorder
C. Once malignant hyperthermia develops, the initial management is to discontinue the inciting anesthetic agent and halt the operation if possible
D. Early presentations of malignant hyperthermia include an increase in end-tidal (CO_2) or tachypnea if the patient is not intubated and ventilated, hypoxia, tachycardia, masseter muscle spasm, or trismus

38. The hypermetabolic response to inhalation anesthetic agents that cause malignant hyperthermia is by all except:

A. Isoflurane
B. Succinylcholine
C. Halothane
D. Etomidate

39. The medication of choice to treat malignant hyperthermia is:

A. Dantrolene an initial dose of 5.0 mg/kg IV should be given and can be repeated according to the response: end-tidal CO_2, tachycardia, muscle rigidity and acidosis
B. Dantrolene an initial dose of 2.5 mg/kg IV should be given and can be repeated according to the response: end-tidal CO_2, tachycardia, muscle rigidity and acidosis
C. Dantrolene an initial dose of 10 mg/kg IV should be given and can be repeated according to the response: end-tidal CO_2, tachycardia, muscle rigidity and acidosis
D. Dantrolene an initial dose of 25 mg/kg IV should be given and can be repeated according to the response: end-tidal CO_2, tachycardia, muscle rigidity and acidosis

40. False about the management of malignant hyperthermia is:

A. Muscle weakness is a side effect from dantrolene so breathing and oxygenation should be monitored and aspiration should be prevented
B. Clotting studies and platelet count should be checked for the possibility of disseminated intravascular coagulation

C. Clotting studies and platelet count should be checked for the possibility of DIC
D. Active cooling with ice packs and 20°C normal saline IV should be initiated if the body temperature is > 40°C but should be stopped when the body temperature decreases to 38.5°C to avoid overcooling and hypothermia

41. False about postoperative fever is:

A. In the postoperative period, the most common infectious causes are wound infections, urinary tract infections (UTIs) and pneumonia
B. Immediate postoperative fever occurring within the first 48 hours after surgery is most likely due to an inflammatory response to surgery
C. Pneumonia is the most common cause of nosocomial bacteremia and septicemia
D. Postoperative UTI is more common in patients with pre-existing prostrate hypertrophy

42. The most common cause of nosocomial bacteremia and septicemia is:

A. Wound infections
B. Catheter-related bloodstream infection (CRBSI)
C. Pneumonia
D. Urinary tract infection

43. False about the management of Catheter-related bloodstream infection (CRBSI) is:

A. The organisms most commonly involved in CRBSI are staphylococci, enterococci, aerobic gram-negative bacilli and fungal species
B. Vancomycin is not recommended for empirical therapy for MRSA
C. Short-term CRBSIs (<10 days) are extraluminal and are preventable as they result from contamination by normal resident flora of the skin at the insertion site
D. The diagnosis of CRBSI requires at least 1 positive blood culture obtained from a peripheral vein, clinical manifestations of infection (e.g., fever, chills, and/or hypotension), and no apparent source for the blood stream infection except the catheter

RESPIRATORY COMPLICATIONS

44. The most common respiratory complication in the postoperative patient is:

A. Pneumonia
B. Atelectasis
C. Acute Respiratory Distress Syndrome
D. Venous Thromboembolism

45. False about postoperative Atelectasis is:

A. Anesthesia, cigarettes, morbid obesity, and pre-existing pulmonary disease also impair mucociliary clearance and decrease the patient's ability to cough and clear secretions, contributing to an increased risk of atelectasis
B. Predisposing factors for atelectasis include general anesthesia and upper abdominal or thoracic surgery with stimulation of GI viscera
C. Atelectasis is the 2nd most common cause of postoperative fever in the early postoperative period
D. It may present with tachypnea, decreased oxygen saturation ± accessory muscle use

46. The CXR after atelectasis may reveal:

A. Air bronchograms
B. Decreased lung volume with tracheal deviation toward the collapsed side in severe cases
C. Loss of the left hemidiaphragm
D. All of the above

47. Atelectasis can be reversed in the first 24 to 48 hours with all except:

A. Incentive spirometry
B. IV antibiotics
C. Deep breathing (5 sequential breaths held for 5–6 seconds)
D. Chest physiotherapy

48. 2nd leading cause of nosocomial infection is:

A. Pneumonia
B. Atelectasis
C. Acute Respiratory Distress Syndrome
D. Venous Thromboembolism

49. After endotracheal intubation, ventilator-associated pneumonia (VAP) is pneumonia developing after:

A. 12–24 hours
B. 24–48 hours
C. 48–72 hours
D. 72–120 hours

50. False about ventilator-associated pneumonia (VAP) is:

A. VAP is polymicrobial in nearly 50% of cases, and the most common organisms include enteric gram-negative bacilli
B. Risk of VAP is greatest during the first 5 days of mechanical ventilation (3%) thereafter, between 5-10 days, the risk declines to 2% per day, further declining to 1%/day after 10 days
C. In surgery, trauma, and critically ill patients, the use of prophylactic antibiotics can alter the microbial flora

D. In late-onset VAP (< 4 days postintubation), the organisms are usually antibiotic resistant

51. Refractory VAP is defined as VAP with failure to improve after:

A. 12 hours
B. 24 hours
C. 48 hours
D. 72 hours

52. Postoperative pneumonia is associated with a mortality rate of:

A. 10%
B. 30%
C. 50%
D. 70%

53. Criteria for suspicion of ventilator associated pneumonia is:

A. Leukocytosis or leukopenia
B. Thrombocytopenia
C. Temperature > 38°C or < 36°C
D. Purulent respiratory secretions

54. Hypoxemia should be treated supportively by increasing the inspired oxygen level or positive end-expiratory pressure to increase the SpO_2 to:

A. 99%
B. 97%
C. 95%
D. 92%

55. Hypoxemia should be treated supportively by increasing the inspired oxygen level or positive end-expiratory pressure to increase the SpO_2 to:

A. 50 mm Hg
B. 65 mm Hg
C. 70 mm Hg
D. 60 mm Hg

56. False about the treatment of ventilator associated pneumonia is:

A. Prompt initiation of appropriate antibiotics within 12 hours of diagnosis leads to improved survival
B. The use of H2 receptor antagonists for stress ulcer prophylaxis is associated with a reduced incidence of pneumonia relative to prophylaxis with sucralfate
C. In patients intubated for 48 to 72 hours, continuous or intermittent endotracheal and oropharyngeal secretions should be suctioned prior to extubation
D. Oropharyngeal decontamination with chlorhexidine may be beneficial in reducing postoperative respiratory infections in cardiac surgery patients

57. False about aspiration pneumonitis is:

A. Aspiration pneumonitis (Mendelson syndrome) refers to an acute inflammatory injury of the lung parenchyma resulting from aspiration of usually sterile acidic gastric contents
B. Bolus feedings possess a higher risk of aspiration than continuous feeding
C. The more acidic (e.g., pH <2.5) and voluminous (e.g., pH 20 mL) the aspirate, the greater the severity of pulmonary damage
D. According to the American Society of Anesthesiology, the routine administration of preoperative medications to reduce gastric pH is not routinely recommended for patients with no increased risk of pulmonary aspiration

58. Critical pH for Aspiration pneumonitis is:

A. 2.0
B. 2.5
C. 3.0
D. 3.5

59. True about aspiration pneumonia is:

A. Aspiration pneumonia is a common infectious complication of enteral nutrition usually resulting either from contamination of the initial aspirate or secondarily from aspiration of colonized oropharyngeal secretions
B. Surgery patients are at increased risk of aspiration pneumonia since tissue injury, hemorrhage, and anesthesia can contribute to impaired host defenses
C. Aspiration pneumonia requires antibiotic treatment
D. All of the above

60. The factors that predispose an individual to increase risk of aspiration include all except:

A. Oropharyngeal or airway instrumentation
B. Chronic debilitating disease
C. Elective surgery
D. Small bowel obstruction

61. The common infectious organisms in aspiration pneumonia are all except:

A. Streptococcus
B. Pseudomonas
C. E. coli
D. Klebsiella

62. False about aspiration pneumonitis is:

A. Hypoxia is the earliest and most reliable sign
B. Gastric aspiration may cause mild, subclinical pneumonitis, or more severe progressive respiratory failure with significant morbidity and mortality
C. The absence of symptoms in the first 30 mins usually correlates with a benign course
D. Aspiration pneumonitis differs from other aspiration sequelae, since it frequently has a rapid onset, is self-limiting, and most radiographic changes of simple toxic aspiration usually clear within 48 hours

63. After an aspiration event, the clinical and radiographic changes begin to appear within the next:

A. 12 - 24 hours B. 24 - 36 hours
C. 36 - 48 hours D. 48 - 72 hours

64. False about management of aspiration pneumonitis is:

A. The risk of aspiration is decreased by reducing the volume of gastric contents, minimizing regurgitation and protecting the airway
B. Antibiotics are required in most cases
C. The administration of corticosteroids to reduce pulmonary inflammation is not routinely recommended
D. Gastric decompression and rapid sequence induction of anesthesia with cricoid pressure has been advocated as the most effective way to prevent aspiration during intubation in high-risk patents but is not 100% effective

65. False about ARDS is:

A. The pathophysiology of ARDS is characterized by inflammation, increased capillary permeability, alveolar edema, and surfactant deactivation
B. Chest radiographs show perihilar haziness, Kerley B lines, septal lines, thickening of the fissures, "batwing" distribution of air space opacification, pleural effusions, and possibly cardiomegaly in cardiogenic pulmonary edema
C. ARDS are characterized by the acute worsening of respiratory symptoms, usually within 1 day of clinical insult
D. Arterial blood gas may show hypoxia with increased $PaCO_2$ or respiratory acidosis

66. The severity of ARDS is categorized as severe, with a PaO_2/FiO_2 ratio:

A. <100 B. <200
C. <300 D. <500

67. False about the management of ARDS is:

A. Diuretics should be given to patients with objective evidence of volume overload, and urine output as well as total fluid intake and output should be monitored
B. The patient's ideal or predicted body weight should be calculated and a tidal volume of 60 mL/kg of predicted body weight with plateau pressure of ≤30 mm H2O should be used initially according to current ARDS net protocols
C. In patients with ARDS, treatment is focused on the underlying cause and the care for lung injury is supportive with mechanical ventilation to optimize oxygenation and allow time for the lungs to recover
D. Because the lung injury in ARDS is frequently heterogeneous, prone positioning can be used to decrease V/Q mismatch in some patients

68. Virchow triad includes all except:

A. Hypothermia
B. Hypercoagulability
C. Venous stasis
D. Endothelial injury

69. Conditions related to increase the risk of clot formation and VTE development is all except:

A. Malignancy
B. Long-distance travel (>24 hours)
C. Pregnancy
D. Nephrotic syndrome

70. False about VTE is:

A. Wells criteria categorize patients into likely or unlikely groups and the revised Geneva score categorizes into high-, moderate-, and low risk group of having VTE
B. D-dimer should be used to screen for VTE in surgery or trauma patients
C. Moderate-risk and low-risk VTE groups should have D-dimer tested and diagnostic imaging if elevated
D. Venous duplex ultrasonography is the imaging of choice for DVT

71. False about the ultrasonography findings in DVT is:

A. Cross-sectional vein incompressibility
B. Normal spectral Doppler
C. Direct thrombus with vein enlargement
D. Abnormal colour Doppler flow

72. The diagnostic imaging procedure of choice for PE is:

A. CT pulmonary angiography
B. Contrast venography
C. Ultrasonography
D. V/Q scan

73. In pulmonary embolism, V/Q scan is sometimes preferred over CT pulmonary angiography in specific situations like all except:

A. IV contrast allergy

B. Children
C. Pregnancy
D. Renal insufficiency

74. False about pulmonary embolism (PE) is:

A. In acute PE, the most common symptoms are dyspnea or shortness of breath
B. Chest radiography and electrocardiography are diagnostic and normal results exclude PE
C. Massive PEs can cause obstruction of pulmonary blood flow and acute right heart strain, leading to hemodynamic compromise
D. The arterial blood gas measurement may show hypoxemia with respiratory alkalosis from hyperventilation

75. Electrocardiography finding in pulmonary embolism (PE) patients is:

A. S1Q3T3
B. Left-axis deviation
C. Nonspecific T-wave change
D. Right bundle branch block

76. Validated scoring systems developed to quantify the VTE risk are all except:

A. California score
B. Padua score
C. IMPROVE score
D. Rogers score

77. False about VTE prophylaxis is:

A. In high-risk VTE patients (Caprini score ≥5), pharmacologic prophylaxis is preferred, if not contraindicated
B. Mechanical prophylaxis is often used in low-risk groups (Rogers score 7–10, Caprini score 1–2) or when patients have high bleeding risk or if anticoagulants are contraindicated
C. Vena cava filters are considered in all high-risk patients
D. In very low risk (Rogers score < 7, Caprini score 0), frequent mobilization and early ambulation are preferred

78. Patients with pulmonary embolism (PE) are considered high risk for mortality in all except:

A. PE severity index score of class II or higher
B. Elevated cardiac biomarkers
C. RV failure by echocardiography or CT
D. Hemodynamic instability

79. True about the management of pulmonary embolism (PE) is:

A. Catheter-directed therapy allows for the administration of fibrinolytic medication at the site of the clot and is associated with fewer systemic bleeding problems
B. Patients may need intubation, mechanical ventilation, and vasopressors to maintain blood pressure and cardiac output
C. Fibrinolytic therapies are usually preferred over the surgical or catheter-based interventions but have a higher incidence of bleeding complications
D. All of the above

80. Complications of catheter-directed therapy includes:

A. Groin hematoma
B. Distal embolization
C. Pulmonary artery injury
D. All of the above

81. True about pharmacotherapy of VTE is:

A. SQ LMWH and fondaparinux are preferred over UFH due to lesser risk of major bleeding and lower incidence of heparin-induced thrombocytopenia (HIT)
B. The medication effect of UFH is monitored by activated partial thromboplastin time (aPTT), with a target of 1.5 to 2.5 times control value or plasma heparin antifactor Xa 0.3 to 0.7 IU/mL
C. IV UFH is preferred in patients whom reperfusion therapy is considered due to its shorter half-life, ease of effect monitoring, availability of rapid discontinuation, and protamine reversal, and UFH should be held during infusion of fibrinolytic medication
D. UFH has better bioavailability and can be given subcutaneously, with a longer half-life

82. True about pharmacotherapy of VTE is/are:

A. Hirudin (0.4 mg/kg IV) is given followed by an infusion of 0.15 mg/kg/h; the dose must be adjusted to renal function, and levels are routinely monitored by aPTT to achieve 1.5 to 2.5 times the laboratory normal value
B. Argatroban is given, 2 μg/kg/min IV, with an aPTT target of 1.5 to 3 times the normal laboratory value
C. Fondaparinux is given daily at a dose of 5 mg SQ if body weight is < 50 kg, 7.5 mg SQ if body weight is between 50 - 75 kg, and 10 mg SQ if body weight is > 100 kg
D. All of the above

CARDIAC COMPLICATIONS

83. According to the Perioperative Ischemia Evaluation (POISE) trial, percentage of patients with perioperative myocardial ischemia and infarction (PMI) that do not experience ischemic symptoms is:

A. 45% B. 50%
C. 65% D. 75%

84. True about perioperative myocardial ischemia and infarction (PMI) is:

A. The causes of PMI are the classic theory of plaque rupture and thrombosis of coronary vessels occluding the blood supply to myocardium and the imbalance between oxygen demand and supply during the perioperative period and postoperative care
B. The stress response to surgery activates the sympathetic nervous system, resulting in elevated catecholamines, which can lead to coronary vasoconstriction and increased myocardial oxygen demand
C. During the perioperative period, alterations in hemodynamics, oxygenation, and ventilation related to surgery can also affect coronary blood flow and cause imbalance of myocardial oxygen demand and supply
D. All of the above

85. Patients at risk for cardiac complications are all except:

A. Peripheral arterial disease
B. Alcohol consumption
C. Recent myocardial infarction or stenting
D. Hyperlipidemia

86. False about perioperative myocardial ischemia and infarction (PMI) is:

A. The 2014 European Society of Cardiology and the European Society of Anaesthesiology guidelines recommend screening every high-risk patient both before surgery and 48 - 72 hours after surgery
B. Changes in electrocardiography are another indication of cardiac ischemia and range from ST-segment elevation, ST depression, T-wave inversion, or Q waves
C. There is insufficient evidence that biomarker screening reduces cardiac events; therefore routine screening is recommended (2014 AHA guideline)
D. Most high-risk patients present with high troponin levels before surgery

87. In patients with signs and symptoms suggestive of myocardial infarction, the 2014 American College of Cardiology and American Heart Association guidelines recommend troponin screening be considered:

A. Before and 12 - 24 hours after surgery
B. Before and 48 - 72 hours after surgery
C. Before and 72 - 96 hours after surgery
D. Before and 6 - 12 hours after surgery

88. After surgery, most patients have perioperative ischemia or infarction within:

A. 6 hours B. 48 hours
C. 12 hours D. 24 hours

89. Risk predictors for the revised cardiac risk index includes all except:

A. History of cerebrovascular disease
B. Preoperative serum creatinine >3 mg/dL
C. History of congestive heart failure
D. High-risk type of surgery (intraperitoneal, intrathoracic, suprainguinal vascular surgery)

90. False about prevention and management of perioperative myocardial ischemia and infarction (PMI) is:

A. Electrocardiography should be done within 3 months before surgery, and patients with unknown dyspnea or change in functional class should have left ventricular function examined
B. 1 MET is equal to the resting oxygen consumption of a 40-year-old and 70 kg man
C. Beta blockers should be discontinued in patients who already take them and initiation of beta blockers should be considered in only high-risk patients (≥1 RCRI)
D. Perioperative beta blockers have been shown to reduce the risk of myocardial infarction and are recommended before surgery

91. True about prevention and management of perioperative myocardial ischemia and infarction (PMI) is:

A. Aspirin should be continued in patients taking aspirin with a history of coronary disease or stenting
B. Statins have been shown to reduce postoperative cardiovascular events and should be continued or initiated especially in vascular surgery patient
C. Thrombotic risk is considered low 4 weeks after balloon angiography, 6 months after bare-metal stents, and 1 year after drug-eluting stents
D. All of the above

92. Once myocardial tissue has been damaged, the median time from PMI to death is approximately:

A. 3 days B. 7 days
C. 12 days D. 14 days

93. As per cardiac risk stratification for noncardiac surgical procedures, level of cardiac risk in breast surgery is:

A. Low B. Intermediate
C. High D. Severe

94. As per cardiac risk stratification for noncardiac surgical procedures, level of cardiac risk in peripheral vascular surgery is:

A. Low B. Intermediate
C. High D. Severe

95. As per cardiac risk stratification for noncardiac surgical procedures, level of cardiac risk in carotid endarterectomy is:

A. Low B. Intermediate
C. High D. Severe

96. As per cardiac risk stratification for noncardiac surgical procedures, level of cardiac risk in intrathoracic surgery is:

A. Low B. Intermediate
C. High D. Severe

97. False about prevention and management of perioperative myocardial ischemia and infarction (PMI) is:

A. Management comes in determining the pathophysiology of PMI between plaque rupture/thrombosis (type I) or imbalance of oxygen demand and supply (type II)
B. Patients suspected of type II injury should have optimal hemodynamics and oxygenation therapy with possible angiography during follow-up after surgery
C. Patients with suspected type I injury should receive aggressive aspirin therapy, with caution exerted for bleeding risk, and statin therapy with consideration of angiography
D. All of the above

98. In patients with >65 years, hypertension is a common problem in surgical patients, with an incidence of approximately:

A. 30% B. 60%
C. 50% D. 80%

99. After surgery, postoperative hypertension is defined as blood pressure:

A. > 180/90 mm Hg in 2 consecutive readings
B. > 190/100 mm Hg in 2 consecutive readings
C. > 180/90 mm Hg in 3 consecutive readings
D. > 190/100 mm Hg in 3 consecutive readings

100. False about management of postoperative hypertension is:

A. Preoperative evaluation of patients with pre-existing hypertension should focus on organ damage related to hypertension
B. The use of antihypertensives with rapid onset and short half-lives is recommended, with an initial target of lowering blood pressure by 25% and then re-evaluating
C. Mild to moderate elevation of blood pressure alone (< 180/110 mm Hg)
D. Stopping ACE inhibitors before surgery has been shown to increase all-cause mortality and vascular events, including myocardial injury and stroke

101. After surgery, postoperative hypertension commonly begins within:

A. 15 minutes B. 30 minutes
C. 60 minutes D. 120 minutes

102. There is an increased risk of cardiac complications in patients with a diastolic blood pressure of:

A. > 90 mm Hg B. > 100 mm Hg
C. > 110 mm Hg D. > 120 mm Hg

103. Risk factors for arrhythmias include all except:

A. Valvular heart disease
B. Female gender
C. Obesity
D. Chronic lung disease

104. False about the management of arrhythmias is:

A. If patients fail to convert to sinus rhythm, long-term anticoagulation should be considered based on the individual patient's risk factors
B. In hemodynamically normal patients, initial treatment involves control of the ventricular rate with beta blockers, calcium channel blockers, or digoxin
C. Chemical cardioversion may be considered to decrease the risk of thromboembolism when the atrial arrhythmia is > 48 hours duration
D. Antiarrhythmic drugs commonly used to convert atrial fibrillation are amiodarone, flecainide, dofetilide, propafenone, or ibutilide

105. The most commonly used thromboembolic risk stratification tool is the CHA_2DS_2-VASc risk score, which recommends routine anticoagulation if the score is:

A. ≥ 1 B. ≥ 2
C. ≥ 3 D. ≥ 4

106. True about the management of arrhythmias is:

A. Narrow complex supraventricular tachycardia can be treated with vagal maneuvers such as carotid sinus massage, with IV adenosine, or cardioversion in case of hemodynamic compromise
B. Treatment of ventricular dysrhythmias includes correction of electrolyte abnormalities (especially potassium and magnesium) and/or medications
C. Medications used to treat symptomatic bradycardias include atropine, aminophylline, or cardiac pacing in patients with sustained symptomatic bradyarrhythmias
D. All of the above

107. As compared to patients with no postoperative heart failure, perioperative heart failure is associated with an increased mortality of:

A. 39% B. 51%
C. 63% D. 75%

108. Patients with diastolic heart failure (preserved LVEF) have lower mortality rate than the ones with systolic heart failure (reduced LVEF), especially LVEF of:

A. < 30% B. < 10%
C. < 50% D. < 70%

109. False about postoperative heart failure is:

A. BNP levels can be used to detect, monitor, and guide therapy in patients with heart failure
B. Patients with LVEF < 45% or QRS complex > 60 ms should be considered for cardiac resynchronization therapy before surgery
C. Surgery patients with heart failure should be medically optimized before surgery using beta blockers, ACE inhibitors/ARBs, aldosterone antagonist, digitalis, and/or diuretics in symptomatic patients as clinically indicated
D. Preoperative BNP and NT proBNP in conjunction with RCRI can help assess perioperative cardiac risk

RENAL AND URINARY COMPLICATIONS

110. As per Kidney Disease: Improving Global Outcomes (KDIGO) criteria definition of acute kidney injury is/are:

A. Increase in serum creatinine by ≥ 0.5 mg/dL within 48 hours
B. Urine volume < 0.5 mL/kg/h for 6 hours
C. Increase in serum creatinine to ≥2.5 times baseline, which is known or presumed to have occurred within the prior 7 days
D. All of the above

111. As per Kidney Disease: Improving Global Outcomes (KDIGO) criteria definition of stage 3 acute kidney injury is all except:

A. Anuria for ≥24 hours
B. In patients <18 years, decrease in eGFR to <35 mL/min/1.73 m^2
C. Initiation of renal replacement therapy
D. Increase in serum creatinine to ≥4.0 mg/dL

112. Risk factors for developing postoperative AKI includes all except:

A. Anaemia
B. Intraoperative transfusion
C. Types of surgery especially hepatic surgery
D. Higher ASA grade

113. Patient risk factors for developing postoperative acute kidney injury include all except:

A. Chronic liver disease
B. Laparoscopic surgery
C. Diabetes
D. Underlying renal insufficiency

114. Renal causes of acute kidney injury include all except:

A. Rhabdomyolysis
B. Nephrotoxic medication
C. NSAIDs
D. Radiocontrast media

115. Prerenal causes of acute kidney injury include all except:

A. Neurogenic bladder B. RAAS blockers
C. Hemorrhage D. Hypotension

116. Diagnostic evaluation of prerenal acute renal failure includes all except:

A. Urine plasma creatinine level >40
B. Urine osmolality >500 mOsm/L
C. Urinary sodium >50 mOsm/L
D. Urine plasma osmolality <1.5

117. Diagnostic evaluation of renal acute renal failure includes all except:

A. Urine plasma creatinine level <20
B. Fractional excretion of sodium <1%

C. Urine osmolality = Plasma
D. Urine plasma osmolality >1.5

118. False about the management of acute renal failure is:

A. During anesthesia, the mean arterial pressure should be maintained > 65 mm Hg or 75 to 80 mm Hg in patients with hypertension
B. Intraoperative urine output should be maintained at ≥0.5 mL/kg/h in the perioperative period if possible
C. Dopamine appears to be more effective than other vasopressors in patients with AKI and vasopressor of choice
D. Hemodialysis is continued until renal function is regained, as noted by a reduction of serum creatinine during stable hemodialysis or an increase in creatinine clearance

119. Strategies used to prevent contrast-induced AKI is/are:

A. Acetylcysteine
B. Diuretic drugs to dilute contrast and reduce exposure time in the renal tubules
C. Vitamin C or bicarbonate
D. All of the above

120. Treatment of contrast-induced AKI is/are:

A. IV fluids of choice include isotonic normal saline or sodium bicarbonate solution and should be started 6 to 12 hours before the procedure and for 4 to 12 hours after the procedure in patients at risk of AKI
B. Volume expansion is the most beneficial intervention possibly by suppression of vasopressin, inhibition of RAAS and dilution of contrast
C. In cases of severe AKI, renal replacement therapy prevents mortality from volume overload, electrolyte imbalance and uremia
D. All of the above

121. Risk factors of urinary retention includes all except:

A. Underlying urinary and neurologic conditions
B. Anesthetic choice
C. Female gender
D. Operative time and intraoperative fluid administration

122. False about presentation and management of urinary retention is:

A. Physical examination may demonstrate a palpable bladder at the lower abdomen
B. Most patients should void within 18 to 24 hours after surgery
C. Bladder volumes of 500 mL or more require intervention, most commonly urinary catheterization, and suprapubic tube placement in cases of urethral stricture or trauma
D. Chronic retention could permanently damage the detrusor muscle and cause long-term complications such as bladder stone, hydronephrosis, incontinence, or renal insufficiency

ENDOCRINE DYSFUNCTION

123. False about adrenal insufficiency (AI) is:

A. The symptoms of AI are nonspecific and include weakness, fatigue, anorexia, weight loss, dizziness, depression, diarrhea and abdominal pain
B. In central AI, hyperpigmentation is observed due to a low corticotropin level, and the mineralocorticoids are not affected
C. Adrenal crisis has no standardized definition or criteria, it is often described as deterioration in general health with absolute or relative hypotension, which resolves after glucocorticoid administration
D. Adrenal crisis has no standardized definition or criteria, it is often described as deterioration in general health with absolute or relative hypotension, which resolves after glucocorticoid administration

124. The most common cause of primary adrenal insufficiency, or Addison disease, is:

A. Autoimmune
B. Adrenal hemorrhage
C. Bilateral adrenal metastasis
D. Infiltrative disease

125. The most common cause of secondary adrenal insufficiency is:

A. Trauma
B. Exogenous glucocorticoids
C. Sheehan syndrome
D. Neurosurgery of pituitary gland

126. True about the management of adrenal crisis is:

A. In patients with adrenal crisis, initial management is to reverse hypotension or shock, correct electrolytes, blood sugar and pH
B. Hydrocortisone (100 mg bolus) is given intravenously with 1 L of normal saline over 60 mins with hemodynamic and electrocardiography monitoring

C. After stabilizing the patient's condition, maintenance hydrocortisone 100 to 200 mg/day is given intravenously or in divided doses of 50 mg intramuscularly
D. All of the above

127. False about hyperthyroid crisis is:

A. Thyroid hormones stimulate metabolism in most tissues, but the cardiovascular manifestations are most characteristic
B. Hyperthyroid crisis may be precipitated by trauma, emergency surgery conditions, childbirth, diabetic ketoacidosis, or an intercurrent illness such as pneumonia
C. The thyroid storm is associated with a high mortality rate (50%–80%)
D. Primary hyperparathyroidism worsens the thyroid storm through its markedly elevated serum calcium level that augments the action of free thyroxine (T4) via the role of a secondary messenger

128. False about presentation and diagnosis of hyperthyroid crisis is:

A. The diagnosis of the thyroid storm is based on clinical signs and symptoms of thyrotoxicosis, including anxiety, palpitations, weight loss, fever (>38°C), tachycardia and tachyarrhythmias, congestive heart failure, GI system dysfunction and central nervous system symptoms
B. Thyroid functions tests differentiate between severe thyrotoxicosis and the thyroid storm
C. As the thyroid storm progresses, coma, hypotension, vascular collapse, and death may ensue unless active therapy is instituted
D. Burch and Wartofsky delineated a scoring system to predict the thyroid storm based on thermoregulatory, cardiovascular, GI, and CNS dysfunction and a score of ≥45 is highly suggestive of the thyroid storm

129. False about management of thyroid crisis is:

A. Intravenous (IV) fluid therapy with continuous evaluation with central venous catheter monitoring is required
B. Salicylates is preferred to acetaminophen since acetaminophen elevates free hormone levels by decreasing T4-binding globin
C. Sedation (chlorpromazine) reduces shivering during the rapid induction
D. IV hydrocortisone, 300 mg initially followed by 100 mg every 8 hours, to prevent adrenal crisis due to relative adrenal insufficiency

130. False about management of thyroid crisis is:

A. Beta blocker oral propranolol (or diltiazem), 60–80 mg every 4 hours, is given to reduce heart rate below 100 beats/min
B. When euthyroidism is achieved, definitive therapy/radioactive ablation must be considered to prevent a second crisis
C. The antithyroid drug Methimazole blocks new hormone synthesis and decreases extrathyroidal conversion of T4 to T3
D. Plasmapheresis and charcoal plasma perfusion or exchange transfusion are reserved for recalcitrant cases if no response in 24–48 hours

131. After the usual therapy, thyroidectomy for thyroid crisis should be considered only if there is no clinical improvement in:

A. 6 - 12 hours B. 12 - 24 hours
C. 24 - 48 hours D. 48 - 72 hours

132. True about Hypothyroidism is:

A. Postoperative hypothyroidism is common after total or near-total thyroidectomy and is correlated with the size of the remnant gland
B. Myxedema coma is an extreme manifestation of severe hypothyroidism that results from a combination of failure of adaptive mechanisms to maintain homeostasis and reduced T3 production
C. Stressors like cold exposure, infection, drugs, trauma, stroke, heart failure, and GI bleeding can precipitate myxedema in patients with previously undiagnosed hypothyroidism
D. All of the above

133. Myxedema coma is the most severe manifestation of hypothyroidism with a mortality rate of:

A. 20%–30% B. 30%–40%
C. 40%–50% D. 60%–80%

134. Management of myxedema coma includes all except:

A. Hypothyroidism: IV T_4 300–500 μg; T_3 in the absence of clinical improvement Or IV 200–300 μg T_4 plus 10–25 μg T_3
B. Hyponatremia: 0.9% normal saline
C. Hypoventilation: Mechanical ventilation
D. Hypocortisolemia: IV hydrocortisone 200–400 mg daily

135. False about syndrome of inappropriate ADH (SIADH) is:

A. SIADH is commonly diagnosed in hospitalized, postoperative patients with hyponatremia (sodium <135 mmol/L) due to the administration of hypotonic fluids, drugs (ACE inhibitors, NSAIDs), and the body's response to stress

B. The syndrome of inappropriate ADH (SIADH) release is caused by unsuppressed vasopressin release from either the pituitary gland or nonpituitary sources

C. Significant neurologic symptoms occur when serum sodium <115 mEq/L and subsequent coma and respiratory arrest develop at 105 - 110 mEq/L

D. Idiopathic SIADH in elderly patients over 65 years of age with mild to moderate hyponatremia are at increased risk of fractures due to risk of falls and gait problems

136. Most common tumor responsible for SIADH is:

A. Small cell lung cancer

B. Head and neck cancers

C. Pheochromocytoma

D. Squamous cell carcinoma of lung

GASTROINTESTINAL COMPLICATIONS

137. Early postoperative (mechanical) bowel obstruction is defined as occurring within:

A. 1 week of surgery

B. 4 weeks of surgery

C. 6 weeks of surgery

D. 12 weeks of surgery

138. Most common cause of early postoperative bowel obstructions is:

A. Intramural hematoma

B. Adhesions

C. Internal herniation

D. Intraabdominal abscess

139. True about postoperative adhesions is:

A. Postoperative adhesions may occur after any intraabdominal surgery but are more likely to cause bowel obstructions after pelvic surgery

B. Adhesions are bridges of collagen tissue caused by fibrin deposition that forms between visceral and/or parietal peritoneum

C. During surgery, peritoneal injury triggers an inflammatory response, causing complement and coagulation cascade activation, exudation of fibrinogen rich-fluid that causes apposition of adjacent surfaces resulting in a band

D. All of the above

140. After surgery, the stomach usually develops contractile activity after:

A. 12 to 24 hours
B. 24 to 48 hours
C. 48 to 72 hours
D. 72 to 96 hours

141. After surgery, the colon usually develops contractile activity after:

A. 1 to 2 days
B. 2 to 3 days
C. 3 to 5 days
D. 5 to 7 days

142. True about postoperative ileus is:

A. The pathophysiology of postoperative ileus is complex and multifactorial in nature: Neurogenic, inflammatory, enteric hormones and neuropeptides, perioperative electrolyte disturbances, and opioids are all contributing factors

B. Postoperative ileus is the most common form of functional bowel obstruction

C. Perioperative electrolyte disturbances, postoperative pain control with opioids, and certain medications can result in reduced GI motility

D. All of the above

143. False about the diagnosis of postoperative bowel obstruction is:

A. CT imaging can help to identify the presence or absence of a focal site of obstruction

B. The use of CT with IV contrast helps to identify vascular patency, and decreased bowel wall enhancement may indicate ischemic bowel

C. The use of enteral contrast with the CT scan is helpful when the diagnosis is uncertain in patients with a nonresolving partial bowel obstruction and to differentiate between partial and complete bowel obstruction

D. Decreased serum amylase, serum D-lactate, and intestinal fatty acid binding protein are associated with intestinal ischemia

144. False about the presentation of postoperative bowel obstruction is:

A. Pain and distention usually precede the nausea and vomiting

B. Closed-loop obstruction presents more rapidly with acute symptoms compared to partial or "open-loop" obstruction

C. Mechanical proximal bowel obstruction typically presents with severe, crampy visceral pain, occurring in short recurrent paroxysms (30 seconds to 2 minutes) in a crescendo/decrescendo pattern

D. The more distal the obstruction, the earlier and more prominent the symptoms of nausea and vomiting (bilious), whereas vomiting with distal bowel obstruction is typically delayed in presentation and feculent in nature

145. False about the treatment of postoperative bowel obstruction is:

A. Early recognition and treatment of early postoperative bowel obstruction prevent irreversible ischemia and transmural necrosis, thereby decreasing morbidity and mortality
B. Minimizing tissue trauma by handling tissues gently, constant bathing of the tissues with saline, avoiding ischemia and desiccation, maintaining hemostasis, and avoiding contamination and infection are conceptually associated with fewer adhesions, but their impact is difficult to quantify
C. Initial management of mechanical obstruction requires appropriate fluid resuscitation, opioid discontinuation, and NG decompression of the obstructed bowel as intraluminal distension results in mucosal ischemia
D. Postoperative physiologic ileus is usually managed by surgical intervention

146. Normal intraabdominal pressure (IAP) in a healthy individual is:

A. < 8 cm of H_2O B. < 8 mm Hg
C. < 12 mm Hg D. < 12 cm of H_2O

147. Abdominal compartment syndrome is defined as sustained increased intraabdominal pressure (IAP) greater than or equal to:

A. 8 cm of H_2O B. 8 mm Hg
C. 12 mm Hg D. 12 cm of H_2O

148. False about abdominal compartment syndrome (ACS) is:

A. Primary ACS develops as a result of intra-abdominal pathology
B. Secondary ACS develops in the absence of abdominal injury and is described in patients with severe burn injury, multiple extremity fractures, and/or septic shock
C. Most patients with Grade III and all patients with Grade IV are managed conservatively
D. ACS-mediated organ dysfunction may be caused by direct compressive effects, inadequate end-organ perfusion, or both

149. Mesenteric and splanchnic hypoperfusion in abdominal compartment syndrome (ACS) is seen at intraabdominal pressure of:

A. >15 mm Hg B. >15 cm H_2O
C. >25 mm Hg D. >25 cm H_2O

150. Grade III abdominal compartment syndrome (ACS) is IAP of:

A. 10–15 cm H_2O B. 20–25 cm H_2O
C. 25–35 cm H_2O D. >35 cm H_2O

151. Grade I abdominal compartment syndrome (ACS) is IAP of:

A. 10–15 cm H_2O B. 15–20 cm H_2O
C. 20–25 cm H_2O D. >25 cm H_2O

152. False about the treatment of abdominal compartment syndrome (ACS) is:

A. Damage control resuscitation has been shown to reduce the development of ACS in patients with severe intraabdominal bleeding
B. Preventive measures include use of neuromuscular relaxants, paracentesis of ascites, and pressure-limiting ventilation strategies to avoid ventilator induced lung injury
C. IAP should still be monitored in "high-risk" patients since recurrent ACS has been reported in up to 10% of patients after damage control laparotomy
D. Damage control resuscitation with fresh whole blood or balanced transfusion of plasma, platelets, and packed RBCs is more commonly used to resuscitate massive hemorrhage than large volumes of crystalloid

153. True about postoperative GI bleeding is:

A. Stress gastritis is more commonly seen in critically ill patients with known risk factors, including mechanical ventilation, coagulopathy (INR >1.5, platelet count 2 times normal), hypoperfusion, significant burn, severe brain or spinal cord injury, multisystem trauma and sepsis
B. Postoperative GI bleeding is associated with significant morbidity; therefore, it is imperative to recognize risk factors prior to operation, as persistent hemorrhage necessitates reoperation in 2% to 5% of patients
C. Flexible endoscopy is the standard of care for localization and control of GI bleeding in the stable patient when UGIB suspicion is high
D. All of the above

154. The risk for hemorrhage from a colorectal anastomosis is generally:

A. < 1% B. < 5%
C. < 10% D. < 20%

155. False about stress ulcers is:

A. Surgery is occasionally needed and may include gastrostomy with oversewing of focal areas of active bleeding, subtotal gastric resection or total gastrectomy in intractable cases

B. Stress ulcers are superficial mucosal lesions which are usually confined to the mucosa of the stomach and proximal duodenum

C. Mechanical ventilation and coagulopathy are associated with decreased risk

D. Intraluminal pH should be maintained above 3.5, and prophylaxis with H_2 blockers, proton pump inhibitors (PPIs), sucralfate, anticholinergics decreases bleeding

156. False about management of postoperative GI bleeding is:

A. The common risk factors for recurrent GI bleeding include older adults (>65 years), malignancy and use of NSAIDs

B. Serial blood counts and coagulation studies (prothrombin time, partial thromboplastin time and bleeding time) should be performed every 24 hours and corrected with appropriate transfusion therapy

C. Aggressive resuscitation with correction of hemodynamics, hemoglobin, and coagulopathy can reduce mortality in patients with postoperative GI bleeding

D. Angiography with selective embolization may be used to treat active LGIB and is successful in >90% of cases

157. The indications for continuous blood transfusions in postoperative GI bleeding are:

A. Unstable vital signs

B. Persistently low hematocrit values (25% to 30%)

C. Continued bleeding

D. Symptoms of tissue hypoxia (shortness of breath, dizziness)

158. In elderly with GI bleeding, patient's hematocrit should be maintained at or above:

A. 35% B. 30%

C. 25% D. 20%

159. Recurrent bleeding in GI bleeding after endoscopic control is seen in:

A. 5% to 10% B. 15% to 20%

C. 25% to 30% D. 30% to 50%

160. Early postoperative stomal complications are defined as those occurring:

A. <1 day postoperatively

B. <1 week postoperatively

C. <1 month postoperatively

D. <3 months postoperatively

161. False about presentation and diagnosis of stomal complications is:

A. Melanosis coli, a brown-black discoloration of the colonic mucosa caused by anthraquinone laxatives, may also cause a dark or even black stoma postoperatively but requires no treatment

B. Mucocutaneous separation of the stoma from the skin occurs as a result of tension, ischemia, infection and poor nutrition

C. Stomal congestion can be caused by bowel edema, a tight abdominal wall trephination, or excess tension on the bowel mesentery, resulting in dark, purple discoloration postoperatively

D. A healthy stoma is always pink but turns dark purple or black usually within the first 1 week when ischemia is present

162. False statement among the following is:

A. Ischemia may be limited to the part of the stoma above the skin level, or it may extend to the fascial level, the peritoneal level, or the proximal intraabdominal ileum

B. Ischemia is associated with stenosis and poor stomal healing

C. Ischemia is more common in a loop stoma relative to an end stoma, due to its tenuous blood supply

D. The presence of arterial bleeding with a pinprick test indicates absence of mucosal necrosis

163. All of the following stomal complications can be late as well as early except:

A. Abscess formation B. Retraction

C. Excoriation D. Dermatitis

164. All of the following are late stomal complication except:

A. Prolapse B. Ischemic necrosis

C. Stenosis D. Dermatoses

165. Patient factors contributing to stoma retraction include all except:

A. Corticosteroid therapy
B. Ulcerative colitis
C. Malnutrition
D. Poor wound healing

166. True about stoma recession/retraction is:

A. Intermittent recession is posture dependent and in the upright position, the stoma length and protrusion are adequate and above the skin level
B. Stoma recession or retraction in the immediate postsurgical period is usually a result of tension on the bowel or its mesentery
C. In intermittent recession when the patient lies supine, the stoma is either flush with the skin or recedes below the skin level, resulting in soiling and leakage of contents due to inadequate appliance seal
D. All of the above

167. Stoma stenosis as a stomal complication has an incidence of:

A. < 1% B. < 5%
C. < 10% D. < 20%

168. False about Osteotomy prolapse is:

A. Fixed prolapse is a common condition in which excessive bowel has been everted during stoma construction and requires treatment
B. Transverse loop colostomies constructed for acute large bowel obstruction are associated with increased risk, especially since the hole in the abdominal fascia needs to be large to accommodate the obstructed bowel
C. Sliding prolapse occurs when a long segment (>50 cm) of ileum or colon protrudes through the stomal orifice intermittently
D. All of the above are true

169. False about parastomal hernias is:

A. The symptoms of parastomal hernia include nausea and vomiting associated with a painful lump or mass adjacent to the stoma
B. Early postoperative parastomal hernias are usually caused by creating a fascial defect that is larger than needed to exteriorize the bowel segment
C. Incarceration and/or strangulation occurs in > 25% of cases
D. Patients may also have difficulty maintaining an appliance seal, pain, small bowel obstruction, stoma outlet obstruction, skin excoriation, and difficulty with stoma irrigation

170. False about peristomal skin irritation is:

A. Appliance leakage and local skin irritation may require more frequent appliance changes, creating a cycle of worsening dermatitis
B. Peristomal skin irritation is more common with colostomies than with ileostomies
C. Traumatic dermatitis also presents with painful, peristomal ulceration
D. Leakage of ileostomy effluent ranges in presentation from contact dermatitis to full-thickness skin necrosis and ulceration

171. False about Stomal dermatitis is:

A. Candida stomal skin infections are characterized by itching and burning bright red primary and satellite papular lesions
B. Infectious dermatitis is the most common type
C. Allergic reactions are caused by sensitivity to skin barriers, adhesives, or tape and are fairly common
D. Leakage of stomal effluent causes proliferation of microorganism under adhesive tape resulting in infectious dermatitis

172. False about the skin conditions associated with stomal leakage is:

A. Pseudoepitheliomatous hyperplasia manifests as painful, wart-like epithelial thickening caused by repeated exposure to highly liquid effluent
B. Psoriasis can develop on the peristomal skin as sharply demarcated, erythematous, weeping, papular lesions or plaques with scales
C. Pyoderma gangrenosum is associated with inflammatory bowel disease or malignancy, presents as a painless, small necrotic ulcers
D. Parastomal varices are abnormal portosystemic vascular collaterals that develop between the mesenteric veins of the intestine and the systemic veins of the peristomal skin

173. Parastomal varices are most commonly seen in patients with portal hypertension caused by:

A. Alcoholic cirrhosis
B. Sclerosing cholangitis
C. Hepatocellular carcinoma
D. Viral hepatitis

174. True about parastomal varices is:

A. Bleeding from stomal varices is usually associated with high mortality due to the patient's underlying liver disease

B. Recurrent bleeding is common and reducing portal pressures with TIPS is the most effective way to stop bleeding
C. Local procedures such as suture ligation or cauterization may be effective for the initial control of bleeding
D. All of the above

175. The ideal stoma site should be:

A. Away from scars, skin creases and bony prominences
B. Centered on a 2-inch flat surface
C. With healthy surrounding skin to provide an adequate pouch seal
D. All of the above

176. Without compromising arterial supply due to submucosal collaterals, the mesentery can usually be detached from the bowel for a distance of up to:

A. 1 cm
B. 2 cm
C. 5 cm
D. 7 cm

177. False about the management of stomal complications is:

A. Skin-level stenosis can be managed by detaching the skin from the mucosa and by excising the stenosed mucocutaneous junction along with a small amount of skin to increase the trephine size, mobilizing the distal intestine and resuturing the fresh, mobilized bowel to the widened skin edge
B. Ischemia limited to mucosa resolves spontaneously and heals by secondary intention
C. A tight stenosis causing subacute intestinal obstruction can be managed with simple and gentle dilatation in conjunction with a high-fiber diet
D. Vascular compromise below the level of the fascia and peritoneum requires immediate laparotomy and colostomy revision to prevent perforation and peritonitis

178. False about management of acute parastomal herniation is:

A. Management of acute parastomal herniation and bowel obstruction in the immediate post-operative period requires urgent reoperation, hernia reduction, resection of nonviable bowel if present, and revision of the fascial opening
B. Strangulation of bowel within a parastomal hernia is an absolute indication for surgery
C. Management of late prolapse depends upon the frequency and severity of symptoms since mild symptomatic, infrequent prolapse does not require repair and can be managed with appliance modification ± a support belt with the aid of a stoma therapist
D. Mesh can't be used due to risk of infection

179. False about the management of stomal complications is:

A. Stoma laceration can be treated by an appropriate size stoma appliance and discontinuing the belt
B. A properly situated stoma has a height of at least 2 cm and can usually be managed with a pouch change every 1 - 2 days
C. Surgical treatment is reserved for ulcerations that extend deep into the ileostomy or extensive, unmanageable peristomal ulcerations
D. A persistent peristomal fistula requires resection of the peristomal disease and construction of a new stoma at a different site to avoid the infection present at the former site

180. False about the technical aspects of stoma construction is:

A. Excision of circular piece of skin ($\approx$2 cm in size)
B. Preservation of subcutaneous fat to provide support for stoma
C. Fascial aperture to admit 3 fingers
D. Small bowel serosa must not be denuded of >5 cm of mesentery

181. False about the management of stomal complications is:

A. Stomal or peristomal skin bleeding may be treated with sodium nitrate
B. Local skin irritation requires more frequent pouch changes, often daily or several times a day
C. Allergic contact dermatitis may be caused by specific stomal products, and patch testing can be used to identify the causative agent and confirm the diagnosis
D. Topical skin management includes providing an adequate appliance seal, controlling wound pain, and infection to enhance skin healing

182. False about Clostridioides difficile Colitis is:

A. Clostridioides difficile spores are resistant to heat, acid, and antibiotics and can be transmitted through the fecal-oral route
B. C difficile colitis is caused by the production of cytotoxin A and enterotoxin B, which damage intestinal epithelia, impair cell function, and promote local inflammation

C. Nearly all antibiotics are associated with CDI, including the ones used to treat the disease (vancomycin, metronidazole)
D. C difficile infection (CDI) is the most common cause of nosocomial diarrhea, although not all patients colonized with C difficile will develop symptoms

183. The risk factors of C difficile infection (CDI) are all except:

A. >45 years old
B. Immunologically compromised host
C. Inflammatory bowel disease
D. Antibiotic exposure

184. False about clinical presentation of C difficile infection (CDI) is:

A. The caecum is most commonly affected
B. CDI symptoms range from asymptomatic, mild to moderate diarrhea, or life-threatening fulminant colitis
C. Rare extracolonic manifestations are reactive arthritis and small intestine infiltration
D. Severe cases of CDI may present with significant dehydration, abdominal distension, ileus, toxic megacolon, bowel ischemia, colonic perforation, peritonitis, renal failure, sepsis, shock and death

185. False about diagnosis of C difficile infection (CDI) is:

A. The gold standard for detecting the C difficile organism is toxigenic culture, but it is time consuming and requires specialized equipment, which delays the diagnosis
B. The gold standard test for toxin detection is a cell cytotoxicity assay, which takes 1 to 2 days, and enzyme immunoassay of the toxin is the most common test
C. Stool testing for C difficile is commonly performed in patients who have 2 or more episodes of unexplained loose or watery stools within 12 hours
D. Leukocytosis >15,000 and serum Cr >1.5 mg/dL suggest severe CDI

186. An abdominal CT scan with oral contrast can evaluate toxic megacolon with cecal diameter:

A. >8 cm B. >10 cm
C. >12 cm D. >14 cm

187. False about management of C difficile infection (CDI) is:

A. The drugs of choice for CDI are vancomycin or fidaxomicin
B. For the initial episode of CDI, vancomycin 250 mg is given orally 4 times/day or fidaxomicin 400 mg orally 2 times/day for 7 days
C. Colectomy may still be required in refractory cases of CDI but is more commonly used for salvage of nonresponders to the fecal diversion and colonic lavage protocol
D. Recently, laparoscopic loop ileostomy and colonic lavage with 8 L of polyethylene glycol (PEG 350) and antegrade vancomycin flushes (500 mg in 500 mL Ringer's lactate every 8 hours) and IV metronidazole for 10 days has been adopted

188. True about the management of recurrent C difficile infection (CDI) is/are:

A. If vancomycin was used in the 1st episode, vancomycin has to be given for a prolonged period in a tapered and pulse manner (125 mg orally 4 times/day for 10–14 days, followed by 2 times/day for 7 days, and then every 2–3 days for 2–8 weeks)
B. Fidaxomicin (200 mg 2 times/day for 10 days) can be used if vancomycin was used for the 1st episode of CDI
C. Fecal microbiota transplantation can be considered in patients with multiple recurrent CDIs
D. All of the above

189. Definitive risk factor associated with anastomotic leak is all except:

A. Technical aspects
B. Tension on suture line
C. Vitamin C deficiency
D. Radiotherapy

190. The tensile strength of an intestinal anastomosis depends on the stapled or sutured collagen fibers in the:

A. Muscularis mucosae B. Submucosa
C. Muscularis propria D. Serosa

191. Anastomotic healing is impaired when arterial oxygen tension falls:

A. <65 mm Hg B. <55 mm Hg
C. <45 mm Hg D. <35 mm Hg

192. Anastomosis considered "high risk" for leak is all except:

A. Colorectal anastomoses
B. Ileocolic anastomoses
C. Esophageal anastomoses
D. Pancreatico enteric anastomoses

193. False statement among the following is:

A. The risk of anastomotic leak is lower if the anastomosis is below the peritoneal reflection

B. Chemotherapy, radiation and cofactor deficiencies (e.g., vitamins A, C and E), which affect the cellular function, proliferation, and tissue repair, can adversely impact the healing process

C. Steroid use impairs healing by lowering transforming growth factor-β, IGF-I and collagen production

D. Zinc deficiency can also affect healing by augmenting matrix metalloproteinase activity, altering collagen-type ratio and reducing cellular proliferation

194. Before an elective colorectal anastomosis, it is recommended that bevacizumab should be administered:

A. 4 weeks before and 28 days after surgery

B. 4 weeks before and 14 days after surgery

C. 6 weeks before and 28 days after surgery

D. 6 weeks before and 14 days after surgery

195. True about optimising patient-related risk factors to decrease the risk of anastomotic leak is/are:

A. Mechanical bowel preparation is not essential for successful anastomotic healing

B. Smoking cessation, nutritional optimization to correct protein malnutrition, and replacement of deficient essential nutrients (e.g., protein, zinc, and copper) and vitamins (e.g., A, C and E)

C. Identifying and treating sleep apnea with continuous positive airway pressure ventilation, preoperative beta blockade or afterload reduction, and/or improving glycemic control in patients with type 2 diabetes mellitus

D. All of the above

196. False about the presentation and diagnosis of anastomotic leak is:

A. Gastrojejunal leaks after gastric bypass surgery usually present early (<24 hours) and small bowel or colon leaks more typically present between 5 - 7 days after surgery

B. On CT Scan, signs of local inflammation like stranding and thickened bowel, large amounts of fluid (>300 mL) around the anastomosis ± free air should raise concern for a leak

C. Laboratory tests like complete blood test, C-reactive protein, and procalcitonin may be elevated with anastomotic leak but are considered relatively specific

D. Fever, tachycardia, increasing abdominal pain, elevated WBC count, decreased urine output, and shortness of breath are commonly seen with intraabdominal leaks

197. False about the treatment of anastomotic leak is:

A. Small leaks (<1 cm) can be managed with simple repair and drainage when there are healthy tissues and minimal inflammation

B. Proximal diverting stoma prevents an anastomotic leak

C. A contained leak, along with an abdominal or pelvic abscess and clinical signs of sepsis, requires drainage of the abscess with broad spectrum antibiotic coverage

D. Anastomotic breakdown in the pelvis is commonly caused by ischemia and frequently results in peritoneal contamination

198. False about intestinal fistulas is:

A. Internal intestinal fistulas, or ICFs, are the most common type

B. Most GI fistulas (75%–85%) are iatrogenic or traumatic

C. Gastric fistulas are mostly iatrogenic (85%), resulting from anastomotic leak

D. Duodenal fistulas occur as a complication of gastric resection, duodenal resection, biliary tract procedures, pancreatic resections, trauma, perforated peptic ulcers and cancer

199. The most common site for an external intestinal fistula (ECF) is:

A. Duodenum B. Jejunum

C. Ileum D. Caecum

200. False among the following is:

A. Aortoenteric fistulas occur due to erosion of prosthetic aortic grafts into the surrounding viscera, usually the jejunum

B. Colocutaneous fistulas may also be seen with diverticulitis, cancer, inflammatory bowel disease, and appendicitis or radiation therapy

C. Crohn's disease is associated with both external fistula and internal fistulas (enteroenteric, enterovesical, or enterocolonic)

D. Low-output fistulas are about 3 times more likely to close spontaneously than high-output fistulas, and postoperative fistulas are about 5 times more likely to close than fistulas associated with inflammatory bowel disease or trauma

201. **High output external intestinal fistula (ECF) is:**
A. >1500 mL/day B. >1000 mL/day
C. >700 mL/day D. >500 mL/day

202. **Low output external intestinal fistula (ECF) is:**
A. <500 mL/day B. <300 mL/day
C. <200 mL/day D. <100 mL/day

203. **Favourable factors affecting healing of external intestinal fistulas includes all except:**
A. Long tract, >2 cm
B. Single tract
C. Non-epithelialized tract
D. End fistula

204. **Unfavourable factors affecting healing of external intestinal fistulas includes all except:**
A. Associated internal fistulas
B. Location: Colon
C. Large enteral defect, >1 cm
D. Malnutrition

205. **False about the presentation and diagnosis of intestinal fistulas is/are:**
A. ECFs may also present with severe abdominal wall infections caused by bacterial invasion and chemical erosion
B. Dehydration, fluid and electrolyte abnormalities and malnutrition are common
C. Most ECFs don't require prolonged hospital stay
D. CT scans of the abdomen and pelvis are commonly obtained in patients with postoperative sepsis and concerning intraabdominal fluid collections are drained with radiographic guidance to treat infected fluid collections

206. **The most common complication seen in patients with an ECF is:**
A. Electrolyte abnormalities
B. Arrythmias
C. Sepsis
D. Diarrhea

207. **True about treatment of intestinal fistulas is:**
A. For low-output and colonic fistulas, the use of enteral nutrition facilitates early fistula closure, reduced pneumonia rate, improved intestinal barrier function and decreased rate of fistula recurrence
B. In patients with high output fistulas and complex intraabdominal pathology, long-term TPN is necessary to provide nutrition support, maintain normovolemia and prevent electrolyte disorders
C. Collection and refeeding of fistula drainage, in combination with enteral feeding to the distal bowel, can decrease the need for TPN, help prevent fluid and electrolyte problems, and maintain nutrition in some patients
D. All of the above

208. **The majority of fistulas that close spontaneously do so in the first:**
A. 1 week B. 2 weeks
C. 4 weeks D. 8 weeks

209. **Indications for surgical management of ECFs include:**
A. Abscess B. Sepsis
C. Persistent drainage D. All of the above

210. **Factors associated with ECF recurrence include:**
A. Small bowel fistula location
B. Inflammatory bowel disease
C. Anastomotic technique
D. All of the above

211. **False about pancreatic fistulas is:**
A. Pancreatico cutaneous/postoperative pancreatic fistula (POPF) develops subsequent to pancreatic anastomotic failure, is noted in nearly 33% of high-risk patients
B. Pancreaticopleural fistulas arise subsequent to pseudocyst fluid tracking into the chest cavity, causing pleural ascites
C. Pancreatico enteric fistula, a rare occurrence, develops when a pseudocyst or abscess ruptures into an adjacent hollow viscus
D. ERCP is recommended in the early period

212. **After distal pancreatectomies pancreatico cutaneous/postoperative pancreatic fistula (POPF) develops subsequent to pancreatic anastomotic failure, is noted in nearly:**
A. 10%–15% B. 20%–30%
C. 5%–10% D. 30%-50%

213. **True about the diagnosis of pancreatic fistula is:**
A. Imaging with CT helps to localize and drain intraabdominal fluid collections.
B. Medical management includes NPO, antisecretagogues (octreotide), nasojejunal feeding, fluid drainage with antibiotics to control the inflammation and potential source of infection, correction of fluid and electrolyte imbalances and skin care

C. MR cholangiopancreatography (MRCP) is noninvasive and delineates the sites of ductal disruption, especially upstream, that are not visible on ERCP
D. All of the above

214. False statement about the treatment of pancreatic fistulas is:

A. Injury near the tail of the pancreas is routinely treated with distal pancreatectomy, whereas injury in the neck is best managed with fistula drainage, allowing a fibrous tract to develop, followed by fistula tract-jejunostomy
B. The use of pancreaticogastrostomy was effective in lowering clinically significant POPF (CR-POPF) rates
C. Persistent fistulas are managed with Roux-en Y fistula tract-jejunostomy, pancreaticojejunostomy, or pancreatic resection
D. Fistulas in the pancreatic head or a small ductal disruption respond to transpapillary stenting

HEPATOBILIARY COMPLICATIONS

215. False about Bile duct injuries (BDIs) is:

A. BDIs during open surgery tend to be more complex than those encountered with laparoscopic surgery
B. Bile duct injury (BDI) is the most common severe and problematic complication associated with gallbladder surgery
C. Inflammation in the area of the triangle of Calot can result in close approximation of the cystic and common bile ducts (CBDs)
D. The CBD is most commonly injured when it is mistaken for the cystic duct

216. False about the presentation and diagnosis of bile duct injuries (BDIs) is:

A. Patients often present with nonspecific symptoms, such as vague abdominal pain, nausea and vomiting, and low-grade fever, usually resulting from uncontrolled bile leakage into the peritoneal cavity
B. Most biliary injuries are diagnosed in a delayed fashion
C. Ultrasound and CT are considered the gold standard for evaluating BDIs
D. Excessive use of cautery or laser in the region of the common duct results in biliary strictures that manifest as recurrent cholangitis, obstructive jaundice, or secondary biliary cirrhosis

217. False about the treatment of bile duct injuries (BDIs) is:

A. The initial management of biliary injuries includes appropriate volume resuscitation and the initiation of antibiotics
B. Immediate detection and repair is not associated with an improved outcome
C. Percutaneous transhepatic cholangiography (PTC) is indicated in cases of complete transection to define the proximal anatomy and site of injury
D. Simple injuries such as cystic duct leak, gallbladder bed leak, and partial duct lacerations can be repaired immediately

218. False about vascular-biliary injury is:

A. Vascular-biliary injury is defined as an injury to both a bile duct and a hepatic artery and/or portal vein
B. Right hepatic artery, accounts for about 90% of vascular-biliary injuries
C. The most common CT scan finding suggestive of hepatic artery injury is enhancement of the right lobe during the venous phase
D. BDIs that include a vascular injury can result in acute hepatic necrosis, abscess formation, or secondary biliary cirrhosis, and in rare cases, liver transplantation may be required

219. True about management of vascular-biliary injury is:

A. Management depends on whether there is evidence of liver injury and the timing of recognition of the hepatic artery injury
B. Patients with hepatic artery injury are more likely to have ischemic biliary mucosa and a higher risk of stricture formation
C. The outcome of patients with major BDIs, combined with arterial disruptions, is worse than in patients with an intact blood supply of the bile ducts
D. All of the above

NEUROLOGIC COMPLICATIONS

220. False about postoperative delirium is:

A. The incidence of postoperative delirium (POD) varies from 15% to 53% in elderly surgical patients and represents a significant cause of morbidity
B. The risk factors for POD include patient-related risk factors, illness-related factors, and interventions triggering POD

C. Patients with higher education level and pre-existing cognitive dysfunction are also at increased risk for POCD

D. Postoperatively, inadequate pain control or impaired oxygenation can increase the risk of POD

221. Patient-related factors for postoperative delirium (POD) includes all except:

A. History of cerebral infarction

B. Advanced age (>55 years)

C. Malnutrition

D. Polypharmacy

222. Postoperatively postoperative delirium (POD) can present early after surgery in the post anaesthetic care unit and, in most cases, presents within:

A. 1 day B. 3 days

C. 5 days D. 7 days

223. False about the prevention and management of postoperative delirium (POD) is:

A. The Confusion Assessment Method and Richmond Agitation-Sedation Scale scoring systems are commonly used to monitor responsiveness and titrate sedation in ICU patients at risk for POD

B. Anticholinergic and benzodiazepine medications should be given

C. Surgical patients should have physical restraints such as Foley catheters, endotracheal tubes, and drains removed and be transferred out of the ICU as soon as possible

D. Prevention of deep sedation by monitoring anesthesia depth during surgery with electroencephalogram (EEG) monitoring or by using dexmedetomidine for light sedation during ICU care reduces the incidence of POD

224. False about perioperative seizure is:

A. Most seizures are followed by changes in consciousness and frequently amnesia

B. The cause of seizures in the perioperative period is often due to preexisting epilepsy or intracranial pathology such as tumor, infarction, hemorrhage, cerebrovascular disease, or traumatic brain injury

C. Initiating preoperative prophylactic AEDs in patients without history of seizure disorder who have never taken AEDs has not been shown to be beneficial

D. Seizures may also result in the loss of autonomic control with bowel or bladder incontinence and may result in decreased intracranial pressure

225. True about the management of perioperative seizure is:

A. Medications should be given to stop seizure activity and prevent progression to status epilepticus, and imaging (e.g., head CT scan) should be performed if clinically indicated

B. Management of perioperative seizures includes monitoring vital signs, electrocardiogram, maintaining airway patency and ventilation, preventing aspiration, and obtaining IV access

C. Brain imaging such as CT or magnetic resonance imaging (MRI) should be done in patients with new-onset seizure or new neurologic symptoms to look for brain tumor, stroke, or intracranial hemorrhage

D. All of the above

226. Perioperative stroke is defined as focal or global loss of cerebral function lasting >24 hours, which occurs during the perioperative period or within:

A. 7 days after surgery

B. 14 days after surgery

C. 30 days after surgery

D. 45 days after surgery

227. False about perioperative stroke is:

A. Embolism is the most common cause of perioperative ischemic stroke causing cerebrovascular occlusion

B. While hemorrhagic strokes are more common, ischemic strokes account for 1% - 4% of perioperative strokes

C. Most perioperative strokes are detected in the hospital and represent a significant portion of all in-hospital strokes

D. Perioperative stroke commonly occurs within 7 days after surgery and presents as an acute neurologic deficit

228. False about the management of perioperative stroke is:

A. Perioperative beta blockers can decrease the risk of stroke

B. Prevention of ischemic stroke requires optimizing cerebral perfusion and decreasing the risk of embolism

C. Patients should be advised to control underlying diseases, such as diabetes and hypertension, quit smoking, and take statins if coronary artery disease is present

D. Treatment of an ischemic stroke is challenging because treating with thrombolytic therapy within 3 to 4.5 hours is a relative contraindication in patients after major surgery due to the risk of bleeding

229. For patients with perioperative stroke, elective surgery should be postponed at least:

A. 1 - 2 months B. 2 - 6 months
C. 6 - 12 months D. 12 - 24 months

EAR, NOSE AND THROAT COMPLICATIONS

230. False about Epistaxis is:

A. The major causes of anterior epistaxis are direct nasal trauma by digital manipulation or iatrogenic injury from nasal tubes

B. The incidence of posterior epistaxis is less in elderly patients with atherosclerosis

C. The anterior septal area is readily accessible, hemorrhage from this region can be managed with direct pressure by pinching the nose over the cartilaginous septum

D. The current management of posterior epistaxis includes combined anterior posterior packing, angiographic embolization, arterial ligation and endoscopic electrocautery

231. False about Nosocomial sinusitis (NS) is:

A. Pseudomonas species and S. aureus are commonly isolated pathogens in patients with NS

B. NS should be suspected in patients with a fever of unknown origin and are endotracheally intubated as the diagnosis of NS is often difficult due to the lack of clinical signs

C. The symptoms of NS are typically masked by more serious illness and the microbiology is more commonly monomicrobial

D. Inflammation and edema of the nasal mucosa decrease sinus ostial patency and impair mucociliary clearance, which favors microbial growth

232. Risk factors for Nosocomial sinusitis (NS) includes all except:

A. Glasgow coma score ≤ 9

B. Corticosteroid use

C. Sepsis-induced inhibition of nitric oxide synthesis in the maxillary sinuses

D. Prolonged oxygen use

233. True about the management of Nosocomial sinusitis (NS) is:

A. Treatment of NS includes antibiotics effective against gram-negative rods and S. aureus, topical decongestants, removal of nasal tubes, and head elevation

B. The CT findings suggestive of sinusitis are sinus opacification, air-fluid levels, sinus wall displacement, and 4 mm or greater mucosal thickening

C. Early detection and treatment of NS is important since delays in diagnosis can lead to the development of VAP, sepsis, and life-threatening complications such as meningitis, mastoiditis, intracranial abscesses, and cavernous sinus thrombosis

D. All of the above

234. Restoration of hearing loss is unlikely if there is no spontaneous recovery within:

A. 1 week B. 2 weeks
C. 4 weeks D. 8 weeks

235. False about Parotitis is:

A. In the absence of clinical improvement with 1 to 2 days of medical treatment, surgical drainage should be considered

B. Parotitis manifests as a sudden painful enlargement of the parotid gland

C. Treatment of parotitis includes topical warm compresses, adequate hydration, and administration of parenteral antibiotics

D. Deep neck space infection is a serious complication that may cause mediastinal empyema, airway compromise, epiglottic/laryngeal edema, and severe sepsis with an associated high mortality rate (20%–40%)

THE GERIATRIC PATIENT AND FRAILTY

236. False statement among the following is:

A. The key characteristics of the frailty cycle are decreased appetite, chronic malnutrition, and progressive loss of skeletal muscle mass, strength and power

B. The Fried criteria are helpful in identifying sarcopenia, which has been linked to increased morbidity and mortality with major surgery

C. No laboratory tests are involved in diagnosing frailty state (FS), the presence of abnormal results in three or more systems was a significant predictor of frailty

D. FS prevalence is higher in surgical preoperative settings, varying from 50% to 70%

237. False about pathophysiologic effects of frailty state on different organ systems includes all except:

A. Immune system: Impaired immunity results with low levels of lymphocytes and CD8 T-cells

B. Coagulation: Procoagulant state with increased plasminogen activator inhibitor-1

C. Endocrine system: Low levels of testosterone, insulin-like growth factor and vitamin D

D. Cognition: Result from a combination of anticholinergic medications and hypoxic injury of the brain during the perioperative period

238. Recommendation for the prevention of frailty complications includes:

A. Assess muscle strength, fall risk, and ability to safely ambulate and perform activities of daily living

B. Promote optimum physiologic status and reduce the risk of complications

C. Rehabilitation (good nutrition and physical therapy) after stressful events is important in preventing frailty state

D. All of the above

ANSWERS

1. **Ans: A. The use of prosthetic mesh in hernia surgery doesn't increase the risk of seroma formation**
Ref: Chapter No.12, Page No.239

2. **Ans: C. Several techniques are used to reduce dead space, including the use of fibrin sealant, quilting sutures and medical talc with consistent results**
Ref: Chapter No.12, Page No.239

3. **Ans: C. 5 days**
Ref: Chapter No.12, Page No.239

4. **Ans: B. 3–5 days**
Ref: Chapter No.12, Page No.239

5. **Ans: C. 5 days**
Ref: Chapter No.12, Page No.239

6. **Ans: C. A hematoma is collection of blood clot and blood at the surgical site and occurs only in the subcutaneous tissue plane**
Ref: Chapter No.12, Page No.239-240

7. **Ans: B. Intermediate risk**
Ref: Chapter No.12, Page No.240

8. **Ans: A. 4 and high risk of bleeding**
Ref: Chapter No.12, Page No.240

9. **Ans: C. Wound dehiscence occurs in 10% - 15% of all surgical procedures**
Ref: Chapter No.12, Page No.240

10. **Ans: A. Wound dehiscence is more common during the 2nd postoperative week**
Ref: Chapter No.12, Page No.240

11. **Ans: C. > 50% cases**
Ref: Chapter No.12, Page No.240

12. **Ans: C. Concepts for fascial closure include accurate approximation of anatomic layers, avoiding excessive tension on the suture line, and avoiding the use of prophylactic mesh or retention sutures in "high-risk" patients**
Ref: Chapter No.12, Page No.241

13. **Ans: C. The use of permanent mesh (polypropylene or polytetrafluoroethylene) is recommended in most cases due to the presence of associated infection or bowel injury**
Ref: Chapter No.12, Page No.241

14. **Ans: B. > 4:1**
Ref: Chapter No.12, Page No.241

15. **Ans: D. All of the above**
Ref: Chapter No.12, Page No.241

16. **Ans: B. Treated osteomyelitis**
Ref: Chapter No.12, Page No.241

17. **Ans: B. Infection occurs within 7 days after the operation**
Ref: Chapter No.12, Page No.242

18. **Ans: D. Infection occurs within 30 days after the operation if implant is left in place**
Ref: Chapter No.12, Page No.242

19. **Ans: B. Hypothermia**
Ref: Chapter No.12, Page No.242

20. **Ans: C. Decreased BMI**
Ref: Chapter No.12, Page No.242

21. **Ans: C. 20–25%**
Ref: Chapter No.12, Page No.242

22. **Ans: B. 5–8%**
Ref: Chapter No.12, Page No.242

23. **Ans: B. Clean contaminated**
Ref: Chapter No.12, Page No.242

24. **Ans: C. Contaminated**
Ref: Chapter No.12, Page No.242

25. **Ans: B. Clean contaminated**
Ref: Chapter No.12, Page No.242

26. **Ans: B. 30–40%**
Ref: Chapter No.12, Page No.242

27. **Ans: B. Decolonizing staphylococcal carriers with 10% mupirocin nasal ointment can reduce the risk of postoperative S. aureus infection in cardiac and orthopedic surgery**
Ref: Chapter No.12, Page No.243

28. **Ans: B. Empiric antibiotics for operations involving axillae, groin, perineum, genital tract, and gastrointestinal (GI) tract should cover gram-positive and aerobic bacteria**
Ref: Chapter No.12, Page No.243-244

29. **Ans: C. < 35°C**
Ref: Chapter No.12, Page No.244

30. **Ans: D. < 28°C**
Ref: Chapter No.12, Page No.244

31. **Ans: B. Hypothermia is not associated with increased risk of SSI**
Ref: Chapter No.12, Page No.244

32. **Ans: C. Prolonged surgeries (>2 hours)**
Ref: Chapter No.12, Page No.244

33. **Ans: C. Shift of oxyhemoglobin-dissociation curve to the right**

Ref: Chapter No.12, Page No.244

34. **Ans: A. Osborn wave**

Ref: Chapter No.12, Page No.244

35. **Ans: A. Hypotension due to shock is the most important impediment to wound oxygenation**

Ref: Chapter No.12, Page No.244

36. **Ans: D. All of the above**

Ref: Chapter No.12, Page No.244-245

37. **Ans: B. It is an autosomal recessive pharmacogenetic disorder**

Ref: Chapter No.12, Page No.245-246

38. **Ans: D. Etomidate**

Ref: Chapter No.12, Page No.245

39. **Ans: B. Dantrolene an initial dose of 2.5 mg/kg IV should be given and can be repeated according to the response: end-tidal CO_2, tachycardia, muscle rigidity, and acidosis**

Ref: Chapter No.12, Page No.246

40. **Ans: D. Active cooling with ice packs and 20°C normal saline IV should be initiated if the body temperature is > 40°C but should be stopped when the body temperature decreases to 38.5°C to avoid overcooling and hypothermia**

Ref: Chapter No.12, Page No.246

41. **Ans: C. Pneumonia is the most common cause of nosocomial bacteremia and septicemia**

Ref: Chapter No.12, Page No.246

42. **Ans: B. Catheter-related bloodstream infection (CRBSI)**

Ref: Chapter No.12, Page No.246

43. **Ans: B. Vancomycin is not recommended for empirical therapy for MRSA**

Ref: Chapter No.12, Page No.246-247

44. **Ans: B. Atelectasis**

Ref: Chapter No.12, Page No.247

45. **Ans: C. Atelectasis is the 2nd most common cause of postoperative fever in the early postoperative period**

Ref: Chapter No.12, Page No.247

46. **Ans: D. All of the above**

Ref: Chapter No.12, Page No.247

47. **Ans: B. IV antibiotics**

Ref: Chapter No.12, Page No.247

48. **Ans: A. Pneumonia**

Ref: Chapter No.12, Page No.247

49. **Ans: C. 48–72 hours**

Ref: Chapter No.12, Page No.247

50. **Ans: D. In early-onset VAP (< 4 days postintubation), the organisms are usually antibiotic resistant**

Ref: Chapter No.12, Page No.247

51. **Ans: D. 72 hours**

Ref: Chapter No.12, Page No.247

52. **Ans: C. 50%**

Ref: Chapter No.12, Page No.247

53. **Ans: B. Thrombocytopenia**

Ref: Chapter No.12, Page No.248

54. **Ans: D. 92%**

Ref: Chapter No.12, Page No.248

55. **Ans: B. 65 mm Hg**

Ref: Chapter No.12, Page No.248

56. **Ans: B. The use of H_2 receptor antagonists for stress ulcer prophylaxis is associated with a reduced incidence of pneumonia relative to prophylaxis with sucralfate**

Ref: Chapter No.12, Page No.248

57. **Ans: B. Bolus feedings possess a higher risk of aspiration than continuous feeding**

Ref: Chapter No.12, Page No.248

58. **Ans: B. 2.5**

Ref: Chapter No.12, Page No.248

59. **Ans: D. All of the above**

Ref: Chapter No.12, Page No.248

60. **Ans: C. Elective surgery**

Ref: Chapter No.12, Page No.248

61. **Ans: A. Streptococcus**

Ref: Chapter No.12, Page No.248

62. **Ans: C. The absence of symptoms in the first 30 mins usually correlates with a benign course**

Ref: Chapter No.12, Page No.248-249

63. **Ans: B. 24 - 36 hours**

Ref: Chapter No.12, Page No.248

64. **Ans: B. Antibiotics are required in most cases**

Ref: Chapter No.12, Page No.249

65. **Ans: C. ARDS are characterized by the acute worsening of respiratory symptoms, usually within 1 day of clinical insult**

Ref: Chapter No.12, Page No.249

66. **Ans: A. <100**

Ref: Chapter No.12, Page No.249

67. **Ans: B. The patient's ideal or predicted body weight should be calculated and a tidal volume of 60 mL/kg of predicted body weight with plateau pressure of ≤30 mm H_2O should be used initially according to current ARDS net protocols**

Ref: Chapter No.12, Page No.249-250

68. **Ans: A. Hypothermia**

Ref: Chapter No.12, Page No.250

69. **Ans: B. Long-distance travel (>24 hours)**

Ref: Chapter No.12, Page No.250

70. **Ans: B. D-dimer should be used to screen for VTE in surgery or trauma patients**

Ref: Chapter No.12, Page No.250

71. **Ans: B. Normal spectral Doppler**

Ref: Chapter No.12, Page No.250

72. **Ans: A. CT pulmonary angiography**

Ref: Chapter No.12, Page No.250

73. **Ans: B. Children**

Ref: Chapter No.12, Page No.251

74. **Ans: B. Chest radiography and electrocardiography are diagnostic and normal results exclude PE**

Ref: Chapter No.12, Page No.250

75. **Ans: B. Left-axis deviation**

Ref: Chapter No.12, Page No.250

76. **Ans: A. California score (Other validated scoring systems include Caprini score, Department of Health VTE risk assessment tool)**

There are 2 PADUA scores

1. The **Padua Prediction Score** is a risk assessment model for the identification of patients at risk of VTE (Patients who are ***high risk (Padua ≥4)*** could benefit from thromboprophylaxis)
2. **PADUA score** in urology assesses the anatomical complexity of a renal tumor with respect to partial nephrectomy

The **IMPROVE score** predicts ***3-month risk of VTE*** in hospitalized patients and ***should not be used in outpatients***

The **Revised Geneva Score (rGeneva)** risk-stratifies patients for pulmonary embolism (PE)

- rGeneva is ***not meant to diagnose*** but to guide workup and testing by predicting pre-test probability of PE
- The rGeneva score ***does not require imaging or serum studies for risk stratification***
- The rGeneva score ***does not require clinical gestalt*** (present in Wells' PE criteria and often subjective) for risk stratification

The **Wells' Criteria** risk stratifies patients for pulmonary embolism (PE), and has been validated in both ***inpatient and emergency department settings***. Its score is often used in conjunction ***with d-dimer testing*** to evaluate for PE. Wells' is ***not meant to diagnose PE*** but to guide workup by predicting pre-test probability of PE and appropriate testing to ***rule out the diagnosis***

Ref: Chapter No.12, Page No.251
https://www.mdcalc.com

77. **Ans: C. Vena cava filters are considered in all high-risk patients**

Ref: Chapter No.12, Page No.251

78. **Ans: A. PE severity index score of class II or higher**

Ref: Chapter No.12, Page No.251

79. **Ans: D. All of the above**

Ref: Chapter No.12, Page No.251

80. **Ans: D. All of the above**

Ref: Chapter No.12, Page No.251

81. **Ans: D. UFH has better bioavailability and can be given subcutaneously, with a longer half-life**

Ref: Chapter No.12, Page No.251-252

82. **Ans: D. All of the above**

Ref: Chapter No.12, Page No.252

83. **Ans: C. 65%**

Ref: Chapter No.12, Page No.252

84. **Ans: D. All of the above**

Ref: Chapter No.12, Page No.252

85. **Ans: B. Alcohol consumption**

Ref: Chapter No.12, Page No.252

86. **Ans: C. There is insufficient evidence that biomarker screening reduces cardiac events; therefore, routine screening is recommended (2014 AHA guideline)**

(AHA doesn't recommend screening if symptoms are not present and the patient is high risk in contrast to European Society of Cardiology which recommends it with all high-risk patients)

Ref: Chapter No.12, Page No.252

87. **Ans: B. Before and 48 - 72 hours after surgery**

Ref: Chapter No.12, Page No.252

88. **Ans: B. 48 hours**

Ref: Chapter No.12, Page No.252

89. **Ans: B. Preoperative serum creatinine >3 mg/dL**

The **RCRI** assesses the ***perioperative risk of major cardiac complications***, including myocardial infarction, pulmonary edema, ventricular fibrillation, or cardiac arrest, and complete heart block based on ***6 patient characteristics***

Patients with ***at least 2*** risk factors are at increased risk for cardiac complications

Ref: Chapter No.12, Page No.253

90. **Ans: C. Beta blockers should be discontinued in patients who already take them and initiation of beta blockers should be considered in only high-risk patients (≥1 RCRI)**

Ref: Chapter No.12, Page No.253

91. **Ans: D. All of the above**

Ref: Chapter No.12, Page No.253

92. **Ans: C. 12 days**

Ref: Chapter No.12, Page No.253

93. **Ans: A. Low**

Ref: Chapter No.12, Page No.253

94. **Ans: C. High**

Ref: Chapter No.12, Page No.253

95. **Ans: B. Intermediate**

Ref: Chapter No.12, Page No.253

96. **Ans: B. Intermediate**

Ref: Chapter No.12, Page No.253

97. **Ans: D. All of the above**

Ref: Chapter No.12, Page No.253-254

98. **Ans: C. 50%**

Ref: Chapter No.12, Page No.254

99. **Ans: B. > 190/100 mm Hg in 2 consecutive readings**

Ref: Chapter No.12, Page No.254

100. **Ans: D. Stopping ACE inhibitors before surgery has been shown to increase all-cause mortality and vascular events, including myocardial injury and stroke**

Ref: Chapter No.12, Page No.255

101. **Ans: B. 30 minutes**

Ref: Chapter No.12, Page No.255

102. **Ans: C. > 110 mm Hg**

Ref: Chapter No.12, Page No.255

103. **Ans: B. Female gender**

Ref: Chapter No.12, Page No.255

104. **Ans: C. Chemical cardioversion may be considered to decrease the risk of thromboembolism when the atrial arrhythmia is > 48 hours duration**

Ref: Chapter No.12, Page No.255

105. **Ans: B. ≥ 2**

Ref: Chapter No.12, Page No.255

106 **Ans: D. All of the above**

Ref: Chapter No.12, Page No.255

107. **Ans: C. 63%**

Ref: Chapter No.12, Page No.256

108. **Ans: A. < 30%**

Ref: Chapter No.12, Page No.256

109. **Ans: B. Patients with LVEF < 45% or QRS complex > 60 ms should be considered for cardiac resynchronization therapy before surgery**

Ref: Chapter No.12, Page No.256

110. **Ans: B. Urine volume < 0.5 mL/kg/h for 6 hours**

Ref: Chapter No.12, Page No.256

111. **Ans: A. Anuria for ≥24 hours**

Ref: Chapter No.12, Page No.256

112. **Ans: C. Types of surgery especially hepatic surgery**

Ref: Chapter No.12, Page No.257

113. **Ans: B. Laparoscopic surgery**

Ref: Chapter No.12, Page No.257

114. **Ans: C. NSAIDs**

Ref: Chapter No.12, Page No.257

115. **Ans: A. Neurogenic bladder**

Ref: Chapter No.12, Page No.257

116. **Ans: C. Urinary sodium >50 mOsm/L**

Ref: Chapter No.12, Page No.257

117. **Ans: B. Fractional excretion of sodium <1%**

Ref: Chapter No.12, Page No.257

118. **Ans: C. Dopamine appears to be more effective than other vasopressors in patients with AKI and vasopressor of choice**

Ref: Chapter No.12, Page No.258

119. **Ans: D. All of the above (Unfortunately, these preventive strategies are still controversial)**

Ref: Chapter No.12, Page No.258

120. **Ans: D. All of the above**

Ref: Chapter No.12, Page No.258

121. **Ans: C. Female gender**

Ref: Chapter No.12, Page No.258

122. **Ans: B. Most patients should void within 18 to 24 hours after surgery**

Ref: Chapter No.12, Page No.258-259

123. **Ans: B. In central AI, hyperpigmentation is observed due to a low corticotropin level, and the mineralocorticoids are not affected**

Ref: Chapter No.12, Page No.259

124. **Ans: A. Autoimmune**

Ref: Chapter No.12, Page No.259

125. **Ans: B. Exogenous glucocorticoids**

Ref: Chapter No.12, Page No.259

126. **Ans: D. All of the above**

Ref: Chapter No.12, Page No.259

127. Ans: C. The thyroid storm is associated with a high mortality rate (50%–80%)

Ref: Chapter No.12, Page No.260

128. Ans: B. Thyroid functions tests differentiate between severe thyrotoxicosis and the thyroid storm

Ref: Chapter No.12, Page No.260

129. Ans: B. Salicylates is preferred to acetaminophen since acetaminophen elevates free hormone levels by decreasing T4-binding globin

Ref: Chapter No.12, Page No.260

130. Ans: C. The antithyroid drug Methimazole blocks new hormone synthesis and decreases extrathyroidal conversion of T4 to T3

Ref: Chapter No.12, Page No.260

131. Ans: B. 12 - 24 hours

Ref: Chapter No.12, Page No.261

132. Ans: D. All of the above

Ref: Chapter No.12, Page No.261

133. Ans: C. 40%–50%

Ref: Chapter No.12, Page No.261

134. Ans: B. Hyponatremia: 0.9% normal saline

Ref: Chapter No.12, Page No.261

135. Ans: C. Significant neurologic symptoms occur when serum sodium <115 mEq/L and subsequent coma and respiratory arrest develop at 105 - 110 mEq/L

Ref: Chapter No.12, Page No.261-262

136. Ans: A. Small cell lung cancer

Ref: Chapter No.12, Page No.262

137. Ans: C. 6 weeks of surgery

Ref: Chapter No.12, Page No.262

138. Ans: B. Adhesions

Ref: Chapter No.12, Page No.262

139. Ans: D. All of the above

Ref: Chapter No.12, Page No.262

140. Ans: B. 24 to 48 hours

Ref: Chapter No.12, Page No.262

141. Ans: C. 3 to 5 days

Ref: Chapter No.12, Page No.262

142. Ans: D. All of the above

Ref: Chapter No.12, Page No.262

143. Ans: D. Decreased serum amylase, serum D-lactate, and intestinal fatty acid binding protein are associated with intestinal ischemia

Ref: Chapter No.12, Page No.263

144. Ans: D. The more distal the obstruction, the earlier and more prominent the symptoms of nausea and vomiting (bilious), whereas vomiting with distal bowel obstruction is typically delayed in presentation and feculent in nature

Ref: Chapter No.12, Page No.262-263

145. Ans: D. Postoperative physiologic ileus is usually managed by surgical intervention

Ref: Chapter No.12, Page No.263

146. Ans: B. < 8 mm Hg

Ref: Chapter No.12, Page No.263

147. Ans: C. 12 mm Hg

Ref: Chapter No.12, Page No.263

148. Ans: C. Most patients with Grade III and all patients with Grade IV are managed conservatively

Ref: Chapter No.12, Page No.263-264

149. Ans: B. >15 cm H_2O

Ref: Chapter No.12, Page No.264

150. Ans: C. 25–35 cm H_2O:

(Remember grades of ACS are in cm H_2O; whereas the definition of ACS involves > 12 mm Hg and not > 12 cm of H_2O)

Ref: Chapter No.12, Page No.264

151. Ans: A. 10–15 cm H_2O

Ref: Chapter No.12, Page No.264

152. Ans: C. IAP should still be monitored in "high-risk" patients since recurrent ACS has been reported in up to 10% of patients after damage control laparotomy

Ref: Chapter No.12, Page No.264

153. Ans: D. All of the above

Ref: Chapter No.12, Page No.265

154. Ans: A. < 1%

Ref: Chapter No.12, Page No.265

155. Ans: C. Mechanical ventilation and coagulopathy are associated with decreased risk

Ref: Chapter No.12, Page No.265

156. Ans: B. Serial blood counts and coagulation studies (prothrombin time, partial thromboplastin time and bleeding time) should be performed every 24 hours and corrected with appropriate transfusion therapy

Ref: Chapter No.12, Page No.265

157. Ans: B. Persistently low hematocrit values (25% to 30%)

Ref: Chapter No.12, Page No.265

158. Ans: B. 30%

Ref: Chapter No.12, Page No.265

159. Ans: B. 15% to 20%

Ref: Chapter No.12, Page No.265

160. Ans: C. <1 month postoperatively

Ref: Chapter No.12, Page No.266

161. Ans: D. A healthy stoma is always pink but turns dark purple or black usually within the first 1 week when ischemia is present

Ref: Chapter No.12, Page No.266

162. Ans: C. Ischemia is more common in a loop stoma relative to an end stoma, due to its tenuous blood supply

Ref: Chapter No.12, Page No.266

163. Ans: C. Excoriation (HARD: High Output, Abscess formation, Retraction, Dermatitis are both early and late complications)

Ref: Chapter No.12, Page No.266

164. Ans: B. Ischemic necrosis

Ref: Chapter No.12, Page No.266

165. Ans: B. Ulcerative colitis

Ref: Chapter No.12, Page No.267

166. Ans: D. All of the above

Ref: Chapter No.12, Page No.267

167. Ans: C. < 10%

Ref: Chapter No.12, Page No.267

168. Ans: A. Fixed prolapse is a common condition in which excessive bowel has been everted during stoma construction and requires treatment

Ref: Chapter No.12, Page No.267

169. Ans: C. Incarceration and/or strangulation occurs in > 25% of cases

Ref: Chapter No.12, Page No.267

170. Ans: B. Peristomal skin irritation is more common with colostomies than with ileostomies

Ref: Chapter No.12, Page No.267

171. Ans: B. Infectious dermatitis is the most common type

Ref: Chapter No.12, Page No.267

172. Ans: C. Pyoderma gangrenosum is associated with inflammatory bowel disease or malignancy, presents as a painless, small necrotic ulcers

Ref: Chapter No.12, Page No.267

173. Ans: B. Sclerosing cholangitis

Ref: Chapter No.12, Page No.267

174. Ans: D. All of the above

Ref: Chapter No.12, Page No.267

175. Ans: D. All of the above

Ref: Chapter No.12, Page No.268

176. Ans: C. 5 cm

Ref: Chapter No.12, Page No.268

177. Ans: C. A tight stenosis causing subacute intestinal obstruction can be managed with simple and gentle dilatation in conjunction with a high-fiber diet

Ref: Chapter No.12, Page No.268

178. Ans: D. Mesh can't be used due to risk of infection

Ref: Chapter No.12, Page No.268

179. Ans: B. A properly situated stoma has a height of at least 2 cm and can usually be managed with a pouch change every 1 - 2 days

Ref: Chapter No.12, Page No.268

180. Ans: C. Fascial aperture to admit 3 fingers

Ref: Chapter No.12, Page No.268

181. Ans: A. Stomal or peristomal skin bleeding may be treated with sodium nitrate

Ref: Chapter No.12, Page No.268

182. Ans: B. C difficile colitis is caused by the production of cytotoxin A and enterotoxin B, which damage intestinal epithelia, impair cell function, and promote local inflammation

Ref: Chapter No.12, Page No.269

183. Ans: A. >45 years old

Ref: Chapter No.12, Page No.269

184. Ans: A. The caecum is most commonly affected

Ref: Chapter No.12, Page No.269

185. Ans: C. Stool testing for C difficile is commonly performed in patients who have 2 or more episodes of unexplained loose or watery stools within 12 hours

Ref: Chapter No.12, Page No.269

186. Ans: C. >12 cm

Ref: Chapter No.12, Page No.269

187. Ans: B. For the initial episode of CDI, vancomycin 250 mg is given orally 4 times/day or fidaxomicin 400 mg orally 2 times/day for 7 days

Ref: Chapter No.12, Page No.269

188. Ans: D. All of the above

Ref: Chapter No.12, Page No.269

189. Ans: C. Vitamin C deficiency

Ref: Chapter No.12, Page No.270

190. Ans: B. Submucosa

Ref: Chapter No.12, Page No.270

191. Ans: D. <35 mm Hg

Ref: Chapter No.12, Page No.270

192. Ans: B. Ileocolic anastomoses

Ref: Chapter No.12, Page No.270

193. Ans: A. The risk of anastomotic leak is lower if the anastomosis is below the peritoneal reflection

Ref: Chapter No.12, Page No.270-271

194. Ans: C. 6 weeks before and 28 days after surgery

Ref: Chapter No.12, Page No.270

195. Ans: D. All of the above

Ref: Chapter No.12, Page No.271

196. Ans: C. Laboratory tests like complete blood test, C-reactive protein, and procalcitonin may be elevated with anastomotic leak but are considered relatively specific

Ref: Chapter No.12, Page No.271

197. Ans: B. Proximal diverting stoma prevents an anastomotic leak

Ref: Chapter No.12, Page No.271-272

198. Ans: A. Internal intestinal fistulas, or ICFs, are the most common type

Ref: Chapter No.12, Page No.272

199. Ans: C. Ileum

Ref: Chapter No.12, Page No.272

200. Ans: A. Aortoenteric fistulas occur due to erosion of prosthetic aortic grafts into the surrounding viscera, usually the jejunum

Ref: Chapter No.12, Page No.272

201. Ans: D. >500 mL/day

Ref: Chapter No.12, Page No.272

202. Ans: C. <200 mL/day

Ref: Chapter No.12, Page No.272

203. Ans: D. End fistula

Ref: Chapter No.12, Page No.272

204. Ans: B. Location: Colon

Ref: Chapter No.12, Page No.272

205. Ans: C. Most ECFs don't require prolonged hospital stay

Ref: Chapter No.12, Page No.272

206. Ans: C. Sepsis

Ref: Chapter No.12, Page No.272-273

207. Ans: D. All of the above

Ref: Chapter No.12, Page No.273

208. Ans: C. 4 weeks

Ref: Chapter No.12, Page No.273

209. Ans: D. All of the above

Ref: Chapter No.12, Page No.273

210. Ans: D. All of the above

Ref: Chapter No.12, Page No.273

211. Ans: D. ERCP is recommended in the early period

Ref: Chapter No.12, Page No.274

212. Ans: B. 20%–30%

Ref: Chapter No.12, Page No.274

213. Ans: D. All of the above

Ref: Chapter No.12, Page No.274

214. Ans: B. The use of pancreaticogastrostomy was effective in lowering clinically significant POPF (CR-POPF) rates

Ref: Chapter No.12, Page No.274

215. Ans: A. BDIs during open surgery tend to be more complex than those encountered with laparoscopic surgery

Ref: Chapter No.12, Page No.274

216. Ans: C. Ultrasound and CT are considered the gold standard for evaluating BDIs

Ref: Chapter No.12, Page No.274-275

217. Ans: B. Immediate detection and repair is not associated with an improved outcome

Ref: Chapter No.12, Page No.275

218. Ans: C. The most common CT scan finding suggestive of hepatic artery injury is enhancement of the right lobe during the venous phase

Ref: Chapter No.12, Page No.275

219. Ans: D. All of the above

Ref: Chapter No.12, Page No.275

220. Ans: C. Patients with higher education level and pre-existing cognitive dysfunction are also at increased risk for POCD

Ref: Chapter No.12, Page No.276

221. Ans: B. Advanced age (>55 years)

Ref: Chapter No.12, Page No.276

222. Ans: C. 5 days

Ref: Chapter No.12, Page No.276

223. Ans: B. Anticholinergic and benzodiazepine medications should be given

Ref: Chapter No.12, Page No.276

224. Ans: D. Seizures may also result in the loss of autonomic control with bowel or bladder incontinence and may result in decreased intracranial pressure

Ref: Chapter No.12, Page No.276-277

225. Ans: D. All of the above

Ref: Chapter No.12, Page No.277

226. Ans: C. 30 days after surgery

Ref: Chapter No.12, Page No.277

227. Ans: B. While hemorrhagic strokes are more common, ischemic strokes account for 1% - 4% of perioperative strokes

Ref: Chapter No.12, Page No.277

228. Ans: A. Perioperative beta blockers can decrease the risk of stroke

Ref: Chapter No.12, Page No.277-278

229. Ans: C. 6 - 12 months

Ref: Chapter No.12, Page No.277

230. Ans: B. The incidence of posterior epistaxis is less in elderly patients with atherosclerosis

Ref: Chapter No.12, Page No.278

231. Ans: C. The symptoms of NS are typically masked by more serious illness and the microbiology is more commonly monomicrobial

Ref: Chapter No.12, Page No.278

232. Ans: A. Glasgow coma score ≤9

Ref: Chapter No.12, Page No.278

233. Ans: D. All of the above

Ref: Chapter No.12, Page No.278

234. Ans: B. 2 weeks

Ref: Chapter No.12, Page No.278

235. Ans: A. In the absence of clinical improvement with 1 to 2 days of medical treatment, surgical drainage should be considered

Ref: Chapter No.12, Page No.279

236. Ans: D. FS prevalence is higher in surgical preoperative settings, varying from 50% to 70%

Ref: Chapter No.12, Page No.279

237. Ans: B. Coagulation: Procoagulant state with increased plasminogen activator inhibitor-1

Ref: Chapter No.12, Page No.280

238. Ans: D. All of the above

Ref: Chapter No.12, Page No.280

13

Surgery in the Geriatric Patient

OUTCOMES OF SURGERY IN OLDER ADULTS

1. **True statement among the following is:**
   A. Mortality from high-risk operations such as esophagectomy or pancreatectomy can be two and three times the mortality in geriatric patients for similar procedures in younger adults
   B. It is now generally accepted that frailty, rather than chronological age, is the most important predictor of traditional surgical outcomes
   C. The American College of Surgeons National Surgical Quality Improvement Program (ACS NSQIP) surgical risk calculator is an extremely useful tool in predicting the likelihood of 30-day mortality and 30-day complications
   D. All of the above

FRAILTY AND PHYSIOLOGIC DECLINE

2. **True about frailty is:**
   A. Frailty is defined as "a biologic syndrome of decreased reserve and resistance to stressors, resulting from cumulative declines across multiple physiologic systems causing vulnerability to adverse outcomes"
   B. The Fried frailty phenotype is the most widely used method to describe frailty
   C. The Edmonton Frail scale is a questionnaire that covers many of the domains of frailty and can be easily administered by support personnel in the office setting
   D. All of the above

3. **False about the cardiovascular changes in geriatric patients is:**
   A. Increased dependence on preload
   B. Decreased diastolic dysfunction
   C. Decrease in ventricular and arterial compliance
   D. Fibrosis of conducting pathways with increased arrhythmias

4. **False about the respiratory changes in geriatric patients is:**
   A. Decrease in PaO_2 and increase in $PaCO_2$
   B. Decrease in lung elasticity (small airway collapse)
   C. Decline in ventilator responses to hypoxemia and hypercapnia
   D. Decreased FVC and FEV_1

5. **False about the renal changes in geriatric patients is:**
   A. Decrease in the number of tubular cells
   B. Decreased renal blood flow
   C. Increase susceptibility to dehydration
   D. Increased glomerular filtration rate

6. **False about the hepatobiliary changes in geriatric patients is:**
   A. Decrease in hepatic blood flow
   B. Decrease in the number of hepatocytes
   C. Decreased synthetic capacity
   D. Increased incidence of gallstones and gallstone-related diseases

7. **False about the immune function changes in geriatric patients is:**
   A. Decrease production and differentiation of naïve T cells
   B. Decrease in inflammatory cytokines
   C. Involution of the thymus gland
   D. Decrease in T cell mitogenic activity

8. **False about the cardiovascular changes in geriatric patients is:**

A. Almost 90% of the autonomic tissue in the sinus node is replaced by fat and connective tissue, and fibrosis interferes with conduction in the intranodal tracts and bundle of His
B. With aging, there is a relative hyposympathetic state in which the heart becomes less responsive to catecholamines, possible secondary to declining receptor function
C. Progressive dilatation of all four valvular annuli is probably responsible for the multivalvular regurgitation demonstrated in healthy older persons
D. Cardiac output and ejection fraction are decreased

9. False about the cardiovascular changes in geriatric patients is:

A. Lifestyle modifications, natural compounds, and hormone therapies are useful for hypertension in elderly
B. Diastolic dysfunction is responsible for up to 50% of cases of heart failure in patients older than 80 years old
C. With aging, there is a progressive decrease in the partial pressure of oxygen
D. Chest pain is still the most common symptom of myocardial infarction, atypical symptoms such as shortness of breath, syncope, acute confusion, or stroke will occur in as many as 40% of older patients

10. False about the respiratory changes in geriatric patients is:

A. Ventilatory responses to hypoxia and hypercapnia fall by 70% and 80%, respectively
B. Respiratory problems are the most common postoperative complications in older patients
C. Forced vital capacity decreases by 14 to 30 mL/year and forced expiratory volume in 1 second decreases by 23 to 32 mL/year (in males)
D. Maximum inspiratory and expiratory forces decrease by as much as 50% as a result of a progressive decrease in the strength of the respiratory muscles

11. False about the renal changes in geriatric patients is:

A. There is urinary incontinence in 10% to 15% of older people living in the community and 50% of those in nursing homes
B. A serum creatinine level of 1.0 mg/dL may represent a CrCl of over 100 mL/ min in a 30-year-old but less than 60 mL/min in an 85-year-old
C. Circulating levels of erythropoietin (EPO) are lower in the healthy elderly as compared to younger individuals
D. Renal blood flow falls by approximately 50%

12. False about the immune function changes in geriatric patients is:

A. With aging, there is a decline in the hematopoietic stem cell pool in the bone marrow that leads to decreased production of naïve T cells from the thymus and of B. cells from the bone marrow
B. Immunoglobulin M (IgM) levels increase, whereas IgG and IgA levels decrease slightly
C. Older patients with major infections frequently have normal white blood cell (WBC) counts, but the differential count will show a profound shift to the left, with a large proportion of immature forms
D. With aging, there is a decline in the hematopoietic stem cell pool in the bone marrow that leads to decreased production of naïve T cells from the thymus and of B. cells from the bone marrow

PREOPERATIVE ASSESSMENT AND DECISION-MAKING

13. Goals of a structured communication include:

A. Place the patient's acute surgical condition in the context of the patient's underlying illness
B. Elicit the patient's goals, priorities, and what is acceptable to the patient regarding life-prolonging and comfort-focused care
C. Describe treatment options—including palliative approaches—in the context of the patient's goals and priorities
D. All of the above

14. False about cognitive assessment of geriatric patients is:

A. Preoperative cognitive status as a risk factor for negative postoperative outcomes in older patients is often overlooked
B. The prevalence of dementia is approximately 1.5% at age 65 years and approximately doubles with every 5 additional years of life
C. Total possible Mini-Cog scores range from 0 to 5 points, with 0 to 3 suggesting high likelihood of cognitive impairment
D. Dementia is the single greatest risk factor for postoperative delirium

15. In order to be considered competent to give consent, the patient must be able to all except:

A. Clearly indicate a treatment choice
B. Understand the relevant information given
C. Appreciate the medical condition and the consequences of treatments
D. All of the above

16. True about Delirium risk in geriatric patient is:

A. Delirium risk can be assessed using a predictive rule that considers the patient's age, comorbidities and type of surgery
B. Delirium is defined as an acute disorder of cognition and attention and is among the most common and potentially devastating complications seen in older surgical patients
C. Delirium risk can also be assessed using the ACS NSQIP Geriatric Surgical Risk Calculator
D. All of the above

17. Risk (predisposing) factors for delirium includes all except:

A. Sensory impairment
B. Functional impairment
C. Good nutritional status
D. Psychotropic medications

18. Precipitating factors for delirium includes all except:

A. Sleep disruption
B. Infection
C. Hypercarbia
D. Use of bladder catheters

19. False about functional assessment in geriatric patients is:

A. For older adults, the ability to perform ADLs (Activities of daily living) and instrumental ADLs has been shown to correlate with postoperative mortality and morbidity
B. ASA classification has been shown to predict postoperative mortality accurately, even in patients older than 80 years old
C. An inability to function >4 METs has been associated with decreased perioperative cardiac events and long-term risk
D. Patients identified as high risk for fall should be considered for preoperative gait and balance training if time allows

20. 1 MET is defined as:

A. 3.5 mL/kg/min, represents the basal oxygen consumption of a 60-kg, 40-year-old man at rest
B. 3.5 mL/kg/min, represents the basal oxygen consumption of a 70-kg, 40-year-old man at rest
C. 4.5 mL/kg/min, represents the basal oxygen consumption of a 60-kg, 40-year-old man at rest
D. 4.5 mL/kg/min, represents the basal oxygen consumption of a 70-kg, 40-year-old man at rest

21. Factors associated with increased risk of malnutrition includes all except:

A. Recent weight loss
B. Disinterest in eating
C. Poor dentition
D. Increased appetite

22. False about Nutritional Status of geriatric patients is:

A. The impact of poor nutrition as a risk factor for perioperative mortality and morbidity such as pneumonia and poor wound healing has long been appreciated
B. Malnutrition is estimated to occur in approximately 0% to 15% of community dwelling older persons, 35% to 65% of older patients in acute care hospitals, and 25% to 60% of institutionalized older adults
C. Malnutrition has been associated with increased risk of falls and hospital admission
D. Standard anthropomorphic measures take into account the changes in body composition and structure that accompany aging

23. False about Nutritional Status of geriatric patients is:

A. Screening tools used include the Subjective Global Assessment (SGA) and Mini Nutritional Assessment (MNA)
B. SGA ratings are most strongly influenced by loss of subcutaneous tissue, muscle wasting, and weight loss
C. Nutritional status, as determined by the SGA and MNA, has been shown to predict outcome in outpatient and hospitalized geriatric medical patients
D. The SGA is used but not been validated in older and critically ill patients

24. The Mini Nutritional Assessment (MNA), measures:

A. 10 factors
B. 12 factors
C. 18 factors
D. 25 factors

25. Patients at high risk for nutritional-related complications include:

A. BMI <18.5 kg/m^2
B. Albumin <3.0 g/dL
C. Unintentional weight loss >10% to 15% within 6 months
D. All of the above

26. Factors associated with swallowing dysfunction include diseases such as:

A. Prior stroke
B. Diabetes
C. GERD
D. All of the above

27. True statement among the following is:

A. The Beer's list is a comprehensive list of medications that should be avoided or used with caution in the older adult
B. The most common drugs to be avoided include all benzodiazepines, the analgesic meperidine (Demerol), and the antihistamines diphenhydramine (Benadryl)
C. For patients with significant cardiac or vascular disease not currently on beta blockers or statin therapy, consideration should be given to starting these medications
D. All of the above

28. ACS–geriatric surgery verification requirements for multimodality pain plan includes all except:

A. Utilize opioid using techniques
B. Titrate medication for increased sensitivity (start low, go slow)
C. Include a prophylactic pharmacologic bowel regimen
D. Avoid Beer's list of drugs (benzodiazepines, meperidine, skeletal muscle relaxants, etc.)

INTRAOPERATIVE AND POSTOPERATIVE MANAGEMENT

29. The most common cause of morbidity and mortality in older patients in the postoperative period is:

A. Delirium
B. Aspiration
C. Renal failure
D. Cardiac arrest

30. Postoperative delirium is associated with all except:

A. Lower overall hospital cost
B. Longer ICU length of stay
C. Higher rates of institutionalization after discharge
D. Higher rates of morbidity (30 days) and mortality (6 months)

31. The incidence of postoperative delirium in older patients after vascular surgery is around:

A. 15%
B. 25%
C. 35%
D. 45%

32. False statement among the following is:

A. No association has been found with the route of anesthesia (epidural vs. general) or the occurrence of intraoperative hemodynamic complications
B. Intraoperative blood loss, need for blood transfusion, and postoperative hematocrit level lower than 30% are associated with a significantly increased risk for postoperative delirium
C. The best treatment for delirium is use of sedatives
D. The use of antipsychotic medications, such as very low-dose haloperidol, should be reserved only for those patients whose behavior presents a danger to themselves or others

33. False about aspiration in older patients in the postoperative period is:

A. The incidence of postoperative aspiration pneumonia increases almost exponentially with increasing age
B. The routine use of nasogastric tubes in patients undergoing colon resection has been correlated with a decreased risk of aspiration pneumonia
C. Poor oral hygiene and the edentulous state are also associated with an overgrowth of pathologic organisms, which predispose to pneumonia following aspiration
D. Prior to feeding patients at risk for aspiration, swallowing function can be assessed by a 3-ounce bedside swallow test

34. As compared to those 18 to 29 years of age, patients >80 years old have a greater risk of aspiration upto:

A. 5-fold
B. 10-fold
C. 20-fold
D. 40-fold

35. Aspiration precautions ordered for any patient thought to be at risk includes all except:

A. Upright position during meals and for 60 - 75 minutes after meals in those on an oral diet

B. 30- to 45-degree upright positioning
C. Careful evaluation of gastrointestinal function prior to starting feeding
D. Careful monitoring of gastric residuals in patients with feeding tubes

36. Organ system effects of bed rest includes all except:

A. Muscles: ↓ Muscle strength, ↓ muscle blood flow
B. Bone: ↑ Bone loss, ↓ bone density
C. Cardiovascular: ↑ Stroke volume, ↑ cardiac output, orthostatic hypotension
D. Respiratory: ↓ Respiratory excursion, ↓ oxygen uptake, ↑ potential for atelectasis

37. True statement about deconditioning during hospitalization in older patients is:

A. Older adult surgical patients who develop functional decline while in the hospital are at greater risk of readmission, complications, and death within 300 days after discharge
B. Risk factor for deconditioning during hospitalization includes 2 or more comorbidities, 5 or more medications, and a hospitalization or emergency room visit in the preceding year
C. Patients who develop delirium while in the hospital are also at greater risk of developing serious functional decline
D. All of the above

SURGERY OF MAJOR ORGAN SYSTEMS

38. False about thyroid disease and geriatric patients is:

A. Medical treatment of hypothyroidism in older adults is like that in younger patients
B. Thyroid nodules are common in the elderly with linear increase with age
C. By ultrasonography, approximately 70% of patients older than 65 years old have nodules
D. Malignant nodules tend to have more aggressive phenotypes in elderly patients, with thyroid cancer specific mortality being about 8%

39. False about thyroid lesions and geriatric patients is:

A. Sporadic papillary thyroid cancer has an almost bell-shaped distribution of age at diagnosis, with a decreasing trend in patients > 60 years old
B. Age is a negative prognostic factor for survival and other outcomes
C. Patients > 60 years old have a decreased risk for local recurrence, and patients < 20 years old and > 60 years old have a lower risk for the development of distant metastasis
D. Increasing patient age correlates with increased risk for death by approximately 2-fold over a span of 20 years.

40. False about Parathyroid disease and geriatric patients is:

A. The most common reason for the finding of hypercalcemia in an elderly outpatient setting is primarily hyperparathyroidism
B. The incidence of primary HPTH increases with age; it affects approximately 2% of older persons, with a 3:1 female preponderance
C. Most cases in older adults are multiple adenomas
D. Elderly patients are less likely to present with kidney stones, but instead, they are more likely to have neuropsychiatric complaints compared to younger patients

41. False about Parathyroid disease and geriatric patients is:

A. Minimally invasive parathyroid surgery should not be offered to elderly patients following the same algorithm as younger patients since the rate of multigland disease is different
B. If surgical treatment had to be done, it would be most cost effective for patients age 50 years or older with an expected life expectancy of 5 years or longer to be surgically treated on
C. There is a significant increase in bone mineral density and a decreased risk of fracture following the surgery
D. Parathyroid hormone surgery in elderly has shown to improve quality of life and increased fracture-free survival

42. False about Breast disease and geriatric patients is:

A. Increasing age is a major risk factor for developing breast cancer, with an estimated 21% of newly diagnosed cases in patients older than age 70 years
B. The painless mass represents the most common symptom of breast cancer
C. Breasts become denser with aging, and this makes the clinical examination difficult in older women

D. The American Cancer Society annual mammography begins at age 45 years, with no upper age limit if a woman remains in good health and the U.S. Preventative Services Task Force (USPSTF) recommends screening up to age 74 years

43. False about Breast cancer and geriatric patients is:

A. Breast cancer in older patients tend to be associated with less favorable pathologic prognostic factors

B. Surgical mortality in elderly women in reasonable health is low (<1%)

C. Omitting surgery exposes patients to a higher risk of local relapse and therefore is considered a suboptimal option, even for unfit older women

D. Older patients with tumor size smaller than 2 to 3 cm and no clinical evidence of axillary involvement should be offered a sentinel lymph node biopsy

44. False about Breast cancer and geriatric patients is:

A. For women 70 years of age or older who have early estrogen-receptor–positive breast cancer, the addition of adjuvant radiation therapy to tamoxifen does not significantly decrease the rate of mastectomy for local recurrence

B. Older women treated with mastectomy should be offered chest wall irradiation if they have tumors > 2 cm or > 10 involved axillary lymph nodes

C. Tamoxifen and aromatase inhibitors, such as anastrozole, improve overall survival, reduce local recurrence, and reduce the risk of contralateral breast cancer for hormone-sensitive tumors in older women

D. Older node-negative patients are unlikely to benefit from chemotherapy unless they have large hormone receptor–positive tumors with adverse pathologic characteristics or hormone receptor–negative tumors > 2 cm

45. Guideline recommendations about screening mammography in older women includes all except:

A. AGS guidelines: Offer screening to women aged ≤85 years who have life expectancy ≥5 years and for healthy women aged and ≥85 years who have excellent functional status or who feel strongly about the benefits of screening

B. ACR guidelines: Offer annual screening to women aged ≥40 years and continue as long as a woman is in good health.

C. ACS guidelines: Offer screening to women aged ≥55 years and continue as long as a woman is in good health and has life expectancy of ≥10 years

D. USPSTF guidelines: Offer biennial screening to women aged 50–74 years. Evidence is insufficient to recommend for or against screening in women >74 years of age

46. False about esophageal changes in geriatric population:

A. Dysfunction of the proximal aspects of swallowing is noted during normal aging

B. Resting upper esophageal sphincter pressure and relaxation are decreased in the older normal population compared with a younger control population

C. Dysmotility of the cricopharyngeus (upper esophageal sphincter) with increasing age can result in Zenker diverticula

D. The duration of oropharyngeal swallowing and the sensory threshold for initiating a swallow are decreased with advancing age

47. False about esophageal disease and geriatric patients is:

A. Older patients with severe esophagitis are more likely to have severe heartburn

B. Due to laxity at the gastroesophageal junction, there is also an increased incidence of sliding hiatal hernia with aging

C. The complications of GERD, including erosive esophagitis, Barrett esophagus, and esophageal adenocarcinoma, are seen with an increased frequency in older patients

D. 90% of older patients, report relief of symptoms, particularly vomiting and aspiration, after a Nissen procedure

48. False about esophageal disease and geriatric patients is:

A. Paraesophageal hernias also increase with advancing age and can reach enormous size without symptoms

B. Patients age 70 years or older compared to younger patients with esophageal cancer have worse overall survival

C. The difference in survival is observed between the elderly and the younger patients if surgical resection is performed

D. Watchful waiting is generally recommended, rather than immediate surgery for asymptomatic paraesophageal hernias

49. False about gastric disease and geriatric patients is:

A. Studies have shown that between 25% - 80% of older adults have fasting achlorhydria
B. Up to 80% of peptic ulcer–related deaths occur in patients > 65 years old
C. When compared with older patients, the use of NSAIDs increases the risk of developing complicated peptic ulcer disease in younger patients
D. 80% of all ulcer-related deaths in older patients are in patients taking NSAIDs

50. Risk factors for operative mortality in a perforated ulcer includes:

A. > 48 hours of perforation
B. The presence of concomitant disease
C. Preoperative shock
D. All of the above

51. False about gastric cancer and geriatric patients is:

A. The incidence of gastric cancer rises progressively with age, with most patients between the ages of 50 and 70 years old at presentation
B. Chronic atrophic gastritis and H. pylori infection are risk factors for gastric lymphoma and its precursor, mucosal-associated lymphoid tissue
C. Older patients who present with a predominance of intestinal-type tumors tend to have the less aggressive diffuse type
D. Between younger and older patients, there is no difference in being able to resect or the rate of positive lymph nodes found at surgery (60%–70%)

52. False about biliary tract disease and geriatric patients is:

A. The prevalence of gallstones increases with increasing age
B. Biliary tract disease is the single most common cause of acute abdominal complaints in patients > 65 years old
C. Even though complications of the disease are less common in those of advanced age, biliary colic is seen more than half as often in older as compared to younger patients
D. Recurrence of CBD stones after sphincterotomy, even with antecedent or subsequent cholecystectomy, is higher in older than in younger patients (20% vs. 4%)

53. Even in the presence of acute cholecystitis, older patients may have no abdominal tenderness in upto:

A. 25%
B. 50%
C. 75%
D. 95%

54. True about Liver disease and geriatric patients is:

A. Tumors of the liver are 20 times more likely to arise from metastatic disease than from primary cancer
B. Patients with colon cancer have a 35% risk for recurrence in the liver, but only 10% to 20% of those identified have resectable disease
C. When determining the appropriateness of resection, it is important to consider the prevalence of insulin, resistance, and non-alcoholic fatty liver disease since it is higher in elderly patients
D. All of the above

55. False about Small bowel obstruction (SBO) and geriatric patients is:

A. Small bowel obstruction (SBO) is the most common and surgically relevant disorder of small intestinal function encountered in older persons
B. Gallstone ileus, accounts for 1% - 3% of all SBOs but has been implicated in as many as 25% of obstructions in patients > 65 years old with no abdominal wall hernia or history of previous surgery
C. Of the deaths associated with SBO, 50% occur in patients > 70 years old
D. Luminal obstruction, other than from deliberately ingested objects, accounts for < 50% of cases and most cases of this type of obstruction occur in older adults

56. False about Appendicitis and geriatric patients is:

A. 5% to 10% of cases present in old age
B. The classic presentation of appendicitis is only present in < 50% of older patients
C. Almost all older patients with acute appendicitis will present with abdominal pain, only 50% - 75% will have pain localized to the right lower quadrant
D. Almost 33% of patients will have diffuse nonlocalizable abdominal pain

57. False about Appendicitis and geriatric patients is:

A. Over 50% of older patients will have perforated appendicitis identified at operation

B. Signs of acute appendicitis are unreliable in older adults

C. The WBC count and temperature are normal in 20% - 50% of older patients with appendicitis

D. Symptoms like nausea, vomiting, and anorexia are also found more frequently in older patients

58. False about management of appendicitis in geriatric patients is:

A. CT scanning has been advocated because of the atypical presentation of appendicitis, which is a high rate of perforation at the time of presentation, and the expanded differential diagnosis in older adults

B. In older adults, recurrent appendicitis after resolution of the abscess is common and interval appendectomy is therefore necessary in all cases

C. When an older patient presents with signs and symptoms of acute appendicitis, but with a longer duration of symptoms and a lower hematocrit than expected, these signs should raise the concern for colon or appendiceal cancer

D. Despite improvements in diagnosis and management of appendicitis in elderly patients, morbidity and mortality for this group remain high

59. False about Colorectal cancer and geriatric patients is:

A. The annual incidence of colon cancer is almost 40 times higher for patients > 85 years old compared with individuals who are 40 - 44 years of age

B. Increasing age is a poor prognostic factor in colorectal cancer

C. Patients > 75 years old have a significantly decreased 5-year, disease-free survival compared with younger patients

D. Compared to younger patients, older patients have an increased incidence of left-sided cancers

60. The USPSTF recommends screening for colorectal cancer in adults beginning at age:

A. 45 years B. 50 years

C. 55 years D. 60 years

61. False about Colorectal cancer and geriatric patients is:

A. Screening trials indicate that a difference in colorectal cancer mortality between screened and unscreened persons does not become noticeable until at least 5 years after screening

B. Coloanal reconstruction can achieve continence in almost 80% of older individuals

C. Cardiopulmonary morbidity appears to be higher in older patients undergoing minimally invasive approach to resection of colorectal cancer

D. Even in patients older than 80 years old, elective operative mortality rates are only approximately 2%

62. False about management of Colorectal cancer and geriatric patients is:

A. When surgery is performed as an emergency, mortality increases 3-fold to 4-fold over elective mortality for similar procedures

B. In older patients with both colon and rectal cancers, the 5-year mortality following surgical resection is 1.5 to 2.5 times greater than for younger patients

C. Mortality rates after liver resection for mets in older adults are > 15%

D. The poorer survival seen in older patients with colorectal cancer may be a result of the reduced use of adjuvant therapy in this group

63. False about abdominal wall hernias in geriatric patients is:

A. The estimated incidence of abdominal wall hernia in persons > 65 years old is 4-fold to 8-fold higher incidence in men than in women

B. Older adults are also at risk for the more occult types of hernias, such as paraesophageal hernias and obturator hernias

C. Intestinal resection is required in up to 12% - 20% of incarcerated inguinal hernias and in as many as 40% of incarcerated femoral hernias

D. Approximately 45% - 60% of hernia repairs for older adults are performed on an emergent basis

64. False about Abdominal Aortic Aneurysm in geriatric patients is:

A. Males 85 years old and older have almost 5 times the perioperative mortality rate of younger men, and females 85 years old and older have over 10 times the mortality rate of younger women

B. Octogenarians are easier to treat by endovascular aneurysm repair (EVAR) than younger patients
C. Emergency open repair for rupture is still associated with an operative mortality rate > 50%
D. In older patients, complications occur in approximately 33% of open AAA repairs with infrarenal clamping and in > 50% of those with suprarenal clamping

65. False about Carotid artery disease in geriatric patients is:

A. In patients > 65 - 80 years old, the stroke rate from surgery is approximately 2.8% and the mortality rate is 2.4%
B. Survival of patients > 80 years old after carotid endarterectomy is less as compares to that in the general population
C. Patients > 75 years old have increased arch calcium deposits and increased arch tortuosity compared with younger patients
D. Carotid stenting has an increased risk of adverse cerebrovascular events in elderly patients, but mortality is equivalent to younger patients

66. False about Peripheral vascular disease in geriatric patients is:

A. It is clear that older patients certainly do better than younger patients after infrageniculate bypass surgery
B. In patients > 80 years old, the mortality rate associated with surgery is < 5%, and limb salvage rates over a period of 3 to 5 years are 50% to almost 90%
C. Treatment of graft infections in older patients is morbid, but aggressive wound care and muscle flap coverage are an option with good results (>50% graft salvage and 90% limb salvage)
D. Amputation can be performed safely in older patients, with rates of perioperative mortality < 10%

67. False about Coronary Artery Disease in geriatric patients is:

A. > 50% of CABG procedures are now performed on patients > 65 years old
B. Older patients referred for cardiac surgery have a higher incidence of advanced disease and more symptomatic disease and require emergency or urgent procedures more often
C. In individuals > 80 years old, coronary artery bypass surgery is associated with an acceptable overall mortality of 7% - 12%
D. The rates of 1-year all-cause death were nearly 10 times higher in octogenarians than in nonoctogenarians

68. Preoperative risk factors for mortality after coronary bypass surgery (CABG) includes all except:

A. NYHA functional class III
B. Severe left ventricular dysfunction
C. Mitral insufficiency requiring a combined procedure
D. Elevated preoperative creatinine level

69. False about Valvular Disease in geriatric patients is:

A. TAVR may be a safe approach in high-risk octogenarians because there is lower likelihood of developing AKI, bleeding, requiring blood transfusion, or transfer to a skilled nursing facility
B. Mitral valve regurgitation occurs in more than 10% of those 75 years old or older, and up to 50% of patients with untreated disease will experience heart failure with 5-year mortality
C. Transcatheter mitral valve replacement and transcatheter mitral valve repair are emerging as an alternative therapy for severe mitral regurgitation in high-risk surgical patients
D. Bioprosthetic valves require anticoagulation and are somewhat less durable, but bioprosthetic valves may suffice for patients with a life expectancy of <10 years

70. False about Lung cancer in geriatric patients is:

A. The incidence of non–small-cell lung cancer (NSCLC) decreases with age
B. Aggressive chemotherapy, particularly platinum-based adjuvant therapy, is often poorly tolerated by older patients
C. There is a significant interaction in poor performance status with age, favouring cisplatin-based treatment in younger patients (<70 years old) and carboplatin-based treatment in older patients
D. 5-year survival in older patients after pulmonary resection for cancer is approximately 35%, with up to 40% survival in patients undergoing just lobectomy

71. False about trauma in geriatric patients is:

A. Persons > 65 years old account for up to 33% of trauma cases and 30% to 40% of trauma deaths

B. Motor vehicle accidents are the most common form of fatal injury in patients < 80 years old, and falls are the most frequent fatal injury after the age of 80 years
C. The incidence of death from motor vehicle accidents in older adults is the same whether they are passengers or pedestrians
D. The incidence of fracture or serious injury from a fall is as high as 80% in an older person

72. In older burns persons, a poor prognosis is estimated when the TBSA involved is:

A. > 20%
B. > 30%
C. > 40%
D. > 50%

73. False about transplantation in geriatric patients is:

A. There is no proven benefit of renal transplantation for the elderly
B. The main cause of organ loss in older patients was death with a functioning kidney
C. The survival rate at 10 years in those > 60 years old is 44% versus 81% for younger patients
D. The high incidence of lymphoproliferative disorders in older transplant patients in general and the high rate of recurrent hepatitis C in older liver transplant patients in particular may be the result of excessive immunosuppression in this already compromised population

ANSWERS

1. **Ans: D. All of the above**

   Ref: Chapter No.13, Page No.284-285

2. **Ans: D. All of the above**

   Ref: Chapter No.13, Page No.285

3. **Ans: B. Decreased diastolic dysfunction**

   Ref: Chapter No.13, Page No.289

4. **Ans: A. Decrease in PaO_2 and increase in $PaCO_2$**

   Ref: Chapter No.13, Page No.289

5. **Ans: D. Increased glomerular filtration rate**

   Ref: Chapter No.13, Page No.289

6. **Ans: C. Decreased synthetic capacity**

   Ref: Chapter No.13, Page No.290

7. **Ans: B. Decrease in inflammatory cytokines**

   Ref: Chapter No.13, Page No.290

8. **Ans: D. Cardiac output and ejection fraction are decreased**

   Ref: Chapter No.13, Page No.286-287

9. **Ans: A. Lifestyle modifications, natural compounds, and hormone therapies are useful for hypertension in elderly**

   Ref: Chapter No.13, Page No.287-288

10. **Ans: A. Ventilatory responses to hypoxia and hypercapnia fall by 70% and 80%, respectively**

    Ref: Chapter No.13, Page No.288

11. **Ans: C. Circulating levels of erythropoietin (EPO) are lower in the healthy elderly as compared to younger individuals**

    Ref: Chapter No.13, Page No.289-290

12. **Ans: B. Immunoglobulin M (IgM) levels increase, whereas IgG and IgA levels decrease slightly**

    Ref: Chapter No.13, Page No.291

13. **Ans: D. All of the above**

    Ref: Chapter No.13, Page No.292

14. **Ans: C. Total possible Mini-Cog scores range from 0 to 5 points, with 0 to 3 suggesting high likelihood of cognitive impairment**

    Ref: Chapter No.13, Page No.293-294

15. **Ans: D. All of the above**

    Ref: Chapter No.13, Page No.294

16. **Ans: D. All of the above**

    Ref: Chapter No.13, Page No.294

17. **Ans: C. Good nutritional status**

    Ref: Chapter No.13, Page No.294

18. **Ans: C. Hypercarbia**

    Ref: Chapter No.13, Page No.294

19. **Ans: C. An inability to function >4 METs has been associated with decreased perioperative cardiac events and long-term risk**

    Ref: Chapter No.13, Page No.294-295

20. **Ans: B. 3.5 mL/kg/min, represents the basal oxygen consumption of a 70-kg, 40-year-old man at rest**

    Ref: Chapter No.13, Page No.294

21. **Ans: D. Increased appetite**

    Ref: Chapter No.13, Page No.295

22. **Ans: D. Standard anthropomorphic measures take into account the changes in body composition and structure that accompany aging**

    Ref: Chapter No.13, Page No.295-296

23. **Ans: D. The SGA is used but not been validated in older and critically ill patients**

    Ref: Chapter No.13, Page No.296

24. **Ans: C. 18 factors**

    Ref: Chapter No.13, Page No.296

25. **Ans: D. All of the above**

    Ref: Chapter No.13, Page No.296

26. **Ans: D. All of the above**

    Ref: Chapter No.13, Page No.296

27. **Ans: D. All of the above**

    Ref: Chapter No.13, Page No.296

28. **Ans: A. Utilize opioid using techniques**

    Ref: Chapter No.13, Page No.296

29. **Ans: B. Aspiration**

    Ref: Chapter No.13, Page No.297

30. **Ans: A. Lower overall hospital cost**

    Ref: Chapter No.13, Page No.296

31. **Ans: C. 35%**

    Ref: Chapter No.13, Page No.296

32. **Ans: C. The best treatment for delirium is use of sedatives**

    Ref: Chapter No.13, Page No.297

33. **Ans: B. The routine use of nasogastric tubes in patients undergoing colon resection has been correlated with a decreased risk of aspiration pneumonia**

    Ref: Chapter No.13, Page No.297

34. **Ans: B. 10-fold**

Ref: Chapter No.13, Page No.297

35. **Ans: A. Upright position during meals and for 60 - 75 minutes after meals in those on an oral diet**

Ref: Chapter No.13, Page No.297

36. **Ans: C. Cardiovascular: ↑ Stroke volume, ↑ cardiac output, orthostatic hypotension**

Ref: Chapter No.13, Page No.297

37. **Ans: D. All of the above**

Ref: Chapter No.13, Page No.297-298

38. **Ans: C. By ultrasonography, approximately 70% of patients older than 65 years old have nodules**

Ref: Chapter No.13, Page No.298-299

39. **Ans: C. Patients > 60 years old have a decreased risk for local recurrence, and patients < 20 years old and > 60 years old have a lower risk for the development of distant metastasis**

Ref: Chapter No.13, Page No.299

40. **Ans: C. Most cases in older adults are multiple adenomas**

Ref: Chapter No.13, Page No.299

41. **Ans: A. Minimally invasive parathyroid surgery should not be offered to elderly patients following the same algorithm as younger patients since the rate of multigland disease is different**

Ref: Chapter No.13, Page No.299

42. **Ans: C. Breasts become denser with aging, and this makes the clinical examination difficult in older women**

Ref: Chapter No.13, Page No.299-300

43. **Ans: A. Breast cancer in older patients tend to be associated with less favorable pathologic prognostic factors**

Ref: Chapter No.13, Page No.300

44. **Ans: B. Older women treated with mastectomy should be offered chest wall irradiation if they have tumors > 2 cm or > 10 involved axillary lymph nodes**

Ref: Chapter No.13, Page No.300-301

45. **Ans: C. ACS guidelines:** Offer screening to women aged ≥55 years and continue as long as a woman is in good health and has life expectancy of ≥10 years
ACR: American College of Radiology; **ACS:** American Cancer Society; **AGS:** American Geriatrics Society; **USPSTF:** US Preventive Services Task Force

Ref: Chapter No.13, Page No.301

46. **Ans: D. The duration of oropharyngeal swallowing and the sensory threshold for initiating a swallow are decreased with advancing age**

Ref: Chapter No.13, Page No.301

47. **Ans: A. Older patients with severe esophagitis are more likely to have severe heartburn**

Ref: Chapter No.13, Page No.301-302

48. **Ans: C. The difference in survival is observed between the elderly and the younger patients if surgical resection is performed**

Ref: Chapter No.13, Page No.302

49. **Ans: C. When compared with older patients, the use of NSAIDs increases the risk of developing complicated peptic ulcer disease in younger patients**

Ref: Chapter No.13, Page No.302

50. **Ans: D. All of the above**

Ref: Chapter No.13, Page No.302

51. **Ans: C. Older patients who present with a predominance of intestinal-type tumors tend to have the less aggressive diffuse type**

Ref: Chapter No.13, Page No.302

52. **Ans: C. Even though complications of the disease are less common in those of advanced age, biliary colic is seen more than half as often in older as compared to younger patients**

Ref: Chapter No.13, Page No.302-303

53. **Ans: A. 25%**
In the presence of ***acute cholecystitis,*** as many as
- 25% of older patients may have ***no abdominal tenderness***
- 33% have ***no elevation in temperature or WBC count***
- 59% have ***no peritoneal signs in the right upper quadrant***

Ref: Chapter No.13, Page No.302-303

54. **Ans: D. All of the above**

Ref: Chapter No.13, Page No.303

55. **Ans: D. Luminal obstruction, other than from deliberately ingested objects, accounts for < 50% of cases and most cases of this type of obstruction occur in older adults**

Ref: Chapter No.13, Page No.303-304

56. **Ans: B. The classic presentation of appendicitis is only present in < 50% of older patients**

Ref: Chapter No.13, Page No.304

57. **Ans: D. Symptoms like nausea, vomiting and anorexia are also found more frequently in older patients**

Ref: Chapter No.13, Page No.304

58. **Ans: B. In older adults, recurrent appendicitis after resolution of the abscess is common and interval appendectomy is therefore necessary in all cases**

Ref: Chapter No.13, Page No.304-305

59. **Ans: D. Older patients have an increased incidence of left-sided cancers**

Ref: Chapter No.13, Page No.305

60. **Ans: B. 50**
The **USPSTF (U.S. Preventive Services Task Force)** recommends screening for colorectal cancer in adults ***beginning at age 50*** and continuing ***until age 75*** for average risk individuals

Recommendations for screening include:

- **Annual fecal occult blood testing and flexible sigmoidoscopy** ***every 5 years***, with a *full colonoscopy for positive occult blood or an adenomatous polyp on flexible sigmoidoscopy* OR
- **Colonoscopy every** 5 to 10 years

Ref: Chapter No.13, Page No.305

61. **Ans: C. Cardiopulmonary morbidity appears to be higher in older patients undergoing minimally invasive approach to resection of colorectal cancer**

Ref: Chapter No.13, Page No.305

62. **Ans: C. Mortality rates after liver resection for mets in older adults are > 15%**

Ref: Chapter No.13, Page No.305-306

63. **Ans: D. Approximately 45% - 60% of hernia repairs for older adults are performed on an emergent basis**

Ref: Chapter No.13, Page No.307

64. **Ans: B. Octogenarians are easier to treat by endovascular aneurysm repair (EVAR) than younger patients**

Ref: Chapter No.13, Page No.307

65. **Ans: B. Survival of patients > 80 years old after carotid endarterectomy is less as compares to that in the general population**

Ref: Chapter No.13, Page No.307-308

66. **Ans: A. It is clear that older patients certainly do better than younger patients after infrageniculate bypass surgery**

Ref: Chapter No.13, Page No.308

67. **Ans: D. The rates of 1-year all-cause death were nearly 10 times higher in octogenarians than in nonoctogenarians**

Ref: Chapter No.13, Page No.309-310

68. **Ans: A. NYHA functional class III**

Ref: Chapter No.13, Page No.309-310

69. **Ans: D. Bioprosthetic valves require anticoagulation and are somewhat less durable, but bioprosthetic valves may suffice for patients with a life expectancy of <10 years**

Ref: Chapter No.13, Page No.310

70. **Ans: A. The incidence of non–small-cell lung cancer (NSCLC) decreases with age**

Ref: Chapter No.13, Page No.310-311

71. **Ans: D. The incidence of fracture or serious injury from a fall is as high as 80% in an older person**

Ref: Chapter No.13, Page No.311

72. **Ans: C. > 40%**

Ref: Chapter No.13, Page No.311

73. **Ans: A. There is no proven benefit of renal transplantation for the elderly**

Ref: Chapter No.13, Page No.312

14

Anesthesiology Principles, Pain Management and Conscious Sedation

PHARMACOLOGIC PRINCIPLES

1. **False among the following is:**
   A. Ether was characterized by notoriously slow induction and equally delayed emergence but could produce unconsciousness, amnesia, analgesia, and lack of movement without the addition of other agents
   B. Both induction and emergence were slower with nitrous oxide
   C. Chloroform was associated with hepatic toxicity and occasionally, fatal cardiac arrhythmias
   D. Isoflurane and sevoflurane have intermediate rates of induction and emergence

2. **Minimum alveolar concentration (MAC) is the concentration of volatile agent required to prevent movement in response to a skin incision in:**
   A. 20% of patients B. 50% of patients
   C. 70% of patients D. 100% of patients

3. **False about minimum alveolar concentration (MAC) is:**
   A. Higher MAC represents a less potent volatile anesthetic
   B. Halothane is the most potent with a MAC of 0.75%
   C. Nitrous oxide has a MAC of 104% at sea level, meaning that nitrous oxide alone is suitable for maintenance of general anesthesia
   D. Desflurane has a MAC of 6%

4. **False about Nitrous oxide is:**
   A. 1-year follow-up of ENIGMA II patients showed an increase in long-term morbidity and mortality with nitrous oxide administration
   B. Nitrous oxide minimally influences respiration and hemodynamics
   C. The most important clinical problem with nitrous oxide is that it is 30 times more soluble than nitrogen and diffuses into closed gas spaces faster than nitrogen diffuses out
   D. ENIGMA II Trial, published in 2014, reported that use of nitrous oxide was not associated with an increased incidence of death, cardiovascular complications, or wound infection in high-risk surgical patients.

5. **Nitrous oxide is contraindicated in:**
   A. Pneumothorax
   B. Small bowel obstruction
   C. Retinal surgery
   D. All of the above

6. **As part of an anesthetic regimen compared to patients randomized to not receive nitrous oxide; The Evaluation of Nitrous Oxide in the Gas Mixture for Anaesthesia (ENIGMA I) Trial, indicated that patients having major surgical procedures had a higher incidence of postoperative complications and severe postoperative nausea and vomiting (PONV) if they received 70% nitrous oxide when the surgery lasts:**
   A. > 1 hour B. > 2 hours
   C. > 4 hours D. > 6 hours

7. **False about isoflurane is:**
   A. Isoflurane has several advantages over halothane, including less reduction in cardiac output, less sensitization to the arrhythmogenic effects of catecholamines, and minimal metabolism
   B. Its pungent odour virtually precludes use for inhalational induction

C. Isoflurane-induced bradycardia, a variable response, can decrease myocardial oxygen consumption
D. In concentrations of 1.0 MAC or less, isoflurane causes little increase in cerebral blood flow and intracranial pressure (ICP) and depresses cerebral metabolic activity more than halothane

8. False about Sevoflurane is:

A. Sevoflurane is pleasant to inhale, thus making it suitable for inhalational induction in children
B. Sevoflurane is associated with faster emergence than isoflurane is, especially in longer cases
C. Sevoflurane is associated with a lower incidence of postoperative somnolence and nausea in the postanaesthetic care unit (PACU)
D. When sevoflurane, halothane, and isoflurane were compared, all 3 of the potent agents increased respiratory resistance in endotracheally intubated non-asthmatics

9. False about Sevoflurane is:

A. The toxicity of Compound A in humans appears clinically important
B. Sevoflurane's cardiovascular side effects are minimal
C. Metabolic transformation of sevoflurane takes place and results in increases in the serum fluoride ion concentration and, in the presence of soda lime or Baralyme, production of compound A
D. Sevoflurane reduced airway resistance more than halothane or isoflurane

10. False about Desflurane is:

A. The most volatile and least potent of the volatile anesthetics, desflurane must be administered through specialized electrically heated vaporizers
B. When exposed to dry CO_2 absorbent, desflurane, isoflurane, and enflurane are partially converted to carbon monoxide
C. Pungent odour precludes inhalational induction
D. Desflurane is associated with tachycardia and hypotension if the inspired concentration is increased too rapidly

11. Which of the following anaesthetic agent is not a potent inhalational anaesthetic agent?

A. Diethyl ether B. Nitrous oxide
C. Halothane D. Sevoflurane

12. Which of the following inhalational agent's speed of induction and emergence is rapid?

A. Diethyl ether B. Isoflurane
C. Halothane D. Sevoflurane

13. Which of the following inhalational agent is suitable for inhalational induction?

A. Enflurane B. Halothane
C. Desflurane D. Isoflurane

14. Which of the following inhalational agent has high sensitization to catecholamines?

A. Enflurane B. Halothane
C. Desflurane D. Isoflurane

15. Among the inhalational anaesthetic agents, minimal decrease in blood pressure is seen in:

A. Enflurane B. Desflurane
C. Sevoflurane D. Isoflurane

16. Among the inhalational anaesthetic agents, marked decrease in blood pressure is seen in:

A. Enflurane B. Desflurane
C. Sevoflurane D. Isoflurane

17. Among the inhalational anaesthetic agents, minimal bronchodilation is seen in:

A. Enflurane B. Desflurane
C. Sevoflurane D. Isoflurane

18. False about propofol is:

A. Propofol is commonly used as a continuous infusion during total IV anesthesia and for sedation during less invasive procedures such as gastrointestinal endoscopy
B. Propofol is a long-acting induction agent that is associated with smooth, nausea-free emergence
C. Limitations of propofol are pain on injection and blood pressure reduction
D. Propofol should be used with caution in patients who may be hypovolemic or who may tolerate hypotension poorly, such as those with severe coronary artery disease

19. The most widely used agent for IV induction of anesthesia is:

A. Etomidate B. Thiopental
C. Propofol D. Ketamine

20. False about Ketamine is:

A. Produces a dissociative state of anesthesia

B. Ketamine is not an appropriate agent for IV induction of asthmatic patients because it increases the bronchomotor tone associated with endotracheal intubation

C. It is the only IV induction agent that increases blood pressure and heart rate and decreases bronchomotor tone

D. Usually associated with increased sympathetic tone, ketamine causes direct cardiac depression that may become evident if given to patients with high pre-anesthetic sympathetic tone, as in patients in hemorrhagic shock

21. False about Ketamine is:

A. In patients in whom ketamine was infused continuously before incision and continued through wound closure, postoperative morphine consumption was significantly lower on postoperative days 1 and 2 than in patients who did not receive ketamine

B. Ketamine causes ventilatory depression and loss of airway reflexes

C. Because of the induction of copious oropharyngeal secretions, a drying agent such as glycopyrrolate is generally administered with ketamine

D. It produces profound amnesia and somatic analgesia & hence, Ketamine can be used as the sole anesthetic for brief, superficial procedures

22. False about Ketamine is:

A. In adults and older children, supplemental benzodiazepines or volatile agents are generally effective in preventing emergence delirium

B. In patients with coronary artery disease, ketamine is usually avoided because tachycardia and increased blood pressure may cause myocardial ischemia

C. Clinically important side effect of ketamine is emergence delirium

D. In patients with increased ICP (e.g., after traumatic brain injury), ketamine may decrease ICP because it is the only IV agent that decreases cerebral blood flow

23. True about Etomidate is:

A. Etomidate is an imidazole compound that produces minimal hemodynamic changes

B. It preserves blood pressure in most patients, etomidate is often chosen as an alternative for induction of patients with cardiovascular disease or severe hypovolemia

C. Major drawbacks include burning pain on injection, abnormal muscular movements (myoclonus), and adrenal suppression when given as a prolonged infusion for sedation of critically ill patients

D. All of the above

24. False about Midazolam is:

A. Its onset of action is acceptably rapid and, even in smaller doses, induces profound amnesia for painful or anxiety-producing events

B. Midazolam is sometimes used for induction but it usually causes marked cardiovascular side effects

C. Midazolam combines powerful anxiolytic and amnesic effects

D. Midazolam is frequently selected for induction of patients for cardiovascular surgery

25. Adrenal suppression is seen with the use of:

A. Etomidate B. Thiopental

C. Propofol D. Ketamine

26. False about Opioids is:

A. As a component of a multifaceted anesthetic, opioids produce profound analgesia and minimal cardiac depression

B. They increase the MAC of potent inhalational agents

C. They provide analgesia that extends through the early post-emergence interval and facilitates smoother awakening from anesthesia

D. In doses 10 to 20 times the analgesic dose, opioids act as complete anesthetics in a high proportion of patients by providing not only analgesia but also hypnosis and amnesia

27. False about Opioids is:

A. Morphine, hydromorphone, and meperidine are inexpensive, intermediate-acting agents that are less commonly used for maintenance of anesthesia than for postoperative analgesia

B. Fentanyl, a synthetic opioid that is 100 to 150 times more potent than morphine

C. Remifentanil accumulates during prolonged infusions and is therefore often used as part of IV anesthetics

D. Methadone is a long-acting opioid that is not only a potent μ-opioid receptor agonist but also interacts with N-methyl-D.-aspartate (NMDA) receptors and alters the reuptake of serotonin and norepinephrine in the brain

28. False about Succinylcholine is:

A. It is the only depolarizing agent still in clinical use, remains popular for endotracheal intubation because of its rapid onset and short duration of action

B. It is associated with serious hazards, including hyperkalemia and malignant hyperthermia, in a small proportion of patients

C. At high doses, onset of muscle relaxation is rapid (60–90 seconds), which facilitates rapid intubation in patients at risk for aspiration

D. A patient who cannot be ventilated by mask after succinylcholine administration will likely resume spontaneous breathing before the onset of life-threatening hypoxemia

29. The side effects of succinylcholine includes all except:

A. Life-threatening hyperkalemia in patients with burns

B. Tachycardia

C. Quadriplegia

D. Paraplegia

30. True about Succinylcholine is:

A. Succinylcholine, alone or when combined with a volatile agent, is also implicated in triggering malignant hyperthermia in susceptible individuals

B. Succinylcholine is a depolarizing agent that causes visible muscle fasciculations, it has been implicated in causing postoperative muscle pain, which can be reduced by pre-treatment with a small, precurarization dose of a non-depolarizing agent

C. Because its duration of action is only 5 minutes, a patient who cannot be successfully intubated can be ventilated by mask for a short time until spontaneous respiration resumes

D. All of the above

31. False about Non-depolarizing relaxants is:

A. If a non-depolarizer is used only after intubation, smaller doses are required

B. Other anesthetic drugs potentiate the actions of non-depolarizing agents

C. Succinylcholine used for intubation decreases subsequent requirements for non-depolarizers

D. The inhalational agent isoflurane potentiates the effects of vecuronium approximately 20% more than desflurane does

32. False about train-of-four (TOF) is:

A. At the conclusion of anesthesia, a TOF ratio > 0.90 has been considered adequate return of neuromuscular function

B. TOF ratio means that the 4th of 4 muscle twitches in response to supramaximal stimuli delivered at 0.5-second intervals to the ulnar nerve is at least 1000% of the magnitude of the first twitch

C. Recent studies show that patients with TOF ratios lower than 0.9 have an increased incidence of postoperative respiratory complications and delayed PACU discharge

D. Satisfactory return of neuromuscular function requires return of the TOF ratio to greater than 0.90 and ideally to 1.0

33. False about Sugammadex among the following is:

A. Sugammadex is a cyclodextrin that directly binds non-depolarizing steroidal neuromuscular blocking agents such as rocuronium and vecuronium

B. Sugammadex rapidly reverses neuromuscular blockade and but doesn't avoid the muscarinic side effects associated with use of anticholinesterases

C. Dosing of sugammadex is based on the depth of neuromuscular blockade

D. Sugammadex administration eliminated residual neuromuscular blockade in the PACU and shortened the time of readiness for discharge from the operating room

PATIENT MONITORING DURING AND AFTER ANESTHESIA

34. The most commonly cannulated artery for invasive blood pressure monitoring is:

A. Ulnar artery

B. Radial artery

C. Femoral artery

D. Posterior tibial artery

35. Indications for invasive blood pressure monitoring include:

A. Morbidly obese patients

B. Need for multiple blood gas analyses

C. During high-risk surgical procedures

D. All of the above

36. Possible complications of intra-arterial monitoring are:

A. Arterial embolization B. Neurologic injury
C. Hematoma D. All of the above

37. False about ventilation monitoring during anaesthesia is:

A. Precordial and esophageal stethoscopes provide continuous input regarding air movement and the development of wheezing
B. The advent of end-tidal CO_2 ($ETCO_2$) monitoring has greatly enhanced the monitoring of ventilation and detection of esophageal intubation
C. $ETCO_2$ will increase during periods of decreased cardiac output and pulmonary perfusion
D. The gradient between end-tidal and arterial CO_2 reflects dead space ventilation, which is increased in cases of decreased pulmonary blood flow, such as pulmonary air embolism or thromboembolism and decreased cardiac output.

38. In normal individuals, the difference between $ETCO_2$ and $PaCO_2$ is:

A. 2 to 5 mm Hg B. 2 to 5 cm of H_2O
C. 5 to 8 mm Hg D. 5 to 8 cm of H_2O

39. During general anaesthesia, the most common site for temperature measurement is:

A. External ear temperature
B. Esophageal temperature
C. Anus temperature
D. Axilla temperature

40. The most common sites of monitoring of neuromuscular monitoring is/are:

A. Masseter muscles
B. Temporalis muscle
C. Orbicularis oculi muscles
D. Brachioradialis

41. Techniques for assessing neuromuscular blockade are all except:

A. Train-of-Four
B. Triple-Burst Stimulation
C. Tetany: Sustained 50- or 100-Hz Burst
D. Accelerometry

42. In Train-of-Four, clinical relaxation requires:

A. 90% to 95% blockade
B. 75% to 95% blockade
C. 50% to 75% blockade
D. 35% to 55% blockade

43. False about central nervous system monitoring during anaesthesia is:

A. Intraoperative electroencephalogram signal processing has resulted in the development of the bispectral index (BIS) array, which is believed to monitor awareness during anesthesia
B. The monitor is essentially a modified electroencephalogram that assesses brain wave activity and reports numbers from 0 to 100, which correlate with the level of awareness
C. A value of 100 represents complete awareness and 0 represents complete suppression of brain wave activity
D. Data suggest that BIS is not an accurate indicator of the depth of anesthesia

44. During general anesthesia, BIS value that may be associated with increased perioperative morbidity, including myocardial infarction and stroke in high-risk patients is:

A. < 50 for more than 2 minutes
B. < 50 for more than 5 minutes
C. < 40 for more than 2 minutes
D. < 40 for more than 5 minutes

PREOPERATIVE EVALUATION

45. Unless a significant change in the patient's medical status has occurred, before surgery laboratory tests need not be repeated if performed within:

A. 1 month B. 3 months
C. 6 months D. 12 months

46. For performing an airway examination mouth opening should be:

A. 2–4 cm B. 4–6 cm
C. 6–8 cm D. 1–2 cm

47. For performing an airway examination thyromental distance should be:

A. 2–4 cm B. 4–6 cm
C. 6–8 cm D. 1–2 cm

48. Important factors in performing an airway examination are:

A. Cervical spine mobility
B. Mallampati classification

C. Neck circumference
D. All of the above

49. Following image shows which class of Mallampati classification:

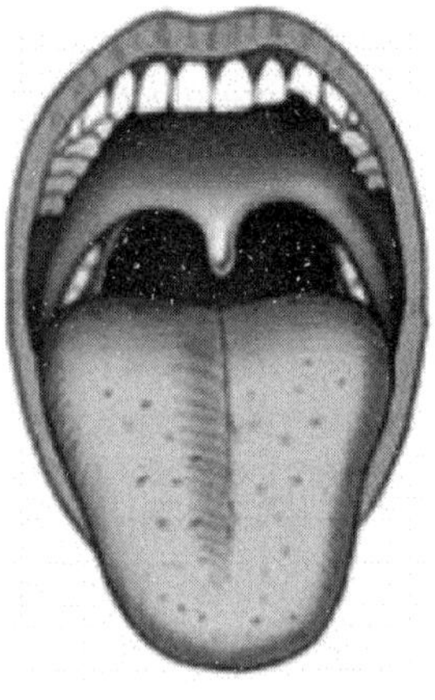

A. Class I
B. Class II
C. Class III
D. Class IV

50. Following image shows which class of Mallampati classification:

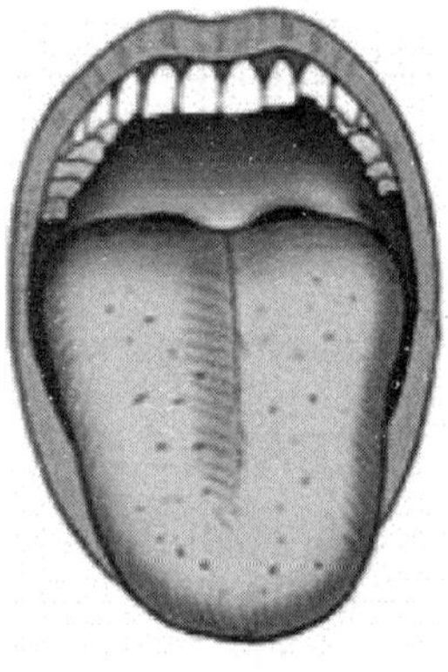

A. Class I
B. Class II
C. Class III
D. Class IV

51. Following image shows which class of Mallampati classification:

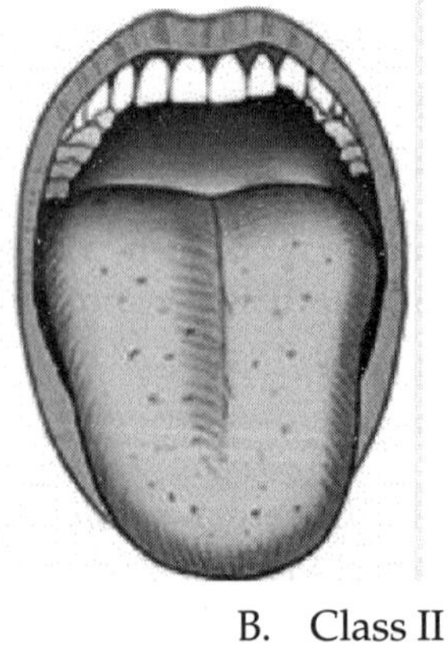

A. Class I
B. Class II
C. Class III
D. Class IV

52. Good functional capacity is defined as:

A. >10 METs
B. 7–10 METs
C. 4–6 METs
D. <4 METs

53. Which of the following is an assessment tool for functional capacity?

A. Duke Activity Status Index
B. Goldman Specific Activity Scale
C. Specific Activity Scale
D. All of the above

54. Recommendations for supplemental preoperative evaluation with 12-Lead ECG is:

A. Preoperative resting 12-lead ECG is reasonable for patients with known coronary heart disease or other significant structural heart disease, except for low-risk surgery
B. Preoperative resting 12-lead ECG may be considered for asymptomatic patients, except for low-risk surgery
C. Routine preoperative resting 12-lead ECG is not useful for asymptomatic patients undergoing low-risk surgical procedures
D. All of the above

55. For patients who have undergone angioplasty, it is recommended that surgery be delayed a minimum of:

A. 10 days
B. 7 days
C. 14 days
D. 30 days

56. For patients who receive bare metal stents (BMSs), it is recommended that surgery be delayed a minimum of:

A. 10 days
B. 7 days
C. 14 days
D. 30 days

57. Recommendations for perioperative medical management with regards to perioperative statin therapy are all except:

A. Continue statins in patients currently taking statins
B. Perioperative initiation of statin use is not reasonable in patients undergoing vascular surgery
C. Perioperative initiation of statins may be considered in patients procedures
D. All of the above are true

58. Recommendations for perioperative medical management with regards to perioperative antiplatelet agents are all except:

A. Continue DAPT in patients undergoing urgent noncardiac surgery during the first 4 to 6 weeks after BMS or DES implantation, unless the risk of bleeding outweighs the benefit of stent thrombosis prevention
B. In patients with stents undergoing surgery that requires discontinuation P2Y12 inhibitors, continue aspirin and restart the P2Y12 platelet receptor–inhibitor as soon as possible after surgery
C. In patients undergoing nonemergency/non-urgent non-cardiac surgery without prior coronary stenting, it may be reasonable to continue aspirin when the risk of increased cardiac events outweighs the risk of increased bleeding
D. Initiation or continuation of aspirin is beneficial in patients undergoing elective non-cardiac non-carotid surgery who have not had previous coronary stenting

59. Recommendations for perioperative medical management with regards to perioperative beta blocker therapy are all except:

A. Continue beta blockers in patients who are on beta blockers chronically
B. In patients with ≥2 RCRI factors, it may be reasonable to begin beta blockers before surgery
C. In patients with a long-term indication but no other RCRI risk factors, it may be reasonable to begin beta blockers
D. Beta-blocker therapy should not be started on the day of surgery

60. After DES implantation, non-cardiac surgery should be delayed for:

A. 30 days B. 60 days
C. 180 days D. 365 days

61. Elective non-cardiac surgery after DES implantation may be considered after:

A. 30 days B. 60 days
C. 180 days D. 365 days

62. False about endocarditis prophylaxis is:

A. Antibiotic prophylaxis is not recommended based solely on an increased lifetime risk of developing IE and should be reserved for patients at highest risk
B. The AHA panel recommends that antibiotic prophylaxis is reasonable for dental procedures that involve manipulation of gingival tissues
C. Antibiotic prophylaxis solely to prevent IE is recommended for genitourinary or gastrointestinal tract procedures
D. Alternative drugs and routes are recommended for patients who are unable to take oral medications or those with penicillin allergy

63. For recommended procedures and indications, for endocarditis prophylaxis the drug of choice is:

A. Oral erythromycin
B. Oral amoxicillin
C. Oral azithromycin
D. Oral clindamycin

64. Cardiac conditions associated with the highest risk of adverse outcome from endocarditis for which prophylaxis with dental procedures is reasonable are all except:

A. Prosthetic cardiac valve or prosthetic material used for cardiac valve repair
B. Previous infective endocarditis
C. Completely repaired congenital heart defect with prosthetic material or device, whether placed by surgery or by catheter intervention, during the first 12 months after the procedure
D. Cardiac transplantation recipients who develop cardiac valvulopathy

65. Relative risk associated with postoperative pulmonary complication is highest with:

A. Age >60 years
B. ASA class >II
C. Congestive heart failure
D. Emergency surgery

66. A strong predictor of pulmonary complications is serum albumin concentration of:

A. < 4.0 g/dL B. < 3.5 g/dL
C. < 3.0 g/dL D. < 2.5 g/dL

67. False about perioperative risk associated with pre-existing pulmonary disease is:

A. Current smoking was a minor predictor of pulmonary complications
B. The presence of obesity or mild to moderate asthma was significantly associated with perioperative pulmonary complications
C. Obstructive sleep apnea (OSA) is an increasingly common condition in surgical patients that requires preoperative evaluation and optimization.

D. Procedures with an increased risk for pulmonary complications include abdominal surgery, thoracic surgery, neurosurgery, head and neck surgery, and vascular surgery

68. Chronic renal insufficiency (CRI) provides many perioperative management challenges, including:

A. Acid-base abnormalities
B. Coagulation disorders
C. Electrolyte disturbances
D. All of the above

69. To avoid the fluid and electrolyte shifts that occur immediately after dialysis, dialysis is performed:

A. 6 to 12 hours before surgery
B. 12 to 18 hours before surgery
C. 18 to 24 hours before surgery
D. 24 to 48 hours before surgery

70. False about perioperative management of diabetic patients undergoing surgery is:

A. Insulin pumps should be continued at sleep basal rates
B. Plasma glucose concentrations should be checked before surgery and before discharge as a minimum
C. Metformin is usually continued on the day of surgery
D. Provide a reduced dose of intermediate-acting or long-acting insulin and hold short-acting insulin on the morning of surgery

71. Perioperative minimum fasting period for clear liquids is:

A. 2 hours B. 4 hours
C. 6 hours D. 8 hours

72. Perioperative minimum fasting period for infant formula is:

A. 2 hours B. 4 hours
C. 6 hours D. 8 hours

73. Perioperative minimum fasting period for breast milk is:

A. 2 hours B. 4 hours
C. 6 hours D. 8 hours

74. Examples of clear liquids are all except:

A. Water
B. Fruit juices with pulp
C. Carbonated beverages
D. Black coffee

75. What is the ASA class of a 53-year-old male who is declared brain-dead?

A. ASA class III B. ASA class IV
C. ASA class V D. ASA class VI

76. A 63-year-old female with unstable angina has an ASA class of:

A. ASA class III B. ASA class IV
C. ASA class V D. ASA class VI

77. A 75-year-old male with uncontrolled hypertension has an ASA class of:

A. ASA class II B. ASA class III
C. ASA class IV D. ASA class V

78. A 58-year-old male with previous myocardial infarction has an ASA class of:

A. ASA class II B. ASA class III
C. ASA class IV D. ASA class V

79. A 75-year-old male with uncomplicated diabetes mellitus an ASA class of:

A. ASA class II B. ASA class III
C. ASA class IV D. ASA class I

80. A 40-year-old male with head injury has intracranial hemorrhage with elevated ICP. What is his ASA class?

A. ASA class II B. ASA class III
C. ASA class IV D. ASA class V

81. A otherwise healthy 22-year-old male patient was undergoing emergency appendectomy. What is his ASA class?

A. ASA class IIE B. ASA class IIIE
C. ASA class IVE D. ASA class IE

82. A 40-year-old male with road traffic accident has ruptured aortic aneurysm. What is his ASA class?

A. ASA class III B. ASA class IV
C. ASA class V D. ASA class VI

83. A 30-year-old man with no past medical history undergoes emergency hernia repair. He has a 10-pack-per-year smoking history. What is his American Society of Anesthesiologists (ASA) physical status classification?

A. ASA class I B. ASA class IIE
C. ASA class III D. ASA class V

SELECTION OF ANESTHETIC TECHNIQUES AND DRUGS

84. Predictors of perioperative adverse events are:

A. Mallampati classification
B. ASA status
C. Anesthetic technique
D. All of the above

85. The risk for cardiac arrest attributable to anesthesia appears to be:

A. < 1 in 1,000 cases
B. < 1 in 10,000 cases
C. < 1 in 100,000 cases
D. < 1 in 1,000,000 cases

GENERAL ANESTHESIA

86. The 4 components of general anesthesia are all except:

A. Inhibition of noxious reflexes
B. Analgesia
C. Paresthesia
D. Skeletal muscle relaxation

REGIONAL ANESTHESIA

87. False about local anesthetic drugs is:

A. The 2 classes of local anesthetic drugs in common use are amino esters and amino amides (often described as esters and amides).
B. The mechanism of action of local anesthetics is dose-dependent blockade of potassium currents in nerve fibers
C. In general, greater hydrophobicity is associated with greater potency
D. Important characteristics are pKa, protein binding and the degree of hydrophobicity

88. False about liposomal bupivacaine is:

A. The development of liposomal bupivacaine has the potential to prolong analgesia after local administration
B. Liposomal bupivacaine is composed of bupivacaine encapsulated in multivesicular liposomes and can provide up to 24 hours of analgesia after local infiltration
C. Liposomal bupivacaine was approved by the FDA for local wound infiltration and for interscalene block
D. All of the above are true

89. Maximal dose of lidocaine without epinephrine is:

A. 2 mg/kg B. 3 mg/kg
C. 5 mg/kg D. 7 mg/kg

90. Maximal dose of lidocaine with epinephrine is:

A. 5 mg/kg B. 7 mg/kg
C. 10 mg/kg D. 15 mg/kg

91. The earliest signs of an overdose or inadvertent intravascular injection of local anesthetic are all except:

A. Metallic taste
B. Numbness or tingling of the tongue or lips
C. Vomiting
D. Light-headedness

92. False about local anesthetic drugs is:

A. In healthy male volunteers, slow IV infusion of levobupivacaine reduced the mean stroke index, acceleration index, and ejection fraction less than racemic bupivacaine did
B. Bupivacaine decreased QRS width during sinus rhythm
C. Ropivacaine, a newer potent amide local anesthetic, was compared to bupivacaine and lidocaine in volunteers receiving a slow IV infusion until CNS symptoms first occurred
D. Regional anesthesia was first produced with cocaine (also a local anesthetic) for subarachnoid block in the late 1800s

93. Lipid emulsion therapy is:

A. American Society of Regional Anesthesia and Pain Medicine recommend bolus injection of 1.5 mL/kg (lean body mass) of 30% lipid emulsion over 1 minute followed by an infusion of 0.25 mL/kg/min
B. American Society of Regional Anesthesia and Pain Medicine recommend bolus injection of 2.5 mL/kg (lean body mass) of 30% lipid emulsion over 1 minute followed by an infusion of 0.25 mL/kg/min
C. American Society of Regional Anesthesia and Pain Medicine recommend bolus injection of 1.5 mL/kg (lean body mass) of 20% lipid emulsion over 1 minute followed by an infusion of 0.25 mL/kg/min
D. American Society of Regional Anesthesia and Pain Medicine recommend bolus injection of 2.5 mL/kg (lean body mass) of 20% lipid emulsion over 1 minute followed by an infusion of 0.25 mL/kg/min

94. False about spinal anesthesia is:

A. Spinal anesthesia is induced by the injection of local anesthetic, with or without opiates, into the subdural space
B. The addition of small doses of fentanyl (e.g., 20 µg) or morphine (e.g., 0.25 mg) will prolong the duration of analgesia and increase the duration of analgesia and tolerance for tourniquet pain
C. Bupivacaine and tetracaine have significantly longer durations of action than lidocaine does
D. The addition of epinephrine or phenylephrine, particularly to short-acting local anesthetics, will increase the duration of action

95. False about spinal anesthesia is:

A. Spinal anesthesia is administered as a single bolus injection; therefore, the block is of limited duration and is not suitable for prolonged procedures
B. The practice of continuous spinal anesthesia with the use of small-bore catheters has largely been abandoned because of neurologic complications associated with local anesthetic toxicity
C. Hypertension occurs as a consequence of sympathectomy
D. Complications of subarachnoid block include hypotension (sometimes refractory), bradycardia, postdural puncture headache, transient radicular neuropathy, backache, urinary retention

96. False statement among the following is:

A. When compared to epidural anesthesia, spinal anesthesia has a slower onset, is less predictably satisfactory for surgery
B. Postdural puncture headache occurs after a small proportion of subarachnoid blocks
C. Transient radicular neuropathy, a painful but usually self-limited condition, recently became evident in association with an increase in enthusiasm for the use of lidocaine for subarachnoid block
D. Epidural analgesia would appear to avoid the complication but, if the dura is inadvertently punctured, it leaves a much larger dural rent

97. Factors that increase the postdural puncture headache's incidence includes all except:

A. Male gender
B. Female gender
C. Younger age
D. Larger needles

98. Absolute contraindications to spinal anesthesia includes all except:

A. Decreased ICP
B. Sepsis, bacteremia
C. Infection at the site of injection
D. Therapeutic anticoagulation

99. False about epidural anesthesia is:

A. Induction of epidural anesthesia or analgesia results from injection of local anesthetics, with or without opiates, into the lumbar or thoracic epidural space
B. Local anesthetics or opiates can be administered for several days to provide postoperative analgesia
C. Epidural anesthesia has not been shown to decrease blood loss and deep venous thrombosis during total joint arthroplasty
D. Postoperative epidural analgesia for thoracic surgery provides superior pain control, less sedation, and better pulmonary function than parenteral opiates do

100. False about epidural anesthesia is:

A. The use of epidural analgesia after general anesthesia decreased the incidence of postoperative pneumonia compared to the use of general anesthesia alone
B. Lumbar epidural anesthesia, appears to be associated with more rapid recovery of gastrointestinal function after major abdominal surgery
C. Because of the risk of spinal hematoma, placement and removal of epidural catheters in patients receiving oral or parenteral anticoagulation are performed in conjunction with an anaesthesiologist
D. Advent of low–molecular-weight heparin (LMWH) for prophylaxis of deep venous thrombosis has resulted in an increase in the incidence of epidural hematomas associated with the removal or placement of epidural catheters

101. After treatment with LMWH, an epidural catheter should not be placed earlier than:

A. 6 hours
B. 12 hours
C. 24 hours
D. 48 hours

102. After epidural catheter placement, LMWH should not be started before:

A. 6 hours
B. 12 hours
C. 24 hours
D. 48 hours

103. After the last dose of LMWH, an epidural catheter should not be removed earlier than:

A. 6 hours B. 12 hours
C. 24 hours D. 48 hours

104. After epidural catheter removal, LMWH should not be restarted earlier than:

A. 1 hour B. 2 hours
C. 6 hours D. 8 hours

105. After administration of epidural anesthesia to the T3 dermatome in a patient with severe COPD undergoing open cholecystectomy, which of the following is least likely to occur?

A. Increased heart rate
B. Decreased venous return
C. Decreased alveolar ventilation
D. Systemic hypotension

106. The advantage of peripheral nerve blocks is/are:

A. Avoidance of airway manipulation and the potential complications associated with endotracheal intubation
B. Reduced physiologic stress in comparison to spinal or epidural anesthesia
C. Avoidance of the potential side effects associated with general anesthesia
D. All of the above

107. Abdominal wall blocks are:

A. Rectus sheath block
B. Ilioinguinal-iliohypogastric block
C. Quadratus lumborum block
D. All of the above

108. Following image shows:

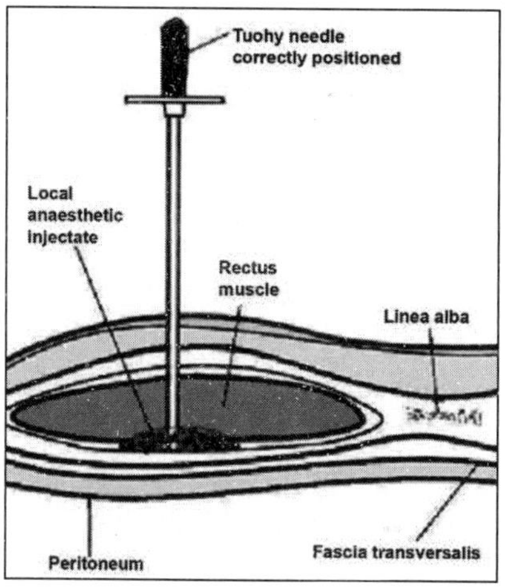

A. Rectus sheath block
B. Ilioinguinal-iliohypogastric block
C. Quadratus lumborum block
D. None of the above

CONSCIOUS SEDATION

109. True statement among the following is/are:

A. Monitored anesthesia care encompasses a wide range of depths of sedation ranging from minimal sedation to brief intervals of complete unconsciousness
B. Drugs used for moderate sedation usually consist of opioids such as fentanyl or morphine, often combined with an anxiolytic such as midazolam
C. When non-anesthesia personnel administer sedation for surgical procedures, the process is generally termed conscious sedation, although the term moderate sedation is preferable
D. All of the above

POSTANESTHESIA CARE

110. In patients > age of 60 who undergo major procedures requiring inpatient care; postoperative delirium is a common complication of surgery and anesthesia that occurs in up to:

A. 20% B. 50%
C. 70% D. 90%

111. True about respiratory problems after anesthesia is/are:

A. Airway obstruction is most commonly due to obstruction of the oropharynx by the tongue or oropharyngeal soft tissues as a result of the residual effects of general anesthetics, pain medications, or muscle relaxants
B. In cases of laryngospasm, continuous positive airway pressure is applied, followed by the administration of 10 to 20 mg of succinylcholine if CPAP is ineffective
C. Refractory obstruction may require the administration of systemic steroids and racemic epinephrine by nebulization
D. All of the above

112. Causes of post operative airway obstruction include:

A. Glottic edema
B. Vocal cord paralysis
C. Laryngospasm
D. All of the above

113. True about postoperative hypoxaemia is:

A. Hypoxemia is a common problem, and administration of supplemental oxygen during transportation to the PACU and during immediate postoperative period decreases the incidence and severity of hypoxemia

B. Treatment of hypoxemia requires the administration of oxygen, assurance of adequate ventilation, and treatment of the underlying causes

C. Hypoxemia must be suspected as an underlying problem in patients exhibiting restlessness, tachycardia, or cardiac irritability

D. All of the above

114. False about postoperative nausea and vomiting (PONV):

A. One of the most annoying problems for both patients and personnel in the PACU is PONV

B. An important complication related to the IV coadministration of ondansetron and metoclopramide has been the production of tachyarrhythmias

C. FDA has placed a so-called black box warning on the use of droperidol in which additional ECG monitoring is required before and after administration of the drug because of an alleged increase in serious cardiac arrhythmias caused by QT prolongation

D. Effective pharmacologic approaches to the treatment of PONV include the use of anticholinergics, serotonin receptor antagonists, antidopaminergics, corticosteroids, and antihistamines

115. Dopamine receptor antagonists (DA-2) among the following are all except:

A. Promethazine B. Chlorpromazine

C. Metoclopramide D. Fluphenazine

116. Anticholinergic drug among the following is:

A. Promethazine B. Chlorpromazine

C. Scopolamine D. Ondansetron

117. Serotonin receptor antagonist among the following is:

A. Promethazine B. Chlorpromazine

C. Scopolamine D. Ondansetron

118. Common side effects of dopamine receptor antagonists (DA-2) among the following are all except:

A. Sedation

B. Dry mouth

C. Extrapyramidal effects

D. Dissociation

119. Important issues related to perioperative hypothermia include all except:

A. Possibility that hypothermia could decrease the rate of surgical infections

B. The risk of increased oxygen consumption postoperatively due to shivering

C. Alterations in drug metabolism

D. Effects on blood coagulation

120. Hypotension in the PACU is most commonly due to all except:

A. Cardiac tamponade

B. Arrhythmias

C. Hypovolemia

D. Left ventricular dysfunction

121. Causes of hypertension in the PACU is/are:

A. Pain B. Anxiety

C. Bladder distention D. All of the above

122. The overall incidence of postoperative visual loss is reported as:

A. 0.2% B. 0.02%

C. 0.5% D. 0.05%

123. Causes of postoperative visual loss include:

A. Cortical blindness:

B. Retinal artery occlusion

C. Ischemic optic neuropathy

D. All of the above

ACUTE PAIN MANAGEMENT

124. False among the following is:

A. The term acute pain refers to pain that is expected to be of relatively short duration and that should resolve with tissue healing or withdrawal of the noxious stimulus

B. Chronic pain, which can persist for years, is defined as pain that persists for at least 1 month beyond the usual course of an acute disease or beyond a reasonable time in which an injury would be expected to heal

C. Chronic pain serves useful function in healing

D. Acute pain generally resolves within minutes, hours, or days

125. **False about the mechanism of acute pain is:**

A. Pain is an unpleasant sensory and emotional experience associated with actual or potential tissue damage or described in terms of such damage

B. Perception, is integral to the subjective and emotional experience

C. Nerve pathways include primary sensory afferents (primarily Aδ and C fibers) that project to the spinal cord, ascending tracts (including the spinothalamic tract) to the brainstem and thalamus

D. Perception, the final step in the nociceptive process, occurs when the pain signal reaches the thalamus

126. **False statement about the methods of analgesia among the following is:**

A. The oral route is the preferred route for analgesic delivery

B. Parenteral administration is preferred for patients experiencing moderate to severe pain, patients who require rapid control of pain, and those who cannot receive agents through the gastrointestinal tract

C. The intramuscular is preferred over IV route and subcutaneous injections when the parenteral route is indicated

D. Intramuscular injections are painful, result in erratic absorption, and lead to variable blood levels of the administered agent

127. **Opioid receptor involved in supraspinal analgesia is:**

A. μ1 receptor B. δ receptor
C. σ receptor D. κ receptor

128. **Opioid receptor involved in spinal analgesia is:**

A. μ1 receptor B. δ receptor
C. σ receptor D. μ2 receptor

129. **False among the following about opioids is:**

A. For moderate to severe pain in patients with renal dysfunction, fentanyl and hydromorphone are not suitable agents

B. Strong opioids are ideal for moderate to severe pain and for pain that is constant in frequency

C. Morphine is metabolized to morphine-3-glucoronide and morphine-6-glucoronide, which can accumulate in patients who have renal impairment

D. Weak opioid agents are suitable for mild to moderate pain that is intermittent in frequency

130. **False among the following about opioids is:**

A. In the setting of acute postoperative pain, the use of opioids has not been shown to be a risk factor for the development of an addiction disorder

B. Meperidine is metabolized to normeperidine, a unique toxic metabolite that can accumulate and cause seizure-like activity

C. Tramadol is an analgesic that is a nonopioid but has some opioid-like effects and is a centrally acting agent that is administered orally and can be used for mild to moderate pain

D. Fentanyl is available in a transdermal preparation, and this route is recommended for acute pain management

131. **False about NSAIDs is:**

A. The mechanism of action is achieved through inhibition of cyclooxygenase (COX) enzyme activity, which results in decreased production of prostaglandins

B. Inhibition of prostaglandin production results in analgesia but can also lead to side effects such as gastric ulceration, bleeding and renal injury

C. Ketorolac is avoided in patients with a history of gastropathy, platelet dysfunction, or thrombocytopenia; in those with a history of allergy to the agent; and in patients with renal impairment or hypovolemia

D. The newer agents (celecoxib, rofecoxib, valdecoxib) are selective COX-1 inhibitors

132. **False about NMDA antagonists is:**

A. Discovery of NMDA antagonists and its role in sensitizing the CNS has led to a re-emergence of this class of agents for the use in management of acute pain in perioperative medicine

B. In the NMDA group, magnesium has also been recognized to possess NMDA antagonist properties

C. If Ketamine is administered via continuous infusion it seems to be ineffective

D. Ketamine has long been recognized as a powerful induction agent with strong analgesic properties, albeit at the expense of psychotropic adverse effects to include dysphoria and, at higher doses of the drug, psychosis

133. **False about Alpha2-Adrenergic agonists:**

A. Aside from analgesic benefits, dexmedetomidine seems to have other preoperative advantages

B. There is a high density of α2-adrenergic receptors in the substantia gelatinosa of the dorsal horn in humans, where it is believed that α2-adrenergic agonists impair the transmission of pain signals
C. Dexmedetomidine has been demonstrated to be effective in perioperative medicine with only transient effects on hemodynamics in exchange for improved analgesia and lower opiate use and lower related opiate side effects
D. Guanfacine is delivered orally and has minimal cardiovascular side effects and is determined to be effective as a perioperative adjunct

134. EMLA cream contains:

A. Prilocaine and bupivacaine
B. Prilocaine and lidocaine
C. Chloroprocaine and bupivacaine
D. Chloroprocaine and lidocaine

135. False statement among the following is:

A. Common analgesia combinations include opioids and NSAIDs in an analgesic regimen or epidural administration of a local anesthetic with an opioid
B. Gabapentin, an anticonvulsant used for the management of chronic neuropathic pain, has shown efficacy for analgesia in the acute postoperative period, including improved pain control and reduced opioid-related side effects
C. Aside from acute pain benefits, gabapentin may play a role in chronic pain as well
D. The goal of pre-emptive analgesia is to influence the analgesic process after initiation of the noxious stimulus (e.g., surgical incision)

136. Effective pre-emptive analgesia results in:

A. Decreased side effects from analgesics
B. Increases postoperative pain
C. Reduced postoperative analgesic requirement
D. Increased compliance with postoperative rehabilitation

137. False about neuraxial analgesia is:

A. Neuraxial routes of administration include the epidural and intrathecal (subarachnoid) routes
B. An important consideration in selecting patients for neuraxial analgesia is the presence of abnormal coagulation, including concurrent use of antiplatelet and anticoagulant agents
C. Opioids, when delivered by the neuraxial route, provide analgesia by their action at opioid receptors located in the anterior horn of the spinal cord
D. Knowledge of coagulation issues is important to minimize the risk for intraspinal bleeding and spinal hematoma formation, which can lead to severe neurologic injury

138. False about neuraxial analgesia is:

A. Morphine is hydrophilic, which accounts for its slow onset of analgesia, long duration of action, ability to provide analgesia over a wide dermatomal distribution, and the risk for late respiratory depression
B. An important determinant of opioid action when delivered by the neuraxial route is the drug's degree of lipid solubility; the drug can travel rostrally to the brain and influence the respiratory centers hours after initial delivery
C. Fentanyl is lipophilic, which accounts for its fast onset and short duration of action, ability to provide segmental analgesia, and limited risk for late respiratory depression
D. A hydrophilic opioid such as morphine, when delivered into the epidural or subarachnoid space, remains in the CSF shorter than a lipophilic opioid does

139. False about intravenous patient-controlled analgesia (PCA) is:

A. Physicians' orders for IV PCA must specify the drug, drug concentration, loading dose, bolus dose, continuous infusion rate (basal rate), lockout interval and dose limits
B. NSAIDs are the agent of choice for IV PCA
C. The preferred agents for IV PCA are opioids, with morphine sulfate most commonly chosen
D. There is an increased risk for complications if staff members are not trained to understand the concept of IV PCA

140. False about chronic pain is:

A. Pain that persists for 3 months beyond the expected time for recovery or initial onset is considered evidence of a chronic pain syndrome
B. Patients with persistent pain frequently use words such as *burning, shooting and shock-like* to describe their pain, which is generally associated with a neuropathic pain syndrome
C. Certain factors that may increase the risk for chronic pain include infection at the surgical site, intraoperative trauma to nerves, diabetes mellitus and nerve entrapment by cancer
D. Treatment modalities include the use of adjuvant medications such as antidepressants and anticonvulsants, nerve blocks, physical therapy and psychological techniques

ANSWERS

1. **Ans: B. Both induction and emergence were slower with nitrous oxide**

   Ref: Chapter No.14, Page No.316

2. **Ans: B. 50% of patients**

   Ref: Chapter No.14, Page No.316

3. **Ans: C. Nitrous oxide has a MAC of 104% at sea level, meaning that nitrous oxide alone is suitable for maintenance of general anesthesia**

   Ref: Chapter No.14, Page No.316

4. **Ans: A. 1-year follow-up of ENIGMA II patients showed an increase in long-term morbidity and mortality with nitrous oxide administration**

   Ref: Chapter No.14, Page No.316

5. **Ans: D. All of the above**

   Ref: Chapter No.14, Page No.316

6. **Ans: B. > 2 hours**

   Ref: Chapter No.14, Page No.316

7. **Ans: C. Isoflurane-induced bradycardia, a variable response, can decrease myocardial oxygen consumption**

   Ref: Chapter No.14, Page No.316-317

8. **Ans: D. When sevoflurane, halothane, and isoflurane were compared, all 3 of the potent agents increased respiratory resistance in endotracheally intubated non-asthmatics**

   Ref: Chapter No.14, Page No.317

9. **Ans: A. The toxicity of compound A. in humans appears clinically important**

   Ref: Chapter No.14, Page No.317

10. **Ans: D. Desflurane is associated with tachycardia and hypotension if the inspired concentration is increased too rapidly**

    Ref: Chapter No.14, Page No.317

11. **Ans: B. Nitrous oxide**

    Ref: Chapter No.14, Page No.316

12. **Ans: D. Sevoflurane**

    Ref: Chapter No.14, Page No.316

13. **Ans: B. Halothane**

    Ref: Chapter No.14, Page No.316

14. **Ans: B. Halothane**

    Ref: Chapter No.14, Page No.316

15. **Ans: B. Desflurane**

    Ref: Chapter No.14, Page No.317

16. **Ans: A. Enflurane**

    Ref: Chapter No.14, Page No.317

17. **Ans: A. Enflurane**

    Ref: Chapter No.14, Page No.317

18. **Ans: B. Propofol is a long-acting induction agent that is associated with smooth, nausea-free emergence**

    Ref: Chapter No.14, Page No.317-318

19. **Ans: C. Propofol**

    Ref: Chapter No.14, Page No.317

20. **Ans: B. Ketamine is not an appropriate agent for IV induction of asthmatic patients because it increases the bronchomotor tone associated with endotracheal intubation**

    Ref: Chapter No.14, Page No.318

21. **Ans: B. Ketamine causes ventilatory depression and loss of airway reflexes**

    Ref: Chapter No.14, Page No.318

22. **Ans: D. In patients with increased ICP (e.g., after traumatic brain injury), ketamine may decrease ICP because it is the only IV agent that decreases cerebral blood flow**

    Ref: Chapter No.14, Page No.318

23. **Ans: D. All of the above**

    Ref: Chapter No.14, Page No.318

24. **Ans: B. Midazolam is sometimes used for induction but it usually causes marked cardiovascular side effects**

    Ref: Chapter No.14, Page No.319

25. **Ans: A. Etomidate**

    Ref: Chapter No.14, Page No.318

26. **Ans: B. They increase the MAC of potent inhalational agents**

    Ref: Chapter No.14, Page No.319

27. **Ans: C. Remifentanil accumulates during prolonged infusions and is therefore often used as part of IV anesthetics**

    Ref: Chapter No.14, Page No.319

28. **Ans: D. A patient who cannot be ventilated by mask after succinylcholine administration will likely resume spontaneous breathing before the onset of life-threatening hypoxemia**

    Ref: Chapter No.14, Page No.319

29. **Ans: B. Tachycardia**

    Ref: Chapter No.14, Page No.319

30. **Ans: D. All of the above**

Ref: Chapter No.14, Page No.319

31. **Ans: D. The inhalational agent isoflurane potentiates the effects of vecuronium approximately 20% more than desflurane does**

Ref: Chapter No.14, Page No.320

32. **Ans: B. TOF ratio means that the 4th of 4 muscle twitches in response to supramaximal stimuli delivered at 0.5-second intervals to the ulnar nerve is at least 1000% of the magnitude of the first twitch**

Ref: Chapter No.14, Page No.320

33. **Ans: B. Sugammadex rapidly reverses neuromuscular blockade and but doesn't avoid the muscarinic side effects associated with use of anticholinesterases**

Ref: Chapter No.14, Page No.320-321

34. **Ans: B. Radial artery**

Ref: Chapter No.14, Page No.322

35. **Ans: D. All of the above**

Ref: Chapter No.14, Page No.322

36. **Ans: D. All of the above**

Ref: Chapter No.14, Page No.322

37. **Ans: C. $ETCO_2$ will increase during periods of decreased cardiac output and pulmonary perfusion**

Ref: Chapter No.14, Page No.322-323

38. **Ans: A. 2 to 5 mm Hg**

Ref: Chapter No.14, Page No.322

39. **Ans: B. Esophageal temperature**

Ref: Chapter No.14, Page No.323

40. **Ans: C. Orbicularis oculi muscles**

Ref: Chapter No.14, Page No.323

41. **Ans: B. Triple-Burst Stimulation**

Ref: Chapter No.14, Page No.323

42. **Ans: B. 75% to 95% blockade**

Ref: Chapter No.14, Page No.323

43. **Ans: D. Data suggest that BIS is not an accurate indicator of the depth of anesthesia**

Ref: Chapter No.14, Page No.323

44. **Ans: D. < 40 for more than 5 minutes**

Ref: Chapter No.14, Page No.323

45. **Ans: C. 6 months**

Ref: Chapter No.14, Page No.324

46. **Ans: C. 6–8 cm**

Ref: Chapter No.14, Page No.325

47. **Ans: C. 6–8 cm**

Ref: Chapter No.14, Page No.325

48. **Ans: D. All of the above**

Ref: Chapter No.14, Page No.325

49. **Ans: A. Class I**

Ref: Chapter No.14, Page No.325

50. **Ans: C. Class III**

Ref: Chapter No.14, Page No.325

51. **Ans: D. Class IV**

Ref: Chapter No.14, Page No.325

52. **Ans: B. 7–10 METs**

Ref: Chapter No.14, Page No.325

53. **Ans: D. All of the above**

Ref: Chapter No.14, Page No.325

54. **Ans: D. All of the above**

Ref: Chapter No.14, Page No.327

55. **Ans: C. 14 days**

Ref: Chapter No.14, Page No.327

56. **Ans: D. 30 days**

Ref: Chapter No.14, Page No.328

57. **Ans: B. Perioperative initiation of statin use is not reasonable in patients undergoing vascular surgery**

Ref: Chapter No.14, Page No.329

58. **Ans: D. Initiation or continuation of aspirin is beneficial in patients undergoing elective non-cardiac non-carotid surgery who have not had previous coronary stenting**

Ref: Chapter No.14, Page No.329

59. **Ans: B. In patients with ≥2 RCRI factors, it may be reasonable to begin beta blockers before surgery**

Ref: Chapter No.14, Page No.329

60. **Ans: D. 365 days**

Ref: Chapter No.14, Page No.329

61. **Ans: C. 180 days**

Ref: Chapter No.14, Page No.329

62. **Ans: C. Antibiotic prophylaxis solely to prevent IE is recommended for genitourinary or gastrointestinal tract procedures**

Ref: Chapter No.14, Page No.329-330

63. **Ans: B. Oral amoxicillin *(2 g single dose 30 to 60 min before procedure)***

Ref: Chapter No.14, Page No.330

64. **Ans: C. Completely repaired congenital heart defect with prosthetic material or device, whether placed by surgery or by catheter intervention, during the first 12 months after the procedure (First 6 months: Prophylaxis is reasonable because *endothelialization of prosthetic material* occurs *within 6 months* after the procedure)**

Ref: Chapter No.14, Page No.330

65. **Ans: B. ASA class >II**

Ref: Chapter No.14, Page No.330

66. **Ans: B. < 3.5 g/dL**

Ref: Chapter No.14, Page No.330

67. **Ans: B. The presence of obesity or mild to moderate asthma was significantly associated with perioperative pulmonary complications**

Ref: Chapter No.14, Page No.330-331

68. **Ans: D. All of the above**

Ref: Chapter No.14, Page No.331

69. **Ans: C. 18 to 24 hours before surgery**

Ref: Chapter No.14, Page No.331

70. **Ans: C. Metformin is usually continued on the day of surgery**

Ref: Chapter No.14, Page No.331-332

71. **Ans: A. 2 hours**

Ref: Chapter No.14, Page No.332

72. **Ans: C. 6 hours**

Ref: Chapter No.14, Page No.332

73. **Ans: B. 4 hours**

Ref: Chapter No.14, Page No.332

74. **Ans: B. Fruit juices with pulp**

Ref: Chapter No.14, Page No.332

75. **Ans: D. ASA class VI**

Ref: Chapter No.14, Page No.332

76. **Ans: B. ASA class IV**

Ref: Chapter No.14, Page No.332

77. **Ans: B. ASA class III**

Ref: Chapter No.14, Page No.332

78. **Ans: B. ASA class III**

Ref: Chapter No.14, Page No.332

79. **Ans: A. ASA class II**

Ref: Chapter No.14, Page No.332

80. **Ans: D. ASA class V**

Ref: Chapter No.14, Page No.332

81. **Ans: D. ASA class IE**

Ref: Chapter No.14, Page No.332

82. **Ans: C. ASA class V**

Ref: Chapter No.14, Page No.332

83. **Ans: B. ASA class IIE**

Ref: Chapter No.14, Page No.332

84. **Ans: D. All of the above**

Ref: Chapter No.14, Page No.333

85. **Ans: B. < 1 in 10,000 cases**

Ref: Chapter No.14, Page No.333

86. **Ans: C. Paresthesia**

Ref: Chapter No.14, Page No.335

87. **Ans: B. The mechanism of action of local anesthetics is dose-dependent blockade of potassium currents in nerve fibers**

Ref: Chapter No.14, Page No.335

88. **Ans: B. Liposomal bupivacaine is composed of bupivacaine encapsulated in multivesicular liposomes and can provide up to 24 hours of analgesia after local infiltration (Up to 72 hours)**

Ref: Chapter No.14, Page No.335

89. **Ans: C. 5 mg/kg**

Ref: Chapter No.14, Page No.335

90. **Ans: B. 7 mg/kg**

Ref: Chapter No.14, Page No.335

91. **Ans: C. Vomiting**

Ref: Chapter No.14, Page No.335

92. **Ans: B. Bupivacaine decreased QRS width during sinus rhythm**

Ref: Chapter No.14, Page No.335-336

93. **Ans: C. American Society of Regional Anesthesia and Pain Medicine recommend bolus injection of 1.5 mL/kg (lean body mass) of 20% lipid emulsion over 1 minute followed by an infusion of 0.25 mL/kg/min**

Ref: Chapter No.14, Page No.336

94. **Ans: A. Spinal anesthesia is induced by the injection of local anesthetic, with or without opiates, into the subdural space**

Ref: Chapter No.14, Page No.336

95. **Ans: C. Hypertension occurs as a consequence of sympathectomy**

Ref: Chapter No.14, Page No.337

96. **Ans: A. When compared to epidural anesthesia, spinal anesthesia has a slower onset, is less predictably satisfactory for surgery**

Ref: Chapter No.14, Page No.337

97. **Ans: A. Male gender**

Ref: Chapter No.14, Page No.337

98. **Ans: A. Decreased ICP**

Ref: Chapter No.14, Page No.337

99. **Ans: C. Epidural anesthesia has not been shown to decrease blood loss and deep venous thrombosis during total joint arthroplasty**

Ref: Chapter No.14, Page No.337

100. Ans: B. Lumbar epidural anesthesia, appears to be associated with more rapid recovery of gastrointestinal function after major abdominal surgery (It is thoracic epidural)

Ref: Chapter No.14, Page No.337

101. Ans: C. 24 hours

Ref: Chapter No.14, Page No.337

102. Ans: A. 6 hours

Ref: Chapter No.14, Page No.337

103. Ans: B. 12 hours

Ref: Chapter No.14, Page No.337

104. Ans: B. 2 hours

Ref: Chapter No.14, Page No.337

105. Ans: A. Increased heart rate

Ref: Chapter No.14, Page No.337

106. Ans: D. All of the above

Ref: Chapter No.14, Page No.338

107. Ans: D. All of the above

Ref: Chapter No.14, Page No.338

108. Ans: A. Rectus sheath block

Ilioinguinal-iliohypogastric block

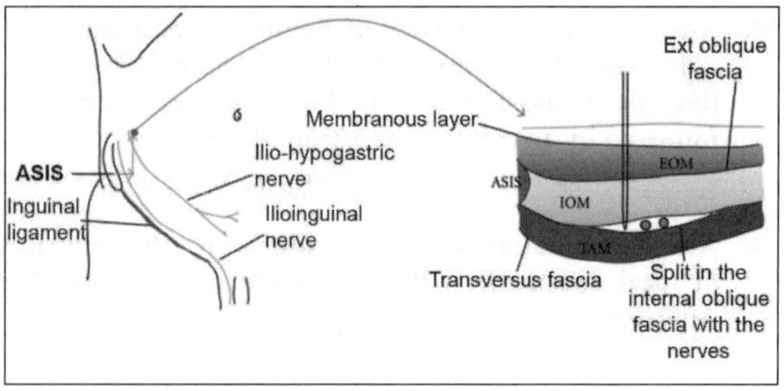

Quadratus lumborum block

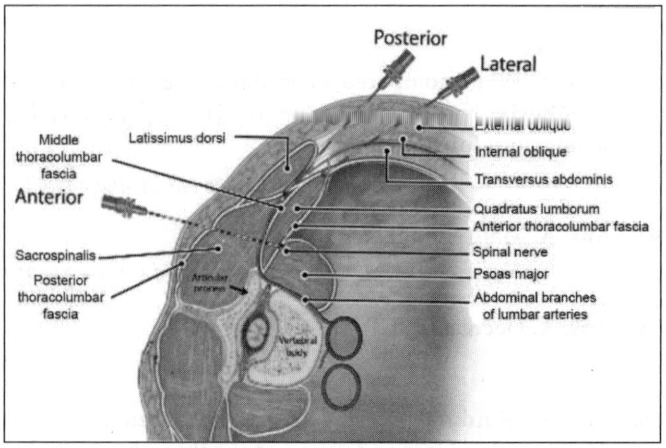

Ref: Chapter No.14, Page No.338

109. Ans: D. All of the above

Ref: Chapter No.14, Page No.338

110. Ans: C. 70%

Ref: Chapter No.14, Page No.339

111. Ans: D. All of the above

Ref: Chapter No.14, Page No.339

112. Ans: D. All of the above

Ref: Chapter No.14, Page No.339

113. Ans: D. All of the above

Ref: Chapter No.14, Page No.339

114. Ans: B. An important complication related to the IV coadministration of ondansetron and metoclopramide has been the production of tachyarrhythmias

Ref: Chapter No.14, Page No.339-340

115. Ans: A. Promethazine

Ref: Chapter No.14, Page No.340

116. Ans: C. Scopolamine

Ref: Chapter No.14, Page No.340

117. Ans: D. Ondansetron

Ref: Chapter No.14, Page No.340

118. Ans: B. Dry mouth

Ref: Chapter No.14, Page No.340

119. Ans: A. Possibility that hypothermia could decrease the rate of surgical infections

Ref: Chapter No.14, Page No.340

120. Ans: A. Cardiac tamponade

Ref: Chapter No.14, Page No.340

121. Ans: D. All of the above

Ref: Chapter No.14, Page No.340

122. Ans: B. 0.02%

Ref: Chapter No.14, Page No.340

123. Ans: D. All of the above

Ref: Chapter No.14, Page No.340

124. Ans: C. Chronic pain serves useful function in healing

Ref: Chapter No.14, Page No.341

125. Ans: D. Perception, the final step in the nociceptive process, occurs when the pain signal reaches the thalamus

Ref: Chapter No.14, Page No.341

126. Ans: C. The intramuscular is preferred over IV route and subcutaneous injections when the parenteral route is indicated

Ref: Chapter No.14, Page No.341

127. Ans: A. μ1 receptor

Ref: Chapter No.14, Page No.341

128. Ans: B. δ receptor (The δ and κ receptors are involved in spinal analgesia)

Ref: Chapter No.14, Page No.341

129. Ans: A. For moderate to severe pain in patients with renal dysfunction, fentanyl and hydromorphone are not suitable agents

Ref: Chapter No.14, Page No.341

130. Ans: D. Fentanyl is available in a transdermal preparation, and this route is recommended for acute pain management

Ref: Chapter No.14, Page No.341

131. Ans: D. The newer agents (celecoxib, rofecoxib, valdecoxib) are selective COX-1 inhibitors

Ref: Chapter No.14, Page No.342-343

132. Ans: C. If Ketamine is administered via continuous infusion it seems to be ineffective

Ref: Chapter No.14, Page No.343

133. Ans: D. Guanfacine is delivered orally and has minimal cardiovascular side effects and is determined to be effective as a perioperative adjunct

Ref: Chapter No.14, Page No.343

134. Ans: B. Prilocaine and lidocaine

Ref: Chapter No.14, Page No.343

135. Ans: D. The goal of pre-emptive analgesia is to influence the analgesic process after initiation of the noxious stimulus (e.g., surgical incision)

Ref: Chapter No.14, Page No.344

136. Ans: B. Increases postoperative pain

Ref: Chapter No.14, Page No.344

137. Ans: C. Opioids, when delivered by the neuraxial route, provide analgesia by their action at opioid receptors located in the anterior horn of the spinal cord

Ref: Chapter No.14, Page No.344

138. Ans: D. A hydrophilic opioid such as morphine, when delivered into the epidural or subarachnoid space, remains in the CSF shorter than a lipophilic opioid does

Ref: Chapter No.14, Page No.344

139. Ans: B. NSAIDs are the agent of choice for IV PCA

Ref: Chapter No.14, Page No.344-345

140. Ans: A. Pain that persists for 3 months beyond the expected time for recovery or initial onset is considered evidence of a chronic pain syndrome

Ref: Chapter No.14, Page No.345

15

Emerging Technology in Surgery: Informatics, Electronics

RECENT SIGNIFICANT ADVANCES IN SURGICAL TECHNOLOGY

1. **False about Minimal-Access Surgery is:**
   A. Minimal-access surgery (such as laparoscopic surgery) provides the means to diminish the trauma of access using image-guided systems to perform the operation without compromising its overall goal
   B. One of the advantages of minimally invasive image-guided surgery is the illumination of target tissues, which conveys a bright, magnified, high-definition image to the surgeon through an attached or incorporated camera system
   C. An important limitation of endoscopic imaging is that it is generally monocular (compared to the binocular view of open surgery), since traditional scopes have a single lens system
   D. With a monocular scope, the surgeon obtains a 3D view of the body displayed on a video monitor

2. **Larger incisions are associated with all except:**
   A. Less postoperative pain
   B. Longer recovery periods
   C. More risk of incisional hernias
   D. Higher rate of symptomatic adhesive bowel obstruction in the future

3. **False among the following is:**
   A. Depth perception is a learned skill, and most surgeons are able to adjust to laparoscopic imaging with adequate training
   B. 3D camera technology shortens the learning curve during the acquisition of laparoscopic skills for novices and may enhance proficiency in complex tasks such as fine dissection and suturing for even experienced surgeons
   C. Laparoscopic images give the surgeon a view of the surface of tissues with the ability for direct manual assessment
   D. Drawback of endoscopic surgery is the limited field of view, requiring the scope to be moved dynamically to maintain an ideal image

4. **NOTES is:**
   A. Natural organ transluminal endoscopic surgery
   B. Natural orifice transluminal endoscopic surgery
   C. Natural orifice transecting endoscopic surgery
   D. Natural organ transecting endoscopic surgery

5. **True among the following is:**
   A. Transoral endoscopic thyroidectomy vestibular approach, in which the thyroid gland is excised endoscopically by obtaining access through the mouth
   B. Transanal total mesorectal excision is an approach, the total mesorectal excision proceeds transanally ("bottom-up"), enhancing the surgeon's view of the total mesorectal excision planes compared to conventional transabdominal total mesorectal excision
   C. Peroral endoscopic myotomy (POEM procedure) is used in achalasia cardia
   D. All of the above

6. **True among the following is:**
   A. The most widely used robotic system in North America uses a proprietary laparoscope with 2 optical systems providing binocular (3D) vision and additional depth perception
   B. Despite the theoretical advantages of providing surgical care to remote regions, the costs and resources required to deploy such a system have limited its practicality and implementation

C. The longer the distance that the data needs to be transmitted from the console to the patient, the greater the latent delay, as even 250 milliseconds can have significant impact on the quality of the operation
D. All of the above

7. **True about Digitization and Augmentation of Surgery is:**
A. Display of preoperatively acquired images or images generated intraoperatively by ultrasound, flexible endoscopy, or fluoroscopy can be very helpful to guide the surgeon and add safety and efficiency to the operation
B. Computer-generated 3D image reconstructions can be acquired and superimposed onto the field of view, providing a digital overlay using image-guided surgery or, more recently, using augmented-reality platform
C. A. method to provide this information is the use of fluorescence markers (such as indocyanine green)
D. All of the above

EVOLVING TECHNOLOGIES IN SURGERY

8. **True among the following is:**
A. Confocal laser endomicrosurgery: microscopic imaging of tissues
B. Chromoendoscopy: using various dyes such as indigo carmine to accentuate dysplastic tissue
C. Optical coherence tomography: cross-sectional tissue imaging using backscattering of light
D. All of the above

ANSWERS

1. **Ans: D. With a monocular scope, the surgeon obtains a 3D view of the body displayed on a video monitor**
Ref: Chapter No.15, Page No.349-350
2. **Ans: A. Less postoperative pain**
Ref: Chapter No.15, Page No.349-350
3. **Ans: C. Laparoscopic images give the surgeon a view of the surface of tissues with the ability for direct manual assessment**
Ref: Chapter No.15, Page No.350
4. **Ans: B. Natural orifice transluminal endoscopic surgery**
Ref: Chapter No.15, Page No.351
5. **Ans: D. All of the above**
Ref: Chapter No.15, Page No.351-352
6. **Ans: D. All of the above**
Ref: Chapter No.15, Page No.353-354
7. **Ans: D. All of the above**
Ref: Chapter No.15, Page No.355
8. **Ans: D. All of the above**
Ref: Chapter No.15, Page No.357

16

Robotic Surgery

PREFACE

1. **False statement among the following is:**
   A. U.S. Food and Drug Administration (FDA) approved da Vinci Surgical System in 2000
   B. Robotic surgery capitalizes on the "master-slave" concept to offer surgeons control over a system that provides enhanced visualization, augmented dexterity and precision, sophisticated articulating instruments, and improved ergonomics
   C. Studies evaluating intraoperative oncologic parameters don't support the reliable use of robotic surgery in the treatment of malignant diseases including gastric, colorectal, pancreatic and liver cancers
   D. Improved patient outcomes with smaller incisions, less pain, less blood loss, shorter length of hospital stay, quicker return of bowel function, and more rapid overall recovery when compared to open procedures

HISTORY

2. **True about the history of robotic surgery is:**
   A. Automated Endoscopic System for Optimal Positioning (AESOP), was the first FDA-approved commercial robot that enabled surgeons to command and manipulate a laparoscopic camera during surgical procedures
   B. AESOP system was soon developed into the Zeus Robotic Surgical System, with the addition of three arms capable of being remotely controlled by the surgeon
   C. The first robot-assisted transatlantic cholecystectomy with the surgeon seated at the robotic manipulator located in New York City with the "patient-side" robot-system in Strasburg, France
   D. All of the above

3. **The latest da Vinci Surgical system is:**
   A. Si System B. Xi System
   C. S System D. X System

PREPARING FOR ROBOTIC SURGERY

4. **The robotic surgery platform offers the surgeon several technological advantages over laparoscopy like:**
   A. Ability to control 4 arms
   B. Enhanced operative view
   C. Increased precision of instrument movements
   D. All of the above

5. **Degrees of freedom in robotic surgical systems is:**
   A. 3 B. 5
   C. 6 D. 7

6. **Enhanced operative view in robotic surgical system is offered by:**
   A. Multiview capabilities
   B. HD 3D camera with up to 10× magnification of surgical anatomy
   C. Ready on and off capability of near-infrared
   D. All of the above

7. **Intraoperative fluorescence-guided identification of surgical anatomy including liver perfusion, vascular perfusion, lymph nodes, and lymphatic drainage in robotic surgical system is by:**
   A. Firefly™ B. Tilepro™
   C. InfraReady™ D. NIR™

8. **Multidisplay imaging capability that allows the surgeon to simultaneously view other images, such as intraoperative ultrasound, endoscopy and radiologic pictures, on the console in real-time during an operation in robotic surgical system is by:**
   A. Firefly™ B. Tilepro™
   C. InfraReady™ D. NIR™

9. **Following image shows:**

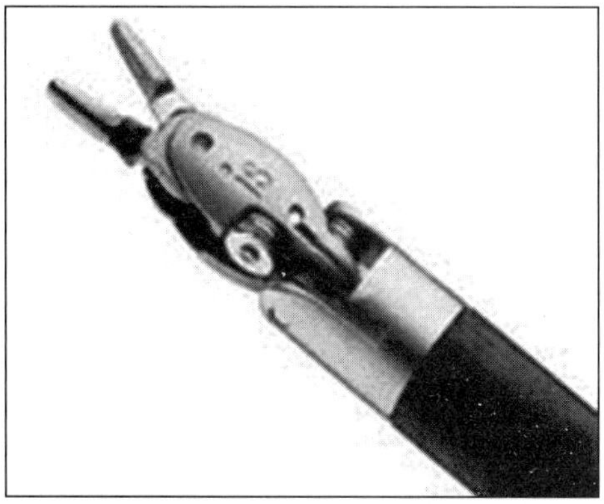

A. Endowristed needle drivers
B. Endowristed energy devices
C. Endowristed staplers
D. Harmonic Ultrasound Shears

10. **Following image shows:**

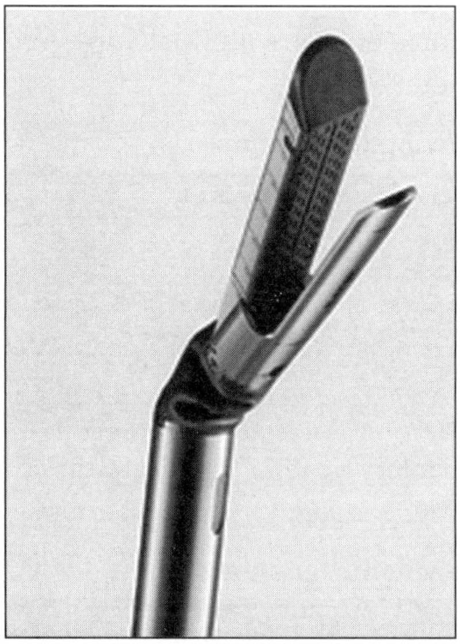

A. Endowristed needle drivers
B. Endowristed energy devices
C. Endowristed staplers
D. Harmonic Ultrasound Shears

11. **False about the operating room setup for robotic surgeries is:**

A. For upper gastrointestinal (GI) operations, there are 2 positions for the patient's cart: (1) brought in straight over the patient's head and docked or (2) brought in off to the left side of the patient's head in a slight angle
B. In lower GI operations, specifically in left sided resections, the Si Robotic System must be brought to the left lower side of the patient
C. In the case of the Xi Surgical System, the docking of the robotic patient-side cart is easier, with the cart's ability to rotate 180 degrees to reach its proper position
D. If stapling is to be performed by the bedside assistant, it is recommended that the bedside assistant be positioned on the patient's left side and the assistant's video monitor placed on the opposite side, facing the assistant

12. **Vessel sealer extension, which is available only on:**

A. Si System　B. Xi System
C. S System　D. X System

13. **True among the following is:**

A. An alternative to the vessel sealer is a Harmonic scalpel (Ethicon, Somerville, NJ) used just as in laparoscopy
B. A. Maryland forceps is ideal for dissection and isolation of vessels with its narrow tip and bipolar energy capabilities to achieve hemostasis around soft tissues
C. Monopolar sheers provide sharp dissection and cause less collateral thermal injury; however, they cannot substitute as a grasper
D. All of the above

14. **The most often used grasper during GI operations in robotic surgeries is the:**

A. ProGrasp forceps　B. Maryland forceps
C. Cadiere forceps　D. Resano forceps

15. **The least traumatic of the graspers and ideal for retraction of stomach, small bowel and pancreas is:**

A. ProGrasp forceps　B. Maryland forceps
C. Cadiere forceps　D. Resano forceps

16. **Following image shows:**

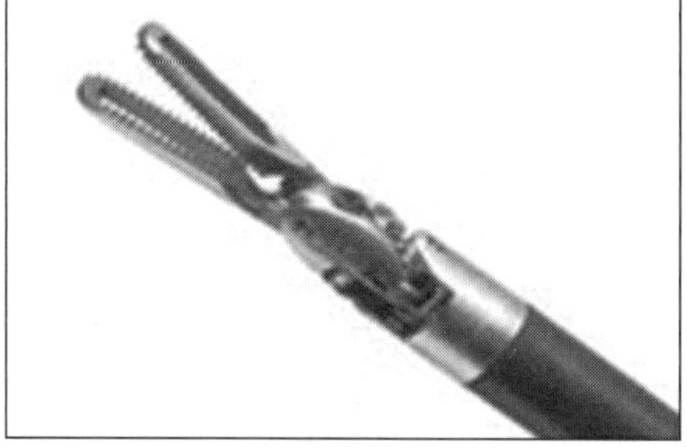

A. ProGrasp forceps　B. Maryland forceps
C. Cadiere forceps　D. Resano forceps

17. Following image shows:

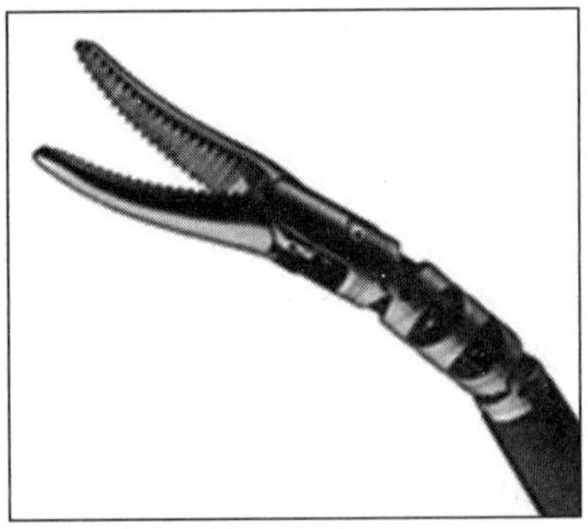

A. ProGrasp forceps B. Maryland forceps
C. Cadiere forceps D. Resano forceps

18. Using data from diagnostic CT imaging, a segmented 3D model of your patient's anatomy is created and then enables the surgeon to consult with your patient and prepare for your case. This system is called:

A. Firefly™ B. Iris™
C. Tilepro™ D. InfraReady™

19. Following image shows:

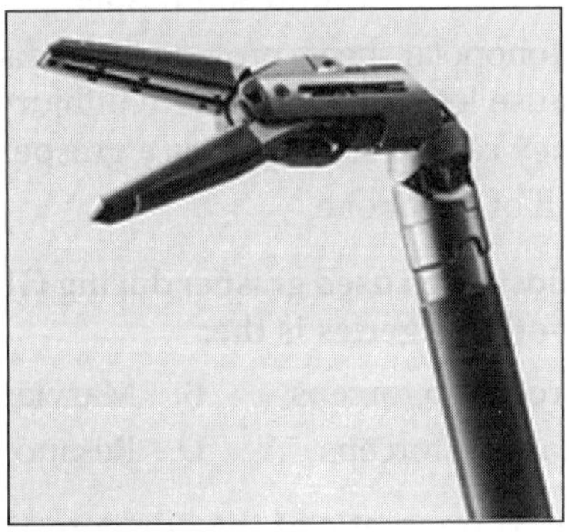

A. Vessel Sealer Extend
B. SynchroSeal
C. Force Bipolar with DualGrip
D. SureForm 45

20. Following image shows:

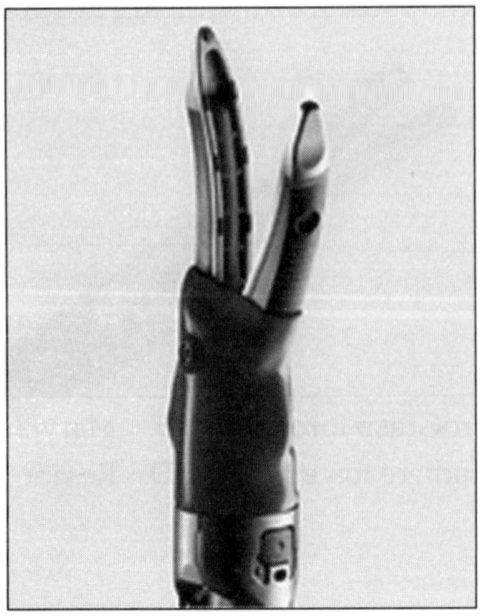

A. Vessel Sealer Extend
B. SynchroSeal
C. Force Bipolar with DualGrip
D. SureForm 45

21. Following image shows:

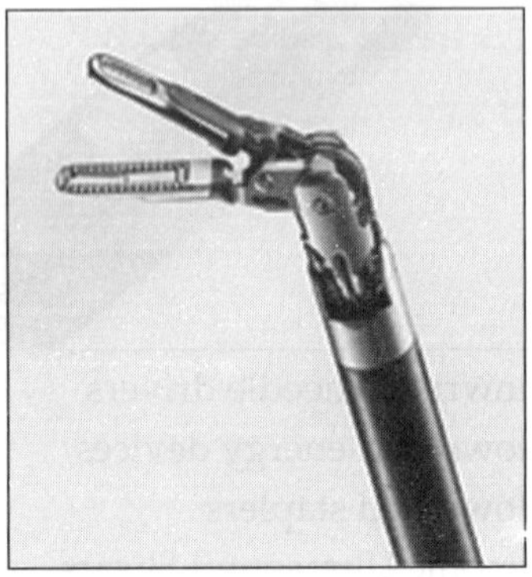

A. Vessel Sealer Extend
B. SynchroSeal
C. Force Bipolar with DualGrip
D. SureForm 45

22. Following image shows:

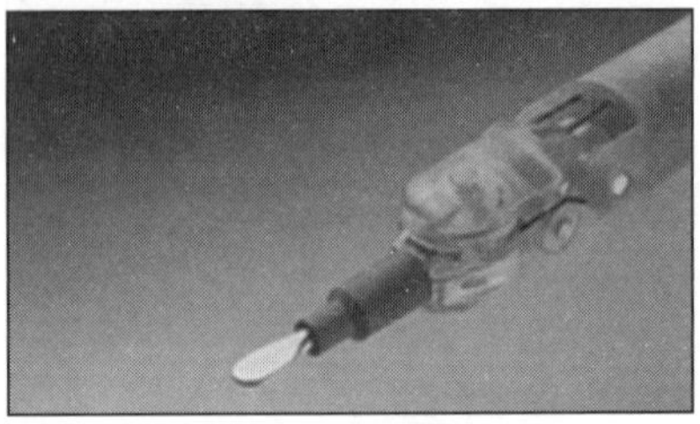

A. Cautery Spatula B. Curved scissors
C. Potts scissors D. Cobra grasper

23. Following image shows:

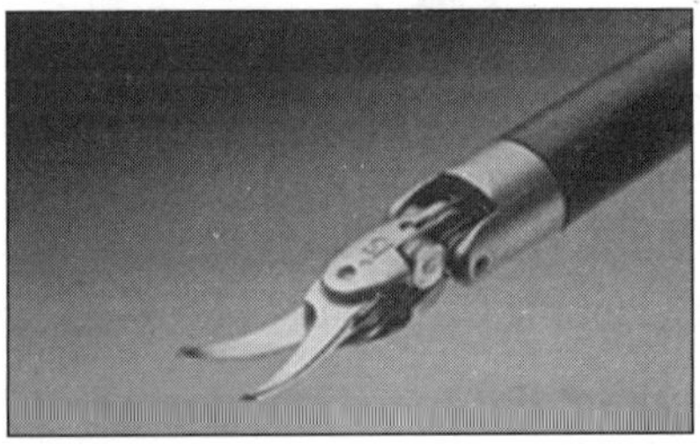

A. Cautery Spatula B. Curved scissors
C. Potts scissors D. Cobra grasper

24. Following image shows:

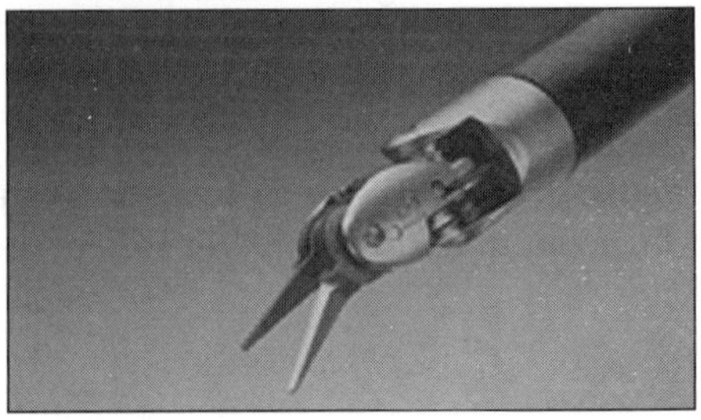

A. Cautery Spatula B. Curved scissors
C. Potts scissors D. Cobra grasper

25. **Following image shows:**

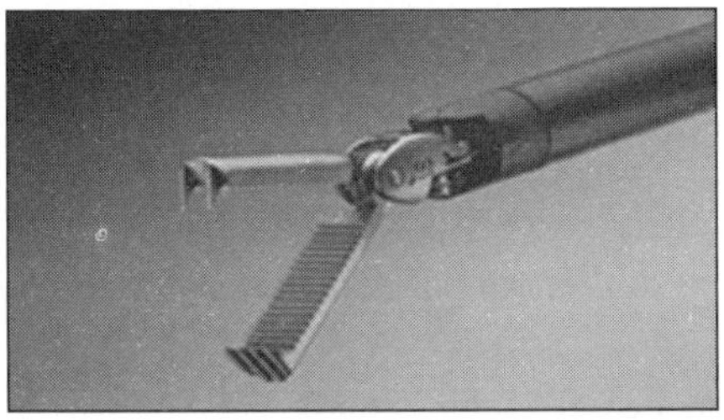

A. Cautery Spatula B. Curved scissors
C. Potts scissors D. Cobra grasper

26. **Following image shows:**

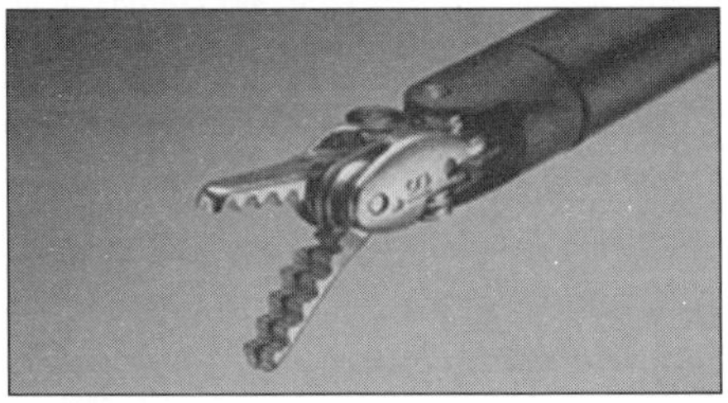

A. ProGrasp forceps B. Maryland forceps
C. Cadiere forceps D. Resano forceps

27. **Following image shows:**

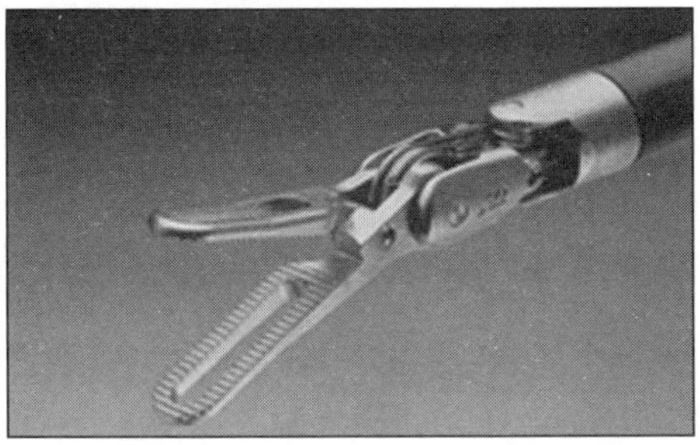

A. ProGrasp forceps B. Maryland forceps
C. Cadiere forceps D. Resano forceps

28. **Following image shows:**

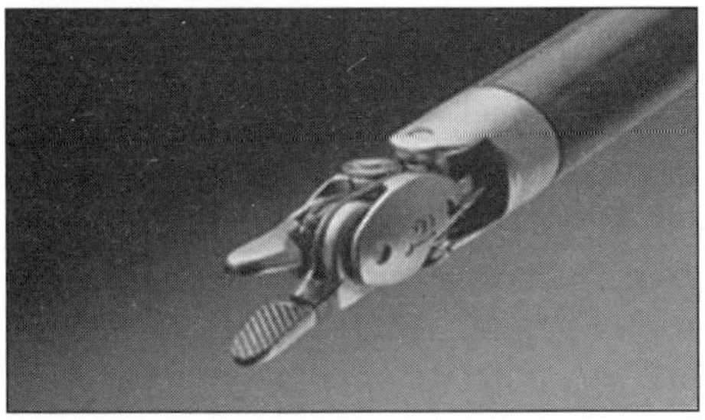

A. Large Needle Driver
B. Suturecut Needle Driver
C. Maryland forceps
D. ProGrasp forceps

29. **A single arm delivering 3 multi-jointed instruments and a fully wristed 3DHD camera for visibility and control in narrow surgical spaces is seen in:**

A. Si System B. Xi System
C. S System D. SP System

CURRENT STATUS OF SELECTED ROBOTIC OPERATIONS

30. **True about robotic ventral hernia repair with mesh is:**

A. Robotic ventral herniorrhaphy addresses the limitations of laparoscopy demonstrating improved clinical outcomes compared to the open approach
B. The highest level of evidence recommends mesh reinforcement in hernias ≥2 cm
C. Robotic techniques in ventral hernia repair have been reported and found to be particularly beneficial in intracorporeal closure of the hernia defect and suturing of the mesh to the fascia
D. All of the above

31. **Elective ventral hernia repairs are not to be done in patients with:**

A. Current smokers B. ≥50 kg/ m^2
C. HbA1C is ≥8% D. All of the above

32. **True about robotic total mesorectal excision for rectal cancer is:**

A. TME is the gold standard and surgical technique of choice for locally advanced rectal cancer
B. There is a relatively short learning curve for rTME, reported to be < 20 cases
C. Obesity didn't have any impact on the operative times, open conversion, estimated blood loss during surgery, and length of hospital stay in rLAR with TME
D. All of the above

ANSWERS

1. **Ans: C. Studies evaluating intraoperative oncologic parameters don't support the reliable use of robotic surgery in the treatment of malignant diseases including gastric, colorectal, pancreatic and liver cancers**

   Ref: Chapter No.16, Page No.362

2. **Ans: D. All of the above**

   Ref: Chapter No.16, Page No.362

3. **Ans: B. Xi System**

   Ref: Chapter No.16, Page No.362

4. **Ans: D. All of the above**

   Ref: Chapter No.16, Page No.377

5. **Ans: D. 7**

   Ref: Chapter No.16, Page No.377

6. **Ans: D. All of the above**

   Ref: Chapter No.16, Page No.377

7. **Ans: A. Firefly™**

   Ref: Chapter No.16, Page No.377

8. **Ans: B. Tilepro™**

   Ref: Chapter No.16, Page No.377

9. **Ans: A. Endowristed needle drivers**

   Ref: https://www.intuitive.com/en-us/products-and-services/da-vinci/instruments

10. **Ans: C. Endowristed staplers**

    Ref: https://www.intuitive.com/en-us/products-and-services/da-vinci/stapling

11. **Ans: D. If stapling is to be performed by the bedside assistant, it is recommended that the bedside assistant be positioned on the patient's left side and the assistant's video monitor placed on the opposite side, facing the assistant**

    Ref: Chapter No.16, Page No.378

12. **Ans: B. Xi System**

    Ref: Chapter No.16, Page No.378

13. **Ans: D. All of the above**

    Ref: Chapter No.16, Page No.378

14. **Ans: C. Cadiere forceps**

    Ref: Chapter No.16, Page No.378

15. **Ans: C. Cadiere forceps**

    Ref: Chapter No.16, Page No.378

16. **Ans: C. Cadiere forceps**

    Ref: https://www.intuitive.com/en-us/products-and-services/da-vinci/instruments

17. **Ans: B. Maryland forceps**

    Ref: https://www.intuitive.com/en-us/products-and-services/da-vinci/instruments

18. **Ans: B. Iris**

    Ref: https://www.intuitive.com/en-us/products-and-services/da-vinci/vision/iris

19. **Ans: A. Vessel Sealer Extend**

    Ref: https://www.intuitive.com/en-us/products-and-services/da-vinci/energy

20. **Ans: B. SynchroSeal**

    Ref: https://www.intuitive.com/en-us/products-and-services/da-vinci/energy

21. **Ans: C. Force Bipolar with DualGrip**

    Ref: https://www.intuitive.com/en-us/products-and-services/da-vinci/instruments

22. **Ans: A. Cautery Spatula**

    Ref: https://www.intuitive.com/en-us/products-and-services/da-vinci/instruments

23. **Ans: B. Curved scissors**

    Ref: https://www.intuitive.com/en-us/products-and-services/da-vinci/instruments

24. **Ans: C. Potts scissors**

    Ref: https://www.intuitive.com/en-us/products-and-services/da-vinci/instruments

25. **Ans: D. Cobra grasper**

    Ref: https://www.intuitive.com/en-us/products-and-services/da-vinci/instruments

26. **Ans: D. Resano forceps**

    Ref: https://www.intuitive.com/en-us/products-and-services/da-vinci/instruments

27. **Ans: A. ProGrasp forceps**

    Ref: https://www.intuitive.com/en-us/products-and-services/da-vinci/instruments

28. **Ans: B. Suturecut Needle Driver**

    Ref: https://www.intuitive.com/en-us/products-and-services/da-vinci/instruments

29. **Ans: D. SP System**

    Ref: https://www.intuitive.com/en-us/products-and-services/da-vinci/systems

30. **Ans: D. All of the above**

    Ref: Chapter No.16, Page No.378

31. **Ans: D. All of the above**

    Ref: Chapter No.16, Page No.378

32. **Ans: D. All of the above**

    Ref: Chapter No.16, Page No.379

17

Management of Acute Trauma

OVERVIEW AND HISTORY

1. **Professional organizations of trauma include:**
   A. American Association for the Surgery of Trauma (AAST)
   B. Eastern Association for the Surgery of Trauma (EAST)
   C. Western Trauma Association (WTA)
   D. All of the above

2. **Establishment of first medical school was during:**
   A. French and Indian War
   B. American Revolutionary War
   C. World War I
   D. Vietnam War

3. **Whole blood transfusion was first used during:**
   A. American Civil War
   B. World War II
   C. World War I
   D. Vietnam War

4. **First blood bank was started during:**
   A. American Civil War
   B. World War II
   C. World War I
   D. Vietnam War

5. **Recognition of Hypovolemic shock was during:**
   A. Korean War
   B. World War II
   C. World War I
   D. Vietnam War

6. **Damage control resuscitation was developed during:**
   A. Vietnam War
   B. World War I
   C. World War II
   D. Operation Enduring Freedom (Iraq)

7. **Use of topical antiseptic agents was started during:**
   A. Vietnam War
   B. Korean War
   C. World War II
   D. American Civil War

8. **Organ dysfunction after injury described during:**
   A. Vietnam War
   B. World War I
   C. World War II
   D. Operation Enduring Freedom (Iraq)

9. **Aeromedical transfer (helicopter) was introduced during:**
   A. Vietnam War
   B. Korean War
   C. World War II
   D. Operation Enduring Freedom (Iraq)

TRAUMA SYSTEMS

10. **Components of comprehensive inclusive trauma system includes:**
    A. Acute care facilities
    B. Postacute care and rehabilitation
    C. Trauma center designation and verification
    D. All of the above

11. **Reduction of in-hospital mortality with care at a trauma center after correction for injury severity, was:**
    A. 10% B. 20%
    C. 40% D. 50%

INJURY SCORING

12. True about Abbreviated Injury Scale (AIS) among the following is:

A. The AIS represents the foundation for other scoring systems that are better able to account for the severity of multiple combined injuries
B. The Abbreviated Injury Scale (AIS) has been the most used anatomic system of injury classification since it was first described in 1971
C. Injuries are characterized by a six-digit taxonomy that includes the body region, type of anatomic structure, and specific anatomic detail of the injury
D. All of the above

13. A 32-year-old male presents after being assaulted by a bat to his head, face and torso. He opens his eyes to sternal rub, localizes to pain, and is only making groaning sounds. What is this patient's GCS?

A. 8 B. 9
C. 10 D. 11

14. A 56-year-old male rubs his abdomen and tells you it really hurts he tells you that he wants to go to the hospital and you help him walk to the stretcher. What is his Glasgow Coma Scale?

A. 11 B. 12
C. 13 D. 15

15. An elderly female in a nursing home is walking around her room and greets you when you enter. She speaks clearly but her answers are confusing. What is her Glasgow Coma score?

A. 11 B. 14
C. 13 D. 15

16. A patient fell while rock climbing. When you apply a deep sternal rub, he extends his arms and legs and shows no other response. What is his Glasgow Coma score?

A. 4 B. 5
C. 6 D. 7

17. A 73-year-old patient looks at spontaneously you when you speak to her. When you ask her the date, she says "blue". You note left-sided weakness when she grips your fingers. What is her Glasgow Coma score?

A. 11 B. 14
C. 13 D. 12

18. A 46-year-old man is found on the ground outside a homeless shelter. When you give him a sternal rub, he opens his eyes, tells you to go away, and pushes your hand away. What is his Glasgow Coma score?

A. 11 B. 14
C. 13 D. 12

19. A 21-year-old male had a road traffic accident. He extends their elbow when you put pressure on the nail bed. They can talk in sentences and are disorientated. He is unable to open their eyes. What is his Glasgow Coma score?

A. 6 B. 7
C. 8 D. 10

20. A 62-year-old female had a road traffic accident. She opens her eyes when you say her name, and speaks to you in words that make no sense. When you apply pressure on her nail bed, she moves her arm away. What is her Glasgow Coma score?

A. 8 B. 10
C. 11 D. 9

21. A 33-year-old male fell from height. He opens his eyes when he hears you shouting for help. He groans and make sounds which you cannot recognize as words. He does not respond to pain. What is his Glasgow Coma score?

A. 6 B. 7
C. 8 D. 9

22. False about Injury severity score (ISS) is:

A. The ISS ranges from 1 to 75
B. The ISS has been commonly used throughout the literature to quantify the overall burden of injury sustained by a patient
C. Minor injury (ISS < 9)
D. Severe injury (ISS > 50)

23. Injury severity score (ISS) of 21 is called:

A. Minor injury
B. Moderate injury
C. Serious injury
D. Severe injury

24. Injury severity score (ISS) of 13 is called:

A. Minor injury
B. Moderate injury
C. Serious injury
D. Severe injury

25. Injury severity score (ISS) of 49 is called:

A. Minor injury
B. Moderate injury
C. Serious injury
D. Severe injury

26. Revised trauma score (RTS) has all the following components except:

A. Heart rate
B. Respiratory rate
C. Systolic blood pressure
D. Glasgow Coma Scale score

27. Maximum Revised trauma score (RTS) is:

A. 6 B. 9
C. 12 D. 15

28. Minimum Glasgow Coma Scale (GCS) score is:

A. 0 B. 1
C. 2 D. 3

29. Minimum Revised trauma score (RTS) is:

A. 0 B. 1
C. 2 D. 3

30. An infant fell from stairs. He flexes his elbow and wrist in response to pain. The infant does not make any response to others around, and does not open its eyes at all. What is his GCS score?

A. 4 B. 5
C. 6 D. 7

31. An infant fell from stairs. She extends her elbows in response to pain, is inconsistently inconsolable and moans, and opens its eyes in response to pain. What is her GCS score?

A. 5 B. 6
C. 7 D. 8

32. An infant fell from stairs. He flexes his elbow and wrist abnormally in response to pain. The infant is inconsolable and agitated. He does not open its eyes spontaneously but does in response to speech. What is his GCS score?

A. 5 B. 6
C. 7 D. 8

33. An infant fell from stairs. She withdraws from touch, can only sometimes be consoled and is often agitated, and opens her eyes in response to pain but not to speech. What is her GCS score?

A. 9 B. 10
C. 11 D. 12

34. An infant fell from stairs. He smiles, is orientated to sounds, and interacts normally. He withdraws his arm when you cause him pain. He spontaneously opens his eyes. What is his GCS score?

A. 12 B. 13
C. 14 D. 15

PREHOSPITAL TRAUMA CARE

35. The "gold standard" for airway maintenance in the severely injured patient is:

A. Cricothyroidotomy
B. Tracheostomy
C. Endotracheal intubation
D. Intercoastal drain

36. A 40-year-old male had a road traffic accident. EMS arrived at the accident scene. On examination, the patient had a GCS score of 11, systolic blood pressure of 100 mm of Hg. What should be the next step in the line of management?

A. Assess anatomy of injury
B. Transport to a trauma center
C. Assess mechanism of injury and evidence of high-energy impact
D. Assess special patient or system considerations

37. High-risk auto crash includes all except:

A. Intrusion, including roof: >6 inches occupant site; >12 inches any site
B. Ejection (partial or complete) from automobile
C. Death in same passenger compartment
D. Vehicle telemetry data consistent with a high risk of injury

38. False among the following is:

A. SBP 110 might represent shock after age 65 years
B. Risk of injury/death increases after age 55 years
C. Evidence of high-energy impact fall for adults is >20 feet
D. Evidence of high-energy impact fall for children is >5 feet or 4 - 5 times the height of the child

INITIAL ASSESSMENT AND MANAGEMENT

39. The primary survey is best described by which sequence of steps?

A. Access, Blood pressure, Chest compressions, Disability, Endotracheal intubation

B. Airway, Blood pressure, Pulses, Breath sounds, Extremities
C. Airway, Breathing, Circulation, Disability, Exposure
D. Airway intubation, Bilateral chest tube placement, Central line placement

40. A middle-aged male is found lying on the ground in an alley and is brought into the trauma bay for additional evaluation. His vital signs are stable. The only sign of trauma is a large scalp laceration. The patient is confused with a Glasgow Coma Scale (GCS) score of 7. The decision is made to intubate the patient. What is the correct order for rapid sequence intubation in trauma?

A. Cervical immobilization, preoxygenation, cricoid pressure, induction, paralysis, intubate, confirm placement with CO_2 detector
B. Cervical immobilization, preoxygenation, cricoid pressure, paralysis, induction, intubate, confirm placement with CO_2 detector
C. Cervical immobilization, preoxygenation, cricoid pressure, induction, intubate, confirm placement with CO_2 detector, paralysis
D. Tilt head back in sniffing position, preoxygenation, cricoid pressure, induction, paralysis, intubate, confirm placement with CO_2 detector

41. False among the following is:

A. Cervical spine protection includes the use of a hard cervical collar and the maintenance of the log roll technique for all movement of the patient
B. After the initial assessment, frequent reassessment for deterioration and the development of airway compromise is paramount
C. Rigid long spine boards may be of value during transport of the patient but should be removed as soon as possible to avoid pressure-related wounds that can occur within a short time
D. The definitive airway of choice for most injured patients remains tracheostomy

42. False about technique of cricothyroidotomy is/are:

A. The cricothyroid membrane is identified by palpation, and a longitudinal incision is first made along the trachea
B. The incision and dissection are continued through the cricothyroid membrane in longitudinal fashion
C. Transversely incising the cricothyroid membrane, which can be palpated between the thyroid cartilage and cricoid ring, followed by insertion of a 6-0 endotracheal tube or tracheostomy appliance
D. All of the above

43. The blind insertion airway device are:

A. Multilumen esophageal airway (Combitube)
B. Laryngeal mask airway
C. Laryngeal tube airway (King LT-D.)
D. All of the above

44. Following image shows:

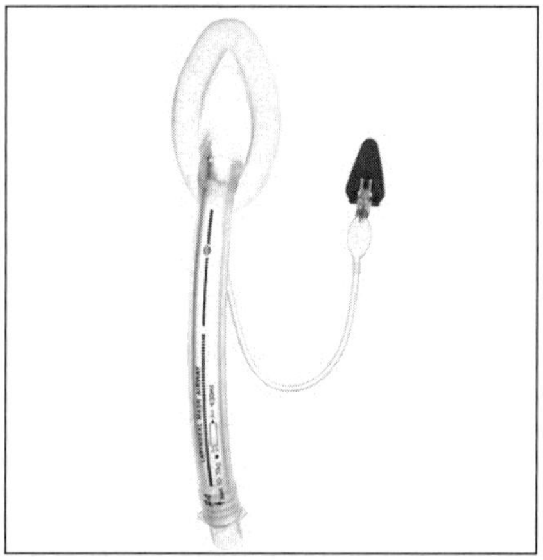

A. Multilumen esophageal airway (Combitube)
B. Laryngeal mask airway
C. Laryngeal tube airway (King LT-D.)
D. Tracheostomy tube

45. Following image shows:

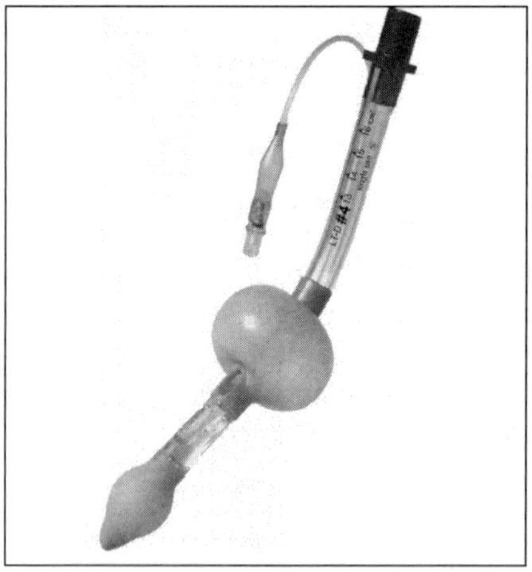

A. Multilumen esophageal airway (Combitube)
B. Laryngeal mask airway
C. Laryngeal tube airway (King LT-D.)
D. Tracheostomy tube

46. **Following image shows:**

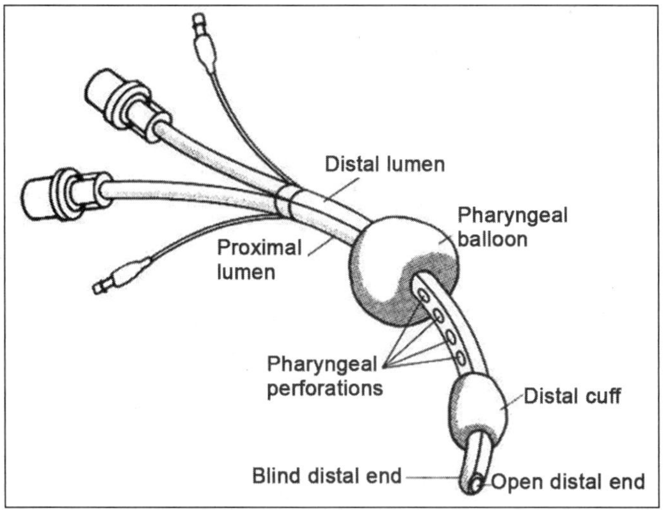

A. Multilumen esophageal airway (Combitube)
B. Laryngeal mask airway
C. Laryngeal tube airway (King LT-D.)
D. Tracheostomy tube

47. **Indicators of shock in the injured patient includes all except:**

A. Warm extremities B. Tachypnea
C. Agitation D. Weak distal pulses

48. **The most common cause of shock in the injured patient is:**

A. Heart failure B. Hemorrhage
C. Renal failure D. Spinal injury

49. **A 45-year-old male patient with head injury had blood loss of around 20%. What is the class of hemorrhagic shock as per ATLS?**

A. Class I B. Class II
C. Class III D. Class IV

50. **A 55-year-old male patient with head injury had blood loss of around 35%. What is the class of hemorrhagic shock as per ATLS?**

A. Class I B. Class II
C. Class III D. Class IV

51. **Tachycardia can be seen in all ATLS hemorrhagic classes except:**

A. Class I B. Class II
C. Class III D. Class IV

52. **A 52-year-old male patient with RTA had base deficit of around -8. What is the class of hemorrhagic shock as per ATLS?**

A. Class I B. Class II
C. Class III D. Class IV

53. **Considering Class I to class IV ATLS hemorrhagic classification on an ascending scale; Respiratory rate increases when the ATLS hemorrhagic shock class reaches:**

A. Class I B. Class II
C. Class III D. Class IV

54. **Considering Class I to class IV ATLS hemorrhagic classification on an ascending scale; Pulse pressure rate decreases when the ATLS hemorrhagic shock class reaches:**

A. Class I B. Class II
C. Class III D. Class IV

55. **Considering Class I to class IV ATLS hemorrhagic classification on an ascending scale; GCS decreases when the ATLS hemorrhagic shock class reaches:**

A. Class I B. Class II
C. Class III D. Class IV

56. **False statement among the following is:**

A. Upon recognizing the presence of shock, ATLS recommends intravenous (IV) access with 2 large-bore, short, peripheral IV catheters, an intraosseous needle, or a central venous catheter and initial resuscitation with 1 L of warmed crystalloid solution
B. Patients who fail to respond appropriately to initial crystalloid resuscitation should undergo product-based resuscitation, recognizing that crystalloid resuscitation beyond 1.5 L increases risk of death
C. The fast abdominal sonography in trauma (FAST) scan is a rapidly obtainable ultrasound examination that assesses for retroperitoneal fluid
D. There are essentially 5 major locations through which exsanguination may occur: chest, abdomen, retroperitoneum, pelvis, and/or long bone fractures

57. **FAST scan is:**

A. Fast abdominal sonography in trauma (FAST) scan
B. Focused abdominal sonography in trauma (FAST) scan
C. First abdominal sonography in trauma (FAST) scan
D. Firm abdominal sonography in trauma (FAST) scan

58. **False statement regarding primary survey among the following is:**

A. During the primary survey, it is valuable to

make a rapid determination of neurologic function

B. Of particular importance is globally characterizing neurologic function to assess for traumatic brain and spinal cord injuries (SCIs)
C. The spinal cord is grossly assessed by visualizing movement of the extremities
D. If a patient is able to move their upper extremities, the likelihood of neurogenic shock is not diminished

59. False about Resuscitative thoracotomy (RT) is:

A. Resuscitative thoracotomy (RT) in the emergency department was first formally described by Cooley and DeBakey over 50 years ago for penetrating cardiovascular trauma
B. Patients with the best outcomes after RT are those with penetrating thoracic injuries and signs of life upon reaching the emergency department
C. Patients presenting after blunt chest mechanism, with and without signs of life, survived better than penetrating chest mechanism
D. RT should only be performed in locations with readily available surgical support for definitive repair of thoracic injuries if return of spontaneous circulation is achieved

60. Resuscitative thoracotomy (RT) provides opportunity for therapeutic maneuvers including all except:

A. Management of intrathoracic bleeding
B. Cross clamping the proximal thoracic aorta
C. Release of cardiac tamponade
D. Temporary repair of cardiac injury

61. False about Resuscitative endovascular balloon occlusion of the aorta (REBOA) is:

A. REBOA has emerged over the past decade as a promising method of obtaining temporary hemorrhage control in the decompensating trauma patient
B. Depending on the zone of trauma, REBOA is introduced through the common femoral artery, advanced proximal to level of injury, and inflated, effectively shunting blood to the heart and brain while also decreasing hemorrhage
C. First described during the Korean War
D. Currently, there is high-grade evidence to support indications or the superiority of REBOA beyond standard care, and a comparison of technique to RT introduces both survival and indication biases

62. Letter A in the image shows:

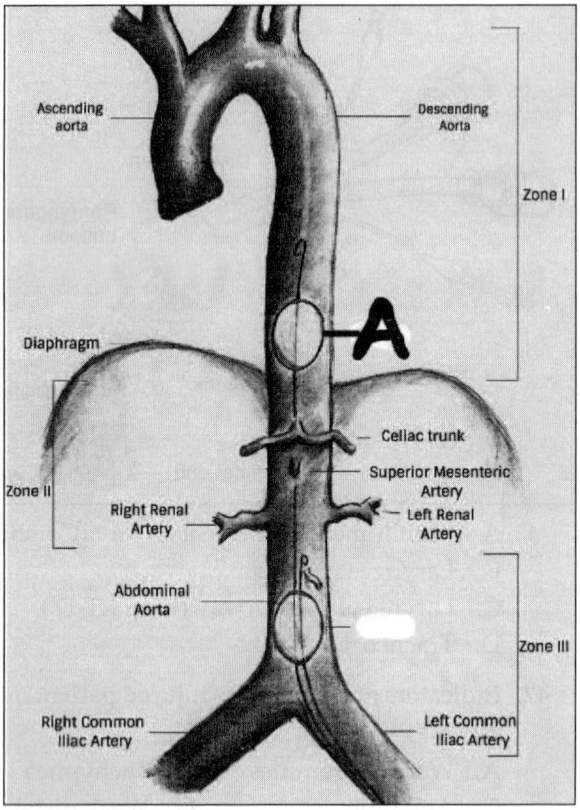

A. Resuscitative endovascular balloon occlusion of the aorta (REBOA)
B. Resuscitative thoracotomy (RT)
C. RIRS
D. PCNL

63. False about secondary survey for trauma as per ATLS is:

A. A rapid determination of neurologic function is done
B. The patient is rolled to evaluate the spine for deformity or tenderness and the long spine board should be removed
C. Seat belt marks or other superficial injury to the neck and abdomen may prompt further evaluation
D. A rectal examination with a nonbloody glove to assess the position of the prostate and the presence of gross gastrointestinal (GI) blood should be included

64. A 20-year-old female presents after a motor vehicle crash. She complains of diffuse abdominal pain. Her HR is 140 beats/min, and blood pressure is 78/42 mmHg. FAST is positive. Which statement is false about the description of the FAST examination?

A. 3.5-MHz convex-array transducer should be used

B. The hepatorenal space, known as the Morison pouch, is viewed between the 10th and 11th ribs in the right midclavicular line
C. The splenorenal space is evaluated between the 9th and 11th ribs in the left posterior axillary line
D. The bladder should preferentially be full before the examination to allow better visualization of fluid in the pelvis

MANAGEMENT OF SPECIFIC INJURIES

65. Following image of Thromboelastogram (TEG) shows:

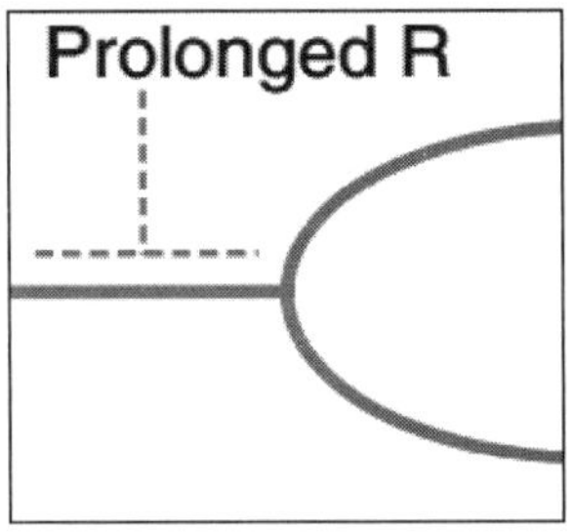

A. Anticoagulation B. Platelet dysfunction
C. Fibrinolysis D. Hypercoagulable

66. To inform initiation of massive transfusion protocol (MTP), the Assessment of Blood Consumption score provides a 4-point metric whereby clinicians may request product coolers based on prehospital (if available) or initial vital signs. All of the following are components except:

A. Positive FAST
B. Blunt mechanism
C. Arrival systolic blood pressure 90 mm Hg
D. Arrival pulse >120 bpm

67. The Clinical Randomization of an Antifibrinolytic in Significant Hemorrhage (CRASH)-2 trial had early administration of TXA within:

A. 3 hours B. 6 hours
C. 8 hours D. 24 hours

68. Following image of Thromboelastogram (TEG) shows:

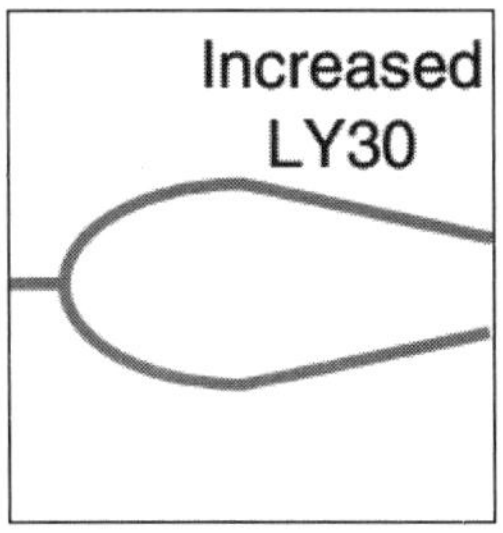

A. Anticoagulation B. Platelet dysfunction
C. Fibrinolysis D. Hypercoagulable

69. Following image of Thromboelastogram (TEG) shows:

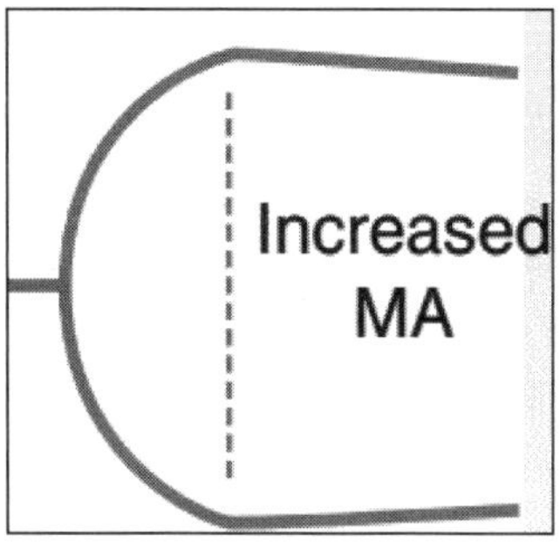

A. Anticoagulation
B. Platelet dysfunction
C. Fibrinolysis
D. Hypercoagulable

70. Following image of Thromboelastogram (TEG) shows:

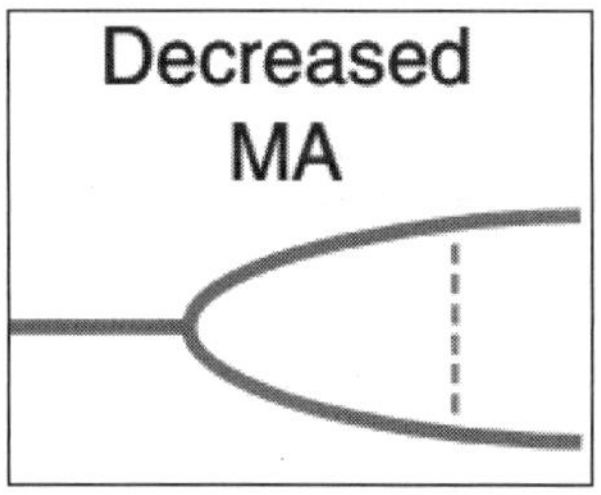

A. Anticoagulation
B. Platelet dysfunction
C. Fibrinolysis
D. Hypercoagulable

INJURIES TO THE BRAIN

71. The most common cause of brain injury is:

A. Road traffic accident
B. Falls
C. Sports injuries
D. Combat injuries

72. Following image shows:

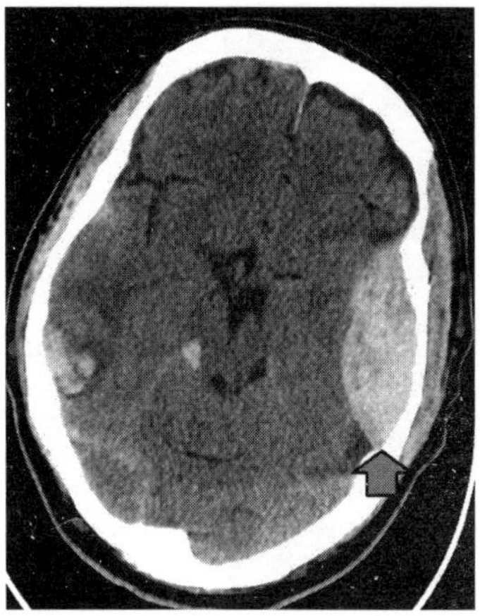

A. Subdural hematoma
B. Epidural hematoma
C. Subarachnoid hemorrhage
D. Intraparenchymal hemorrhage

73. Epidural hematomas typically result from bleeding from the:

A. Tearing of the bridging veins
B. Middle meningeal artery
C. Bleeding from brain tissue
D. Anterior communicating artery

74. Subdural hematomas typically result from bleeding from the:

A. Tearing of the bridging veins
B. Middle meningeal artery
C. Bleeding from brain tissue
D. Anterior communicating artery

75. Following image shows:

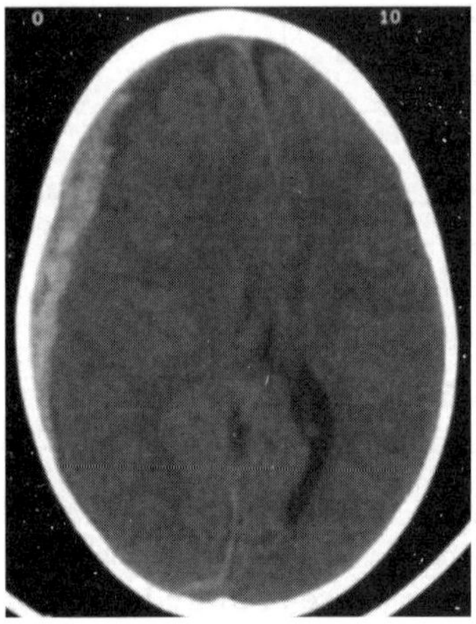

A. Subdural hematoma
B. Epidural hematoma
C. Subarachnoid hemorrhage
D. Brain contusion

76. Following image shows:

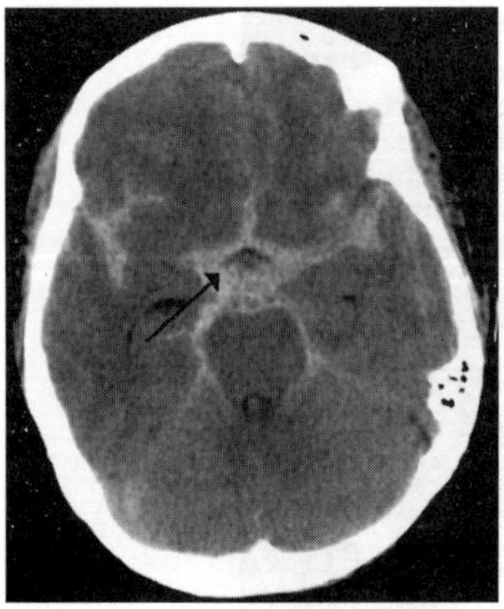

A. Subdural hematoma
B. Epidural hematoma
C. Subarachnoid hemorrhage
D. Brain contusion

77. Following image shows:

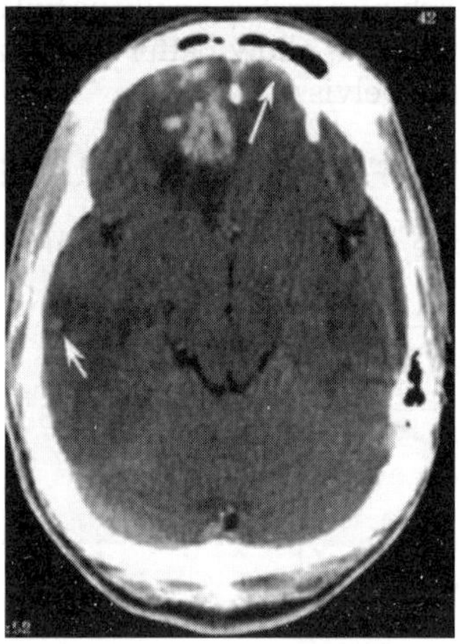

A. Subdural hematoma
B. Epidural hematoma
C. Subarachnoid hemorrhage
D. Brain contusion

78. False statement among the following is:

A. The underlying brain tissue is severely injured in the setting of an epidural hematoma
B. Bleeding within the subarachnoid space is indicative of diffuse bleeding from brain tissue and in itself is not deleterious
C. Diffuse axonal injury describes the phenomenon of axonal disruption of from the neuronal body secondary to severe rotational forces
D. Imaging often underestimates the severity of diffuse axonal injury, revealing only punctate hemorrhages and loss of gray and white matter differentiation

79. CRASH-3 trial suggest a mortality benefit in mild-moderate but not severe TBI patients receiving TXA:

A. Within 3 hours of injury
B. Within 6 hours of injury
C. Within 8 hours of injury
D. Within 12 hours of injury

80. False statement among the following is:

A. As the primary brain injury process cannot be reversed or corrected, outcomes after TBI are dictated by how well secondary injury is prevented

B. Airway control and ventilatory support are critical immediately after TBI, as transient episodes of hypoxia may increase mortality up to 10-fold
C. In the hypotensive polytrauma patient with severe TBI, military guidelines recommend 3% saline 250 mL bolus followed by 50 to 100 mL infusion for hemodynamic resuscitation and ICP reduction, possibly conferring survival benefit
D. Prevention of secondary brain injury, or treatment of recoverable cells (penumbra) around the traumatic focus, is the primary goal of TBI management

81. Amongst the components of GCS, the most predictive of future neurologic outcome is:

A. Eye opening
B. Motor function
C. Vocal response
D. All of the above

82. The most important diagnostic study during the initial evaluation of TBI is:

A. MRI
B. USG
C. CT brain without contrast
D. CT brain with contrast

83. A 53-year-old male had a road traffic accident. He was severe injury with presumed TBI. Urgent cranial CT was done was done and an ICP monitor was placed. ICP was elevated. All of the following should be done next except:

A. HOB elevation
B. Drainage of CSF
C. Mild hypoventilation
D. Hypertonic saline

84. False about the management of Traumatic brain injury (TBI) is:

A. In the setting of medically recalcitrant severe intracranial hypertension, patients may be considered for decompressive craniectomy, operative salvage has recently been shown to improve mortality and functional outcomes
B. Most commonly, epidural and subdural hematomas with mass effect benefit from immediate decompression in the OR
C. The necessity of invasive monitoring has been called into question by the Benchmark Evidence from South American Trials - Treatment of Intracranial Pressure (BEST-TRIP) trial data, suggesting noninferiority with serial imaging and clinical exam
D. As ICP tends to peak at 48 to 72 hours, patients who respond to management will experience a subsequent slow decrease in ICP with reductions in tissue edema and improvement in neurologic function

85. The goal of ICP in management of TBI is:

A. < 15 mm Hg
B. < 22 mm Hg
C. < 25 mm Hg
D. < 30 mm Hg

86. Indication for ICP monitor placement include GCS of:

A. < 5
B. < 8
C. < 10
D. < 12

87. CPP, the difference between the mean arterial pressure (MAP) and ICP, is also commonly used to guide severe TBI management with goal of:

A. 40 to 50 mm Hg
B. 50 to 60 mm Hg
C. 60 to 70 mm Hg
D. 70 to 80 mm Hg

88. Increased ventilation results in an optimal therapeutic vasoconstriction, when the PCO_2 is:

A. 20 to 25 mm Hg
B. 25 to 30 mm Hg
C. 30 to 35 mm Hg
D. 35 to 40 mm Hg

INJURIES TO THE SPINAL CORD AND THE VERTEBRAL COLUMN

89. False statement among the following is:

A. In blunt trauma patients, vertebral column fracture alone is over 10 times more frequent than SCIs
B. Mortality associated with to blunt vertebral spine injuries is approximately 8%
C. The 5th to 6th thoracic vertebrae are within the zone of greatest mobility and hence most susceptible to injury
D. In the cervical spine, where mobility is maximal, incidence of SCI is highest (55%)

90. True statement among the following is:

A. Chance fractures occur most commonly with motor vehicle accidents and have a high association with retroperitoneal or abdominal visceral injury
B. Penetrating mechanisms either directly lacerate the spinal cord or cause indirect injury through ischemia or vertebral fracture
C. The thoracic and lumbar spines are more limited in mobility and mechanisms of injury to this region include axial loading

(anterior wedge compression, burst injury) and flexion-extension (Chance fracture, fracture-dislocations)

D. All of the above

91. False about immediate management of SCI (Spinal Cord Injury) is:

A. In neurogenic shock patients, intravascular volume expansion and vasopressor support is needed

B. All blunt trauma patients are assumed to have an injury to the spine until a proper evaluation can exclude the diagnosis

C. The classic presentation of neurogenic shock is hypotension in the setting of cold, poorly-perfused extremities in the paralyzed patient

D. High cervical SCI (C3–C5) may have immediate respiratory suppression requiring airway management and ventilatory support due to paresis of the phrenic nerves

92. As per American Spinal Injury Association impairment scale, A on the scale is:

A. Complete injury

B. Sensory incomplete

C. Motor incomplete

D. Normal

93. As per American Spinal Injury Association impairment scale, D on the scale is:

A. Complete injury

B. Sensory incomplete

C. Motor incomplete

D. Normal

94. As per American Spinal Injury Association impairment scale, E on the scale is:

A. Complete injury

B. Sensory incomplete

C. Motor incomplete

D. Normal

95. False about the evaluation of SCI (Spinal Cord Injury) is:

A. Plain radiograph of the spine (anteroposterior, lateral, odontoid) is the modality of choice in most emergency departments for evaluate of vertebral column injury

B. Prehospital screening tools, such as the Canadian C-spine Rule or the National Emergency X-Radiography Utilization Study (NEXUS), provide a means by which patients who have no findings on examination, demonstrate no decreased level of consciousness, and have no distracting injuries can undergo clearance of the spine by clinical means alone

C. Sagittal and coronal reconstruction of CT imaging of the spine provides better anatomic visualization

D. MRI is often needed to better characterize soft tissue injury, particularly in the setting of neck pain and normal radiography, if performed within the first 72 hours of trauma

96. False about the management of SCI (Spinal Cord Injury) is:

A. As a general rule, the spine should be protected from further injury by maintaining strict immobilization until injuries can be ruled out

B. Cervical SCIs with neurogenic shock require resuscitation with volume expansion and often vasopressor/inotropic therapy

C. Brief periods of hypotension (<90 mm Hg), not unlike TBI, have been not shown previously to be detrimental to long-term outcomes in SCI; thus, shock can be treated non aggressively

D. Society guidelines include recommendations for MAP goals 85 to 90 mm Hg for 7 days following injury

97. True about Corticosteroid therapy for SCI:

A. Short-duration steroids remain a potentially therapeutic option following SCI, although they should be considered in consultation between trauma and neurosurgical services

B. Several large randomized trials (National Acute Spinal Cord Injury Study series) have demonstrated motor improvement at 6 weeks and 6 months following methylprednisolone administration if initiated within 8 hours of injury

C. Functional recovery is similar whether methylprednisolone is administered as bolus-infusion for a duration of 24 or 48 hours in patients receiving treatment within 3 hours or 3 to 8 hours after injury, respectively

D. All of the above

98. Disruption of C1 ring in multiple locations; blow-out of ring is called:

A. Odontoid fractures B. Jefferson fracture

C. Hangman fracture D. Chance fracture

99. Avulsion of posterior elements of lumbar vertebrae seen with high seat belt use is:

A. Odontoid fractures B. Jefferson fracture

C. Hangman fracture D. Chance fracture

100. Hangman fracture is:

A. Bilateral C1 pedicles with spondylolisthesis
B. Bilateral C2 pedicles with spondylolisthesis
C. Unilateral C1 pedicles with spondylolisthesis
D. Unilateral C2 pedicles with spondylolisthesis

101. Following image shows image of a C2 vertebrae. Which type of fracture is shown and the treatment of the #?

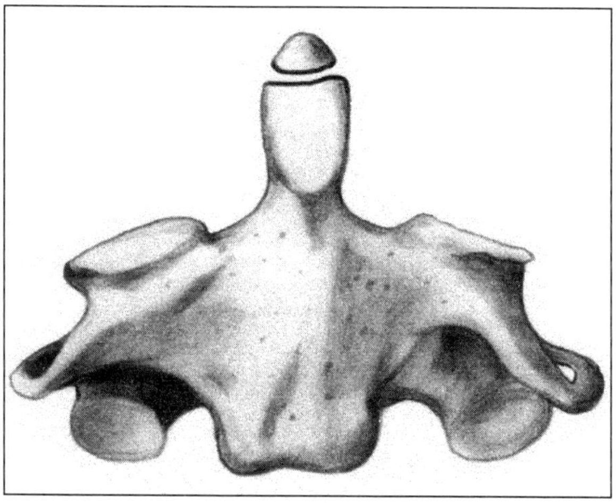

A. Type I Odontoid #; hard collar
B. Type II Odontoid #; hard collar
C. Type I Odontoid #; halo vest
D. Type II Odontoid #; halo vest

102. Following image shows image of a C2 vertebrae. Which type of fracture is shown and the treatment of the #?

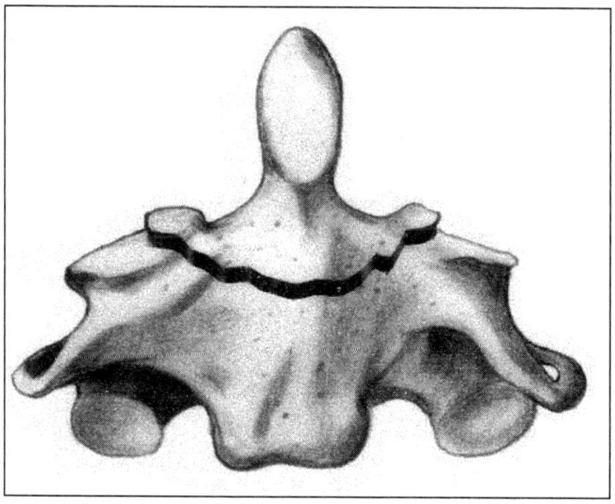

A. Type I Odontoid #; hard collar
B. Type II Odontoid #; hard collar
C. Type II Odontoid #; halo vest
D. Type III Odontoid #; halo vest

103. Following image shows image of a C2 vertebrae. Which type of fracture is shown?

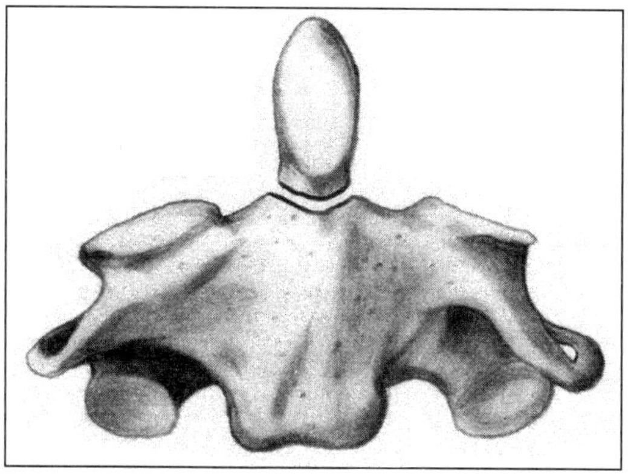

A. Type I Odontoid #
B. Type II Odontoid #
C. Type III Odontoid #
D. Type IV Odontoid #

104. Following image shows which Le Fort's class of facial fracture?

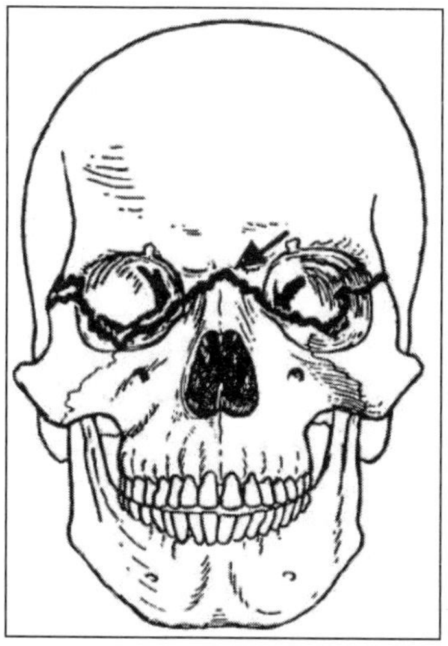

A. Type 1 B. Type 2
C. Type 3 D. Type 4

105. Following image shows which Le Fort's class of facial fracture?

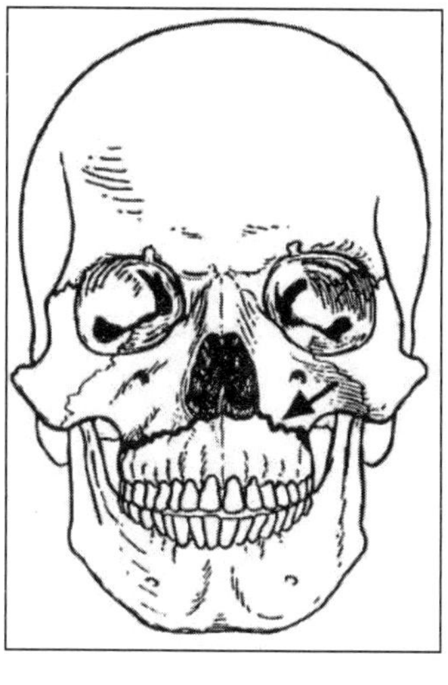

A. Type 1
B. Type 2
C. Type 3
D. Type 4

INJURY TO THE MAXILLOFACIAL REGION

106. False about injury to the maxillofacial region is:

A. Injury to the face requires prompt assessment and management of the airway, particularly when lower face soft tissue and bone involvement is present
B. Due to the vascularity of the face, bleeding can be an immediate concern and should be managed with direct pressure, suture ligature, and the initiation of resuscitation
C. Bleeding from deep vessels or fractured bone may require angioembolization for definitive control to be obtained
D. Imaging of the face should be performed immediately, as management of facial trauma is time sensitive in the majority of cases

107. False about evaluation of injury to the maxillofacial region is:

A. The condition of the globe and the surrounding orbit requires careful evaluation for rupture or extraocular muscle entrapment, which requires urgent treatment
B. CT is indicated when any external injury is identified on primary survey
C. Midface and mandibular stability, proper occlusion, and quality of the dentition are assessed
D. When fractures or soft tissue injuries are identified, the motor function of the face should be assessed to evaluate facial nerve function

108. False about management of injury to the maxillofacial region is:

A. Before wound closure, jagged or nonviable skin edges should be debrided, followed by irrigation of the wound with sterile fluid
B. Lacerations can frequently be closed with local anesthesia using deep absorbable sutures followed by closure of the skin with 5-0 or 6-0 interrupted or running sutures
C. Large open wounds and fractures involving sinuses or the aerodigestive tract never require antibiotics
D. Mandibular fractures can be treated with maxillary-mandibular fixation, although significant fracture displacement may require internal fixation with plating

109. Parade ground fracture is also called as:

A. Le Fort's class IV #
B. Fracture of the symphysis of mandible
C. Guardsman fracture
D. Le Fort's class I #

INJURIES TO THE NECK

110. False about injuries to neck is:

A. Trauma to the neck is relatively uncommon but results in the highest mortality of all body regions (17% mortality for AIS $\geq$3 injuries in the NTDB)
B. Blunt cerebrovascular injuries (BCVIs) result from seat belt compression or severe flexion-extension mechanisms
C. Blunt mechanisms can cause sudden compression, with subsequent fracture of the larynx or trachea and is the most common mechanism of injury
D. Blunt pharyngeal or esophageal injuries are even less common but can result in tissue devitalization, leakage into the surrounding soft tissues with consequent abscess, or mediastinitis

111. Grade III BCVI among the following is:

A. Intimal tears
B. Pseudoaneurysm formation
C. Arterial occlusion
D. Arterial transection

112. Arterial occlusion is BCVI:

A. Grade II
B. Grade III
C. Grade IV
D. Grade V

113. False about immediate management of injuries to neck is:

A. Immediate intubation should occur in the setting of an expanding neck hematoma or if there is concern for impending airway compromise
B. Direct injury to the larynx or trachea is the most common cause of airway compromise and presents one of the most challenging circumstances to airway management
C. The surgical airway of choice for an upper airway injury is a cricothyroidotomy
D. Direct pressure with either finger or Foley balloon effectively manages most bleeding from the neck during transport to the OR

114. Zone 2 of neck injury is:

A. Between the cricoid cartilage and the base of skull
B. Between the cricoid cartilage and the angle of the mandible
C. Extends from the angle of the mandible to the skull base
D. Extends from the thoracic inlet to the cricoid cartilage

115. Zone 3 of neck injury is:

A. Between the cricoid cartilage and the base of skull
B. Between the cricoid cartilage and the angle of the mandible
C. Extends from the angle of the mandible to the skull base
D. Extends from the thoracic inlet to the cricoid cartilage

116. False about neck injury is:

A. Zone I extends from the thoracic inlet to the cricoid cartilage and contains large vascular structures as well as the trachea and esophagus
B. Stretching from the cricoid cartilage to the angle of the mandible, zone II is the most accessible surgically and contains the carotid and vertebral arteries, jugular veins, and structures of the aerodigestive tract
C. Zone III includes the neck between the angle of the mandible and the base of the skull
D. Structures within zone III include blood vessels that are easy to expose surgically

117. False about the evaluation of neck injury is:

A. DSA is the study of choice for diagnosis of BCVI
B. CT angiographic evaluation of the neck, performed in the emergency department, has become readily available and decreased the rate of negative neck explorations for penetrating injury
C. DSA confirmed BCVI in 30% of high-risk cohort
D. All of the above are true

118. Indicator of high risk for blunt cerebrovascular injury includes all except:

A. Expanding neck hematoma
B. Arterial hemorrhage from neck, nose or mouth
C. Focal neurologic deficit
D. Cervical bruit (patient >50 years old)

119. Indicator of high risk for blunt cerebrovascular injury includes all except:

A. Diffuse axonal injury and GCS score ≤ 6
B. Le Fort I
C. Significant soft tissue injury to anterior neck (i.e., seat belt mark)
D. Basilar skull fracture involving the carotid canal

120. False about the management of neck injury is:

A. An injured internal jugular vein may require direct repair with Prolene suture or ligation, if closure is not possible
B. Most commonly, structures of the neck are exposed by an incision along the anterior border of the sternocleidomastoid on the side of the injury
C. Short-segment carotid artery injuries should require reconstruction with a synthetic graft or autologous vein
D. A collar incision may be more versatile, especially if a bilateral neck exploration is required

121. False about the management of neck injury is:

A. Injuries to the esophagus should be debrided to expose the entirety of the mucosal perforation
B. Tracheal lacerations can be primarily closed with absorbable suture if the injury is small and will approximate in a tension-free fashion
C. Large tracheal defects may require resection and anastomosis, although some anterior tracheal injuries can be managed by creating a tracheostomy through the injury
D. All of the above

122. False about the management of BCVI is:

A. To decrease the risk of thromboembolic stroke (37%–4.8%), anticoagulation or antiplatelet therapy is initiated, although neither has demonstrated superiority
B. Anticoagulation with heparin should be started with the goal of achieving a partial thromboplastin time between 40 and 50 seconds, although daily 325 mg aspirin (ASA) presents an equivalent therapeutic option
C. Endovascular stenting may be considered in select circumstances involving pseudoaneurysm and dissection with 50% flow limitation
D. MDCTA may be repeated in 24 to 48 hours if findings are indeterminate on initial scan and all confirmed injuries should undergo repeat imaging at 7 to 10 days to evaluate

for progression or resolution and subsequent discontinuation of therapy

123. A 32-year-old female had a road traffic accident. She had a penetrating neck trauma. She was hemodynamically stable and has no hard signs of arterial injury. There was zone 1 neck injury. She underwent CTA which was normal. There was concern for TE injury. What is the next line of management?

A. Esophagography B. Esophagoscopy
C. Bronchoscopy D. All of the above

124. A 40-year-old male was caught in a brawl and was brought to hospital. On examination he has BCVI and risk factors for BCVI. He underwent CTA and was found to have grade 1 BCVI. What is the next step of management?

A. Send him home and repeat CT angiogram or DSA in 7–10 days
B. Start antithrombotic therapy (Heparin with PTT 40–50 sec)
C. Operative or endovascular treatment
D. Repeat CTA neck in 24–48h or DSA

125. A 30-year-old female has RTA and was brought to hospital. On examination she has BCVI and risk factors for BCVI. She underwent CTA and was found to have grade 5 BCVI. What is the next step of management?

A. Send him home and repeat CT angiogram or DSA in 7–10 days
B. Start antithrombotic therapy (Heparin with PTT 40–50 sec)
C. Operative or endovascular treatment
D. Repeat CTA neck in 24–48h or DSA

126. A 35-year-old male presents after being stabbed in the neck. A 3 cm wound is present at the base of the neck, just right of midline above the sternum. An expanding hematoma is noted. The patient is intubated for airway protection and taken to the operating room for exploration. What is the best initial incision to expose and control this injury?

A. Anterior border of the sternocleidomastoid muscle
B. Median sternotomy
C. Right anterolateral thoracotomy
D. Collar incision

INJURIES TO THE CHEST

127. False about chest trauma is:

A. Chest trauma with pulmonary compromise requires immediate management of the airway and ventilatory assistance
B. Falls and motor vehicle crashes comprise the majority of blunt chest injuries via transmission of energy to the chest wall and direct compression or deceleration forces to underlying structures.
C. Although hemodynamic instability most commonly indicates hemorrhage until proven otherwise, cardiac dysfunction secondary to pericardial tamponade, cardiac contusion, or coronary air embolism may represent other possible sources
D. Patients with persistent shock despite resuscitation and ongoing blood loss from the chest rarely require operative intervention

128. Blunt trauma to the chest requiring surgical management is:

A. < 5% B. < 10%
C. < 20% D. < 50%

129. False about the evaluation of chest injury is:

A. Chest wall tenderness and paradoxical movement can be identified to reflect segmental injuries to the ribs (flail) and sternum
B. Thoracic MDCTA has become the standard approach to evaluation of the chest and provides superior visualization of the chest wall, vasculature, pleural spaces, and lung parenchyma
C. Deviation of the trachea at the sternal notch may reveal intrathoracic tension on the side opposite the trachea
D. MDCTA is reliable for evaluation of pericardium

130. Boundaries of "the cardiac box" are all except:

A. Sternum medially
B. Sternal notch superiorly
C. The costal margin inferiorly
D. The nipples laterally

131. True about the evaluation of chest injury is:

A. CT angiography has become accepted as sufficient to guide operative intervention without the need for standard angiography of the chest
B. As with blunt trauma, the great vessels are evaluated for injury with MDCTA
C. Depending on the trajectory of the penetrating object, the trachea and proximal airways may require evaluation with bronchoscopy and a

combination of esophagoscopy with contrast esophagography are diagnostic for esophageal injuries
D. All of the above

132. Percentage of thoracic injuries that are successfully treated with tube thoracostomy alone is up to:

A. 80% B. 85%
C. 90% D. 95%

133. True about the management of thoracic injuries is:

A. To avoid the development of an empyema, the chest should be prepared appropriately by wide preparation with chlorhexidine as well as wide draping to maintain the sterility of the field
B. Chest tube sizing for trauma has typically ranged from 32 to 36 Fr
C. Chest tube is connected to an underwater drainage device providing 20 cm H_2O suction
D. All of the above

134. Overall incidence of chest empyema in chest trauma is:

A. 1% B. 3%
C. 8% D. 15%

135. Boundary of triangle of safety is:

A. Spine posteriorly
B. Scapula posteriorly
C. Coastal margin inferiorly
D. Nipple or inframammary fold inferiorly

136. The traditional indications for emergency thoracotomy in blunt trauma chest is:

A. > 500 mL of blood drained on chest tube insertion
B. Persistent hemodynamic stability in the setting of ongoing transfusion requirement
C. 100 mL/hr of drainage for 2 to 4 consecutive hours
D. > 1500 mL of blood drained on chest tube insertion

137. Access to the lungs, pulmonary vasculature, and hemidiaphragm in emergency thoracotomy is achieved through a:

A. Anterolateral thoracotomy
B. Posterolateral thoracotomy
C. Median sternotomy
D. Clamshell incision

138. A median sternotomy can be a highly versatile approach, providing exposure to all except:

A. Left subclavian artery
B. Right side of the heart
C. Aortic arch with right sided arch vessels
D. Ascending aorta

139. Pulmonary vasculature exposure is best provided by:

A. Anterolateral thoracotomy
B. Posterolateral thoracotomy
C. Median sternotomy
D. Clamshell incision

140. Descending aorta exposure is best provided by:

A. Anterolateral thoracotomy
B. Posterolateral thoracotomy
C. Median sternotomy
D. Clamshell incision

141. The most common thoracic injury is:

A. Aortic rupture
B. Rib fracture
C. Esophageal injury
D. Pulmonary contusion

142. True about chest wall injuries is:

A. Some volume of air (pneumothorax) or blood (hemothorax) is commonly associated with chest injury, owing to compressive forces upon the lung or penetrating mechanisms
B. Rib fractures typically occur secondary to compression of the thoracic cage in an anteroposterior or lateral direction
C. CT easily recognizes significant chest wall deformities, such as flail segment, displaced ribs, and sternal fractures, and may be used to guide considerations of chest wall reconstruction
D. All of the above

143. Flail chest is:

A. 1 or more adjacent ribs fractured in 2 or more locations
B. 3 or more adjacent ribs fractured in 1 or more locations
C. 2 or more adjacent ribs fractured in 2 or more locations
D. 3 or more adjacent ribs fractured in 2 or more locations

144. False about pleural injuries is:

A. Although large-volume pneumothoraces are typically detected on X-ray, up to half are subsequently discovered on CT chest
B. All pneumo- or hemothoraces visible on a chest radiograph should be considered for tube thoracostomy
C. Recent data suggest that observation for pneumothoraces with CT radial diameter of up to 55 mm may be safe for both blunt and penetrating trauma
D. Occult pneumothoraces not accompanied by respiratory compromise can be managed with observation and a repeated chest radiograph 12 to 24 hours later to demonstrate stability

145. Hemothoraces visible on upright chest X-ray represent an approximate volume of:

A. 50–100 mL B. 100–150 mL
C. 200–300 mL D. 400–500 mL

146. True about hemothorax is:

A. Chest tubes may be safely removed following demonstrated pleural space evacuation, on underwater seal, with < 300 mL output over prior 24 hours
B. Residual hemothorax that does not resolve after insertion of a chest tube should be considered for video-assisted thoracoscopic (VATS) drainage
C. Timing of VATS intervention is best undertaken in days 3 to 7 of hospitalization to reduce the risk of conversion to thoracotomy
D. All of the above

147. Risk of empyema in retained hemothorax following chest tube placement is approximately:

A. 33% B. 25%
C. 66% D. 50%

148. A 26-year-old male presents with a stab wound to the right chest about 1 cm lateral to the sternum between the second and third ribs. The patient is awake but confused, his HR is 100 beats/min, and his blood pressure is 102/54 mm Hg. He is taken to the operating room after initial resuscitation. What is the best approach to expose this injury?

A. Median sternotomy
B. Right anterolateral thoracotomy
C. Right posterolateral thoracotomy
D. Right supraclavicular incision

149. A 41-year-old male falls from a 12-foot ladder and lands on his left side. He fractures left ribs 2 to 9 with a flail segment, resulting in pneumothorax. After the chest tube is placed, what is the next best step in management?

A. Pain control with an epidural
B. Incentive spirometer
C. Early ambulation
D. All of the above

150. A 21-year-old man is taken to the ED with a gunshot wound to the right side of his chest. HR is 126 beats/min and blood pressure is 88/46 mm Hg. A right-sided chest tube is placed, with the return of 1200 mL of blood. He is resuscitated with 2 L of lactated Ringer's solution, and his vital signs return to within normal limits. His chest tube output is rechecked 4 h later, and the total amount in the collection container is 2300 ml. What is the next most appropriate step in management?

A. Chest CT
B. Stat hemoglobin/hematocrit
C. Right thoracotomy
D. Left anterolateral thoracotomy

151. A 23-year-old man is receiving positive-pressure ventilation in the ICU after sustaining multiple trauma in an automobile collision. The patient has sudden onset of hypotension and dyspnea. Which of the following is the most appropriate immediate management?

A. Catheter aspiration
B. Chest X-ray
C. Needle decompression
D. Tube thoracostomy

152. A pneumothorax that causes mediastinal shift and compression of the functioning lung is called:

A. Primary pneumothorax
B. Secondary pneumothorax
C. Traumatic pneumothorax
D. Tension pneumothorax

153. 50-year-old who fell from 3 meters. Which of the following best accounts for the increased density of the left hemithorax?

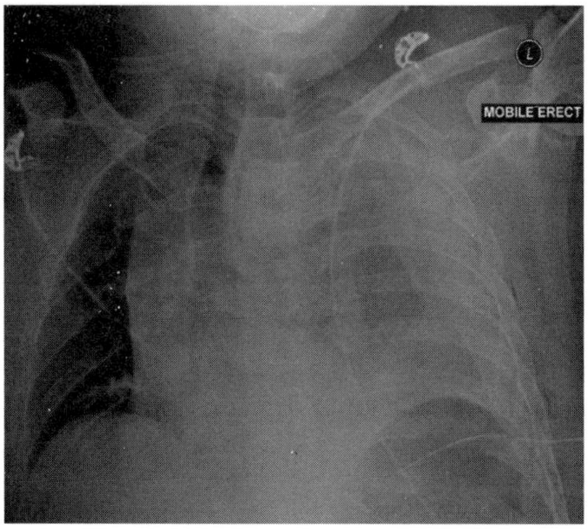

A. Diaphragmatic rupture
B. Hemothorax
C. Lung contusion
D. Lung collapse

154. A 25-year-old male was involved in a fight. He was brought to emergency department with complaints of pain on the right side of the chest. There was decreased air entry on the right side of the chest on auscultation. His chest X-ray is as given below. What is the diagnosis?

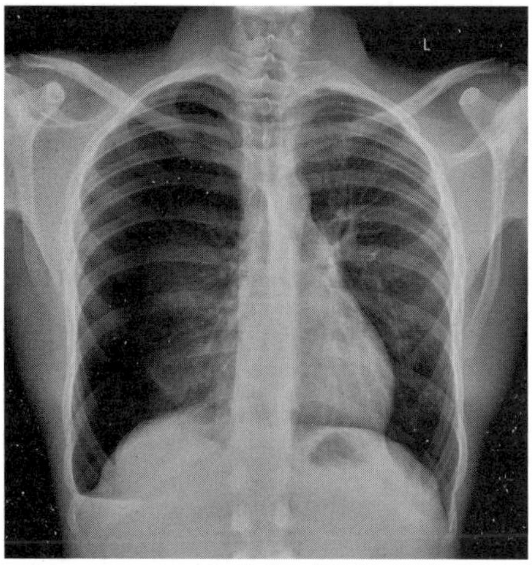

A. Left sided pneumothorax
B. Right sided pneumothorax
C. Left sided hemothorax
D. Right sided hemothorax

155. False about pulmonary injuries is:

A. Approximately 1 in 5 patients in the NTDB sustains a pulmonary contusion after chest trauma
B. Trauma to the lung is caused by energy transfer through the chest wall to the pulmonary parenchyma, resulting in tissue damage as well as hemorrhage into the alveolar and interstitial spaces
C. Lung contusions are occasionally present on the initial chest radiograph, but typically require time (24–48 hours) to become visualized
D. Pulmonary contusion occurs with a flail segment and is often more clinically important than the bony trauma

156. False about pulmonary injuries is:

A. Injured lung tissue on CT appears as a lesser density
B. Thoracic CT is valuable for the identification of pulmonary contusion, although it can be challenging at times to differentiate contusion from atelectasis.
C. Pulmonary contusion is typically managed with supportive care (aggressive pulmonary toilet, adequate pain control)
D. Patients should be monitored for hypoxemia, increased work of breathing, and agitation, the sum of which indicates respiratory decompensation

157. The most common indication for ECMO following chest trauma is:

A. Pulmonary contusion
B. ARDS
C. Pulmonary embolism
D. Pneumothorax

158. False about the management of pulmonary injuries is:

A. In most cases, tube thoracostomy alone with lung expansion adequately manages low pressure lung bleeding and small air leaks
B. Trauma pneumonectomy is morbid with mortality (< 30%)
C. Hilar control with either clamp or "hilar twist" should be the initial maneuver performed if significant bleeding is encountered upon entry into the chest
D. Anatomic lobectomy and pneumonectomy are more commonly performed if resection is required in association with blunt trauma

159. False about cardiac injuries is:

A. Mortality among patients arriving to a trauma center with a penetrating cardiac injury ranges from 17% to 58%
B. Penetrating injury to the heart occurred in 10% to 20% of patients with penetrating trauma in the NTDB and in > 50% of the subset with penetrating chest trauma alone
C. For cardiac injuries that cause cardiovascular collapse, a left anterolateral thoracotomy is

performed in the emergency department and may be extended to a contralateral ("clamshell") incision if need be

D. Ultrasound is a valuable tool for quickly assessing the pericardium for fluid and should be performed in all patients with hemodynamic instability

160. Beck triad includes all except:

A. Distended neck veins
B. Muffled heart sounds
C. Hypotension
D. Decreased air entry on auscultation

161. When time permits, most cardiac injuries are best approached through:

A. Median sternotomy
B. Right anterolateral thoracotomy
C. Right posterolateral thoracotomy
D. Right supraclavicular incision

162. False about blunt cardiac injury (BCI) is:

A. Most of the cases represent a contusion of the myocardium that results in arrhythmias and is frequently need intervention
B. A new abnormality on the electrocardiogram (ECG), most commonly tachyarrhythmia, should result in admission for continuous ECG monitoring
C. Cardiogenic shock may require treatment with inotropic support and right ventricular afterload reduction, given the frequent involvement of the right side of the heart
D. Patients who demonstrate structural abnormalities, such as valvular incompetence, may require urgent operation for repair

163. A 19-year-old male presents after a high-speed head-on motor vehicle crash into a tree. He was the unrestrained driver and hit the steering wheel with his chest. He has a sternal fracture, broken left clavicle, and a left pneumothorax. A left chest tube is placed with a resolution of the pneumothorax. What is the best initial evaluation for a blunt cardiac injury (BCI)?

A. Serial electrocardiogram (ECG) only
B. Serial troponins only
C. Echocardiogram only
D. Admission ECG and troponin

164. A 37-year-old female comes in with a stab wound to the right chest just lateral to the sternal border. HR is 130 beats/min, blood pressure is 74/58 mm Hg, and jugular venous distention is noted on examination with muffled heart sounds. Which option provides the appropriate diagnosis and treatment?

A. Tension pneumothorax: right thoracotomy
B. Tension pneumothorax: right tube thoracostomy
C. Tension pneumothorax: median sternotomy
D. Cardiac tamponade: pericardial window

165. Percentage of trauma patients with blunt traumatic aortic injury (BTAI) that die before they reach a hospital is:

A. 10%
B. 30%
C. 50%
D. 80%

166. False about blunt thoracic aortic injury (BTAI) is:

A. Chest radiograph may demonstrate findings such as a widened mediastinum, apical capping, loss of the aortic knob, or deviation of the left mainstem bronchus
B. Because of a high rate of missed injuries with use of chest radiography as a screening study, most patients involved in high-energy injury mechanisms undergo helical CT angiography of the chest to evaluate for aortic injury
C. BTAI with pseudoaneurysm will require operative repair, as the natural history of these injuries is slow expansion to free aortic rupture.
D. When open surgical repair is required, the aorta is exposed through a right thoracotomy

167. On CT angiography of the chest after blunt thoracic aortic injury (BTAI), Grade III injury is:

A. Pseudoaneurysm
B. Intramural hematoma
C. Rupture
D. Disruption in the intima

168. On CT angiography of the chest after blunt thoracic aortic injury (BTAI), Grade II injury is:

A. Pseudoaneurysm
B. Intramural hematoma
C. Rupture
D. Disruption in the intima

169. False about tracheobronchial tree injuries is:

A. Penetrating mechanisms are the most common cause
B. Penetrating tracheobronchial injuries are predominantly a result of gun shot wounds that cause direct laceration of the tracheobronchial tree

C. Distal airway injuries may result in large amounts of pneumomediastinum identified by chest radiography or CT imaging
D. Diagnosis is made with either rigid or flexible bronchoscopy, depending on the location of the injury and the ability to manipulate the neck

170. False about management of tracheobronchial tree injuries is:

A. Management includes humidified oxygen, careful suctioning, and close observation to monitor for infectious sequelae that may develop
B. Operative management of the trachea, right-sided airways, and proximal left mainstem bronchus is best approached through a left posterolateral thoracotomy
C. Coverage of the repair with a tissue pedicle, such intercostal muscle flap, may improve healing
D. Devitalized tissue should be debrided and injures closed with absorbable monofilament suture

171. False about esophageal injuries is:

A. Penetrating injury is slightly more common; however, historically, less than 1% of chest injuries in the NTDB had involvement of the esophagus by blunt or penetrating mechanism
B. The esophagus is best evaluated through a combination of contrast esophagography (water-soluble first, followed by thin barium) and esophagoscopy; these 2 modalities result in a sensitivity of almost 100% for esophageal injury
C. In the absence of contrast, chest CT reveals air adjacent to the esophagus but outside the lumen with surrounding soft tissue inflammation
D. High-resolution CT imaging rarely demonstrates an esophageal wall defect

172. The mortality associated with penetrating esophageal injuries is substantial:

A. 15% B. 35%
C. 55% D. 75%

173. False about the management of esophageal injuries is:

A. Esophageal injuries require operative repair to close the esophageal defect, ideally in 2 layers (mucosal/muscular), with provision of adequate drainage
B. Creation of a vascularized intercostal muscle flap on entry into the chest will allow excellent coverage of the repair
C. Following repair, an esophagram may be performed at day 14 to confirm healing and liberalization of oral intake
D. Esophageal repairs at the gastroesophageal junction can be covered with a fundoplication of gastric tissue

174. The upper and midthoracic esophagus is best approached through a:

A. Right posterolateral thoracotomy
B. Left posterolateral thoracotomy
C. Right anterolateral thoracotomy
D. Left anterolateral thoracotomy

175. The lower esophagus is best approached through a:

A. Right posterolateral thoracotomy
B. Left posterolateral thoracotomy
C. Right anterolateral thoracotomy
D. Left anterolateral thoracotomy

176. False about traumatic diaphragmatic injuries is:

A. Penetrating trauma was more common than blunt
B. The right side of the diaphragm is the injured location in approximately 75% of the cases
C. The chest radiograph may demonstrate the presence of abdominal viscera, most commonly the stomach, within the chest
D. The morbidity related to diaphragmatic injuries is occasionally identified months to years later when the perforation was not initially repaired

177. False about the management of traumatic diaphragmatic injuries is:

A. It is important to obtain hemostasis because diaphragmatic injuries can bleed significantly from branches of the phrenic artery that can be exposed at the edges of the tear
B. Diaphragmatic injuries are typically repaired by debriding nonviable tissue and then closing the defect
C. Closure is performed with a single layer of absorbable suture incorporating large full-thickness bites of healthy diaphragmatic tissue
D. A peripheral detachment of the diaphragm from the wall of the torso can be repaired by reinserting the injured tissue 1 or 2 interspaces superior

178. A 38-year-old car mechanic is taken to the ED after having been pinned underneath a car. On chest radiography, multiple rib fractures are noted, as well as an air-fluid level consistent with the stomach being above the level of the left diaphragm. Which of the following statements regarding this injury is true?

A. Right-sided diaphragmatic rupture is more common than left-sided rupture
B. There is a 30% incidence of coexisting pelvic fractures
C. The best initial radiographic assessment for this type of injury is FAST
D. In most acute diaphragmatic ruptures, repair can be completed with primary repair

179. An 18-year-old man is brought to the emergency department with a stab wound just to the right of the sternum in the sixth intercostal space. His blood pressure is 80 mm Hg. Faint heart sounds and pulsus paradoxus are noted. Auscultation of the right chest reveals decreased breath sounds. The initial management of this patient should be which of the following?

A. Drainage of the right chest cavity
B. Insertion of central venous access line
C. Aspiration of the pericardium
D. Echocardiogram

180. An 18-year-old man presents to the emergency department with a gunshot wound to the left chest in the anterior axillary line in the seventh intercostal space. A rushing sound is audible during inspiration. Immediate management is which of the following?

A. Exploratory thoracotomy
B. Closure of the hole with sterile dressing
C. Pleurocentesis
D. Exploratory laparotomy

181. A 25-year-old man is shot in the left lateral chest. In the emergency department, his blood pressure is 120/90 mm Hg, pulse rate is 104 beats per minute (bpm), and respiration rate is 36 breaths per minute. Chest X-ray shows air and fluid in the left pleural cavity. Nasogastric aspiration reveals blood-stained fluid. What is the best step to rule out esophageal injury?

A. Contrast esophagography and esophagoscopy
B. Peritoneal lavage
C. Insertion of chest tube
D. Insertion of nasogastric tube

182. A 26-year-old man is stabbed in the right intercostal space in the midclavicular line and presents to the emergency department. On examination, subcutaneous emphysema of the right chest wall, absent breath sounds, and a trachea shifted to the left are noted. What is the most likely serious diagnosis?

A. Pneumothorax
B. Hemopneumothorax
C. Tension pneumothorax
D. Massive hemothorax

183. A 31-year-old man is shot in the back of the left chest, and the bullet exits the left anterior chest. The patient's blood pressure is 130/90 mm Hg, respiration rate is 28 breaths per minute, and pulse is 110 bpm. A chest X-ray reveals hemothorax. A chest tube is inserted and yields 800 mL of blood; the first- and second-hour drainage is 200 mL/h and 240 mL/h, respectively. What is the next step in management?

A. Collect the blood for autotransfusion
B. Perform a left thoracotomy
C. Insert a Swan-Ganz catheter
D. Place a 2nd chest tube

184. A 60-year-old man is in a car crash in which he is the driver. He did not have a seat belt or an airbag. He is found to have multiple rib fractures over his right chest. His pulse is weaker during inspiration. What are the most likely diagnoses?

A. Flail chest
B. Diaphragm rupture
C. Pectus excavation
D. Cervical rib

185. A 23-year-old man, tall and thin, was jogging one evening when he suddenly felt a sharp pain in the left chest, worse on taking a deep breath and shortness of breath. What is the most likely diagnosis?

A. Tension pneumothorax
B. Spontaneous pneumothorax
C. Massive hemothorax
D. Open pneumothorax

186. A 45-year-old man was a passenger in a car when he was T-boned by a truck at a high speed. He is short in breath, complains of severe pain in the chest, and is hypoxic on the pulse oximeter. The breath sounds are diminished on the left and the percussion note is completely dull. He rapidly

becomes tachycardic and hypotensive. What is the most likely diagnosis?

A. Rupture diaphragm
B. Cardiac tamponade
C. Massive hemothorax
D. Open pneumothorax

187. A 25-year-old woman was stabbed by her boyfriend in the left chest. On examination, she has a 1 cm stab wound just inferior to her left breast in the mid-clavicular line. There is jugular venous distension and breath sounds are completely absent on the left side. She is becoming extremely dyspneic and hypoxic. What is the most likely diagnosis?

A. Tension pneumothorax
B. Massive hemothorax
C. Rupture diaphragm
D. Spontaneous pneumothorax

INJURIES TO THE ABDOMEN

188. True about blunt trauma abdomen is:

A. FAST is limited by operator familiarity, body habitus, and subcutaneous emphysema/bowel gas
B. Ultrasound for trauma evaluates the pericardium, hepatorenal fossa, splenorenal fossa, and retrovesicular space (pouch of Douglas)
C. Abdominal CT for trauma is typically performed with IV administration of a contrast agent additionally timed to capture the portal venous phase, which best demonstrates the perfusion of the solid abdominal organs
D. All of the above

189. False about penetrating abdominal trauma is:

A. GSWs involving the thoracoabdomen may also require evaluation of the chest for mediastinal, pleural, or pulmonary injuries
B. Thoracoabdominal stab wounds should employ a chest X-ray for evaluation of pneumothorax and pericardial ultrasound for effusion
C. Stab wounds to the left upper quadrant and right upper quadrant will always require laparoscopy for diaphragmatic assessment
D. Patients without any fascial penetration can be considered for discharge

190. In patients who are not examinable after penetrating abdominal injury, evaluation for peritoneal violation may be conducted via:

A. Local wound exploration
B. Ultrasound
C. CT or diagnostic laparoscopy
D. All of the above

191. 22-year-old woman presents to the emergency department with a chief complaint of severe left upper quadrant (LUQ) pain after being punched by her husband. Her blood pressure is 110/70 mm Hg, pulse is 100 bpm, and respiration rate is 24 breaths per minute. The best means to establish a diagnosis is which of the following?

A. FAST
B. CT scan
C. Upper gastrointestinal (GI) series
D. Peritoneal lavage

192. A 17-year-old girl presents to the emergency department with a stab wound to the abdomen and a blow to the head that left her groggy. Her blood pressure is 80/30 mm Hg, pulse is 120 bpm, and respiration rate is 28 breaths per minute. Her abdomen has a stab wound in the anterior axillary line at the right costal margin. Two large-bore intravenous lines, a nasogastric tube, and a Foley catheter are inserted. The systolic blood pressure rises to 85 mm Hg after 2 L of Ringer's lactate. The appropriate management is which of the following?

A. Exploratory laparotomy
B. Laparoscopic assessment of the peritoneal cavity
C. Ultrasound of the abdomen
D. Peritoneal lavage

193. A 19-year-old man presents to the emergency department with a gunshot wound through the umbilicus. The systolic blood pressure is 70 mm Hg on palpation and his abdomen is tightly distended. Large-bore intravenous lines are placed, and Ringer's lactate is infused. What should be the next step?

A. Peritoneal lavage
B. CT scan of the abdomen
C. Exploratory laparotomy
D. Transfusion of the patient until the systolic blood pressure reaches 90 mm Hg

194. A 40-year-old woman is brought to the emergency department following a car crash in which she was the driver. In the emergency department, her blood pressure is 80/60 mm Hg, pulse is 128 bpm, and respiratory rate is 32 breaths per minute. She

complains of right lower chest wall and severe right upper quadrant (RUQ) tenderness. Her breath sounds are questionably diminished. The immediate priority is to perform which of the following?

A. Peritoneal lavage
B. Chest X-ray
C. CT scan of chest and abdomen
D. Thoracentesis

195. A 26-year-old man is brought to the emergency department with a stab wound to the right side of the back just medial to the posterior axillary line. His blood pressure is 120/80 mm Hg, pulse rate is 98 bpm, and respiration rate is 22 breaths per minute. Physical examination reveals no abdominal tenderness, guarding, or neurologic changes. Local exploration of the stab wound is performed using local anesthesia. The track to the wound ends in the paraspinal muscles. What would be the next step in management?

A. Perform peritoneal lavage
B. Admit the patient for 24 hours of observation
C. Perform CT scan with rectal and intravenous contrast
D. Discharge to outpatient clinic for follow-up monitoring

196. A 20-year-old woman presents to the emergency department with a stab wound to the abdomen. There is minimal abdominal tenderness. Local wound exploration indicates that the knife penetrated the peritoneum. What is the ideal use of antibiotic administration?

A. Intraoperatively, if a colon injury is found
B. Postoperatively, based on culture and sensitivity of fecal contamination found at the time of surgery
C. Preoperatively
D. Postoperatively, if the patient develops fever

197. A 47-year-old woman involved in a skiing accident suffered a severe blow to the middle upper abdomen. Physical examination revealed diffuse tenderness, but there was no evidence of rebound tenderness or guarding. What test would be performed to rule out traumatic pancreatitis?

A. Peritoneal lavage
B. CT scan with oral and intravenous contrast
C. Serum amylase
D. Upper GI study

198. The injury most often missed by selective nonoperative management of abdominal stab wounds is to which of the following?

A. Colon
B. Spleen
C. Ureter
D. Diaphragm

199. A 16-year-old boy presents to the emergency department with a gunshot wound to the anterior abdominal wall. Fascial violation was present on local wound examination. What is the next line of management?

A. FAST
B. Peritoneal lavage
C. CT with intravenous and oral contrast
D. Exploratory laparotomy

200. A 60-year-old woman presents with a stab wound to the back just above the iliac crest. She is in stable condition. What is the next line of management?

A. FAST
B. Peritoneal lavage
C. CT with intravenous and oral contrast
D. Exploratory laparotomy

201. A 26-year-old man presents with a tangential small-caliber gunshot wound of the anterior abdominal wall. What is the next line of management?

A. Exploratory laparotomy
B. Wound exploration
C. Peritoneal lavage
D. FAST

202. The most common abdominal organ injured in trauma is:

A. Liver
B. Spleen
C. Small intestine
D. Stomach

203. False about splenic injury is:

A. In blunt trauma, direct compression of the spleen with parenchymal fracture is a common pathophysiologic mechanism at the tissue level
B. Rates of nonoperative management in splenic trauma has increased from roughly 40% - 70% with coincident decreases in mortality among the higher grades of injury
C. Unstable patients with abdominal trauma who are taken emergently to the OR may have a splenic injury identified at the time of laparotomy (50% of blunt splenic injury)
D. Patients who respond to resuscitation with normalized physiology can often be managed nonoperatively, although this group is at

risk for delayed reinitiation of hemorrhage (majority < 72 hours)

204. True about splenic injury is:

A. Active bleeding can be identified by visualizing extravasation of contrast material (i.e., high-density blush or accumulation of contrast-laden blood)
B. Abdominal CT with IV administration of a contrast agent is the most valuable study for identifying and characterizing splenic injuries (sensitivity/specificity 96%–100%)
C. Splenic injuries appear as disruptions in the normal splenic parenchyma, frequently with surrounding hematoma and free intraabdominal blood
D. All of the above

205. The overall success rate for nonoperative management in blunt splenic trauma is approximately:

A. 60% B. 70%
C. 80% D. 90%

206. True about the management of splenic injury is:

A. Due to the increasing use of splenic angiography and embolization over the past decade, nonoperative management failure rates of 5% are achievable in AAST Grades III to V
B. High-grade injuries (III–V) are also evaluated by interventional radiology and proceed to angiography and embolization within 24 hours
C. Patients with high-grade injures should undergo intensive care monitoring on admission, maintaining a low threshold for surgical management in the setting of decline
D. All of the above

207. A 48-year-old woman was brought to the emergency department after sustaining a stab wound to the left side of the abdomen. Exploration of the abdomen shows 1000 mL of blood, clot and faeces. There is a bleeding laceration across the middle third of the spleen but not involving the pedicle, a 3 cm laceration of the left transverse colon, and through-and-through lacerations of the stomach and the left lobe of the liver. What should be the management of the splenic injury?

A. Packing
B. Splenectomy
C. Splenorrhaphy with Dexon mesh
D. Partial splenectomy

208. 1 week following splenectomy, a 12-year-old girl presents with nausea, vomiting, headache, high grade fever and confusion. What is the most worrisome diagnosis?

A. Left lower lobe pneumonia
B. Subphrenic abscess
C. Postsplenectomy sepsis
D. Pancreatitis

209. 14 days following splenectomy, a 13-year-old patient presents with fever and leukocytosis. The chest X-ray shows free air under the diaphragm. What is the most likely diagnosis?

A. Left colon perforation
B. Subphrenic abscess
C. Left lower lobe pneumonia
D. Postsplenectomy sepsis

210. A 25-year-old man fell down from his bicycle and hit a concrete wall on his left side. An ultrasound examination showed free fluid in the abdomen. A CT scan confirmed a grade III splenic injury. The most important contraindication for a nonoperative management of the splenic injury is:

A. Hemodynamic instability
B. Active bleeding on CT scan
C. Adult patient
D. Lack of availability of blood for transfusion

211. A 47-year-old male had a road traffic accident. He was brought to the trauma bay. On examination he was vitally stable and had splenic injury on CT scan. Diagrammatic representation of the injury is as shown below. What is the grade of the injury as per AAST?

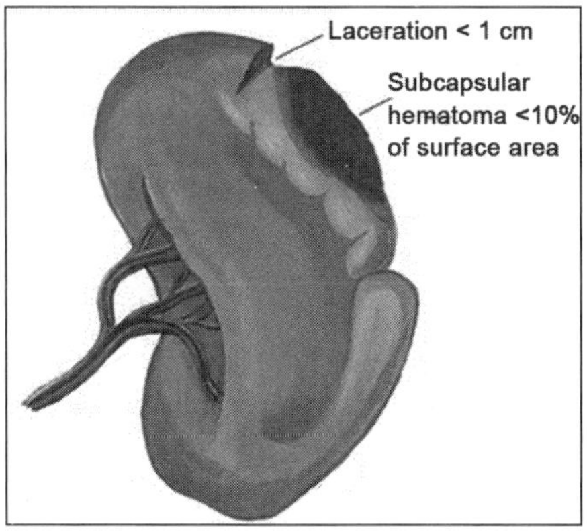

A. Grade I B. Grade II
C. Grade III D. Grade IV

212. A 29-year-old male had a road traffic accident. He was brought to the trauma bay. CT scan of abdomen showed active bleeding confined within the splenic capsule. What is the grade of the injury as per AAST?

A. Grade II B. Grade III
C. Grade IV D. Grade V

213. What is the grade of the splenic injury as per AAST?

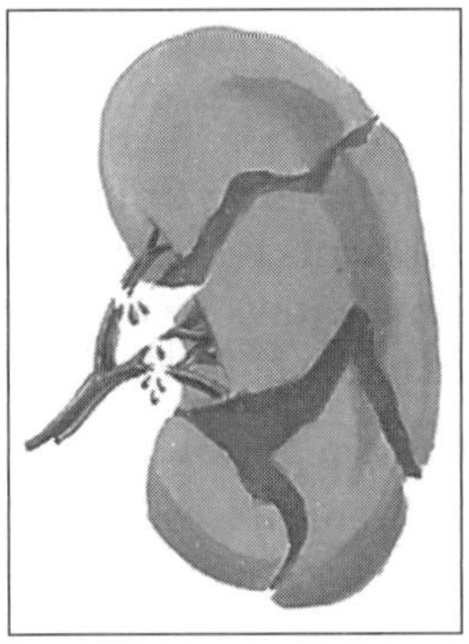

A. Grade II B. Grade III
C. Grade IV D. Grade V

214. A 32-year-old female had a road traffic accident. She was brought to the trauma bay. CT scan of abdomen showed a 5 cm splenic laceration. What is the grade of the injury as per AAST?

A. Grade II B. Grade III
C. Grade IV D. Grade V

215. A 45-year-old female had a road traffic accident. She was brought to the trauma bay. CT scan of abdomen showed active bleeding extending beyond the spleen into the peritoneum. What is the grade of the injury as per AAST?

A. Grade II B. Grade III
C. Grade IV D. Grade V

216. A 65-year-old female had a road traffic accident. She was brought to the trauma bay. CT scan of abdomen showed ruptured splenic subcapsular hematoma. What is the grade of the injury as per AAST?

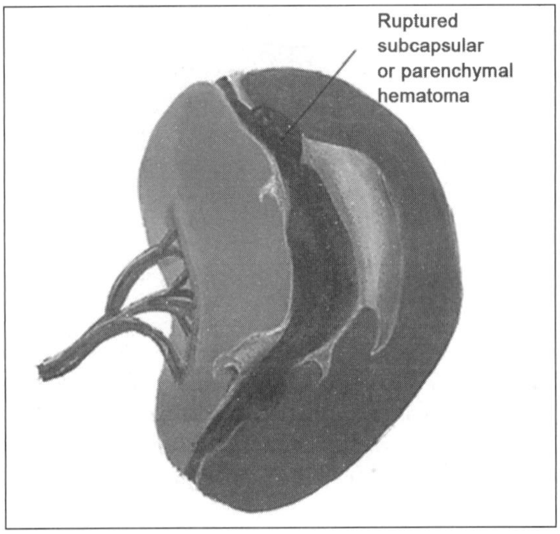

A. Grade I B. Grade II
C. Grade III D. Grade IV

217. A 25-year-old male had a fight. He was hit on the abdomen. He was brought to the trauma bay. CT scan of abdomen showed shattered spleen. What is the grade of the injury as per AAST?

A. Grade II B. Grade III
C. Grade IV D. Grade V

218. The most commonly injured abdominal organ after penetrating trauma is:

A. Small intestine B. Colon
C. Spleen D. Liver

219. True about liver injuries is:

A. Liver injuries are often first diagnosed on entering the abdomen in the unstable patient explored for free fluid on FAST examination
B. CT is capable of providing excellent anatomic detail that allows highly accurate characterization of injuries.
C. Common findings on CT indicative of liver injury include disruption of the hepatic parenchyma with perihepatic blood or hematoma and hemoperitoneum
D. All of the above

220. False about the management of liver injuries is:

A. The majority of patients with Grades I to III injuries being successfully managed nonoperatively, while 10% of Grades IV and V residually require surgical care
B. Patients who are hemodynamically stable in the setting of blunt and penetrating liver trauma should be considered primarily for nonoperative management
C. Parenchymal bleeding or pseudoaneurysm on contrasted imaging should prompt consultation to interventional radiology for evaluation
D. In appropriately selected patients, the use of angioembolization has improved the rate of successful nonoperative management with a reduction in conversion to surgical treatment

221. False about the management of liver injuries and its complications is:

A. CT or ultrasound imaging can be valuable in evaluating for abscess and biloma
B. Endoscopic retrograde cholangiopancreatography (ERCP) with stent placement is occasionally required to decompress the biliary tree and to promote healing of a bile leak
C. Hemobilia is managed with angiography, which includes embolization of the hepatic vessel that is communicating with the biliary tree

D. Biliary ascites amenable to percutaneous drainage mostly needs laparoscopy or laparotomy for adequate drainage to be obtained

222. False about the operative management of liver injuries is:

A. When operative management is required, a Kocher's incision is the most versatile approach for managing any liver injury that might be encountered

B. When needed, perihepatic packing and manual compression can temporize bleeding to provide the opportunity to catch up with the resuscitation

C. Mild injuries with minimal ongoing bleeding may be managed with further compression, topical hemostatic agents, or suture hepatorrhaphy

D. When more severe bleeding from the liver is present, a Pringle maneuver is a valuable adjunct to slow blood flow enough to visualize the injury.

223. False about the operative management of liver injuries is:

A. A vascularized pedicle of omentum may reduce parenchymal bleeding and promote healing of the laceration when it is packed within the liver injury

B. Hepatic parenchyma that appears to be devitalized should be debrided and drains placed when injuries appear to be at risk for a bile leak

C. Liver injuries in the vicinity of the retrohepatic vena cava that are not actively bleeding should be packed and explored

D. An atriocaval (Schrock) shunt is one method that includes isolation of the retrohepatic vena cava by placing an intravascular shunt between the right atrium and infrahepatic vena cava used for repair of retrohepatic vena cava injuries

224. During exploratory laparotomy in a patient with multiple gunshot wounds to the abdomen, a through-and-through gunshot wound is noted in the left lobe of the liver. Brisk bleeding is seen from the bullet track. Which is an appropriate operative maneuver for this injury?

A. Pringle maneuver

B. Large mattress sutures traversing the bullet track

C. Omental packing

D. All of the above

225. A 32-year-old female is a restrained passenger in a high-speed motor vehicle crash. Initial workup shows an HR of 95 beats/min, blood pressure of 110/82 mm Hg, and hemoglobin of 12.2 g/dL. On FAST, a moderate amount of fluid is seen in the RUQ, between the liver, kidney and diaphragm. A grade IV liver laceration is seen on CT with no active extravasation. Her vital signs 6 h after admission are an HR of 100 beats/min and blood pressure of 105/80 mm Hg. What is the next most appropriate step?

A. Exploratory laparotomy

B. Angiography

C. Repeated hemoglobin determination

D. Diagnostic laparoscopy

226. The patient in the previous scenario is discharged home on hospital day 4 without needing operative intervention. She returns to the clinic 2 months after discharge with persistent dull continuous RUQ pain. She denies any fevers or chills, and all laboratory studies, including a hepatic function panel, are within normal limits. CT of the abdomen and pelvis is performed and reveals a localized homogeneous fluid collection directly adjacent to the liver. What is the correct diagnosis and treatment?

A. Hemobilia: exploratory laparotomy and ligation of bleeding vessel

B. Hemobilia: ERCP with stent placement

C. Biloma: image-guided percutaneous drainage

D. Biloma: exploratory laparotomy with external drainage

227. A 22-year-old construction worker falls off of a ladder and lands on his left side. He fractures left ribs 6 to 12 and has a grade II splenic laceration. HR is 88 beats/min, and blood pressure is 110/76 mmHg. Hemoglobin is 12.3 g/dL. The patient is admitted to the ICU for serial hemoglobins and monitoring. 6 hours later, the HR is 104 beats/min, blood pressure is 100/68 mmHg, and hemoglobin is 9.1 g/dL. What is the next step in management?

A. Exploratory laparoscopy

B. Transfuse two units, and continue serial examinations

C. Angiography

D. Continue serial examinations

228. A patient presents with multiple gunshot wounds to the extremity and right lower quadrant. In the operating room, upon entry into the abdomen, a large amount of hemoperitoneum is encountered and all quadrants are packed immediately. Upon reinspection, the patient is noted to have an injury to the infrahepatic vena cava. How can you best expose this injury?

A. Transect the right renal artery
B. Right medial visceral rotation
C. Left medial visceral rotation
D. Transect the pancreas

229. A 65-year-old female had a road traffic accident. She was brought to the trauma bay. CT scan of abdomen showed hepatic injury showing active bleeding extending beyond the liver parenchyma into the peritoneum. What is the grade of the injury as per AAST?

A. Grade II B. Grade III
C. Grade IV D. Grade V

230. A 42-year-old female had a road traffic accident. She was brought to the trauma bay. CT scan of abdomen showed hepatic injury showing ruptured subcapsular hematoma. What is the grade of the injury as per AAST?

A. Grade II B. Grade III
C. Grade IV D. Grade V

231. A 22-year-old male had a road traffic accident. He was brought to the trauma bay. CT scan of abdomen showed a 3 cms hepatic laceration with the presence of a liver vascular injury. What is the grade of the injury as per AAST?

A. Grade II B. Grade III
C. Grade IV D. Grade V

232. A patient presents with multiple gunshot wounds to the extremity and right lower quadrant. In the operating room, upon entry into the abdomen, a large amount of hemoperitoneum is encountered and all quadrants are packed immediately. Upon reinspection, the patient is noted to have an injury to the infrahepatic vena cava. What is the grade of the injury as per AAST?

A. Grade II B. Grade III
C. Grade IV D. Grade V

233. A 60-year-old man is brought into the emergency department after being hit by a car. His blood pressure is 70 mm Hg palpable, and abdomen is massively distended and tender. A large, stellate fracture of the right lower liver is noted, and despite repeated attempts at suturing, bleeding persists. The anaesthesiologist notes that the pH of arterial blood is 7.2 and that the patient has become hypothermic. A total of 8 U of blood have been transfused. What is the next step in management?

A. Insert an atriocaval shunt
B. Perform a right hepatic lobectomy
C. Perform a right hepatic artery ligation
D. Firmly pack the RUQ, close the abdomen, and plan to return to the OR within 24–48 hours

234. A 60-year-old man is attacked with a baseball bat and sustains multiple blows to the abdomen. He presents to the emergency department in shock and is brought to the operating room (OR), where a laparotomy reveals massive hemoperitoneum and a stellate fracture of the right and left lobes of the liver. Which of the following techniques should be used immediately?

A. Pringle's maneuver
B. Packing the liver
C. Suture ligation
D. Ligation of the right and left hepatic artery

235. Following image shows:

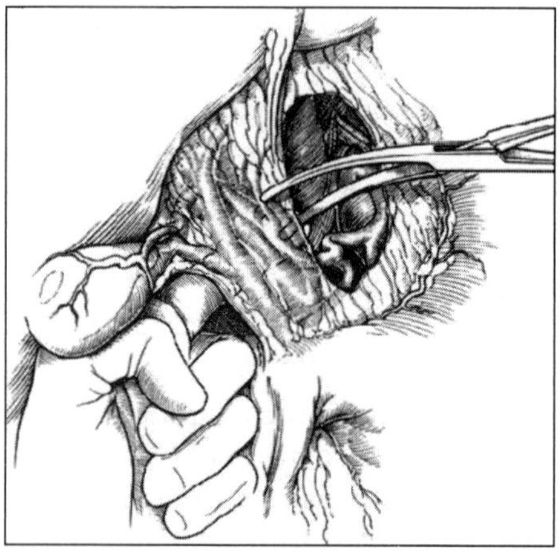

A. The liver hanging maneuver
B. Cattell braasch maneuver
C. Pringle's maneuver
D. Kocher's maneuver

236. Following diagrammatic representation of hepatic injury shows intraparenchymal hematoma, subcapsular hematoma 10%–50% surface area and laceration of 1–3 cm in depth and ≤10 cm length. What is the grade of the injury as per AAST?

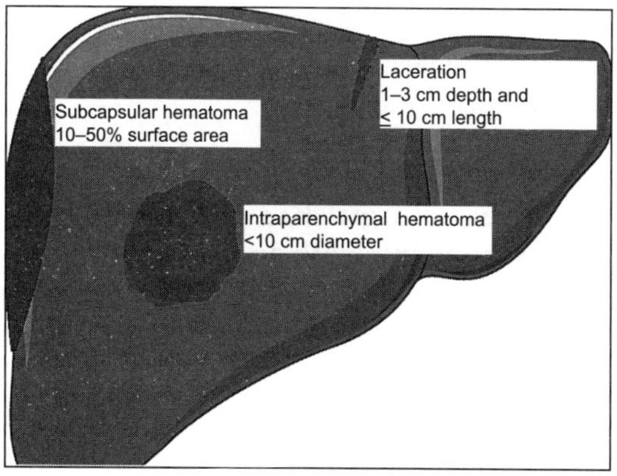

A. Grade II
B. Grade III
C. Grade IV
D. Grade V

237. An 18-year-old man presents to the emergency department with a stab wound to the abdomen. His blood pressure is 80/50 mm Hg. He is brought immediately to the OR, where an enlarged hemoperitoneum is found at laparotomy. Primary repair of the hepatic artery is performed, but because of ongoing blood loss resulting in an unstable hemodynamic situation, the portal vein injury is simply ligated. Bleeding is well controlled. The patient is brought to the recovery room, where his blood pressure drops to 80/60 mm Hg and central venous pressure is 2 cm H_2O. What should be the next step in management?

A. Ringer's lactate to increase blood pressure
B. Reexploration to repair portal vein
C. Transfusion of whole blood to elevate blood pressure
D. Vasopressor to increase blood pressure

238. False about gastric injury is:

A. Penetrating gastric injuries often cause full-thickness perforations with spillage of gastric contents into the abdomen
B. The overall sensitivity and specificity for hollow visceral injury on CT are limited (sensitivity 55%–95%, specificity 48%–92%)
C. A full evaluation of the stomach includes visualization of the anterior and posterior walls, requiring entry into the lesser sac
D. Hematomas within the gastric wall should not be evacuated to ensure the absence of perforation.

239. True about the operative management of stomach injury is:

A. Injuries involving the gastroesophageal junction, lesser curve, fundus, and posterior wall may be more challenging to approach and require better exposure of the upper abdomen
B. Injuries that are full thickness should have all nonviable tissue debrided; the gastric wall is then closed in 1 or 2 layers
C. Reconstruction could require Billroth I or II gastroenterostomy or creation of a Roux-en-Y esophagojejunostomy, depending on the extent of the resection
D. All of the above

240. False about duodenal injuries is:

A. Because of the retroperitoneal location of the duodenum, most injuries are due to blunt modalities in approximately 50% of cases
B. The classic description includes abdominal impact by a steering wheel or, in children, a bicycle handlebar
C. Morbidity in duodenal injury is most commonly related to septic complications, particularly in the setting of repair failure
D. Penetrating duodenal injuries are commonly first diagnosed at laparotomy, initiated on the basis of penetrating wound location

241. False about the management of duodenal injuries is:

A. Hematomas of the duodenal wall will often resolve without intervention and are an issue only if they cause a gastric outlet obstruction
B. Duodenal hematomas identified incidentally during laparotomy should be intentionally opened as there is a high concern for full-thickness injury
C. If the duodenal obstruction persists after approximately 14 days, operative exploration is warranted to evacuate hematoma evaluate for perforation, stricture, or associated pancreatic injury
D. Treatment of obstructing hematomas consists of gastric decompression, initiation of total parenteral nutrition, and reevaluation of gastric emptying with a contrast study after 5 to 7 days

242. False about the management of duodenal injuries is:

A. Longer segments of duodenal injury or areas adjacent to the ampulla may require enteric bypass with a Roux-en-Y reconstruction
B. Duodenal wall perforations can be repaired by a single- or double layer approach after debridement of devitalized tissue
C. Drain placement following definitive repair is mandatory
D. All of the above are true

243. An 8-year-old child hits a curb with his bicycle, which causes him to flip over the handlebars. He had no initial symptoms and was monitored at home by his parents. However, 2 days after the incident, he begins having nonbilious emesis. He is brought to the ED and undergoes CT of the abdomen and pelvis, which demonstrates a duodenal hematoma. What is the next step in management?

A. Initiation of NPO status and gastric decompression with a nasogastric tube
B. EGD to assess for luminal compromise
C. Drainage of the hematoma via laparoscopy
D. Resection of the injured portion of the duodenum with primary anastomoses

244. A 20-year-old unrestrained driver was involved in a motor-vehicle crash. A computed tomography (CT) of the abdomen revealed a large hematoma in the second portion of duodenum. The rest of the abdomen is normal. The initial management of this duodenal hematoma should be:

A. Operative evacuation
B. Nasogastric decompression, intravenous fluids, and gradual resumption of oral diet
C. Endoscopic retrograde cholangiopancreatography (ERCP)
D. Laparotomy, pyloric exclusion and gastrojejunostomy

245. A 70-year-old woman is hit by a car and injures her mid abdomen. The best way to rule out a rupture of the second part of the duodenum is by which mode?

A. CT with oral and intravenous contrast
B. Repeated physical examinations
C. Ultrasound
D. Repeated amylase levels

246. A 35-year-old woman was punched in the right side of the abdomen and chest. There was some right upper abdomen tenderness but no guarding or rebound. Results of a gastrografin upper GI study showed a coiled-spring (stack of coins) appearance of the second and third part of the duodenum. What is the most likely diagnosis?

A. Intraluminal blood clot
B. Duodenal hematoma
C. Retroperitoneal hematoma
D. Contusion to the head of the pancreas

247. Which would be the appropriate management of the patient described in Q. 246?

A. Exploratory laparotomy and drainage
B. Duodenal diverticulization
C. Pyloric exclusion
D. Repeat upper GI series at 5- to 7-day interval

248. A 15-year-old girl had an injury to the right retroperitoneum with duodenal contusion. What is the test required to exclude a rupture of the duodenum?

A. Serum amylase
B. Gastrografin study
C. Upper GI with barium
D. ERCP

249. False about pancreatic injuries is:

A. True pancreatic trauma-related mortality is difficult to identify, as deaths are often attributable to associated pathology
B. A blunt mechanism is more commonly the cause
C. True pancreatic trauma-related mortality is difficult to identify, as deaths are often attributable to associated pathology
D. A common mechanism of blunt pancreatic injury involves crushing of the body of the pancreas between a rigid structure, such as a steering wheel or seat belt and the vertebral column

250. False about pancreatic injuries is:

A. CT provides the best view of the pancreas and associated injury
B. The retroperitoneal location of the pancreas makes physical examination findings less helpful for diagnosis
C. CT alone is always satisfactory to rule out a clinically significant pancreatic injury
D. On abdominal CT, findings suggestive of pancreatic injuries include malperfusion of the pancreatic parenchyma, surrounding fluid, or hematoma and stranding in the adjacent soft tissue

251. Reported incidence of missed pancreatic trauma on CT approximates:

A. 5%
B. 15%
C. 25%
D. 45%

252. False about the management of pancreatic injuries is:

A. A closed suction drain should be placed to manage any pancreatic enzyme leak

B. When obtained > 1 hour after injury occurrence, an elevated serum amylase level may reflect pancreatic trauma
C. Exposure of the entire pancreas is required to evaluate for injury and to develop an effective surgical plan
D. Imaging of the pancreatic ducts with ERCP or magnetic resonance cholangiopancreatography may increase diagnostic yield, especially for those patients who have a suggestion of pancreatic injury cholangiopancreatography may increase diagnostic yield, especially for those patients who have a suggestion of pancreatic injury

253. A 42-year-old male unrestrained driver struck his steering wheel against his abdomen during a motor vehicle crash. He is hemodynamically stable but complains of abdominal pain. CT of the abdomen demonstrates a moderate amount of free fluid with no solid organ injuries. He undergoes an exploratory laparotomy, at which time complete transection of the pancreatic neck is found. What is the most appropriate management of this injury?

A. Roux-en-Y pancreaticojejunostomy to the distal end of the pancreas with oversewing of the proximal pancreatic stump
B. Distal pancreatectomy with oversewing of the proximal pancreatic stump
C. Primary repair and drainage of the pancreatic duct
D. Pancreaticoduodenectomy

254. False about the management of pancreatic injuries is:

A. Less severe pancreatic injuries that do not involve the pancreatic duct (Grades I and II), including hematomas, parenchymal contusions, and lacerations of the capsule or superficial parenchyma, should be managed with external drainage
B. Closed suction systems are associated with a increased rate of abscess development compared with open-style drains
C. Massive destruction of the pancreatic head with devitalized parenchyma (Grade V) or combined pancreatic and duodenal injuries may require a pancreaticoduodenectomy (Whipple procedure)
D. When tissue destruction is limited, managing these injuries with drainage alone often diverts the leakage of pancreatic fluid externally, creating a controlled fistula that frequently will close spontaneously

255. A 25-year-old man presents to the emergency department with a gunshot wound to the abdomen. On exploratory laparotomy, he is found to have multiple small-bowel enterotomies, transverse colon enterotomy, and a partial injury just to the left of the midline of the pancreas. The pancreatic duct appears intact. What is the appropriate management of the pancreatic injury?

A. Drain with sump drains
B. Operative pancreatogram followed by distal pancreatectomy if ductal injury is noted
C. Closed-suction drainage and lavage
D. Transection of injured area of pancreas with Roux-en-Y (jejunal) anastomosis to the transected tail of the pancreas

256. Distal transection or pancreatic parenchymal injury with ductal injury was seen in a patient with abdominal trauma. What is the AAST grade of injury?

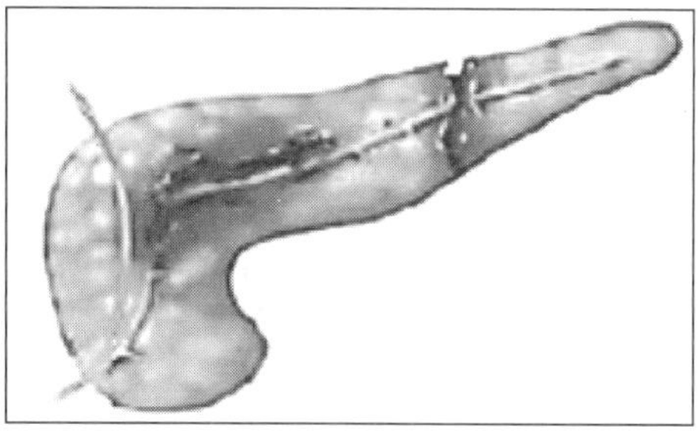

A. Grade II B. Grade III
C. Grade IV D. Grade V

257. Proximal transection and pancreatic parenchymal injury involving the ampulla was seen in a patient with abdominal trauma. What is the AAST grade of injury?

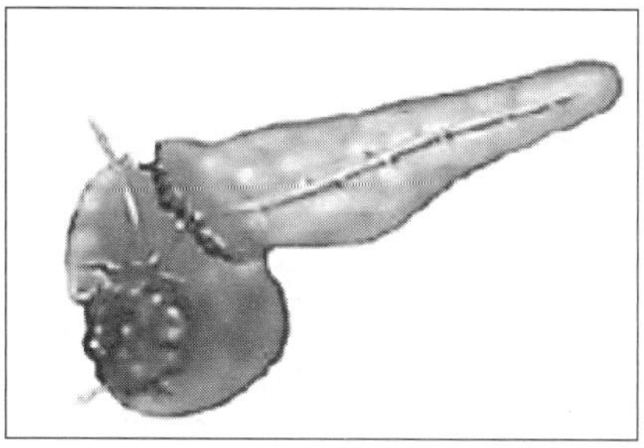

A. Grade II B. Grade III
C. Grade IV D. Grade V

258. Major contusion without ductal injury or tissue loss was seen in a patient with abdominal trauma. What is the AAST grade of injury?

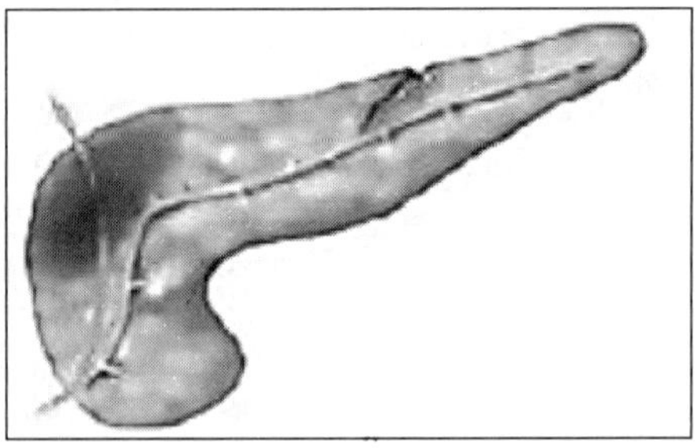

A. Grade I
B. Grade II
C. Grade III
D. Grade V

259. A 30-year-old woman involved in a car crash is brought into the emergency department. Her blood pressure is 100/60 mm Hg, pulse rate is 120 bpm, and respiration rate is 18 breaths per minute. On peritoneal lavage, she is noted to have free blood in the peritoneal cavity. At the time of exploratory laparotomy, a liver laceration is noted, and there is a 2.5-cm-diameter contusion to an area of small bowel. How should the small-bowel contusion be treated?

A. Transillumination evaluation of hematoma with meticulous hemostasis
B. Observation (no surgical therapy)
C. Resection of the bowel and ileostomy
D. Resection of the bowel with single-layer anastomosis

260. False about small bowel trauma is:

A. Deceleration mechanisms can result in a shearing of the serosa or muscularis throughout a segment of small bowel
B. Mortality rates range from 50% to 70%, with most caused by associated vascular injuries
C. Injuries to the intestinal serosa can be reinforced with interrupted nonabsorbable suture, which imbricates the injury
D. Injuries to the small bowel mesentery can result in devascularization and subsequent intestinal necrosis without direct tissue injury

261. In injuries involve of the small intestine, bowel resection with anastomosis should be performed if the circumference is:

A. > 30%
B. > 50%
C. > 75%
D. > 90%

262. Destructive injury in penetrating trauma is defined by all except:

A. Wounds > 50% of the colonic circumference
B. Presence of devascularized segments.
C. Wounds > 25% of the colonic circumference
D. Complete transection

263. False about colonic injuries is:

A. Colon and rectal injuries occur most commonly after penetrating abdominal trauma and rarely after blunt mechanisms
B. In blunt injury, serosal tears > 25% colon circumference and mesenteric devascularization are considered destructive
C. Peritonitis may be present on exam in the setting of free perforation, yet the retroperitoneal location of the right and left colon may obscure this finding
D. Colonic injuries may first be identified at the time of laparotomy prompted by hemodynamic instability or a suggestive penetrating mechanism

264. False about the management colonic injuries is:

A. WTA guidelines suggest bias toward ostomy creation in patients with ongoing shock, concomitant abdominal injuries, chronic illness, immunosuppression, or inability to close fascia
B. Abdominal CT has very good capabilities in the diagnosis
C. Distal injuries require segmental resection with colocolonic anastomosis
D. Primary repair (one or two layers) in all nondestructive injuries, resection, and anastomosis for destructive injury in the healthy patient without extremis and diversion for destructive injury in the comorbid patient requiring resuscitation

265. False about rectal injuries is:

A. Positive digital rectal examination for gross blood or a penetrating pelvic trajectory requires further evaluation with imaging
B. Even if the CT is negative for injury, clinically relevant trauma is much likely
C. If the imaging results are indeterminate or there is clinical concern, an exam under anesthesia with rigid proctosigmoidoscopy can be valuable to provide visualization of the rectum and distal sigmoid colon
D. Upper rectal injuries, especially those on the anterior or lateral surfaces, may be first identified during visualization of the pelvic structures at the time of laparotomy

266. Destructive rectal injury defined by:

A. Wound > 25% of the rectal circumference
B. Wound > 33% of the rectal circumference
C. Wound > 50% of the rectal circumference
D. Wound > 66% of the rectal circumference

267. **True about the management rectal injuries is:**
   A. Destructive rectal injuries (>25% circumference) are predominantly managed with fecal diversion (loop ileostomy or colostomy) and consideration of presacral drainage until healing has occurred
   B. A rectal contrasted enema will serve to define wound resolution with subsequent ostomy reversal
   C. If an extraperitoneal rectal injury is found at laparotomy, management should convert to treatment of intraperitoneal colon trauma
   D. All of the above

268. **Which is true of intraperitoneal colon injuries?**
   A. Most can be treated by debridement and repair
   B. They should always be treated with resection and colocolostomy
   C. They always require drainage after repair
   D. They should never be repaired primarily

269. **A 44-year-old male presents with a single gunshot wound to the abdomen. He is hemodynamically stable and taken to the operating room. On exploration, his injuries are found to be limited to four small bowel injuries 8 cm apart, each with destruction of 50% of the bowel wall, and a through-and through injury to the ascending colon with destruction of 30% of the bowel wall. How should these injuries be managed?**
   A. Resection and anastomosis of the small bowel injuries and primary repair of the colon injury
   B. Primary repair of both the small bowel and colon injuries
   C. Primary repair of the small bowel injuries, primary repair of the colon injury, and creation of a diverting ileostomy
   D. Resection of the small bowel injuries and exteriorization of the colon injury as a colostomy

270. **A 23-year-old man is shot with a handgun and found to have a through-and-through injury to the right transverse colon. There is little ileotransverse fecal contamination and no bowel devascularization. At operation, what does he require?**
   A. Debridement and closure of wounds with exteriorization of colon
   B. Right hemicolectomy with ileotransverse colon anastomosis
   C. Right hemicolectomy with ileostomy and mucous fistula
   D. Debridement and closure of wounds

271. **A 29-year-old woman is brought to the emergency department with a gunshot wound to the abdomen. Her blood pressure is 80/60 mm Hg, pulse rate is 118 bpm, and respiration rate is 24 breaths per minute. She is brought immediately to the OR, where a large amount of blood and clots are found within the abdomen. After initial packing of the abdomen and stabilization of the patient, a retroperitoneal hematoma is found just above the renal veins. Proximal and distal control of the inferior vena cava is obtained and the blood pressure comes up to 100/60 mm Hg. Which is the most appropriate management?**
   A. Packing of the area with a definitive plan to return to the OR in 48 hours
   B. Vascular repair of the injury
   C. Ligation of the inferior vena cava
   D. Use of intracaval shunt to allow venous return while repairing the injury

272. **False statement is:**
   A. Most commonly, major abdominal vascular injuries are secondary to penetrating mechanisms
   B. Abdominal vascular injuries are often first recognized at the time of laparotomy being performed for penetrating abdominal trauma
   C. Hematomas of the infrarenal vasculature or the right renal hilum are exposed with a right medial visceral mobilization, also known as the Mattox maneuver
   D. All of the above are true

273. **Following image shows:**

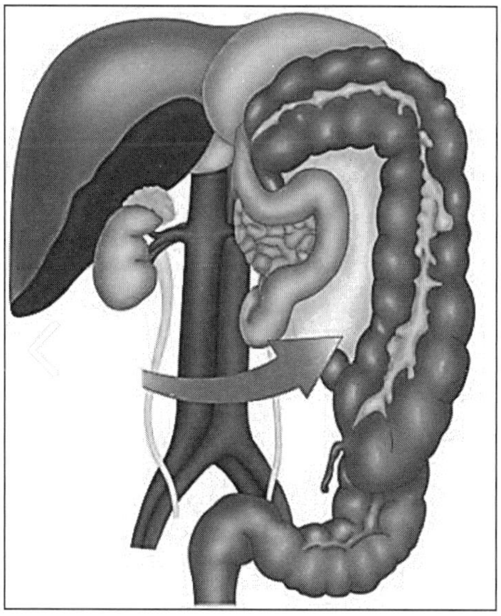

   A. Mattox maneuver
   B. Cattell-Braasch maneuver

C. Kocher's maneuver
D. Pringle's maneuver

274. Following image shows:

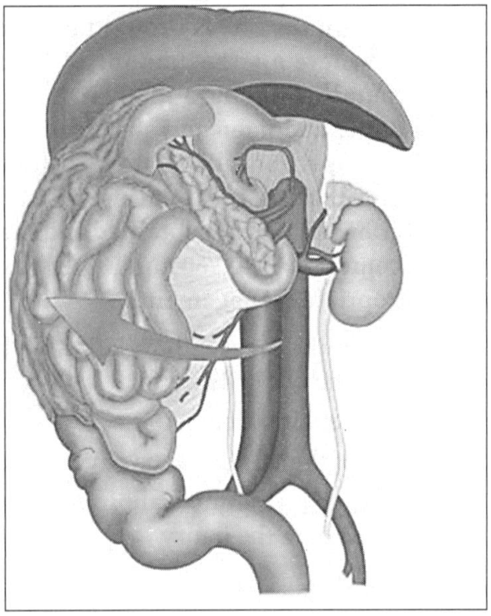

A. Mattox maneuver
B. Cattell-Braasch maneuver
C. Kocher's maneuver
D. Pringle's maneuver

275. Following image shows:

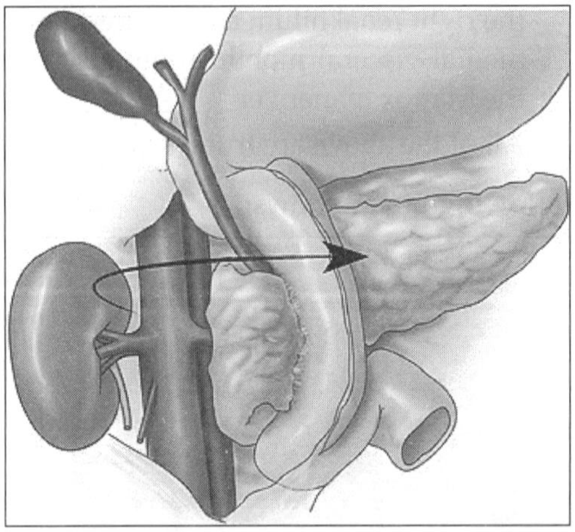

A. Mattox maneuver
B. Cattell-Braasch maneuver
C. Kocher's maneuver
D. Pringle's maneuver

276. True about the management of retroperitoneal hematoma is:

A. Zone 1 hematomas require exploration
B. A hematoma in the region of zone 2, which predominantly contains the kidneys, should be explored only if it appears that the hematoma is expanding and continuing to lose blood
C. Hematoma in zone 3 is usually secondary to pelvic fracture bleeding and should not be explored unless exsanguinating hemorrhage is obvious
D. All of the above

277. True about genitourinary injuries is:

A. The typical mechanism for bladder injuries is the transmission of significant energy to the urine-filled bladder, resulting in wall rupture
B. The presence of gross hematuria is the most valuable screen for injuries to the genitourinary organs and should prompt further evaluation.
C. In male patients, blood at the urethral meatus or a displaced prostate on rectal examination is suggestive of a urethral injury and requires evaluation
D. All of the above

278. Which option provides the most appropriate management for the injury described?

A. Blunt mechanism: zone 3 nonexpanding retroperitoneal hematoma: exploration
B. Blunt mechanism: zone 2 expanding retroperitoneal hematoma: angiogram
C. Penetrating mechanism: zone 1 expanding hematoma: observation
D. Penetrating mechanism: zone 1 nonexpanding hematoma: exploration

279. The patient is a 52-year-old male involved in a high-speed head-on motor vehicle crash. He arrives to the ED unstable with BP 80/60 mmHg and HR 125 beats/min. Initial X-ray workup reveals an open-book pelvis fracture. Despite 2 L of crystalloid, the patient remains tachycardic and hypotensive. What techniques can be used to control bleeding in this patient?

A. Interventional radiology (IR) angiogram
B. Preperitoneal packing
C. Pelvic binder
D. All of the above

280. For the patient in the previous scenario, a pelvic binder is placed and blood pressure and HR improves. A negative urethrogram is completed, and a Foley catheter is inserted. The urine output is bloody, and a cystogram demonstrates a bladder injury. Which combination of injury and management is correct?

A. Extraperitoneal bladder injury = operating room for primary repair

B. Extraperitoneal bladder injury = suprapubic catheter placement
C. Intraperitoneal bladder injury = operating room for primary repair
D. Intraperitoneal bladder injury = maintain Foley catheter

281. A 40-year-old man is hit by a car and sustains an injury to the pelvis. Which of the following is most indicative of a urethral injury?

A. Hematuria
B. Scrotal ecchymosis
C. High-riding prostate on rectal examination
D. Intravenous pyelography (IVP) showing dye extravasation in the pelvis

282. A 30-year-old man sustained a pelvic fracture with a large pelvic hematoma. Rectal examination reveals a large laceration in the rectal wall and a nonpalpable prostate. His vital signs have stabilized with multiple transfusions. This patient requires which of the following?

A. Resuscitation, blood transfusions, external fixature and exploratory laparotomy
B. ORIF of pelvic fracture by a posterior approach, colostomy and suprapubic cystostomy
C. Exploratory laparotomy, urinary diversion, sigmoid colostomy, presacral drainage and debridement of the rectal wall
D. Resuscitation, angiography, embolization of the pelvic bleeders, exploratory laparotomy

283. Zones of the retroperitoneum visualized at the time of laparotomy are:

A. Zone 1 includes the central vascular structures, such as the aorta and vena cava
B. Zone 2 includes the kidneys and adjacent adrenal glands
C. Zone 3 describes the retroperitoneum associated with the pelvic vasculature
D. All of the above

284. A 26-year-old woman in her sixth month of pregnancy is brought to the emergency department. She had been punched in the abdomen. She is found to have generalized abdominal pain, tenderness, abdominal distention, ileus, and absent fetal heart sounds. The patient's blood pressure is 80/60 mm Hg; despite administration of 3 L of Ringer's lactate, her blood pressure only comes up to 90/60 mm Hg. What is the next step in management?

A. Transfusion of 2 U of blood and reevaluate
B. Application of pneumatic antishock garment (PASG)
C. Exploratory laparotomy with evacuation of the uterus and closure of the uterus disruption
D. CT scan of the abdomen

ANSWERS

1. **Ans: D. All of the above**
Ref: Chapter No.17, Page No.386-387

2. **Ans: B. American Revolutionary War**
Ref: Chapter No.17, Page No.387

3. **Ans: A. American Civil War**
Ref: Chapter No.17, Page No.387

4. **Ans: C. World War I**
Ref: Chapter No.17, Page No.387

5. **Ans: A. Korean War**
Ref: Chapter No.17, Page No.387

6. **Ans: D. Operation Enduring Freedom (Iraq)**
Ref: Chapter No.17, Page No.387

7. **Ans: D. American Civil War**
Ref: Chapter No.17, Page No.387

8. **Ans: C. World War II**
Ref: Chapter No.17, Page No.387

9. **Ans: A. Vietnam War**
Ref: Chapter No.17, Page No.387

10. **Ans: D. All of the above**
Ref: Chapter No.17, Page No.388

11. **Ans: B. 20%**
Ref: Chapter No.17, Page No.388

12. **Ans: D. All of the above**
Ref: Chapter No.17, Page No.388-389

13. **Ans: B. 9 (E2V2M5)**
Ref: Chapter No.17, Page No.389

14. **Ans: D. 15 (E4V5M6)**
Ref: Chapter No.17, Page No.389

15. **Ans: B. 14 (E4V4M6)**
Ref: Chapter No.17, Page No.389

16. **Ans: A. 4 (E1V1M2)**
Ref: Chapter No.17, Page No.389

17. **Ans: C. 13 (E4V3M6)**
Ref: Chapter No.17, Page No.389

18. **Ans: D. 12 (E2V5M5)**
Ref: Chapter No.17, Page No.389

19. **Ans: B. 7 (E1V4M2)**
Ref: Chapter No.17, Page No.389

20. **Ans: B. 10 (E3V3M4)**
Ref: Chapter No.17, Page No.389

21. **Ans: A. 6 (E3V2M1)**
Ref: Chapter No.17, Page No.389

22. **Ans: D. Severe injury (ISS > 50)**
Ref: Chapter No.17, Page No.389

23. **Ans: C. Serious injury**
Ref: Chapter No.17, Page No.389

24. **Ans: B. Moderate injury**
Ref: Chapter No.17, Page No.389

25. **Ans: D. Severe injury**
Ref: Chapter No.17, Page No.389

26. **Ans: A. Heart rate**
    - **GCS** (Glasgow Coma Score) - Eye opening, best motor and verbal response **(EVM)**
    - **RTS** (Revised Trauma Score) - Physiological score of GCS, **S**ystolic BP and **R**espiratory frequency **(RTS)**. ***RTS <4 proposed for transfer to trauma center***
    - Injury Severity Score **(ISS)** - Anatomical score and is based on the AIS (Abbreviated Injury Scale). The 3 most severely injured body regions have their score squared and added together to produce the ISS score. Based on scores of ***9 anatomic regions***.
    - New Injury Severity Score **(NISS)** - 3 most severe injuries squared ***regardless of the body region***. More predictive of complications and mortality than ISS
    - Modified Injury Severity Score **(MISS)**- similar to ISS but for ***pediatric*** trauma categorizes body into ***5 areas, instead of 9.***
    - **TRISS = RTS + ISS**
    - Mangled extremity severity score **(MESS)** - used to predict necessity of amputation after lower extremity trauma. ***Score of > 7*** is predictive of amputation. Variables used:
        (a) Skeletal and soft tissue injury (graded 1-4)
        (b) Limb ischemia (graded 1-3)
        (c) Shock (graded 0-2)
        (d) Age (graded 0-2)

Ref: Chapter No.17, Page No.389

27. **Ans: C. 12**
Ref: Chapter No.17, Page No.389

28. **Ans: D. 3**
Ref: Chapter No.17, Page No.389

29. **Ans: A. 0**
Ref: Chapter No.17, Page No.389

30. **Ans: B. 5 (E1V1M3)**
Ref: Use pediatric GCS score

Holmes JF, Palchak MJ, MacFarlane T, Kuppermann N. Performance of the pediatric Glasgow coma scale in children with blunt head trauma. Acad Emerg Med 2005; 12:814

	Child	Infant	Score
Eye opening	Spontaneous To speech To pain only No response	Spontaneous To speech To pain only No response	4 3 2 1
Best verbal response	Oriented, appropriate Confused Inappropriate words Incomprehensible sounds No response	Coos and babbles Irritable cries Cries to pain Moans to pain No response	5 4 3 2 1
Best motor response*	Obeys commands Localizes painful stimulus Withdraws in response to pain Flexion in response to pain Extension in response to pain No response	Moves spontaneously and purposefully Withdraws to touch Withdraws to response in pain Abnormal flexion posture to pain Abnormal extension posture to pain No response	6 5 4 3 2 1

31. **Ans: C. 7 (E2V2M3)**

Ref: Use pediatric GCS score from reference in Q.30

32. **Ans: D. 8 (E3V3M2)**

Ref: Use pediatric GCS score from reference in Q.30

33. **Ans: C. 11 (E2V4M5)**

Ref: Use pediatric GCS score from reference in Q.30

34. **Ans: B. 13 (E4V5M4)**

Ref: Use pediatric GCS score from reference in Q.30

35. **Ans: C. Endotracheal intubation**

Ref: Chapter No.17, Page No.389-391

36. **Ans: B. Transport to a trauma center**

Ref: Chapter No.17, Page No.390

37. **Ans: A. Intrusion, including roof: >6 inches occupant site; >12 inches any site**

Ref: Chapter No.17, Page No.390

38. **Ans: D. Evidence of high-energy impact fall for children is >5 feet or 4 - 5 times the height of the child**

Ref: Chapter No.17, Page No.390

39. **Ans: C. Airway, Breathing, Circulation, Disability, Exposure**

Ref: Chapter No.17, Page No.391

40. **Ans: A. Cervical immobilization, preoxygenation, cricoid pressure, induction, paralysis, intubate, confirm placement with CO_2 detector**

Ref: Chapter No.17, Page No.391

41. **Ans: D. The definitive airway of choice for most injured patients remains tracheostomy**

Ref: Chapter No.17, Page No.392

42. **Ans: B. The incision and dissection are continued through the cricothyroid membrane in longitudinal fashion**

Ref: Chapter No.17, Page No.393

43. **Ans: D. All of the above**

Ref: Chapter No.17, Page No.393

44. **Ans: B. Laryngeal mask airway**

Ref: Chapter No.17, Page No.393

45. **Ans: C. Laryngeal tube airway (King LT-D.)**

Ref: Chapter No.17, Page No.393

46. **Ans: A. Multilumen esophageal airway (Combitube)**

Ref: Chapter No.17, Page No.393

47. **Ans: A. Warm extremities**

Ref: Chapter No.17, Page No.394

48. **Ans: B. Hemorrhage**

Ref: Chapter No.17, Page No.394

49. **Ans: B. Class II**

Ref: Chapter No.17, Page No.394

50. **Ans: C. Class III**

Ref: Chapter No.17, Page No.394

51. **Ans: A. Class I**

Ref: Chapter No.17, Page No.394

52. **Ans: C. Class III**

Ref: Chapter No.17, Page No.394

53. **Ans: C. Class III**

Ref: Chapter No.17, Page No.394

54. **Ans: B. Class II**

Ref: Chapter No.17, Page No.394

55. **Ans: C. Class III**

Ref: Chapter No.17, Page No.394

56. **Ans: C. The fast abdominal sonography in trauma (FAST) scan is a rapidly obtainable ultrasound examination that assesses for retroperitoneal fluid**

Ref: Chapter No.17, Page No.394

57. **Ans: B. Focused abdominal sonography in trauma (FAST) scan**

Ref: Chapter No.17, Page No.394

58. **Ans: D. If a patient is able to move their upper extremities, the likelihood of neurogenic shock is not diminished**

Ref: Chapter No.17, Page No.394-395

59. **Ans: C. Patients presenting after blunt chest mechanism, with and without signs of life, survived better than penetrating chest mechanism**

Ref: Chapter No.17, Page No.395

60. **Ans: B. Cross clamping the proximal thoracic aorta**

Ref: Chapter No.17, Page No.395

61. **Ans: D. Currently, there is high-grade evidence to support indications or the superiority of REBOA beyond standard care, and a comparison of technique to RT introduces both survival and indication biases**

Ref: Chapter No.17, Page No.395

62. **Ans: A. Resuscitative endovascular balloon occlusion of the aorta (REBOA)**

Ref: Chapter No.17, Page No.395

63. **Ans: A. A rapid determination of neurologic function is done**

Ref: Chapter No.17, Page No.395

64. **Ans: B. The hepatorenal space, known as the Morison pouch, is viewed between the 10th and 11th ribs in the right midclavicular line (*between 11th and 12th rib in midaxillary line*)**

FAST

Patient is in supine position

3.5-5.0 MHz convex transducer is used

5 regions may be scanned:

- **Pericardial view:** commonly referred to as the **subcostal** or **subxiphoid** view to examine the ***pericardium***, the ***liver*** in the epigastric region is most commonly used as a sonographic window to the heart. The potential space between the visceral and parietal pericardium is examined for a ***pericardial effusion*** if anatomical factors preclude epigastric probe placement, parasternal or apical 4-chamber views may be used
- **Right flank view:** commonly referred to as the ***perihepatic*** view, ***Morison pouch view*** or ***right upper quadrant view***. 4 potential spaces are sequentially examined for the accumulation of free fluid:
  1. The ***hepatorenal interface (Morison pouch)*** is first identified
  2. With subsequent assessment of the ***more cephalad subphrenic and pleural spaces***
  3. Visualization of the ***inferior pole of the kidney***, which is a continuation of the right paracolic gutter, defines the caudad extent of an adequate view
- **Left flank view:** commonly referred to as the ***perisplenic*** or ***left upper quadrant view***. 4 potential spaces are sequentially examined in an analogous fashion to the right flank, albeit the ***splenorenal interface*** is assessed on the left
- **Pelvic view** commonly referred to as the ***suprapubic view***, this space is the ***most dependent peritoneal space*** in the supine trauma patient a transverse sweep, using the bladder as a sonographic window, the pouch of Douglas or rectovesical space is explored for free fluid.

An **extended FAST or "eFAST"** scan is now standard of care, and is performed by incorporating 2 views assessing the anterior thorax

- **Anterior pleural views:** the anterior pleura is assessed for the presence or absence of ***lung sliding*** as a sensitive, ***but non-specific***, indicator of a traumatic **pneumothorax**
- The probe is placed in a sagittal orientation in the midclavicular line between the clavicle and diaphragm

  Anterior and lateral interrogation of ***interspaces 5-8*** bilaterally is recommended

Causes of **false positive** FAST:

1. **Epicardial fat pads,** the **descending aorta**, and **pericardial cysts** have been mistakenly identified as an effusion
2. Pre-existing **ascites**, pleural, and pericardial effusions due to medical conditions
3. **Seminal vesicles** mistaken for pelvic free fluid in the young male patient

Causes of **false negative** FAST:

1. **Obesity:** severely limits assessment of the peritoneal cavity
2. **Subcutaneous emphysema**
3. Posterior acoustic enhancement caused by the **fluid-filled bladder** can result in free fluid being missed in the pelvic view

Ref: Chapter No.17, Page No.395

https://radiopaedia.org/articles/focussed-assessment-with-sonography-for-trauma-fast-scan

65. **Ans: A. Anticoagulation**

Ref: Chapter No.17, Page No.396

66. **Ans: B. Blunt mechanism**

A. score of **at least 2** was **predictive of MTP need** (75% sensitivity, 86% specificity) and a delay in initiation is associated with a **5% increase in mortality per minute**

Ref: Chapter No.17, Page No.396

67. **Ans: C. 8 hours**

Ref: Chapter No.17, Page No.396

68. **Ans: C. Fibrinolysis**

Ref: Chapter No.17, Page No.396

69. **Ans: D. Hypercoagulable**

Ref: Chapter No.17, Page No.396

70. **Ans: B. Platelet dysfunction**

Ref: Chapter No.17, Page No.396

71. **Ans: B. Falls**

Ref: Chapter No.17, Page No.396

72. **Ans: B. Epidural hematoma**

Ref: Chapter No.17, Page No.397

73. **Ans: B. Middle meningeal artery**

Ref: Chapter No.17, Page No.397

74. **Ans: A. Tearing of the bridging veins**

Ref: Chapter No.17, Page No.397

75. **Ans: A. Subdural hematoma**

Ref: Chapter No.17, Page No.397

76. **Ans: C. Subarachnoid hemorrhage**

Ref: Chapter No.17, Page No.397

77. **Ans: D. Brain contusion**

Ref: Chapter No.17, Page No.397

78. **Ans: A. The underlying brain tissue is severely injured in the setting of an epidural hematoma**

Ref: Chapter No.17, Page No.397

79. **Ans: A. Within 3 hours of injury**

Ref: Chapter No.17, Page No.397

80. **Ans: B. Airway control and ventilatory support are critical immediately after TBI, as transient episodes of hypoxia may increase mortality up to 10-fold**

Ref: Chapter No.17, Page No.396

81. **Ans: B. Motor function**

Ref: Chapter No.17, Page No.397

82. **Ans: C. CT brain without contrast (Magnetic resonance imaging (MRI) may be able to provide better anatomic detail, but it has no role in the initial evaluation of the brain-injured patient)**

Ref: Chapter No.17, Page No.397

83. **Ans: C. Mild hypoventilation**

Ref: Chapter No.17, Page No.398

84. **Ans: A. In the setting of medically recalcitrant severe intracranial hypertension, patients may be considered for decompressive craniectomy, operative salvage has recently been shown to improve mortality and functional outcomes**

Ref: Chapter No.17, Page No.398

85. **Ans: B. < 22 mm Hg**

Ref: Chapter No.17, Page No.398

86. **Ans: B. < 8**

Ref: Chapter No.17, Page No.398

87. **Ans: C. 60 to 70 mm Hg**

Ref: Chapter No.17, Page No.398

88. **Ans: C. 30 to 35 mm Hg**

Ref: Chapter No.17, Page No.399

89. **Ans: C. The 5th to 6th thoracic vertebrae are within the zone of greatest mobility and hence most susceptible to injury**

Ref: Chapter No.17, Page No.399

90. **Ans: D. All of the above**

Ref: Chapter No.17, Page No.399

91. **Ans: C. The classic presentation of neurogenic shock is hypotension in the setting of cold, poorly-perfused extremities in the paralyzed patient**

Ref: Chapter No.17, Page No.399

92. **Ans: A. Complete injury**

Ref: Chapter No.17, Page No.399

93. **Ans: C. Motor incomplete**

Ref: Chapter No.17, Page No.399

94. **Ans: D. Normal**

Ref: Chapter No.17, Page No.399

95. **Ans: A. Plain radiograph of the spine (anteroposterior, lateral, odontoid) is the modality of choice in most emergency departments for evaluate of vertebral column injury**

   1. **The Canadian C-Spine Rule** is a well-validated decision rule that can be used to safely rule out cervical spine injury (CSI) in alert, stable trauma patients without the need to obtain radiographic images
      - CCR is ***highly sensitive for CSI,*** with the majority of studies finding it catches ***99-100%*** of these types of injuries
      - Applying the Canadian C.-Spine Rule would allow healthcare providers to safely ***decrease the need for imaging among this patient population by over 40%***
      - Subsequent studies have found a sensitivity of 90-100% for CSI with majority finding 99-100% sensitivity.

Mnemonic:

a. **High** risk features: ***Sixty-five, Fast drive, Sense deprive? Image, if alive***

b. **Low** risk features: ***Slow wreck, Slow neck, Sitting down, Walking 'round, C.-spine fine? Range the spine!***

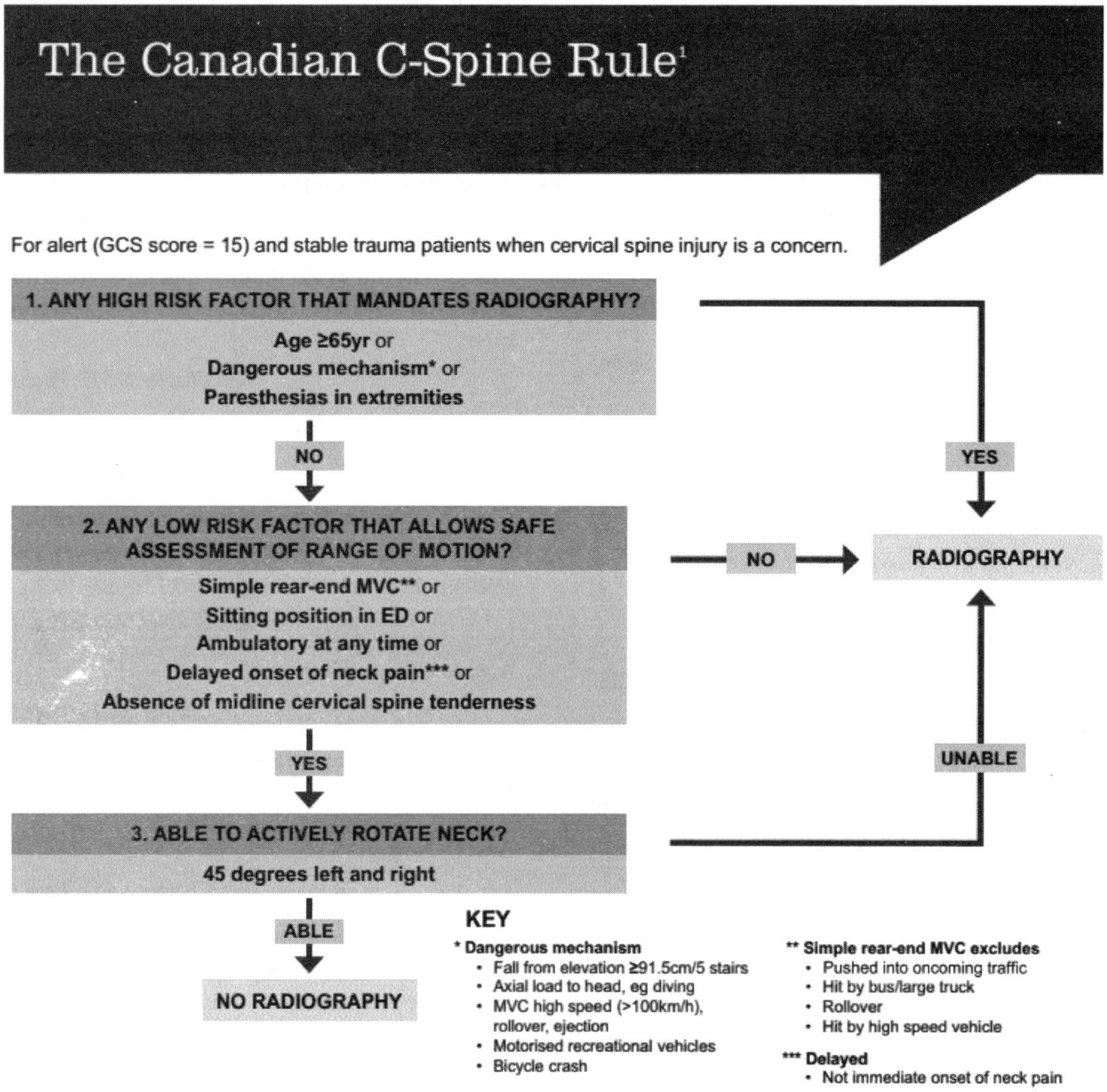

Instructions for using the Canadian C-Spine Rule

1. Define whether any high risk factors are present such as age (≥65 years) or dangerous mechanism (includes high speed or roll over or ejection, motorised recreation vehicle or bicycle crash). If this is the case, an X-ray of the cervical spine should be performed.
2. Define low risk factors that allow safe assessment of neck ROM. If the low risk factors shown in the flow chart are not present, an X-ray of the neck should be performed.
3. Assess rotation of the neck to 45 degrees in people who have low risk factors shown in the QTF Classification of Grades of WAD. If people are able to rotate their neck to 45 degrees, they do not require an X-ray of the neck.

This rule has been validated across several different populations and has been shown to have a sensitivity of 99.4 per cent and a specificity of 42.5 per cent. Essentially, physicians who follow this rule can be assured that a fracture will not be missed (95% CI 98–100%).[2] Further a systematic review investigated the diagnostic accuracy of the Canadian C-Spine Rule and the National Emergency, X-Radiography Utilization Study (NEXUS) criteria and found that the Canadian C-Spine Rule had better accuracy.[3]

2. **NEXUS (National Emergency X-Radiography Utilization Study)** is a set of validated criteria used to decide which trauma patients ***do not require cervical spine imaging***

   Trauma patients who do not require cervical spine imaging require all of the following:

   - Alert and stable
   - No focal neurologic deficit
   - No altered level of consciousness
   - Not intoxicated
   - No midline spinal tenderness
   - No distracting injury

The **NEXUS criteria** have a sensitivity of 99.6% for ruling out cervical spine injury in the original study validating the criteria (95% confidence interval, 98.6-100%)

The NEXUS criteria may ***not be reliable with patient >65 years of age***.

Mnemonic: **NEXUS**

1. **N**eurologic deficit (focal)
2. **E**thanol/Intoxication
3. e**X**treme distracting injury (painful injury elsewhere that could distract patient from recognizing the pain associated with a neck injury)
4. **U**nable to provide history (altered mental status)
5. **S**pinal tenderness (midline)

Mnemonic: **NSAID**

- **N**eurologic deficit (focal)
- **S**pinal tenderness (midline)
- **A**ltered mental status
- **I**ntoxication

Ref: Chapter No.17, Page No.400

https://www.sira.nsw.gov.au/resources-library/motor-accident-resources/publications/for-professionals/whiplash-resources/SIRA08109-Canadian-C.-Spine-Rule1117-396476.pdf https://www.ncbi.nlm.nih.gov/pmc/articles/PMC6214507/

96. Ans: C. Brief periods of hypotension (<90 mm Hg), not unlike TBI, have been not shown previously to be detrimental to long-term outcomes in SCI; thus, shock can be treated non aggressively

Ref: Chapter No.17, Page No.400

97. Ans: D. All of the above

Ref: Chapter No.17, Page No.400

98. Ans: B. Jefferson fracture

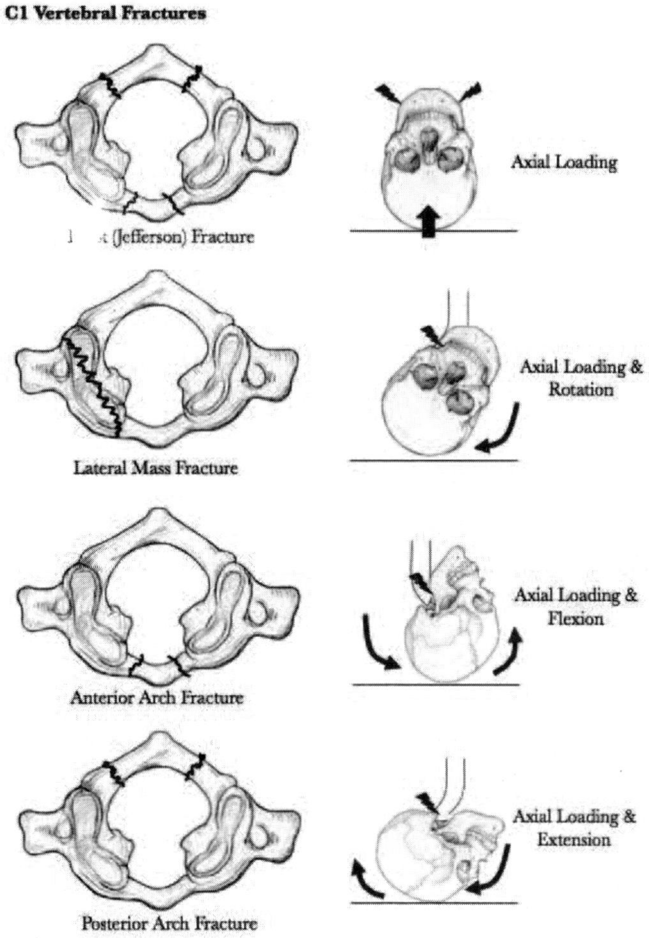

Ref: Chapter No.17, Page No.401

99. Ans: D. Chance fracture

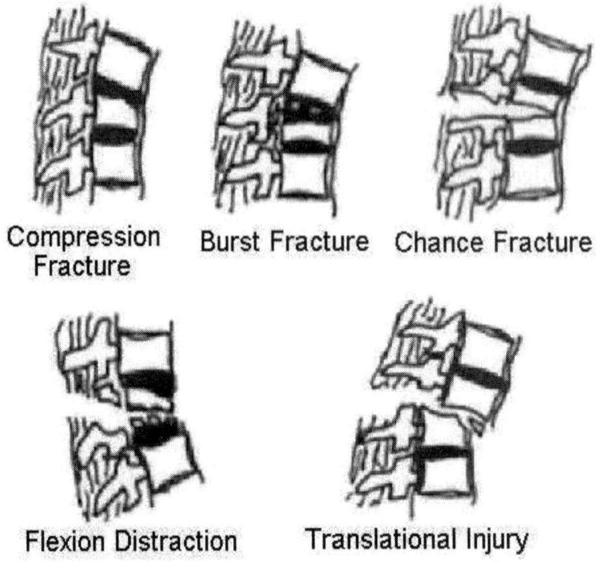

Ref: Chapter No.17, Page No.401

100. Ans: B. Bilateral C2 pedicles with spondylolisthesis

Hangman's fracture classification

Classification	Definition	Mechanism
Effendi		
Type I	Isolated hairline fracture of ring of axis	Axial loading and hyperextension
Type II	Displacement of anterior fragment and abnormal disk below axis	Further hyperextension and rebound flexion
Type III	Displacement of anterior fragment and locked facet at C2–C3	Flexion and rebound extension
Levine and Edwards		
Type I	Nondisplaced fracture (<3 mm)	Hyperextension and axial loading
Type II	Significant angulation (>11 degrees) and translation (>3 mm)	Hyperextension, axial loading and rebound flexion
Type IIa	Very severe angulation without translation	Flexion-distraction
Type III	Severe angulation and displacement with facet dislocation	Flexion-compression

Ref: Chapter No.17, Page No.401
https://www.ncbi.nlm.nih.gov/pmc/articles/PMC4836940/

101. Ans: A. Type I Odontoid #; hard collar

Ref: Chapter No.17, Page No.401

102. Ans: D. Type III Odontoid #; halo vest

Ref: Chapter No.17, Page No.401

103. Ans: B. Type II Odontoid #

Ref: Chapter No.17, Page No.401

104. Ans: C. Type 3

Ref: Chapter No.17, Page No.401

105. Ans: A. Type 1

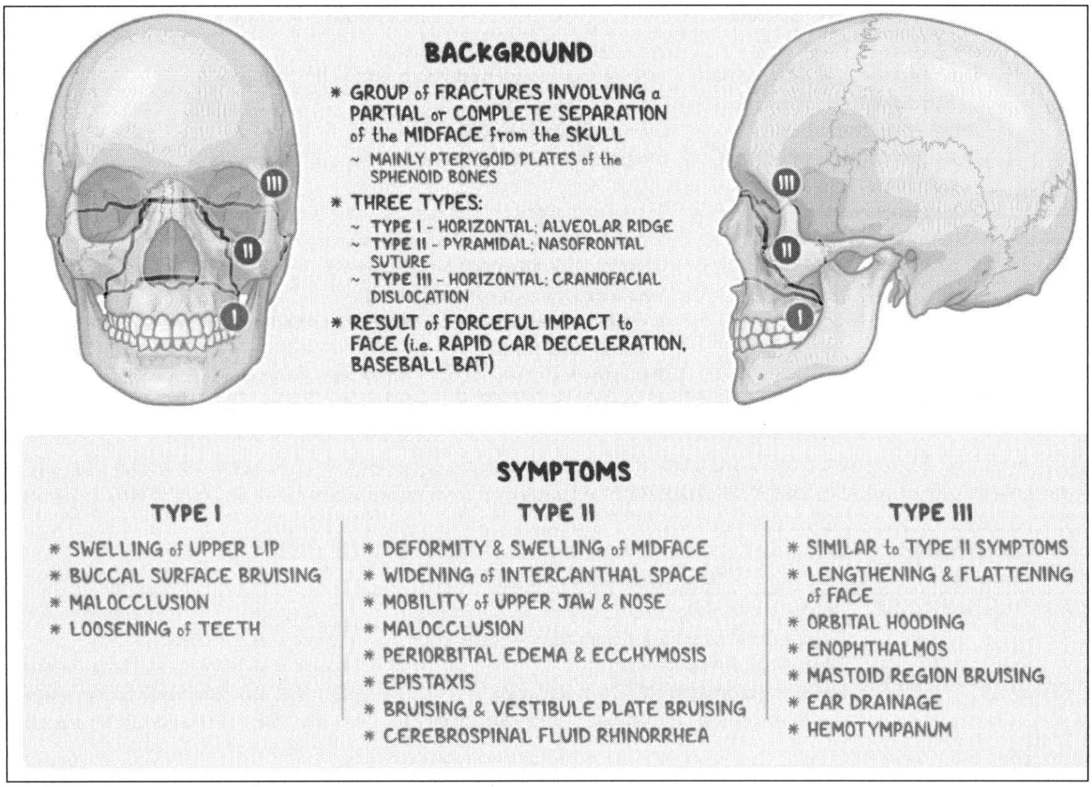

Ref: Chapter No.17, Page No.401

106. Ans: D. Imaging of the face should be performed immediately, as management of facial trauma is time sensitive in the majority of cases

Ref: Chapter No.17, Page No.401

107. Ans: B. CT is indicated when any external injury is identified on primary survey

Ref: Chapter No.17, Page No.401

108. Ans: C. Large open wounds and fractures involving sinuses or the aerodigestive tract never require antibiotics

Ref: Chapter No.17, Page No.401-402

109. Ans: C. Guardsman fracture

- A **guardsman fracture**, also referred to as **parade ground fracture**, is one of the common forms of mandibular fracture which is caused by a fall on the ***midpoint of the chin*** resulting in fracture of the ***symphysis as well as both condyles***
- It is usually seen in **epileptics, elderly patients** and occasionally in **soldiers** (fall forwards due to syncope) and is known as guardsman fracture

Ref: https://link.springer.com/chapter/10.1007/978-981-15-1346-6_52

110. Ans: C. Blunt mechanisms can cause sudden com-pression, with subsequent fracture of the larynx or trachea and is the most common mechanism of injury

Ref: Chapter No.17, Page No.402

111. Ans: B. Pseudoaneurysm formation

Ref: Chapter No.17, Page No.402

112. Ans: C. Grade IV

1. The **Denver criteria** are a set of *screening criteria* used to determine when *CT angiography* of the neck is indicated to detect **blunt cerebrovascular injury** (***BCVI) in trauma patients***.

Grade of Injury	Denver Grading System[31]	CTA Findings	Stroke Incidence (%)[9,48] (CAI/VAI)
I	Irregularity of vessel wall Dissection or IMH with <25% narrowing	Nonstenotic luminal irregularity Intimal flap or wall thickening with <25% stenosis	3/6
II	Intraluminal thrombus Dissection or IMH with >25% narrowing	Luminal hypodensity Intimal flap or wall thickening with >25% stenosis	14/38
III	Pseudoaneurysm	Eccentric contrast-filled outpouching limited by periarterial tissue	26/27
IV	Occlusion	Lack of any intraluminal enhancement Carotid occlusions: abrupt or tapered Vertebral occlusion: usually abrupt	50/28
V	Transection	Irregular extravascular collection of contrast, not limited by periarterial tissue Increases in density on delayed images, if obtained	100/100

Note:—CAI indicates carotid artery injury; VAI, vertebral artery injury; IMH, intramural hematoma.

2. The **modified Memphis criteria** are a set of screening criteria for <u>blunt</u> ***cerebrovascular injury*** (BCVI) in trauma. The presence of ***one or more of these criteria makes necessary a complementary CTA or DSA study*** to exclude a BCVI

Name of Screening Criteria	Patients to Be Screened	
	Signs/Symptoms of BCVI	Risk Factors of BCVI
Modified[a] Denver Criteria[14]	Arterial hemorrhage (from neck, nose, or mouth) Cervical bruit (in younger than 50 yr of age) Expanding cervical hematoma Focal neurologic defect: TIA, hemiparesis, vertebrobasilar symptoms, Horner syndrome Stroke on CT or MRI Neurologic deficit inconsistent with head CT	High-energy transfer mechanism with the following: LeFort II or III fracture Basilar skull fracture involving carotid canal Cervical vertebral body or transverse foramen fracture, subluxation, or ligamentous injury at any level; any fracture at C1–C3 Closed head injury consistent with DAI and GCS <6 Near-hanging with anoxia Clothesline-type injury or seat belt abrasion with significant swelling, pain, or altered mental status
Memphis Criteria[16]	Cervical spine fracture Neurologic exam not explained by brain imaging Horner syndrome LeFort II or III facial fractures Skull base fractures involving the foramen lacerum Neck soft-tissue injury (eg, seat belt injury or hanging)	

Ref: Chapter No.17, Page No.402

https://www.researchgate.net/figure/Denver-grading-system-corresponding-CTA-findings-and-grade-based-stroke-incidence_tbl2_320374305

https://www.researchgate.net/figure/Published-screening-criteria-for-BCVI_tbl1_320374305

113. Ans: C. The surgical airway of choice for an upper airway injury is a cricothyroidotomy

Ref: Chapter No.17, Page No.402

114. Ans: B. Between the cricoid cartilage and the angle of the mandible

Ref: Chapter No.17, Page No.402

115. Ans: C. Extends from the angle of the mandible to the skull base

Ref: Chapter No.17, Page No.402

116. Ans: D. Structures within zone III include blood vessels that are easy to expose surgically

Ref: Chapter No.17, Page No.402

117. Ans: A. DSA is the study of choice for diagnosis of BCVI

Ref: Chapter No.17, Page No.402-403

118. Ans: D. Cervical bruit (patient >50 years old)

Ref: Chapter No.17, Page No.403

119. Ans: B. Le Fort I

Ref: Chapter No.17, Page No.403

120. Ans: C. Short-segment carotid artery injuries should require reconstruction with a synthetic graft or autologous vein

Ref: Chapter No.17, Page No.403

121. Ans: D. All of the above

Ref: Chapter No.17, Page No.403

122. Ans: C. Endovascular stenting may be considered in select circumstances involving pseudoaneurysm and dissection with 50% flow limitation

Ref: Chapter No.17, Page No.403-404

123. Ans: D. All of the above

Ref: Chapter No.17, Page No.404

124. Ans: B. Start antithrombotic therapy (Heparin with PTT 40–50 sec)

Ref: Chapter No.17, Page No.405

125. Ans: C. Operative or endovascular treatment

Ref: Chapter No.17, Page No.405

126. Ans: A. Anterior border of the sternocleidomastoid muscle

Ref: Chapter No.17, Page No.403

127. Ans: D. Patients with persistent shock despite resuscitation and ongoing blood loss from the chest rarely require operative intervention

Ref: Chapter No.17, Page No.404

128. Ans: B. < 10%

Ref: Chapter No.17, Page No.404

129. Ans: D. MDCTA is reliable for evaluation of pericardium

Ref: Chapter No.17, Page No.405

130. Ans: A. Sternum medially

Ref: Chapter No.17, Page No.405

131. Ans: D. All of the above

Ref: Chapter No.17, Page No.406

132. Ans: B. 85%

Ref: Chapter No.17, Page No.406

133. Ans: D. All of the above

Ref: Chapter No.17, Page No.406

134. Ans: B. 3%

Ref: Chapter No.17, Page No.406

135. Ans: D. Nipple or inframammary fold inferiorly

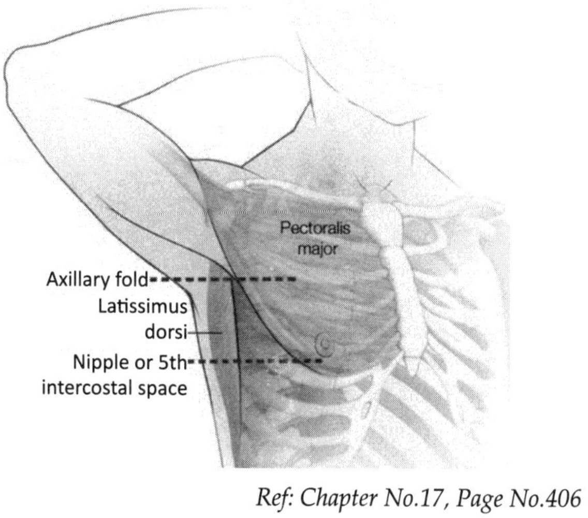

Ref: Chapter No.17, Page No.406

https://www.researchgate.net/figure/British-Thoracic-Societys-triangle-of-safety-detailing-anatomic-borders-for-placement-of_fig1_301685988

136. Ans: D. > 1500 mL of blood drained on chest tube insertion

Other indications for thoracotomy include a ***massive air leak with associated pneumothorax*** and ***drainage of esophageal or gastric contents from the chest tube***

Ref: Chapter No.17, Page No.407

137. Ans: B. Posterolateral thoracotomy

Ref: Chapter No.17, Page No.407

138. Ans: A. Left subclavian artery

Ref: Chapter No.17, Page No.407

139. Ans: C. Median sternotomy

Ref: Chapter No.17, Page No.407

140. Ans: B. Posterolateral thoracotomy

Ref: Chapter No.17, Page No.407

141. Ans: B. Rib fracture

Ref: Chapter No.17, Page No.407

142. Ans: D. All of the above

Ref: Chapter No.17, Page No.407

143. Ans: C. 2 or more adjacent ribs fractured in 2 or more locations

Ref: Chapter No.17, Page No.407

144. Ans: C. Recent data suggest that observation for pneumothoraces with CT radial diameter of up to 55 mm may be safe for both blunt and penetrating trauma

Ref: Chapter No.17, Page No.407

145. Ans: D. 400–500 mL

Ref: Chapter No.17, Page No.407

146. Ans: D. All of the above

Ref: Chapter No.17, Page No.407

147. Ans: A. 33%

Ref: Chapter No.17, Page No.407

148. Ans: A. Median sternotomy

Ref: Chapter No.17, Page No.407

149. Ans: D. All of the above

Ref: Chapter No.17, Page No.407-408

150. Ans: C. Right thoracotomy

Ref: Chapter No.17, Page No.407

151. Ans: C. Needle decompression (Choice D. is the next best step after needle decompression is done)

Ref: Chapter No.17, Page No.407

152. Ans: D. Tension pneumothorax

Ref: Chapter No.17, Page No.407

153. Ans: B. Hemothorax

Ref: Chapter No.17, Page No.407

154. Ans: B. Right sided pneumothorax

Ref: Chapter No.17, Page No.407

155. Ans: A. Approximately 1 in 5 patients in the NTDB sustains a pulmonary contusion after chest trauma

Ref: Chapter No.17, Page No.408

156. Ans: A Injured lung tissue on CT appears as a lesser density

Ref: Chapter No.17, Page No.408

157. Ans: B. ARDS

Ref: Chapter No.17, Page No.408

158. Ans: B. Trauma pneumonectomy is morbid with mortality (< 30%)

Ref: Chapter No.17, Page No.408

159. Ans: B. Penetrating injury to the heart occurred in 10% to 20% of patients with penetrating trauma in the NTDB and in > 50% of the subset with penetrating chest trauma alone

Ref: Chapter No.17, Page No.408-409

160. Ans: D. Decreased air entry on auscultation

Ref: Chapter No.17, Page No.409

161. Ans: A. Median sternotomy

Ref: Chapter No.17, Page No.409

162. Ans: A. Most of the cases represent a contusion of the myocardium that results in arrhythmias and is frequently need intervention

Ref: Chapter No.17, Page No.409

163. Ans: D. Admission ECG and troponin

Patients suspected of having a blunt cardiac injury should undergo electrocardiography and troponin I evaluation at the time of initial workup

Ref: Chapter No.17, Page No.409

164. Ans: D. Cardiac tamponade: pericardial window

Ref: Chapter No.17, Page No.409

165. Ans: D. 80%

Ref: Chapter No.17, Page No.409

166. Ans: D. When open surgical repair is required, the aorta is exposed through a right thoracotomy

Ref: Chapter No.17, Page No.409-410

167. Ans: A. Pseudoaneurysm

Ref: Chapter No.17, Page No.409

168. Ans: B. Intramural hematoma

Ref: Chapter No.17, Page No.409

169. Ans: C. Distal airway injuries may result in large amounts of pneumomediastinum identified by chest radiography or CT imaging

Ref: Chapter No.17, Page No.410

170. Ans: B. Operative management of the trachea, right-sided airways, and proximal left mainstem bronchus is best approached through a left posterolateral thoracotomy

Ref: Chapter No.17, Page No.410

171. Ans: D. High-resolution CT imaging rarely demonstrates an esophageal wall defect

Ref: Chapter No.17, Page No.410

172. Ans: B. 35%

Ref: Chapter No.17, Page No.410

173. Ans: C. Following repair, an esophagram may be performed at day 14 to confirm healing and liberalization of oral intake

Ref: Chapter No.17, Page No.410-411

174. Ans: A. Right posterolateral thoracotomy (4th or 5th interspace)

Ref: Chapter No.17, Page No.411

175. Ans: B. Left posterolateral thoracotomy (6th or 7th interspace)

Ref: Chapter No.17, Page No.411

176. Ans: B. The right side of the diaphragm is the injured location in approximately 75% of the cases

Ref: Chapter No.17, Page No.411

177. Ans: C. Closure is performed with a single layer of absorbable suture incorporating large full-thickness bites of healthy diaphragmatic tissue

Ref: Chapter No.17, Page No.411

178. Ans: D. In most acute diaphragmatic ruptures, repair can be completed with primary repair.

Ref: Chapter No.17, Page No.411

179. Ans: A. Drainage of the right chest cavity

Ref: Chapter No.17, Page No.407

180. Ans: B. Closure of the hole with sterile dressing

- The immediate treatment is the ***closure of the hole by any means available***.
- Sucking chest wounds allow shift of the mediastinum to the opposite side leading to ***tension pneumothorax***
- A ***chest tube will be required,*** following closure of the sucking wound

Ref: Chapter No.17, Page No.407

181. Ans: A. Contrast esophagography and esophagoscopy

Nasogastric tube aspiration showing blood is suggestive of an esophageal injury in this patient but is not specific, hence contrast esophagography and esophagoscopy will be needed for confirmation of esophageal injury.

Ref: Chapter No.17, Page No.410

182. Ans: C. Tension pneumothorax

Ref: Chapter No.17, Page No.407

183. Ans: B. Perform a left thoracotomy

Ref: Chapter No.17, Page No.407

184. Ans: A. Flail chest

Ref: Chapter No.17, Page No.407

185. Ans: B. Spontaneous pneumothorax

Ref: Chapter No.17, Page No.407

186. Ans: C. Massive hemothorax

Ref: Chapter No.17, Page No.407

187. Ans: A. Tension pneumothorax

Ref: Chapter No.17, Page No.407

188. Ans: D. All of the above

Ref: Chapter No.17, Page No.412

189. Ans: C. Stab wounds to the left upper quadrant and right upper quadrant will always require laparoscopy for diaphragmatic assessment

(Optional in right upper quadrant)

Ref: Chapter No.17, Page No.412

190. Ans: D. All of the above

Ref: Chapter No.17, Page No.412

191. Ans: B. CT scan (best means to establish a diagnosis is asked)

Ref: Chapter No.17, Page No.413

192. Ans: A. Exploratory laparotomy

Ref: Chapter No.17, Page No.412

193. Ans: C. Exploratory laparotomy

Ref: Chapter No.17, Page No.414

194. Ans: D. Thoracentesis

Ref: Chapter No.17, Page No.414

195. Ans: D. Discharge to outpatient clinic for follow-up monitoring

Ref: Chapter No.17, Page No.413

196. Ans: C. Preoperatively

Ref: Chapter No.17, Page No.413

197. Ans: B. CT scan with oral and intravenous contrast

Ref: Chapter No.17, Page No.413

198. Ans: D. Diaphragm

Missed diaphragmatic injuries may cause late diaphragmatic hernias with potential morbidity and mortality

Ref: Chapter No.17, Page No.411

199. Ans: D. Exploratory laparotomy

Ref: Chapter No.17, Page No.414

200. Ans: C. CT with intravenous and oral contrast

Ref: Chapter No.17, Page No.414

201. Ans: B. Wound exploration

Ref: Chapter No.17, Page No.414

202. Ans: B. Spleen

Ref: Chapter No.17, Page No.414

203. Ans: C. Unstable patients with abdominal trauma who are taken emergently to the OR may have a splenic injury identified at the time of laparotomy (50% of blunt splenic injury)

Ref: Chapter No.17, Page No.414

204. Ans: D. All of the above

Ref: Chapter No.17, Page No.414

205. Ans: D. 90%

Ref: Chapter No.17, Page No.415

206. Ans: D. All of the above

Ref: Chapter No.17, Page No.415-416

207. Ans: B. Splenectomy

Ref: Chapter No.17, Page No.416

208. Ans: C. Postsplenectomy sepsis

Ref: Chapter No.17, Page No.416

209. Ans: A. Left colon perforation

Ref: Chapter No.17, Page No.416

210. Ans: A. Hemodynamic instability

Ref: Chapter No.17, Page No.416

211. Ans: A. Grade I

Ref: Chapter No.17, Page No.415

212. Ans: C. Grade IV

Ref: Chapter No.17, Page No.415

213. Ans: D. Grade V

Ref: Chapter No.17, Page No.415

214. Ans: B. Grade III

Ref: Chapter No.17, Page No.415

215. Ans: D. Grade V

Ref: Chapter No.17, Page No.415

216. Ans: C. Grade III

Ref: Chapter No.17, Page No.415

217. Ans: D. Grade V

Ref: Chapter No.17, Page No.415

218. Ans: D. Liver

Ref: Chapter No.17, Page No.416

219. Ans: D. All of the above

Ref: Chapter No.17, Page No.416

220. Ans: A. The majority of patients with Grades I to III injuries being successfully managed nonoperatively,

while 10% of Grades IV and V residually require surgical care

Ref: Chapter No.17, Page No.416

221. **Ans: D. Biliary ascites amenable to percutaneous drainage mostly needs laparoscopy or laparotomy for adequate drainage to be obtained**

Ref: Chapter No.17, Page No.417

222. **Ans: A. When operative management is required, a Kocher's incision is the most versatile approach for managing any liver injury that might be encountered**

Ref: Chapter No.17, Page No.417

223. **Ans: C. Liver injuries in the vicinity of the retrohepatic vena cava that are not actively bleeding should be packed and explored**

Ref: Chapter No.17, Page No.418

224. **Ans: D. All of the above**

Ref: Chapter No.17, Page No.418

225. **Ans: C. Repeated hemoglobin determination**

Ref: Chapter No.17, Page No.417

226. **Ans: C. Biloma: image-guided percutaneous drainage**

Ref: Chapter No.17, Page No.418

227. **Ans: C. Angiography**

Ref: Chapter No.17, Page No.415

228. **Ans: B. Right medial visceral rotation**

Ref: Chapter No.17, Page No.418

229. **Ans: C. Grade IV**

- Active bleeding extending beyond the ***spleen*** into the peritoneum is ***grade V***
- Active bleeding extending beyond the ***liver*** parenchyma into the peritoneum is ***grade IV***

Ref: Chapter No.17, Page No.417

230. **Ans: B. Grade III**

Ref: Chapter No.17, Page No.417

231. **Ans: B. Grade III**

- Any injury in the presence of a ***splenic vascular*** injury is ***grade IV***
- Any injury in the presence of a ***liver vascular*** injury is ***grade III***

Ref: Chapter No.17, Page No.417

232. **Ans: D. Grade V**

Ref: Chapter No.17, Page No.417

233. **Ans: D. Firmly pack the RUQ, close the abdomen, and plan to return to the OR within 24–48 hours**

Ref: Chapter No.17, Page No.418

234. **Ans: B. Packing the liver**

Ref: Chapter No.17, Page No.418

235. **Ans: C. Pringle's maneuver**

- **The liver hanging maneuver:** It is a technique of passing a ***tape along the retrohepatic avascular space and suspending the liver during parenchymal transection,*** facilitates anterior approach of major hepatectomy.

Ref: Chapter No.17, Page No.418

https://www.ncbi.nlm.nih.gov/pmc/articles/PMC1867932/

236. **Ans: A. Grade II**

Ref: Chapter No.17, Page No.417

237. **Ans: C. Transfusion of whole blood to elevate blood pressure**

Ref: Chapter No.17, Page No.417-418

238. **Ans: D. Hematomas within the gastric wall should not be evacuated to ensure the absence of perforation.**

Ref: Chapter No.17, Page No.418-419

239. **Ans: D. All of the above**

Ref: Chapter No.17, Page No.419

240. **Ans: A. Because of the retroperitoneal location of the duodenum, most injuries are due to blunt modalities in approximately 50% of cases**

Ref: Chapter No.17, Page No.419

241. **Ans: B. Duodenal hematomas identified incidentally during laparotomy should be intentionally opened as there is a high concern for full-thickness injury**

Ref: Chapter No.17, Page No.419

242. **Ans: C. Drain placement following definitive repair is mandatory**

Ref: Chapter No.17, Page No.419

243. **Ans: A. Initiation of NPO status and gastric decompression with a nasogastric tube**

Ref: Chapter No.17, Page No.419

244. **Ans: B. Nasogastric decompression, intravenous fluids, and gradual resumption of oral diet**

Ref: Chapter No.17, Page No.419

245. **Ans: A. CT with oral and intravenous contrast**

Ref: Chapter No.17, Page No.419

246. **Ans: B. Duodenal hematoma**

- **Stack of coins sign** refers to the appearance of small bowel folds that are smoothly and uniformly thickened. The margins between the folds are sharply delineated and the arrangement of clearly demarcated parallel folds is likened to a stack of coins or a picket fence.

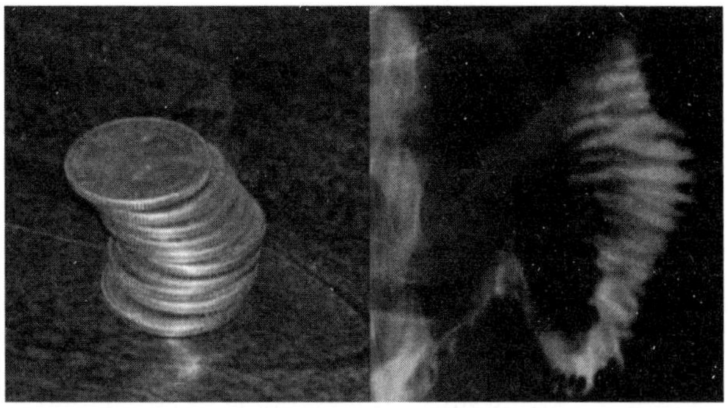

Ref: 1. Chapter No.17, Page No.419
2. Eisenberg R. Thickening of Small Bowel Folds. AJR Am J Roentgenol. 2009;193(1):W1-W6. doi:10.2214/ajr.09.2762

247. Ans: D. Repeat upper GI series at 5- to 7-day interval

Ref: Chapter No.17, Page No.419

248. Ans: B. Gastrografin study

Ref: Chapter No.17, Page No.419

249. Ans: B. A blunt mechanism is more commonly the cause

Ref: Chapter No.17, Page No.420

250. Ans: C. CT alone is always satisfactory to rule out a clinically significant pancreatic injury

Ref: Chapter No.17, Page No.420

251. Ans: B. 15%

Ref: Chapter No.17, Page No.420

252. Ans: B. When obtained > 1 hour after injury occurrence, an elevated serum amylase level may reflect pancreatic trauma

Ref: Chapter No.17, Page No.420

253. Ans: B. Distal pancreatectomy with oversewing of the proximal pancreatic stump

Ref: Chapter No.17, Page No.420

254. Ans: B. Closed suction systems are associated with a increased rate of abscess development compared with open-style drains

Ref: Chapter No.17, Page No.420

255. Ans: C. Closed-suction drainage and lavage

Ref: Chapter No.17, Page No.420

256. Ans: B. Grade III

Ref: Chapter No.56, Page No.1563

257. Ans: C. Grade IV

Ref: Chapter No.56, Page No.1563

258. Ans: B. Grade II

Ref: Chapter No.56, Page No.1563

259. Ans: D. Resection of the bowel with single-layer anastomosis

Ref: Chapter No.17, Page No.421

260. Ans: B. Mortality rates range from 50% to 70%, with most caused by associated vascular injuries.

Ref: Chapter No.17, Page No.421

261. Ans: B. > 50%

Ref: Chapter No.17, Page No.421

262. Ans: C. Wounds > 25% of the colonic circumference

Ref: Chapter No.17, Page No.422

263. Ans: B. In blunt injury, serosal tears > 25% colon circumference and mesenteric devascularization are considered destructive

Ref: Chapter No.17, Page No.422

264. Ans: B. Abdominal CT has very good capabilities in the diagnosis

Ref: Chapter No.17, Page No.422

265. Ans: B. Even if the CT is negative for injury, clinically relevant trauma is much likely

Ref: Chapter No.17, Page No.422

266. Ans: A. Wound > 25% of the rectal circumference

Ref: Chapter No.17, Page No.422

267. Ans: D. All of the above

Ref: Chapter No.17, Page No.423

268. Ans: A. Most can be treated by debridement and repair

Ref: Chapter No.17, Page No.422

269. Ans: A. Resection and anastomosis of the small bowel injuries and primary repair of the colon injury

Ref: Chapter No.17, Page No.422

270. Ans: D. Debridement and closure of wounds

Ref: Chapter No.17, Page No.422

271. Ans: B. Vascular repair of the injury

Ref: Chapter No.17, Page No.423

272. Ans: C. Hematomas of the infrarenal vasculature or the right renal hilum are exposed with a right medial visceral mobilization, also known as the Mattox maneuver

Ref: Chapter No.17, Page No.423

273. Ans: B. Cattell-Braasch maneuver

Ref: Chapter No.17, Page No.423

274. Ans: A. Mattox maneuver

Ref: Chapter No.17, Page No.423

275. Ans: C. Kocher's maneuver

Extended Kocher's manoeuvre is a part of Cattel–Braasch manoeuvre and generally consists of full exposition of the inferior vena cava (IVC), renal veins, abdominal aorta, and superior mesenteric artery (SMA)

Ref: Chapter No.17, Page No.423

276. Ans: D. All of the above

Ref: Chapter No.17, Page No.423

277. Ans: D. All of the above

Ref: Chapter No.17, Page No.423-424

278. Ans: D. Penetrating mechanism: zone 1 nonexpanding hematoma: exploration

Ref: Chapter No.17, Page No.423

279. Ans: D. All of the above

Ref: Chapter No.17, Page No.424

280. Ans: C. Intraperitoneal bladder injury = operating room for primary repair

Ref: Chapter No.17, Page No.424

281. Ans: C. High-riding prostate on rectal examination

Ref: Chapter No.17, Page No.424

282. Ans: C. Exploratory laparotomy, urinary diversion, sigmoid colostomy, presacral drainage, and debridement of the rectal wall

Ref: Chapter No.17, Page No.422-424

283. Ans: D. All of the above

Ref: Chapter No.17, Page No.424

284. Ans: C. Exploratory laparotomy with evacuation of the uterus and closure of the uterus disruption

Ref: https://www.ncbi.nlm.nih.gov/pmc/articles/PMC7273360/

18

The Difficult Abdominal Wall

SUTURE MATERIAL

1. **As compared to absorbable sutures, use of nonabsorbable sutures for abdominal closure (e.g., polypropylene) has been associated with all except:**
   A. Decreased wound dehiscence
   B. Increased patient pain and sinus tract formation wound dehiscence
   C. No significant difference in the incidence surgical site infection (SSI)
   D. No significant difference in the incidence of incisional hernia formation

2. **The ideal suture material for abdominal wall closure is one that:**
   A. Minimizes tissue damage
   B. Nonabsorbable
   C. Provides adequate tensile strength to prevent abdominal wall disruption
   D. Resists infection

3. **Polydioxanone has an advantage over polyglactin like:**
   A. May resist infection to a greater degree than the braided suture
   B. Longer absorption time
   C. Longer strength retention profile
   D. Shorter absorption time

4. **False about barbed sutures is:**
   A. Barbed sutures are increasingly being used for fascial closure
   B. Barbed sutures have also been shown to have a less hernia recurrence rate in fascial plication for rectus diastasis
   C. This suture has tiny barbs in a helical arrangement that allow an even distribution of tension across the incision rather than just at the knots
   D. They are secured without knots, thus allowing for faster placement, and eliminate the knot as a nidus for infection

CLOSURE TECHNIQUE

5. **For the closure of the abdominal wall, ratio of suture to wound length has been advocated is:**
   A. 3:1 B. 4:1
   C. 6:1 D. 2:1

6. **Strategy of taking smaller bites, with smaller space between them is associated with a lower rate of incisional hernia. Current recommendation is:**
   A. 3 mm B. 5 mm
   C. 7 mm D. 10 mm

7. **False about abdominal closure is:**
   A. A continuous suture of slowly absorbable suture material is the recommended method of closure in elective abdominal surgery
   B. Retention sutures have been associated with increased pain, increased wound inflammation, wound complications and skin breakdown, and problems with ostomy appliance placement
   C. Layered closure is preferred
   D. Patients at high risk of acute fascial dehiscence may benefit from some method of evisceration prophylaxis, and some have promoted the use of synthetic mesh in high-risk abdominal wall closures

PROPHYLACTIC MESH

8. **False among the following is:**
   A. In multiple studies, there is a decrease in incisional hernia rates when a mesh is utilized, with no increase in surgical site occurrence (SSO) rates

B. Both the onlay and sublay positions have been utilized for this purpose
C. Postoperative seroma rates are increased in the population that undergoes mesh placement, particularly in the onlay position
D. Prophylactic mesh placement has not been shown to be cost effective

ABDOMINAL FASCIAL DEHISCENCE

9. The risk of fascial dehiscence may persist beyond 3 weeks postoperatively; the usual time frame is within the first _______ after primary closure.

A. 5 days B. 7 days
C. 10 days D. 14 days

10. Patient risk factors for abdominal wall suture complications includes all except:

A. Age >50
B. Diabetes mellitus
C. Obesity
D. Cigarette use/chronic obstructive pulmonary disease

11. Patient risk factors for abdominal wall suture complications includes:

A. Steroid use B. Ascites
C. Malnutrition D. All of the above

12. Surgical risk factors for abdominal wall suture complications includes all except:

A. Ruptured abdominal aortic aneurysm
B. Wound Class II
C. Pancreatitis
D. Peritonitis/sepsis

13. Surgical risk factors for abdominal wall suture complications includes all except:

A. Abdominal wall defect >5 cm width
B. Bowel occlusion surgery with resection or suture
C. Presence of enterocutaneous fistula
D. Synthetic mesh infection

TEMPORARY ABDOMINAL CLOSURE

14. Indications for temporary abdominal closure are all except:

A. Major abdominal and/or retroperitoneal tissue edema
B. Intraabdominal hypertension or compartment syndrome
C. Unplanned acute reoperation
D. Triage

15. Two opposing Velcro sheets with hooks and loops sutured to facial edges is:

A. Negative pressure wound therapy
B. Dynamic retention systems
C. Wittmann Patch
D. Vacuum-assisted closure

16. Artificial burr is also known as:

A. Vacuum-assisted closure
B. Wittmann Patch
C. Negative pressure wound therapy
D. Dynamic retention systems

17. ABTHERA VAC, false statement is:

A. Doesn't decrease bowel edema
B. Negative pressure wound therapy
C. Unique capsulated foam extension system incorporated into polyethylene sheet placed over abdominal viscera
D. Extension runs deep into paracolic gutters to allow more efficient suctioning of ascites fluid

18. Which of the following is a method of temporary abdominal closure?

A. Artificial burr
B. Vacuum pack
C. Dynamic retention sutures
D. All of the above

19. In Five-stage proposed algorithm for management of the open abdomen, fascial closure is done in which stage?

A. Stage 1 B. Stage 2
C. Stage 3 D. Stage 4

20. To minimize complications related to the open abdomen management, the goal of delayed primary fascial closure is to have the fascia closed as soon as possible, ideally within the first:

A. 7 days B. 8 days
C. 10 days D. 14 days

MANAGEMENT OF THE OPEN ABDOMEN AND ASSESSING READINESS FOR ABDOMINAL CLOSURE

21. The primary goal in the initial resuscitation of the patient with an open abdomen is correction of hypothermia, coagulopathy and acidosis; this can usually be accomplished within:

A. 12 to 24 hours B. 24 to 36 hours
C. 36 to 48 hours D. 48 to 72 hours

22. Timing of initial reexploration can usually be achieved within:

A. 12 to 24 hours B. 24 to 36 hours
C. 36 to 48 hours D. 24 to 72 hours

23. During attempts at fascial closure are warning signs of high fascial tension with the potential for compromise to the abdominal wall is rise of peak inspiratory pressure of:

A. 5 cm H_2O B. 5 cm mm Hg
C. 10 cm H_2O D. 10 cm mm Hg

24. Which of the following approaches can be used to address small and large bowel injuries in a definitive management phase of damage control surgery?

A. Resection of devitalized tissue
B. Primary repair
C. Externalization with creation of a stoma
D. All of the above

25. Planned ventral hernia delayed abdominal reconstruction is done at:

A. 3-4 months B. 6-12 months
C. 12-24 months D. 24-36 months

PHARMACOLOGIC ADJUNCTS TO CLOSURE

26. Which of the following mesh products should not be used in the open abdomen setting because they have very high rates of intestinal fistula formation and mesh infection?

A. Human dermal acellular dermis
B. PTFE
C. Porcine dermal matrix
D. All can be used

27. False about synthetic mesh is:

A. Infections should be eradicated before considering any major repair, and measures should be taken to heal open wounds, as the bacterial colonization may be significant even in the absence of a frank infection
B. The use of synthetic prosthetic mesh can provide a long-lasting repair with low recurrence rates
C. Lighter-weight, macroporous meshes carry a higher risk of infection compared to the heavier microporous meshes such as extended polytetrafluoroethylene (ePTFE)
D. Synthetic mesh may variably become infected dependent on the degree of contamination of the wound and the nature of the prosthetic material utilized

CHALLENGES IN THE CONTAMINATED FIELD

28. False about biological mesh among the following is:

A. The theoretical benefits of biologic mesh over synthetic mesh include more adhesion formation
B. The donor sites for biological mesh include dermis, intestinal mucosa and pericardium
C. A variety of biologic mesh material currently used includes sources from human, porcine, and bovine species with variable amounts of elastin and collagen and may or may not be cross-linked
D. All of the above are true

29. The Ventral Hernia Working Group and a recent systematic review and meta-analysis recommend consideration of biologic mesh in:

A. Grades 2 B. Grades 3
C. Grades 4 D. Both B and C

SEROMA AND SKIN NECROSIS

30. Suction drains should be stripped regularly during the early postoperative period and are typically removed when less than ____ in 24 hours.

A. 80 to 100 mL B. 50 to 80 mL
C. 25 to 30 mL D. 30 to 50 mL

31. Methods that have been described in the literature to decrease seroma formation include all except:

A. Surgical tissue adhesive application under skin flaps
B. Talc application
C. Quilting stiches
D. Faster operative times

32. False among the following is:

A. The perforators' density is highest around the periumbilical area, and thus it is important to spare a circular distance of about 3 cm around the umbilicus area during dissection
B. Full-thickness wounds require skin and subcutaneous sharp debridement
C. Full-thickness wounds can be treated locally with hydrating gels or enzymatic debriding agents
D. Aspiration or reoperative drainage may be required if the seroma enlarges or shows signs of infection

PREPARATION FOR ABDOMINAL WALL RECONSTRUCTION

33. Every effort should be made to control diabetes and obtain a hemoglobin A1C less than:

A. 6.5 B. 7.5
C. 8.0 D. 8.5

34. Mandatory cigarette smoking cessation is required for at least ____ before repair.

A. 1 to 2 weeks
B. 2 to 4 weeks
C. 4 to 6 weeks
D. 6 to 10 weeks

DEFINITIVE REPAIR—CREATING A DYNAMIC ABDOMINAL WALL

35. False among the following is:

A. The most important factor in preventing postoperative complications is placement of the mesh in the retrorectus space utilizing a onlay technique
B. Ramirez's technique has high wound morbidity and is, in general, not recommended for high-risk patients
C. There is now widespread belief that a tension-free, fascia-to-fascia closure utilizing component separation techniques combined with underlay reinforcement with mesh is the ideal method for abdominal wall reconstruction
D. The retrorectus repair and the sublay placement of mesh have resulted in the lowest complication rate as compared to the onlay or inlay techniques

RIVES-STOPPA-WANTZ AND TRANSVERSUS ABDOMINIS RELEASE TECHNIQUES

36. False among the following is:

A. The retrorectus plane is then developed to the lateral extent of the dissection: The linea semilunaris
B. If the dissection is insufficient to close the posterior rectus fascia, an extension of Rives Stoppa's technique includes the transversus abdominis release
C. The posterior rectus sheath is incised approximately one half of a centimeter from the fascial edge of the defect
D. Both procedures need a major subcutaneous dissection and leads to damage of neurovascular bundle

PERIOPERATIVE CONSIDERATIONS

37. Postoperative respiratory complications have been found to be significantly increased when the plateau pressure was raised above:

A. 2 mm Hg B. 4 mm Hg
C. 6 mm Hg D. 10 mm Hg

38. Intraoperative and postoperative monitoring of abdominal pressures indirectly using bladder pressure measurements is routinely recommended when the abdominal wall defect is:

A. >100 cm^2 B. >200 cm^2
C. >400 cm^2 D. >600 cm^2

39. It is not advisable to attempt delayed primary fascial closure if there is undue tension on the fascia or if the peak inspiratory pressure rises:

A. >15 cm H_2O B. >4 cm H_2O
C. >6 cm H_2O D. >10 cm H_2O

ANSWERS

1. **Ans: A. Decreased wound dehiscence**
Ref: Chapter No.18, Page No.429

2. **Ans: B. Nonabsorbable**
Ref: Chapter No.18, Page No.429

3. **Ans: D. Shorter absorption time**
Ref: Chapter No.18, Page No.429

4. **Ans: B. Barbed sutures have also been shown to have a less hernia recurrence rate in fascial plication for rectus diastasis**
Ref: Chapter No.18, Page No.429

5. **Ans: B. 4:1**
Ref: Chapter No.18, Page No.429

6. **Ans: B. 5 mm**
Ref: Chapter No.18, Page No.429

7. **Ans: C. Layered closure is preferred**
Ref: Chapter No.18, Page No.429

8. **Ans: D. Prophylactic mesh placement has not been shown to be cost effective**
Ref: Chapter No.18, Page No.430

9. **Ans: B. 7 days**
Ref: Chapter No.18, Page No.430

10. **Ans: A. Age >50**
Ref: Chapter No.18, Page No.430

11. **Ans: D. All of the above**
Ref: Chapter No.18, Page No.430

12. **Ans: B. Wound Class II**
Ref: Chapter No.18, Page No.430

13. **Ans: A. Abdominal wall defect >5 cm width**
Ref: Chapter No.18, Page No.430

14. **Ans: C. Unplanned acute reoperation**
Ref: Chapter No.18, Page No.431

15. **Ans: C. Wittmann Patch**
Ref: Chapter No.18, Page No.431

16. **Ans: B. Wittmann Patch**
Ref: Chapter No.18, Page No.431

17. **Ans: A. Doesn't decrease bowel edema**
Ref: Chapter No.18, Page No.431

18. **Ans: D. All of the above**
Ref: Chapter No.18, Page No.431

19. **Ans: C. Stage 3**
Ref: Chapter No.18, Page No.432

20. **Ans: B. 8 days**
Ref: Chapter No.18, Page No.432

21. **Ans: B. 24 to 36 hours**
Ref: Chapter No.18, Page No.432

22. **Ans: D. 24 to 72 hours**
Ref: Chapter No.18, Page No.432

23. **Ans: C. 10 cm H_2O**
Ref: Chapter No.18, Page No.432

24. **Ans: D. All of the above**
Ref: Chapter No.18, Page No.432

25. **Ans: B. 6-12 months**
Ref: Chapter No.18, Page No.432

26. **Ans: B. PTFE**
Ref: Chapter No.18, Page No.433

27. **Ans: C. Lighter-weight, macroporous meshes carry a higher risk of infection compared to the heavier microporous meshes such as extended polytetrafluoroethylene (ePTFE)**
Ref: Chapter No.18, Page No.433.

28. **Ans: A. The theoretical benefits of biologic mesh over synthetic mesh include more adhesion formation**
Ref: Chapter No.18, Page No.433-434

29. **Ans: D. Both B and C**
Ref: Chapter No.18, Page No.434

30. **Ans: C. 25 to 30 mL**
Ref: Chapter No.18, Page No.434

31. **Ans: D. Faster operative times**
Ref: Chapter No.18, Page No.435

32. **Ans: C. Full-thickness wounds can be treated locally with hydrating gels or enzymatic debriding agents**
Ref: Chapter No.18, Page No.435

33. **Ans: C. 8.0**
Ref: Chapter No.18, Page No.435

34. **Ans: C. 4 to 6 weeks**
Ref: Chapter No.18, Page No.435

35. **Ans: A. The most important factor in preventing postoperative complications is placement of the mesh in the retrorectus space utilizing a onlay technique**
Ref: Chapter No.18, Page No.435

36. **Ans: D. Both procedures need a major subcutaneous dissection and leads to damage of neurovascular bundle**
Ref: Chapter No.18, Page No.436

37. **Ans: C. 6 mm Hg**
Ref: Chapter No.18, Page No.436

38. **Ans: D. >600 cm^2**
Ref: Chapter No.18, Page No.436

39. **Ans: D. >10 cm H_2O**
Ref: Chapter No.18, Page No.437

19

Emergency Care of Musculoskeletal Injuries

TERMINOLOGY

1. **False among the following is:**
   A. Radiographically, acute fractures can be differentiated from older fractures by the identification of sharp, well-defined edges of the fragments
   B. Older fractures will have evidence of callus formation and a blunting of the fracture edges
   C. Subacute and chronic fractures, while frequently needing treatment and do require emergent care
   D. Chronic fractures can be radiographically dramatic because of bony hypertrophy and/ or adjacent structure destruction

2. **Axial loads of long bones in children can lead to buckling of the cortex without a visible fracture line, appropriately termed as:**
   A. Greenstick fractures
   B. Buckle fracture
   C. Physeal fracture
   D. Butterfly fracture

3. **When a bone fails through an area weakened by pre-existing disease, it is termed a:**
   A. Insufficiency fracture
   B. Comminuted fracture
   C. Pathologic fracture
   D. Spiral fracture

4. **In children, incomplete disruptions of the cortex are termed:**
   A. Greenstick fractures B. Buckle fracture
   C. Physeal fracture D. Butterfly fracture

5. **False among the following is:**
   A. Final grading of open fractures occurs in the operating room, after thorough debridement and evaluation of the soft tissue envelope
   B. Open fractures can range from small poke-holes to severe soft tissue degloving
   C. The Tscherne's classification is typically used to grade open fractures
   D. A fracture is considered open when an overlying wound produces communication between the fracture site and the outside environment

6. **Salter-Harris classification was described for fractures:**
   A. Diaphyseal B. Physeal
   C. Metaphyseal D. Epiphyseal

7. **False among the following is:**
   A. Articular fractures may be partially reduced in order to achieve the good possible long-term outcome
   B. A fracture that extends into a joint is termed intra-articular
   C. Intra-articular injuries are normally caused by an axial load across the joint
   D. Intra-condylar injuries are between the articular condyles

8. **False among the following is:**
   A. Butterfly # - Separate fragment at the fracture
   B. Spiral # - Torsional failure
   C. Transverse # - Parallel to the long axis of the bone
   D. Oblique # - Angular to the long axis of the bone

9. **According to Salter-Harris classification, the following image represents:**

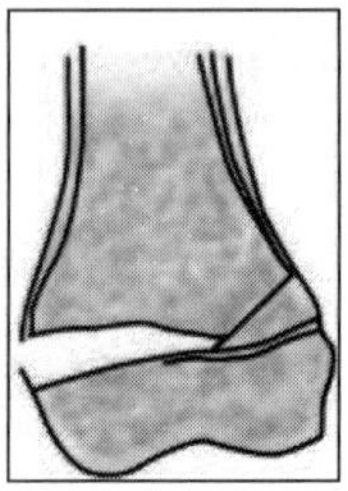

A. Type I
B. Type II
C. Type III
D. Type IV

10. According to Salter-Harris classification, the following image represents:

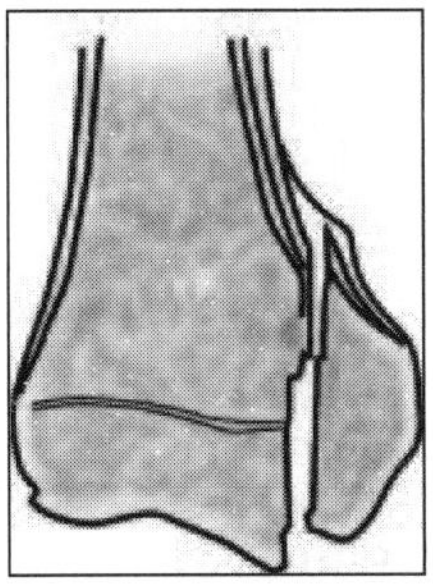

A. Type V
B. Type VI
C. Type III
D. Type IV

11. According to Salter-Harris classification, the following image represents:

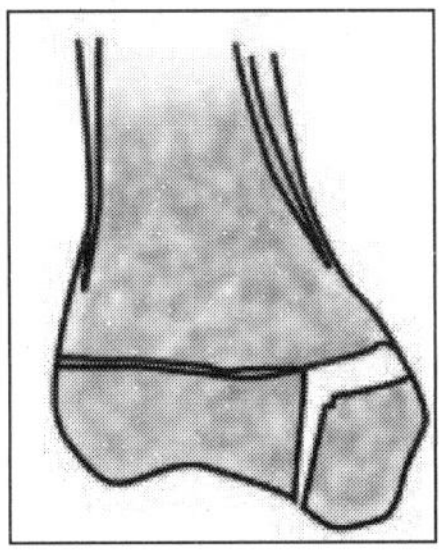

A. Type I
B. Type II
C. Type III
D. Type IV

12. Regarding ligamentous injury false among the following:

A. Grade I ligamentous injuries are caused by stretching of a ligament or ligament complex
B. When a ligament is damaged but is still in continuity, it is termed a sprain
C. Partial ruptures of ligaments can result in minor instability and are considered Grade II injuries
D. Complete ruptures aka Grade IV injuries, lead to significant instability at the associated joint

13. Regarding strain false among the following:

A. Rest, ice, compression, and elevation are the mainstays of treatment for a strain
B. A strain is an injury to a muscle or tendon
C. More urgent orthopaedic management is not necessary for a rupture
D. Strain injuries are most commonly of an overuse nature

14. Regarding joint injury false among the following:

A. Small osteochondral defects can be asymptomatic; however, many of these lesions can lead to chronic pain and joint degeneration
B. Articular contusions, or bone bruises, usually heal with a period of rest and restricted weight bearing but can lead to late degenerative changes in the joint
C. If the osteochondral fragment is large enough, it is important to immobilize the joint to minimize joint damage from the free-floating bone fragment
D. Disc herniations always needs surgical intervention

15. Type of fracture in the following image is:

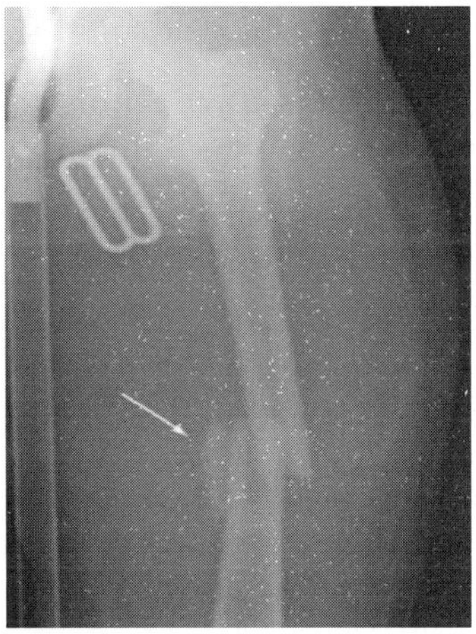

A. Butterfly #
B. Spiral #
C. Comminuted #
D. Oblique #

FIXATION PRINCIPLES

16. Regarding skeletal traction false among the following is:

A. Transosseous pin with traction weight
B. Permanent stabilization of femur and pelvis fractures
C. Helps control pain and bleeding, maintains length
D. Indirect control of the bone, does not allow for patient mobilization

17. Regarding external fixation false among the following is:

A. Risk of pin-site infection; indirect reduction of fracture
B. Can't be used for complex deformities
C. Multiple transosseous pins/wires with attached external rings
D. Definitive fixation with the ability to manipulate the bones

18. Regarding intramedullary nailing false among the following is:

A. Limited soft tissue disruption and poor mechanical stability

B. Uses intraosseous nail
C. Long bone fracture treatment
D. Indirect reduction of fracture & limited utility in articular injuries

19. Regarding splinting false among the following is:

A. Plaster or fiberglass is used
B. Indirect control of the bone, not length stable
C. Temporary stabilization of acute extremity injuries
D. Can't accommodate soft tissue swelling

20. Regarding closed reduction and percutaneous pins false among the following is:

A. Small bone fixation; pediatric fixation
B. Transosseous pins across a fracture site
C. Risk of pin-site infection; indirect reduction of fracture
D. Extensive soft tissue disruption; removed once fracture healed

21. Regarding open reduction and internal fixation false among the following is:

A. Plates and screws are used
B. Limited soft tissue disruption; mechanically more stable than nails
C. Direct reduction and absolute stability feasible
D. Used in articular fractures; upper extremity long bone fractures

22. False among the following is:

A. The primary goal of long bone fracture fixation is reestablishment of the mechanical axis
B. Intra-articular fractures almost always require direct visualization of the fracture for fixation
C. Any fracture that is not intraarticular does not necessarily require anatomic fixation
D. All of the above are true

23. Which is the easiest and most common form of limb stabilization?

A. External fixation
B. Splinting
C. Skeletal traction
D. Closed reduction and percutaneous pins

24. The only form of fixation that does not directly attach to the bone is:

A. External fixation
B. Splinting
C. Skeletal traction
D. Closed reduction and percutaneous pins

PATIENT EVALUATION

25. After fall on outstretched hand, all of the following #s can occur except:

A. Vertebral burst fracture
B. Distal radius fracture
C. Supracondylar humerus fracture
D. Posterior elbow dislocation

26. Examination and management of the extremities are deferred to the:

A. Primary survey
B. Secondary survey
C. Tertiary survey
D. Quaternary survey

27. Unstable pelvic fractures are addressed in the:

A. Primary survey
B. Secondary survey
C. Tertiary survey
D. Quaternary survey

28. Traumatic spine injuries with associated neurologic compromise are addressed in the:

A. Primary survey
B. Secondary survey
C. Tertiary survey
D. Quaternary survey

29. False among the following is:

A. Diagnostic peritoneal lavage has increased sensitivity in detecting intraperitoneal bleeding in patients with a pelvic fracture; however, false-positives in patients with pelvic fractures can occur
B. FAST scanning has been shown to have high sensitivity in detecting intraperitoneal bleeding in patients with a pelvic fracture
C. The current recommendation for hemodynamically stable patients with a pelvic fracture is to undergo CT of the abdomen and pelvis with intravenous (IV) administration of a contrast agent to evaluate for intraperitoneal bleeding, regardless of FAST results
D. All of the above are true

30. Morel-Lavallée lesion is:

A. An ecchymotic lesion over the gluteal region that represents a subcutaneous degloving injury
B. An ecchymotic lesion over the greater trochanter that represents a subcutaneous degloving injury
C. An ecchymotic lesion over the lesser trochanter that represents a subcutaneous degloving injury

D. An ecchymotic lesion over the thigh that represents a subcutaneous degloving injury

31. **Morel-Lavallée lesion is frequently associated with:**

A. Shaft of femur fractures
B. Neck of femur fractures
C. Acetabular fractures
D. Disruption of pubic symphysis

32. **It has been shown that the standard plain films fail to identify _______of clinically relevant fractures identified by multislice CT.**

A. 55.5% B. 45.5%
C. 35.5% D. 65.5%

33. **False among the following is:**

A. CT of the thoracic, lumbar, and sacral spine is faster and more accurate than radiography at identifying traumatic injury
B. Plain radiographs of the cervical spine, including AP, lateral, and open-mouth odontoid views, were previously considered part of the standard trauma series of radiographs
C. It has been shown that the standard plain films fail to identify 55.5% of clinically relevant fractures identified by multislice CT and add no clinically relevant data
D. Plain films are still indicated

34. **Regarding the examination of the extremities, false among the following is:**

A. Deformity, edema, ecchymosis, crepitus, tenderness, and pain with motion are the cardinal signs of an acute fracture
B. When an isolated extremity injury is the primary reason for evaluation, the entire skeleton need not be examined
C. Doppler signals are obtained when palpable pulses are not present or are weak
D. Measuring the ankle-brachial index (ABI) is important when vascular injury is suspected

35. **False about diagnostic imaging is:**

A. CT scan should be ordered when finer detail is necessary - such as in the assessment of an intraarticular injury or to confirm the findings of an equivocal radiograph
B. Cervical spine radiographs should be deferred for a CT scan of the cervical spine (if available)
C. MRI is now commonly used for the diagnosis of acute fractures even when plain films are positive
D. In filming long bone injuries, it is important to verify the integrity of adjacent limb segments because of the relatively high incidence of concurrent articular injuries

36. **Modified axillary view that provides orthogonally equivalent images is called as:**

A. Bloom Obata view B. Judet view
C. Velpeau view D. Both A and C

37. **Velpeau view: while wearing a sling, the patient leans:**

A. Forward 60 degrees over the cassette on the table
B. Backward 60 degrees over the cassette on the table
C. Backward 30 degrees over the cassette on the table
D. Forward 30 degrees over the cassette on the table

38. **False about imaging of the elbow is:**

A. The presence of an anterior fat pad sign is strongly suggestive of occult fracture
B. Internal and external oblique views are included in a complete elbow series
C. CT scan is sometimes ordered if there is a question of intraarticular extension
D. The sail sign can be noted when hemarthrosis from an intraarticular fracture forces the anterior and posterior fat pads out of the coronoid and olecranon fossae, respectively

39. **Positive fat pad or sail sign is seen in:**

A. Hip radiograph
B. Elbow radiograph
C. Pelvis radiograph
D. Shoulder radiograph

40. **False about diagnostic imaging about forearm and wrist is:**

A. The wrist should be imaged in the AP, oblique and lateral views
B. The forearm should be imaged in 2 cassettes in both the AP and lateral planes
C. Injuries at the wrist can sometimes affect the elbow joint
D. Any wrist fracture that undergoes a closed reduction should have postreduction imaging as well

41. **Judet views are used to evaluate:**

A. Acetabulum B. Pelvis
C. Neck of femur D. Shaft of femur

42. **Judet views, aka:**
A. 30-degree oblique views of the pelvis
B. 45-degree oblique views of the pelvis
C. 60-degree oblique views of the pelvis
D. 75-degree oblique views of the pelvis

43. **Inlet views of the pelvis is taken with the beam:**
A. Angled 30-degree cephalad
B. Angled 60-degree cephalad
C. Angled 30-degree caudad
D. Angled 60-degree caudad

44. **Outlet views of the pelvis is a:**
A. 30-degree lateral view
B. 30-degree oblique view
C. 60-degree lateral view
D. 60-degree oblique view

45. **Imaging modality of choice for suspected osteomyelitis or pelvic abscess:**
A. CT scan B. MRI
C. X-ray D. PET scan

46. **False about hip imaging is:**
A. In an adult patient with acute groin pain and inability to bear weight, an occult hip fracture should be ruled out with an MRI
B. A hip series consists of AP and cross-table lateral radiographs
C. In patients with femoral shaft fractures, the incidence of ipsilateral femoral neck fracture is as high as 9%
D. All of the above true

47. **False about knee imaging is:**
A. CT angiography or MR angiography should be strongly considered in the setting of an acute knee dislocation
B. If there is any doubt as to the degree of articular involvement, displacement, or depression, a CT scan should be ordered
C. AP, lateral and internal or external oblique plain films allow visualization of most traumatic osseous abnormalities of the knee
D. CT Scan is helpful in the acute setting, evaluation of ligamentous derangement

48. **False about ankle imaging is:**
A. A positive stress X-ray is demonstrative of an unstable ankle joint that requires operative fixation
B. With AP, mortise, and lateral radiographs, disruptions in the bone anatomy can be visualized directly
C. Pilon fractures almost always must be placed in an external-fix for 7–14 days to allow for soft tissue recovery prior to definitive treatment
D. In a positive stress exam, either or both the medial clear space and the tibia-fibula clear space will be narrowed

49. **An angle formed by the bisection of a line drawn from the superior aspect of the calcaneal tuberosity to the superior aspect of the posterior facet and a line drawn from the tip of the anterior process to the superior aspect of the posterior facet, evaluated in the lateral view:**
A. Harris angle B. Bohler angle
C. Canale angle D. Broden angle

50. **A normal Bohler angle is between:**
A. 10 and 20 degrees B. 20 and 40 degrees
C. 40 and 50 degrees D. 40 and 60 degrees

51. **Which view should be added to evaluate the varus-valgus alignment of the tuberosity as well as any sagittal splits in the bone?**
A. Harris axial view B. Bohler axial view
C. Canale axial view D. Broden axial view

52. **Specialized view of the bone like canale view is for the evaluation of:**
A. Tibiotalar joint B. Talar neck
C. Talonavicular joint D. Subtalar joint

53. **Specialized view of the bone like broaden view is for evaluation of:**
A. Tibiotalar joint B. Talar neck
C. Talonavicular joint D. Subtalar joint

54. **False about spine imaging is:**
A. CT is useful for defining bone anatomy
B. If ligamentous injury or neurologic compromise is suspected, CT scan should be performed
C. CT myelography can be used to look for compromise of the spinal canal or intervertebral foramina
D. If MRI is contraindicated, a bone scan can be considered if occult fracture is suspected

55. **Vascular injury after traumatic knee dislocation has a reported rate of:**
A. 10% B. 15%
C. 40% D. 30%

56. **A volar or ulnar gutter splint is used for:**
A. Wrist or forearm fractures
B. Fractures of the hand

C. Fractures about the elbow
D. Foot and ankle

57. **A sugar tong splint is used for:**
A. Fractures about the elbow
B. Foot and ankle
C. Wrist or forearm fractures
D. Fractures of the hand

58. **Posterior long arm splint is used for:**
A. Fractures about the elbow
B. Foot and ankle
C. Fractures of the hand
D. Wrist or forearm fractures

59. **Posterior slab and a U or stirrup component together is used for disease of the:**
A. Fractures of the hand
B. Wrist or forearm fractures
C. Foot and ankle
D. Fractures about the elbow

60. **False among the following is:**
A. Open splint maintains a reduction more effectively than an bi-valved cast which still allows soft tissue swelling
B. Because swelling of the injured extremity increases for 48 to 72 hours, a circular cast can be too constrictive and may lead to pressure necrosis or compartment syndrome
C. The role of circumferential casting in the acute setting is questionable
D. All of the above are true

61. **Traction may be applied through the skin using a Buck traction boot; any extended period causes skin damage when the traction is more than:**
A. 4 pounds B. 8 pounds
C. 14 pounds D. 18 pounds

62. **False about skeletal traction is:**
A. Neurovascular structures must be avoided during placement of the pins
B. Pins should be placed from the posterior side of the extremity
C. Skeletal traction may be maintained for longer periods with more weight than that possible with skin traction
D. It is applied using Steinmann pins or Kirschner wires

63. **In the distal femur, the pin should be passed from:**
A. Medial to lateral
B. Lateral to medial
C. Anterior to posterior
D. Any of the above

64. **In the proximal tibia, the pin should be passed from:**
A. Medial to lateral B. Lateral to medial
C. Anterior to posterior D. Any of the above

65. **In the calcaneus, the pin should be passed:**
A. Medial to lateral B. Lateral to medial
C. Anterior to posterior D. Any of the above

66. **False among the following about skeletal traction is:**
A. While pin track infections are a rare complication, they can lead to osteomyelitis or septic arthritis in the worst cases
B. In the distal femur, the pin should be passed from lateral to medial
C. The ideal pin placement is parallel to the joint, approximately 2 cm distal and 2 cm posterior to the top of the tibial tubercle
D. Pin site care should be performed twice daily with a half-strength hydrogen peroxide solution and sterile dressings

67. **Limb-threatening vascular injuries are managed on an emergency basis as we want to limit the warm ischemia time to:**
A. 8 hours B. 4 hours
C. 6 hours D. 12 hours

68. **Regarding prioritization of surgical care of extremity injuries, false statement is:**
A. Decisions about limb viability, compartment syndrome, and the need for amputation of a mangled extremity are made in concert with all services involved
B. Limb-threatening vascular injuries are managed on an emergency basis because limiting the warm ischemia time to 6 hours is essential for optimal recovery
C. Consideration must also be given to unreduced joint dislocations and time-sensitive fractures, such as fractures of the spine, pelvic ring, acetabulum, or proximal and diaphyseal femur
D. All of the above are true

TIME-DEPENDENT ORTHOPEDIC INJURIES

69. **Gustilo-Anderson classification is used for:**
A. Open fractures B. Closed fractures
C. Vascular injuries D. All of the above

70. **For Grade III fractures, infection rate is:**
A. 0% to 2% B. 2% to 10%
C. 10% to 50% D. 50% to 90%

71. **For Grade II fractures, infection rate is:**
A. 0% to 2% B. 2% to 10%
C. 10% to 20% D. 20% to 50%

72. **Open fracture with a vascular injury is seen in:**
A. Type II B. Type IIIA
C. Type IIIB D. Type IIIC

73. **Gunshot injuries are seen in:**
A. Type II B. Type IIIA
C. Type IIIB D. Type IIIC

74. **Simple transverse or short oblique fracture with minimal comminution is seen in:**
A. Type I B. Type II
C. Type IIIA D. Type IIIB

75. **Segmental fractures are seen in:**
A. Type I B. Type II
C. Type IIIA D. Type IIIB

76. **Extensive soft tissue damage with periosteal stripping and bone exposure necessitating formal soft tissue coverage is:**
A. Type II B. Type IIIA
C. Type IIIB D. Type IIIC

77. **The general expectation is that antibiotics should be administered within _____ of a patient arriving to the ED.**
A. 15 minutes B. 60 minutes
C. 30 minutes D. 90 minutes

78. **After closure in Grade I fractures, antibiotics should be delivered for:**
A. 12 hours B. 24 hours
C. 48 hours D. 72 hours

79. **False about the management of open fractures is:**
A. All grades of open fracture should receive gram-positive coverage, usually in the form of Cefazolin
B. For patients with Grades II and III open fractures, it is standard practice to add an aminoglycoside for gram-negative coverage
C. A recent prospective study showed piperacillin-tazobactam to be as ineffective as compared to aminoglycosides in preventing deep infection
D. Antibiotics should be delivered for 24 hours after closure in Grade I and 48 to 72 hours for Grade III fractures

80. **Muscle viability is assessed by the "4 C's" of:**
A. Contractility B. Colour
C. Comparability D. Capacity to bleed

81. **True among the following is:**
A. Expert consensus is to use 3 L of normal saline for Grade I fractures, 6 L for Grade II fractures, and 9 L for Grade III fractures
B. It is thought that high-pressure irrigation may push contamination deeper into the wound bed
C. Irrigation is typically performed using gravity and regular surgical tubing
D. All of the above are true

82. **Planning for wound coverage begins with the initial debridement, if skin grafting or muscle flap coverage is necessary, it should be performed within the first:**
A. 24 hours B. 48 hours
C. 72 hours D. 12 hours

83. **Treatment goals of the open fractures is/are:**
A. Antibiotic therapy initiated within 1 hour of arrival
B. Operative debridement within 6–24 hours
C. When necessary, soft tissue coverage within 7 days of injury
D. All of the above

84. **Prophylactic antibiotic recommended after marine contamination is:**
A. Vancomycin B. Levaquin
C. Penicillin D. Flagy

85. **Prophylactic antibiotic recommended after gunshot injury with fracture is:**
A. Vancomycin B. Levaquin
C. Penicillin D. Flagy

86. **False among the following is:**
A. High-grade (III) tibia fractures - ex-fix followed by unreamed nail or Ilizarov
B. Calcaneus fractures - often treated with debridement alone
C. Pelvic ring - almost always treated with internal fixation in the front
D. Upper extremities - often treated definitively at initial debridement

87. Transcolonic injuries will require ____ days of vancomycin/cefepime/flagyl.

A. 2 days
B. 5 days
C. 7 days
D. 14 days

88. False among the following is:

A. Limb salvage was related to vascular status, age of the patient, duration of ischemia, and absorbed energy
B. The Mangled Extremity Severity Score (MESS) is the most widely validated classification systems
C. LEAP study and METALS study are studies done for patients with severe lower extremity injuries
D. All of the above are true

89. In fractures secondary to firearm injury, high-energy injury is:

A. >3000 ft/s projectile velocity
B. >2000 ft/s projectile velocity
C. >1000 ft/s projectile velocity
D. >500 ft/s projectile velocity

90. False about injuries secondary to firearm injury is:

A. Bullets traversing the intraabdominal cavity are associated with fractures of the hip, pelvis, and spine
B. Bullets or fragments that remain lodged in a joint can lead to plumbism or systemic lead toxicity
C. For periarticular gunshots, a CT scan can be a useful adjunct to determine if any fragments remain in the joint
D. Retained fragments with an incomplete or evolving spinal cord injury or evolving neurologic exam should be left alone

91. False about injuries secondary to firearm injury is:

A. Gunshot wounds at the metaphysis may have nondisplaced intraarticular extension and thus may warrant further imaging with CT
B. Fractures caused by high-velocity weapons are treated per an open fracture protocol
C. Bullets that traverse the joint without retention of the bullet are also associated with increased infection rates
D. Temporary stabilization with external fixation is employed to allow soft tissue management until definitive fixation can occur

92. True about skeletal stabilisation is/are:

A. IM nailing is the fixation of choice for open tibial fractures
B. External fixation minimizes dissection and avoids the insertion of large metallic implants
C. IM canal before insertion of the nail allows placement of a larger diameter nail and forces bone marrow in between the fractured bone ends, which facilitates healing
D. All of the above are true

93. False about IM nailing is:

A. The increased infection rate was believed to be caused by destruction of cortical blood flow by reaming
B. Reaming the IM canal before insertion of the nail allows placement of a larger diameter nail and forces bone marrow in between the fractured bone ends, which facilitates healing
C. Studies have shown a higher risk of reoperation when reamed IM nails are used
D. Definitive fracture care usually can be accomplished in a multiple operations

ACUTE COMPARTMENT SYNDROME

94. The most common cause of increased volume in compartment syndrome is:

A. Bleeding
B. Hypertrophy
C. Edema secondary to muscle injury
D. Both A and B

95. False about acute compartment syndrome is:

A. The most important attribute of treating this very morbid condition is maintaining vigilance
B. Missed or delayed diagnosis of compartment syndrome is one of the most common causes of malpractice litigation for orthopedic surgeons
C. Volkmann was the first to describe the sequelae of postischemic contracture more than a century ago
D. All of the above are true

96. The most common method of measurement of compartmental pressure is:

A. Fiber optic devices
B. Stryker Intra-Compartmental Pressure Monitor System
C. Wick catheter
D. Slit catheter

97. If a fracture is present, measure of compartmental pressure should occur within ____of the fracture.

A. 15 cm B. 10 cm
C. 5 cm D. 8 cm

98. Fasciotomies are performed for a persistent ΔP is:

A. Less than 20 mm Hg
B. Less than 30 mm Hg
C. Less than 25 mm Hg
D. Less than 10 mm Hg

99. False statement about surgical treatment of acute compartment syndrome is:

A. The two-incision approach to fasciotomy of the lower part of the leg is a reliable
B. The anterolateral incision in lower limb fasciotomy is centered halfway between the fibular shaft and tibia
C. The posteromedial incision is made approximately 2 cm posterior to the tibial shaft
D. Secondary closure may be attempted when limb swelling has been reduced (7–14 days)

100. Nerve to be protected during the release of the medial compartment is:

A. The sural nerve
B. The popliteal nerve
C. The saphenous nerve
D. The femoral nerve

PELVIC RING DISRUPTION

101. False about pelvic ring disruption is:

A. Higher ISS scores, shock on arrival, greater transfusion requirements, and patient age are risk factors to mortality in patients with pelvic ring fractures
B. Pelvic ring disruption is a major cause of morbidity and mortality in multiply injured patients with a high rate of associated injuries
C. In combination with a head or abdominal injury that requires surgical intervention or if the pelvis fracture is open, mortality increases to 90%
D. Mortality rates vary from 15% to 25%, resulting from uncontrolled hemorrhage or other associated injuries

102. In a pelvic ring disruption, when the patient is hypotensive mortality increases almost:

A. 5 times B. 8 times
C. 13 times D. 15 times

103. In a pelvic ring disruption, long-term disability includes all except:

A. Impotence B. Pelvic pain
C. Dyspareunia D. Haematuria

104. False among the following is:

A. Stability depends on the integrity of the only the osseous structures
B. Instability can be divided into rotational and vertical components
C. A stable pelvis is defined as one that can withstand normal physiologic forces without being displaced
D. Early recognition of an unstable pelvic ring is essential because pelvic instability is associated with potentially fatal hemorrhage

105. Stable injuries have been defined by less than _______of translation of the anterior structures.

A. 1 cm B. 1.5 cm
C. 2.5 cm D. 3.5 cm

106. Instability in the vertical plane is translation of more than ____through either a sacral fracture or the sacroiliac joint.

A. 1 cm B. 1.5 cm
C. 2.5 cm D. 3.5 cm

107. False among the following is:

A. Vertical instability may be appreciated with push-pull radiographs
B. An anterior defect can sometimes be detected by palpation at the symphysis pubis
C. Anterior injuries are easily identified on this projection and are the most unstable
D. In the vast majority of cases, the physical examination and AP pelvic radiograph are sufficient to assess stability and to guide initial treatment

108. According to the Young and Burgess classification, Type A results from:

A. Vertical shear forces
B. Lateral compression force
C. AP compression force
D. None

109. According to the Young and Burgess classification, Type C results from:

A. Vertical shear forces
B. Lateral compression force
C. AP compression force
D. None

110. According to the Young and Burgess classification, Type B results from:

A. Vertical shear forces
B. Lateral compression force
C. AP compression force
D. None

111. Open-book pelvis is:

A. Type B III
B. Type A III
C. Type C
D. Type B II

112. False among the following is:

A. Type A I, a posteriorly directed force causing a sacral crushing injury and horizontal pubic ramus fractures ipsilaterally
B. Type A III, an anteriorly directed force that is continued and leads to a type I or type II ipsilateral fracture with an external rotation component to the contralateral side; the sacroiliac joint is opened posteriorly, and the sacrotuberous and spinous ligaments are disrupted
C. Type B II, continuation of a type I fracture with disruption of the sacrospinous and potentially the sacrotuberous ligaments and an anterior sacroiliac joint opening. This fracture is rotationally unstable
D. Intrapelvic visceral injuries are also more common with the Lateral Compression patterns

113. Mortality in APC injuries is related to:

A. Intra-abdominal and head injuries
B. Combination of retroperitoneal bleeding and visceral injuries
C. Closed head trauma
D. Pulmonary embolism

114. LC and vertical shear fractures are associated with:

A. Combination of retroperitoneal bleeding and visceral injuries
B. Closed head trauma
C. Intra-abdominal and head injuries
D. Pulmonary embolism

115. The most common cause of death in a patient with this lateral compression pattern is associated:

A. Combination of retroperitoneal bleeding and visceral injuries
B. Closed head trauma
C. Intra-abdominal and head injuries
D. Pulmonary embolism

116. Most bleeding resulting from pelvic fracture comes from the:

A. Femoral veins
B. Presacral venous plexus
C. Internal iliac veins
D. Inferior epigastric vessels

117. False among the following is:

A. In patients who remain hemodynamically unstable after initial resuscitation and stabilization, a source of arterial bleeding must be considered
B. In most pelvic fractures, hemorrhage results from disruption of the pelvic venous plexus posteriorly and bleeding cancellous bone
C. CT angiography is another useful tool to evaluate patients who may benefit from angiographic or open control of pelvic bleeding
D. Factors predicting arterial bleeding included a base deficit of 2 mmol/L, a systolic blood pressure less than 90 mm Hg, and the need for transfusion in the ED

118. The negative predictive value of CT angiography in pelvic injuries is much higher, typically greater than:

A. 60%
B. 70%
C. 80%
D. 90%

119. False about initial stabilisation after pelvic ring fracture is:

A. When field personnel detect unstable pelvic ring disruptions on physical examination, they can begin treatment by binding the pelvis with a rolled sheet, pelvic binder, or applying pneumatic antishock garments (PASGs)
B. If they are applied in the field, PASGs should be deflated as soon as the patient is in the tertiary care center
C. A PASG has the advantage of ease of use, application in the field and reusability
D. PASG blocks access to the patient and restricts excursion of the diaphragm, and there have been reports of gluteal and thigh compartment syndromes developing after extended use of PASGs in hypotensive patients

120. False about pelvic binders after pelvic ring fracture is:

A. Binders or sheets are properly applied by centering them over the umbilicus and applying pressure
B. In LC-type pelvic injuries, the binder may

theoretically over-reduce the fracture and injure intrapelvic structures

C. Patients who do not respond to binder or sheet placement may necessitate other interventions including pelvic artery embolization (PAE) or pelvic packing

D. Internally rotating both legs and holding this position with tape across the ankles or knees also assist in pelvic reduction

121. False about pelvic artery embolization after pelvic ring fracture is:

A. Pelvic artery embolization (PAE) can be performed in either the external iliac artery (nonselective) or distal to the external iliac artery (selective)

B. Complications of PAE include muscle necrosis, surgical wound breakdown, infection, and impotence

C. Complication rates are particularly high when associated with bilateral or nonselective PAE

D. All of the above are true

122. False about pelvic packing after pelvic ring fracture is:

A. If the patient has a pelvic hematoma and remains unstable after abdominal exploration and intervention, pelvic packing may be considered

B. Six to nine laps are placed, starting posteriorly at the sacrum and moving anteriorly to the pub

C. Pelvic packing can be considered in the patient who does not respond to resuscitation efforts in the ED/ICU

D. Packing should be removed after resuscitation in 72 hours

123. False about definitive management of pelvic ring disruption is:

A. Complex anterior fracture patterns or patient anatomy may preclude fixation of the anterior pelvis with plates and or screws

B. The exact timing of definitive fixation of the pelvis is in debate with institutional variations, but it should generally be performed within the first month

C. The sacroiliac joint or sacral fractures can be secured with plates, bars, or percutaneously inserted cannulated screws

D. Stable fracture patterns usually require no more than protected weight bearing

SPINAL INJURIES

124. False about the evaluation of spinal injuries is:

A. If midline neck pain or tenderness is present, MRI evaluation is indicated

B. Level 1 evidence suggests that the awake, sober, neurologically intact patient without distracting injury should have the collar removed as soon as possible if certain criteria are met

C. MRI may be used to identify injury to the posterior ligamentous structures

D. All trauma patients are typically placed in a cervical collar in the prehospital or ED phase of care

125. Spinal shock resolves, usually within:

A. 12 hours
B. 24 hours
C. 48 hours
D. 72 hours

126. Which reflex is tested for diagnosis of spinal shock?

A. Hoffmann's reflex

B. Bulbocavernosus reflex

C. Knee reflex

D. Babinski's reflex

127. False about Denis's model of the spine is:

A. The spinal cord is divided into three columns

B. The posterior column includes all bone and ligamentous structures posterior to the posterior longitudinal ligament

C. The anterior column consists of the anterior two-thirds of the vertebral body and anterior longitudinal ligament

D. The middle column includes the posterior two-third of the vertebral body and posterior longitudinal ligament

128. By definition, compression fractures of spine are:

A. Injuries involving the posterior and middle columns

B. Injuries involving the anterior and middle columns

C. Injuries involving the anterior and posterior columns

D. Injuries involving the anterior, posterior and middle columns

129. Compression fractures involve the:

A. Anterior column

B. Middle column

C. Posterior column

D. Anterior and middle columns

130. According to ASIA classification, maximum motor score is:

A. 25 B. 50
C. 100 D. 200

131. According to ASIA classification, maximum pin prick score is:

A. 28 B. 56
C. 112 D. 224

132. Whether complete vs incomplete spinal cord injury, which segments are assessed?

A. Complete = any sensory or motor function in S4-S5
B. Incomplete = any sensory or motor function in S4-S5
C. Complete = any sensory or motor function in S1-S2
D. Incomplete = any sensory or motor function in S1-S2

133. Sensory supply of posterior aspect of thigh is by:

A. S1 B. S2
C. S3 D. S4-5

134. Motor supply of elbow extensors is by:

A. C5 B. C6
C. C7 D. C8

135. Sensory supply of umbilical area is:

A. T8 B. T10
C. T12 D. T9

136. Sensory supply of lateral aspect of foot:

A. L5 B. S1
C. S2 D. S3

137. Motor supply of finger abductors is by:

A. C6 B. C7
C. C8 D. T1

138. Motor supply of ankle dorsiflexors is by:

A. L3 B. L4
C. L5 D. S1

139. Motor supply of knee extensors is by:

A. L3 B. L4
C. L5 D. S1

140. Thoracolumbar Injury Classification and Severity score, max score is:

A. 8 B. 9
C. 10 D. 12

141. False about treatment of spine injury is:

A. Treatment of all injuries begins with strict immobilization and spine precautions
B. Compression fractures are typically managed nonoperatively if there is not a significant (>50%) loss of height
C. Depending on the fracture pattern, treatment of spine injuries may range from observation with bracing to surgical fixation or external halo fixation
D. Bracing or kyphoplasty may be offered if pain limits a patient's recovery

142. Indications for surgical decompression and stabilization of a lumbar burst fracture include all except:

A. Retropulsion of more than 50% of the spinal canal
B. 30 degrees of focal kyphosis
C. 25% body height loss
D. All of the above are true

143. False about cauda equina syndrome is:

A. The classic symptoms of cauda equina syndrome include varying degrees of back pain, bladder dysfunction saddle anesthesia, lower extremity numbness, and weakness and reduced rectal tone
B. When a diagnosis of cauda equina syndrome is confirmed, surgical exploration and decompression should be performed in a few days
C. If MRI is not available or the patient cannot undergo MRI, CT myelography can be performed
D. If cauda equina syndrome is suspected, MRI should be ordered immediately to look for canal compromise

DISLOCATIONS

144. False about dislocation is:

A. All dislocated joints should be reduced as soon as an experienced provider and adequate analgesia or sedation is available
B. A neurovascular exam should be performed with careful attention to structures known to be at risk with certain dislocations
C. The shoulder usually dislocates with the humerus posterior to the glenoid
D. A dislocated joint is considered an orthopedic emergency

145. The femoral head dislocates, relative to the acetabulum:

A. Posteriorly
B. Anteriorly
C. Laterally
D. Medially

146. In knee joint dislocation, false is:

A. Risk of popliteal artery injury
B. Risk of sciatic nerve injury
C. Multiligamentous knee injury
D. Risk of common peroneal nerve injury

147. In shoulder joint injury, false is:

A. In patients >40 years old, risk of rotator cuff tear
B. In patients <40 years old, risk of labral tear
C. Axillary nerve injury
D. Brachial artery injury

148. False among the following is:

A. Knee dislocations should be evaluated for popliteal artery injury
B. Avascular necrosis and the subsequent femoral head collapse are devastating sequela that lead to significant dysfunction and, in many cases, total hip arthroplasty
C. Up to 50% of knee dislocations will reduce spontaneously, but if the knee presents dislocated, it should be reduced promptly
D. Delay in the reduction of a dislocated hip can lead to femoral nerve injury, cartilage cell death and avascular necrosis

149. False about vascular workup after dislocation is:

A. A common protocol uses sequentially timed vascular exams at presentation, 4 to 6 hours later and then 12 hours later
B. Current evidence supports the use of selective arteriography, reserved for patients with abnormal exams
C. The exam includes symmetry of distal pulses, gross evaluation of colour and temperature, and the ABI
D. When the vascular exam is normal, CT angiography has been shown to be an effective and efficient next step in diagnosing the injury

150. False about treatment of dislocation is:

A. Knee dislocation usually occur with the tibia posterior to the femur
B. A neurovascular exam should be performed before reduction to provide a baseline for comparison after reduction
C. Skin furrowing at the anteromedial aspect of the femur, also known as the "dimple sign," suggests femoral condyle protrusion through the soft tissue
D. IV sedation is very helpful in reducing muscle tone that can resist reduction and is always necessary

VASCULAR INJURIES

151. Blunt trauma generally causes:

A. Complete transection with hemorrhage or occlusion
B. Arteriovenous fistulas
C. Intimal injury
D. Spasm

152. With vascular injury normal pulses are present in:

A. 1% to 5%
B. 5% to 15%
C. 15% to 25%
D. 25% to 40%

153. For lower extremity trauma, an ABI of _____ warrants further workup for vascular injury.

A. Less than 0.7
B. Less than 0.9
C. Less than 1.0
D. Less than 0.5

154. False about management of vascular injuries is:

A. The vascular procedure should be performed first if there is cold ischemia
B. It is recommended that the orthopedic procedure be always performed first
C. Prophylactic fasciotomies should be considered in all patients who have restored blood flow after a vascular procedure
D. All major vein injuries are repaired to increase the patency rate of the arterial repair and to prevent the sequelae of chronic venous congestion

COMMON LONG BONE FRACTURES

155. False about femur fractures is:

A. With the exception of pathologic or insufficiency fractures in older patients, these fractures are the result of a high-energy injury
B. Not all femur fractures need to be immobilized before the patient is transported from the scene of the accident
C. The treating team should have a high suspicion of concomitant femoral neck fractures for all patients with femoral shaft fractures
D. In closed femoral shaft fracture is considered a major injury in calculating the ISS

156. Regarding definitive management of femur fracture all are true except:

A. The evidence has consistently held the standard of care for a stable femoral shaft patient to be ETC within 48 hours

B. DCO primarily consists of the placement of an external fixator on the femur to hold the fracture fragments in good alignment and out to length

C. If DCO is performed, it is best to wait for longer than 5 days before performing definitive fixation to avoid any second hit

D. The goals of DCO include provisional fracture fixation that allows mobilization of the patient, hemorrhage control, soft tissue management, and the important avoidance of a major surgery

157. False about tibial shaft fractures is:

A. Tibial shaft fractures tend to be slow healing as a result of their tenuous blood supply and limited soft tissue envelope

B. The incidence of compartment syndrome in tibial shaft fractures is as high as 50%

C. Common mechanisms are bumper injuries, gunshot wounds, and bending or torsional injuries with a firmly planted foot

D. There is some contribution from the penetrating branches of the periosteal arteries that supply the outer third of the cortex, a diaphyseal fracture can easily compromise the nutrient arterial blood supply

158. Regarding the management of tibial shaft fractures all are true except:

A. Reamed IM nailing is the technique of choice, when appropriate

B. Plate fixation has fallen treatment of choice for diaphyseal fractures

C. Closed fracture with minimal displacement can be treated by cast immobilization and functional bracing

D. External fixation is an option for a patient who is unstable or when soft tissue injury precludes definitive fixation

159. False about Humerus Shaft Fractures is:

A. Operative management is the mainstay of treatment for fractures that maintain acceptable alignment

B. Functional (Sarmiento) brace is used for conservative management

C. Radial nerve injuries occur in up to 6% to 18% of these fractures, especially mid-shaft fractures with significant displacement

D. In the trauma setting, right-sided humeral shaft fractures can be predictive of concomitant injury to the liver and other intraabdominal organs

160. Regarding the management of humeral shaft fractures all are true except:

A. The most common treatment is an initial coaptation splint followed by transition to functional brace at clinic follow-up

B. The mainstay of surgical management is compression plating with four bicortical screws on each side of the fracture

C. If a coaptation splint is placed and the patient develops a radial nerve palsy afterward, then the splint should be promptly reduced

D. During the functional brace stage, patients are allowed free elbow flexion-extension and arm abduction to 30 degrees

161. When a radial nerve injury is encountered, it is likely a neuropraxia and will recover spontaneously within:

A. 1 to 2 months
B. 3 to 4 months
C. 5 to 6 months
D. 6 to 10 months

162. A 35 years old male has at RTA and had humeral shaft fracture with radial nerve palsy. On examination it was a non-operative fracture; what should be the next line of management?

A. Surgical exploration
B. Observe for 4 months
C. ORIF or IM nail
D. Nerve grafting

163. A 35 years old male has at RTA and had humeral shaft fracture without radial nerve palsy. Patient has an operative fracture and underwent ORIF. Post operatively radial nerve palsy was present. Next line of management is:

A. Surgical exploration
B. Observe for 4 months
C. ORIF or IM nail
D. Nerve grafting

CHALLENGES AND COMPLICATIONS

164. Cocaine can also facilitate cardiac arrhythmias when it is combined with:

A. Nitrous oxide
B. Ketamine
C. Halothane
D. Etomidate

165. Clinical reassessment of trauma patients within 24 hours has reduced the incidence of missed injuries by almost:

A. 20% B. 30%
C. 40% D. 50%

166. The incidence of drug and alcohol use in patients with musculoskeletal injuries has been reported to be as high as:

A. 20% B. 30%
C. 40% D. 50%

167. False about Drug and Alcohol Use is:

A. Alcohol and drug use result in more severe orthopedic injuries and more frequent injuries requiring longer hospitalization
B. Prophylaxis for delirium tremens in post-operative patients should be performed when indicated
C. ISS have been poorly correlated with higher inpatient opioid use
D. Associated complications include those from cocaine use, such as fever, hypertension, acute myocardial ischemia, arrhythmias and stroke

168. False about Thromboembolic Complications is:

A. There is no clinical benefit to routine chemo-prophylaxis after hospitalization in lower extremity fractures of the tibia
B. DVT risk factors include trauma, lower extremity fractures, immobilization, hospitalization, and recent surgery
C. It is estimated that patients remain at increased risk for a DVT or PE for up to 60 days following major orthopedic surgery about the hip
D. Orthopedic and trauma patients are at significantly higher rate of developing deep venous thrombosis (DVT) and pulmonary embolism (PE)

169. Following total hip arthroplasty, total knee arthroplasty, or hip fracture surgery the American Academy of Chest Surgeons has a strong recommendation for chemoprophylaxis for:

A. 14 days B. 28 days
C. 35 days D. 56 days

170. Incidence of Fat emboli syndrome (FES) is:

A. 1% to 2% B. 10% to 20%
C. 5% to 10% D. 10% to 20%

171. ARDS is a pulmonary failure state defined as all except:

A. PaO_2/FiO_2 ratio < 200
B. Pulmonary artery occlusion pressure of </=18 mm Hg
C. B/L diffuse infiltrates on chest radiographs in the absence of congestive heart failure
D. B/L diffuse infiltrates on chest radiographs in the presence of congestive heart failure

172. False about postoperative mobilisation is:

A. When excessive loads are anticipated, such as with heavy or obese patients, the typical fixation is adequate
B. Stable fixation of the fracture must be achieved
C. There must be bone-to-bone contact at the fracture site as demonstrated intraoperatively or on post reduction radiograph
D. Mobilization is transfer of the patient from the supine position, either under the patient's own power or with the help of nurses or therapists

173. False among the following is:

A. Crutch walking with the foot off the floor (non–weight bearing) leads to a significant increase in force across the hip joint because of contraction of the muscles around the hip
B. Touch-down weight bearing allows the patient to place the foot of the affected extremity flat on the floor, without bearing any of the patient's body weight
C. Joint motion is necessary for the good health of articular cartilage
D. Cartilage is nourished from synovial fluid most efficiently when the joint is stable

ANSWERS

1. **Ans: C. Subacute and chronic fractures, while frequently needing treatment and do require emergent care**

   Ref: Chapter No.19, Page No.441

2. **Ans: B. Buckle fracture**

   Ref: Chapter No.19, Page No.441

3. **Ans: C. Pathologic fracture**

   Ref: Chapter No.19, Page No.442

4. **Ans: A. Greenstick fractures**

   Ref: Chapter No.19, Page No.441

5. **Ans: C. The Tscherne's classification is typically used to grade open fractures**

   Ref: Chapter No.19, Page No.442

6. **Ans: B. Physeal**

   Ref: Chapter No.19, Page No.443

7. **Ans: A. Articular fractures may be partially reduced in order to achieve the good possible long-term outcome**

   Ref: Chapter No.19, Page No.442

8. **Ans: C. Transverse # - Parallel to the long axis of the bone**

   Ref: Chapter No.19, Page No.441

9. **Ans: B. Type II**

   Ref: Chapter No.19, Page No.444

10. **Ans: D. Type IV**

    Ref: Chapter No.19, Page No.444

11. **Ans: C. Type III**

    Ref: Chapter No.19, Page No.444

12. **Ans: D. Complete ruptures aka Grade IV injuries, lead to significant instability at the associated joint**

    Ref: Chapter No.19, Page No.444

13. **Ans: C. More urgent orthopaedic management is not necessary for a rupture**

    Ref: Chapter No.19, Page No.444

14. **Ans: D. Disc herniations always needs surgical intervention**

    Ref: Chapter No.19, Page No.445

15. **Ans: A. Butterfly #**

    Ref: Chapter No.19, Page No.445

16. **Ans: B. Permanent stabilization of femur and pelvis fractures**

    Ref: Chapter No.19, Page No.446

17. **Ans: B. Can't be used for complex deformities**

    Ref: Chapter No.19, Page No.446

18. **Ans: A. Limited soft tissue disruption and poor mechanical stability**

    Ref: Chapter No.19, Page No.446

19. **Ans: D. Can't accommodate soft tissue swelling**

    Ref: Chapter No.19, Page No.446

20. **Ans: D. Extensive soft tissue disruption; removed once fracture healed**

    Ref: Chapter No.19, Page No.446

21. **Ans: B. Limited soft tissue disruption; mechanically more stable than nails**

    Ref: Chapter No.19, Page No.446

22. **Ans: D. All of the above are true**

    Ref: Chapter No.19, Page No.446

23. **Ans: B. Splinting**

    Ref: Chapter No.19, Page No.446

24. **Ans: B. Splinting**

    Ref: Chapter No.19, Page No.446

25. **Ans: A. Vertebral burst fracture**

    Ref: Chapter No.19, Page No.447

26. **Ans: B. Secondary survey**

    Ref: Chapter No.19, Page No.447

27. **Ans: A. Primary survey**

    Ref: Chapter No.19, Page No.447

28. **Ans: A. Primary survey**

    Ref: Chapter No.19, Page No.447

29. **Ans: B. FAST scanning has been shown to have high sensitivity in detecting intraperitoneal bleeding in patients with a pelvic fracture**

    Ref: Chapter No.19, Page No.447

30. **Ans: B. An ecchymotic lesion over the greater trochanter that represents a subcutaneous degloving injury**

    Ref: Chapter No.19, Page No.448

31. **Ans: C. Acetabular fractures**

    Ref: Chapter No.19, Page No.448

32. **Ans: A. 55.5%**

    Ref: Chapter No.19, Page No.448

33. **Ans: D. Plain films are still indicated**

    Ref: Chapter No.19, Page No.448

34. **Ans: B. When an isolated extremity injury is the primary reason for evaluation, the entire skeleton need not be examined**

    Ref: Chapter No.19, Page No.448

35. **Ans: C. MRI is now commonly used for the diagnosis of acute fractures even when plain films are positive**

Ref: Chapter No.19, Page No.448-449

36. **Ans: D. Both A and C**

Ref: Chapter No.19, Page No.449

37. **Ans: C. Backward 30 degrees over the cassette on the table**

Ref: Chapter No.19, Page No.449

38. **Ans: A. The presence of an anterior fat pad sign is strongly suggestive of occult fracture**

Ref: Chapter No.19, Page No.449

39. **Ans: B. Elbow radiograph**

Ref: Chapter No.19, Page No.449

40. **Ans: B. The forearm should be imaged in 2 cassettes in both the AP and lateral planes**

Ref: Chapter No.19, Page No.450

41. **Ans: A. Acetabulum**

Ref: Chapter No.19, Page No.451

42. **Ans: B. 45-degree oblique views of the pelvis**

Ref: Chapter No.19, Page No.451

43. **Ans: D. Angled 60-degree caudad**

Ref: Chapter No.19, Page No.451

44. **Ans: B. 30-degree oblique view**

Ref: Chapter No.19, Page No.451

45. **Ans: B. MRI**

Ref: Chapter No.19, Page No.451

46. **Ans: D. All of the above true**

Ref: Chapter No.19, Page No.451

47. **Ans: D. CT Scan is helpful in the acute setting, evaluation of ligamentous derangement**

Ref: Chapter No.19, Page No.451

48. **Ans: D. In a positive stress exam, either or both the medial clear space and the tibia-fibula clear space will be narrowed**

Ref: Chapter No.19, Page No.451-452

49. **Ans: B. Bohler angle**

Ref: Chapter No.19, Page No.453.

50. **Ans: B. 20 and 40 degrees**

Ref: Chapter No.19, Page No.453

51. **Ans: A. Harris axial view**

Ref: Chapter No.19, Page No.453

52. **Ans: B. Talar neck**

Ref: Chapter No.19, Page No.453

53. **Ans: D. Subtalar joint**

Ref: Chapter No.19, Page No.453

54. **Ans: B. If ligamentous injury or neurologic compromise is suspected, CT scan should be performed**

Ref: Chapter No.19, Page No.453

55. **Ans: D. 30%**

Ref: Chapter No.19, Page No.453

56. **Ans: B. Fractures of the hand**

Ref: Chapter No.19, Page No.454

57. **Ans: C. Wrist or forearm fractures**

Ref: Chapter No.19, Page No.454

58. **Ans: A. Fractures about the elbow**

Ref: Chapter No.19, Page No.454

59. **Ans: C. Foot and ankle**

Ref: Chapter No.19, Page No.454

60. **Ans: A. Open splint maintains a reduction more effectively than an bi-valved cast which still allows soft tissue swelling**

Ref: Chapter No.19, Page No.454

61. **Ans: B. 8 pounds**

Ref: Chapter No.19, Page No.454

62. **Ans: B. Pins should be placed from the posterior side of the extremity**

Ref: Chapter No.19, Page No.454

63. **Ans: A. Medial to lateral**

Ref: Chapter No.19, Page No.454

64. **Ans: B. Lateral to medial**

Ref: Chapter No.19, Page No.454

65. **Ans: A. Medial to lateral**

Ref: Chapter No.19, Page No.454

66. **Ans: B. In the distal femur, the pin should be passed from lateral to medial**

Ref: Chapter No.19, Page No.454-455

67. **Ans: C. 6 hours**

Ref: Chapter No.19, Page No.456

68. **Ans: D. All of the above are true**

Ref: Chapter No.19, Page No.456

69. **Ans: A. Open fractures**

Ref: Chapter No.19, Page No.457

70. **Ans: C. 10% to 50%**

Ref: Chapter No.19, Page No.457

71. **Ans: B. 2% to 10%**

Ref: Chapter No.19, Page No.457

72. **Ans: D. Type IIIC**

Ref: Chapter No.19, Page No.457

73. **Ans: B. Type IIIA**

Ref: Chapter No.19, Page No.457

74. **Ans: B. Type II**

Ref: Chapter No.19, Page No.457

75. **Ans: C. Type IIIA**

Ref: Chapter No.19, Page No.457

76. **Ans: C. Type IIIB**

Ref: Chapter No.19, Page No.457

77. **Ans: B. 60 minutes**

Ref: Chapter No.19, Page No.457

78. **Ans: B. 24 hours**

Ref: Chapter No.19, Page No.457

79. **Ans: C. A recent prospective study showed piperacillin-tazobactam to be as ineffective as compared to aminoglycosides in preventing deep infection**

Ref: Chapter No.19, Page No.457

80. **Ans: C. Comparability**

Ref: Chapter No.19, Page No.457

81. **Ans: D. All of the above are true**

Ref: Chapter No.19, Page No.457

82. **Ans: C. 72 hours**

Ref: Chapter No.19, Page No.457

83. **Ans: D. All of the above**

Ref: Chapter No.19, Page No.459

84. **Ans: B. Levaquin**

Ref: Chapter No.19, Page No.459

85. **Ans: A. Vancomycin**

Ref: Chapter No.19, Page No.459

86. **Ans: C. Pelvic ring - almost always treated with internal fixation in the front**

Ref: Chapter No.19, Page No.459

87. **Ans: C. 7 days**

Ref: Chapter No.19, Page No.459

88. **Ans: D. All of the above are true**

Ref: Chapter No.19, Page No.460

89. **Ans: B. >2000 ft/s projectile velocity**

Ref: Chapter No.19, Page No.460

90. **Ans: D. Retained fragments with an incomplete or evolving spinal cord injury or evolving neurologic exam should be left alone**

Ref: Chapter No.19, Page No.461

91. **Ans: C. Bullets that traverse the joint without retention of the bullet are also associated with increased infection rates**

Ref: Chapter No.19, Page No.461

92. **Ans: D. All of the above are true**

Ref: Chapter No.19, Page No.461

93. **Ans: D. Definitive fracture care usually can be accomplished in a multiple operations**

Ref: Chapter No.19, Page No.461

94. **Ans: C. Edema secondary to muscle injury**

Ref: Chapter No.19, Page No.461

95. **Ans: D. All of the above are true**

Ref: Chapter No.19, Page No.461

96. **Ans: B. Stryker Intra-Compartmental Pressure Monitor System**

Ref: Chapter No.19, Page No.463

97. **Ans: C. 5 cm**

Ref: Chapter No.19, Page No.463

98. **Ans: B. Less than 30 mm Hg**

Ref: Chapter No.19, Page No.463

99. **Ans: D. Secondary closure may be attempted when limb swelling has been reduced (7–14 days)**

Ref: Chapter No.19, Page No.463

100. **Ans: C. The saphenous nerve**

Ref: Chapter No.19, Page No.463

101. **Ans: C. In combination with a head or abdominal injury that requires surgical intervention or if the pelvis fracture is open, mortality increases to 90%**

Ref: Chapter No.19, Page No.464

102. **Ans: C. 13 times**

Ref: Chapter No.19, Page No.464

103. **Ans: D. Haematuria**

Ref: Chapter No.19, Page No.464

104. **Ans: A. Stability depends on the integrity of the only the osseous structures**

Ref: Chapter No.19, Page No.464

105. **Ans: C. 2.5 cm**

Ref: Chapter No.19, Page No.464

106. **Ans: A. 1 cm**

Ref: Chapter No.19, Page No.464

107. **Ans: C. Anterior injuries are easily identified on this projection and are the most unstable**

Ref: Chapter No.19, Page No.464

108. **Ans: B. Lateral compression force**

Ref: Chapter No.19, Page No.466

109. **Ans: A. Vertical shear forces**

Ref: Chapter No.19, Page No.466

110. **Ans: C. AP compression force**

Ref: Chapter No.19, Page No.466

111. **Ans: A. Type B III**

Ref: Chapter No.19, Page No.466

112. Ans: D. Intrapelvic visceral injuries are also more common with the Lateral Compression patterns

Ref: Chapter No.19, Page No.467

113. Ans: B. Combination of retroperitoneal bleeding and visceral injuries

Ref: Chapter No.19, Page No.466

114. Ans: C. Intra-abdominal and head injuries

Ref: Chapter No.19, Page No.466

115. Ans: B. Closed head trauma

Ref: Chapter No.19, Page No.466

116. Ans: B. Presacral venous plexus

Ref: Chapter No.19, Page No.466

117. Ans: D. Factors predicting arterial bleeding included a base deficit of 2 mmol/L, a systolic blood pressure less than 90 mm Hg, and the need for transfusion in the ED

Ref: Chapter No.19, Page No.466

118. Ans: D. 90%

Ref: Chapter No.19, Page No.466

119. Ans: B. If they are applied in the field, PASGs should be deflated as soon as the patient is in the tertiary care center

Ref: Chapter No.19, Page No.467

120. Ans: A. Binders or sheets are properly applied by centering them over the umbilicus and applying pressure

Ref: Chapter No.19, Page No.468

121. Ans: A. Pelvic artery embolization (PAE) can be performed in either the external iliac artery (nonselective) or distal to the external iliac artery (selective)

Ref: Chapter No.19, Page No.468

122. Ans: D. Packing should be removed after resuscitation in 72 hours

Ref: Chapter No.19, Page No.468-469

123. Ans: B. The exact timing of definitive fixation of the pelvis is in debate with institutional variations, but it should generally be performed within the first month

Ref: Chapter No.19, Page No.469

124. Ans: A. If midline neck pain or tenderness is present, MRI evaluation is indicated

Ref: Chapter No.19, Page No.469

125. Ans: C. 48 hours

Ref: Chapter No.19, Page No.469

126. Ans: B. Bulbocavernosus reflex

Ref: Chapter No.19, Page No.469

127. Ans: D. The middle column includes the posterior two-third of the vertebral body and posterior longitudinal ligament

Ref: Chapter No.19, Page No.471

128. Ans: B. Injuries involving the anterior and middle columns

Ref: Chapter No.19, Page No.471

129. Ans: A. Anterior column

Ref: Chapter No.19, Page No.471

130. Ans: C. 100

Ref: Chapter No.19, Page No.470

131. Ans: C. 112

Ref: Chapter No.19, Page No.470

132. Ans: B. Incomplete = any sensory or motor function in S4-S5

Ref: Chapter No.19, Page No.470

133. Ans: B. S2

Ref: Chapter No.19, Page No.470

134. Ans: C. C7

Ref: Chapter No.19, Page No.470

135. Ans: B. T10

Ref: Chapter No.19, Page No.470

136. Ans: B. S1

Ref: Chapter No.19, Page No.470

137. Ans: D. T1

Ref: Chapter No.19, Page No.470

138. Ans: B. L4

Ref: Chapter No.19, Page No.470

139. Ans: A. L3

Ref: Chapter No.19, Page No.470

140. Ans: C. 10

Ref: Chapter No.19, Page No.472

141. Ans: B. Compression fractures are typically managed nonoperatively if there is not a significant (>50%) loss of height

Ref: Chapter No.19, Page No.471

142. Ans: C. 25% body height loss

Ref: Chapter No.19, Page No.472

143. Ans: B. When a diagnosis of cauda equina syndrome is confirmed, surgical exploration and decompression should be performed in a few days

Ref: Chapter No.19, Page No.472

144. Ans: C. The shoulder usually dislocates with the humerus posterior to the glenoid

Ref: Chapter No.19, Page No.472

145. Ans: A. Posteriorly

Ref: Chapter No.19, Page No.472

146. Ans: B. Risk of sciatic nerve injury

Ref: Chapter No.19, Page No.473

147. Ans: D. Brachial artery injury

Ref: Chapter No.19, Page No.473

148. Ans: D. Delay in the reduction of a dislocated hip can lead to femoral nerve injury, cartilage cell death, and avascular necrosis

Ref: Chapter No.19, Page No.473

149. Ans: A. A common protocol uses sequentially timed vascular exams at presentation, 4 to 6 hours later, and then 12 hours later

Ref: Chapter No.19, Page No.473

150. Ans: D. IV sedation is very helpful in reducing muscle tone that can resist reduction and is always necessary

Ref: Chapter No.19, Page No.473

151. Ans: C. Intimal injury

Ref: Chapter No.19, Page No.474

152. Ans: B. 5% to 15%

Ref: Chapter No.19, Page No.474

153. Ans: B. less than 0.9

Ref: Chapter No.19, Page No.474

154. Ans: B. It is recommended that the orthopedic procedure be always performed first

Ref: Chapter No.19, Page No.474

155. Ans: B. Not all femur fractures need to be immobilized before the patient is transported from the scene of the accident

Ref: Chapter No.19, Page No.474

156. Ans: A. The evidence has consistently held the standard of care for a stable femoral shaft patient to be ETC within 48 hours

Ref: Chapter No.19, Page No.475

157. Ans: B. The incidence of compartment syndrome in tibial shaft fractures is as high as 50%

Ref: Chapter No.19, Page No.475

158. Ans: B. Plate fixation has fallen treatment of choice for diaphyseal fractures

Ref: Chapter No.19, Page No.475-476

159. Ans: A. Operative management is the mainstay of treatment for fractures that maintain acceptable alignment

Ref: Chapter No.19, Page No.476

160. Ans: D. During the functional brace stage, patients are allowed free elbow flexion-extension and arm abduction to 30 degrees

Ref: Chapter No.19, Page No.476

161. Ans: B. 3 to 4 months

Ref: Chapter No.19, Page No.476

162. Ans: B. Observe for 4 months

Ref: Chapter No.19, Page No.477

163. Ans: B. Observe for 4 months

Ref: Chapter No.19, Page No.477

164. Ans: D. Etomidate

Ref: Chapter No.19, Page No.477

165. Ans: C. 40%

Ref: Chapter No.19, Page No.476

166. Ans: D. 50%

Ref: Chapter No.19, Page No.477

167. Ans: C. ISS have been poorly correlated with higher inpatient opioid use

Ref: Chapter No.19, Page No.477

168. Ans: C. It is estimated that patients remain at increased risk for a DVT or PE for up to 60 days following major orthopedic surgery about the hip

Ref: Chapter No.19, Page No.477-478

169. Ans: C. 35 days

Ref: Chapter No.19, Page No.478

170. Ans: D. 10% to 20%

Ref: Chapter No.19, Page No.478

171. Ans: D. B/L diffuse infiltrates on chest radiographs in the presence of congestive heart failure

Ref: Chapter No.19, Page No.478

172. Ans: A. When excessive loads are anticipated, such as with heavy or obese patients, the typical fixation is adequate

Ref: Chapter No.19, Page No.478

173. Ans: D. Cartilage is nourished from synovial fluid most efficiently when the joint is stable

Ref: Chapter No.19, Page No.479

20

Burns

GENERAL CONSIDERATIONS

1. **False among the following is:**
   A. The number of burns in the elderly has actually increased, likely in association with the growing percentage of the population
   B. Burn deaths generally occur in a unimodal distribution
   C. Two-thirds of all burns occur at home and commonly involve children less than 10 years of age, adult males, and increasingly the elderly
   D. Interestingly, the cause of fire with the highest mortality is from cigarette smoking, which leads to 22% of house-fire–related deaths

2. **Seventy-five percent of all burn-related deaths occur in house fires commonly associated with:**
   A. Cigarette smoking
   B. Food preparation or heating equipment
   C. Motor vehicle problems
   D. Bomb blasts

3. **False among the following is:**
   A. Young adults are frequently burned with flammable liquids, whereas toddlers are often scalded by hot liquids
   B. A significant percentage of burns in children are due to child abuse
   C. Risk factors include low socioeconomic class and unsafe environments
   D. All of the above are true

4. **Patients with the following criteria should be referred to a designated burn center except:**
   A. Any full-thickness burn
   B. Partial-thickness burns greater than 20% TBSA
   C. Burns in patients with pre-existing medical disorders that could complicate management, prolong recovery, or affect outcome
   D. Burned children in hospitals without qualified personnel or equipment to care for children

5. **Patients with the following criteria should be referred to a designated burn center:**
   A. Chemical burns B. Inhalation injury
   C. Electrical burns D. All of the above

6. **Thermal conductivity is the ability to transfer heat; for water, it is:**
   A. 0.21 W/m/°C B. 0.41 W/m/°C
   C. 0.61 W/m/°C D. 0.81 W/m/°C

7. **Thermal conductivity of hot cooking oil is:**
   A. 2.2 joule/g °C B. 4.2 joule/g °C
   C. 6.2 joule/g °C D. 8.2 joule/g °C

8. **Thermal conductivity of grease is:**
   A. 1.0 joule/g °C B. 1.4 joule/g °C
   C. 1.8 joule/g °C D. 2.8 joule/g °C

9. **Damage from contact with hot liquids is called as:**
   A. None B. Flame burns
   C. Chemical burns D. None

10. **Burns injury to the epidermis and papillary dermis is called as:**
    A. Superficial
    B. Superficial partial-thickness burns
    C. Deep partial-thickness burns
    D. Full-thickness burns

11. **The necrotic area of burn where cells were directly disrupted is termed:**
    A. Zone of coagulation
    B. Zone of stasis
    C. Zone of hypᵔraemia
    D. Zone of death

12. The area immediately surrounding the necrotic zone has a moderate degree of insult with decreased tissue perfusion is termed:

A. Zone of coagulation
B. Zone of stasis
C. Zone of hyperaemia
D. Zone of death

13. Which zone is associated with vascular damage and vessel leakage?

A. Zone of coagulation
B. Zone of stasis
C. Zone of hyperaemia
D. Zone of death

14. Which zone is characterized by vasodilatation from inflammation surrounding the burn wound?

A. Zone of coagulation
B. Zone of stasis
C. Zone of hyperaemia
D. Zone of death

15. Which zone has irreversibly damaged at the time of injury?

A. Zone of coagulation
B. Zone of stasis
C. Zone of hyperaemia
D. Zone of death

16. Which degree of burn is painful, erythematous, and blanch to the touch with an intact epidermal barrier?

A. Superficial burns
B. Superficial partial-thickness
C. Deep partial-thickness burns
D. Full-thickness burns

17. False about superficial burns is:

A. Superficial burns are, by definition, injury confined to the epidermis
B. Previously termed "first-degree"
C. Sunburn or a very minor scald from a kitchen incident
D. Treatment is aimed at dressings

18. False about Superficial partial-thickness burns:

A. Erythematous, painful, blanch to touch and often blister
B. Hair follicles are not viable and intact
C. Scald injuries sustained in kitchen incidents and flash flame burns
D. After healing, these burns may have some slight skin discoloration and textural differences without other significant scarring

19. Superficial partial-thickness burns spontaneously reepithelialise from retained epidermal structures in:

A. 5 to 10 days B. 7 to 14 days
C. 15 to 21 days D. 21 to 28 days

20. Deep partial-thickness burns heal in:

A. 5 to 10 days B. 7 to 14 days
C. 15 to 21 days D. 21 to 28 days

21. False about deep partial-thickness burns is:

A. Appear more pale and mottled
B. Not painful to pinprick
C. Do not blanch to touch
D. These burns heal in 15 to 21 days by reepithelialisation from deep hair follicles and sweat gland keratinocytes, often with severe scarring as a result of loss of dermal integrity

22. False statement about full thickness burns is:

A. Characterized by a hard leathery eschar that is painless and black, white, or cherry red in colour
B. Deep dermal and full-thickness burns benefit from excision of the eschar with autologous skin grafting in order to heal in a timely fashion and minimize contraction
C. No epidermal or dermal keratinocytes remain thus, these wounds must heal by reepithelialisation from the wound edges
D. Full-thickness burns can extend below the superficial fat, but doesn't involve other structures, such as muscle and bone

23. Burns depth is most accurately assessed by:

A. Laser Doppler flowmetry
B. Judgment of experienced practitioners
C. Laser speckle imaging
D. Optical coherence with or without artificial intelligence techniques

24. The perineum and genitalia are assumed to be:

A. 1% of the TBSA B. 2% of the TBSA
C. 3% of the TBSA D. 4% of the TBSA

25. In infants the head and neck is about:

A. 13% of the TBSA B. 18% of the TBSA
C. 21% of the TBSA D. 25% of the TBSA

26. In infants each leg is about:

A. 13% of the TBSA B. 18% of the TBSA
C. 21% of the TBSA D. 25% of the TBSA

27. Which formula is used to accurately determine burn size in children?

A. Rule of 9s′ B. Berkow
C. Parkland D. Brooke

28. Immediately after burns, which of the following decreases the resuscitation fluid needs?

A. High-dose steroid therapy
B. High-dose vitamin D therapy
C. High-dose vitamin C therapy
D. High-dose vitamin A therapy

29. Which of the following is not true about the effects of burns injury on the Renal System?

A. With the use of continuous venovenous hemofiltration compared to intermittent hemodialysis controls, 28-day mortality and in-hospital mortality in the severely burned with renal failure decreased by 50% and 25%
B. Result in oliguria, which, if left untreated, will cause acute tubular necrosis and renal failure
C. Stress induced hormones and mediators such as angiotensin, aldosterone, vasopressin, and thromboxane B2 further reduce renal blood flow immediately after the injury
D. All of the above are true

30. With burns of _______, impairment of immune functions is proportional to burn size:

A. More than 10% TBSA
B. More than 15% TBSA
C. More than 20% TBSA
D. More than 25% TBSA

31. Which of the following is false about effects of a burns injury on immune system?

A. Burned patients are then at great risk for a number of infectious complications, including bacterial wound infection, pneumonia, and fungal and viral infections
B. Macrophage production after burn is relatively diminished, which is related to spontaneous elaboration of negative regulators of myeloid growth
C. Total neutrophil counts are initially decreased after burn by demargination and decreased cell death by apoptosis
D. After 48 to 72 hours, neutrophil counts decrease somewhat like macrophages with similar causes

32. Which of the following is false about effects of a burns injury on T cells?

A. T-cell function is depressed after a severe burn
B. Early burn wound excision decreases cytotoxic T-cell activity
C. The Th17 phenotype is likely to play a significant role in the burn wound given its association with adaptive immunity on mucosal surfaces and the skin
D. Burns also impairs cytotoxic T lymphocyte activity as a function of burn size, thus increasing the risk of infection, particularly from fungi and viruses

33. True about the metabolism in burns injury is:

A. After severe burn and resuscitation, typically 3 to 4 days after injury, the condition of hypermetabolism develops
B. Hypermetabolism may be sustained for months, leading to massive weight loss and decreased strength
C. Changes in metabolic activity are due in part to the release of catabolic hormones
D. All of the above

INITIAL TREATMENT OF BURNS

34. To decrease the depth of the wound to improve healing and scarring, room temperature water should be copiously poured on the wound within:

A. 1 hour of the injury B. 2 hours of the injury
C. 3 hours of the injury D. 4 hours of the injury

35. Prophylactic intubation should be done for patients with TBSA of:

A. >20% TBSA B. >30% TBSA
C. >40% TBSA D. >50% TBSA

36. Which of the following is false in the initial assessment of burns patient?

A. Most burn patients remain tachycardic even with adequate resuscitation
B. Pulse rate can be used as an indirect measure of circulation
C. In those who have been in an explosion or deceleration incident, a possibility exists for spinal cord injury and other fractures
D. The presence of pulses or Doppler signals in the distal extremities may not be adequate to determine adequate circulation of blood

37. False about wound care in burns patient is:

A. Application of a clean dry dressing or sheet to cover the involved part
B. Damp dressings can be used
C. Intramuscular or subcutaneous narcotic injections for pain should never be used because drug absorption is decreased as a result of the peripheral vasoconstriction

D. The first step in diminishing pain is to cover the wounds to prevent contact to exposed nerve endings

38. The fluid of choice for burns patient's resuscitation is:

A. Normal Saline
B. Lactated Ringer's solution without dextrose
C. 5% dextrose Ringer's lactate
D. Hypertonic saline

39. The fluid of choice for burns patient's resuscitation in children younger than 2 years is:

A. Normal Saline
B. Lactated Ringer's solution without dextrose
C. 5% dextrose Ringer's lactate
D. Hypertonic saline

40. Parkland's formula for crystalloid calculation for resuscitation is:

A. 2 cc/kg/% TBSA burned
B. 4 cc/kg/% TBSA burned
C. 6 cc/kg/% TBSA burned
D. 8 cc/kg/% TBSA burned

41. Brooke's formula for crystalloid calculation for resuscitation is:

A. 2 cc/kg/% TBSA burned
B. 4 cc/kg/% TBSA burned
C. 6 cc/kg/% TBSA burned
D. 8 cc/kg/% TBSA burned

42. Galveston's formula for crystalloid calculation for resuscitation is:

A. 5000 cc/m^2 burned + 1500 cc/m^2 total surface area
B. 5000 cc/m^2 burned + 2500 cc/m^2 total surface area
C. 4000 cc/m^2 burned + 1500 cc/m^2 total surface area
D. 4000 cc/m^2 burned + 2500 cc/m^2 total surface area

43. All patients with burns of greater than ___TBSA should receive 0.5 mL tetanus toxoid.

A. 10% B. 20%
C. 30% D. 40%

44. False among the following is:

A. Extremities at risk are identified either on clinical examination or on measurement of tissue pressures greater than 30 mm Hg
B. When deep partial-thickness or full-thickness burns encompass the circumference of an extremity, peripheral circulation to the limb can be compromised
C. Increased muscle compartment pressures after escharotomies may indicate fasciotomies
D. The most common complications associated with fasciotomy is infection

INHALATION INJURY

45. False statement about inhalational injury is:

A. Inhalation injury increases the amount of time spent on mechanical ventilation, a strong predictor of mortality
B. Early diagnosis and prevention of complications are of interest to decrease morbidity and mortality rates related to this condition
C. Direct thermal damage to the lung is seen because of dispersal of the heat in the pharynx
D. All of the above are true

46. Definitive diagnosis of inhalational injury should be clarified by the use of:

A. Radiography B. Bronchoscopy
C. CT scan D. MRI

47. False statement about carbon monoxide (CO) in inhalational injury is:

A. CO also causes a conformational change to hemoglobin that diminishes oxygen off-loading ability in peripheral tissues
B. Intracellularly, CO also has been shown to bind cytochrome c oxidase, disrupting the electron transport chain in mitochondria
C. The impact of CO is most apparent in organ systems with high metabolic output such as the brain and heart
D. Initial treatment is 80% oxygen

48. Carbon monoxide (CO) is all of the following except:

A. Colorless B. Foul smelling
C. Tasteless D. Nonirritating

49. CO poisoning therefore most commonly manifests as:

A. Respiratory arrest
B. Neurologic changes
C. Renal failure
D. Skin changes

50. Which of the following is false?

A. Cyanide is a potent and rapidly acting poison, which, under normal conditions, is converted into thiocyanide that is excreted through the urine

B. The cyanide ion interferes with cellular energy production, leading to rapid depletion of ATP stores and the subsequent development of lactic acidosis

C. For cyanide toxicity, removal from the source is indicated as well as hydroxocobalamin might be given intravenously

D. All of the above are true

51. Carbon Monoxide's affinity to hemoglobin as compared to oxygen:

A. 50 times B. 100 times
C. 200 times D. 300 times

52. CO poisoning is measured by carboxyhaemoglobin levels; dizziness and impaired judgment is seen with:

A. Levels above 5% B. Levels above 10%
C. Levels at 20% D. Levels above 30%

53. CO poisoning is measured by carboxyhaemoglobin levels; dyspnoea is seen with:

A. Levels above 5% B. Levels above 10%
C. Levels at 20% D. Levels above 30%

54. In the clinical course of patients with inhalation injury during the second stage occurs from 72 to 96 hours after injury and is associated with:

A. Hypoxia
B. Increased extravascular lung water
C. Development of diffuse lobar infiltrates
D. All of the above

55. In the clinical course of patients with inhalation injury during the third stage all of the following are true except:

A. Clinical bronchopneumonia dominates and appears in up to 60% of these patients

B. The differentiation of pneumonia from tracheobronchitis is difficult at this stage, and bronchoscopy with lavage may be of assistance

C. Early pneumonias are usually caused by Pseudomonas and Klebsiella

D. Ball-valve effects and ventilator-associated barotrauma are also hallmarks of this period.

56. Inhalation treatments of smoke inhalation injury includes:

A. Nebulized heparin - 5000 units in 3 cc normal saline q4h
B. Bronchodilators - q2h
C. Nebulized acetylcysteine - 20%, 3 cc q4h
D. All of the above

57. False statements among the following is:

A. Prophylactic antibiotics for inhalation injury are indicated

B. Inhalation treatments have been effective in improving the clearance of tracheobronchial secretions and decreasing bronchospasm

C. Steroids are not of benefit in inhalation injury and should not be given unless the patient is steroid dependent before injury

D. All of the above are true

WOUND CARE

58. False among the following is:

A. All treatments are aimed at slow and less painful healing

B. It should protect the damaged epithelium, minimize bacterial and fungal colonization, and provide splinting action to maintain the desired position of function

C. The dressing should be occlusive to reduce evaporative heat loss and minimize cold stress

D. The dressing should provide comfort over the painful wound

59. Organisms proliferate and may penetrate into viable tissue when wound counts are:

A. >10^2 organisms per gram of tissue
B. >10^3 organisms per gram of tissue
C. >10^4 organisms per gram of tissue
D. >10^5 organisms per gram of tissue

60. True about the following is:

A. Salves are generally applied directly to the wound with cotton dressings placed over them

B. Soaks are solutions poured into cotton dressings on the wound

C. Antimicrobial dressings contain active agents to inhibit microbial growth

D. All of the following

61. Silver sulfadiazine, false statement is:

A. Painful daily dressing changes
B. Does not penetrate eschar
C. Inhibition of epithelialization
D. It must be changed once in 3-4 days

62. Transient leukopenia as a side effect is seen in:

A. Mafenide acetate B. Silver sulfadiazine
C. Silver nitrate 0.5% D. Dakin's solution

63. True about transient leukopenia is/are:

A. Develops 3 to 5 days
B. Following continued use
C. Harmless and resolves with or without treatment cessation
D. All of the above

64. Metabolic acidosis as a side effect is seen in:

A. Mafenide acetate B. Silver sulfadiazine
C. Silver nitrate 0.5% D. Dakin's solution

65. False about Mafenide acetate is:

A. 0.5 % Mafenide acetate is used
B. Broad spectrum of activity owing to its sulfa moiety
C. It can penetrate eschar
D. Painful application on skin

66. Petroleum-based antimicrobial ointments, false statement is:

A. Polymyxin B, neomycin and bacitracin are clear on application and allow for easy wound observation
B. Painful application
C. Commonly used for treatment of facial burns, graft sites, healing donor sites, and small partial-thickness burns
D. Mupirocin is a petroleum based ointment that has improved activity against gram-positive bacteria, particularly methicillin-resistant S. aureus

67. Combination of which of the following should not be used?

A. Nystatin and Bacitracin
B. Nystatin and Polymyxin B
C. Nystatin and Mafenide acetate
D. Nystatin and Silver sulfadiazine

68. Mafenide acetate as a solution is available in:

A. 1% solution B. 5% solution
C. 10% solution D. 11% solution

69. Which among the following is associated with methemoglobinemia?

A. Mafenide acetate B. Silver sulfadiazine
C. Silver nitrate 0.5% D. Dakin's solution

70. Dakin's solution is:

A. 0.5% sodium hypochlorite
B. 0.05% sodium hypochlorite
C. 0.25% acetic acid
D. 0.025% acetic acid

71. Domboro's solution is:

A. 0.5% sodium hypochlorite
B. 0.05% sodium hypochlorite
C. 0.25% acetic acid
D. 0.025% acetic acid

72. Biofilm formation is inhibited by:

A. 0.25% acetic acid
B. 0.5% sodium hypochlorite
C. 5% Mafenide acetate
D. Silver nitrate 0.5%

73. Which of the following stains contacted areas?

A. 0.25% acetic acid
B. 0.5% sodium hypochlorite
C. 5% Mafenide acetate
D. Silver nitrate 0.5%

74. False about Synthetic and biologic dressings is:

A. Dressings provide for stable coverage without painful dressing changes, provide a barrier to evaporative losses, and decrease pain in the wounds
B. Do not inhibit epithelialization, which is a feature of all topical antimicrobials
C. Most often, synthetic and biologic dressings are used to cover second degree wounds
D. Should generally be applied within 24 hours of the injury

75. To avoid high bacterial colonization of the wound, synthetic and biologic dressings should generally be applied within:

A. 12 hours of the injury
B. 24 hours of the injury
C. 48 hours of the injury
D. 72 hours of the injury

76. False statement about biologic dressings among the following is:

A. Particularly well suited to massive partial-thickness injuries (>50% TBSA) to close the wound and allow for healing to take place underneath the dressing
B. Possible transmission of viral diseases with allograft and the possibility that a residual

mesh pattern will be left from engrafted cadaver dermis if meshed allograft is used
C. Biologic dressings can be used to cover any wound as a temporary dressing
D. Severely burned patients are immunosuppressed, and biologic dressings that have adhered will get rejected

77. False among the following is:

A. Biobrane consists of collagen-coated silicone manufactured into a sheet
B. Biobrane has antimicrobial activities
C. Suprathel is another like formulation
D. When the epithelium is complete under the sheet, it is easily peeled off the wound

78. False about Integra among the following is:

A. Integra combine a collagen matrix (dermal substitute) with a silicone sheet outside layer (epidermal substitute)
B. It takes two operations for wound coverage, as the silicone layer simulating the epidermis must be replaced 2 to 3 weeks after application with autograft
C. The collagen matrix engrafts into the wound, and after 2 weeks, the silicone layer is removed and replaced with available autograft
D. The disadvantage of Integra is that it can't be used in full thickness burns to close the wound

79. False about Excision and Grafting is:

A. These excisions can be performed with tourniquet control or with application of topical epinephrine and thrombin to minimize blood loss
B. Wounds covering 20% to 30% TBSA can usually be closed at one operation with autograft split-thickness skin taken from the patient's available donor sites
C. A typical method of treatment is to use widely expanded autografts (4:1 or greater) covered with cadaver allograft to completely close the wounds for which autograft is available
D. The 2:1 skin heals underneath the cadaver skin in approximately 14 days, and the cadaver skin falls off

80. Loss of skin grafts is due to the following reasons except:

A. Fluid collection over the graft
B. Shearing forces that disrupt the adhered graft
C. Presence of infection causing graft lysis
D. Inadequate excision of the wound bed

81. Most common cause of loss of skin grafts:

A. Fluid collection under the graft
B. Shearing forces that disrupt the adhered graft
C. Presence of infection causing graft lysis
D. Inadequate excision of the wound bed

82. False about cultured epithelial autografts is:

A. Cultured epithelial autografts are of use in truly massive burns (>80% TBSA) because of their limited donor sites
B. Keratinocytes can be cultured in sheets from full-thickness skin biopsies, which are used as autografts
C. Technologies like cultured epithelial autografts hold the promise to radically limit donor sites
D. All of the above

83. The disadvantages of cultured epithelial autografts are all except:

A. Length of time required to grow the autografts is long (2–3 weeks)
B. 20% to 30% take up rate of the grafts after initial application
C. These grafts are also very expensive to produce
D. There is a potential for squamous cell cancer

MINIMIZING COMPLICATIONS

84. False statement about prevention burns wound complications:

A. The current recommendations are to prevent the development of organ dysfunction and to provide optimal support to avoid conditions that promote the onset
B. The best solution is likely delayed wound closure
C. One of the most important contributors to survival was the time to starting intravenous resuscitation, regardless of the initial volume given
D. Removal of devitalized tissue prevents wound infections and decreases inflammation associated with the wound

85. Recommendation is to complete early excision of clearly full-thickness wounds within:

A. 24 hours B. 48 hours
C. 72 hours D. 96 hours

86. Perioperative antibiotics clearly benefit patients with injuries greater than:

A. 20% TBSA burns B. 30% TBSA burns
C. 40% TBSA burns D. 50% TBSA burns

87. The most common source of sepsis in burns wound is:

A. Renal failure
B. Tracheobronchial trees
C. Mesenteric ischemia
D. Cardiac arrest

88. Adequate measure of renal perfusion in the absence of underlying renal disease in children is:

A. 0.5 mL/kg/hr
B. 1 mL/kg/hr
C. 2 mL/kg/hr
D. 4 mL/kg/hr

89. Increased insensible losses from the wounds, can be roughly calculated at:

A. 2500 mL/m^2 TBSA +3750 mL/m^2 TBSA burned
B. 2500 mL/m^2 TBSA +5750 mL/m^2 TBSA burned
C. 1500 mL/m^2 TBSA +3750 mL/m^2 TBSA burned
D. 1500 mL/m^2 TBSA +5750 mL/m^2 TBSA burned

90. False statement about renal failure after burns injury is:

A. Renal failure is hallmarked by decreasing urine output, hypervolemia, electrolyte abnormalities
B. Urine output of more than 1 mL/kg/hr in children and 30 cc/ hr in adults is an adequate measure of renal perfusion
C. Almost invariably, severely burned patients receive exogenous potassium
D. Hyperkalemia is seen with renal insufficiency

91. The first sign of impending pulmonary failure is:

A. Raised PCO_2 levels
B. Decline in oxygenation
C. Cyanosis
D. Paleness

92. Decrease in saturation to less than ___ is indicative of pulmonary failure.

A. 88%
B. 90%
C. 92%
D. 95%

93. False statement about the hematological changes in burns among the following is:

A. Burn patients may become coagulopathic
B. Platelet counts of less than 50,000 requires treatment
C. Severely burned patients are also at risk for thrombotic and embolic complications likely related to immobilization
D. Complications of deep venous thrombosis was associated with increasing age, weight, and TBSA burned

NUTRITION

94. As per Curreri formula, caloric needs in burns patients can be calculated by:

A. 25 kcal/kg/day plus 40 kcal per percent TBSA burned per day
B. 25 kcal/kg/day plus 30 kcal per percent TBSA burned per day
C. 35 kcal/kg/day plus 40 kcal per percent TBSA burned per day
D. 25 kcal/kg/day plus 50 kcal per percent TBSA burned per day

95. Predict the maintenance calorie needs (in severely burned children) for adolescents (12–18 years):

A. 2100 kcal/% TBSA burned/24 hours
B. 1800 kcal/% TBSA burned/24 hours
C. 1500 kcal/% TBSA burned/24 hours
D. 1200 kcal/% TBSA burned/24 hours

ELECTRICAL BURNS

96. False among the following is:

A. The skin has a relatively high resistance to electrical current and is therefore mostly spared
B. The bone itself does sustain any increase in temperature or injury
C. Low voltage injury is similar to thermal burns without transmission to the deeper tissues
D. Heat generated by the transfer of electrical current and passage of the current itself then injures the tissues

97. Most household currents (110–220 volts) produce low voltage type of injury, which causes only local damage. Worst of these injuries are at:

A. Fingers
B. Hands
C. Feet
D. Edge of the mouth

98. The syndrome of high-voltage injury includes all except:

A. These patients also have cutaneous burns associated with ignition of clothing from the discharge of electrical current
B. The most serious derangements occur in the first 4 hours after injury
C. If patients with electrical injuries have no cardiac dysrhythmias on initial electrocardiogram or

recent history of cardiac arrest, no further monitoring is necessary

D. The burns on the skin are mostly thermal, and not electrical

99. **False among the following is:**

A. The most significant injury is within the deep tissue, and subsequent edema formation can cause vascular compromise to any area distal to the injury

B. Tissue that has questionable viability should be debrided during fasciotomy

C. If the muscle compartment is extensively injured and necrotic, such that the prospects for eventual function are dismal, early amputation may be necessary

D. Fasciotomies should be complete and may include nerve decompressions

100. **Neurologic deficits after electric injury can occur upto:**

A. Up to 3 months after injury

B. Up to 9 months after injury

C. Up to 1 year after injury

D. Up to 6 months after injury

101. **Neurologic deficits after electric injury can occur upto:**

A. 10% B. 20%

C. 30% D. 40%

CHEMICAL BURNS

102. **The degree of tissue damage, as well as the level of toxicity, is determined by:**

A. Chemical nature of the agent

B. Concentration of the agent

C. Duration of skin contact

D. All of the above

103. **False about the treatment of chemical burns is:**

A. Speed is essential in the management of chemical burns

B. For all chemicals, lavage with copious quantities of clean water should not be done immediately after removing all clothing

C. Early irrigation dilutes the chemical, which is already in contact with the skin, and timeliness increases effectiveness of irrigation

D. Dry powders should be brushed from the affected areas before irrigation

104. **For significant chemical injuries, a reasonable rule of thumb is to lavage with _____of tap water.**

A. 5 to 10 L B. 10 to 15 L

C. 15 to 20 L D. 20 to 30 L

105. **Factors involved in the mechanism of alkali burns are:**

A. Saponification of fat

B. Alkalis dissolve and unite with the proteins of the tissues to form alkaline proteinates

C. Massive extraction of water from cells

D. All of the above

106. **False about alkali burns is:**

A. The critical substance responsible for the skin damage is the hydrogen ion

B. Treatment consists of removing all clothing and irrigating the affected area with water and soap until all the alkali is removed and the effluent has a pH of less than 8

C. Injuries tend to be deep because of exposure times, and surgical excision and grafting of the resultant eschar may be indicated

D. All of the above are true

107. **False about acid burns is:**

A. Acids induce protein breakdown by hydrolysis and coagulative necrosis

B. Acid induced burns result in a hard eschar that does not penetrate as deeply as the alkalis

C. Acid induces thermal injury by heat generation with contact of the skin

D. All of the above are true

108. **False about formic acid injuries is:**

A. Electrolyte abnormalities are of great concern for patients who have sustained extensive formic acid injuries

B. With metabolic acidosis, renal failure, intravascular hemolysis, and pulmonary complications being common

C. Acidemia detected by a metabolic acidosis on arterial blood gas analysis should be corrected with intravenous sodium bicarbonate

D. A formic acid wound typically has a brownish appearance

109. **False about Hydrofluoric acid burns is:**

A. Hydrofluoric acid is a toxic substance used widely in both industrial and domestic settings and is the strongest inorganic acid known

B. Hydrofluoric acid produces dehydration and corrosion of tissue with free hydrogen ions

C. All patients with hydrofluoric acid burns should be admitted for cardiac monitoring, with particular attention paid to prolongation of the QT interval

D. All of the above are true

110. About management of Hydrofluoric acid burns is all except:

A. Wounds in general are very painful because of the calcium chelation and associated potassium release; this finding can be used to determine the effectiveness of treatment

B. Beyond initial copious irrigation with clean water, the burned area should be treated immediately with copious 2.5% calcium gluconate gel

C. If pain relief is incomplete after several applications or symptoms recur, intradermal injections of 10% calcium gluconate (0.5 mL/cm^2 affected)

D. The gel should be changed at 60-minute intervals until the pain subsides, an indication of removal of the active fluoride ion

ANSWERS

1. **Ans: B. Burn deaths generally occur in a unimodal distribution**
Ref: Chapter No.20, Page No.484-485

2. **Ans: B. Food preparation or heating equipment**
Ref: Chapter No.20, Page No.485

3. **Ans: D. All of the above are true**
Ref: Chapter No.20, Page No.485

4. **Ans: B. Partial-thickness burns greater than 20% TBSA**
Ref: Chapter No.20, Page No.485

5. **Ans: D. All of the above**
Ref: Chapter No.20, Page No.485

6. **Ans: C. 0.61 W/m/°C**
Ref: Chapter No.20, Page No.486

7. **Ans: B. 4.2 joule/g °C**
Ref: Chapter No.20, Page No.486

8. **Ans: C. 1.8 joule/g °C**
Ref: Chapter No.20, Page No.486

9. **Ans: D. None**
Ref: Chapter No.20, Page No.486

10. **Ans: B. Superficial partial-thickness burns**
Ref: Chapter No.20, Page No.486

11. **Ans: A. Zone of coagulation**
Ref: Chapter No.20, Page No.486

12. **Ans: B. Zone of stasis**
Ref: Chapter No.20, Page No.486

13. **Ans: B. Zone of stasis**
Ref: Chapter No.20, Page No.486

14. **Ans: C. Zone of hyperaemia**
Ref: Chapter No.20, Page No.486

15. **Ans: A. Zone of coagulation**
Ref: Chapter No.20, Page No.486

16. **Ans: A. Superficial burns**
Ref: Chapter No.20, Page No.486

17. **Ans: D. Treatment is aimed at dressings**
Ref: Chapter No.20, Page No.486

18. **Ans: B. Hair follicles are not viable and intact**
Ref: Chapter No.20, Page No.486

19. **Ans: B. 7 to 14 days**
Ref: Chapter No.20, Page No.486

20. **Ans: C. 15 to 21 days**
Ref: Chapter No.20, Page No.486

21. **Ans: B. Not painful to pinprick**
Ref: Chapter No.20, Page No.486

22. **Ans: D. Full-thickness burns can extend below the superficial fat, but doesn't involve other structures, such as muscle and bone**
Ref: Chapter No.20, Page No.486

23. **Ans: B. Judgment of experienced practitioners**
Ref: Chapter No.20, Page No.486

24. **Ans: A. 1% of the TBSA**
Ref: Chapter No.20, Page No.487

25. **Ans: C. 21% of the TBSA**
Ref: Chapter No.20, Page No.487

26. **Ans: A. 13% of the TBSA**
Ref: Chapter No.20, Page No.487

27. **Ans: B. Berkow**

Ref: Chapter No.20, Page No.487

28. **Ans: C. High-dose vitamin C. therapy**

Ref: Chapter No.20, Page No.488

29. **Ans: D. All of the above are true**

Ref: Chapter No.20, Page No.488

30. **Ans: C. More than 20% TBSA**

Ref: Chapter No.20, Page No.488

31. **Ans: C. Total neutrophil counts are initially decreased after burn by demargination and decreased cell death by apoptosis**

Ref: Chapter No.20, Page No.488

32. **Ans: B. Early burn wound excision decreases cytotoxic T-cell activity**

Ref: Chapter No.20, Page No.488-489

33. **Ans: D. All of the above**

Ref: Chapter No.20, Page No.489

34. **Ans: C. 3 hours of the injury**

Ref: Chapter No.20, Page No.490

35. **Ans: C. >40% TBSA**

Ref: Chapter No.20, Page No.491

36. **Ans: D. The presence of pulses or Doppler signals in the distal extremities may not be adequate to determine adequate circulation of blood**

Ref: Chapter No.20, Page No.491

37. **Ans: B. Damp dressings can be used**

Ref: Chapter No.20, Page No.491

38. **Ans: B. Lactated Ringer's solution without dextrose**

Ref: Chapter No.20, Page No.491

39. **Ans: C. 5% dextrose Ringer's lactate**

Ref: Chapter No.20, Page No.491

40. **Ans: B. 4 cc/kg/% TBSA burned**

Ref: Chapter No.20, Page No.492

41. **Ans: A. 2 cc/kg/% TBSA burned**

Ref: Chapter No.20, Page No.492

42. **Ans: A. 5000 cc/m^2 burned + 1500 cc/m^2 total surface area**

Ref: Chapter No.20, Page No.492

43. **Ans: A. 10%**

Ref: Chapter No.20, Page No.492

44. **Ans: D. The most common complications associated with fasciotomy is infection**

Ref: Chapter No.20, Page No.492

45. **Ans: D. All of the above are true**

Ref: Chapter No.20, Page No.492-493

46. **Ans: B. Bronchoscopy**

Ref: Chapter No.20, Page No.493

47. **Ans: D. Initial treatment is 80% oxygen**

Ref: Chapter No.20, Page No.493

48. **Ans: B. Foul smelling**

Ref: Chapter No.20, Page No.493

49. **Ans: B. Neurologic changes**

Ref: Chapter No.20, Page No.493

50. **Ans: D. All of the above are true**

Ref: Chapter No.20, Page No.493-494

51. **Ans: C. 200 times**

Ref: Chapter No.20, Page No.493

52. **Ans: C. Levels at 20%**

Ref: Chapter No.20, Page No.494

53. **Ans: D. Levels above 30%**

Ref: Chapter No.20, Page No.494

54. **Ans: D. All of the above**

Ref: Chapter No.20, Page No.494

55. **Ans: C. Early pneumonias are usually caused by Pseudomonas and Klebsiella**

Ref: Chapter No.20, Page No.494

56. **Ans: D. All of the above**

Ref: Chapter No.20, Page No.494

57. **Ans: A. Prophylactic antibiotics for inhalation injury are indicated**

Ref: Chapter No.20, Page No.494

58. **Ans: A. All treatments are aimed at slow and less painful healing**

Ref: Chapter No.20, Page No.494-495

59. **Ans: D. >10^5 organisms per gram of tissue**

Ref: Chapter No.20, Page No.495

60. **Ans: D. All of the following**

Ref: Chapter No.20, Page No.495

61. **Ans: D. It must be changed once in 3-4 days**

Ref: Chapter No.20, Page No.495-496

62. **Ans: B. Silver sulfadiazine**

Ref: Chapter No.20, Page No.496

63. **Ans: D. All of the above**

Ref: Chapter No.20, Page No.495

64. **Ans: A. Mafenide acetate**

Ref: Chapter No.20, Page No.495

65. **Ans: A. 0.5 % Mafenide acetate is used**

Ref: Chapter No.20, Page No.495-496

66. **Ans: B. Painful (Not painful dressing changes but application)**

Ref: Chapter No.20, Page No.495

67. **Ans: C. Nystatin and Mafenide acetate**

Ref: Chapter No.20, Page No.495

68. **Ans: B. 5% solution**

Ref: Chapter No.20, Page No.495

69. **Ans: C. Silver nitrate 0.5%**

Ref: Chapter No.20, Page No.496

70. **Ans: A. 0.5% sodium hypochlorite**

Ref: Chapter No.20, Page No.496

71. **Ans: C. 0.25% acetic acid**

Ref: Chapter No.20, Page No.496

72. **Ans: A. 0.25% acetic acid**

Ref: Chapter No.20, Page No.496

73. **Ans: D. Silver nitrate 0.5%**

Ref: Chapter No.20, Page No.496

74. **Ans: D. Should generally be applied within 24 hours of the injury**

Ref: Chapter No.20, Page No.496

75. **Ans: D. 72 hours of the injury**

Ref: Chapter No.20, Page No.496

76. **Ans: D. Severely burned patients are immuno-suppressed, and biologic dressings that have adhered will get rejected**

Ref: Chapter No.20, Page No.496

77. **Ans: B. Biobrane has antimicrobial activities**

Ref: Chapter No.20, Page No.496

78. **Ans: D. The disadvantage of Integra is that it can't be used in full thickness burns to close the wound**

Ref: Chapter No.20, Page No.496-497

79. **Ans: D. The 2:1 skin heals underneath the cadaver skin in approximately 14 days and the cadaver skin falls off**

Ref: Chapter No.20, Page No.497

80. **Ans: A. Fluid collection over the graft**

Ref: Chapter No.20, Page No.497

81. **Ans: D. Inadequate excision of the wound bed**

Ref: Chapter No.20, Page No.497

82. **Ans: D. All of the above**

Ref: Chapter No.20, Page No.497-498

83. **Ans: B. 20% to 30% take up rate of the grafts after initial application**

Ref: Chapter No.20, Page No.498

84. **Ans: B. The best solution is likely delayed wound closure**

Ref: Chapter No.20, Page No.498-499

85. **Ans: B. 48 hours**

Ref: Chapter No.20, Page No.498

86. **Ans: B. 30% TBSA burns**

Ref: Chapter No.20, Page No.499

87. **Ans: B. Tracheobronchial trees**

Ref: Chapter No.20, Page No.499

88. **Ans: B. 1 mL/kg/hr**

Ref: Chapter No.20, Page No.499

89. **Ans: C. 1500 mL/m^2 TBSA +3750 mL/m^2 TBSA burned**

Ref: Chapter No.20, Page No.499

90. **Ans: D. Hyperkalemia is seen with renal insufficiency**

Ref: Chapter No.20, Page No.499

91. **Ans: B. Decline in oxygenation**

Ref: Chapter No.20, Page No.499

92. **Ans: C. 92%**

Ref: Chapter No.20, Page No.499

93. **Ans: B. Platelet counts of less than 50,000 requires treatment**

Ref: Chapter No.20, Page No.500

94. **Ans: A. 25 kcal/kg/day plus 40 kcal per percent TBSA burned per day**

Ref: Chapter No.20, Page No.500

95. **Ans: C. 1500 kcal/% TBSA burned/24 hours**

Ref: Chapter No.20, Page No.501

96. **Ans: B. The bone itself does sustain any increase in temperature or injury**

Ref: Chapter No.20, Page No.501

97. **Ans: D. Edge of the mouth**

Ref: Chapter No.20, Page No.501

98. **Ans: B. The most serious derangements occur in the first 4 hours after injury**

Ref: Chapter No.20, Page No.501

99. **Ans: B. Tissue that has questionable viability should be debrided during fasciotomy**

Ref: Chapter No.20, Page No.501

100. **Ans: B. Upto 9 months after injury**

Ref: Chapter No.20, Page No.501

101. **Ans: C. 30%**

Ref: Chapter No.20, Page No.501

102. Ans: D. All of the above

Ref: Chapter No.20, Page No.502

103. Ans: B. For all chemicals, lavage with copious quantities of clean water should not be done immediately after removing all clothing

Ref: Chapter No.20, Page No.502

104. Ans: C. 15 to 20 L

Ref: Chapter No.20, Page No.502

105. Ans: D. All of the above

Ref: Chapter No.20, Page No.502

106. Ans: A. The critical substance responsible for the skin damage is the hydrogen ion

Ref: Chapter No.20, Page No.502

107. Ans: D. All of the above are true

Ref: Chapter No.20, Page No.502

108. Ans: D. A formic acid wound typically has a brownish appearance

Ref: Chapter No.20, Page No.502

109. Ans: D. All of the above are true

Ref: Chapter No.20, Page No.502-503

110. Ans: D. The gel should be changed at 60-minute intervals until the pain subsides, an indication of removal of the active fluoride ion

Ref: Chapter No.20, Page No.502-503

21

Bites and Stings

SNAKEBITES

1. **False among the following is:**
   A. Crotalinae are more commonly known as pit vipers
   B. Pit vipers are named for their infrared sensing facial pit
   C. Upper extremity bites are more common when the victim is not intentionally handling the snake
   D. All of the above are true

2. **Crotalinae includes all except:**
   A. Rattlesnakes
   B. Texas coral snake
   C. Copperheads
   D. Cottonmouths/water moccasins

3. **Crotalinae have all except:**
   A. Elliptical pupils
   B. Triangular heads
   C. Retractable posterior fangs
   D. Heat-sensing facial pits

4. **Most patients with Crotalinae envenomation present with:**
   A. Cardiac arrest
   B. Renal failure
   C. Swelling and pain to the site of injury
   D. Psychological disturbances

5. **False about pathophysiology of snakebites is:**
   A. Crotalinae venom typically contains zinc-dependent metalloproteinases
   B. Elapidae venom contains alpha neurotoxin, which results in a direct neurotoxic effect
   C. Crotalinae envenomation is typically deposited into the subcutaneous tissue by the fangs of the viper
   D. Rattlesnake envenomation are typically less severe and less likely to require antivenin therapy

6. **False about clinical features of snakebites is:**
   A. Pain is reported as a burning that starts within minutes of envenomation
   B. Coral snake envenomation, which primarily causes neurotoxicity, may present with respiratory failure or neurologic symptoms with minimal local findings
   C. Patients report initial nausea, perioral paraesthesia, metallic taste, and muscle twitching
   D. Swelling, if progressive, rarely develops into compartment syndrome

7. **False about management of snakebites is:**
   A. All patients with signs of envenomation should be observed for at least 72 hours in the hospital
   B. Animals should not be handled because bite reflex can occur for up to 1 hour after the snake has been dead
   C. Patients with Crotalinae bites without signs of envenomation or laboratory abnormalities can be discharged after 6 to 8 hours of observation
   D. The area of the bite should be marked, and the affected area should be assessed every 15 minutes for progression until the progression has stabilized

8. **Animals should not be handled because bite reflex can occur for upto ____ after the snake has been dead.**
   A. 15 mins B. 30 mins
   C. 60 mins D. 90 mins

9. **As per snakebite severity grading scale paralysis:**
   A. Grade 1 B. Grade 2
   C. Grade 3 D. Grade 4

10. As per snakebite severity grading scale disseminated intravascular coagulopathy is seen in:

A. Grade 2 B. Grade 3
C. Grade 4 D. Both B and C

11. As per snakebite severity grading scale minimal pain and tenderness is seen in:

A. Grade 0 B. Grade 1
C. Grade 2 D. Grade 3

12. As per snakebite severity grading scale swelling and erythema of 30 cm is seen in:

A. Grade 0 B. Grade 1
C. Grade 2 D. Grade 3

13. A 45 years old farmer had a snakebite with signs of envenomation and meets the criteria for CroFab administration, all of the following can be done except:

A. Control envenomation: Give 4-6 vials of CroFab and assess for progression of swelling/pain/systemic effects
B. If no progression is seen after giving CroFab: Start maintenance dosing of 2 vials at hours 6, 12 and 18
C. If progression is seen after giving CroFab: Redose 4-6 vials of CroFab until there is improvement with no progression of envenomation symptoms
D. All of the above are true

14. False about antivenin therapy is:

A. CroFab, as its name implies, consists of fragment antigen-binding segments of the antibodies (Fab)
B. Antivenin therapy is the mainstay of treatment for significant envenomations from Crotalinae and Elapidae species
C. Pregnancy is a contraindication to CroFab
D. The initial standard dosing is four to six vials in pediatric and adult patients

15. Elective surgery must be avoided after evenomation upto:

A. 2 weeks B. 4 weeks
C. 6 weeks D. 8 weeks

16. False about fasciotomy after snakebites is:

A. There is a role for Prophylactic fasciotomy
B. Antivenin is effective in reducing compartment syndrome
C. One must refrain from debridement of injured muscle groups
D. Children and patients with bites to the hands or fingers are most likely to sustain intramuscular injection of venom

MAMMALIAN BITES

17. Most common animal responsible for animal bite is:

A. Cats B. Dogs
C. Tiger D. Rat

18. High risk factors for infection are all except:

A. >50 years old
B. Chronic alcoholism
C. Asplenic
D. Hypertension

19. Low risk factors for infection are all except:

A. Large, clean lacerations that can be thoroughly irrigated
B. Face
C. Wrist
D. Scalp

20. False about wound care after animal bite is:

A. Primary closure is appropriate for head and neck wounds that are initially seen within 72 hours of the bite
B. The clinician should be alert to the fact that significant dog bites may have extensive undermined areas created by the large canine teeth
C. Early wound cleaning is the most important therapy for preventing infection and zoonotic diseases such as rabies
D. All of the above are true

21. Primary closure can also be used for low-risk wounds to the arms, legs and trunk if seen within ____of the bite.

A. 12 to 24 hours B. 6 to 12 hours
C. 24 to 36 hours D. 24 to 48 hours

22. Wounds prone to the development of infection are covered with moist dressings and undergo delayed primary closure after:

A. 3 to 5 days B. 5 to 7 days
C. 8 to 10 days D. 10 to 14 days

23. Most hand lacerations are recommended to undergo:

A. Primary intention healing
B. Secondary intention healing

C. Tertiary intention healing
D. None

24. Clenched fist injury (fight bite), false statement is:

A. Clenched fist injury (fight bite) results from striking the tooth of another person's mouth
B. All bite injuries are re-evaluated in 1 or 2 days to rule out secondary infection
C. Regardless of the history obtained, injuries over the dorsum of the metacarpophalangeal joints are treated as clenched fist injuries
D. Minor injuries require exploration and debridement in the operating room and administration of IV antibiotics

25. Most common bacterial pathogen, found in dog bites and cat bites is:

A. Pasteurella spp B. Staphylococcus
C. Streptococcus D. Anaerobes

26. In addition to the microorganisms found after dog and cat bites, human bite wounds are typically contaminated with:

A. Staphylococcus epidermidis
B. Veillonella parvula
C. Eikenella corrodens
D. Fusobacterium spp.

27. Infections developing within 24 hours of the bite are generally caused by:

A. Pasteurella spp B. Staphylococcus
C. Streptococcus D. Anaerobes

28. False about Rabies among the following is:

A. Bats have been the main source of human rabies reported in the United States
B. If rabies exposure is strongly suspected, consider closing the wound open
C. Rabies is caused by a rhabdovirus found in the saliva of animals and is transmitted through bites or scratches
D. The more common encephalitic or furious form is typified by fever and hyperactivity that can be stimulated by internal or external factors

29. True about rabies prophylaxis is all except:

A. Passive immunization consists of administering 20 IU/kg body weight of rabies immune globulin
B. Rabies prophylaxis involves passive (with rabies immune globulin) and active (with rabies vaccine) immunization
C. Patients with preexposure immunization do not require passive immunization and need active immunization only on days 0 and 3
D. If the human rabies immune globulin is not given immediately, it can still be administered for up to 3 days

ARTHROPOD BITES AND STINGS

30. Female black widow spider has a leg span of:

A. 1 to 4 cms B. 4 to 7 cms
C. 7 to 10 cms D. 10 to 15 cms

31. The major component of black widow spider is:

A. Alpha-latrotoxin
B. Alpha-guanosine
C. Alpha-adenosine
D. Sphingomyelinase D

32. After the bite of black widow spider neuromuscular symptoms occurs after:

A. 5 minutes B. 15 minutes
C. 30 minutes D. 60 mintues

33. False about treatment of black widow spider is:

A. IV calcium gluconate is recommended as a first-line drug to relieve muscle spasms after widow spider bites
B. Antivenin has been shown to reduce or eliminate symptoms of latrodectism
C. Narcotics and benzodiazepines are more effective agents to relieve muscular pain
D. Patients about to receive antivenom may be pre-treated with antihistamines to reduce the likelihood or severity of a systemic reaction to the serum

34. Antivenom after black widow spider bite is currently recommended for:

A. Pregnant women
B. Children younger than 10 years
C. Adults older than 60 years
D. Patients with uncontrolled hypertension

35. Typical violin-shaped marking on the cephalothorax is seen on:

A. Scorpions
B. Ticks
C. Black Widow Spiders
D. Brown Recluse Spiders

36. The major deleterious factor in Brown Recluse Spider's venom is:

A. Sphingomyelinase A
B. Sphingomyelinase B
C. Sphingomyelinase C
D. Sphingomyelinase D

37. True about the clinical manifestations of Brown Recluse Spider's bite are all except:

A. In more severe bites, the central area turns purple as a result of microvascular thrombosis
B. Peripheral vasoconstriction can also create a pale border surrounding the central region of necrosis
C. Systemic features include headache, nausea and vomiting, fever, malaise, arthralgia and maculopapular rash
D. Systemic loxoscelism is more common in adults and can occur with minimal local findings

38. After Brown Recluse Spider's bite necrosis is the most severe in areas such as the:

A. Breast B. Abdomen
C. Upper limbs D. Neck

39. False statement about the treatment of Brown Recluse Spider's bite is:

A. Brown spider bites in which necrosis does not develop within 72 hours generally heal well and require no additional therapy
B. Heat therapy inhibits venom activity and has been reported to reduce inflammation and necrosis
C. Dapsone may reduce local inflammation and necrosis by inhibiting neutrophil function
D. Diphenhydramine has been suggested to be of benefit and is associated with a much more favourable risk profile

40. Dapsone can cause methemoglobinemia and is contraindicated in patients with:

A. Lactose intolerant
B. G6PD deficiency
C. Alcohol dehydrogenase deficiency
D. All of the above

41. Dapsone is not approved for use in:

A. Adults B. Elderly
C. Children D. None of the above

42. In the treatment of Brown Recluse Spider's bite all of the following are true except:

A. In severe cases, wide excision and split-thickness skin grafting are necessary while dapsone therapy is continued
B. Early surgical intervention, other than simple conservative debridement of obviously necrotic tissue, is done
C. Pyoderma gangrenosum, manifested as nonhealing ulcers and failure of skin grafts, occurs more often in patients undergoing early excision and debridement
D. Primary staphylococcal soft tissue infections are much more prevalent than brown recluse spider bites and are often attributed to "spider bites"

43. False statement about scorpion bite is:

A. The bark scorpion is a yellow-to-brown crablike arthropod up to 5 cm in length
B. If systemic signs are present, an equine-derived Fab antivenin approved by the FDA is available for use
C. Scorpions tend to be diurnal and sting when threatened
D. Neurotoxic scorpion venoms can cause rapid systemic toxicity and potentially death

44. False about ticks is:

A. Proper removal involves grasping the tick by the body as close to the skin surface as possible with an instrument and applying gradual, gentle axial traction, without twisting
B. Crushing the tick can be done in some cases
C. If the tick was embedded for less than 24 hours, the risk of transmitting infection is very low
D. Any retained mouthparts of the tick are removed with the tip of a needle

45. The most common vector-borne disease in the United States is:

A. Colorado tick fever B. Lyme disease
C. Babesiosis D. Relapsing fever

46. Incubation period of Borrelia burgdorferi is:

A. 30 to 60 days B. 7 to 10 days
C. 3 to 30 days D. 45 to 60 days

47. False about the rash in Lyme's disease is:

A. The rash is erythema migrans, is typically a round or oval erythematous lesion that begins at the bite site and expands at a relatively rapid rate, up to 1 cm/day, to a median size of 15 cm in diameter
B. Without treatment, the rash fades in approximately 2 weeks
C. Fatigue, myalgia, headache, fever, nausea, vomiting, regional lymphadenopathy, sore

throat, photophobia, anorexia, and arthralgia may accompany the rash

D. All of the following are true

48. Neuroborreliosis occurs in approximately _______ of untreated patients.

A. 15% B. 5%
C. 25% D. 60%

49. Cardiac findings occur in approximately _______ of untreated patients.

A. 15% B. 5%
C. 25% D. 60%

50. Oligoarticular arthritis is a common finding in early disseminated Lyme disease and occurs in approximately ____ of untreated victims.

A. 15% B. 5%
C. 25% D. 60%

51. First-line treatment of early or disseminated Lyme disease, in the absence of neurologic involvement, is:

A. Oral azithromycin for 3 to 5 days
B. Oral erythromycin for 14 to 21 days
C. Oral doxycycline for 14 to 21 days
D. Oral doxycycline for 7 to 14 days

52. The second-line agent for use in children 8 years of age or younger and pregnant women is:

A. Doxycycline B. Amoxicillin
C. Erythromycin D. Ceftriaxone

53. Neuroborreliosis or patients with cardiac manifestations, treatment consists of:

A. Daily IV ceftriaxone for 7 to 14 days
B. Daily IV ceftriaxone for 14 to 28 days
C. Daily IV Amoxicillin for 7 to 14 days
D. Daily IV Amoxicillin for 14 to 28 days

54. Tick bite prophylaxis to prevent Lyme disease is:

A. Single dose of doxycycline 100 mg orally given within 72 hours of a tick bite
B. Single dose of doxycycline 200 mg orally given within 24 hours of a tick bite
C. Single dose of doxycycline 100 mg orally given within 24 hours of a tick bite
D. Single dose of doxycycline 200 mg orally given within 72 hours of a tick bite

55. False about Hymenoptera is:

A. Stings from fire ants characteristically produce isolated pustules from repetitive stings at the same site
B. Hymenoptera venom contains vasoactive compounds such as histamine and serotonin
C. A positive IgE mediated skin test to Hymenoptera extract helps predict an allergic sting reaction
D. The stingers of most Hymenoptera are attached to venom sacs located on the abdomen and can be used repeatedly

56. Regarding the treatment of hymenoptera, all of the following are true except:

A. Blisters and pustules (typically sterile) from fire ant stings are left intact
B. Mild anaphylaxis can be treated with 0.01 mg/kg (up to 0.5 mg) of 1:10000 (1 mg/mL, or 0.1%) intramuscular (mid-anterolateral thigh) epinephrine and an oral or parenteral antihistamine
C. If an offending bee has left behind a stinger, it is removed as quickly as possible to prevent continued injection of venom
D. Venom immunotherapy effectively prevents recurrent anaphylaxis from subsequent stings in patients with positive skin tests

MARINE BITES AND STINGS

57. False about injuries from marine organisms is:

A. Immersion in cold water predisposes patients to hypothermia and near-drowning
B. Anaphylactic reaction to venom may further complicate an envenomation
C. Late complications include unique infections caused by a wide variety of aquatic microorganisms and immune mediated phenomena
D. All of the above are true

58. General management in marine bites includes all except:

A. Computed tomography is more useful than ultrasound or MRI to identify small spine fragments
B. For large shark wounds, postoperative management may be prolonged, and common complications and sequelae of shock, massive blood transfusion, myoglobinuria and respiratory failure may occur
C. Antivenom is available for several types of envenomation, including from the box jellyfish, sea snake and stonefish
D. Large or complex wounds require exploration and management in the operating room

59. **False statement about shark injuries is:**
   A. Most incidents occur at the surface of shallow water within 100 feet of the shore
   B. Sharks locate prey by detecting motion, electrical fields, and sounds and by sensing body fluids through smell and taste
   C. Most wounds require exploration and repair in the operating room
   D. Most injuries occur to the hands

60. **False about Coelenterates is/are:**
   A. One of the most venomous creatures on earth, found primarily off the coast of northern Australia, is the box jellyfish Chironex fleckeri (sea wasp)
   B. To decontaminate other jellyfish stings, ethyl alcohol is used only if vinegar is ineffective
   C. Therapy consists of detoxification of nematocysts and systemic support
   D. Medical care providers need to wear gloves for self-protection

61. **False about the treatment of sponges is/are:**
   A. Treatment consists of gently washing and drying the affected area
   B. Dilute (5%) acetic acid (vinegar) is applied for 60 minutes four times daily
   C. Any remaining spicules can be removed with adhesive tape
   D. A steroid cream can be applied to the skin after decontamination

62. **False about Echinodermata is/are:**
   A. Starfish, sea urchins and sea cucumbers are members of the phylum Echinodermata
   B. Sea urchins are covered with venomous spines capable of causing local and systemic reactions similar to those from coelenterates
   C. A spine is always removed
   D. Retained spines may cause the formation of granulomas that are amenable to excision or intralesional injection with triamcinolone hexacetonide, 5 mg/mL

63. **False about Mollusks is:**
   A. Octopuses and cone snails are the primary envenoming species in the phylum Mollusca
   B. Blue ringed octopuses can bite and inject tetrodotoxin, a hemolytic agent
   C. Envenomation occurs from a detachable harpoon-like dart injected via an extensible proboscis into the victim
   D. Management of the bite site is best achieved by pressure and immobilization to contain the venom

64. **False about Stingrays is:**
   A. Venom is stored in whiplike caudal appendages
   B. Stingrays react defensively by thrusting their spines into a victim, causing puncture wounds and lacerations
   C. The wound is irrigated and soaked in non-scalding hot water (up to 45°C [113°F]) for 1 hour
   D. The venom is often paralytic

65. **The most common site of injury by stingrays is:**
   A. Neck
   B. Top of the foot
   C. Upper extremities
   D. Back

ANSWERS

1. **Ans: C. Upper extremity bites are more common when the victim is not intentionally handling the snake**

   Ref: Chapter No.21, Page No.506

2. **Ans: B. Texas coral snake**

   Ref: Chapter No.21, Page No.506

3. **Ans: C. Retractable posterior fangs**

   Ref: Chapter No.21, Page No.506

4. **Ans: C. Swelling and pain to the site of injury**

   Ref: Chapter No.21, Page No.506

5. **Ans: D. Rattlesnake envenomation are typically less severe and less likely to require antivenin therapy**

   Ref: Chapter No.21, Page No.506-507

6. **Ans: D. Swelling, if progressive, rarely develops into compartment syndrome**

   Ref: Chapter No.21, Page No.507-508

7. **Ans: A. All patients with signs of envenomation should be observed for at least 72 hours in the hospital**

   Ref: Chapter No.21, Page No.508

8. **Ans: C. 60 mins**

   Ref: Chapter No.21, Page No.508

9. **Ans: D. Grade 4**

   Ref: Chapter No.21, Page No.508

10. **Ans: D. Both B and C**

    Ref: Chapter No.21, Page No.508

11. **Ans: A. Grade 0**

    Ref: Chapter No.21, Page No.508

12. **Ans: C. Grade 2**

    Ref: Chapter No.21, Page No.508

13. **Ans: D. All of the above are true**

    Ref: Chapter No.21, Page No.509

14. **Ans: C. Pregnancy is a contraindication to CroFab**

    Ref: Chapter No.21, Page No.509

15. **Ans: A. 2 weeks**

    Ref: Chapter No.21, Page No.509

16. **Ans: A. There is role for Prophylactic fasciotomy**

    Ref: Chapter No.21, Page No.509

17. **Ans: B. Dogs**

    Ref: Chapter No.21, Page No.510

18. **Ans: D. Hypertension**

    Ref: Chapter No.21, Page No.510

19. **Ans: C. Wrist**

    Ref: Chapter No.21, Page No.510

20. **Ans: A. Primary closure is appropriate for head and neck wounds that are initially seen within 72 hours of the bite**

    Ref: Chapter No.21, Page No.510-511

21. **Ans: B. 6 to 12 hours**

    Ref: Chapter No.21, Page No.510

22. **Ans: A. 3 to 5 days**

    Ref: Chapter No.21, Page No.510

23. **Ans: B. Secondary intention healing**

    Ref: Chapter No.21, Page No.511

24. **Ans: D. Minor injuries require exploration and debridement in the operating room and administration of IV antibiotics**

    Ref: Chapter No.21, Page No.511

25. **Ans: A. Pasteurella spp**

    Ref: Chapter No.21, Page No.511

26. **Ans: C. Eikenella corrodens**

    Ref: Chapter No.21, Page No.511

27. **Ans: A. Pasteurella spp**

    Ref: Chapter No.21, Page No.511

28. **Ans: B. If rabies exposure is strongly suspected, consider closing the wound open**

    Ref: Chapter No.21, Page No.512

29. **Ans: D. If the human rabies immune globulin is not given immediately, it can still be administered for up to 3 days**

    Ref: Chapter No.21, Page No.512

30. **Ans: A. 1 to 4 cms**

    Ref: Chapter No.21, Page No.512

31. **Ans: A. Alpha-latrotoxin**

    Ref: Chapter No.21, Page No.513

32. **Ans: C. 30 minutes**

    Ref: Chapter No.21, Page No.513

33. **Ans: A. IV calcium gluconate is recommended as a first-line drug to relieve muscle spasms after widow spider bites**

    Ref: Chapter No.21, Page No.513

34. **Ans: B. Children younger than 10 years**

    Ref: Chapter No.21, Page No.513

35. **Ans: D. Brown Recluse Spiders**

Ref: Chapter No.21, Page No.513

36. **Ans: D. Sphingomyelinase D**

Ref: Chapter No.21, Page No.513

37. **Ans: D. Systemic loxoscelism is more common in adults and can occur with minimal local findings**

Ref: Chapter No.21, Page No.513-514

38. **Ans: B. Abdomen**

Ref: Chapter No.21, Page No.513

39. **Ans: B. Heat therapy inhibits venom activity and has been reported to reduce inflammation and necrosis**

Ref: Chapter No.21, Page No.514

40. **Ans: B. G6PD deficiency**

Ref: Chapter No.21, Page No.514

41. **Ans: C. Children**

Ref: Chapter No.21, Page No.513

42. **Ans: B. Early surgical intervention, other than simple conservative debridement of obviously necrotic tissue, is done**

Ref: Chapter No.21, Page No.514

43. **Ans: C. Scorpions tend to be diurnal and sting when threatened**

Ref: Chapter No.21, Page No.514

44. **Ans: B. Crushing the tick can be done in some cases**

Ref: Chapter No.21, Page No.514-515

45. **Ans: B. Lyme disease**

Ref: Chapter No.21, Page No.515

46. **Ans: C. 3 to 30 days**

Ref: Chapter No.21, Page No.515

47. **Ans: B. Without treatment, the rash fades in approximately 2 weeks**

Ref: Chapter No.21, Page No.515

48. **Ans: A. 15%**

Ref: Chapter No.21, Page No.515

49. **Ans: B. 5%**

Ref: Chapter No.21, Page No.515

50. **Ans: D. 60%**

Ref: Chapter No.21, Page No.515

51. **Ans: C. Oral doxycycline for 14 to 21 days**

Ref: Chapter No.21, Page No.515

52. **Ans: B. Amoxicillin**

Ref: Chapter No.21, Page No.515

53. **Ans: B. Daily IV ceftriaxone for 14 to 28 days**

Ref: Chapter No.21, Page No.515

54. **Ans: D. Single dose of doxycycline 200 mg orally given within 72 hours of a tick bite**

Ref: Chapter No.21, Page No.515

55. **Ans: A. Stings from fire ants characteristically produce isolated pustules from repetitive stings at the same site**

Ref: Chapter No.21, Page No.515-516

56. **Ans: B. Mild anaphylaxis can be treated with 0.01 mg/kg (up to 0.5 mg) of 1:10000 (1 mg/mL, or 0.1%) intramuscular (mid-anterolateral thigh) epinephrine and an oral or parenteral antihistamine**

Ref: Chapter No.21, Page No.516

57. **Ans: D. All of the above are true**

Ref: Chapter No.21, Page No.516

58. **Ans: A. Computed tomography is more useful than ultrasound or MRI to identify small spine fragments**

Ref: Chapter No.21, Page No.516-517

59. **Ans: D. Most injuries occur to the hands**

Ref: Chapter No.21, Page No.517

60. **Ans: B. To decontaminate other jellyfish stings, ethyl alcohol is used only if vinegar is ineffective**

Ref: Chapter No.21, Page No.517

61. **Ans: B. Dilute (5%) acetic acid (vinegar) is applied for 60 minutes four times daily**

Ref: Chapter No.21, Page No.518

62. **Ans: C. A spine is always removed**

Ref: Chapter No.21, Page No.518

63. **Ans: B. Blue ringed octopuses can bite and inject tetrodotoxin, a hemolytic agent**

Ref: Chapter No.21, Page No.518

64. **Ans: D. The venom is often paralytic**

Ref: Chapter No.21, Page No.518

65. **Ans: B. Top of the foot**

Ref: Chapter No.21, Page No.518

22

Surgical Critical Care

NEUROLOGIC SYSTEM

1. **False about opioids is:**
   A. Have a slower onset of action
   B. Highly effective for nonneuropathic pain
   C. Opioids have traditionally been the first-line therapy for pain as they are centrally acting
   D. Can be administered via multiple routes

2. **All of the following are true about opioids except:**
   A. Prolonged use can also result in physiologic dependence, tolerance and opioid-induced hyperalgesia
   B. Opioids are often under-prescribed
   C. Deleterious side effects including nausea, vomiting, pruritis, sedation, respiratory depression
   D. The use of multimodal pain medications has become the standard of care to reduce opioid reliance and should be implemented widely

3. **Agitation is quantified using various scoring systems to include the:**
   A. Alan Agitation-Sedation Scale
   B. Richmond Agitation-Sedation Scale
   C. Richard Agitation-Sedation Scale
   D. Raymond Agitation-Sedation Scale

4. **The most commonly used sedatives in the ICU include all except:**
   A. Benzodiazepines B. Propofol
   C. Ketamine D. Dexmedetomidine

5. **False about propofol is all except:**
   A. Rapid clearance of propofol makes it the ideal drug for daily sedation weans to assess a patient's neurologic status
   B. Propofol is a highly protein-bound, lipophilic molecule that is frequently utilized in the ICU
   C. Hypotension and cardiovascular depression are commonly seen with propofol administration, especially in the hypovolemic patient
   D. Propofol is highly lipophilic, it readily traverses the blood-brain barrier and results in rapid onset of action in <1 hr as well as a short duration of action

6. **False about propofol infusion syndrome is:**
   A. Common complication associated with prolonged and/or high doses of propofol administration that is thought to be caused by mitochondrial respiratory chain inhibition
   B. Treatment is fairly limited to supportive care and discontinuing propofol administration
   C. Clinical features include bradycardia, rhabdomyolysis, hyperlipidemia, hepatomegaly and renal failure
   D. Early recognition is critical because it has a high mortality rate

7. **The most serious potential side effects of propofol infusion include all except:**
   A. Hypertriglyceridemia
   B. Propofol infusion syndrome
   C. Hypertension
   D. Pancreatitis

8. **False about benzodiazepines is:**
   A. All benzodiazepines can be administered intermittently and have rapid onsets of action
   B. Treatment is limited to dialysis and discontinuing the offending agent
   C. Benzodiazepines are GABA receptor agonists that produce anxiolysis at low doses and sedation, amnesia, and cardiorespiratory depression at higher doses
   D. Propylene glycol is used as the solvent for IV lorazepam and diazepam, and toxicity is rare

9. The US Food and Drug Administration (FDA) states the use of dexmedetomidine for initial sedation should be limited to:

A. 6 hours B. 12 hours
C. 24 hours D. 48 hours

10. False about dexmedetomidine is:

A. Studies have also demonstrated that dexmedetomidine usage results in extubation almost 2 days sooner compared to midazolam use
B. The main disadvantage of dexmedetomidine is that it has an effect on respiratory drive, so patients on sedation need mechanical ventilation
C. It has a relatively quick onset of action between 5 and 15 minutes and a duration of action between 60 and 120 minutes
D. The adverse effects of dexmedetomidine use include bradycardia, hypotension, atrial fibrillation, and reflex hypertension with abrupt cessation of administration

11. False about delirium among the following is:

A. New-onset delirium has been documented to result in a statistically significant increase in the 90-day mortality rate
B. The elderly and patients with prior mental illness or decreased cognition are at lower risk for developing hypoactive delirium
C. The basis of treatment includes identifying and reversing any potential organic causes and providing supportive measures that bring the patient's behavioural alterations back to baseline
D. Delirium is defined as confusion along with a disturbance in focus, attention, or awareness that occurs over a short period of time

12. False about encephalopathy is:

A. Acute encephalopathy can potentially be reversed with a return to baseline functional status if the inciting insult is removed or treated in a timely fashion
B. Chronic encephalopathy is slow to progress and results in structural changes in the brain that are usually reversible
C. Encephalopathy is a term to describe an altered mental state per the underlying pathophysiologic process
D. Encephalopathy develops as a syndrome of overall brain dysfunction and can occur from many organic and inorganic causes that directly induce brain injury or remotely affect the brain from other systemic causes

13. When comatose patients have a GCS score of______, their brain injury or dysfunction is deemed severe and they should be intubated as they cannot reliably protect their airway.

A. 12 or lower B. 10 or lower
C. 8 or lower D. 6 or lower

14. Most common cause of death and disability in people between the ages of 15 and 30 is:

A. Chest trauma
B. Traumatic brain injury
C. Spine injury
D. Extremity trauma

15. False about traumatic brain injury is:

A. Management and treatments are focused on optimizing intracranial pressure and blood pressure in order to maintain adequate cerebral perfusion, avoiding hypoxia, and maintaining normothermia and normoglycemia
B. Long-term prognosis and recovery are good
C. Primary brain injury occurs during the initial insult, whereas the focus of critical care management of TBI is to limit secondary brain injury
D. Secondary brain injury is a consequence of pathologic and physiologic alterations that manifest after the initial injury usually due to concomitant multiorgan injury

16. Approximately______of patients with severe TBI (GCS <8) are discharged in a vegetative state.

A. 5% to 10% B. 10% to 15%
C. 20% to 30% D. 30% to 50%

CARDIOVASCULAR SYSTEM

17. False among the following is:

A. The heart's primary node is the sinoatrial node, which is influenced by sympathetic stimulation from the sympathetic trunk mainly arising from the T1–T4 spinal levels
B. CO is 4 to 6 L/min
C. CO is defined as the blood flow put out by the heart per unit time, typically expressed in liters/min
D. During diastole, the subendocardial vessels experience retrograde flow, and thus the heart is primarily supplied during systole

18. False about cardiac arrythmias is:

A. Amiodarone is favoured in the context of heart failure, as it does not depress cardiac function as is done by beta blockers and calcium channel blockers

B. While all drugs used to treat atrial fibrillation may induce cardioversion into sinus rhythm, amiodarone is especially prone to do so
C. Acutely, digoxin alone is recommended
D. Traditionally, it was held that cardioversion of an atrial rhythm into sinus could safely occur up to 48 hours after initiation of the rhythm

19. **Drugs contraindicated in Wolf-Parkinson-White syndrome is/are all except:**
A. Amiodarone
B. Beta blockers
C. Calcium channel blockers
D. Ibutilide

20. **Wolf-Parkinson-White syndrome recommended drug is:**
A. Procainamide B. Amiodarone
C. ACE inhibitor D. Diuretics

21. **Multifocal atrial tachycardia is most commonly associated with:**
A. Hypocalcaemia B. Hypokalaemia
C. Hypomagnesemia D. Hyponatremia

22. **False about multifocal atrial tachycardia is:**
A. Empiric push of 6 mg of IV magnesium sulfate terminated multifocal atrial tachycardia
B. Pulmonary insufficiency, hypokalaemia, and coronary artery disease are known precipitating factors
C. Multifocal atrial tachycardia is most commonly associated with hypomagnesemia
D. If correcting hypokalemia and hypomagnesemia (in that order) are not effective, then beta blockers should not be tried

23. **FDA approved for the conversion of atrial flutter to normal sinus rhythm is:**
A. Amiodarone
B. Ibutilide
C. Calcium channel blockers
D. Procainamide

24. **False about atrial flutter is:**
A. It is not infrequent following the treatment of atrial fibrillation with amiodarone
B. IV magnesium given alongside ibutilide both enhance its ability to break atrial flutter and prevent torsade de pointes
C. Ibutilide is FDA approved for the conversion of atrial flutter to normal sinus rhythm and has not shown to be superior to amiodarone and procainamide
D. The management of atrial flutter is similar to that of atrial fibrillation, with rate and rhythm control options, but electrocardioversion is the preferred therapy

25. **Most common paroxysmal supraventricular tachycardia is:**
A. Atrioventricular re-entrant tachycardia
B. Atrioventricular nodal re-entrant tachycardia
C. Paroxysmal atrial tachycardia
D. Supraventricular Ectopy

26. **False about bradycardia is:**
A. Sinus bradycardia associated with MI, commonly seen in inferior wall infarctions due to involvement of the sinoatrial node
B. Sinus bradycardia secondary to a spinal cord injury can occur in high (cervical) spinal cord injuries
C. Bradycardia is most prevalent in general ICU populations, as it is a sign of profound cardiac dysfunction and sometimes a periarrest rhythm
D. Sinus bradycardia secondary to the use of dexmedetomidine; atropine and epinephrine will be effective

27. **False about neurogenic shock is:**
A. Spinal cord injuries, below C5, the hypotension causes an appropriate reflex bradycardia
B. The overall etiology is decreased vascular resistance
C. Treatment consists of vasopressor support to maintain blood pressure
D. Neurogenic shock occurs secondary to the loss of sympathetic tone after a spinal cord injury

28. **In higher spinal cord injuries, C5 and above, the patient is often:**
A. Tachycardic B. Bradycardic
C. Hypertensive D. None of the above

29. **False about septic shock is:**
A. Organ dysfunction represented by an increase in SOFA score of 3 or more represents sepsis
B. Vasopressors are the first choice for septic shock
C. Septic shock arises from inflammatory mediators released by the body in response to bacterial or fungal pathogens and is considered a dysregulated immune response
D. Septic shock was then sepsis unresponsive to fluid resuscitation requiring vasopressor support to maintain the blood pressure

30. **False about Surviving Sepsis Campaign guidelines in 2017 is:**
    - A. It is recommended continued close monitoring, a target mean arterial pressure of 75 mm Hg
    - B. Recommends the use of so-called dynamic parameters, including passive leg raise, fluid challenges, pulse pressure variation in response to mechanical ventilation instead of central lines
    - C. Clinical judgment must still be used to guide fluid resuscitation and vasopressor therapy in septic shock states
    - D. Using lactate as a measure of tissue hypo-perfusion and as a guide to resuscitation

31. **False about Surviving Sepsis Campaign guidelines in 2017 is:**
    - A. Phenylephrine has been associated with lower in-hospital mortality in septic shock
    - B. The current recommendation by the Surviving Sepsis Campaign is for low-dose steroids in vasopressor-dependent, volume-replete septic shock
    - C. High-dose vasopressin is not recommended
    - D. Dobutamine may also be used to augment tissue perfusion if the CO is low

32. **True about hemorrhagic shock is/are:**
    - A. Crystalloid administration leads to increased coagulopathy and can increase the blood pressure, resulting in more bleeding
    - B. It should be noted that a strict 1:1:1 ratio was shown to be no better than a 1:1:2 ratio of FFP to platelets to PRBCs in patients with severe trauma
    - C. In hemorrhagic shock, blood products are the resuscitative fluid of choice
    - D. All of the above

33. **False about right heart failure:**
    - A. Inodilators both dilate the vasculature, reducing blood pressure, and promote CO by increasing contractility
    - B. Inodilators in conjunction with vasopressors such as norepinephrine are a commonly pursued strategy
    - C. Inodilators are ideal choices when the CO is low and the SVR low
    - D. The mainstay of right heart failure therapy is fluid boluses until the central venous pressure is above 15 mm Hg, followed by inodilator therapy with dobutamine or milrinone

34. **False about myocardial ischemia is:**
    - A. The treatment of a type I MI in the postoperative period focuses on a percutaneous coronary intervention with thrombolysis as an option
    - B. Type 2 MI is based upon a mismatch of the supply of blood and the heart's demand for it and is also commonly referred to as demand ischemia
    - C. Type I MI is based upon atherosclerotic plaque rupture, and consequent ischemia and infarction of muscle that was being supplied by that blood vessel
    - D. The treatment for type 1 MI is reduction of cardiac oxygen demand

35. **In NSTEMI, intervention can be delayed in some cases up to:**
    - A. 12 hours
    - B. 24 hours
    - C. 48 hours
    - D. 72 hours

RESPIRATORY SYSTEM

36. **False about oxygen therapy is:**
    - A. In intubated and mechanically ventilated patients, a target FiO_2 should be less than 50% if tolerated
    - B. 100% FiO_2 can be lethal to SCUBA divers, and supplemental oxygen given to heart attack patients who did not have hypoxia (O_2 saturation >94%) caused increased infarct size at 6 months and no mortality benefit
    - C. It must be emphasized that oxygen itself is a drug, with risks and benefits
    - D. All of the above are true

37. **False about volume assist control ventilation is:**
    - A. The four basic settings in this mode include respiratory rate, tidal volume, PEEP and FiO_2
    - B. Two parameters multiplied (respiratory rate and tidal volume) equal the minute ventilation
    - C. Volume assist control delivers a set tidal volume at a variable respiratory rate
    - D. It is adjustment in minute ventilation that affects clearance of CO_2 from the bloodstream

38. **Peak airway pressures greater than _____ are potentially deleterious.**
    - A. 25 mm Hg
    - B. 20 mm Hg
    - C. 35 mm Hg
    - D. 30 mm Hg

39. **In SIMV, fifth parameter is:**
    - A. Respiratory rate
    - B. Pressure support
    - C. PEEP
    - D. Tidal volume

40. Following deflation the endotracheal tube cuff, a loss of ________ of the ventilated volume should be observed.

A. 5% to 10%
B. 10% to 20%
C. 20% to 25%
D. 30% to 40%

41. A spontaneous breathing trial is performed by placing the patient on pressure support ventilation 5/5 at:

A. 70% FiO_2
B. 60% FiO_2
C. 50% FiO_2
D. 40% FiO_2

42. While a rapid shallow breathing index a value _____ is essentially a guarantee of extubation failure.

A. <105
B. >105
C. <110
D. >110

43. Which of the following is not indicative of successful extubation?

A. Respiratory rate <25
B. Tidal volume >5 cc/kg
C. Minute ventilation <10 L/min
D. Minute ventilation 10 cc/kg

44. Pneumonia is diagnosed by infiltrate on chest radiograph together with all except:

A. Fever
B. Hemoptysis
C. Leucocytosis
D. Purulent secretions

45. The recommendation is for direct ICU admission in community acquired pneumonia is three of the following factors except:

A. PaO_2/FiO_2 ratio <250
B. Thrombocytopenia
C. Multilobar infiltrates
D. Hyperthermia

46. The mainstay of the treatment of community-acquired pneumonia is:

A. Tetracycline + Macrolide
B. Beta-lactam + Macrolide
C. Beta-lactam + Metronidazole
D. Tetracycline + Beta-lactam

47. The diagnoses of health care-associated pneumonias (HAPs) and ventilator-associated pneumonias (VAPs) are loosely defined as pneumonia diagnosed within _____ of hospital admission and intubation.

A. 12 hours
B. 24 hours
C. 48 hours
D. 72 hours

48. Multidrug resistant pathogens, defined as prior antibiotics within:

A. 30 days
B. 60 days
C. 90 days
D. 120 days

49. Hospital acquired pneumonia should be treated with a regimen of all except:

A. Cefepime
B. Metronidazole
C. Levaquin
D. Vancomycin

50. False among the following is:

A. But the ultimate prevention measure for VAP is liberation from the mechanical ventilator as early as safely possible
B. All patients should have the head of their bed elevated to 30 degrees, a measure that can prevent HAPs, along with incentive spirometry and early mobilization
C. Prior to initiating therapy in both HAP and VAP, it is critical to send cultures (bronchoalveolar lavage or by endotracheal aspirate)
D. A key in managing HAPs and VAPs is antibiotics

51. Diagnosis of ARDS includes all except:

A. PaO_2/FiO_2 ratio <300
B. Bilateral infiltrates on chest radiograph or CT scan
C. An inciting factor within 3 days prior to the diagnosis
D. Rule-out of hydrostatic edema as a cause of the bilateral infiltrates

52. PaO_2/FiO_2 ratio in severe ARDS is:

A. <300
B. <200
C. <100
D. <50

53. The mainstay of treatment was lung protective ventilation; it includes:

A. Plateau pressure $\leq$30 cm H_2O
B. Requires lower PEEP settings
C. 4 to 6 cc/kg tidal volumes
D. SpO_2 88% to 95%

54. False about ARDS is:

A. Fluid diuresis and optimization of fluid status to reduce any extrapulmonary edema are a sensible first step
B. Steroids, inhaled nitric oxide, inhaled epoprostenol, and high frequency oscillatory ventilation techniques have all been shown to have no mortality benefit

C. Prone positioning is one of the few options that has not been shown to reduce mortality
D. ECMO serves as a final option for refractory ARDS

GASTROINTESTINAL SYSTEM

55. **The components of a patient's overall energy expenditure include all except:**
A. Thermic effect of food (10%–15%)
B. Physical activity and exercise (20%–30%)
C. Resting energy expenditure (60%–70%)
D. Resting energy expenditure (40%–55%)

56. **Variables that can affect the accuracy of indirect calorimetry measurements include:**
A. Continuous renal replacement therapy
B. Supplemental oxygen administration
C. Presence of air leaks or chest tubes
D. All of the above

57. **According to guidelines published in 2016 by Society of Critical Care Medicine and the American Society of Parenteral and Enteral Nutrition, optimal nutrition requirements for the critically ill patient are roughly:**
A. 20 to 30 kcal/kg/day
B. 25 to 30 kcal/kg/day
C. 30 to 40 kcal/kg/day
D. 20 to 25 kcal/kg/day

58. **Serum albumin has a half-life of approximately:**
A. 2 days B. 2 weeks
C. 20 days D. 20 hours

59. **Serum transferrin has a half-life of approximately:**
A. 8 hours B. 8 days
C. 4 hours D. 4 days

60. **Prealbumin has a half-life of:**
A. 2 to 3 days B. 2 to 3 weeks
C. 2 to 3 hours D. 5 to 6 days

61. **Cross-sectional imaging at the _______ vertebrae provides precise estimates of total body composition.**
A. T10 B. T12
C. L3 D. L5

62. **Investigations into alterations of which muscle's quality and density correlate with changes in a patient's nutritional status and length of hospital stay:**
A. Pectoralis major B. Psoas muscle
C. Quadratus femoris D. Soleus muscle

63. **Before starting parenteral nutrition in well-nourished patients, it is typical to wait up to:**
A. 2 days B. 5 days
C. 7 days D. 10 days

64. **The most common organism of central line associated bloodstream infection (CLABSI) is:**
A. Pseudomonas B. Streptococcus
C. Staphylococci D. E coli

65. **Strongest risk factor for nosocomial candidemia is:**
A. Foley's catheter
B. Parenteral nutrition
C. Central line insertion
D. Tracheostomy

66. **False about refeeding syndrome is:**
A. Overfeeding results in electrolyte imbalances, hyperglycemia, and hypertriglyceridemia and complicates weaning from mechanical ventilation
B. Disuse of the GI tract results in intestinal mucosal atrophy and loss of microvilli, bile stasis, cholelithiasis and hepatic steatosis
C. Refeeding syndrome occurs secondary to full caloric administration after a period of starvation
D. Refeeding syndrome resulting in hypercalcemia, hypophosphatemia and hypomagnesemia

67. **Gastric ulcerations can be found in up to _____ of patients after severe trauma or hypotension.**
A. 50% B. 60%
C. 80% D. 90%

68. **Main risk factor associated with the formation of GI ulcerations and GI bleeding is:**
A. Mechanical ventilation for greater than 24 hours
B. Development of coagulopathy
C. Hypotension
D. Burns

69. **Cushing ulcer is seen in:**
A. Burns
B. Elevated intracranial pressures
C. Cardiogenic shock
D. High-dose corticosteroid use

70. **Curling ulcer is seen in:**
A. Burns
B. Elevated intracranial pressures
C. Cardiogenic shock
D. High-dose corticosteroid use

HEPATIC SYSTEM

71. **Clinical features that should raise suspicion for underlying liver disease include:**
A. Splenomegaly B. Temporal wasting
C. Testicular atrophy D. All of the above

72. **False about radiologic examination of liver is:**
A. Ultrasound is, however, limited by the patient's body habitus and the variability in quality of images obtained that can occur as it is technician dependent
B. MRI can be obtained if the patient has a metal device or implant
C. Started with a right upper quadrant ultrasound with duplex
D. Contrast enhanced cross-sectional imaging using CT or MRI allows for very detailed visualization of the entire liver, spleen and portal system

73. **The mortality rate at 1 year with decompensated cirrhosis is:**
A. 10% B. 20%
C. 30% D. 40%

74. **The Child-Pugh Turcot Score includes all except:**
A. International normalized ratio [INR]
B. Serum direct bilirubin
C. Prothrombin time (PT)
D. Serum albumin

75. **Perioperative mortality for abdominal surgery as per Child-Pugh-Turcot class A is:**
A. 10% B. 30%
C. 80% D. 50%

76. **Perioperative mortality for abdominal surgery as per Child-Pugh-Turcot class C is:**
A. 10% B. 30%
C. 80% D. 50%

77. **Child-Pugh-Turcot class C has a score of:**
A. 5-6 B. 7-9
C. 10-15 D. 12-15

78. **Child-Pugh-Turcot class B has how many points?**
A. 5-6 B. 7-9
C. 10-12 D. 12-15

79. **Diuretic refractory ascites has a score of:**
A. 0 B. 1
C. 2 D. 3

80. **Grade 1 has a score of:**
A. 0 B. 1
C. 2 D. 3

81. **After a transjugular intrahepatic portosystemic shunt procedure used to treat cirrhosis induced portal hypertension, the MELD score was developed as a means of predicting the:**
A. 1-month mortality rate
B. 3-month mortality rate
C. 6-month mortality rate
D. 12-month mortality rate

82. **Not used in MELD score is:**
A. Serum albumin B. INR level
C. Serum creatinine D. Serum total bilirubin

83. **MELD Score 20–29, has a 3-month mortality rate of:**
A. 6.0% B. 19.6%
C. 52.6% D. 71.3%

84. **For high-risk procedures, platelet count goals prior to surgery are ______. If not present it should be corrected.**
A. < 10,000/μL B. < 20,000/μL
C. < 50,000/μL D. < 100,000/μL

85. **The most commonly injured abdominal organ in blunt trauma is:**
A. Kidney B. Liver
C. Spleen D. Stomach

86. **The second most common in penetrating injuries is:**
A. Liver B. Intestine
C. Spleen D. Stomach

87. **Complications of nonoperative management of liver injuries include:**
A. Hemobilia B. Bile leak and biloma
C. Delayed hemorrhage D. Malnutrition

88. **False about liver injury and its management is:**
A. Preferred management of delayed bile peritonitis or rupture of subcapsular hematoma is with laparoscopy with early ERCP for suspected bile leak
B. Bile leak and biloma formation may be managed by percutaneous drainage, with ERCP with stenting strongly encouraged

C. Patients who develop hepatic necrosis may be managed by only observation
D. Hemobilia, often presenting as upper GI bleeding, should be initially managed with angiography and embolization but may require surgical intervention if uncontrolled

RENAL SYSTEM

89. Normal or nonanion gap acidosis is most commonly associated with:
A. Ketosis
B. Methanol poisoning
C. Diarrhea
D. Retention of a strong acid

90. The most common electrolyte disorder seen in the hospitalized population, including the ICU is:
A. Hypokalemia B. Hyponatremia
C. Hyperkalemia D. Hypernatremia

91. The most common cause of hyponatremia in the hospital and ICU is the:
A. SIADH
B. Diabetes Insipidus
C. Use of hypotonic maintenance solutions
D. Sepsis

92. The goal is to correct the hyponatremia no quicker than:
A. 0.5 mEq/hr B. 1.0 mEq/hr
C. 1.5 mEq/hr D. 2.0 mEq/hr

93. Correction of chronic severe (serum sodium <120 mEq) hyponatremia too quickly may result in:
A. Central medullary myelinolysis
B. Central pontine myelinolysis
C. Spinal myelolysis
D. None of the above

94. Free H_2O Deficit is calculated as:
A. Free H_2O Deficit = (Total Body H_2O)[(Serum K/4) -1]
B. Free H_2O Deficit = (Total Body H_2O)[(Serum Na/140) -1]
C. Free H_2O Deficit = (Total Body H_2O)[(Serum Ca/10) -1]
D. Free H_2O Deficit = (Total Body H_2O)[(Serum Cl/100) -1]

95. The Kidney Disease: Improving Global Outcomes criteria includes:
A. Increase in serum creatinine by ≥0.3 mg/dL (≥26.5 µmol/L) within 48 hours
B. Urine volume < 0.5 mL/kg/hr for 6 hours
C. Increase in serum creatinine to ≥1.5 times baseline, which is known or presumed to have occurred within the prior 7 days
D. All of the above

96. Intrarenal AKI is most commonly caused by:
A. Nephrolithiasis
B. Acute tubular necrosis
C. SLE
D. Hypotension

97. The gold standard for potassium removal from the body is:
A. Dialysis
B. Calcium gluconate
C. Insulin
D. Sodium polystyrene sulfonate

98. Risk for serious metabolic effects such as left ventricular depression and hemodynamic instability is seen in metabolic acidosis when pH is:
A. <7.25 B. <7.2
C. <7.15 D. <7.1

HEMATOLOGIC SYSTEM

99. False about TEG is:
A. Thromboelastogram provides a functional assay of clotting and clot lysis that can be used to guide resuscitation and treatment efforts
B. TEG was used to guide resuscitation during transplant and cardiac surgeries and was found to decrease the total administration of blood products and mortality
C. It can't accurately predict the need for transfusion for the first 24 hours after a penetrating injury
D. There are three phases of coagulation that are measured with TEG: clot initiation, clot strength, and clot stability

100. The initial results from a TEG require:
A. 10 to 15 minutes B. 15 to 30 minutes
C. 30 to 45 minutes D. 45 to 60 minutes

101. A standard PT, INR, PTT and platelet count require roughly:
A. 10 to 15 minutes B. 15 to 30 minutes
C. 30 to 45 minutes D. 45 to 60 minutes

102. False about type 1 heparin induced thrombocytopenia is:

A. Platelet counts typically nadir at approximately 100,000/µL and recover to normal levels without intervention

B. Thrombocytopenia occurs due to a nonimmune-mediated direct effect of heparin on platelets, causing aggregation

C. Type 1 HIT generally has clinical significance, causes thrombosis

D. Type 1 HIT is a mild, transient thrombocytopenia that affects approximately 10% of patients within 2 days of heparin exposure

103. False about type 2 heparin induced thrombocytopenia is:

A. The development of type 2 HIT usually occurs approximately 5 to 7 days after heparin administration

B. Type 2 HIT is a serious and life-threatening immune mediated thrombocytopenia that affects 1% to 5% of patients exposed to heparin

C. 20% to 68% of patients who develop type 2 HIT will also have arterial and venous thromboembolic events

D. Heparin will bind to circulating platelet factor 2 molecules and form immunogenic complexes that can be bound by immunoglobulin G antibodies

104. Gold standard of the laboratory assessment of HIT is:

A. ELISA

B. Serotonin release assay

C. 4 Ts score

D. None of the above

105. False about venous thromboembolism:

A. Approximately 70% of patients at risk of VTE remain untreated

B. VTE is a preventable cause of death that is common but often undiagnosed and clinically silent

C. Approximately 10% to 30% of patients with VTE die within 1 month of diagnosis

D. Omission of thromboprophylaxis after 24 hours conveys an attributable mortality of approximately 3.9% to 15.4% in patients with major trauma, sepsis, cardiac arrest, or heavy cancer burden

106. After major trauma, delays in initiating pharmacologic VTE prophylaxis after ICU admission by over 24 hours are associated with ______ increase in VTE formation.

A. Twofold B. Threefold

C. Fourfold D. Fivefold

107. Sudden death is the first symptom in ______ of pulmonary embolism.

A. 12.5% B. 25%

C. 50% D. 75%

108. Absolute contraindications to chemical thromboprophylaxis includes all except:

A. Intracranial hemorrhage

B. Mild thrombocytopenia

C. Active bleeding

D. Coagulopathy

109. For all hemodynamically stable patients including the critically ill, currently the American Association of Blood Banks (AABB) strongly recommends a restrictive transfusion threshold of a hemoglobin level of:

A. 6 g/dL B. 7 g/dL

C. 8 g/dL D. 9 g/dL

110. For patients undergoing orthopedic or cardiac surgery, a slightly more liberal transfusion threshold of hemoglobin level of _____ is recommended by the AABB.

A. 6 g/dL B. 7 g/dL

C. 8 g/dL D. 9 g/dL

ENDOCRINE SYSTEM

111. Now the standard of care of blood glucose in critically ill patients is:

A. 180 - 220 mg/dL B. 140 - 180 mg/dL

C. 120 - 150 mg/dL D. 100 - 150 mg/dL

112. Which trial demonstrated that corticosteroid administration had no effect on survival or reversal of shock in the setting of sepsis but did quicken shock reversal in patients who recovered?

A. NICE-SUGAR trial

B. CORTICUS trial

C. STEROID-SHOCK trial

D. OPTIMUS trial

113. Thyroid storm, a life-threatening condition has a mortality rate of approximately:

A. 5% to 10% B. 10% to 30%

C. 30% to 50% D. 50% to 70%

114. False about the management of thyroid storm is:

A. Glucocorticoids can also be given to decrease peripheral conversion of thyroxine to triiodothyronine and may help treat an underlying Graves' disease as the cause of thyroid storm
B. Propylthiouracil inhibit new thyroid hormone synthesis
C. Beta blockers such as propranolol or esmolol control the tachycardia and hypertension and reduce anxiety
D. When thyroid storm is suspected, treatment should be started after confirmation of diagnosis

INFECTIOUS DISEASES

115. False about Central Line Associated Bloodstream Infections is:

A. If the line is to be removed, catheter tip cultures are to be obtained, as they are often diagnostic
B. The duration of treatment varies by organism and ranges from 7 days to 6 weeks
C. Attempts at catheter salvage with antibiotics alone are not recommended in the critically ill population
D. By definition, a CLABSI is a laboratory confirmed bloodstream infection in a patient with a central line, where the cultured organism is unaffiliated with an infection from a different site

116. False about Catheter Associated Urinary Tract Infections is:

A. Optimal duration of treatment is not firmly established, yet 7 to 14 days is widely accepted based on the organism
B. CAUTI is a UTI in which the positive urinary culture is from an indwelling urinary catheter that has been in place for more than 2 calendar days
C. The diagnosis of a CAUTI is per urinalysis and urine culture with 10^4 colony forming units
D. The best treatment of CAUTI is prevention

117. The most commonly reported health care-associated infection is:

A. Central Line Associated Bloodstream Infections
B. Diarrhoea
C. Urinary Tract Infections
D. Intra-abdominal Infections

118. False about C difficile infections is:

A. Indications to sample include 5 or more watery stools in 24 hours, or significantly increased ostomy quantity and output
B. The severe metabolic derangements and end-organ failure that occur with toxic megacolon often mandate a total colectomy and end-ileostomy
C. Initial bouts of mild disease are managed with oral vancomycin over oral metronidazole
D. Factors such as antibiotic exposure, older age, and recent hospitalizations increase the risk for patients to develop C difficile diarrhea

SPECIAL ISSUES

119. The open abdomen is most commonly seen due to:

A. Acute compartment syndrome
B. Perforative peritonitis
C. Pancreatitis
D. Intestinal Obstruction

120. False about the management of open abdomen is:

A. Failure of the vacuum-assisted closure therapy system often requires replacement either at the bedside or in the operating room
B. Vacuum assisted closure therapy provides a temporarily closed environment where negative-pressure is applied to the wound
C. Vacuum assisted closure therapy systems are changed at 48-hour intervals until the abdomen is closed
D. Patients with an open abdomen need to remain intubated and on the mechanical ventilator

ANSWERS

1. **Ans: A. Have a slower onset of action**

Ref: Chapter No.22, Page No.522

2. **Ans: B. Opioids are often under-prescribed**

Ref: Chapter No.22, Page No.522

3. **Ans: B. Richmond Agitation-Sedation Scale**

Ref: Chapter No.22, Page No.522

4. **Ans: C. Ketamine**

Ref: Chapter No.22, Page No.522

5. **Ans: D. Propofol is highly lipophilic, it readily traverses the blood-brain barrier and results in rapid onset of action in <1 hr as well as a short duration of action**

Ref: Chapter No.22, Page No.522

6. **Ans: A. Common complication associated with prolonged and/or high doses of propofol administration that is thought to be caused by mitochondrial respiratory chain inhibition**

Ref: Chapter No.22, Page No.522

7. **Ans: C. Hypertension**

Ref: Chapter No.22, Page No.522

8. **Ans: A. All benzodiazepines can be administered intermittently and have rapid onsets of action**

Ref: Chapter No.22, Page No.522

9. **Ans: C. 24 hours**

Ref: Chapter No.22, Page No.522

10. **Ans: B. The main disadvantage of dexmedetomidine is that it has an effect on respiratory drive, so patients on sedation need mechanical ventilation**

Ref: Chapter No.22, Page No.522

11. **Ans: B. The elderly and patients with prior mental illness or decreased cognition are at lower risk for developing hypoactive delirium**

Ref: Chapter No.22, Page No.523

12. **Ans: B. Chronic encephalopathy is slow to progress and results in structural changes in the brain that are usually reversible**

Ref: Chapter No.22, Page No.523

13. **Ans: C. 8 or lower**

Ref: Chapter No.22, Page No.523

14. **Ans: B. Traumatic brain injury**

Ref: Chapter No.22, Page No.523

15. **Ans: B. Long-term prognosis and recovery are good**

Ref: Chapter No.22, Page No.524

16. **Ans: B. 10% to 15%**

Ref: Chapter No.22, Page No.524

17. **Ans: D. During diastole, the subendocardial vessels experience retrograde flow, and thus the heart is primarily supplied during systole**

Ref: Chapter No.22, Page No.524

18. **Ans: C. Acutely, digoxin alone is recommended**

Ref: Chapter No.22, Page No.524-525

19. **Ans: D. Ibutilide**

Ref: Chapter No.22, Page No.525

20. **Ans: A. Procainamide**

Ref: Chapter No.22, Page No.525

21. **Ans: C. Hypomagnesemia**

Ref: Chapter No.22, Page No.525

22. **Ans: D. If correcting hypokalemia and hypomagnesemia (in that order) are not effective, then beta blockers should not be tried**

Ref: Chapter No.22, Page No.525

23. **Ans: B. Ibutilide**

Ref: Chapter No.22, Page No.525

24. **Ans: C. Ibutilide is FDA approved for the conversion of atrial flutter to normal sinus rhythm and has not shown to be superior to amiodarone and procainamide**

Ref: Chapter No.22, Page No.525

25. **Ans: B. Atrioventricular nodal re-entrant tachycardia**

Ref: Chapter No.22, Page No.525

26. **Ans: D. Sinus bradycardia secondary to the use of dexmedetomidine; atropine and epinephrine will be effective**

Ref: Chapter No.22, Page No.526

27. **Ans: A. Spinal cord injuries, below C5, the hypotension causes an appropriate reflex bradycardia**

Ref: Chapter No.22, Page No.526

28. **Ans: B. Bradycardic**

Ref: Chapter No.22, Page No.526

29. **Ans: A. Organ dysfunction represented by an increase in SOFA score of 3 or more represents sepsis**

Ref: Chapter No.22, Page No.526

30. **Ans: A. It is recommended continued close monitoring, a target mean arterial pressure of 75 mm Hg**

Ref: Chapter No.22, Page No.526

31. **Ans: A. Phenylephrine has been associated with lower in-hospital mortality in septic shock**

Ref: Chapter No.22, Page No.527

32. **Ans: D. All of the above**

Ref: Chapter No.22, Page No.527

33. **Ans: C. Inodilators are ideal choices when the CO is low and the SVR low**

Ref: Chapter No.22, Page No.527

34. **Ans: D. The treatment for type 1 MI is reduction of cardiac oxygen demand**

Ref: Chapter No.22, Page No.528

35. **Ans: D. 72 hours**

Ref: Chapter No.22, Page No.528

36. **Ans: D. All of the above are true**

Ref: Chapter No.22, Page No.529

37. **Ans: C. Volume assist control delivers a set tidal volume at a variable respiratory rate**

Ref: Chapter No.22, Page No.529-530

38. **Ans: C. 35 mm Hg**

Ref: Chapter No.22, Page No.530

39. **Ans: B. Pressure support**

Ref: Chapter No.22, Page No.530

40. **Ans: B. 10% to 20%**

Ref: Chapter No.22, Page No.530

41. **Ans: D. 40% FiO_2**

Ref: Chapter No.22, Page No.531

42. **Ans: B. >105**

Ref: Chapter No.22, Page No.531

43. **Ans: B. Tidal volume >10 cc/kg**

Ref: Chapter No.22, Page No.531

44. **Ans: B. Hemoptysis**

Ref: Chapter No.22, Page No.531

45. **Ans: D. Hyperthermia**

Ref: Chapter No.22, Page No.531

46. **Ans: B. Beta-lactam + Macrolide**

Ref: Chapter No.22, Page No.531

47. **Ans: C. 48 hours**

Ref: Chapter No.22, Page No.531

48. **Ans: C. 90 days**

Ref: Chapter No.22, Page No.531

49. **Ans: B. Metronidazole**

Ref: Chapter No.22, Page No.531

50. **Ans: D. A key in managing HAPs and VAPs is antibiotics**

Ref: Chapter No.22, Page No.531

51. **Ans: C. An inciting factor within 3 days prior to the diagnosis**

Ref: Chapter No.22, Page No.531

52. **Ans: C. <100**

Ref: Chapter No.22, Page No.531

53. **Ans: B. Requires lower PEEP settings**

Ref: Chapter No.22, Page No.531-532

54. **Ans: C. Prone positioning is one of the few options that has not been shown to reduce mortality**

Ref: Chapter No.22, Page No.532-533

55. **Ans: D. Resting energy expenditure (40%–55%)**

Ref: Chapter No.22, Page No.533

56. **Ans: D. All of the above**

Ref: Chapter No.22, Page No.533

57. **Ans: B. 25 to 30 kcal/kg/day**

Ref: Chapter No.22, Page No.533

58. **Ans: C. 20 days**

Ref: Chapter No.22, Page No.533

59. **Ans: B. 8 days**

Ref: Chapter No.22, Page No.533

60. **Ans: A. 2 to 3 days**

Ref: Chapter No.22, Page No.533

61. **Ans: C. L3**

Ref: Chapter No.22, Page No.534

62. **Ans: B. Psoas muscle**

Ref: Chapter No.22, Page No.534

63. **Ans: C. 7 days**

Ref: Chapter No.22, Page No.534

64. **Ans: C. Staphylococci**

Ref: Chapter No.22, Page No.534

65. **Ans: B. Parenteral nutrition**

Ref: Chapter No.22, Page No.534

66. **Ans: D. Refeeding syndrome resulting in hypercalcemia, hypophosphatemia and hypomagnesemia**

Ref: Chapter No.22, Page No.534

67. **Ans: D. 90%**

Ref: Chapter No.22, Page No.535

68. **Ans: B. Development of coagulopathy**

Ref: Chapter No.22, Page No.535

69. Ans: B. Elevated intracranial pressures

Ref: Chapter No.22, Page No.535

70. Ans: A. Burns

Ref: Chapter No.22, Page No.535

71. Ans: D. All of the above

Ref: Chapter No.22, Page No.535

72. Ans: B. MRI can be obtained if the patient has a metal device or implant

Ref: Chapter No.22, Page No.535

73. Ans: B. 20%

Ref: Chapter No.22, Page No.535

74. Ans: B. Serum direct bilirubin

Ref: Chapter No.22, Page No.536

75. Ans: A. 10%

Ref: Chapter No.22, Page No.536

76. Ans: C. 80%

Ref: Chapter No.22, Page No.536

77. Ans: C. 10-15

Ref: Chapter No.22, Page No.536

78. Ans: B. 7-9

Ref: Chapter No.22, Page No.536

79. Ans: D. 3

Ref: Chapter No.22, Page No.536

80. Ans: C. 2

Ref: Chapter No.22, Page No.536

81. Ans: B. 3-month mortality rate

Ref: Chapter No.22, Page No.536

82. Ans: A. Serum albumin

Ref: Chapter No.22, Page No.536

83. Ans: B. 19.6%

Ref: Chapter No.22, Page No.536

84. Ans: D. < 100,000/μL

Ref: Chapter No.22, Page No.537

85. Ans: B. Liver

Ref: Chapter No.22, Page No.537

86. Ans: A. Liver

Ref: Chapter No.22, Page No.537

87. Ans: D. Malnutrition

Ref: Chapter No.22, Page No.537

88. Ans: C. Patients who develop hepatic necrosis may be managed by only observation

Ref: Chapter No.22, Page No.537

89. Ans: C. Diarrhea

Ref: Chapter No.22, Page No.537

90. Ans: B. Hyponatremia

Ref: Chapter No.22, Page No.538

91. Ans: C. Use of hypotonic maintenance solutions

Ref: Chapter No.22, Page No.538

92. Ans: A. 0.5 mEq/hr

Ref: Chapter No.22, Page No.538

93. Ans: B. Central pontine myelinolysis

Ref: Chapter No.22, Page No.538

94. Ans: B. Free H_2O Deficit = (Total Body H_2O)[(Serum Na/140) -1]

Ref: Chapter No.22, Page No.538

95. Ans: D. All of the above

Ref: Chapter No.22, Page No.538

96. Ans: B. Acute tubular necrosis

Ref: Chapter No.22, Page No.538

97. Ans: A. Dialysis

Ref: Chapter No.22, Page No.539

98. Ans: D. <7.1

Ref: Chapter No.22, Page No.539

99. Ans: C. It can't accurately predict the need for transfusion for the first 24 hours after a penetrating injury

Ref: Chapter No.22, Page No.539

100. Ans: A. 10 to 15 minutes

Ref: Chapter No.22, Page No.539

101. Ans: D. 45 to 60 minutes

Ref: Chapter No.22, Page No.539

102. Ans: C. Type 1 HIT generally has clinical significance, causes thrombosis

Ref: Chapter No.22, Page No.540

103. Ans: D. Heparin will bind to circulating platelet factor 2 molecules and form immunogenic complexes that can be bound by immunoglobulin G antibodies

Ref: Chapter No.22, Page No.540

104. Ans: B. Serotonin release assay

Ref: Chapter No.22, Page No.540

105. Ans: A. Approximately 70% of patients at risk of VTE remain untreated

Ref: Chapter No.22, Page No.540-541

106. Ans: B. Threefold

Ref: Chapter No.22, Page No.540

107. Ans: B. 25%

Ref: Chapter No.22, Page No.541

108. Ans: B. Mild thrombocytopenia

Ref: Chapter No.22, Page No.541

109. Ans: B. 7 g/dL

Ref: Chapter No.22, Page No.541

110. Ans: C. 8 g/dL

Ref: Chapter No.22, Page No.541

111. Ans: B. 140 - 180 mg/dL

Ref: Chapter No.22, Page No.541

112. Ans: B. CORTICUS trial

Ref: Chapter No.22, Page No.541

113. Ans: B. 10% to 30%

Ref: Chapter No.22, Page No.542

114. Ans: D. When thyroid storm is suspected, treatment should be started after confirmation of diagnosis

Ref: Chapter No.22, Page No.542

115. Ans: A. If the line is to be removed, catheter tip cultures are to be obtained, as they are often diagnostic

Ref: Chapter No.22, Page No.542

116. Ans: C. The diagnosis of a CAUTI is per urinalysis and urine culture with 10^4 colony forming units

Ref: Chapter No.22, Page No.542

117. Ans: C. Urinary Tract Infections

Ref: Chapter No.22, Page No.542

118. Ans: A. Indications to sample include 5 or more watery stools in 24 hours, or significantly increased ostomy quantity and output

Ref: Chapter No.22, Page No.543

119. Ans: A. Acute compartment syndrome

Ref: Chapter No.22, Page No.543

120. Ans: D. Patients with an open abdomen need to remain intubated and on the mechanical ventilator

Ref: Chapter No.22, Page No.543

23

Bedside Surgical Procedures

SAFETY PRACTICES FOR BEDSIDE SURGICAL PROCEDURES

1. **False among the following about the 10 safety objectives outlined in the WHO Guidelines for Safe Surgery 2009 are:**
   A. The team will operate on the correct patient at the correct site
   B. The team will recognize and effectively prepare for life-threatening loss of airway or respiratory function
   C. The team will recognize and effectively prepare for risk of high blood loss
   D. All of the above are true

2. **Fundamentals vital to the success of bedside surgical procedures are all except:**
   A. Procedure support personnel
   B. Management guidelines
   C. Skills of surgeon
   D. Supply chain

SELECTION OF PATIENTS FOR BEDSIDE SURGICAL PROCEDURES

3. **Which of the following is an indication for bedside procedures?**
   A. Decompressive celiotomy for abdominal compartment syndrome
   B. Exploratory celiotomy to rule out intra-abdominal sepsis in a patient with ventilatory requirements that prohibit safe transport to the operating room (OR)
   C. Exploratory celiotomy for intra-abdominal hemorrhage after damage control and packing
   D. All of the above

4. **Which of the following is not an indication to proceed to OR?**
   A. Surgical bleeding
   B. Need to open another body cavity
   C. Dead bowel
   D. Patient's preference

5. **Which of the following is not done for laparotomies as a bedside procedure?**
   A. The ICU attending physician will oversee anaesthetic management of the patient
   B. Preoperative antibiotics are always indicated
   C. A 4-L warm irrigation with normal saline will be used
   D. A povidone-iodine (Betadine)–chlorhexidine abdominal preparation will be used

6. **Which of the following is a commonly performed bedside procedure?**
   A. Placement of inferior vena cava filters
   B. Damage control orthopedic procedures
   C. Bronchoscopy
   D. All of the above

BEDSIDE LAPAROTOMY

7. **Common emergent indications of bedside laparotomy are all except:**
   A. Decompressive laparotomy for ACS
   B. Management of traumatic abdominal defects
   C. Suspicion of intraabdominal infection in patients too critically ill to be transported
   D. Control and packing for recurrent bleeding after a previous damage control laparotomy

8. **Common semi elective indications of bedside laparotomy are:**
   A. Pack removal after damage control laparotomy
   B. Source control for sepsis resulting from intra-abdominal pathology
   C. Irrigation and debridement of the open abdomen
   D. All of the above

9. **The most common emergent indication for bedside laparotomy:**
   A. Irrigation and debridement of the open abdomen
   B. Pack removal after damage control laparotomy
   C. Decompression of abdominal hypertension
   D. Management of traumatic abdominal defects

10. **Grade IV abdominal compartment syndrome is pressure of:**
    A. 15-20 mm Hg B. 21-25 mm Hg
    C. >25 mm Hg D. >30 mm Hg

11. **Open abdominal approach is applied to the general surgery population, most commonly for the management of:**
    A. Necrotizing soft tissue infection of the abdominal wall
    B. Mesenteric ischemia
    C. Necrotizing pancreatitis
    D. All of the above

12. **Patients who require an emergent bedside laparotomy have an extremely high rate of death, with over _____ mortality.**
    A. 20% B. 30%
    C. 50% D. 80%

TRACHEOSTOMY

13. **Indications for tracheostomy in critically ill patients include:**
    A. Upper airway obstruction
    B. Neurologic condition preventing safe extubation
    C. Prolonged mechanical ventilation
    D. All of the above

14. **Indication of tracheostomy is all except:**
    A. Severe agitation or delirium
    B. Significant maxillofacial trauma
    C. Prolonged altered mental status
    D. Fraction of inspired oxygen >70%

15. **Indication of tracheostomy is all except:**
    A. Difficult airway
    B. Angioedema
    C. Upper airway tumors
    D. Local infection or malignancy at proposed site

16. **Contraindication of tracheostomy is all except:**
    A. Recent anterior neck surgery (<7 days)
    B. Positive end expiratory pressure >10 cm H_2O
    C. Spinal cord injury
    D. Elevated intracranial pressure

17. **Contraindication of tracheostomy is all except:**
    A. Significant maxillofacial trauma
    B. Predicted early mortality
    C. Hemodynamic instability
    D. Significant bleeding risk

18. **The most common surgical procedure in critically ill patients requiring prolonged mechanical ventilation is:**
    A. Bronchoscopy
    B. Tracheostomy
    C. Cricothyroidotomy
    D. Intercoastal drain insertion

19. **False about complications of tracheotomy is:**
    A. Bronchoscopic guidance does not eliminate severe tracheal injuries
    B. Long-term, the incidence of serious tracheal stenosis after percutaneous tracheostomy is low with reports of 6%
    C. Dedicated multidisciplinary tracheostomy teams have been shown to reduce time to decannulation, length of stay and adverse events
    D. The use of preprocedure ultrasound to identify the neck anatomy is not helpful in decreasing potential risk of bleeding from crossing veins

20. **Subclinical tracheal stenosis is found in _____ of patients.**
    A. 20% B. 30%
    C. 40% D. 50%

PERCUTANEOUS ENDOSCOPIC GASTROSTOMY

21. **False about PEG is:**
    A. PEG tubes have been associated with increasing overall hospital cost

B. Accepted primary indications for a PEG or PEGJ include inability to swallow, high risk of aspiration, severe facial trauma
C. Newer PEGJ tubes combine gastric and jejunal ports to allow distal feeding and proximal decompression
D. PEG tubes may be placed in the presence of a ventriculoperitoneal shunt or a dialysis catheter

22. Indication of PEG is mechanical ventilation for longer than:

A. 1 week B. 2 weeks
C. 4 weeks D. 6 weeks

23. Although feeding can be started on the same day as the PEG is placed, most critically ill patients are not started on feedings for:

A. 12 hours B. 24 hours
C. 48 hours D. 72 hours

24. Contraindications for PEG placement include all of the following except:

A. Survival less than 10 weeks
B. Severe immunosuppression
C. Significant ascites
D. Gastric bypass surgery

25. False among the following is:

A. The tube may necrose through the stomach wall, if this occurs before development of a fibrous tract during the initial 10 to 14 days, it should be considered a surgical emergency because gastric contents would spill into the abdominal cavity
B. History of a previous or recent laparotomy is a contraindication for PEG
C. PEG is thought to be a safe procedure whether it is performed in the gastrointestinal laboratory, the OR, or at bedside in the ICU
D. Dislodgement may occur acutely through the application of traction on the gastrostomy tube, pulling it partially or completely through the abdominal wall

26. Free intraperitoneal air after PEG is common and can persist for:

A. 1 week B. 2 weeks
C. 4 weeks D. 6 weeks

27. The most popular method used for PEG insertion is:

A. Laparoscopic technique
B. Introducer technique
C. Push technique
D. Pull technique

BRONCHOSCOPY

28. False among the following is:

A. Diagnostic bronchoscopy is most commonly used for obtaining pulmonary specimens for diagnosis and management of pneumonia
B. The risks of the procedure itself are pneumothorax, hypoxia, airway hyperreactivity, pulmonary hemorrhage
C. The risk associated with diagnostic bronchoscopy is related to surgical skills
D. Medication use could possibly result in depressed mental status progressing to hypoventilation, airway vulnerability and the risk of aspiration

29. Therapeutic indications of bronchoscopy includes:

A. Removal of foreign bodies inadvertently aspirated
B. Insertion of an endotracheal tube
C. Diagnosis of obstructive pneumonia
D. All of the above

ANSWERS

1. **Ans: D. All of the above are true**
Ref: Chapter No.23, Page No.546

2. **Ans: C. Skills of surgeon**
Ref: Chapter No.23, Page No.547

3. **Ans: D. All of the above**
Ref: Chapter No.23, Page No.548

4. **Ans: D. Patient's preference**
Ref: Chapter No.23, Page No.548

5. **Ans: B. Preoperative antibiotics are always indicated**
Ref: Chapter No.23, Page No.548

6. **Ans: D. All of the above**
Ref: Chapter No.23, Page No.548-549

7. **Ans: B. Management of traumatic abdominal defects**
Ref: Chapter No.23, Page No.550

8. **Ans: D. All of the above**
Ref: Chapter No.23, Page No.550

9. **Ans: C. Decompression of abdominal hypertension**
Ref: Chapter No.23, Page No.550

10. **Ans: C. >25 mm Hg**
Ref: Chapter No.23, Page No.550

11. **Ans: D. All of the above**
Ref: Chapter No.23, Page No.550

12. **Ans: C. 50%**
Ref: Chapter No.23, Page No.550

13. **Ans: D. All of the above**
Ref: Chapter No.23, Page No.550

14. **Ans: D. Fraction of inspired oxygen >70%**
Ref: Chapter No.23, Page No.551

15. **Ans: D. Local infection or malignancy at proposed site**
Ref: Chapter No.23, Page No.551

16. **Ans: C. Spinal cord injury**
Ref: Chapter No.23, Page No.551

17. **Ans: A. Significant maxillofacial trauma**
Ref: Chapter No.23, Page No.551

18. **Ans: B. Tracheostomy**
Ref: Chapter No.23, Page No.551

19. **Ans: D. The use of preprocedure ultrasound to identify the neck anatomy is not helpful in decreasing potential risk of bleeding from crossing veins**
Ref: Chapter No.23, Page No.551

20. **Ans: C. 40%**
Ref: Chapter No.23, Page No.551

21. **Ans: A. PEG tubes have been associated with increasing overall hospital cost**
Ref: Chapter No.23, Page No.551

22. **Ans: C. 4 weeks**
Ref: Chapter No.23, Page No.551

23. **Ans: B. 24 hours**
Ref: Chapter No.23, Page No.551

24. **Ans: A. Survival less than 10 weeks**
Ref: Chapter No.23, Page No.551

25. **Ans: B. History of a previous or recent laparotomy is a contraindication for PEG**
Ref: Chapter No.23, Page No.552

26. **Ans: C. 4 weeks**
Ref: Chapter No.23, Page No.552

27. **Ans: D. Pull technique**
Ref: Chapter No.23, Page No.551

28. **Ans: C. The risk associated with diagnostic bronchoscopy is related to surgical skills**
Ref: Chapter No.23, Page No.552

29. **Ans: D. All of the above**
Ref: Chapter No.23, Page No.552

24

The Surgeon's Role in Mass Casualty Incidents

1. **False among the following is:**
   A. The hallmarks of almost all MASCAL events is the presence of major traumatic injuries that require rapid triage, evaluation and surgical or other procedural interventions
   B. Among the earliest changes in the way that patients are managed during a MASCAL event is the "sifting and sorting" into categories and their priorities for receiving emergent/urgent care
   C. The surgeon has a critical and obvious role in nearly every aspect of MASCAL management
   D. Mass casualty (MASCAL) incidents or events are characterized by a small number of people becoming injured or ill in a specific event or series of related events

HISTORY

2. **The term "triage" was coined by:**
   A. WHO
   B. Napoleon Bonaparte
   C. Dr. Baron Larrey
   D. Both B and C

3. **No. of patients who will have severe or immediately life-threatening injuries in mass casualty:**
   A. 50% B. 20%
   C. 30% D. 40%

KEY DEFINITIONS

4. **When seriously injured patients are transported to non-trauma centers or centers that do not have the expertise or capability to manage the severity of the injury, it is called as:**
   A. Overtriage B. Undertriage
   C. Field triage D. Hospital triage

5. **When patients with minor or nonurgent injuries are transported to major trauma centers or triaged to an immediate care bed, it is called as:**
   A. Overtriage B. Undertriage
   C. Field triage D. Hospital triage

6. **The most common trauma incidents that occur in rural and urban trauma centers are:**
   A. MASCAL incident
   B. Standard trauma incident
   C. Disaster incident
   D. MCI

7. **When the number of injured patients or the resources required to care for the patients exceed what is available and put a significant stress on the trauma system, hospital and providers, it is called as:**
   A. MASCAL incident
   B. Standard trauma incident
   C. Disaster incident
   D. MCI

8. **Large-scale natural or manmade MASCAL event that often results in overwhelming numbers of patients injured or ill, as well as frequent destruction or degradation of local infrastructure, which may include the health care facilities is called as:**
   A. MASCAL incident
   B. Standard trauma incident
   C. Disaster incident
   D. MCI

9. **The surge capacity of the hospital trauma service line is the:**
   A. Minimum critical casualty load that can be managed without a precipitous drop in the level of care

B. Maximal critical casualty load that can be managed without a precipitous drop in the level of care
C. Minimal critical casualty load that can be managed with a precipitous drop in the level of care
D. Maximal critical casualty load that can be managed with a precipitous drop in the level of care

MASCAL KEY PRINCIPLES

10. **Which among the following is not a MASCAL key principle?**
A. For in-hospital or single hospital triage, patients should be triaged through one entry point and with one-way only flow into the facility
B. Triage is a dynamic process and should be happening at each level of care from the point of injury/scene to the final receiving hospital or other facility
C. There must be duplication of action, not redundancy of capability, to avoid inefficiencies in an already stressed system
D. Success of failure during an MCI or MASCAL depends on accurate and effective triage

11. **The MASCAL goal is:**
A. Do the best for the most, not everything for everyone
B. Do the best for everyone, everything for everyone
C. Do the best for the most and everything for everyone
D. Do the little for the most, not everything for everyone

CRITICAL MASCAL LESSONS LEARNED

12. **False among the following is:**
A. Triage officer is usually best performed by an experienced trauma surgeon or emergency medicine provider
B. A widely accepted "best practice" for achieving this goal is the performance of in-depth after-action reviews (AARs) as soon as possible after any multiple casualty or MASCAL event
C. Triage at the hospital level is arguably the most important of the key clinical leadership roles during the initial phases of any true MASCAL event
D. All of the above are true

MASCAL MANAGEMENT AND THE SURGEON'S ROLE IN TRIAGE

13. **False among the following is about management of MASCAL event is:**
A. T - Training (in-hospital response/local)
B. R - Readiness
C. E - Exsanguination Control (along the continuum)
D. I - Intelligence

14. **Triage by classic ABCs takes _____ per casualty.**
A. 10-15 seconds B. 20-30 seconds
C. 30-40 seconds D. 45-60 seconds

15. **True about classic triage is:**
A. 1st sweep: Assess/treat two As': Arterial Hemorrhage and an Airway
B. 2nd sweep: Breathing and Circulation and document injuries, vital signs, treatments and times on casualty card or trauma form
C. 3rd sweep: Disability with rapid neurological exam and GCS and Exposure to look for missed injuries and protect from hypothermia
D. All of the above

16. **In a classic triage, to prevent end-organ damage while reducing blood loss from a higher circulatory pressure, treat shock with IV and careful hypotensive resuscitation, titrating fluid to mentation to keep systolic BP:**
A. ~ 60 mm Hg B. ~ 65 mm Hg
C. ~ 90 mm Hg D. ~ 100 mm Hg

17. **Commonly utilized triage systems is/are:**
A. Sort, assess, lifesaving interventions and treatment/transport (SALT)
B. Simple Treatment and Rapid Transport (START)
C. Secondary Assessment of Victim Endpoint (SAVE)
D. All of the above

18. **Pediatric version of START is:**
A. KickSTART B. JumpSTART
C. RunSTART D. ChildSTART

19. **According to NATO DIME triage categorization system, injury that may be life-threatening, but intervention may be delayed for several hours with frequent reassessment is:**
A. Minimal (green tag)
B. Delayed (yellow tag)

C. Expectant (black tag)
D. Immediate (red tag)

20. According to NATO DIME triage categorization system; ambulatory, minor injuries such as lacerations, minor burns or musculoskeletal injuries and can wait for definitive attention is:

A. Minimal (green tag)
B. Delayed (yellow tag)
C. Expectant (black tag)
D. Immediate (red tag)

21. According to NATO DIME triage categorization system; immediate attention required to prevent death which usually have "AABC" issue – airway, arterial bleed, ventilation, circulatory is:

A. Minimal (green tag)
B. Delayed (yellow tag)
C. Expectant (black tag)
D. Immediate (red tag)

22. Key bullet points related to hospital level triage is/are:

A. Patients in the minimal category can undergo a secondary and tertiary survey and usually be discharge
B. Retriage is a crucial component of the triage process
C. As the situation changes and resources become more or less available, retriage of delayed and expectant patients should occur
D. All of the above

23. In triage triad card and patient tag, red tag has which of the following?

A. Rabbit B. Tortoise
C. Ambulance D. Cross

24. In triage triad card and patient tag, yellow tag has which of the following?

A. Rabbit B. Tortoise
C. Ambulance D. Cross

25. True among the following is/are:

A. For local (in-hospital) triage, the most important protection that the security team provides is not from enemies, but rather from media, frenzied families and onlookers
B. Backup communications such as pagers and even alerts through social media should be considered as contingency plans
C. The ACS COT sets nation benchmarks for the measurement of Field Triage accuracy
D. All of the above

CONCLUSIONS

26. False about the core and critical concepts to successful mass casualty (MASCAL) planning and execution is:

A. Minimize chaos: Remain calm and confident
B. Assess: Perform accurate, ongoing triage; assess weather, supply status, personnel, etc.
C. Safety: Create additional patients and take care of everyone
D. Communication: Can never be enough; make it clear and concise

ANSWERS

1. **Ans: D. Mass casualty (MASCAL) incidents or events are characterized by a small number of people becoming injured or ill in a specific event or series of related events**
Ref: Chapter No.24, Page No.555

2. **Ans: C. Dr. Baron Larrey**
Ref: Chapter No.24, Page No.556

3. **Ans: B. 20%**
Ref: Chapter No.24, Page No.556

4. **Ans: B. Undertriage**
Ref: Chapter No.24, Page No.556

5. **Ans: A. Overtriage**
Ref: Chapter No.24, Page No.556

6. **Ans: B. Standard trauma incident**
Ref: Chapter No.24, Page No.557

7. **Ans: A. MASCAL incident**
Ref: Chapter No.24, Page No.557

8. **Ans: C. Disaster incident**
Ref: Chapter No.24, Page No.557

9. **Ans: B. Maximal critical casualty load that can be managed without a precipitous drop in the level of care**
Ref: Chapter No.24, Page No.557

10. **Ans: C. There must be duplication of action, not redundancy of capability, to avoid inefficiencies in an already stressed system**
Ref: Chapter No.24, Page No.558

11. **Ans: A. Do the best for the most, not everything for everyone**
Ref: Chapter No.24, Page No.558

12. **Ans: D. All of the above are true**
Ref: Chapter No.24, Page No.558-559

13. **Ans: D. I - Intelligence**
Ref: Chapter No.24, Page No.559

14. **Ans: A. 10-15 seconds**
Ref: Chapter No.24, Page No.560

15. **Ans: D. All of the above**
Ref: Chapter No.24, Page No.560

16. **Ans: A. ~ 60 mm Hg**
Ref: Chapter No.24, Page No.560

17. **Ans: D. All of the above**
Ref: Chapter No.24, Page No.560

18. **Ans: B. JumpSTART**
Ref: Chapter No.24, Page No.560

19. **Ans: B. Delayed (yellow tag)**
Ref: Chapter No.24, Page No.561

20. **Ans: A. Minimal (green tag)**
Ref: Chapter No.24, Page No.561

21. **Ans: D. Immediate (red tag)**
Ref: Chapter No.24, Page No.561

22. **Ans: D. All of the above**
Ref: Chapter No.24, Page No.561

23. **Ans: A. Rabbit**
Ref: Chapter No.24, Page No.563

24. **Ans: B. Tortoise**
Ref: Chapter No.24, Page No.563

25. **Ans: D. All of the above**
Ref: Chapter No.24, Page No.562-565

26. **Ans: C. Safety: Create additional patients and take care of everyone**
Ref: Chapter No.24, Page No.567

25

Transplantation Immunobiology and Immunosuppression

1. **Following image shows a technique of vascular anastomosis. Who developed the technique?**

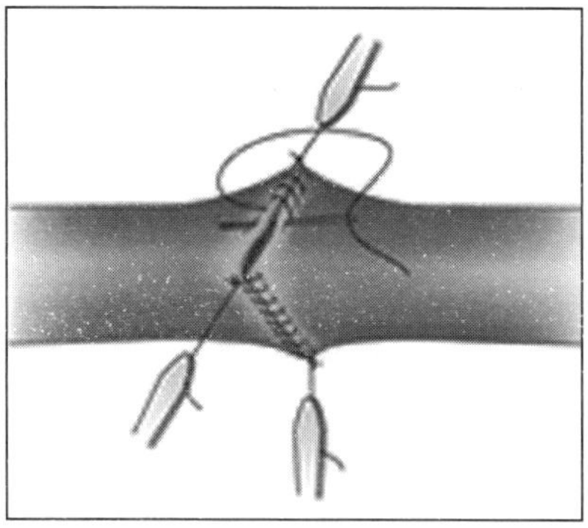

A. Roy Calne B. Joseph Murray
C. Alexis Carrel D. Gertrude Elion

2. **The first successful renal transplant was performed by:**

A. Roy Calne B. Joseph Murray
C. Alexis Carrel D. Gertrude Elion

3. **Who developed 6-mercaptopurine and azathioprine?**

A. Roy Calne
B. Peter Medawar
C. Frank Macfarlane Burnet
D. Gertrude Elion

THE IMMUNE RESPONSE

4. **False about the innate immune system is:**

A. Danger-associated molecular pattern molecules (DAMPs) are nuclear or cytosolic proteins or even DNA that is released or exposed in the setting of cell injury
B. The receptors of innate immunity are the same from one individual to another within a species and, in general, do play a role in the direct recognition of a transplanted organ
C. DAMP receptors include some of the TLRs, including TLR2 and TLR4, but also a variety of other proteins, such as receptor for advanced glycosylation end-products (RAGE) and triggering receptor expressed on myeloid cells 1 (TREM-1)
D. Toll-like receptors (TLRs) has been described to play an important role as activation molecules for innate APCs

5. **True about monocytes is:**

A. Their function is to acquire, process, and present antigen as well as to serve as effector cells in certain situations
B. They play a significant role in facilitating the acquired T cell response through antigen presentation, and their cytokines induce substantial tissue dysfunction in sites of inflammation
C. Mononuclear phagocytes are bone marrow–derived cells that initially emerge as monocytes within peripheral blood
D. All of the above

6. **False about Dendritic cells is:**

A. Plasmacytoid dendritic cells are less tolerogenic
B. Dendritic cells are specialized macrophages that are regarded as professional APCs
C. Myeloid dendritic cells are more immunogenic
D. Immature dendritic cells can be found along the gut mucosa, within the skin, and in other sites of antigen entry

7. **False about natural killer (NK) cells is:**

A. NK cells also play an important role in the immune response after bone marrow transplantation and xenotransplantation
B. NK cells are large granular lymphocytes with potent cytolytic function that constitute a critical component of innate immunity
C. NK cells lyse cell targets that lack expression of self-class II MHC, termed the missing self-hypothesis

D. NK cells produce various cytokines, including interferon γ (IFN-γ), which may function to activate macrophages, which can in turn eliminate host cells infected by intracellular microbes

8. **False about acquired immune system is:**

A. The B-cell receptor or antibody can identify its epitope directly after preparation of the antigen
B. The term antigen is used to describe a molecule that can be recognized by the acquired immune system
C. The 2 main types of receptors that the immune system employs to recognize any given epitope are the TCR and B-cell receptor or antibody
D. An epitope is the portion of the antigen, generally a carbohydrate or peptide moiety, that actually serves as the binding site for the immune system receptor and is the base unit of antigen recognition

9. **Location and organization of the HLA complex is on human chromosome no:**

A. 2 B. 6
C. 11 D. 17

10. **False about human histocompatibility complex is:**

A. Class I molecules includes HLA-A, B and C
B. Class II molecules includes HLA-DP, DQ and DR
C. Class III molecules includes TNF-α, lymphotoxin β, components of the complement cascade, nuclear transcription factor-β and heat shock protein 70
D. The blood group antigens of the ABO system must not be considered transplant antigens

11. **False among the following is:**

A. Class II molecules are found almost exclusively on cells associated with the immune system
B. HLA class I molecules are present on all nucleated cells
C. Isografts are organs are immunologically distinguishable and thus are naturally rejected
D. Donor recipient pairings that are matched at these HLA loci are referred to as HLA-identical allografts, and those matched at half of the HLA loci are termed haploidentical

12. **False about Class I MHC is:**

A. The critical structural feature of class I molecules is the presence of a groove formed by two α helices mounted on a β pleated sheet in the α1 and α2 domains
B. The α3 immunoglobulin (Ig)-like domain, which is the domain closest to the membrane and interacts with the CD4 molecule on the T cell
C. The α chain has three domains, α1, α2 and α3
D. The assembly of class I is dependent on association of the α chain with β2-microglobulin and native peptide within the groove

13. **Following image shows structure of:**

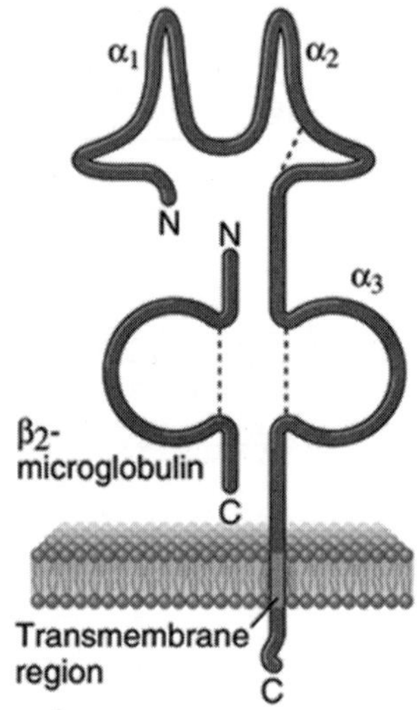

A. MHC Class I B. MHC Class II
C. MHC Class III D. MHC Class IV

14. **True about MHC Class II is:**

A. The trauma of surgery and ischemia upregulate class II on all cells of the allograft, making nonself MHC more abundant
B. Class II molecules, in contrast to class I molecules, are confined to cells related to the immune response, particularly APCs (macrophages, dendritic cells, B cells and monocytes)
C. After binding class II molecules, CD4+ T cells participate in APC-mediated activation of CD8+ T cells and antibody-producing B cells
D. All of the above

15. **The most commonly employed technique for class II typing:**

A. Polymerase chain reaction with sequence-specific primers
B. Serologic techniques
C. Restriction fragment length polymorphism
D. Oligonucleotide hybridization

16. The predominant method for class I typing is:

A. Polymerase chain reaction with sequence-specific primers
B. Serologic techniques
C. Restriction fragment length polymorphism
D. Oligonucleotide hybridization

17. False about the implications of HLA for transplantation is:

A. The current immunosuppressive regimens negate much of the impact of matching, several studies have demonstrated better renal allograft survival when the 6 primary alleles (A, B and DR) are matched between donor and recipient, a so-called 6-antigen match or zero-antigen mismatch
B. Humans potentially have two different HLA-A, B and DR alleles
C. MHC compatibility had been defined using two cellular assays: the lymphocytotoxicity assay and the mixed lymphocyte reaction
D. The use of the mixed lymphocyte reaction as a prospective typing assay is limited to dead donors

18. True about Acquired Immune System is:

A. The development of the lymphoid system begins with pluripotent stem cells in the liver and bone marrow of the fetus
B. T cells are responsible for cell-mediated immunity and of necessity must interact with cells in the periphery to neutralize and to eliminate foreign antigens
C. B cells are structured to respond to whole antigen and in response synthesize and secrete antibody that can interact with antigen at distant sites
D. All of the above

19. False about T-Cell Receptor is:

A. Most T cells are γδ T cells
B. αβ T cells are more typically limited to recognition of MHC complexed with processed peptide
C. T cells first attempt to recombine the γ and δ TCR genes and then, if recombination fails to yield a properly formed receptor, resort to the more diverse α and β TCR genes
D. T cells expressing the γδ TCR have more primitive functions, including recognition of heat shock proteins and activity similar to NK cells as well as MHC recognition

20. False about T-Cell Receptor is:

A. It is estimated that approximately 10^9 naïve T-cell clonotypes (i.e., T cells with the same TCR specificity) are present at any point in time
B. The frequency of naïve T cells available to respond to any given pathogen is relatively small, estimated to be between 1 in 200,000 and 1 in 500,000
C. The frequency specific for a similar, nonself MHC (i.e., alloreactive) is estimated to be between 10% and 20% of all T cells
D. All of the above

21. Source of Interleukin-6 is all except:

A. T cells B. B cells
C. Macrophages D. Endothelial cells

22. Biologic effects of IL-4 are all except:

A. Liver: ↑ synthesis of acute-phase proteins
B. B cells: Isotype switching to IgE
C. Mast cells: Stimulates proliferation
D. T cells: Th2 differentiation, proliferation

23. Biologic effects of IL-2 are all except:

A. B cells: Proliferation, antibody synthesis (in vitro)
B. NK cells: Proliferation, activation
C. Hypothalamus: Fever
D. T cells: Proliferation, ↑ cytokine synthesis, survival, potentiates Fas-mediated apoptosis, promotes regulatory T-cell development

24. Source of Interleukin-1 is:

A. Macrophages B. T cells
C. B cells D. NK cells

25. Source of Tumor necrosis factor is:

A. Macrophages B. Fibroblasts
C. B cells D. NK cells

26. Source of Interferon-γ is:

A. Macrophages B. Fibroblasts
C. B cells D. NK cells

27. Biologic effects of Interferon-γ are all except:

A. T cells: Th1 differentiation
B. Lymphoid organogenesis
C. B cells: Isotype switching to IgG subclasses that facilitate complement fixation and opsonization
D. Macrophages: Activation (increased microbicidal functions)

28. **Biologic effects of Tumor necrosis factor is all except:**
   A. Fibroblasts: Increased collagen synthesis
   B. Liver: ↑ synthesis of acute-phase proteins
   C. Muscle, fat: Catabolism (cachexia)
   D. Hypothalamus: Fever

29. **B cell isotype switching to IgE is by:**
   A. Interleukin-1 B. Interleukin-4
   C. Interleukin-5 D. Interleukin-2

30. **B cell-inhibition of proliferation and ↑ IgA production is by:**
   A. Lymphotoxin
   B. Type I interferons
   C. Transforming growth factor-β
   D. Interleukin-10

31. **Lymphoid organogenesis is done by:**
   A. Interleukin-12 B. IFN-β
   C. Lymphotoxin D. IFN-α

32. **False about the source and the cytokine is:**
   A. Interleukin-3 - B cells
   B. APRIL (CD256) - T cells, follicular dendritic cells, monocytes
   C. IFN-α - Macrophages
   D. BAFF (CD257) - Follicular dendritic cells, monocytes, B cells

33. **Eosinophil activation, ↑ production is done by:**
   A. Interleukin-1 B. Interleukin-4
   C. Interleukin-5 D. Interleukin-2

34. **Driving the development of Th17 and Tfh is:**
   A. Interleukin-17 B. Interleukin-21
   C. Interleukin-22 D. Interleukin-27

35. **Biologic effects of Interleukin-27 is:**
   A. T cells: Inhibits production of IL-17/Th17 cells, promotes Th1 differentiation
   B. T cells: Maintenance of IL-17–producing T cells
   C. Th2 development and cytokine production
   D. T cells: Proliferation (memory CD8+ T cells)

36. **Biologic effects of Interleukin-11 is/are:**
   A. Megakaryocytes: Thrombopoiesis
   B. B cells: Stimulates T-dependent antibody production
   C. Liver: Induces acute-phase proteins
   D. All of the above

37. **False about NK cells is:**
   A. Type I interferons - NK: Cell activation
   B. Interleukin-12 - NK: Increased cytotoxic activity
   C. Interleukin-27 - NK cells: Functional maturation
   D. Interleukin-15- NK cells: Proliferation

38. **CD28 receptor is present on:**
   A. Soluble platelets B. Activated APCs
   C. T cells D. All of the above

39. **Ligand of CD40 is:**
   A. CD80/CD86 B. CD153
   C. CD154 D. CD70

40. **CD80/CD86 is present on:**
   A. Soluble platelets B. Activated APCs
   C. T cells D. All of the above

41. **Ligand of CD30 is:**
   A. CD80/CD86 B. CD153
   C. CD154 D. CD70

42. **Ligand of CD95 is:**
   A. CD252 B. CD254
   C. CD178 D. CD70

43. **CD40 is present on all except:**
   A. Macrophages B. T cells
   C. Dendritic cells D. B cells

44. **CD265 (RANK) on dendritic cells has a ligand on activated T cells called:**
   A. CD252 B. CD254
   C. CD178 D. CD70

45. **PD-1 (Programmed death 1) is:**
   A. CD279 B. CD274
   C. CD275 D. CD273

46. **PD-L1 (Programmed death ligand 1) is:**
   A. CD279 B. CD274
   C. CD275 D. CD273

47. **ICOSL (inducible costimulator ligand) is:**
   A. CD278 B. CD274
   C. CD275 D. CD273

48. **PD-L2 (Programmed death ligand 2) is:**
   A. CD278 B. CD274
   C. CD275 D. CD273

49. **Role in allergies is played by:**
A. Th1 B. Th2
C. Th17 D. Tfh

50. **Defining cytokines in Th2 are all except:**
A. IL-5 B. IL-4
C. IL-21 D. IL-13

51. **Host defence against helminths is via:**
A. Th1 B. Th2
C. Th17 D. Tfh

52. **Host defence against extracellular bacteria and fungi is via:**
A. Th1 B. Th2
C. Th17 D. Tfh

53. **B cells are the principal targets of:**
A. Th1 B. Th2
C. Th17 D. Tfh

54. **Macrophages are the principal targets of:**
A. Th1 B. Th2
C. Th17 D. Tfh

55. **Neutrophils are the principal targets of:**
A. Th1 B. Th2
C. Th17 D. Tfh

56. **Role in chronic inflammation is played by:**
A. Th1 B. Th2
C. Th17 D. Tfh

57. **True about chemokines is:**
A. Chemokines, or chemotactic cytokine chemokines, are a unique set of cytokines that are structurally homologous, 8- to 10-kDa polypeptides that have a varying number of cysteine residues in conserved locations that are key to forming their 3-dimensional shape
B. Chemokines or their receptors have been exploited by viruses such as human immunodeficiency virus (HIV) (CCR5 and CXCR4 expressed on CD4 T cells are used as entry coreceptors) or used as therapeutic targets, such as CCR7 (FTY720 or fingolimod)
C. Chemokine receptors are G protein–coupled receptors containing seven transmembrane domains
D. All of the above

58. **In an antibody, 5 different heavy chain loci (μ, γ, α, ε and δ) are found on:**
A. Chromosome 2 B. Chromosome 6
C. Chromosome 14 D. Chromosome 17

59. **In an antibody, 2 light chain loci (κ and λ) are located on:**
A. Chromosome 2
B. Chromosome 6
C. Chromosome 14
D. Chromosome 17

60. **False among the following is:**
A. In humans, there are 9 different Ig subclasses or isotypes: IgM, IgD, IgG1, IgG2, IgG3, IgG4, IgA1, IgA2 and IgE
B. Light chain use defines the subtype of any given antibody
C. IgM and IgG antibodies provide a pivotal role in the endogenous or intravascular immune response
D. IgA is primarily responsible for mucosal immunity and is largely confined to the gastrointestinal and respiratory tracts

61. **False among the following is:**
A. Resting B cells that have not yet been exposed to antigen express IgD and IgM on their cell surface
B. The threshold for B-cell activation can be lowered 100-fold by costimulatory signals received by the transmembrane complex CD19-CD21
C. After interaction with antigen, the first isotype produced is IgM
D. B cells express CD30, and when bound by CD154 expressed on activated T cells, the result is upregulation of B7 molecules on the B cell and delivery of important costimulatory signals to T cells as well

TRANSPLANT IMMUNITY

62. **False among the following is:**
A. With the use of cyclosporine A. and newer agents such as tacrolimus, 1-year graft survival has exceeded 70% for virtually all organs except the small intestine
B. Paul Terasaki developed the microlymphocyte cytotoxicity test, allowing pretransplantation detection of recipient-derived antidonor antibody
C. Jean-François Borel identified an active metabolite, cyclosporine A (CsA), that showed selective in vitro inhibition of lymphocyte cultures but no significant myelotoxic effects
D. Joseph Murray performed the first successful kidney transplant between identical twins

63. False about mechanism of rejection of a graft is:

A. Acute rejection is a process mediated most commonly by B cells
B. Hyperacute rejection occurs within minutes to days after transplantation and is primarily mediated by preformed antibody
C. Chronic rejection is a common contributing cause of long-term allograft loss and is an indolent fibrotic process that occurs over months to years
D. All of the above are true

64. False about hyperacute graft rejection is:

A. This form of rejection occurs when preformed antibodies against the donor, commonly referred to as donor-specific antibodies, are present in the recipient's system before transplantation
B. This type of rejection is not avoidable with pretransplantation testing
C. On histologic evaluation, there may be platelet and fibrin thrombi, early neutrophil infiltration, and positive staining for the complement product C4d on the endothelial lining of small blood vessels
D. All of the above are true

65. True about hyperacute graft rejection is:

A. Panel reactive antibody (PRA) assay is a technique for screening a patient's sensitization status is to screen a potential recipient's serum against a panel of random donor cells representing the anticipated regional donor pool
B. In the event a compatible donor is not available for a highly sensitized recipient, clinical protocols exist to attempt desensitization that uses plasmapheresis or intravenous immune globulin (IVIG) to reduce circulating antibody and prevent hyperacute rejection
C. A negative crossmatch assay coupled with proper ABO matching will effectively prevent hyperacute rejection in 99.5% of transplants
D. All of the above

66. The type of rejection that can be reversed once established is:

A. Hyperacute Rejection
B. Acute Rejection
C. Chronic Rejection
D. All of the above

67. False about acute graft rejection is:

A. T cells constitute the core element responsible for acute rejection, often termed T cell–mediated rejection
B. It most commonly occurs within the first 3 months after transplantation
C. In an effort to prevent acute cellular rejection, induction therapy is generally used during the initial stages after transplantation
D. Histology shows cellular rejection of kidney with inflammatory cells within the connective tissue around the tubules (peritubular) and between tubular epithelial cells

68. In transplants, T cell specific treatments lead to the prevention of acute rejection in approximately:

A. 50% B. 30%
C. 70% D. 90%

69. In acute graft rejection, T-cell presensitization will result in an accelerated form of cellular rejection mediated by memory T cells and after transplantation generally occurs within first:

A. 2-3 days B. 21-28 days
C. 7-14 days D. 3-10 days

70. True about chronic rejection of grafts is/are:

A. Kidney: Interstitial fibrosis and tubular atrophy
B. Heart: Chronic coronary vasculopathy
C. Liver: Vanishing bile duct syndrome
D. All of the above

IMMUNOSUPPRESSION

71. True about immunosuppressive therapies in transplantation is:

A. Immunosuppression is extremely intense in the early postoperative period and normally tapered thereafter
B. The most critical time for immune protection is the first few days to months after transplantation
C. Immunosuppressants used to reverse an acute rejection episode are called rescue agents
D. All of the above

72. False about antithymocyte globulin is:

A. These preparations are used as induction agents as well as rescue treatment for acute rejection episodes
B. The two most commonly used preparations are rabbit antithymocyte globulin (RATG) and horse antithymocyte globulin (ATGAM)

C. Recently, RATG has been used as a key component of newer steroid minimization or calcineurin inhibitor free regimens
D. ATGAM seems to be more effective than RATG at reducing the incidence of acute rejection episodes

73. False about antithymocyte globulin is:

A. Overimmunosuppression is a concern; given that these preparations are extremely effective at T-cell depletion, there is an increase in viral reactivation and primary viral infections
B. Chills and fevers occur in up to 50% of patients, and this cytokine release syndrome usually needs to stop the drugs
C. A major side effect is profound thrombocytopenia secondary to platelet-specific antibodies within the polyclonal preparation
D. The effect on EBV specific T cells also predisposes treated patients to a higher incidence of EBV associated lymphoid malignant neoplasms

74. False about Anti–IL-2 Receptor Antibodies is:

A. Daclizumab has since been discontinued as a result of diminished demand, leaving basiliximab as the sole anti-IL-2 receptor option
B. The α chain, CD25, is a type I transmembrane protein that is responsible for the high-affinity binding of IL-2 on activated T cells and is critical for T-cell clonal expansion
C. Basiliximab is humanized and Daclizumab is a mouse-human chimeric antibody
D. Daclizumab and Basiliximab are 2 nondepleting monoclonal antibodies specific for CD25, developed and approved for use in transplantation

75. False about Anti–IL-2 Receptor Antibodies is:

A. In contradistinction to lymphocyte depleting agents, daclizumab and basiliximab confer less risk of infection and malignancy posttransplant
B. Cytokine release syndrome can be seen as a side effect
C. Both daclizumab and basiliximab are the products of genetic engineering, with the some or all of the structural components of the mouse antibody having been replaced with human IgG
D. Daclizumab and Basiliximab are much less likely to invoke neutralizing antibody responses themselves

76. The first commercially available monoclonal antibody preparation for use in organ transplantation with T-cell specificity devoid of the unintended bystander effects observed with polyclonal preparations is:

A. Muromonab-CD3 B. OKT3
C. Daclizumab D. Both A and B

77. Anti-CD20 chimeric monoclonal antibody is:

A. Rituximab B. Alemtuzumab
C. Belatacept D. Basiliximab

78. Anti-CD52 humanized monoclonal antibody is:

A. Rituximab B. Alemtuzumab
C. Belatacept D. Basiliximab

79. High-affinity homologue of CTLA-4–Ig is:

A. Rituximab B. Alemtuzumab
C. Belatacept D. Basiliximab

80. False about Alemtuzumab is:

A. It is a humanized antibody against human CD52, a cell surface protein expressed on most mature lymphocytes and monocytes and on their stem cell precursors
B. Administration of alemtuzumab is extremely effective at reducing the number of T cells both in the peripheral blood and in secondary lymphoid organs
C. It depletes, to a lesser extent, both B cells and monocytes
D. Its optimal use in transplantation remains to be established

81. False about Corticosteroids is:

A. Glucocorticoids, remain one of the most commonly employed medications to prevent rejection
B. They may also be used in higher doses as induction or rescue therapy for acute rejection episodes
C. Steroids possess potent immunosuppressive properties but they can contribute significantly to the morbidity of transplantation by their effects on wound healing and propensity to cause diabetes, hypertension and osteoporosis
D. High-dose steroids remain a common component of current standard immunosuppressive regimens

82. False about steroid's mechanism against immune response is:

A. Phospholipase A2, and consequently the entire arachidonic acid cascade, is inhibited

B. Steroids act to diminish transcription of IL-1 and TNF-α by APCs as well as to prevent upregulation of MHC expression

C. Steroids increase the leukocyte response to various chemokines and chemotactins and by stimulating vasodilators, such as histamine and prostacyclin, they dampen the inflammatory response globally

D. Steroids inhibits the function of NF-κB, a key activator of proinflammatory cytokines and an important transcription factor involved in T-cell activation

83. **The most commonly used oral glucocorticoid formulation is:**

A. Methylprednisolone B. Prednisone
C. Dexamethasone D. Cortisone

84. **False about Azathioprine is:**

A. It is a nucleotide analogue that targets cells undergoing rapid division; in the case of an immune response, its goal is to limit the clonal expansion of T and B cells

B. Azathioprine undergoes hepatic conversion to several active metabolites, including 6-mercaptopurine and 6-thioinosine monophosphate

C. The effects of azathioprine are relatively specific and unlike other antiproliferative agents

D. It has largely been replaced by MMF as the first-line antiproliferative agent

85. **The agent of choice during pregnancy is:**

A. MMF B. Azathioprine
C. Tacrolimus D. Sirolimus

86. **False about Mycophenolate mofetil (MMF) is:**

A. The major clinical side effects include thrombocyopenia

B. Mycophenolic acid inhibits inosine monophosphate dehydrogenase

C. MMF exploits a critical difference between lymphocytes and other body tissues, resulting in relatively lymphocyte-specific immunosuppressive effects

D. MMF has been shown to decrease the rate of biopsy proven rejection and the need for rescue therapy compared with azathioprine

87. **False about Cyclosporine A (CsA) is:**

A. It is a cyclic, nonribosomal peptide of 11 amino acids produced by the fungus Tolypocladium inflatum

B. The mechanism of action of CsA is mediated primarily through its ability to bind the cytoplasmic protein cyclophilin

C. CsA is used as a maintenance agent, blocking the initiation of an immune response, but it is ineffective as a rescue agent once IL-2 has already been produced

D. CsA acts to decrease transcription of TGF-β

88. **False about Cyclosporine A (CsA) is:**

A. CsA has good water solubility

B. CsA is metabolized by the hepatic cytochrome P450 enzymes, and blood levels are therefore influenced by agents that affect the P450 system

C. CsA induces the expression of TGF-β, and much of CsA toxicity can be linked to increased TGF-β activity

D. CsA has a significant vasoconstrictor effect on proximal renal arterioles, resulting in a 30% decrease in renal blood flow

89. **Higher CsA levels are seen due to P450 inhibitors, which includes all except:**

A. Grapefruit juice
B. Ketoconazole
C. Phenytoin
D. Calcium channel blockers

90. **Side effects of Cyclosporine A is/are:**

A. Gingival hyperplasia B. Renal toxicity
C. Hypertrichosis D. All of the above

91. **Hypertrichosis (increased hair growth) is a frequent side effect of Cyclosporine A, seen in up to:**

A. 10% B. 30%
C. 50% D. 70%

92. **False about Tacrolimus is:**

A. It is a macrolide produced by the fungus Streptomyces tsukubaensis

B. The intracellular target is an immunophilin protein distinct from cyclophilin known as FK-binding protein (FK-BP)

C. The side effect profile for tacrolimus is similar to that of CsA with regard to renal toxicity and cosmetic side effects such as abnormal hair growth and gingival hyperplasia

D. Neurotoxicity, including tremors and mental status changes, is more pronounced with tacrolimus, as is its diabetogenic effect

93. **False about mTOR inhibitors is:**
A. It is a macrolide derived from the bacterium Streptomyces hygroscopicus with potent immunosuppressive properties
B. Sirolimus has demonstrated activity against EBV
C. Sirolimus and tacrolimus can act synergistically to impair rejection, but the combination can result in intolerable clinical toxicity
D. mTOR inhibitors have been shown to have promising antitumor effects as well

94. **False about mTOR inhibitors is:**
A. These agents may play an important role in the prevention of posttransplantation lymphoproliferative disorder (PTLD)
B. There is an increased incidence of hypercholesterolemia and hypertriglyceridemia with these agents but rarely needs treatment
C. Oral ulcers, wound healing complications (in particular an increased incidence of lymphoceles), elevated levels of proteinuria, and thrombocytopenia remain frequent problems
D. Sirolimus and everolimus have been used in the development of drug-eluting coronary stents to limit the rate of in-stent restenosis because of their antiproliferative properties

95. **True about Belatacept is:**
A. Higher than-expected acute rejection rates and logistic challenges related to intravenous infusion administration requirements have slowed large-scale uptake of belatacept
B. LEA29Y (belatacept) is a second-generation CTLA-4–Ig molecule that differs by two amino acid residues within the ligand binding domain, resulting in increased affinity for CD80 and CD86
C. FDA approved for use in kidney transplantation
D. All of the above

96. **False about Rituximab is:**
A. CD20 is a cell surface protein expressed on all mature B cells and on plasma cells
B. Rituximab is a murine antihuman CD20 chimeric antibody that was initially developed for the treatment of B-cell lymphoma and has since been used in the treatment of PTLD
C. Rituximab has been used in a wide variety of autoimmune disorders and as a component in some investigational strategies designed as induction therapy in highly sensitized transplant recipients undergoing kidney transplantation or even in ABO-incompatible pairings
D. Rituximab binds to CD20 and facilitates antibody-dependent cellular cytotoxicity and complement-dependent cytotoxicity of B cells as well as promoting programmed cell death

97. **True about daratumumab is:**
A. CD38 is expressed on the surface of short- and long-lived plasma cells
B. Daratumumab is anti-CD38 mAb
C. Daratumumab mediates potent depletion of not only plasma cells but also potentially beneficial immunoregulatory T- and B-cell subsets
D. All of the above

98. **True about Eculizumab is:**
A. Its binding to C5 inhibits the formation of complement components downstream, including the split product C5a and membrane attack complex
B. It is approved to treat patients with paroxysmal nocturnal hemoglobinuria and atypical hemolytic uremic syndrome
C. Eculizumab is a humanized monoclonal antibody targeting the complement component C5
D. All of the above

99. **JAK3 inhibitor is:**
A. Bortezomib B. Tofacitinib
C. Carfilzomib D. Fingolimod

100. **Sphingosine 1-phosphate receptor modulator is:**
A. Bortezomib B. Tofacitinib
C. Carfilzomib D. Fingolimod

101. **Bortezomib and carfilzomib are:**
A. Anti-CD154 mAbs
B. Proteasome inhibitors
C. JAK3 inhibitor
D. CD28/B7 pathway blockers

102. **True about the risk of infections after immunosuppression is:**
A. In the setting of induction and maintenance immunosuppressive therapy in transplantation, CMV reactivation can occur, resulting in pneumonitis, hepatitis, pancreatitis or colitis
B. Recipient-derived infections are much more common after transplantation than donor-derived infections
C. Detection of BK viral DNA in blood and urine has been useful for monitoring response to

therapy, which includes minimizing immunosuppression and treatment with antiviral therapies

D. All of the above

103. After transplantation, the risk for reactivation of infections is highest at approximately:

A. 1 - 2 weeks B. 2 - 4 weeks
C. 6 - 12 weeks D. 12 - 18 weeks

104. True about prophylaxis of infections after immunosuppression is:

A. Clotrimazole troche or nystatin for oral and esophageal fungal infections
B. Ganciclovir or valganciclovir for CMV infections
C. Trimethoprim-sulfamethoxazole for Pneumocystis pneumonia and urinary tract infections
D. All of the above

105. JC virus has been associated with:

A. Progressive nephropathy
B. Ureteral obstruction
C. Progressive multifocal leukoencephalopathy
D. Progressive neuropathy

106. The most common malignant condition in transplant recipients is:

A. Squamous cell cancer B. Leukemia
C. Basal cell carcinoma D. Kaposi sarcoma

107. Which of the following is associated with the development of PTLD?

A. Human papillomavirus
B. Human herpesvirus 8
C. Epstein bar virus
D. Hepatitis B

108. False about side effects of immunosuppressants is:

A. New onset diabetes after transplantation is an important problem, particularly in individuals receiving tacrolimus or steroids
B. The incidence of new-onset immunosuppressive-related diabetes mellitus approaches 50% in the first 1 year after renal transplantation
C. Histologic evidence of calcineurin inhibitor–associated nephrotoxicity is essentially universal in renal transplants by 10 years
D. Immunosuppressive therapy can lead to hyperlipidemia, anemia, and accelerated cardiovascular disease, which is a leading cause of death in long term transplant survivor

XENOTRANSPLANTATION

109. True about Concordant xenografts is:

A. Concordant xenografts refer to transplants between closely related species; for humans, these include Old World monkeys and apes
B. Similar to humans, concordant species lack galactosyltransferase, and as a result, their carbohydrates are the typical blood group antigens and they lack the N-linked disaccharide galactose-α (1-3)-galactose (α Gal)
C. The typical mechanisms of graft rejection remain, including acute cellular rejection, acute vascular rejection and presumably, chronic rejection
D. All of the above

110. True about Discordant xenografts is:

A. Transplant concordance among species is predominantly determined on the basis of the expression of the enzyme galactosyltransferase
B. When organs from discordant species are transplanted into humans, they rapidly undergo hyperacute rejection
C. The primary mechanism of rejection relies on the presence of preformed IgM antibodies against cell surface carbohydrate moieties, particularly α-Gal
D. All of the above

NEW AREAS OF TRANSPLANTATION

111. True about Vascularized composite tissue transplantation is:

A. The first successful hand transplantation was performed in Lyon, France, in 1998
B. Vascularized composite tissue transplantation involves the transfer of multiple tissue types, including skin, fat, muscle, nerves, blood vessels, tendon, and bone, within one functional unit, such as a hand or face
C. The first successful face composite allograft was reported by a group of surgeons from France in 2005
D. All of the above

112. True about uterine transplant is:

A. The first technically successful uterus transplant was performed in 2011
B. The first functionally successful transplanted uterus to lead to a healthy live birth occurred in 2014
C. Uterus transplantation introduces the unique considerations of cyclical physiologic function and undulating periods of immunological activity and potential for hosting a fetus
D. All of the above

ANSWERS

1. **Ans: C. Alexis Carrel**

   Ref: Chapter No.25, Page No.572-573

2. **Ans: B. Joseph Murray**

   Ref: Chapter No.25, Page No.572

3. **Ans: D. Gertrude Elion**

   Ref: Chapter No.25, Page No.572-573

4. **Ans: B. The receptors of innate immunity are the same from one individual to another within a species and, in general, do play a role in the direct recognition of a transplanted organ**

   Ref: Chapter No.25, Page No.573-574

5. **Ans: D. All of the above**

   Ref: Chapter No.25, Page No.574-575

6. **Ans: A. Plasmacytoid dendritic cells are less tolerogenic**

   Ref: Chapter No.25, Page No.575

7. **Ans: C. NK cells lyse cell targets that lack expression of self-class II MHC, termed the missing self-hypothesis**

   Ref: Chapter No.25, Page No.575

8. **Ans: A. The B-cell receptor or antibody can identify its epitope directly after preparation of the antigen**

   Ref: Chapter No.25, Page No.575

9. **Ans: B. 6**

   Ref: Chapter No.25, Page No.576

10. **Ans: D. The blood group antigens of the ABO system must not be considered transplant antigens**

    Ref: Chapter No.25, Page No.576

11. **Ans: C. Isografts are organs are immunologically distinguishable and thus are naturally rejected**

    Ref: Chapter No.25, Page No.576

12. **Ans: B. The α_3 immunoglobulin (Ig)-like domain, which is the domain closest to the membrane and interacts with the CD4 molecule on the T cell**

    Ref: Chapter No.25, Page No.577

13. **Ans: A. MHC Class I**

    Ref: Chapter No.25, Page No.577

14. **Ans: D. All of the above**

    Ref: Chapter No.25, Page No.577

15. **Ans: A. Polymerase chain reaction with sequence-specific primers**

    Ref: Chapter No.25, Page No.579

16. **Ans: B. Serologic techniques**

    Ref: Chapter No.25, Page No.579

17. **Ans: D. The use of the mixed lymphocyte reaction as a prospective typing assay is limited to dead donors**

    Ref: Chapter No.25, Page No.578

18. **Ans: D. All of the above**

    Ref: Chapter No.25, Page No.579

19. **Ans: A. Most T cells are γδ T cells**

    Ref: Chapter No.25, Page No.579

20. **Ans: C. The frequency specific for a similar, nonself MHC (i.e., alloreactive) is estimated to be between 10% and 20% of all T cells**

    Ref: Chapter No.25, Page No.579-581

21. **Ans: B. B cells**

    Ref: Chapter No.25, Page No.580

22. **Ans: A. Liver: ↑ synthesis of acute-phase proteins**

    Ref: Chapter No.25, Page No.580

23. **Ans: C. Hypothalamus: fever**

    Ref: Chapter No.25, Page No.580

24. **Ans: A. Macrophages**

    Ref: Chapter No.25, Page No.580

25. **Ans: A. Macrophages (Also T cells)**

    Ref: Chapter No.25, Page No.580

26. **Ans: D. NK cells (Also T cells- Th1)**

    Ref: Chapter No.25, Page No.580

27. **Ans: B. Lymphoid organogenesis**

    Ref: Chapter No.25, Page No.580

28. **Ans: A. Fibroblasts: increased collagen synthesis**

    Ref: Chapter No.25, Page No.580

29. **Ans: B. Interleukin-4 (Also IL-13)**

    Ref: Chapter No.25, Page No.580

30. **Ans: C. Transforming growth factor-β**

    Ref: Chapter No.25, Page No.580

31. **Ans: C. Lymphotoxin**

    Ref: Chapter No.25, Page No.580

32. **Ans: A. Interleukin-3 - B cells**

    Ref: Chapter No.25, Page No.580

33. **Ans: C. Interleukin-5**

    Ref: Chapter No.25, Page No.580

34. **Ans: B. Interleukin-21**

    Ref: Chapter No.25, Page No.581

35. **Ans: A. T cells: inhibits production of IL-17/Th17 cells, promotes Th1 differentiation**

Ref: Chapter No.25, Page No.581

36. **Ans: D. All of the above**

Ref: Chapter No.25, Page No.580

37. **Ans: C. Interleukin-27 - NK cells: functional maturation (It is by IL-21)**

Ref: Chapter No.25, Page No.580-581

38. **Ans: C. T cells**

Ref: Chapter No.25, Page No.586

39. **Ans: C. CD154**

Ref: Chapter No.25, Page No.586

40. **Ans: B. Activated APCs**

Ref: Chapter No.25, Page No.586

41. **Ans: B. CD153**

Way to remember

CD30, take the first digit 3, hence CD153

CD40, take the first digit 4, hence CD154

CD28, take the last digit 8, hence CD80/86

CD27, take the last digit 7, hence CD70

Ref: Chapter No.25, Page No.586

42. **Ans: C. CD178 (FasL)**

Ref: Chapter No.25, Page No.586

43. **Ans: B. T cells**

Ref: Chapter No.25, Page No.586

44. **Ans: B. CD254 (TRANCE)**

Ref: Chapter No.25, Page No.586

45. **Ans: A. CD279**

Ref: Chapter No.25, Page No.586

46. **Ans: B. CD274**

Ref: Chapter No.25, Page No.586

47. **Ans: C. CD275**

Ref: Chapter No.25, Page No.586

48. **Ans: D. CD273**

Way to remember:

The addition of the last digits is always 13! (except for PD-L2)

E.g., CD278 (ICOS) and CD275 (ICOSL) - 8+5=13

CD279 (PD-1) and CD274 (PD-L1) – 9+4=13

Also PD-L1 has more effect on Th1 > Th2 and PD-L2 has more effect on Th2 > Th1

Ref: Chapter No.25, Page No.586

49. **Ans: B. Th2**

Ref: Chapter No.25, Page No.588

50. **Ans: C. IL-21**

Ref: Chapter No.25, Page No.588

51. **Ans: B. Th2**

Ref: Chapter No.25, Page No.588

52. **Ans: C. Th17**

Ref: Chapter No.25, Page No.588

53. **Ans: D. Tfh**

Ref: Chapter No.25, Page No.588

54. **Ans: A. Th1**

Ref: Chapter No.25, Page No.588

55. **Ans: C. Th17**

Ref: Chapter No.25, Page No.588

56. **Ans: A. Th1**

Ref: Chapter No.25, Page No.588

57. **Ans: D. All of the above**

Ref: Chapter No.25, Page No.589

58. **Ans: C. Chromosome 14**

Ref: Chapter No.25, Page No.590

59. **Ans: A. Chromosome 2**

Ref: Chapter No.25, Page No.590

60. **Ans: B. Light chain use defines the subtype of any given antibody**

Ref: Chapter No.25, Page No.591

61. **Ans: D. B cells express CD30, and when bound by CD154 expressed on activated T cells, the result is up-regulation of B7 molecules on the B. cell and delivery of important costimulatory signals to T cells as well**

Ref: Chapter No.25, Page No.591

62. **Ans: A. With the use of cyclosporine A and newer agents such as tacrolimus, 1-year graft survival has exceeded 70% for virtually all organs except the small intestine**

Ref: Chapter No.25, Page No.592

63. **Ans: A. Acute rejection is a process mediated most commonly by B cells**

Ref: Chapter No.25, Page No.592-594

64. **Ans: B. This type of rejection is not avoidable with pre-transplantation testing**

Ref: Chapter No.25, Page No.594

65. **Ans: D. All of the above**

Ref: Chapter No.25, Page No.594

66. **Ans: B. Acute Rejection**

Ref: Chapter No.25, Page No.594

67. **Ans: B. It most commonly occurs within the first 3 months after transplantation**

Ref: Chapter No.25, Page No.594-595

68. **Ans: C. 70%**

Ref: Chapter No.25, Page No.595

69. **Ans: A. 2-3 days**

Ref: Chapter No.25, Page No.595

70. **Ans: D. All of the above**

Ref: Chapter No.25, Page No.595-596

71. **Ans: D. All of the above**

Ref: Chapter No.25, Page No.597-598

72. **Ans: D. ATGAM seems to be more effective than RATG at reducing the incidence of acute rejection episodes**

Ref: Chapter No.25, Page No.598

73. **Ans: B. Chills and fevers occur in up to 50% of patients, and this cytokine release syndrome usually needs to stop the drugs**

Ref: Chapter No.25, Page No.598

74. **Ans: C. Basiliximab is humanized and Daclizumab is a mouse-human chimeric antibody**

Ref: Chapter No.25, Page No.598

75. **Ans: B. Cytokine release syndrome can be seen as a side effect**

Ref: Chapter No.25, Page No.598

76. **Ans: D. Both A and B**

Ref: Chapter No.25, Page No.598

77. **Ans: A. Rituximab**

Ref: Chapter No.25, Page No.599

78. **Ans: B. Alemtuzumab**

Ref: Chapter No.25, Page No.599

79. **Ans: C. Belatacept**

Ref: Chapter No.25, Page No.599

80. **Ans: A. It is a humanized antibody against human CD52, a cell surface protein expressed on most mature lymphocytes and monocytes and on their stem cell precursors**

Ref: Chapter No.25, Page No.600-601

81. **Ans: D. High-dose steroids remain a common component of current standard immunosuppressive regimens**

Ref: Chapter No.25, Page No.601

82. **Ans: C. Steroids increase the leukocyte response to various chemokines and chemotactins and by stimulating vasodilators, such as histamine and prostacyclin, they dampen the inflammatory response globally**

Ref: Chapter No.25, Page No.601

83. **Ans: B. Prednisone**

Ref: Chapter No.25, Page No.601

84. **Ans: C. The effects of azathioprine are relatively specific, and unlike other antiproliferative agents**

Ref: Chapter No.25, Page No.601

85. **Ans: B. Azathioprine**

Ref: Chapter No.25, Page No.601

86. **Ans: A. The major clinical side effects include thrombocyopenia**

Ref: Chapter No.25, Page No.601

87. **Ans: D. CsA acts to decrease transcription of TGF-β**

Ref: Chapter No.25, Page No.601-602

88. **Ans: A. CsA has good water solubility**

Ref: Chapter No.25, Page No.602

89. **Ans: C. Phenytoin**

Ref: Chapter No.25, Page No.602

90. **Ans: D. All of the above**

Ref: Chapter No.25, Page No.602

91. **Ans: C. 50%**

Ref: Chapter No.25, Page No.602

92. **Ans: C. The side effect profile for tacrolimus is similar to that of CsA with regard to renal toxicity and cosmetic side effects such as abnormal hair growth and gingival hyperplasia**

Ref: Chapter No.25, Page No.602

93. **Ans: B. Sirolimus has demonstrated activity against EBV**

Ref: Chapter No.25, Page No.602

94. **Ans: B. There is an increased incidence of hypercholesterolemia and hypertriglyceridemia with these agents but rarely needs treatment**

Ref: Chapter No.25, Page No.602

95. **Ans: D. All of the above**

Ref: Chapter No.25, Page No.603

96. **Ans: A. CD20 is a cell surface protein expressed on all mature B cells and on plasma cells**

Ref: Chapter No.25, Page No.604

97. **Ans: D. All of the above**

Ref: Chapter No.25, Page No.604

98. **Ans: D. All of the above**

Ref: Chapter No.25, Page No.604

99. **Ans: B. Tofacitinib**

Ref: Chapter No.25, Page No.604

100. **Ans: D. Fingolimod**

Ref: Chapter No.25, Page No.604

101. **Ans: B. Proteasome inhibitors**

Ref: Chapter No.25, Page No.604

102. Ans: D. All of the above

Ref: Chapter No.25, Page No.605

103. Ans: C. 6 - 12 weeks

Ref: Chapter No.25, Page No.605

104. Ans: D. All of the above

Ref: Chapter No.25, Page No.605

105. Ans: C. Progressive multifocal leukoencephalopathy

Ref: Chapter No.25, Page No.605

106. Ans: A. Squamous cell cancer

Ref: Chapter No.25, Page No.606

107. Ans: C. Epstein bar virus

Ref: Chapter No.25, Page No.606

108. Ans: B. The incidence of new-onset immunosuppressive-related diabetes mellitus approaches 50% in the first 1 year after renal transplantation

Ref: Chapter No.25, Page No.606

109. Ans: D. All of the above

Ref: Chapter No.25, Page No.608

110. Ans: D. All of the above

Ref: Chapter No.25, Page No.608

111. Ans: D. All of the above

Ref: Chapter No.25, Page No.609

112. Ans: D. All of the above

Ref: Chapter No.25, Page No.609-610

26

Liver Transplantation

HISTORY

1. **Who discovered that graft loss is due to immunological factors?**
   A. Alexis Carrel
   B. Sir Peter Medawar
   C. Gertrude Eillion
   D. Joseph Murray

2. **The first attempt at human liver transplantation was done by:**
   A. Jean Borel
   B. Joseph Murray
   C. Thomas Starzl
   D. Koichi Tanaka

3. **Who discovered that cyclosporine, initially investigated as an antifungal agent, had immunosuppressive properties?**
   A. Jean Borel
   B. Joseph Murray
   C. Thomas Starzl
   D. Koichi Tanaka

INDICATIONS

4. **Cholestatic Cirrhotic disease states causing liver failure that may be successfully treated with transplant include all except:**
   A. Primary sclerosing cholangitis (PSC)
   B. Caroli disease
   C. Non-alcoholic fatty liver disease
   D. Choledochal cyst

5. **The most common reason for listing for liver transplantation is:**
   A. Alcoholic liver disease
   B. Non-alcoholic steatohepatitis (NASH)
   C. Hepatitis C
   D. Biliary atresia

6. **False about alcoholic liver disease is:**
   A. Current recommendations for referral for transplant is, if the model for end-stage liver disease (MELD) is > 26 given high short-term mortality
   B. Chronic alcohol ingestion is the most common indication for liver transplantation, responsible for approximately 25% of all listings
   C. Alcoholic hepatitis is a subset of alcohol-associated liver disease that occurs in patients with a long history of alcohol use who present with an acute inflammatory syndrome with a bilirubin of greater than 1.5
   D. Ingestion of 30 g of alcohol per day seems to be a relevant threshold and will cause chronic liver damage in approximately 6% of people

7. **Not seen in alcoholic liver disease is:**
   A. Alanine aminotransferase (ALT)/Aspartate aminotransferase (AST) ratio is > 2
   B. Aspartate aminotransferase (AST)/alanine aminotransferase (ALT) ratio is > 2
   C. Mild transaminase elevation (<500)
   D. Pericentral fibrosis progresses to pan lobar fibrosis with associated manifestations of cirrhosis

8. **The second most common indication for liver transplantation in the United States is:**
   A. Alcoholic liver disease
   B. Non-alcoholic steatohepatitis (NASH)
   C. Hepatitis C
   D. Biliary atresia

9. **Biopsy in NASH demonstrates all except:**
   A. Ballooning degeneration
   B. Lobular inflammation most commonly in zone 3

C. Hepatocyte steatosis
D. Lobular inflammation most commonly in zone 1

10. True about Hepatitis C is:

A. Patients who present with advanced cirrhosis should be considered for liver transplantation consistent with usual clinical indications
B. Even patients who achieve a sustained virologic response to therapy remain at a 3% per year risk of the development of hepatocellular cancer or disease progression
C. Hepatitis C has gone from the most common to the 3rd most common indication for liver transplantation in the United States
D. All of the above

11. Cryptogenic cirrhosis is generally now thought to be:

A. Advanced alcoholic cirrhosis
B. Advanced NASH cirrhosis
C. Advanced viral cirrhosis
D. All of the above

12. For type I autoimmune hepatitis, an inflammatory disease of the liver occurs mostly in women at ratio of:

A. 2:1 B. 4:1
C. 10:1 D. 40:1

13. False about autoimmune hepatitis is:

A. In the initial stages of the disease, fibrosis may be absent
B. Characteristic findings on laboratory evaluation include high elevations in AST and ALT with lesser elevations in alkaline phosphatase and elevated gamma globulins
C. Histologic findings include a mononuclear cell infiltrate primarily in the portal regions, and piecemeal necrosis may be present at the periportal region
D. The course is always self-limited

14. False about Hepatitis B is:

A. Patients who develop fulminant hepatic failure, should be considered for emergent liver transplantation
B. 60% will develop jaundice
C. For perinatal acquired infection, 90% will progress to chronic infection, with rates decreasing as the age of transmission increases
D. Acute infection with hepatitis B is subclinical in 70% of patients

15. False among the following is:

A. Positive antimitochondrial antibodies are the hallmark of primary biliary cholangitis
B. Most commonly, Caroli's disease is transmitted as an autosomal dominant fashion with polycystic renal disease
C. Patients with PSC carry significant risk of cholangiocarcinoma of 13%
D. All of the above are true

16. From the symptom onset, hyperacute liver failure occurs within:

A. 3 days B. 7 days
C. 14 days D. 21 days

17. The most common cause of acute liver failure is:

A. Acetaminophen overdose
B. Autoimmune
C. Drug ingestion
D. Hepatitis B

18. False about acute liver failure is:

A. Acute liver failure is a clinical syndrome of hepatic encephalopathy and elevated prothrombin time (PT)/international normalized ratio (INR) due to injury to the liver in patients without preexisting liver disease
B. Progression of hepatic encephalopathy to stage III can be used as a guideline to move forward with transplant
C. The presence of encephalopathy is required for the diagnosis and for listing in the most urgent category for liver transplant, a status 1A designation
D. Use of serial computed tomography (CT) scans or an intracranial pressure monitor (bolt) can help guide therapy and, importantly, the decision to proceed with transplantation

19. In a patient with acetaminophen overdose, King's College criteria suggesting the need for transplant is all except:

A. Grade III or IV encephalopathy
B. High creatinine
C. Arterial pH < 7.3 after resuscitation
D. High bilirubin

20. Milan Criteria includes:

A. One lesion 2 to 5 cm in diameter
B. Patients with up to 3 lesions
C. Each of the 3 lesions between 1 - 3 cm in diameter
D. All of the above

21. **The amount of liver to be preserved to ensure adequate synthetic function is:**
    A. 20%
    B. 30%
    C. 35%
    D. 40%

22. **False about Budd-Chiari syndrome is:**
    A. Budd-Chiari syndrome is a rare condition that occurs when hepatic venous outflow is occluded, typically due to thrombosis of the hepatic veins or vena cava at the level of the hepatic veins
    B. Approximately 50% of patients will present with acute liver failure
    C. An underlying hypercoagulable or other reason is identified in over 80% of patients and should be actively sought with a hypercoagulable workup
    D. In patients with established fibrosis or cirrhosis, liver transplantation should be considered

CONTRAINDICATIONS

23. **Following statements are true except:**
    A. Portopulmonary hypertension uncorrectable to < 50 mm Hg is generally considered a contraindication, as is hepatopulmonary syndrome if the PaO_2 cannot be corrected on 100% oxygen
    B. Patients with human immunodeficiency virus (HIV), are an absolute contraindication to transplant
    C. Patients with advanced cardiac disease are usually excluded from consideration of transplant
    D. Patients with coronary heart disease are at risk for intraoperative myocardial infarction and may have accelerated progression of atherosclerosis due to immunosuppression after transplant

MELD AND ALLOCATION

24. **False about MELD score is:**
    A. Currently, the MELD score determines priority for liver transplantation
    B. Originally developed to predict 3-month mortality in patients after transjugular porto-systemic shunt placement
    C. Serum potassium has recently been added to improve the predictive value of the score
    D. In its original formulation, it was based on serum creatinine, INR and bilirubin

25. **True about MELD score is:**
    A. Status 1 patients suffer from fulminant liver failure with expected death on the order of days and these patients are prioritized above patients with MELD scores
    B. Patients with hepatocellular cancer can be cured with liver transplantation but typically have low MELD scores and would likely not come to transplant prior to disease progression
    C. There is general agreement that most patients with low MELD scores (< 15) do not benefit from transplantation
    D. All of the above

26. **Common indications for exception points for liver transplant includes all except:**
    A. Primary hyperoxaluria
    B. Portopulmonary hypertension (provided the mean arterial pressure can be maintained at >35 mm Hg with treatment)
    C. Hepatopulmonary syndrome
    D. Cystic fibrosis

27. **Diagnoses that may be appropriate for exception points includes:**
    A. Portal hypertensive gastropathy leading to chronic blood loss
    B. Refractory ascites
    C. Refractory hepatic encephalopathy
    D. All of the above

DONOR SELECTION

28. **False about liver donor is:**
    A. The ideal liver donor is young, healthy, and thin with normal liver function tests and no history of liver disease or risk factors for infectious disease
    B. Older donors carry additional risk of short- and long-term graft loss, and older age is an independent risk factor for mortality
    C. Livers > 30% steatosis or with significant fibrosis for any reason should be used with caution
    D. The use of hepatitis C infected donors is becoming routine given the success of specific antiviral therapy

PREOPERATIVE EVALUATION

29. **True about preoperative evaluation is:**
    A. Liver transplantation requires long-term follow-up and medications to prevent rejection and other complication

B. Cardiac and pulmonary workup is similarly essential including stress testing and pulmonary function tests in patients with appropriate risk factors
C. All screening testing should be up-to-date, including mammography, colonoscopy, prostate cancer screening, etc.
D. All of the above

SURGICAL CONSIDERATIONS

30. False about the liver transplant operation is:

A. Difficult biliary anastomoses can be managed with a Roux-en-Y technique or even direct choledochoduodenostomy
B. In the piggyback technique, the caudate is dissected off of the retrohepatic cava, and the recipient cava is ligated
C. In recipients with portal vein thrombosis, first attempts should be to open the vein with thrombectomy catheters and thrombo-endovenectomy if needed
D. If thromboendovenectomy fails, inflow can be obtained from the superior mesenteric vein, nearby varices, and even the left renal vein in patients in whom there is significant splenorenal shunting

POSTOPERATIVE MANAGEMENT

31. True about postoperative management in liver transplantation is:

A. Feeding should begin as early as is safe, and there should be a low threshold for placing a feeding tube should the patient demonstrate an inability to consume adequate calories after normal gastrointestinal (GI) function returns
B. If the patient is massively volume overloaded but hypotensive, a vasopressor may mitigate the need for massive ongoing fluid resuscitation
C. The best way to determine total body volume status is an accurate patient weight taking into account preoperative ascites
D. All of the above

COMPLICATIONS AND THEIR TREATMENT

32. False about early complications of transplantation is:

A. Postoperative hypotension can be caused by many factors, but bleeding must always be considered
B. Frequent assessment of graft function is essential and quick action must be taken when indicated
C. Ongoing hemorrhage requiring continuous blood replacement is generally managed conservatively
D. Patients who develop a compartment syndrome must return to the operating room

33. False about primary nonfunction of liver after transplantation is:

A. Primary nonfunction is a serious complication but rarely requires retransplantation
B. The most common causes are an unrecognized procurement error, use of certain types of higher-risk grafts (fatty, fibrotic, DCDD), or arterial complication after the transplant
C. Typically, the patient will not wake up, the lactate will remain very high, bilirubin will continue to rise, and the AST and ALT will rise into the 5000 to 10,000 range
D. An ultrasound should be obtained to interrogate the artery

34. The most common complication in the post-operative period after liver transplantation is:

A. Portal vein stenosis
B. Biliary issues
C. Arterial complications
D. Portal vein thrombosis

35. False about arterial complications after liver transplantation is:

A. Arterial complications not producing primary nonfunction occur in approximately 2% to 4% of patients
B. It usually manifests as increased AST and ALT, high bilirubin, and poor synthetic function with elevated INR
C. Early arterial thrombosis, even if not associated with primary nonfunction, can be managed conservatively
D. Arterial stenosis or thrombosis can be diagnosed on ultrasound or contrast CT and must be addressed as soon as possible if discovered

36. False about biliary issues after liver transplantation is:

A. Modern management of bile duct issues employs endoscopic management for stent placement and dilations
B. It can present as bile in the drain in the case of a leak or in a patient who returns with a biloma
C. Early major biliary issues should prompt an ultrasound to ensure vessel patency and reoperation to check for bile duct ischemia and to consider reanastomosis

D. Stricture leads to decreased bilirubin and alkaline phosphatase

37. Biliary issues, the most common complication in the postoperative period of liver transplantation and occur in approximately:

A. 10% B. 20%
C. 30% D. 50%

IMMUNOSUPPRESSION

38. False about immunosuppression after liver transplantation is:

A. Distinct from renal transplantation, liver transplantation does not require matching between donor and recipient human leukocyte antigen
B. Hepatocytes express low levels of class I antigen and high levels of class II antigen
C. Steroids inhibit transcription of cytokines, the most important of which is IL-2, which downregulates the immunological response to antigen
D. Mycophenolate mofetil inhibits purine synthase, which decreases proliferation of T and B cells. The major side effect is GI upset

39. Major side effect of mycophenolate mofetil is:

A. Hypertension B. Renal toxicity
C. GI upset D. Cataracts

40. Side effects of Calcineurin is/are all except:

A. Renal toxicity
B. Hypertension
C. Osteoporosis
D. Lipid abnormalities

41. The mainstay of immunosuppression for liver transplantation is:

A. Calcineurin inhibitors
B. Tacrolimus
C. Mycophenolate mofetil
D. Steroids

42. The incidence of acute rejection by 1-year post-transplant is approximately:

A. 2% B. 5%
C. 10% D. 20%

LIVING DONOR LIVER TRANSPLANTATION INCLUDING DONOR SELECTION

43. True about living donor liver transplantation (LDLT) is:

A. The first LDLT consisted of an adult segment II/III graft including the left hepatic vein, left hepatic artery, left portal vein and left hepatic duct
B. Adult-to-adult liver transplantation is with right lobe grafts consisting of segments V/VI/VII/VIII along with the right hepatic veins, right hepatic arteries, right portal veins
C. The left lobe grafts consist of segments II/III/IV along with the left hepatic vein, left hepatic arteries, left portal vein, and left hepatic ducts
D. All of the above

44. False about liver donor is:

A. Donors with acute or chronic liver diseases or extrahepatic disease that may subsequently impair regeneration are excluded from becoming living liver donors
B. A donor should be left with a residual liver volume of no < 40%
C. Donation is associated with a mortality rate of 1 in 400 to 1 in 500
D. While laparoscopic live liver donation has been reported, most centers perform an open hepatectomy

45. The most frequent complication in liver donor is:

A. Infection B. Hernia
C. Bile leak/biloma D. Reoperation

46. False about recipient of liver transplantation is:

A. Recipient's metabolic needs as determined by the donor graft-recipient weight ratio (GRWR)
B. A GRWR of 0.8% to 1% is generally accepted as safe
C. Donor steatosis, donor age > 50 years old, and high recipient MELD score frequently necessitate higher GRWR up to or in excess of 1
D. All of the above

47. In the liver recipient, the biliary reconstructions are particularly complication prone with biliary structuring occurring in approximately:

A. 5% B. 10%
C. 20% D. 30%

48. LDLT is currently associated with 1-year patient survival of:

A. 75% B. 80%
C. 90% D. 95%

PEDIATRIC LIVER TRANSPLANTATION

49. The most common cause of end-stage liver disease in children which account for one third of all pediatric liver transplants is:

A. Hepatoblastoma
B. Biliary atresia
C. Hepatocellular carcinoma
D. Maple Syrup Urine disease

50. False about pediatric liver transplantation is:

A. Infants and small children utilize the left lateral section of an adult liver based on the vasculobiliary anatomy of the left lobe
B. Most pediatric recipients who undergo orthotopic liver transplantation are younger than 5 years of age
C. Long-term results for pediatric liver transplantation are excellent, with a 5-year graft survival of 75% for biliary atresia
D. The transplantation of left lateral segment and live donor grafts necessitates the utilization of a cava-preserving technique

51. Machine perfusion may be a superior alternative to cold storage and can be beneficial in a number of different ways as:

A. Perfusion can be used to extend the viability of the organ to improve logistics and allow safer transportation
B. Perfusion can allow for assessment of the quality of the graft
C. Perfusion can be used either to rehabilitate grafts from ongoing oxygenation or to administer drugs to enhance function
D. All of the above

ANSWERS

1. **Ans: B. Sir Peter Medawar**
Ref: Chapter No.26, Page No.614

2. **Ans: C. Thomas Starzl**
Ref: Chapter No.26, Page No.614

3. **Ans: A. Jean Borel**
Ref: Chapter No.26, Page No.614

4. **Ans: C. Non-alcoholic fatty liver disease**
Ref: Chapter No.26, Page No.615

5. **Ans: A. Alcoholic liver disease**
Ref: Chapter No.26, Page No.615

6. **Ans: C. Alcoholic hepatitis is a subset of alcohol-associated liver disease that occurs in patients with a long history of alcohol use who present with an acute inflammatory syndrome with a bilirubin of greater than 1.5**
Ref: Chapter No.26, Page No.615

7. **Ans: A. Alanine aminotransferase (ALT)/Aspartate aminotransferase (AST) ratio is > 2**
Ref: Chapter No.26, Page No.615

8. **Ans: B. Non-alcoholic steatohepatitis (NASH)**
Ref: Chapter No.26, Page No.615

9. **Ans: D. Lobular inflammation most commonly in zone 1**
Ref: Chapter No.26, Page No.615

10. **Ans: D. All of the above**
Ref: Chapter No.26, Page No.615

11. **Ans: B. Advanced NASH cirrhosis**
Ref: Chapter No.26, Page No.616

12. **Ans: B. 4:1**
Ref: Chapter No.26, Page No.616

13. **Ans: D. The course is always self-limited**
Ref: Chapter No.26, Page No.616

14. **Ans: B. 60% will develop jaundice**
Ref: Chapter No.26, Page No.616

15. **Ans: D. All of the above are true**
Ref: Chapter No.26, Page No.616

16. **Ans: B. 7 days**
Ref: Chapter No.26, Page No.616

17. **Ans: A. Acetaminophen overdose**
Ref: Chapter No.26, Page No.616

18. **Ans: B. Progression of hepatic encephalopathy to stage III can be used as a guideline to move forward with transplant**
Ref: Chapter No.26, Page No.616-617

19. **Ans: D. High bilirubin**
Ref: Chapter No.26, Page No.617

20. **Ans: D. All of the above**
Ref: Chapter No.26, Page No.617

21. **Ans: B. 30%**
Ref: Chapter No.26, Page No.617

22. **Ans: B. Approximately 50% of patients will present with acute liver failure**

Ref: Chapter No.26, Page No.617

23. **Ans: C. Patients with advanced cardiac disease are usually excluded from consideration of transplant**

Ref: Chapter No.26, Page No.618

24. **Ans: C. Serum potassium has recently been added to improve the predictive value of the score**

Ref: Chapter No.26, Page No.618-619

25. **Ans: D. All of the above**

Ref: Chapter No.26, Page No.619

26. **Ans: B. Portopulmonary hypertension (provided the mean arterial pressure can be maintained at >35 mm Hg with treatment)**

Ref: Chapter No.26, Page No.619

27. **Ans: D. All of the above**

Ref: Chapter No.26, Page No.619

28. **Ans: C. Livers > 30% steatosis or with significant fibrosis for any reason should be used with caution**

Ref: Chapter No.26, Page No.619

29. **Ans: D. All of the above**

Ref: Chapter No.26, Page No.619-620

30. **Ans: B. In the piggyback technique, the caudate is dissected off of the retrohepatic cava, and the recipient cava is ligated**

Ref: Chapter No.26, Page No.620

31. **Ans: D. All of the above**

Ref: Chapter No.26, Page No.620-621

32. **Ans: C. Ongoing hemorrhage requiring continuous blood replacement is generally managed conservatively**

Ref: Chapter No.26, Page No.621

33. **Ans: A. Primary nonfunction is a serious complication but rarely requires retransplantation**

Ref: Chapter No.26, Page No.621

34. **Ans: B. Biliary issues**

Ref: Chapter No.26, Page No.621

35. **Ans: C. Early arterial thrombosis, even if not associated with primary nonfunction, can be managed conservatively**

Ref: Chapter No.26, Page No.621

36. **Ans: D. Stricture leads to decreased bilirubin and alkaline phosphatase**

Ref: Chapter No.26, Page No.621

37. **Ans: B. 20%**

Ref: Chapter No.26, Page No.621

38. **Ans: B. Hepatocytes express low levels of class I antigen and high levels of class II antigen**

Ref: Chapter No.26, Page No.621-622

39. **Ans: C. GI upset**

Ref: Chapter No.26, Page No.622

40 **Ans: C. Osteoporosis**

Ref: Chapter No.26, Page No.622

41. **Ans: B. Tacrolimus**

Ref: Chapter No.26, Page No.622

42. **Ans: C. 10%**

Ref: Chapter No.26, Page No.622

43. **Ans: D. All of the above**

Ref: Chapter No.26, Page No.622

44. **Ans: B. A donor should be left with a residual liver volume of no < 40%**

Ref: Chapter No.26, Page No.622

45. **Ans: A. Infection**

Ref: Chapter No.26, Page No.622

46. **Ans: D. All of the above**

Ref: Chapter No.26, Page No.622

47. **Ans: D. 30%**

Ref: Chapter No.26, Page No.622

48. **Ans: C. 90%**

Ref: Chapter No.26, Page No.622

49. **Ans: B. Biliary atresia**

Ref: Chapter No.26, Page No.622-623

50. **Ans: C. Long-term results for pediatric liver transplantation are excellent, with a 5-year graft survival of 75% for biliary atresia**

Ref: Chapter No.26, Page No.623

51. **Ans: D. All of the above**

Ref: Chapter No.26, Page No.623

27

Kidney and Pancreas Transplantation

HISTORICAL PERSPECTIVE

1. **The first successful renal transplantation was performed by:**
   A. Joseph Murray B. William Kelly
   C. Alexis Carrel D. Richard Lillehei

2. **The first successful human pancreas transplantation was performed by:**
   A. Joseph Murray B. William Kelly
   C. Alexis Carrel D. Hedon

3. **Who develop University of Wisconsin Solution?**
   A. Scharp and Lacy
   B. Borel and Calne
   C. Belzer and Southard
   D. Kelly and Lillehei

4. **The first successful human clinical islet transplantation was reported by:**
   A. Scharp and Lacy
   B. Borel and Calne
   C. Belzer and Southard
   D. Kelly and Lillehei

KIDNEY TRANSPLANTATION

5. **Absolute contraindications to renal transplantation include all except:**
   A. Active infection
   B. Active malignant disease
   C. Unreconstructable peripheral vascular disease
   D. Morbid obesity

6. **Relative contraindications to renal transplantation include all except:**
   A. Morbid obesity
   B. Renal disease with high recurrence rate
   C. Active intravenous drug abuse
   D. Frailty

7. **Glomerular disease recurrence rate after kidney transplantation is highest with:**
   A. FSGS
   B. IgA nephropathy
   C. MPGN type 2
   D. Hemolytic uremic syndrome

8. **Which primary renal disease has highest chances of graft loss after renal transplantation?**
   A. Systemic lupus
   B. IgA nephropathy
   C. Membranous nephropathy
   D. Hemolytic uremic syndrome

9. **Which primary renal disease has least chances of graft loss after renal transplantation?**
   A. Systemic lupus
   B. IgA nephropathy
   C. Membranous nephropathy
   D. Hemolytic uremic syndrome

10. **True about renal transplantation is:**
    A. The HIV Organ Policy Equity (HOPE) Act passed by Congress in 2015 has allowed organs from HIV-positive donors to be transplanted to HIV-positive recipients
    B. The length of time on dialysis has been noted to be an independent risk factor for poorer outcomes
    C. The death rate is highest in the first year after transplant and survival benefit is gained by 2 years after transplant
    D. All of the above

11. **False about the evaluation for renal transplantation is:**

A. Patients should have a baseline electrocardiogram, recognizing that nearly 75% will have evidence of left ventricular hypertrophy
B. Routine age-appropriate screening examinations, such as Papanicolaou smears, mammograms, colonoscopy, prostate specific antigen, dental prophylaxis, and bone density, should be obtained as recommended by clinical practice guidelines
C. Dobutamine stress echocardiography has been shown to have superiority in accuracy and predictability for perioperative cardiac events
D. Patients with chronic kidney disease (CKD) are 50 to 60 times more likely to have significant cardiovascular disease compared to the general population

12. True about renal transplantation patients is:

A. Low-risk patients include those who have good functional capacity and no cardiac disease previously identified
B. Moderate-risk patients include those without cardiac symptoms but who have diabetes, a prior history of heart disease, or two or more other risk factors for coronary disease
C. High-risk patients include those with a positive result on noninvasive testing, long-standing diabetes, or history of severe congestive heart failure
D. All of the above

13. As compared to general population, renal failure patients are at increased risk for cerebrovascular events, and the stroke risk upto:

A. 5 times B. 10 times
C. 20 times D. 40 times

14. Kidney donor profile index score components includes all except:

A. Height B. Age
C. Ethnicity D. BMI

15. Kidney donor profile index score components includes all except:

A. Stroke B. Hepatitis B
C. Diabetes D. Hypertension

16. Currently accepted eligibility criteria of renal transplantation includes all except:

A. No cancer or active infection
B. 18 to 70 years
C. Body mass index (BMI) < 40
D. Age

17. Relative contraindications for renal transplantation includes all except:

A. GFR of 70 to 80 mL/min/1.72 m^2
B. BMI < 35
C. Renal stones
D. Impaired glucose tolerance with a family history of type 1 diabetes

18. Cardiac risk factors for renal transplantation includes all except:

A. DM
B. RBBB
C. CVA or TIA
D. Current smoker or >10 pack years

19. Electroencephalography for confirmatory testing for a determination of brain death includes all except:

A. The sensitivity should be increased to at least 2μV for 30 minutes with inclusion of appropriate calibrations
B. A minimum of 4 scalp electrodes should be used
C. Electroencephalography should demonstrate a lack of reactivity to intense somatosensory or audio-visual stimuli
D. The distance between electrodes should be at least 10 cm

20. Contraindications to living kidney donation includes all except:

A. Horseshoe kidney
B. Diabetes
C. BMI >35
D. Active malignant disease

21. The most common perioperative complication in potential kidney donors is:

A. Gastrointestinal B. Bleeding
C. Liver failure D. Hypertension

22. The most common complication after renal transplantation is:

A. Bleeding B. Urinary retention
C. Rhabdomyolysis D. DVT/PE

23. The most common complication after renal transplantation is:

A. Injury to the bowel or bladder
B. Ileus
C. Injury to the spleen
D. DVT/PE

24. Preoperative components of Duke enhanced recovery after donor nephrectomy protocol include all except:

A. Carbohydrate drink 2 hours preoperatively
B. Cefazolin 1–2 g IV
C. Heparin 5000 units SC
D. Fentanyl patch

25. False about preservation and storage of kidneys for transplantation is:

A. The predominant storage solutions currently used are Viaspan (Dupont, University of Wisconsin Solution) and Custodial (histidine-tryptophan-ketoglutarate)
B. Kidneys may be stored in static cold solution
C. Delayed graft function significantly increases at 24 hours
D. If delayed graft function developed, the duration was 7 days shorter in machine-perfused kidneys

26. Increased risk CDC donor includes all except:

A. A child who is ≤24 months of age and born to a mother known to be infected with or at increased risk for HIV, HBV, or HCV infection
B. People who have had sex with a person who has injected drugs by intravenous, intramuscular, or subcutaneous route for nonmedical reasons in the preceding 12 months
C. People who have been newly diagnosed with or have been treated for syphilis, gonorrhea, chlamydia, or genital ulcers in the preceding 12 months
D. People who have been in lockup, jail, prison, or a juvenile correctional facility for more than 72 hours in the preceding 12 months

27. False about KDPI and kidney donation is:

A. Kidneys with a KDPI greater than 85% will be an "opt in" system that will require recipients to sign prior consent for these kidneys
B. Kidneys with the top 10% KDPI are preferentially allocated to the top 10% Estimated Post Transplant Survival score candidates
C. Kidneys with a KDPI greater than 85% will be allocated on the basis of waiting time and local or regional area
D. All of the above are true

28. The overall rate of technical complications in kidney transplantation is:

A. 2%-5%
B. 5%-10%
C. 10%-20%
D. 1%-2%

29. In hemorrhage after kidney transplant, all statements are false except:

A. Patients will commonly present with the acute onset of flank pain, and there may be a palpable mass at the incision site
B. Risk factors include increased mid abdominal circumference, antiplatelet agents, and anticoagulation
C. Tachycardia is a reliable sign
D. Because of compression of the kidney parenchyma, patients will sometimes present with hypertension rather than with the expected hypotension

30. Venous thrombosis after renal transplantation occurs in:

A. < 1%
B. < 3%
C. < 5%
D. < 10%

31. False about venous thrombosis after renal transplantation is:

A. Usually is manifested within the 1st week postoperatively
B. Dialysis patients also have a high incidence of hypercoagulable states
C. The graft is usually salvageable after renal vein thrombosis
D. The patient may develop sudden hematuria or a decrease in urine output

32. False about arterial thrombosis after renal transplantation is:

A. The kidney will tolerate warm ischemia, and a transplant nephrectomy is rarely warranted
B. The patient may have sudden cessation of urine output, or the failure of the β2-microglobulin levels to fall after transplantation
C. If a lower pole artery is thrombosed, the ureter becomes ischemic, and a urine leak may develop from ureteral necrosis
D. Ultrasound is diagnostic

33. Arterial thrombosis after renal transplantation occurs in:

A. < 1%
B. < 3%
C. < 5%
D. < 10%

34. False about stenosis of the renal artery after renal transplantation is:

A. The ultrasound is diagnostic if the renal artery velocity is ≥100 cm/sec, spectral broadening is seen (indicating turbulence), and tardus parvus waveforms are present
B. Balloon angioplasty of transplant renal artery stenosis has success rates varying between 20% and 80%
C. If the native iliac artery is diseased, balloon angioplasty has been successful, demonstrates native iliac artery atherosclerotic disease
D. Patients usually present with an asymptomatic rise in creatinine concentration

35. False about urologic complications after renal transplantation is/are:

A. Long stricture or very proximal stricture will need to be repaired by performing a ureteropyelostomy and using the native ureter
B. Graft loss is rare with urologic complications
C. Polyomavirus (BK) is a cause of late multiple strictures
D. Use of a stent at the time of implantation has not been associated with fewer mechanical urologic complications

36. Golden triangle in periureteric tissue is defined by all except:

A. Descending aorta
B. Renal artery
C. The lower pole of the kidney
D. The ureter

37. Of all urologic complications, urine leak is about:

A. 5% B. 25%
C. 40% D. 50%

38. False about Lymphocele after renal transplantation is:

A. The treatment of symptomatic lymphoceles is surgical, with a peritoneal communication being established either by open techniques or laparoscopically
B. Drain placement at the time of the transplant prevents the complication
C. Percutaneous aspiration has poor results with a high rate of recurrence and carries the risk of infecting the fluid collection
D. The lymphocele fluid should be sent for creatinine levels at the time of surgery to ensure that there is no occult urine leak

39. Recipients experiencing a urinary tract infection after renal transplantation is up to:

A. 20% B. 40%
C. 60% D. 80%

40. False about infectious complications after renal transplantation is:

A. Viral infections are also common in the first 1 month after transplantation as this is the time that the patient is receiving the highest levels of maintenance immunosuppression
B. There is a 1% to 10% chance of wound infections immediately after surgery
C. Many transplant centers will treat patients in the early post transplantation phase with antivirals including ganciclovir, acyclovir and valganciclovir
D. Diabetes, obesity and the use of steroids increase the risk

41. Prophylaxis for common opportunistic infection in Pneumocystis jiroveci is:

A. Erythromycin
B. Trimethoprim sulfamethoxazole
C. Ceftriaxone
D. Azithromycin

PANCREAS TRANSPLANTATION

42. Leading cause of blindness worldwide is:

A. Hypertension B. Diabetes
C. Stroke D. Trauma

43. True about patient selection for pancreatic transplantation is:

A. In pancreas after kidney transplant candidates, a GFR of more than 50 mL/min/1.72 m^2 is required to maintain renal function with a temporary increase in immunosuppression
B. Patients requiring pancreas transplantation are usually type 1 diabetics with a clear C-peptide deficiency
C. Because the patients will require calcineurin inhibitor therapy after PTA, a GFR of more than 70 to 80 mL/min/1.72 m^2 and proteinuria of < 1 g are required in our program
D. All of the above

44. The leading cause of death among type 1 diabetics is:

A. Renal failure
B. Cardiovascular disease

C. Peripheral vascular disease
D. Stroke

45. Pancreas donor risk index donor components includes all except:

A. Terminal amylase B. Height
C. Race D. Sex

46. Pancreas donor risk index donor components includes all except:

A. Preservation time
B. Warm ischemia time
C. Cause of death
D. DCD

47. In DCD, the recommended warm ischemia time is:

A. < 30 minutes B. < 45 minutes
C. < 60 minutes D. < 120 minutes

48. False about pancreas procurement and preparation is:

A. It is most common to procure the liver and pancreas en bloc and then to separate the organs in ice to minimize warm ischemia time
B. The aorta is cross-clamped, and 2 L of University of Wisconsin solution (ViaSpan) is flushed through the organs
C. Histidine-tryptophan-ketoglutarate preservation solution remains the preferred solution as University of Wisconsin solution has been associated with increased risk of thrombosis
D. At least 1 cm of portal vein should be preserved for the pancreas anastomosis

49. False about pancreatic transplantation is:

A. The iliac artery graft is sutured to the common iliac artery of the recipient
B. The pancreas transplant is usually placed on the right side to prevent undue stretching of the venous anastomosis
C. For systemic venous drainage, the portal vein is anastomosed to the distal vena cava in an side-to-side fashion
D. For portal drainage, the donor portal vein is anastomosed to the recipient proximal superior mesenteric vein (SMV)

50. False about bladder drainage of exocrine secretion is:

A. There is a high incidence of urinary tract infections, dysuria, urethritis and even urethral disruption
B. Bladder drainage offers the advantages of decreasing the risk of enteric content contamination from the native enterotomy and allowing monitoring of urinary amylase level as an early diagnostic tool for dysfunction or rejection of the transplant
C. A leak from the bladder anastomosis can be managed nonoperatively by placement of a Foley catheter and but commonly leads to graft loss
D. Urinary anastomotic leaks can be diagnosed with a bladder contrast-enhanced CT scan with delayed images

51. The incidence of enteric leak after pancreatic transplantation is:

A. 0.5% to 1% B. 2% to 10%
C. 15% to 20% D. 40% to 50%

52. False about leak after pancreatic transplantation is:

A. Leak from the enteric anastomosis was the Achilles heel of early attempts at pancreas transplantation
B. As a consequence of immunosuppression, transplant patients may not display overt signs of infection or leak, and a high index of suspicion is critical to timely diagnosis and treatment
C. Enteric leak rarely requires reoperation
D. Early leaks are most often anastomotic, and treatment depends on the size of the leak and the condition of the donor duodenum

53. False about bleeding after pancreatic transplantation is:

A. Delayed gastrointestinal bleeding can also occur from the enteric anastomosis
B. Immediate posttransplantation bleeding can occur from the pancreatic parenchyma, particularly near the SMA or splenic arteries
C. Endoscopy or radiographic studies are usually diagnostic
D. This usually is manifested from postoperative days 6 - 10 and is self-limited

54. Late gastrointestinal bleeding after pancreatic transplantation is/are:

A. Rejection or development of pseudoaneurysms
B. Duodenal ulcers of the duodenal stump from ischemia
C. CMV infection
D. All of the above

55. False about late gastrointestinal bleeding after pancreatic transplantation is:

A. Findings on angiography of the celiac trunk and superior and inferior mesenteric arteries may be normal as the source of the fistula is the iliac vessel

B. Most cases of late bleeding are associated with graft loss

C. The source of bleeding can be identified on upper and lower endoscopy

D. Both aortoenteric fistulas and pseudoaneurysms are prone to develop in cases of chronic rejection, infection, or in proximity to already failed organs

56. False about thrombosis after pancreatic transplantation is:

A. Graft thrombosis represents the most common nonimmunologic cause of pancreas transplant failure

B. The risk factors for graft thrombosis are multifactorial and include donor factors such as injury during procurement and reperfusion injury

C. Patients with arterial thrombosis may have an acute rise in glucose concentration with pain as the graft is swollen

D. Coagulopathy related to uremia may confer protection from thrombosis in recipients of SPK transplants, whereas the diabetic state is known to be associated with hypercoagulability

57. Surgical site infection after pancreatic transplantation, most commonly from gram-positive organisms, may occur in up to:

A. 10% B. 30%

C. 50% D. 70%

58. Graft pancreatitis is common after transplantation, occurring in:

A. 15% B. 25%

C. 35% D. 45%

59. False about pancreatitis after pancreatic transplantation is:

A. Early pancreatitis is likely to be related to reperfusion injury to the graft

B. It is important to rule out the possibility of acute rejection, as abdominal pain is more likely with rejection

C. Most cases of pancreatitis are self-limited

D. CT imaging of the graft reveals a swollen, hypervascular organ, often with a significant amount of surrounding fluid

60. The major cause of death in pancreas transplant recipients is:

A. Renal failure

B. Cardiovascular disease

C. Acute pancreatitis

D. Stroke

61. False about pancreatic transplantation outcomes is:

A. Normoglycemia is restored, and patients demonstrate normal hemoglobin A1c levels and patients do not suffer from hypoglycemic unawareness

B. Those with severe disease before transplantation never progress to blindness

C. A major consideration for pancreas transplantation is the potential for prevention of the secondary complications of diabetes

D. Peripheral neuropathy is improved with improvements seen in motor and sensory nerve conduction

ISLET TRANSPLANTATION

62. Islets can be cultured for up to:

A. 12 hours B. 24 hours

C. 72 hours D. 48 hours

63. The main risk related to pancreatic islet transplantation, intra-abdominal bleeding occurs in:

A. 1% - 5% B. 3% - 15%

C. 20% - 25% D. 30% - 45%

64. False about pancreatic islet transplantation is:

A. Fatty organs from donors with a BMI > 32 might go directly to islet centers with high isolation yields

B. The pancreas is dissociated during enzymatic digestion with collagenase, and then the islets are separated from acinar tissue during gradient purification

C. It should be highlighted that 90% of patients maintained islet function more than 5 years after the procedure, expressing normal levels of C peptide in the bloodstream

D. Islets are infused into the IVC by an interventional radiologist

ANSWERS

1. **Ans: A. Joseph Murray**

Ref: Chapter No.27, Page No.627

2. **Ans: B. William Kelly**

Ref: Chapter No.27, Page No.627

3. **Ans: C. Belzer and Southard**

Ref: Chapter No.27, Page No.628

4. **Ans: A. Scharp and Lacy**

Ref: Chapter No.27, Page No.628

5. **Ans: D. Morbid obesity**

Ref: Chapter No.27, Page No.628

6. **Ans: C. Active intravenous drug abuse**

Ref: Chapter No.27, Page No.628

7. **Ans: C. MPGN type 2**

Ref: Chapter No.27, Page No.628

8. **Ans: D. Hemolytic uremic syndrome**

Ref: Chapter No.27, Page No.628

9. **Ans: A. Systemic lupus**

Ref: Chapter No.27, Page No.628

10. **Ans: D. All of the above**

Ref: Chapter No.27, Page No.628-629

11. **Ans: D. Patients with chronic kidney disease (CKD) are 50 to 60 times more likely to have significant cardiovascular disease compared to the general population**

Ref: Chapter No.27, Page No.629

12. **Ans: D. All of the above**

Ref: Chapter No.27, Page No.629

13. **Ans: B. 10 times**

Ref: Chapter No.27, Page No.629

14. **Ans: D. BMI**

Ref: Chapter No.27, Page No.631

15. **Ans: B. Hepatitis B**

Ref: Chapter No.27, Page No.631

16. **Ans: C. Body mass index (BMI) < 40**

Ref: Chapter No.27, Page No.629

17. **Ans: D. Impaired glucose tolerance with a family history of type 1 diabetes**

Ref: Chapter No.27, Page No.629

18. **Ans: B. RBBB**

Ref: Chapter No.27, Page No.630

19. **Ans: B. A minimum of 4 scalp electrodes should be used**

Ref: Chapter No.27, Page No.631

20. **Ans: C. BMI >35**

Ref: Chapter No.27, Page No.631

21. **Ans: A. Gastrointestinal**

Ref: Chapter No.27, Page No.631

22. **Ans: B. Urinary retention**

Ref: Chapter No.27, Page No.631

23. **Ans: B. Ileus**

Ref: Chapter No.27, Page No.632

24. **Ans: D. Fentanyl patch**

Ref: Chapter No.27, Page No.632

25. **Ans: D. If delayed graft function developed, the duration was 7 days shorter in machine-perfused kidneys**

Ref: Chapter No.27, Page No.633

26. **Ans: A. A child who is ≤24 months of age and born to a mother known to be infected with or at increased risk for HIV, HBV, or HCV infection**

Ref: Chapter No.27, Page No.633

27. **Ans: B. Kidneys with the top 10% KDPI are preferentially allocated to the top 10% Estimated Post Transplant Survival score candidates**

Ref: Chapter No.27, Page No.634

28. **Ans: B. 5%–10%**

Ref: Chapter No.27, Page No.634

29. **Ans: C. Tachycardia is a reliable sign**

Ref: Chapter No.27, Page No.634

30. **Ans: B. < 3%**

Ref: Chapter No.27, Page No.634

31. **Ans: C. The graft is usually salvageable after renal vein thrombosis**

Ref: Chapter No.27, Page No.634

32. **Ans: A. The kidney will tolerate warm ischemia, and a transplant nephrectomy is rarely warranted**

Ref: Chapter No.27, Page No.634

33. **Ans: A. < 1%**

Ref: Chapter No.27, Page No.634

34. **Ans: A. The ultrasound is diagnostic if the renal artery velocity is ≥100 cm/sec, spectral broadening is seen (indicating turbulence), and tardus parvus waveforms are present**

Ref: Chapter No.27, Page No.634-635

35. **Ans: D. Use of a stent at the time of implantation has not been associated with fewer mechanical urologic complications**

Ref: Chapter No.27, Page No.635

36. **Ans: A. Descending aorta**

Ref: Chapter No.27, Page No.635

37. **Ans: B. 25%**

Ref: Chapter No.27, Page No.635

38. **Ans: B. Drain placement at the time of the transplant prevents the complication**

Ref: Chapter No.27, Page No.635

39. **Ans: D. 80%**

Ref: Chapter No.27, Page No.636

40. **Ans: A. Viral infections are also common in the first 1 month after transplantation as this is the time that the patient is receiving the highest levels of maintenance immunosuppression**

Ref: Chapter No.27, Page No.636

41. **Ans: B. Trimethoprim sulfamethoxazole**

Ref: Chapter No.27, Page No.636

42. **Ans: B. Diabetes**

Ref: Chapter No.27, Page No.636

43. **Ans: D. All of the above**

Ref: Chapter No.27, Page No.637

44. **Ans: B. Cardiovascular disease**

Ref: Chapter No.27, Page No.637

45. **Ans: A. Terminal amylase**

Ref: Chapter No.27, Page No.637

46. **Ans: B. Warm ischemia time**

Ref: Chapter No.27, Page No.637

47. **Ans: B. < 45 minutes**

Ref: Chapter No.27, Page No.637

48. **Ans: C. Histidine-tryptophan-ketoglutarate preservation solution remains the preferred solution as University of Wisconsin solution has been associated with increased risk of thrombosis**

Ref: Chapter No.27, Page No.637-638

49. **Ans: C. For systemic venous drainage, the portal vein is anastomosed to the distal vena cava in a side-to-side fashion**

Ref: Chapter No.27, Page No.638

50. **Ans: C. A leak from the bladder anastomosis can be managed nonoperatively by placement of a Foley catheter and but commonly leads to graft loss**

Ref: Chapter No.27, Page No.638

51. **Ans: B. 2% to 10%**

Ref: Chapter No.27, Page No.639

52. **Ans: C. Enteric leak rarely requires reoperation**

Ref: Chapter No.27, Page No.639

53. **Ans: C. Endoscopy or radiographic studies are usually diagnostic**

Ref: Chapter No.27, Page No.639

54. **Ans: D. All of the above**

Ref: Chapter No.27, Page No.639

55. **Ans: C. The source of bleeding can be identified on upper and lower endoscopy**

Ref: Chapter No.27, Page No.639

56. **Ans: C. Patients with arterial thrombosis may have an acute rise in glucose concentration with pain as the graft is swollen**

Ref: Chapter No.27, Page No.639

57. **Ans: C. 50%**

Ref: Chapter No.27, Page No.640

58. **Ans: C. 35%**

Ref: Chapter No.27, Page No.640

59. **Ans: B. It is important to rule out the possibility of acute rejection, as abdominal pain is more likely with rejection**

Ref: Chapter No.27, Page No.640

60. **Ans: B. Cardiovascular disease**

Ref: Chapter No.27, Page No.640

61. **Ans: B. Those with severe disease before transplantation never progress to blindness**

Ref: Chapter No.27, Page No.640

62. **Ans: C. 72 hours**

Ref: Chapter No.27, Page No.641

63. **Ans: B. 3% - 15%**

Ref: Chapter No.27, Page No.641

64. **Ans: D. Islets are infused into the IVC by an interventional radiologist**

Ref: Chapter No.27, Page No.640-641

28

Small Bowel Transplantation

HISTORY

1. **Short bowel syndrome and lack of enteral autonomy are expected after resection of:**
   A. > 50% of the native intestine
   B. > 60% of the native intestine
   C. > 75% of the native intestine
   D. > 90% of the native intestine

2. **Intestinal failure associated liver disease (IFALD):**
   A. It is often biochemically characterized as a conjugated bilirubin level > 2 mg/dL in patients who have been on TPN for > 2 weeks
   B. Once IFALD develops, it is associated with a 43% 5-year mortality in patients with remnant jejunum and ileum length of less than 50 cm
   C. IFALD develops in approximately 50% of pediatric patients and is closely related to the duration of TPN (>3 months)
   D. Risk of IFALD induced steatosis in adults receiving home parenteral nutrition is high, with reported rates of 50% to 80%

3. **The first successful human isolated intestine allograft (with the achievement of enteral autonomy) was reportedly performed by:**
   A. Grant and colleagues
   B. Deltz and colleagues
   C. Murray and colleagues
   D. Richards and colleagues

4. **The first cadaveric combined liver-intestine transplant to achieve complete enteral autonomy was reportedly performed by:**
   A. Grant and colleagues
   B. Deltz and colleagues
   C. Murray and colleagues
   D. Richards and colleagues

5. **Indications for transplantation of the intestine are irreversible intestinal failure and:**
   A. Overt or impending liver failure caused by PNALD
   B. Single episode of fungal line infection
   C. > 2 episodes of catheter-related infection requiring hospitalization in any year
   D. All of the above

6. **Most common pediatric condition necessitating intestinal transplantation is:**
   A. Necrotizing enterocolitis
   B. Motility disorders
   C. Volvulus
   D. Gastroschisis

7. **Most common adult condition necessitating intestinal transplantation is:**
   A. Tumor
   B. Crohn's disease
   C. Ischemia
   D. Motility disorders

EVALUATION

8. **False about donor evaluation of patient for intestinal transplantation is:**
   A. Prolonged cold storage of the graft may lead to loss of mucosal integrity, and thus, bacterial translocation or intestinal perforation early after implantation
   B. Size is a significant consideration for the intestine donor because substantial loss of abdominal domain is common in the recipients who have typically undergone extensive resection
   C. An ideal donor should have a body weight 75% to 90% that of the recipient
   D. An appropriate cadaveric donor is selected on the basis of compatible blood type and size of the donor compared with the recipient

9. Many protocols advise a maximum cold ischemia time for small intestine of:

A. 6 - 8 hours
B. 8 - 12 hours
C. 12 - 18 hours
D. 18 - 36 hours

10. False about diagnostic studies for evaluation of the intestine transplant candidate is:

A. Immunologic evaluation: HLA typing, HLA antibody, panel reactive antibody (PRA)
B. Serologic tests for infectious diseases: CMV immunoglobulin G/immunoglobulin M, EBV antibodies, hepatitis B virus, hepatitis C virus, HIV
C. Pathology: Percutaneous Lymph nodal biopsy
D. Radiographic evaluation: Computed tomography of abdomen and pelvis, liver ultrasound

11. True about Intestinal Transplantation is:

A. Carotid or iliac arteries and iliac or jugular veins are also procured from the cadaveric donor to allow vascular reconstruction in the recipient
B. Isolated intestine (or small bowel) allografts typically include the entire jejunum and ileum with the associated vasculature, that is, the superior mesenteric artery (SMA) and vein (SMV)
C. The donor jejunum is divided with a surgical stapler just distal to the ligament of Treitz, and the ileum is transected proximal to the ileocecal valve
D. All of the above

12. The term modified multivisceral has been used to describe a multiorgan intestine containing graft that:

A. Includes donor spleen when the donor kidney is excluded
B. Includes donor stomach when the donor liver is excluded
C. Includes donor stomach when the donor kidney is excluded
D. Includes donor spleen when the donor liver is excluded

13. The cluster graft was used primarily for the transplantations performed for:

A. Trauma
B. Ischemia
C. Tumor
D. Congenital abnormalities

IMMUNOSUPPRESSION

14. True about the immunosuppression for intestinal transplantation is:

A. The introduction of cyclosporine was the key to the successful introduction of intestine transplantation
B. No specific maintenance regimen has proved to be superior to another
C. Belatacept (Nulojix) has also been successfully employed as maintenance therapy in intestinal transplant recipients who did not tolerate tacrolimus due to nephrotoxic side effects
D. All of the above

COMPLICATIONS

15. Intestinal transplantation remains a surgical procedure with high morbidity and reported complication rates approach:

A. 10%
B. 30%
C. 50%
D. 70%

16. The most common types of technical complications are:

A. Intestine perforations
B. Wound complications
C. Bowel anastomotic leaks
D. All of the above

17. False about complications after intestinal transplantation is:

A. Vascular complications are common and include both bleeding and thrombosis
B. Postoperative hemorrhage may result from recipient coagulopathy and be amplified by the extensive dissection usually required as a result of multiple adhesions from previous surgeries
C. Thrombosis of arterial inflow or venous outflow conduits is typically associated with devastating sudden graft necrosis and results in patient or graft loss
D. Biliary complications can be largely avoided in liver-intestine transplantations by including the duodenum and pancreas, thus avoiding any hilar dissection as noted before

18. False about monitoring after intestinal transplantation is:

A. Ileoscopy through the ostomy provides a method of visualizing the mucosa and directly obtaining tissue for pathologic examination

B. Acute cellular rejection usually occurs within the 1st year after transplantation but can occur at any time
C. Like in hepatic or renal transplantation, convenient serochemicals marker exists to monitor intestinal function
D. Routine ileoscopy and biopsy typically begin between postoperative days 5 and 7, and most centers will obtain biopsy specimens once or twice weekly for the first 1 to 3 months and as needed for symptoms thereafter

19. False about donor specific antibodies (DSAs) is:

A. These antibodies bind donor human leukocyte antigen (HLA) and are present in 11% to 31% of patients before transplant and develop de novo in up to 18% to 25% of patients posttransplant
B. DSA has been measured at 1-, 3-, 6- and 12-month intervals following transplant
C. Their presence indicates up to 50% risk of graft loss within 1 year
D. Monitoring DSA is accomplished via enzyme linked immunosorbent assay or HLA bound microbead assay (Luminex)

20. Moderate acute cellular rejection is defined by:

A. Increased apoptotic bodies within the crypts
B. Markedly increased inflammation within the lamina propria
C. Blunting or distortion of the villous architecture
D. All of the above

21. True about treatment of rejection after intestinal transplantation is:

A. Resistant cases may be treated with potent immunosuppression, such as rabbit anti-thymocyte globulin with or without additional immunosuppressive medications (e.g., sirolimus, mycophenolate mofetil)
B. During treatment for rejection, the combination of increased immunosuppression and potential compromise of the gut mucosal barrier can lead to secondary infections
C. Once rejection has been established, treatment usually consists of large steroid doses and an increase in the target levels of maintenance immunosuppression
D. All of the above

22. Leading cause of morbidity and mortality after intestinal transplantation and the most common cause of graft loss is:

A. Cardiovascular disorders
B. Infection
C. Respiratory failure
D. Electrolyte abnormalities

23. False about infections after intestinal transplantation is:

A. Bacterial infections can be manifested as intra-abdominal infection, catheter-related infections, pneumonia, or wound infections, with central line infections being the most common
B. CMV is a common pathogen with infection rates from 18% to 25%, and a 7% incidence of invasive disease
C. Ischemia-reperfusion injury may also lead to loss of the gut mucosal barrier and bacterial translocation or intestinal anastomotic leak in the immediate postoperative period
D. Transplanting bowel from the CMV positive donor to a CMV negative recipient doesn't facilitate transmission

24. Viral infections are common in patients receiving intestine transplants, affecting approximately:

A. 33% B. 50%
C. 66% D. 80%

25. True about CMV infection after intestine transplants is:

A. The presence of CMV inclusion bodies on hematoxylin and eosin stain or identification of CMV by immunohistochemistry or stool electron microscopy confirms the diagnosis of CMV enteritis
B. The symptoms of CMV infection may mimic those of intestine allograft rejection, biopsy of the allograft may be needed to differentiate the two causes of graft injury
C. With appropriate antimicrobial treatment, typically IV ganciclovir alone or in combination with CMV immune globulin, and reduction in immunosuppression, graft loss can be avoided in most cases
D. All of the above

26. In intestine transplant recipients, the reported incidence of PTLD is:

A. 1% - 2% B. 5% - 10%
C. 10% - 20% D. 20% - 40%

27. False about PTLD after intestinal transplants is:

A. EBV-associated PTLD is more common after primary infection and therefore more common in children than in adults

B. PTLD usually is manifested within the 10 years after intestine transplantation and has a variable presentation, ranging from mild to moderate symptoms of infection

C. Routine screening for seroconversion by a serum quantitative EBV polymerase chain reaction assay is common to try to identify primary infections before severe symptoms occur

D. Surgical excision of localized disease, if possible (e.g., tonsillectomy, splenectomy, lobectomy, or enterectomy), is highly effective

28. EBV-associated PTLD has a mortality rate:

A. > 5% B. > 15%

C. > 25% D. > 45%

OUTCOMES

29. Leading cause of graft loss after intestinal transplants is:

A. Rejection

B. Sepsis

C. PTLD

D. Cardiovascular events

30. Children < 18 years are more likely than adults to lose grafts due to:

A. Rejection

B. Sepsis

C. PTLD

D. Cardiovascular events

ANSWERS

1. **Ans: C. > 75% of the native intestine**

   Ref: Chapter No.28, Page No.644

2. **Ans: D. Risk of IFALD induced steatosis in adults receiving home parenteral nutrition is high, with reported rates of 50% to 80%**

   Ref: Chapter No.28, Page No.645

3. **Ans: B. Deltz and colleagues**

   Ref: Chapter No.28, Page No.645

4. **Ans: A. Grant and colleagues**

   Ref: Chapter No.28, Page No.645

5. **Ans: D. All of the above**

   Ref: Chapter No.28, Page No.645

6. **Ans: D. Gastroschisis**

   Ref: Chapter No.28, Page No.646

7. **Ans: C. Ischemia**

   Ref: Chapter No.28, Page No.646

8. **Ans: C. An ideal donor should have a body weight 75% to 90% that of the recipient**

   Ref: Chapter No.28, Page No.646

9. **Ans: A. 6 - 8 hours**

   Ref: Chapter No.28, Page No.646

10. **Ans: C. Pathology: Percutaneous Lymph nodal biopsy**

    Ref: Chapter No.28, Page No.646

11. **Ans: D. All of the above**

    Ref: Chapter No.28, Page No.646

12. **Ans: B. Includes donor stomach when the donor liver is excluded**

    Ref: Chapter No.28, Page No.648

13. **Ans: C. Tumor**

    Ref: Chapter No.28, Page No.648-649

14. **Ans: D. All of the above**

    Ref: Chapter No.28, Page No.649

15. **Ans: C. 50%**

    Ref: Chapter No.28, Page No.649

16. **Ans: D. All of the above**

    Ref: Chapter No.28, Page No.649

17. **Ans: A. Vascular complications are common and include both bleeding and thrombosis**

    Ref: Chapter No.28, Page No.649

18. **Ans: C. Like in hepatic or renal transplantation, convenient serochemical marker exists to monitor intestinal function**

    Ref: Chapter No.28, Page No.649

19. **Ans: C. Their presence indicates up to 50% risk of graft loss within 1 year**

    Ref: Chapter No.28, Page No.650

20. **Ans: D. All of the above**

    Ref: Chapter No.28, Page No.650

21. **Ans: D. All of the above**

    Ref: Chapter No.28, Page No.650

22. **Ans: B. Infection**

    Ref: Chapter No.28, Page No.650

23. **Ans: D. Transplanting bowel from the CMV positive donor to a CMV negative recipient doesn't facilitate transmission**

    Ref: Chapter No.28, Page No.650

24. **Ans: C. 66%**

    Ref: Chapter No.28, Page No.650

25. **Ans: D. All of the above**

    Ref: Chapter No.28, Page No.650

26. **Ans: C. 10% - 20%**

    Ref: Chapter No.28, Page No.650

27. **Ans: B. PTLD usually is manifested within the 10 years after intestine transplantation and has a variable presentation, ranging from mild to moderate symptoms of infection**

    Ref: Chapter No.28, Page No.650

28. **Ans: C. > 25%**

    Ref: Chapter No.28, Page No.651

29. **Ans: B. Sepsis**

    Ref: Chapter No.28, Page No.651

30. **Ans: A. Rejection (Also Lymphoma)**

    Ref: Chapter No.28, Page No.651

29

Tumor Biology and Tumor Markers

EPIDEMIOLOGY

1. **In women, the most common cancers are all except:**
   A. Lung/bronchus B. Breast
   C. Colorectal D. Urinary bladder

2. **In men, the most common cancers are all except:**
   A. Lung/bronchus B. Esophagus
   C. Prostate D. Urinary bladder

3. **The most commonly diagnosed cancer worldwide and the leader in cancer death is:**
   A. Breast cancer B. Prostate cancer
   C. Lung cancer D. Esophageal cancer

4. **False statement among the following is:**
   A. The incidence of cancer increases with age
   B. Worldwide, approximately 50% of cancers are diagnosed in people 50 years of age or older
   C. In people > 70 years old, the incidence of invasive cancer is 1 in 3 for males and 1 in 4 for females
   D. The major mechanism driving increased cancer with aging relies on the accumula-tion of mutations over time that confer a growth advantage to the cell

5. **False about obesity and physical exercise with cancer is:**
   A. Increased physical activity was associated with decreased risk of melanoma and prostate cancer
   B. With bariatric surgery, it has been demonstrated to have the potential to offset some of the cancer risk in this population, with a recent study demonstrating a 33% reduction in cancer risk for obese patients undergoing bariatric surgery
   C. Globally, increased BMI is third, only behind infection and smoking, as a risk factor for cancer and contributes to up to 20% of cancer-related deaths
   D. The cancers where increased exercise is most protective are esophageal adenocarcinoma, gallbladder, and liver cancer

6. **False about obesity and physical exercise with cancer is:**
   A. Physical activity has been shown to upregulate cell cycle and deoxyribonucleic acid (DNA) repair pathways in male patients undergoing surveillance for prostate cancer
   B. Mechanistically, immune, metabolic, endocrine, and inflammatory properties of excess adipose tissue appear to lead to the increased incidence of malignancy in overweight/obese individuals
   C. Cancer outcomes have been shown to be inferior in sedentary individuals, with cancer mortality being increased by ~20% for individuals in the least active quartile of the population
   D. Circulating levels of estrogens are poorly related to adiposity

TUMOR BIOLOGY

7. **False about sustained proliferative signaling in development of cancer is:**
   A. Tumor cells and stroma produce factors (autocrine and paracrine factors) that, in cell-bound, matrix-bound, or soluble form, directly or indirectly influence tumor development
   B. Most tumors are characterized by infiltrating immune cells, such as lymphocytes, polymorphonuclear cells, mast cells and macrophages
   C. Paracrine growth mechanisms are dominant during the later stages of development of tumor
   D. Tumor cells secrete paracrine factors that act on host cells or ECMs, generating a supportive microenvironment

8. **Epidermal growth factor receptor family (ErbB) includes:**
   A. BRAF
   B. HER2/neu receptor
   C. KRAS
   D. BRCA

9. **Therapy for breast cancer includes all except:**
   A. Olaparib B. Tamoxifen
   C. Gefitinib D. Trastuzumab

10. **PARP inhibitor among the following is:**
    A. Olaparib B. Tamoxifen
    C. Gefitinib D. Dabrafenib

11. **Anti EGFR among the following is:**
    A. Rituximab B. Cetuximab
    C. Crizotinib D. Pembrolizumab

12. **Anti PD1 drug is:**
    A. Rituximab B. Cetuximab
    C. Crizotinib D. Pembrolizumab

13. **Anti CD20 drug is:**
    A. Rituximab B. Cetuximab
    C. Crizotinib D. Gefitinib

14. **Tyrosine kinase inhibitor among the following is:**
    A. Dabrafenib B. Cetuximab
    C. Crizotinib D. Trastuzumab

15. **All of the following are tyrosine kinase inhibitor except:**
    A. Gefitinib B. Dabrafenib
    C. Crizotinib D. Imatinib

16. **Anti BRAF drug is:**
    A. Trametinib B. Dabrafenib
    C. Trastuzumab D. Tamoxifen

17. **Anti MEK drug is:**
    A. Trametinib B. Dabrafenib
    C. Trastuzumab D. Tamoxifen

18. **False about evading growth suppressors in cancer development is:**
    A. In quiescent cells, pRb is hypophosphorylated and blocks cell division by binding E2F transcription factors that control the expression of many genes essential for progression from G1 into S phase
    B. Disruption of the pRb pathway liberates E2Fs and thus allows cell proliferation, rendering cells insensitive to antigrowth factors that normally operate along this pathway to block advance through the G1 phase of the cell cycle
    C. TGF-β responsiveness is lost through down regulation of TGF-β receptors or through expression of mutant, dysfunctional receptors
    D. TGF-β prevents the phosphorylation of pRb, which activates pRb and thereby blocks advance through G1

19. **False about resisting cell death in cancer development is:**
    A. The 2 best described receptor pathways of apoptosis are the Fas receptor and death receptor 5 that bind the extracellular Fas ligand and TRAIL, respectively
    B. p53 is a key regulator of apoptosis by sensing DNA damage that cannot be repaired and subsequent activation of the apoptotic pathway
    C. The intrinsic pathway is triggered by various extracellular and intracellular stresses, such as growth factor withdrawal, hypoxia, DNA damage, and oncogene induction
    D. Membrane-bound death receptors osteoprotegerin and DcR1 neutralize death inducing ligands such as TRAIL and FAS ligand in breast cancer, and a high fraction of lung and colon cancers

20. **Non apoptotic types of cell death that can promote tumor growth includes:**
    A. Ferroptosis B. Autophagy
    C. Mitotic catastrophe D. All of the above

21. **False among the following is:**
    A. Necrosis is normally induced by pathophysiologic conditions such as infection, inflammation and ischemia
    B. Autophagy is triggered by growth factor withdrawal, hypoxia, DNA damage, and differentiation and developmental triggers
    C. Aberrant mitosis caused by failure of the G1 checkpoint to block mitosis when DNA is damaged can lead to cell death, known as mitotic catastrophe
    D. Ferroptosis is a recently discovered form of cell death that results from iron-dependent lipid peroxide accumulation

22. Autophagy is particularly important for growth of RAS-mutated cancers such as all except:

A. Lung cancers B. Esophageal cancer
C. Pancreatic cancers D. Colon cancers

23. Deletion of the autophagy-regulating gene beclin-1 is seen in high percentages of:

A. Breast cancers B. Ovarian cancers
C. Prostrate cancers D. All of the above

24. False about enabling replicative immortality in cancer development is:

A. When the critical length is bridged, the unprotected chromosomal ends participate in end-to-end chromosomal fusions, yielding a karyotype disarray that almost inevitably results in the death of the affected cell
B. Telomeres prevent end-to-end chromosomal fusion
C. Each DNA replication is associated with a loss of 500 to 1000 base pairs of telomeric DNA from the ends of every chromosome
D. By maintaining a telomere length above a critical threshold, the tumor cells have unlimited proliferative potential and are considered immortal

25. Cell surface markers used to define Cancer stem cells (CSCs) are:

A. CD44 B. CD133
C. CXCR4 D. All of the above

26. False about Cancer stem cells (CSCs) is:

A. Characteristic of CSCs is the exponentially enhanced ability to seed new tumors
B. Various cell surface markers have been used to define CSCs, such as CD44, CD133 and CXCR4
C. CSCs may generate tumors through self-renewal as well as through differentiation into multiple cell types
D. CSCs are more sensitive to traditional therapeutic modalities, such as chemotherapy and radiation

27. False about inducing angiogenesis in cancer development is:

A. Both primary and metastatic tumors may be nonangiogenic, and are most commonly observed in lung, liver and brain lesions
B. Microscopic tumors lack the ability to induce angiogenesis, and only an estimated 1 in 600 acquire angiogenic activity
C. Bevacizumab significantly prolongs the survival of some patients with advanced cancer
D. Bcl-2 inactivation leads to significantly increased expression of VEGF and angiogenesis

28. Angiogenesis inhibitors are all except:

A. VEGF B. Tumstatin
C. Thrombospondin D. IFN-α

29. Progressing tumors give rise to distant metastases that are the cause of ___ human cancer deaths.

A. 60% B. 70%
C. 80% D. 90%

30. True about activating invasion and metastasis in cancer development is:

A. The growth factor theory, proposes that tumor cells in the blood or lymphatics invade organs at similar frequency, but only those that find favorable growth factors multiply
B. The adhesion theory, proposes that endothelial cells lining the blood vessels in certain organs express adhesion molecules that bind tumor cells and permit extravasation
C. Increased concentrations of transferrin are found in lung, bone, and the brain and are associated with elevated levels of transferrin receptors on metastasizing tumor cells
D. All of the above

31. True about activating invasion and metastasis in cancer development is:

A. Chemokines secreted by the target organ can enter the circulation and selectively attract tumor cells that express receptors for the chemokines
B. Melanoma cells that were found to express elevated levels of the receptors CXCR4, CCR7, and CCR10 compared with normal melanocytes & lymph nodes, lung, liver, bone marrow, and skin express the highest levels of the ligands for these receptors and are the preferred sites for metastatic spread of melanomas
C. The chemokine receptor-ligand axis between elevated levels of CXCR4 on breast cancer cells and CXCL12 secreting bone marrow, liver, lymph nodes, and lung explains why these organs are preferred sites for breast cancer metastasis
D. All of the above

32. False about activating invasion and metastasis in cancer development is:

A. E-cadherin function is gained in most epithelial tumors during progression to tumor malignancy and may in fact be a prerequisite for tumor cell invasion and metastasis formation

B. Cancer cells use EMT to become invasive and to metastasize

C. E–cadherin is the prototype cadherin responsible for cell polarity and organization of epithelium

D. Expression of the protease tenascin, which neutralizes adhesion to fibronectin, is increased 10 fold in invasive breast carcinoma compared with normal breast tissue

33. True about avoiding immune destruction in cancer development is:

A. Local disruption of tissue that occurs as a result of expansion of transformed cells is associated with release of chemokines and proinflammatory cytokines such as interferons, IL-1, IL-6, and tumor necrosis factor-α that trigger innate immunity

B. Tumors infiltrated with abundant myeloid cells, particularly macrophages, correlate with worse prognosis in many types of cancers, such as pancreas and breast

C. The continuous pressure of the immune system in an immunocompetent host determines to a great degree if and how tumors evolve, a process called immunoediting

D. All of the above

34. False about deregulating cellular energetics and metabolomics in cancer development is:

A. Cancer cells limit their energy metabolism to glycolysis, even in the presence of oxygen (aerobic glycolysis) is termed the Warburg effect

B. Warburg effect is used to diagnose or to stage cancers, such as visualizing glucose uptake by positron emission tomography with 18F-fluorodeoxyglucose

C. Cancer cells must dramatically upregulate the rate of glycolysis (up to 200-fold higher than normal cells) to keep up with the rapid metabolism of rapidly dividing neoplastic cells

D. Tumor cells increase the rate of glycolysis to upregulate the expression of glucose transporters, such as GLUT4

35. False about genomic instability and mutation in cancer development is:

A. 2 recently described classes of tumor genomic rearrangements include chromothrypsis and chromopexy

B. In chromopexy there is coordinated rearrangement across multiple chromosomes

C. In chromothrypsis, a massive chromosomal rearrangement event occurs in a localized genomic region

D. All of the above

36. False among the following is:

A. Inflammation is an early event in tumorigenesis and can incite the conversion of a premalignant lesion into a full-blown cancer

B. Immune cells don't play an important role in antitumor defense

C. Macrophages isolated from tumors, such as pancreatic cancer, are potently immunosuppressive and prevent antitumor immune responses by T cells

D. Tumors can alter the functionality of infiltrating immune cells, causing functional leukocytes to become anergic or even immunosuppressive

37. Model of solid tumor metastasis depicted in the image shown below is:

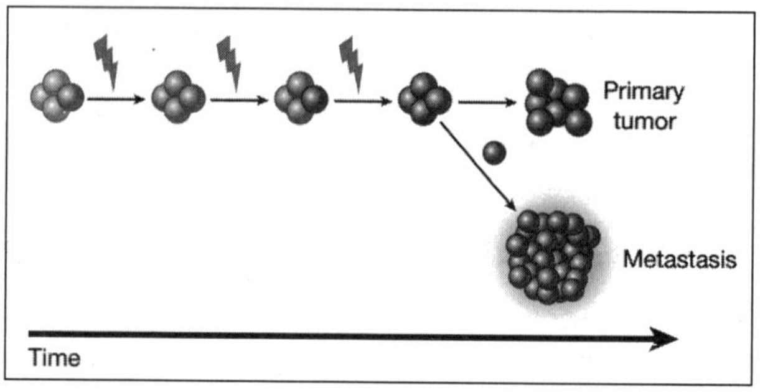

A. Early dissemination with early distant metastasis and parallel evolution

B. Linear evolution model with late metastasis

C. Late distant metastasis from multiple late-occurring subclones in the primary tumor

D. Late dissemination from a late-arising subclone that has the propensity to see multiple metastases

38. Model of solid tumor metastasis depicted in the image shown below is:

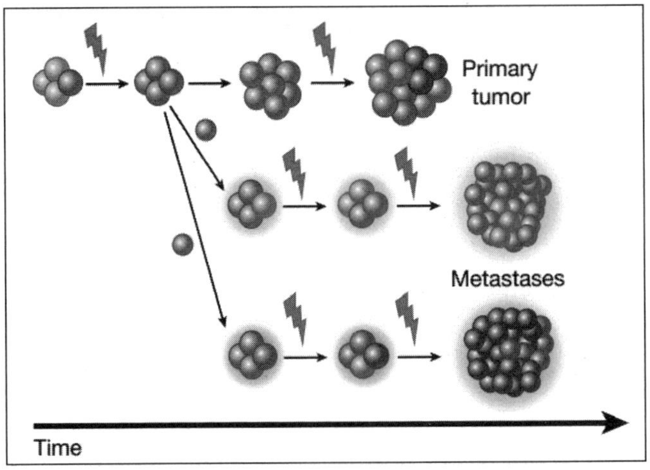

A. Early dissemination with early distant metastasis and parallel evolution
B. Linear evolution model with late metastasis
C. Late distant metastasis from multiple late-occurring subclones in the primary tumor
D. Late dissemination from a late-arising subclone that has the propensity to see multiple metastases

CARCINOGENESIS

39. False about the following is:

A. Genetic mutations that are inherited from one's parents and are present in all cells of the body are called germline
B. Somatic mutations are acquired during an individual's lifetime and cannot be passed on to one's children
C. Genetic mutations account for most mutations in cancer
D. In hereditary cases, a germline mutation is responsible for the predisposition to neoplasia

40. Autosomal recessive inheritance among the following is:

A. Ataxia-telangiectasia
B. Carney complex
C. Beckwith-Wiedemann syndrome
D. Cowden disease

41. BRCA1 gene is on chromosome no:

A. 17q21 B. 13p21
C. 17p21 D. 13q21

42. Carney complex is associated with:

A. CDKN1C B. PRKAR1A gene
C. PDGFRA D. PTCH

43. BRCA2 gene is on chromosome no:

A. 13q12 B. 13p12
C. 17p12 D. 17q12

44. Beckwith-Wiedemann syndrome is associated with all except:

A. Adrenal carcinoma B. Wilms tumor
C. Schwannoma D. Hepatoblastoma

45. Ataxia-telangiectasia's ATM gene is on chromosome no:

A. 9q22 B. 9p22
C. 11q22 D. 11p22

46. Carney complex is associated with all except:

A. Myxoid tumors
B. Medulloblastoma
C. Mammary fibroadenoma
D. Pituitary adenoma

47. Cowden disease is associated with:

A. PTCH B. PTEN
C. MET D. hCHK2

48. PTEN gene is on chromosome no:

A. 10q23 B. 10p23
C. 7q31 D. 7p31

49. Melanoma cancer syndrome is associated with all except:

A. Melanoma B. Basal cell cancer
C. Atypical moles D. Dysplastic nevi

50. Familial gastrointestinal stromal tumor is associated with:

A. CDKN2A B. CDH1
C. c-KIT D. PTCH

51. Gene associated with Gorlin syndrome is:

A. CDKN2A/p16 B. CDH1
C. SDHB D. PTCH

52. Gorlin syndrome is associated with all except:

A. Medulloblastoma
B. Ovarian cancer
C. Gastric cancer
D. Basal cell cancer

53. Gene associated with Melanoma cancer syndrome is:

A. CDKN2A/p16 B. CDH1
C. SDHB D. PTCH

54. Gene associated with Hereditary papillary renal cell carcinoma is:

A. SDHD B. BMPRIA
C. MET D. MYH

55. Chromosome not associated with Hereditary papillary renal cell carcinoma is:

A. 7p31 B. 7q31
C. 10p31 D. 10q31

56. Chromosome not associated with Gorlin syndrome is:

A. 9q22 B. 9p22
C. 13q22 D. 13p22

57. Gene associated with Li-Fraumeni is:

A. RB B. RET
C. p53 D. MYH

58. Chromosome associated with p53 is:

A. 17p13 B. 17q13
C. 13p14 D. 13q14

59. Chromosome associated with Multiple endocrine neoplasia type 1 is:

A. 11p13 B. 11q13
C. 10p11 D. 10q11

60. MYH-associated adenomatous polyposis is associated with all except:

A. Colon cancer B. Breast cancer
C. Rectum cancer D. Prostate cancer

61. Which of the following doesn't have autosomal recessive inheritance:

A. Retinoblastoma
B. MYH-associated adenomatous polyposis
C. Werner syndrome
D. Xeroderma pigmentosum

62. Chromosome associated with Neurofibromatosis type 1 is:

A. 17q11 B. 22q12
C. 17p11 D. 22p12

63. Neurofibromatosis type 2 is associated with all except:

A. Ependymomas B. Neurofibrosarcoma
C. Meningiomas D. Acoustic neuromas

64. Chromosome associated with Peutz-Jeghers syndrome is:

A. 9q34 B. 9p34
C. 19p13 D. 19q13

65. Retinoblastoma is associated with all except:

A. Pheochromocytoma B. Melanoma
C. Retinoblastoma D. Sarcomas

66. Chromosome associated with retinoblastoma is:

A. 13p14 B. 13q14
C. 17p13 D. 17q13

67. Chromosome associated with Tuberous sclerosis gene TSC1 is:

A. 9p34 B. 9q34
C. 16p13 D. 16q13

68. Chromosome associated with Tuberous sclerosis gene TSC2 is:

A. 9p34 B. 9q34
C. 16p13 D. 16q13

69. Chromosome associated with von Hippel-Lindau syndrome is:

A. 3p25 B. 3q25
C. 8q12 D. 8p12

70. Chromosome associated with WAGR is:

A. 11q13 B. 11p13
C. 17q11 D. 17p11

71. WAGR is associated with:

A. Wilms tumor
B. Astrocytoma
C. Genitourinary abnormalities
D. Mental retardation

72. False about Werner syndrome is:

A. Associated with chromosome 8p12
B. Meningioma
C. Sarcoma/osteosarcoma
D. Autosomal dominant inheritance

73. The first tumor suppressor gene to be cloned is:

A. p53 B. PTEN
C. RB1 D. BRCA1

74. False about retinoblastoma is:

A. Distinct sporadic and hereditary forms of retinoblastoma have long been recognized, with predisposition conferred by a germline mutation in approximately 40% of cases
B. Most affected children with an affected parent develop tumors unilaterally
C. In children with unilateral disease and no family history, both mutations are somatic

D. The RB1 protein product is a key regulator of the cell cycle, and its loss results in failure of retinoblasts to differentiate properly

75. False about Li-Fraumeni Syndrome is:

A. Chompret criteria is used to identify clinical scenarios where there should be high suspicion for Li-Fraumeni syndrome and genetic counseling and testing should be offered
B. Approximately 30% of Li Fraumeni kindreds have mutations in TP53 gene, which produces the protein p53
C. Penetrance is nearly 100% by the age of 70 years
D. Inheritance is in an autosomal dominant fashion

76. The most common malignant neoplasm in Li-Fraumeni Syndrome is:

A. Brain tumors
B. Adrenocortical carcinomas
C. Breast cancers
D. Leukemias

77. Chompret criteria includes all except:

A. Patients with adrenocortical carcinoma, choroid plexus carcinoma or embryonal anaplastic subtype rhabdomyoscarcoma (independent of family history)
B. A proband diagnosed with a Li-Fraumeni spectrum tumor prior to the age of 46 years, and at least 1 first or second degree relative with a Li-Fraumeni syndrome spectrum tumor
C. Proband with multiple malignancies (except 2 breast cancers), of which at least 2 are considered Li-Fraumeni syndrome associated, before 46 years of age
D. Breast cancer before the age of 40 years old

78. False about Familial Adenomatous Polyposis is:

A. Penetrance is extremely high, with colorectal cancer incidence approaching 100% by age 50
B. Untreated individuals typically present with colorectal cancer at 35 - 40 years of age, around 30 years earlier than the median age for sporadic colorectal cancer
C. Polyps of the duodenum most commonly occur in the periampullary region
D. FAP accounts for ~5% of the total colorectal cancer burden

79. Most common extracolonic manifestations of FAP is:

A. Thyroid cancer
B. Duodenal adenomas
C. CHPRE
D. Gastric adenomas

80. Patients who have attenuated polyposis but who test negative for APC mutations are MYH-associated polyposis (MAP) accounting for about:

A. 10% B. 20%
C. 30% D. 50%

81. MAP-associated colorectal cancer typically presents with an attenuated polyposis phenotype, often with:

A. < 10 polyps B. < 100 polyps
C. > 100 polyps D. > 1000 polyps

82. False about MYH-associated polyposis (MAP) is:

A. The polyps are distributed throughout the colon
B. Penetrance is estimated at 80% by age 60
C. MYH-associated polyposis (MAP) is a syndrome caused by mutations in the human MutY homologue (MYH) gene
D. The mutations Y179C on exon 7 and G396D on exon 13 account for ~80% of all cases

83. False about HNPCC is:

A. Also known as Lynch syndrome
B. The broad phenotype of HNPCC is of right-sided predominance of colonic cancers that appear at an earlier age
C. Lifetime risk of colorectal cancer is nearly 100% in males and just > 80% in females
D. A colonic adenoma may progress to carcinoma within 2 to 3 years

84. False about BRCA1/ BRCA2 is:

A. Male carriers of BRCA1 and BRCA2 are at greater risk for prostate cancer, while breast cancer in males is most commonly attributed to BRCA2
B. In families with a history of hereditary breast and ovarian cancer, it is estimated that 90% are attributable to BRCA1 or BRCA2 mutations
C. BRCA1 mutation conferred a 6.2 times increased risk of pancreatic cancer
D. For instance, for BRCA1 the c.68_69delAG mutation, the most frequent mutation among Ashkenazi Jews, confers an 84% risk of breast cancer by age 70

85. The cumulative breast cancer risk at age 80 for a female BRCA1 carrier is:

A. 44%	B. 72%
C. 69%	D. 17%

86. Cumulative risk through age 80 for ovarian cancer in a female who is a carrier for BRCA1 is:

A. 44%	B. 72%
C. 69%	D. 17%

87. The cumulative breast cancer risk at age 80 for a female BRCA1 carrier is:

A. 44%	B. 72%
C. 69%	D. 17%

88. False about von Hippel-Lindau (VHL) is:

A. Tumors associated with VHL include hemangioblastomas of the retina and central nervous system, renal cysts that develop into clear cell renal cell cancer, pheochromocytomas, endolymphatic sac tumors of the middle ear, and epididymal or round ligament cysts
B. Penetrance is 50% by the age of 65 years
C. VHL affects approximately 1 in 35,000 live births
D. pVHL functions as a tumor suppressor and is part of the cell's response mechanism to hypoxia

89. True about epigenetic changes is:

A. CpG island methylator phenotype can lead to silencing of the tumor suppressor p16 and of DNA mismatch repair genes
B. MGMT encodes a DNA repair factor, and in some colorectal tumors hypermethylation of MGMT has been implicated
C. Mutant IDH generates an oncometabolite that inhibits hydroxylases, and specifically TET enzymes, which function normally to catalyze demethylation
D. All of the above

90. False among the following is:

A. Loss of methylation is particularly severe in pericentromeric satellite sequences, and cancers of the ovary and breast
B. Genomic imprinting refers to the conditioning of the maternal and paternal genomes during gametogenesis, such that a specific parental allele is more abundantly expressed in the offspring
C. The modification of histones (e.g., by acetylation, methylation, or phosphorylation) is important in the compaction of chromatin structure and but is not crucial in cancer pathogenesis
D. In Wilms tumors, loss of imprinting has been demonstrated to lead to pathologic biallelic expression of IGF2

91. False about cancer microbiome is:

A. It has been shown that colorectal cancers often have decreased abundance of Bacteroidetes
B. It has been shown that colorectal cancers often have overrepresentation of Firmicutes species
C. It is now believed that microbial pathogens drive tumorigenesis in 15% to 20% of cancers
D. Dysbiosis of the gastrointestinal tract involves shifts in the abundance of commensal bacteria

92. Which bacteria was found in pancreatic cancer specimens, was shown to metabolize gemcitabine and convert it to an inactive form?

A. Fusobacterium
B. Gammaproteobacteria
C. Bacteroidetes
D. Helicobacter pylori

93. False among the following regarding carcinogens is:

A. Light smokers with the susceptible genotype of CYP1A1 have a 10 fold higher risk for development of lung cancer compared with smokers without the permissive genotype
B. Age, sex and nutritional status also have an effect on the metabolism of carcinogens and thus their probability of inducing malignancy
C. Most of the known carcinogens are metabolized by cytochrome P450–dependent monooxygenases
D. The Ames test is the most common method for evaluating mutagenic potential and measures the ability of a chemical to induce mutations in the bacterium Salmonella typhimurium

94. Agents that are probably not carcinogenic to humans are:

A. Group 2A	B. Group 3
C. Group 2B	D. Group 4

95. Agents that are probable human carcinogens for which there is limited evidence of carcinogenicity in humans but sufficient evidence to prove carcinogenicity in experimental animal are:

A. Group 2A	B. Group 3
C. Group 2B	D. Group 4

96. Agents that are possibly carcinogenic to humans for which there is limited evidence of carcinogenicity in humans and less than sufficient

evidence of carcinogenicity in experimental animals are:

A. Group 2A B. Group 3
C. Group 2B D. Group 4

97. **Predominant tumor type associated with Aflatoxins is:**

A. Leukemia
B. Hepatocellular carcinoma
C. Hepatic angiosarcoma
D. Lung cancer

98. **Predominant tumor type associated with Asbestos is:**

A. Mesothelioma
B. Cancer of the urinary bladder
C. Skin cancer
D. Scrotal cancer

99. **Which of the following chemical carcinogen is associated with scrotal cancer?**

A. Beryllium B. Benzidine
C. Benzene D. Coal tars

100. **Arsenic is associated with all except:**

A. Hepatic angiosarcoma
B. Skin cancer
C. Leukemia
D. Lung cancer

101. **Which of the following is not associated with lung cancer?**

A. Benzidine B. Radon
C. Silica D. Nickel

102. **Diethylstilbestrol is associated with:**

A. Clear cell adenocarcinoma of the vagina
B. Squamous cell carcinoma of the vagina
C. Sarcoma of the vagina
D. Melanoma of the vagina

103. **Thorium-232/Thorotrast is associated with all except:**

A. Lung cancer
B. Hepatocellular carcinoma
C. Pancreatic cancer
D. Bile duct cancer

104. **Which of the following is not associated with Hepatic angiosarcoma?**

A. Alcohol
B. Thorium-232/Thorotrast
C. Vinyl chloride
D. Arsenic

105. **All of the following is associated with Alcohol except:**

A. Breast cancer
B. Cancer of urinary bladder
C. Squamous cell carcinoma of the oropharynx and esophagus
D. Intrahepatic cholangiocarcinoma

106. **All of the following are seen with Cyclosporine except:**

A. Nonmelanoma skin cancer
B. Leukemia
C. Cancer of the urinary bladder
D. Lymphoma

107. **Tamoxifen use can cause:**

A. Endometrial cancer
B. Cancer of the breast
C. Ovarian cancer
D. Non-Hodgkin lymphoma

108. **Azathioprine use can cause all except:**

A. Squamous cell cancer of the skin
B. Melanoma
C. Non-Hodgkin lymphoma
D. Hepatocellular carcinoma

109. **True about Radiation Carcinogenesis is:**

A. The two most important forms of radiation causing malignant change in humans are ultraviolet (UV) radiation and ionizing radiation (IR)
B. UV radiation has been found to cause a variety of cancers, IR is principally implicated in the causation of skin cancers
C. There is typically a small latency period between radiation exposure and clinical development of cancer
D. All of the above

110. **Severe sunburn events are associated with:**

A. Basal cell carcinoma
B. Squamous cell carcinoma
C. Malignant melanoma
D. All of the above

111. **Spectrum of UVB is:**
A. 340 - 400 nm
B. 280 - 400 nm
C. 280 - 320 nm
D. 200 - 260 nm

112. **False about UV radiation and carcinogenesis is:**
A. The carcinogenicity of UVB is due to its formation of pyrimidine dimers in DNA
B. UVC is the most important carcinogen
C. The degree of risk depends on the type of UV rays, the intensity of exposure, and the quantity of melanin present in the individual's skin
D. Xeroderma pigmentosum, characterized by extreme photosensitivity and a 2000-fold increased risk of skin cancer, is caused by mutations in the genes involved in nucleotide excision repair

113. **True about Ionizing radiation (IR) and carcinogenesis is:**
A. IR works via directly causing single and double stranded DNA breaks, as well as indirectly by causing radiolysis of water inside cells, leading to ROS generation
B. IR is composed of electrically charged particles that pass through tissue and deposit energy, with the goal being that they will lead to death of rapidly dividing cancer cells
C. IR also works indirectly by inducing the cytosolic Rac1/NADPH oxidase system, which further leads to ROS formation and resultant DNA damage
D. All of the above

114. **False about Ionizing radiation (IR) and carcinogenesis is:**
A. The goal of IR is to kill tumor cells while sparing as much of the normal cell mass as possible
B. ATM biallelic mutation, as seen in patients with ataxia telangiectasia, is considered an indication to radiation therapy
C. Normal cells are often able to upregulate DNA damage repair enzymes, such as PARP1, which recognizes single cell DNA breaks and recruits enzymes to repair the damage
D. Double-stranded breaks are recognized by ATM, together with MRE-RAD50 and NBS1 and repaired

115. **Epstein-Barr virus is associated with all except:**
A. Kaposi sarcoma
B. Nasopharyngeal carcinoma
C. Burkitt lymphoma
D. Hodgkin disease

116. **Kaposi sarcoma can be due to:**
A. HSV 1
B. HHV 8
C. HSV 2
D. HPV

117. **AIDS defining malignancies after HIV infection are all except:**
A. Non-Hodgkin lymphoma
B. Anal cancer
C. Kaposi sarcoma
D. Cervical cancer

118. **Non-AIDS defining malignancies after HIV infection are all except:**
A. Lung cancer
B. Non-Hodgkin lymphoma
C. Hodgkin lymphoma
D. Penile cancer

119. **Helicobacter pylori is associated with all except:**
A. Gastric neuroendocrine tumor
B. Gastric MALT lymphoma
C. Gastric adenocarcinoma
D. Gastric diffuse large B cell lymphoma

120. **Which infectious agent is associated with cancer of the urinary bladder?**
A. Clonorchis sinensis
B. Opisthorchis viverrini
C. Helicobacter pylori
D. Schistosoma haematobium

121. **Which infectious agent is associated with cholangiocarcinoma?**
A. Clonorchis sinensis
B. Opisthorchis viverrini
C. Both A and B
D. None of the above

122. **Regarding principles and strategies of viral carcinogenesis, all are true except:**
A. Oncoviruses are necessary and usually sufficient for viral carcinogenesis
B. Viral-related cancers occur in the context of persistent infection and only many years after initial infection
C. The immune system can play a provirus or an antivirus role
D. All of the above are true

123. **False about HBV and carcinogenesis is:**
A. HBx can also promote HCC invasion and distant metastasis by increasing expression of matrix metalloproteinases

B. HBx decreases the formation of ROS while promoting cell survival via upregulation of HIF1α, which activates angiogenesis
C. Major player in chronic HBV-mediated HCC carcinogenesis is HBV-encoded X Ag (HBx)
D. HBx stimulates cell division and growth by activating both cyclins and cyclin-dependent kinases and also by directly suppressing p53 (via direct binding) and Rb (by phosphorylation)

124. To lead to potential AIDS-defining malignancies CD4+ T-cell counts should be:

A. < 50 cells/mm^3
B. < 100 cells/mm^3
C. < 200 cells/mm^3
D. < 400 cells/mm^3

125. In cases of Merkel cell carcinoma, Merkel cell polyomavirus is associated with up to:

A. 20%
B. 40%
C. 60%
D. 80%

126. False about H. pylori and carcinogenesis is:

A. Infection with strains of H pylori that carry the cytotoxin-associated antigen A (cagA) gene is associated with gastric carcinoma
B. H pylori infection is the only bacterial infection listed as a level I carcinogen by the IARC
C. H pylori was the second bacterium ever directly linked to human cancer
D. CagA is tyrosine phosphorylated by SRC family kinases and then is able to specifically bind and activate the oncogenic phosphatase SHP2

TUMOR MARKERS

127. True about tumor markers is:

A. They are surrogate measures of the biology of the cancer, providing insight into the clinical behavior of the tumor
B. Tumor markers found in body fluids, particularly blood and urine, have the greatest potential for clinical application
C. Protein biomarkers and DNA mutational analysis are part of FDA and CLIA approved laboratory testing that are routinely used for clinical evaluation of patients with various solid tumors
D. All of the above

128. False about Carcinoembryonic antigen (CEA) is:

A. It is probably the most studied cancer tumor marker and is predominantly used clinically in patients with colorectal cancers
B. CEA has been shown to be involved in cell adhesion and is able to inhibit apoptosis induced by loss of anchorage to the ECM
C. Serum levels of less than 2.5 ng/mL are normal
D. CEA is useful as a screening test in colorectal cancers

129. Smoking increases CEA levels; normal levels in smokers should be upto:

A. 2 ng/mL
B. 3.5 ng/mL
C. 5 ng/mL
D. 8 ng/mL

130. False about Carcinoembryonic antigen (CEA) is:

A. Preoperative serum CEA is an independent predictor of survival
B. Elevated CEA levels rarely reflect the burden of tumor present
C. The most common application of CEA is in monitoring of patients for recurrent disease
D. A CEA level of greater than 5 ng/mL in any patient who has undergone treatment for colorectal adenocarcinoma should be considered tumor recurrence unless proven otherwise

131. True about Carcinoembryonic antigen (CEA) is:

A. CEA is not useful in monitoring response to chemotherapy in patients with metastatic colorectal cancer
B. An elevated CEA level is an independent factor associated with poor survival and progression on 5-fluorouracil-based chemotherapy in patients with metastatic colorectal cancer
C. Patients with advanced cancer whose CEA levels fall during chemotherapy survive significantly shorter than those patients whose CEA levels do not change or increase
D. All of the above

132. False about α-Fetoprotein (AFP) is:

A. α-Fetoprotein (AFP) is used in the detection and management of HCC
B. Levels are elevated in the fetus, fall to low levels after birth, and are elevated during pregnancy
C. The upper limit of normal for a healthy, nonpregnant adult is < 100 ng/mL
D. It is synthesized by hepatocytes and endodermally derived gastrointestinal tissues

133. False about α-Fetoprotein (AFP) is:

A. In a recent metaanalysis of HCC screening for cirrhotic patients, ultrasound and AFP had a sensitivity of 97% picking up HCC

B. For screening purposes in high-risk populations, AFP is used in addition to ultrasound imaging
C. AFP on its own is a good screening tool, with a sensitivity of 70%
D. AFP concentration reflects tumor size, with levels > 400 ng/mL associated with larger tumors

134. False about α-Fetoprotein (AFP) is:

A. AFP has been shown to decline after resection or ablation of tumor, and levels after complete resection should be < 100 ng/mL
B. Monitoring of AFP avoids prolonged use of ineffective chemotherapy
C. AFP levels usually decline in response to effective chemotherapy
D. AFP is part of the standard surveillance regimen for HCC patients on the transplant list

135. False about Carbohydrate antigen 19-9 (CA 19-9) is:

A. Biliary tract disease, both acute and chronic, can elevate serum CA 19-9 levels
B. CA 19-9 is detected by an immunoassay, with the upper limit of normal for a healthy adult being 37 U/mL
C. CA 19-9 is considered to be useful as a screening tool
D. Patients with negative Lewis[a] blood group antigen (10% of population) cannot synthesize CA 19-9, and therefore it should not be used as a serologic marker in these individuals

136. CA 19-9 levels are elevated in patients with cancers of:

A. Testis
B. Biliary tree
C. Stomach
D. Colon

137. False about Carbohydrate antigen 19-9 (CA 19-9) is:

A. Serial measurement of CA 19-9 is used to monitor response to therapy
B. In patients with unresectable or metastatic disease, failure of CA 19-9 levels to fall with chemotherapy reflects poor tumor response
C. In symptomatic patients, increasing levels of CA 19-9 make the diagnosis of pancreatic cancer more accurate
D. Positive predictive value for pancreatic cancer when used as a screening modality in the general population is 90%

138. False about Prostate-specific antigen (PSA) is:

A. Prostate-specific antigen (PSA) is a serine protease that is formed in the prostatic epithelium and is secreted into the prostatic ducts
B. PSA is considered a tissue-specific rather than a prostate cancer-specific marker
C. Women have small detectable PSA levels
D. Its function is to digest the gel that is formed in seminal fluid after ejaculation

139. False about Prostate-specific antigen (PSA) is:

A. Serum PSA levels may be elevated include prostatitis, prostatic massage, prostatic biopsy
B. Elevation after digital rectal examination is seen and testing for PSA level can't be done after a digital rectal examination in the same clinic visit
C. Levels greater than 10 ng/mL suggestive of malignancy
D. The ratio of free to total PSA has also been found to improve the specificity of prostate cancer diagnosis in the PSA range of 4 - 10 ng/mL, with a free to total PSA ratio of < 10% being considered abnormal

140. After operative resection, the PSA level is expected to normalize after:

A. 1 to 2 weeks
B. 2 to 3 weeks
C. 4 to 6 weeks
D. 8 to 12 weeks

141. After radiotherapy the PSA levels normalize after:

A. 1 - 2 months
B. 3 - 5 months
C. 6 - 8 months
D. 8 - 12 months

142. False about Carbohydrate antigen 125 is:

A. Carbohydrate antigen 125 is a carbohydrate epitope on a glycoprotein carcinoma antigen
B. Ovarian epithelium does normally express some CA 125
C. It is also known as MUC16
D. It is present in the fetus and in derivatives of the coelomic epithelium, including peritoneum, pleura, pericardium and amnion

143. False about Carbohydrate antigen 125 is:

A. Elevated levels are detected in 50% of patients with early stage and 80% of patients with later stage ovarian cancer
B. CA 125 is useful as a screening tool for ovarian cancer
C. Patients with elevated CA 125 levels at the time of diagnosis have a worse prognosis compared with those patients with normal levels
D. When rising CA 125 levels are used as an

indication for secondlook laparotomies, recurrent disease is found approximately 90% of the time

144. In stage III ovarian cancer patients, percentage of patients having elevated CA 125 levels is:

A. 50% B. 70%
C. 90% D. 95%

145. Percentage of teratomas with elevated AFP is:

A. 10% B. 20%
C. 40% D. 60%

146. Percentage of embryonal carcinomas with elevated AFP is:

A. 10% B. 20%
C. 40% D. 60%

147. False about Proteomic Profiling is:

A. Proteomics is the study of all the proteins expressed by the genome
B. Clinically, proteomics offers the potential to allow for enhanced cancer diagnosis and treatment decision making
C. Detection and measurement of these proteins rarely provides information about the clinical behavior of the cancer
D. Proteomic profiling uses mass spectrometry technologies to generate complex fingerprints of ion peaks corresponding to protein concentrations that can be correlated with disease states

148. False about RNA-Based Markers is:

A. Micro RNAs are often carried in exosomes, tumor-educated platelets, apoptotic bodies, or proteins
B. Oncotype DX includes 16 tumor-associated genes and 15 reference genes
C. Multigene panel: Decision-Dx-UM for uveal melanoma
D. The Oncotype Dx score was incorporated as part of the most recent AJCC 8th edition breast cancer staging systems

149. The NETest was developed based on isolated messenger RNA from a whole blood sample, with:

A. 37 genes B. 51 genes
C. 63 genes D. 75 genes

150. False among the following is:

A. MammaPrint and PAM 50: Breast cancer
B. Oncotype DX: Colon cancer
C. ColoPrint: Stomach cancer
D. Decision-Dx-UM: Uveal melanoma

151. True about Circulating Tumor DNA is:

A. FDA-approved Cologuard uses a combination of stool DNA and fecal immunochemical testing to identify colorectal cancers and advanced adenomas
B. The cobase EGFR Mutation test uses cfDNA to identify the T790M gatekeeper mutation that can be seen in patients with progressive disease after treatment with EGFR inhibitors
C. Patients with colorectal cancer, cfDNA drawn several weeks after curative surgery could identify patients with residual disease and predict future relapse
D. All of the above

ANSWERS

1. **Ans: D. Urinary bladder**

Ref: Chapter No.29, Page No.656

2. **Ans: B. Esophagus**

Ref: Chapter No.29, Page No.656

3. **Ans: C. Lung cancer**

Ref: Chapter No.29, Page No.657

4. **Ans: B. Worldwide, approximately 50% of cancers are diagnosed in people 50 years of age or older**

Ref: Chapter No.29, Page No.657-658

5. **Ans: A. Increased physical activity was associated with decreased risk of melanoma and prostate cancer**

Ref: Chapter No.29, Page No.658-659

6. **Ans: D. Circulating levels of estrogens are poorly related to adiposity**

Ref: Chapter No.29, Page No.659-660

7. **Ans: C. Paracrine growth mechanisms are dominant during the later stages of development of tumor**

Ref: Chapter No.29, Page No.661

8. **Ans: B. HER2/neu receptor**

Ref: Chapter No.29, Page No.661

9. **Ans: C. Gefitinib**

Ref: Chapter No.29, Page No.662

10. **Ans: A. Olaparib**

Ref: Chapter No.29, Page No.662

11. **Ans: B. Cetuximab**

Ref: Chapter No.29, Page No.662

12. **Ans: D. Pembrolizumab**

Ref: Chapter No.29, Page No.662

13. **Ans: A. Rituximab**

Ref: Chapter No.29, Page No.662

14. **Ans: C. Crizotinib**

Ref: Chapter No.29, Page No.662

15. **Ans: B. Dabrafenib**

Ref: Chapter No.29, Page No.662

16. **Ans: B. Dabrafenib**

Ref: Chapter No.29, Page No.662

17. **Ans: A. Trametinib**

Ref: Chapter No.29, Page No.662

18. **Ans: D. TGF-β prevents the phosphorylation of pRb, which activates pRb and thereby blocks advance through G1**

Ref: Chapter No.29, Page No.662-663

19. **Ans: D. Membrane-bound death receptors osteoprotegerin and DcR1 neutralize death inducing ligands such as TRAIL and FAS ligand in breast cancer, and a high fraction of lung and colon cancers**

Ref: Chapter No.29, Page No.663-664

20. **Ans: D. All of the above (Also necrosis)**

Ref: Chapter No.29, Page No.664

21. **Ans: C. Aberrant mitosis caused by failure of the G1 checkpoint to block mitosis when DNA is damaged can lead to cell death, known as mitotic catastrophe (It is G2 checkpoint)**

Ref: Chapter No.29, Page No.664

22. **Ans: B. Prostate cancer**

Ref: Chapter No.29, Page No.664

23. **Ans: D. All of the above**

Ref: Chapter No.29, Page No.664

24. **Ans: C. Each DNA replication is associated with a loss of 500 to 1000 base pairs of telomeric DNA from the ends of every chromosome**

Ref: Chapter No.29, Page No.664

25. **Ans: D. All of the above**

Ref: Chapter No.29, Page No.665

26. **Ans: D. CSCs are more sensitive to traditional therapeutic modalities, such as chemotherapy and radiation**

Ref: Chapter No.29, Page No.665

27. **Ans: D. BCL-2 inactivation leads to significantly increased expression of VEGF and angiogenesis**

Ref: Chapter No.29, Page No.665

28. **Ans: A. VEGF**

Ref: Chapter No.29, Page No.665

29. **Ans: D. 90%**

Ref: Chapter No.29, Page No.665

30. **Ans: D. All of the above**

Ref: Chapter No.29, Page No.665-666

31. **Ans: D. All of the above**

Ref: Chapter No.29, Page No.666

32. **Ans: A. E-cadherin function is gained in most epithelial tumors during progression to tumor malignancy and may in fact be a prerequisite for tumor cell invasion and metastasis formation**

Ref: Chapter No.29, Page No.666-667

33. **Ans: D. All of the above**

Ref: Chapter No.29, Page No.667-668

34. **Ans: D. Tumor cells increase the rate of glycolysis to upregulate the expression of glucose transporters, such as GLUT4**

Ref: Chapter No.29, Page No.668-669

35. **Ans: D. All of the above**

Ref: Chapter No.29, Page No.669

36. **Ans: B. Immune cells don't play an important role in antitumor defense**

Ref: Chapter No.29, Page No.669

37. **Ans: B. Linear evolution model with late metastasis**

Ref: Chapter No.29, Page No.670

38. **Ans: A. Early dissemination with early distant metastasis and parallel evolution**

Ref: Chapter No.29, Page No.670

39. **Ans: C. Genetic mutations account for most mutations in cancer**

Ref: Chapter No.29, Page No.671

40. **Ans: A. Ataxia-telangiectasia**

Ref: Chapter No.29, Page No.672

41. **Ans: A. 17q21**

Ref: Chapter No.29, Page No.672

42. **Ans: B. PRKAR1A gene**

Ref: Chapter No.29, Page No.672

43. **Ans: A. 13q12**

Ref: Chapter No.29, Page No.672

44. **Ans: C. Schwannoma**

Ref: Chapter No.29, Page No.672

45. **Ans: C. 11q22**

Ref: Chapter No.29, Page No.672

46. **Ans: B. Medulloblastoma**

Ref: Chapter No.29, Page No.672

47. **Ans: B. PTEN**

Ref: Chapter No.29, Page No.672

48. **Ans: A. 10q23**

Ref: Chapter No.29, Page No.672

49. **Ans: B. Basal cell cancer**

Ref: Chapter No.29, Page No.672

50. **Ans: C. c-KIT**

Ref: Chapter No.29, Page No.672

51. **Ans: D. PTCH**

Ref: Chapter No.29, Page No.672

52. **Ans: C. Gastric cancer**

Ref: Chapter No.29, Page No.672

53. **Ans: A. CDKN2A/p16**

Ref: Chapter No.29, Page No.672

54. **Ans: C. MET**

Ref: Chapter No.29, Page No.672

55. **Ans: B. 7q31**

Ref: Chapter No.29, Page No.672

56. **Ans: A. 9q22**

Ref: Chapter No.29, Page No.672

57. **Ans: C. p53**

Ref: Chapter No.29, Page No.672

58. **Ans: A. 17p13**

Ref: Chapter No.29, Page No.672

59. **Ans: B. 11q13**

Ref: Chapter No.29, Page No.672

60. **Ans: D. Prostate cancer**

Ref: Chapter No.29, Page No.672

61. **Ans: A. Retinoblastoma**

Ref: Chapter No.29, Page No.672

62. **Ans: A. 17q11**

Ref: Chapter No.29, Page No.672

63. **Ans: B. Neurofibrosarcoma**

Ref: Chapter No.29, Page No.672

64. **Ans: C. 19p13**

Ref: Chapter No.29, Page No.672

65. **Ans: A. Pheochromocytoma**

Ref: Chapter No.29, Page No.672

66. **Ans: B. 13q14**

Ref: Chapter No.29, Page No.672

67. **Ans: B. 9q34**

Ref: Chapter No.29, Page No.672

68. **Ans: C. 16p13**

Ref: Chapter No.29, Page No.672

69. **Ans: A. 3p25**

Ref: Chapter No.29, Page No.672

70. **Ans: B. 11p13**

Ref: Chapter No.29, Page No.672

71. **Ans: B. Astrocytoma**

Ref: Chapter No.29, Page No.672

72. **Ans: D. Autosomal dominant inheritance**

Ref: Chapter No.29, Page No.672

73. Ans: C. RB1

Ref: Chapter No.29, Page No.671

74. Ans: B. Most affected children with an affected parent develop tumors unilaterally

Ref: Chapter No.29, Page No.671-673

75. Ans: B. Approximately 30% of Li Fraumeni kindreds have mutations in TP53 gene, which produces the protein p53

Ref: Chapter No.29, Page No.673

76. Ans: C. Breast cancers

Ref: Chapter No.29, Page No.673

77. Ans: D. Breast cancer before the age of 40 years old

Ref: Chapter No.29, Page No.673

78. Ans: D. FAP accounts for ~5% of the total colorectal cancer burden

Ref: Chapter No.29, Page No.673

79. Ans: B. Duodenal adenomas

Ref: Chapter No.29, Page No.673

80. Ans: B. 20%

Ref: Chapter No.29, Page No.674

81. Ans: B. < 100 polyps

Ref: Chapter No.29, Page No.674

82. Ans: B. Penetrance is estimated at 80% by age 60

Ref: Chapter No.29, Page No.674

83. Ans: C. Lifetime risk of colorectal cancer is nearly 100% in males and just > 80% in females

Ref: Chapter No.29, Page No.674

84. Ans: C. BRCA1 mutation conferred a 6.2 times increased risk of pancreatic cancer

Ref: Chapter No.29, Page No.674-675

85. Ans: B. 72%

Ref: Chapter No.29, Page No.674

86. Ans: A. 44%

Ref: Chapter No.29, Page No.674

87. Ans: C. 69%

Ref: Chapter No.29, Page No.674

88. Ans: B. Penetrance is 50% by the age of 65 years

Ref: Chapter No.29, Page No.675

89. Ans: D. All of the above

Ref: Chapter No.29, Page No.675

90. Ans: C. The modification of histones (e.g., by acetylation, methylation, or phosphorylation) is important in the compaction of chromatin structure and but is not crucial in cancer pathogenesis

Ref: Chapter No.29, Page No.675-676

91. Ans: B. It has been shown that colorectal cancers often have overrepresentation of Firmicutes species

Ref: Chapter No.29, Page No.676

92. Ans: B. Gammaproteobacteria

Ref: Chapter No.29, Page No.676

93. Ans: A. Light smokers with the susceptible genotype of CYP1A1 have a 10-fold higher risk for development of lung cancer compared with smokers without the permissive genotype

Ref: Chapter No.29, Page No.676

94. Ans: D. Group 4

Ref: Chapter No.29, Page No.676

95. Ans: A. Group 2A

Ref: Chapter No.29, Page No.676

96. Ans: C. Group 2B

Ref: Chapter No.29, Page No.676

97. Ans: B. Hepatocellular carcinoma

Ref: Chapter No.29, Page No.677

98. Ans: A. Mesothelioma

Ref: Chapter No.29, Page No.677

99. Ans: D. Coal tars

Ref: Chapter No.29, Page No.677

100. Ans: C. Leukemia

Ref: Chapter No.29, Page No.677

101. Ans: A. Benzidine

Ref: Chapter No.29, Page No.677

102. Ans: A. Clear cell adenocarcinoma of the vagina

Ref: Chapter No.29, Page No.677

103. Ans: B. Hepatocellular carcinoma

Ref: Chapter No.29, Page No.677

104. Ans: A. Alcohol

Ref: Chapter No.29, Page No.677

105. Ans: B. Cancer of urinary bladder

Ref: Chapter No.29, Page No.677

106 Ans: C. Cancer of the urinary bladder

Ref: Chapter No.29, Page No.677

107. Ans: A. Endometrial cancer

Ref: Chapter No.29, Page No.677

108. Ans: B. Melanoma

Ref: Chapter No.29, Page No.677

109. Ans: A. The two most important forms of radiation causing malignant change in humans are ultraviolet (UV) radiation and ionizing radiation (IR)

Ref: Chapter No.29, Page No.677

110. Ans: C. Malignant melanoma

Ref: Chapter No.29, Page No.677

111. Ans: C. 280 - 320 nm

Ref: Chapter No.29, Page No.677

112. Ans: B. UVC is the most important carcinogen

Ref: Chapter No.29, Page No.677-678

113. Ans: D. All of the above

Ref: Chapter No.29, Page No.678

114. Ans: B. ATM biallelic mutation, as seen in patients with ataxia telangiectasia, is considered an indication to radiation therapy

Ref: Chapter No.29, Page No.678

115. Ans: A. Kaposi sarcoma

Ref: Chapter No.29, Page No.678

116. Ans: B. HHV 8

Ref: Chapter No.29, Page No.678

117. Ans: B. Anal cancer

Ref: Chapter No.29, Page No.678

118. Ans: B. Non-Hodgkin lymphoma

Ref: Chapter No.29, Page No.678

119. Ans: A. Gastric neuroendocrine tumor

Ref: Chapter No.29, Page No.678

120. Ans: D. Schistosoma haematobium

Ref: Chapter No.29, Page No.678

121. Ans: C. Both A and B

Ref: Chapter No.29, Page No.678

122. Ans: A. Oncoviruses are necessary and usually sufficient for viral carcinogenesis

Ref: Chapter No.29, Page No.679

123. Ans: B. HBx decreases the formation of ROS while promoting cell survival via upregulation of HIF1α, which activates angiogenesis

Ref: Chapter No.29, Page No.679

124. Ans: C. < 200 cells/mm^3

Ref: Chapter No.29, Page No.679

125. Ans: D. 80%

Ref: Chapter No.29, Page No.679

126. Ans: C. H pylori was the second bacterium ever directly linked to human cancer

Ref: Chapter No.29, Page No.680

127. Ans: D. All of the above

Ref: Chapter No.29, Page No.680-681

128. Ans: D. CEA is useful as a screening test in colorectal cancers

Ref: Chapter No.29, Page No.681

129. Ans: C. 5 ng/mL

Ref: Chapter No.29, Page No.681

130. Ans: B. Elevated CEA levels rarely reflect the burden of tumor present

Ref: Chapter No.29, Page No.681

131. Ans: B. An elevated CEA level is an independent factor associated with poor survival and progression on 5-fluorouracil–based chemotherapy in patients with metastatic colorectal cancer

Ref: Chapter No.29, Page No.681

132. Ans: C. The upper limit of normal for a healthy, non-pregnant adult is < 100 ng/mL

Ref: Chapter No.29, Page No.681

133. Ans: C. AFP on its own is a good screening tool, with a sensitivity of 70%

Ref: Chapter No.29, Page No.681

134. Ans: A. AFP has been shown to decline after resection or ablation of tumor, and levels after complete resection should be < 100 ng/mL

Ref: Chapter No.29, Page No.681

135. Ans: C. CA 19-9 is considered to be useful as a screening tool

Ref: Chapter No.29, Page No.681-682

136. Ans: A. Testis

Ref: Chapter No.29, Page No.682

137. Ans: D. Positive predictive value for pancreatic cancer when used as a screening modality in the general population is 90%

Ref: Chapter No.29, Page No.682

138. Ans: C. Women have small detectable PSA levels

Ref: Chapter No.29, Page No.682

139. Ans: B. Elevation after digital rectal examination is seen and testing for PSA level can't be done after a digital rectal examination in the same clinic visit

Ref: Chapter No.29, Page No.682

140. Ans: B. 2 to 3 weeks

Ref: Chapter No.29, Page No.682

141. Ans: B. 3 - 5 months

Ref: Chapter No.29, Page No.682

142. Ans: B. Ovarian epithelium does normally express some CA 125

Ref: Chapter No.29, Page No.682

143. Ans: B. CA 125 is useful as a screening tool for ovarian cancer

Ref: Chapter No.29, Page No.682-683

144. Ans: C. 90%

Ref: Chapter No.29, Page No.683

145. Ans: B. 20%

Ref: Chapter No.29, Page No.683

146. Ans: A. 10%

Ref: Chapter No.29, Page No.683

147. Ans: C. Detection and measurement of these proteins rarely provides information about the clinical behavior of the cancer

Ref: Chapter No.29, Page No.683

148. Ans: B. Oncotype DX includes 16 tumor-associated genes and 15 reference genes

Ref: Chapter No.29, Page No.683

149. Ans: B. 51 genes

Ref: Chapter No.29, Page No.683

150. Ans: C. ColoPrint: Stomach cancer

Ref: Chapter No.29, Page No.683

151. Ans: D. All of the above

Ref: Chapter No.29, Page No.683

30

Tumor Immunology and Immunotherapy

OVERVIEW OF TUMOR IMMUNOLOGY

1. **False statement about T Lymphocytes among the following is:**
   A. CD8+ T cells recognize antigen in the context of MHC class I molecules, express αβ TCRs, are commonly referred to as cytotoxic T cells
   B. CD4+ T cells recognize antigen in the context of MHC class II molecules
   C. Th1 cells assist in the stimulation of B. cells for antibody production, allergic responses and addressing extracellular pathogens
   D. Treg cells constitute 5% to 10% of CD4+ cells, express the transcription factor Foxp3 and dominantly suppress autoimmune responses

2. **False statement about T Lymphocytes among the following is:**
   A. Recombination events could potentially yield a repertoire exceeding 10^{12} unique TCRs
   B. PD-1/PD-L1 axis in which the inhibitory ligand (PD-L1), commonly expressed in many cancers, can engage T-cell PD-1, thereby abrogating lymphocyte activation
   C. The activation of resting T cells requires engagement of the correct MHC-peptide complex by the TCR (so-called signal 1) and additional costimulatory signals (signal 2)
   D. Engagement of CTLA-4 induces a stimulatory signal that upregulates T-cell activation

3. **False about antigen-presenting cells (Dendritic cells: DCs) is:**
   A. Immature DCs are migratory and highly efficient in antigen capture, whereas mature DCs are less mobile but more efficient in processing and presenting antigen in an immunostimulatory context
   B. Dendritic cells in the gastrointestinal tract can sample bacteria in the intestinal lumen and initiate secretory immunoglobulin M (IgM) responses
   C. Mature DCs patrol their environment, sampling by pinocytosis and receptor-mediated endocytosis
   D. DC function is powerfully modulated by a variety of receptors including Toll-like receptors (TLRs) and surface C-type lectin receptors

4. **Cancer cell defense mechanisms includes:**
   A. T regulatory (Treg) cells: CD4+-CD25+ T-cell population, which inhibits T-cell function and proliferation
   B. Cytotoxic T lymphocyte–associated antigen 4 (CTLA-4) (CD152): Inhibitory receptor induced by T-cell activation that binds to CD80 and CD86 ligands
   C. Programmed cell death receptor 1 (PD-1) (CD279; programmed death 1): Another inhibitory receptor on T cells, prevalent on lymphocytes in the tumor microenvironment
   D. All of the above

IMMUNOTHERAPY

5. **False about cytokine therapy is:**
   A. IFN-α was the first cytokine to demonstrate reproducibly curative outcomes in patients with several types of widely metastatic cancer
   B. Toxicity of IL-2 is managed by judicious limitations on IL-2 dosing, fluid management, and supportive care because these toxicities are almost always self-limited and fully reversible
   C. For patients with metastatic disease, IL-2 therapy has an objective response rate (partial and complete) for melanoma and renal cell cancer were approximately 15% and 20%, respectively

D. The U.S. Food and Drug Administration (FDA) has approved the use of high-dose IFN-α after resection of node-positive melanoma on the basis of a randomized prospective study showing a delay in time to progression and borderline improved overall survival

6. **True about use of Vaccines in immunotherapy is:**
   A. The application of multiple vaccination approaches against cancer-associated antigens has not led to consistent success in causing cancer regression
   B. Initial crude adjuvants such as alum and the tuberculosis vaccine bacille Calmette-Guérin (BCG) have been replaced by molecules such as imiquimod or unmethylated CpG dinucleotides, which stimulate antigen-presenting cells through TLRs
   C. The application of multiple vaccination approaches against cancer-associated antigens has not led to consistent success in causing cancer regression
   D. All of the above

7. **Monoclonal antibodies that block CTLA-4 in humans have been developed and is called:**
   A. Nivolumab B. Pembrolizumab
   C. Ipilimumab D. All of the above

8. **Monoclonal antibodies that block CTLA-4; a fully human IgG2 monoclonal antibody is called:**
   A. Ipilimumab B. Tremelimumab
   C. Pembrolizumab D. Nivolumab

9. **The FDA has approved PD-1/PD-L1 inhibitors for all except:**
   A. Non-Hodgkin lymphoma (NHL)
   B. Non-small cell lung cancer
   C. Colorectal cancer
   D. Merkel cell carcinoma

10. **False statement among the following is:**
    A. There is higher incidence and severity of adverse events are observed with combination therapy and with PD-1 monotherapy greater than CTLA-4
    B. The majority of patients receiving CTLA-4, PD-1 checkpoint inhibitors
    C. While PD-L1 expression is associated with a higher likelihood of response to PD-1/PD-L1 blockade, its absence does not preclude a response
    D. These immune therapies had overall response rates from between 10% and 70% depending on the cancer type, with improvement in relapse-free and overall survival

11. **False about T-Cell Adoptive Therapy is:**
    A. The basic approach is to isolate, expand, and readminister tumor-reactive T cells as a means to overcome the weak expansion of cells in vivo by vaccination
    B. Patients undergoing CD19 CAR treatment also generally develop B-cell aplasia because CD19 is expressed by normal B cells; this can be successfully managed with immunoglobulin infusion and infection control and is considered an acceptable toxicity
    C. An overall objective response rate of 70% was seen
    D. The most successful CAR effort to date has been in targeting the CD19 molecule on B-cell malignant neoplasms

12. **Bispecific antibodies (BsAbs) among the following is:**
    A. Adalimumab B. Blinatunomab
    C. Secukinumab D. Ramucirumab

13. **Anti PD-1 monoclonal antibody among the following is:**
    A. Vedolizumab B. Pembrolizumab
    C. Adalimumab D. Situximab

14. **Anti-RANK-L monoclonal antibody is:**
    A. Abciximab B. Basiliximab
    C. Denosumab D. Palivizumab

15. **Anti-HER2 monoclonal antibody is:**
    A. Alemtuzumab B. Ranibizumab
    C. Ustekinumab D. Pertuzumab

16. **Anti-IL-6R monoclonal antibody is:**
    A. Belimumab B. Tocilizumab
    C. Obinutuzumab D. Raxibacuzumab

17. **Anti-TNF monoclonal antibody is:**
    A. Gemtuzumab B. Adalimumab
    C. Ofatumumab D. Obinutuzumab

18. **Anti-CD52 monoclonal antibody is:**
    A. Alemtuzumab B. Ranibizumab
    C. Ustekinumab D. Obinutuzumab

19. **Anti-CD33 monoclonal antibody is:**
    A. Ustekinumab B. Gemtuzumab
    C. Raxibacuzumab D. Obinutuzumab

20. Anti-GPIIb/IIIa monoclonal antibody is:

A. Abciximab
B. Ustekinumab
C. Raxibacuzumab
D. Obinutuzumab

21. True among the following is:

A. The first application of passive serotherapy in the treatment of cancer was performed in 1895 by Hericourt and Richet, when they immunized dogs with human sarcoma and transferred the serum to patients in an attempt to provide cancer immunity
B. To date, the FDA has approved more than 76 monoclonal antibodies/antibody-based therapeutics to treat various diseases
C. A chimeric IgG molecule is approximately 75% human and 25% murine
D. All of the above

22. A humanized murine monoclonal antibody is approximately:

A. 75% human
B. 85% human
C. 95% human
D. 100% human

23. After the last dose of bevacizumab, it is customary to delay elective surgical procedures until:

A. 1 week
B. 4 weeks
C. 6 weeks
D. 8 weeks

24. Bevacizumab has received FDA approval for use in patients with cancers, such as:

A. Astrocytoma
B. Breast cancer
C. Renal cell cancer (combined with IFN-α)
D. Non-small cell lung cancer

25. Radionuclide considered high-energy beta emitters is:

A. Iodine-131
B. Lutetium-177
C. Yttrium-90
D. All of the above

26. High-energy beta emitters (yttrium-90 and rhenium-188), and the path length of cytotoxic radiation can penetrate a tumor up to a distance of:

A. 1 mm
B. 5 mm
C. 1 cm
D. 5 cm

27. Radionuclide considered medium-energy beta emitters is:

A. Lutetium-177
B. Rhenium-188
C. Yttrium-90
D. All of the above

28. Radionuclides such as lutetium-177 and iodine-131 are considered medium-energy beta emitters whose energy can traverse approximately:

A. 1 mm
B. 5 mm
C. 1 cm
D. 5 cm

29. Anti-CD20 IgG radioimmunoconjugate currently FDA approved for the treatment of non-Hodgkin lymphoma is:

A. Ibritumomab is conjugated to iodine-131
B. Ibritumomab is conjugated to yttrium-90
C. Tositumomab is conjugated to yttrium-90
D. All of the above

ANSWERS

1. **Ans: C. Th1 cells assist in the stimulation of B cells for antibody production, allergic responses, and addressing extracellular pathogens**

Ref: Chapter No.30, Page No.688

2. **Ans: D. Engagement of CTLA-4 induces a stimulatory signal that upregulates T-cell activation**

Ref: Chapter No.30, Page No.688-689

3. **Ans: C. Mature DCs patrol their environment, sampling by pinocytosis and receptor-mediated endocytosis**

Ref: Chapter No.30, Page No.689-690

4. **Ans: D. All of the above**

Ref: Chapter No.30, Page No.691

5. **Ans: A. IFN-α was the first cytokine to demonstrate reproducibly curative outcomes in patients with several types of widely metastatic cancer**

Ref: Chapter No.30, Page No.692

6. **Ans: D. All of the above**

Ref: Chapter No.30, Page No.692-693

7. **Ans: C. Ipilimumab**

Ref: Chapter No.30, Page No.694

8. **Ans: B. Tremelimumab**

Ref: Chapter No.30, Page No.694

9. **Ans: A. Non-Hodgkin lymphoma (NHL)**

Ref: Chapter No.30, Page No.694-695

10. **Ans: A. There is higher incidence and severity of adverse events are observed with combination therapy, and with PD-1 monotherapy greater than CTLA-4**

Ref: Chapter No.30, Page No.695

11. **Ans: C. An overall objective response rate of 70% was seen**

Ref: Chapter No.30, Page No.696

12. **Ans: B. Blinatunomab (A BsAb (Blinatunomab), bispecific for CD3a and CD19, is FDA approved for certain *B cell malignancies*)**

Ref: Chapter No.30, Page No.697

13. **Ans: B. Pembrolizumab**

Ref: 20th Edition, Chapter No.29, Page No.719

14. **Ans: C. Denosumab**

Ref: 20th Edition, Chapter No.29, Page No.719

15. **Ans: D. Pertuzumab**

Ref: 20th Edition, Chapter No.29, Page No.719

16. **Ans: B. Tocilizumab**

Ref: 20th Edition, Chapter No.29, Page No.719

17. **Ans: B. Adalimumab**

Ref: 20th Edition, Chapter No.29, Page No.719

18. **Ans: A. Alemtuzumab**

Ref: 20th Edition, Chapter No.29, Page No.719

19. **Ans: B. Gemtuzumab**

Ref: 20th Edition, Chapter No.29, Page No.719

20. **Ans: A. Abciximab**

Ref: 20th Edition, Chapter No.29, Page No.719

21. **Ans: D. All of the above**

Ref: Chapter No.30, Page No.699

22. **Ans: C. 95% human**

Ref: Chapter No.30, Page No.701

23. **Ans: C. 6 weeks**

Ref: Chapter No.30, Page No.701

24. **Ans: A. Astrocytoma**

Ref: Chapter No.30, Page No.701

25. **Ans: C. Yttrium-90**

Ref: Chapter No.30, Page No.702

26. **Ans: C. 1 cm**

Ref: Chapter No.30, Page No.702

27. **Ans: A. Lutetium-177**

Ref: Chapter No.30, Page No.702

28. **Ans: A. 1 mm**

Ref: Chapter No.30, Page No.702

29. **Ans: B. Ibritumomab is conjugated to yttrium-90**

Ref: Chapter No.30, Page No.702

31

Melanoma and Cutaneous Malignancies

MELANOMA

1. **The most common cause of skin cancer–related death is:**
   A. Basal cell carcinoma
   B. Melanoma
   C. SCC
   D. Merkel cell carcinoma

2. **The first modern published account of the surgical treatment of melanoma was by:**
   A. René Laennec
   B. John Hunter
   C. Hippocrates
   D. Bernard

3. **False about the epidemiology of melanoma is:**
   A. Melanoma causes the majority of skin cancer–related deaths
   B. The degree of pigmentation in the skin is a relative protective factor against cutaneous melanoma; those with lighter skin tones are at increased risk
   C. Patients with a fair complexion, blonde or red hair, and blue eyes are at increased risk, as are those who sunburn easily, have a tendency to develop freckles, or have an inability to tan
   D. Melanoma is slightly more common in women across most races/ethnicities

4. **Genetic risk factors for melanoma includes all except:**
   A. Family history of melanoma
   B. Fitzpatrick type I
   C. Fitzpatrick type III
   D. Xeroderma pigmentosum

5. **Environmental risk factors for melanoma includes all except:**
   A. Lower socioeconomic status
   B. Upper socioeconomic status
   C. Immunosuppression
   D. Episodes of intense intermittent sun exposure associated with severe blistering sunburns

6. **False about the epidemiology of melanoma is:**
   A. Chronic sun exposure (UV radiation) exposure appears to be a strong causative factor for melanoma
   B. Recommendations for reducing the risk of melanoma include avoidance of sunbathing and tanning beds, use of sun-protective clothing and use of sunscreens
   C. UVA is the predominant wavelength in tanning beds and as a cause of melanoma skin cancer and NMSC
   D. A UV signature consistent with mutations caused by UV damage was found in over 90% of three of the four melanoma subtypes identified in The Cancer Genome Atlas project

7. **The chief cause of sunburns is:**
   A. UVA B. UVB
   C. UVC D. UVD

8. **Melanomas arising within pre-existing lesions is upto:**
   A. 20% B. 40%
   C. 60% D. 80%

9. **Melanoma patients that have a family history of the disease is:**
   A. 1-5% B. 5-10%
   C. 10-20% D. 20-40%

10. **False about dysplastic nevus is:**
    A. A dysplastic nevus is a 6- to 15-mm macular (flat) pigmented skin lesion with indistinct margins and variable colour

B. Most nevi are benign, but some may reflect early atypia associated with increased intracellular growth signaling and can progress to invasive disease with the accumulation of additional mutations
C. The risk of melanoma in those patients with congenital nevi is proportional to the size and number of nevi
D. Small- or medium-sized congenital nevi represent a moderate risk and therefore are observed

11. Giant congenital nevi has a diameter of:

A. >5 cm B. >10 cm
C. >20 cm D. >40 cm

12. With regard to ultraviolet (UV) radiation, which of the following statements is correct?

A. Type A UV (UVA) radiation is responsible for most of the sun damage to human skin
B. UVA is within the photoabsorption spectrum of DNA, whereas UVB is not
C. The melanin content of the skin is the single best intrinsic factor for protecting the skin from the harmful effects of UV radiation
D. UV radiation acts as a tumor promoter but not a tumor initiator

13. False about Spitzoid melanocytic lesion is:

A. Benign Spitz nevi are most common in children, lesions in adults are more likely to have atypical features or to represent melanoma with spitzoid features
B. A Spitz nevus is a slow growing, pink or brown, benign skin lesion with risk for further progression to melanoma
C. Although complete excision with negative margins is adequate for an unequivocal Spitz nevus, the diagnosis is often unclear
D. Sentinel lymph node (SLN) biopsy is appropriate for invasive spitzoid melanomas and can be used as a prognostic measure in indeterminate cases

14. Atypical features of spitz nevus includes all except:

A. >10 mm
B. Poor circumscription
C. Symmetry
D. Ulceration

15. The most common genomic subtype in cutaneous melanoma is:

A. Mutant RAS
B. Mutant BRAF
C. Mutant NF1
D. Triple-wild-type

16. The most common BRAF mutation is the:

A. V600K B. V600E
C. V600D D. V600A

17. The second most common subtype in cutaneous melanoma is:

A. Mutant RAS B. Mutant BRAF
C. Mutant NF1 D. Triple-wild-type

18. Which statement correctly describes increased risk for the development of malignant melanoma?

A. Melanoma accounts for 50% of all skin cancer diagnoses but accounts for 10% of deaths due to skin cancer
B. An inactivating mutation in the gene CDKN2A occurs in 25% to 40% of familial melanomas
C. A genetic component has been implicated in the pathogenesis of melanoma, with nearly 25% of all patients diagnosed with melanoma reporting a positive family history
D. Populations that reside at further distances from the equator have a higher incidence of melanoma

19. In nonfamilial melanomas, loss of PTEN occurs in approximately:

A. <25% B. 25% to 50%
C. 50% to 75% D. >75%

20. The ABCDE criteria are used to guide diagnosis and the decision to perform a biopsy of suspicious cutaneous lesions includes all except:

A. Asymmetry B. Irregular Borders
C. Colour variegation D. Diameter >10 mm

21. False statement about melanoma among the following is:

A. Most melanomas occur de novo but some can arise within a congenital or acquired nevus
B. Amelanotic melanomas are these lesions are not pigmented and present as a raised pink or flesh-coloured skin lesion
C. If a patient presents with a skin lesion that has changed in size, colour, or shape and/or is itching or bleeding, there should be a low threshold for biopsy
D. 25% of patients will present with regional disease, while up to 50% may present with metastases

22. The most common benign pigmented skin lesions are:

A. Freckles
B. Lentigines
C. Seborrheic keratoses
D. Melasma

23. True about Seborrheic keratoses is:

A. The characteristic appearance usually is completely diagnostic and these lesions do not need to be removed
B. The most common benign pigmented skin lesions are seborrheic keratoses. Known for their propensity to accumulate over time in elderly patients
C. Typically these are scaly, waxy, raised lesions with a stuck-on look that makes them appear as if they could easily be scraped off with a fingernail
D. All of the above

24. False about excisional biopsy of melanoma is:

A. Transverse orientation of incision on the extremities is best
B. An excisional biopsy completely removes a pigmented skin lesion and is particularly well suited to diagnosis and completely remove small lesions
C. The depth of excision should extend to the subcutaneous fat to ensure a full-thickness biopsy
D. Incisions should allow closure with the least tension and best cosmetic outcome in the event wider excision is needed

25. False about punch biopsy of melanoma is:

A. In a punch biopsy, a sharp disposable instrument is twisted into the anesthetized skin to remove a 2-mm to 8-mm cylinder of skin and subcutaneous tissue
B. Punch biopsies of at least 4 mm should be performed, since smaller tissue samples often do not provide adequate tissue for pathologic evaluation
C. Multiple punch biopsies should not be performed to sample larger lesions
D. The punch biopsy should be performed through the thickest or most suspicious-looking area of the lesion

26. The most common technique by which melanomas are biopsied and diagnosed is:

A. Shave biopsy
B. Punch biopsy
C. Excisional biopsy
D. True cut biopsy

27. False about shave biopsy of melanoma is:

A. Drawback to the use of a shave biopsy to diagnose melanoma is that the lesion may be transected, compromising the ability to accurately assess tumor thickness
B. Shave biopsy is the most common technique by which melanomas are biopsied and diagnosed
C. Shave biopsy is performed by elevating the skin lesion with forceps or inserting a small needle beneath the lesion, followed by shaving the lesion with a razor blade or scalpel
D. Deep shave or saucerization biopsies, completely remove the lesion down to dermis but not the subcutaneous fat

28. False statement among the following is:

A. All melanomas initially proliferate in the basal layer of the skin
B. As melanoma cells multiply, these cells expand radially in the epidermis and superficial dermal layer, termed the radial growth phase
C. The vertical growth phase allows invasion into the deeper layers of the skin, where the tumor may ultimately achieve metastatic potential by invasion of blood vessels and lymphatic channels
D. Histologic subtype is a major factor in prognosis

29. The most common melanoma histologic subtype is:

A. Superficial spreading melanoma
B. Lentigo maligna melanoma
C. Acral lentiginous melanoma
D. Nodular melanomas

30. False about superficial spreading melanoma is:

A. It is not necessarily associated with sun exposed skin
B. Superficial spreading melanoma initially appears as a flat-pigmented lesion growing radially
C. Untreated, these melanomas will subsequently develop a vertical growth phase, invade more deeply into the skin and possibly ulcerate
D. It most commonly appears on the neck and distal extremities

31. False about Lentigo maligna melanoma is:

A. Lentigo maligna melanoma occurs most commonly on the sun-exposed areas of older individuals and presents as a flat, dark,

variably pigmented lesion, with irregular borders and a history of slow development
B. Lentigo maligna melanomas may become relatively large prior to diagnosis, as the slow progression can escape the patient's notice
C. The prognosis of lentigo maligna melanoma is worse than for the other subtypes given the deep nature of these tumors
D. Before proceeding with complex tissue flaps for closure, it is prudent to ensure negative margins

32. False about Acral lentiginous melanoma is:

A. These tumors develop in the subungual areas beneath fingernails and toenails and on the palms of the hands and soles of the feet
B. The histologic appearance of acral lentiginous melanomas is similar to melanomas arising on the mucous membranes
C. The diagnosis is often made at an early stage
D. The distinguishing feature of subungual melanomas is that they do not change in position underneath the nail, while a hematoma should migrate distally with growth of the nail

33. The most common type of melanoma in non-white patients is:

A. Superficial spreading melanoma
B. Lentigo maligna melanoma
C. Acral lentiginous melanoma
D. Nodular melanomas

34. False about Nodular melanomas is:

A. Nodular melanomas often have a good prognosis
B. Nodular melanomas are raised papular lesions that can occur anywhere on the body
C. These melanomas can have atypical presentations that do not always conform to ABCDE criteria, including a higher rate of amelanotic lesions compared to the other subtypes
D. They tend to develop a vertical growth pattern early in their course

35. False about Desmoplastic melanomas is:

A. It is characterized by a combination of melanoma cells with a prominent stromal fibrosis
B. Desmoplastic melanomas are classified as either pure or mixed depending upon the degree of desmoplasia present
C. Pure desmoplastic melanomas have a high risk of lymph node metastases
D. Mixed desmoplastic melanomas have lymph node metastatic rates that are similar to other histologic subtypes; therefore, SLN biopsy should be considered for the usual indications in these lesions

36. Melanomas are commonly referred to as thin if the thickness is:

A. <1 mm Breslow thickness
B. <2 mm Breslow thickness
C. <4 mm Breslow thickness
D. <5 mm Breslow thickness

37. Melanomas are commonly referred to as thin if the thickness is:

A. >1 mm Breslow thickness
B. >2 mm Breslow thickness
C. >4 mm Breslow thickness
D. >5 mm Breslow thickness

38. A melanoma with thickness of 3 mm and without ulceration has T staging as:

A. T2b B. T3b
C. T3a D. T2a

39. A melanoma with thickness of 7 mm and with ulceration has T staging as:

A. T3a B. T3b
C. T4a D. T4b

40. A metastatic melanotic lesion was found without known primary. What is the T staging?

A. TX B. T0
C. Tis D. T4

41. A completely regressed melanoma has a T staging of:

A. TX B. T0
C. Tis D. T4

42. A melanoma with thickness of 0.9 mm without ulceration has a T staging of:

A. Tis B. T1a
C. T1b D. T2a

43. A melanoma with distant metastasis to lung has M staging as:

A. M1a B. M1b
C. M1c D. M1d

44. A melanoma with distant metastasis to CNS has M staging as:

A. M1a
B. M1b
C. M1c
D. M1d

45. A melanoma with 2 or more clinically occult or clinically detected and/or presence of any number of matted nodes with presence of in-transit nodes has N staging as:

A. N2c
B. N3a
C. N3b
D. N3c

46. False statement about melanoma among the following is:

A. Older patients have a greater risk of melanoma mortality than younger patients, despite the fact that younger patients are more likely to have nodal metastasis
B. Patients with axial (trunk, head and neck) melanomas have a worse prognosis than those with extremity tumors
C. Men have a better prognosis than women
D. The number of mitoses per square millimetres is an important predictor of survival across all thickness categories

47. False about Workup and Imaging of melanoma is:

A. Patients clinically staged with localized stage I or II disease do not require any further tests unless symptoms prompt further evaluation
B. Patients with thick primary tumors (stage IIA) can be considered for imaging to detect metastatic disease
C. The probability of detecting actual disease in patients with microscopic nodal metastasis using radiographic studies such as positron emission tomography (PET) and computed tomography (CT) scanning is low
D. For stage IV advanced presentations, PET/CT or CT scans of the chest, abdomen, and pelvis and magnetic resonance imaging (MRI) of the brain are generally recommended

48. False about WLE for melanoma treatment is:

A. WLE can be performed under local anesthesia in most cases, although general anesthesia is preferred for patients who will also undergo SLN biopsy or lymphadenectomy
B. Excision of the fascia is necessary in most cases
C. There is no evidence that margins >2 cm are beneficial; however, greater margins may be considered for advanced melanomas when local recurrence risk is high
D. The appropriate margins of excision are measured from the edge of the lesion or previous biopsy scar

49. In melanoma the recommended margin of wide local excision (WLE) for thickness of 3 mm is:

A. 0.5 cm
B. 1 cm
C. 1–2 cm
D. 2 cm

50. In melanoma the recommended margin of wide local excision (WLE) for in situ lesions is:

A. 0.5 cm
B. 1 cm
C. 1–2 cm
D. 2 cm

51. False statement about the management of melanoma among the following is:

A. For fingers, ray amputations are unnecessary because the melanoma commonly involves only the distal phalanx, and amputation at the distal interphalangeal joint is sufficient
B. Subungual melanomas are treated with amputation of the distal digit
C. It is necessary to reexcise the melanoma if the final pathology report indicates that the measured distance from the melanoma to the edge of the excised skin is less than the recommended margin
D. Mohs micrographic surgery (MMS) is preferred for cosmetically sensitive areas such as the face, where it may minimize the skin defect while still achieving negative margins of excision

52. Sentinel lymph node biopsy was introduced by:

A. Cabana
B. Donald Morton
C. Pettway
D. Kumar and Anandakrishnan

53. False about Sentinel lymph node biopsy is:

A. The accuracy of the technique has been well validated and it is now a required part of staging for melanoma >1.0 mm in thickness according to the AJCC
B. Features of the primary lesion that have been linked to an increased risk of nodal metastasis include ulceration and mitotic rate (≥1 mitosis/mm^2)
C. The status of the SLNs is the single most important prognostic factor in melanoma patients without clinical evidence of nodal metastases
D. SLN biopsy is recommended for thin melanomas

54. The NCCN guidelines recommend consideration of SLN biopsy in all patients with:

A. T1 or greater (>0.8 mm) melanomas
B. T2 or greater (>1.0 mm) melanomas
C. T3 or greater (>2.0 mm) melanomas
D. T4 or greater (>4.0 mm) melanomas

55. False about Sentinel lymph node biopsy is:

A. All patients should undergo preoperative lymphoscintigraphy, typically performed on the same day as the operation to perform SLN biopsy and WLE
B. Technetium-99 sulfur colloid (0.5 mCi) should be injected into the dermis, raising a wheal in four aliquots around the melanoma or biopsy site
C. It is important to inject the tracer into the normal skin approximately 0.5 cm away from the melanoma or scar from the biopsy and not into the melanoma itself or biopsy scar
D. Interval nodes have the less risk of harbouring melanoma cells than sentinel nodes in traditional nodal basins; therefore, it is not recommended to be removed at the time of sentinel node biopsy

56. False about Sentinel lymph node biopsy is:

A. At operation, a vital blue dye (e.g., isosulfan blue) is injected into the dermis around the melanoma site in a manner similar to that for injection of the radioactive tracer
B. A sentinel node is defined as any lymph node that is the most radioactive node in the nodal basin, any node that is blue, any node that has a radioactive count of 50% or higher of the most radioactive node in that basin
C. Because the blue dye will not persist in the sentinel nodes for prolonged periods, it is injected just before the operation; 1 to 5 mL is used, depending on the size of the melanoma
D. Because blue dye will persist in the skin for many months after injection; it is best to inject it within the margins of the planned WLE

57. False about Sentinel lymph node biopsy is:

A. Immediate frozen section histology should be done
B. There is often a poor correlation between the number of nodes visualized on the lymphoscintigram and the number of SLNs identified
C. In general, the average number of sentinel nodes identified is 2 per nodal basin
D. Sentinel nodes should be sent for permanent section histopathology with immunohistochemical stains for melanoma markers

58. IHC markers for melanoma is/are:

A. HMB-40
B. S-100
C. Melan-2
D. All of the above

59. False about Multicentre Selective Lymphadenectomy Trial (MSLT-I) is:

A. The trial randomized patients with intermediate-thickness melanoma (1.2–3.5 mm thick) and patients with thick melanoma (>3.5 mm thick) to either SLN biopsy or observation
B. No difference in 10-year melanoma-specific survival was found between SLN biopsy and observation group in either the intermediate thickness or thick melanoma groups
C. No improvement in 10-year disease-free was observed with SLN biopsy in both intermediate and thick melanomas
D. The status of the sentinel node was the strongest predictor of recurrence or death from melanoma: in patients with intermediate thickness melanoma

60. False about Completion Lymphadenectomy (CLND) is:

A. Completion lymphadenectomy or CLND is used to remove the remaining lymph nodes in a regional nodal basin that is found to have metastatic melanoma by SLN biopsy
B. CLND may have a potential therapeutic benefit by removing additional lymph nodes with micrometastatic disease, improving disease-free survival as seen in MSLT-I
C. In general, the maximum diameter of the largest tumor deposit is the most prognostically significant tumor burden measure that can predict survival and non-SLN metastases
D. Around 30% to 50% of patients with SLN-positive micrometastatic lymph node disease have additional micrometastatic nonsentinel nodes after CLND

61. Complications of CLND include:

A. Permanent lymphedema
B. Paresthesias
C. Wound complications
D. All of the above

62. False about Multicentre Selective Lymphadenectomy Trial II is:

A. In MSLT-II, 1939 patients with a tumor-positive SLN biopsy were randomized to a CLND or observation, which consisted of ultrasound-based surveillance of the involved nodal basin
B. There was no difference in the primary endpoint, melanoma-specific survival, between the two groups
C. The 3-year disease-free survival rate was numerically and statistically greater in the CLND group compared to the observation group
D. MSLT-II study firmly establish that it is safe and reasonable to avoid CLND for the vast majority of patients with positive SLN

63. True about German Dermatologic Cooperative Group Trial (DeCOGSLT) is:

A. 483 patients with a positive SLN biopsy were randomized to either a CLND of the positive lymph node basin or observation
B. With a median follow-up of 35 months, there were no differences in the primary endpoint or distant metastasis-free survival between the two groups
C. It is an important study that establishes the safety of an observation strategy with SLN-positive melanoma
D. All of the above

64. True about Therapeutic Lymph Node Dissection is:

A. It is a lymphadenectomy of a regional nodal basin with clinically apparent nodal metastases
B. It is an excellent procedure for achieving locoregional disease control, and given the findings of MSLT-II and DeCOGSLT, it will likely be the most common reason for performing a lymphadenectomy in the future
C. In a patient with cutaneous melanoma, palpable lymph nodes should be concerning for metastatic disease until proven otherwise
D. All of the above

65. The first successful targeted therapy developed for melanoma was:

A. Ipilimumab B. Vemurafenib
C. Pembrolizumab D. Nivolumab

66. Dual BRAF (dabrafenib) and MEK (trametinib) inhibition therapy Vs placebo for 12 months after resection was observed in:

A. EORTC 18071 trail
B. CheckMate 238 trail
C. COMBI-AD trail
D. EORTC 1325 trail

67. Nivolumab every 2 weeks Vs Ipilimumab 10 mg/kg every 3 weeks × 4, then every 12 weeks for 12 months was observed in:

A. EORTC 18071 trail
B. CheckMate 238 trail
C. COMBI-AD trail
D. EORTC 1325 trail

68. The first immunotherapy agent to gain approval for adjuvant therapy of melanoma was:

A. Ipilimumab B. Vemurafenib
C. Pembrolizumab D. Nivolumab

69. Which trial demonstrated that adjuvant nivolumab was more effective than ipilimumab at preventing recurrence in resected stage III and stage IV melanoma?

A. EORTC 18071 trail
B. CheckMate 238 trail
C. COMBI-AD trail
D. EORTC 1325 trail

70. True statement among the following is:

A. Like nivolumab, pembrolizumab was effective across multiple subgroups, including PD-1 ligand (PD-L1) expression, gender, stage (IIIA, IIIB, IIIC), number of positive lymph node, micro- versus macrometastatic lymph node disease, ulceration, and BRAF mutation status
B. Nivolumab and pembrolizumab have become the preferred adjuvant immunotherapy option for patients with resected stage III and IV melanoma
C. The majority of patients with nodal metastases detected by SLN biopsy have a single microscopically positive lymph node
D. All of the above

71. False about radiation therapy in melanoma is:

A. ANZMTG 01.02/TROG 02.01 trial, adjuvant radiation therapy after regional lymphadenectomy reduced the cumulative incidence of lymph node field relapse from 36% to 21%
B. Adjuvant radiation therapy appears to offer some improvement in control of regional lymph node disease in high-risk patients after lymphadenectomy

C. Several newer studies suggest that there may be role for radiation treatment in the adjuvant and palliative settings as well as a potential adjunct to systemic immunotherapy
D. All of the above are true

72. Compared to the general population, increased risk of a subsequent melanoma in melanoma survivors is:

A. 1-fold B. 5-fold
C. 10-fold D. 20-fold

73. Compared to the general population, a cumulative risk of the development of a second primary melanoma in melanoma survivors is approximately:

A. 1% B. 5%
C. 10% D. 20%

74. False about Local recurrence of melanoma is:

A. Recurrences within 5 cm of the WLE scar or skin graft are considered local recurrences
B. Recurrence risk increases with tumor thickness and has been estimated as 0.2%, 2%, 6% and 13% for melanomas less than 0.75 mm, 0.75 to 1.5 mm, 1.5 to 4 mm, and larger than 4 mm, respectively
C. Although WLE guidelines for primary tumors do not apply, at least a 5-cm margin should be attempted with complete resection of the prior WLE scar
D. The rate of a positive SLN biopsy when performed for recurrence may be as high as 40%

75. False about In-transit disease is:

A. In-transit tumors, either at presentation or as a recurrence after initial local therapy, are subcutaneous or cutaneous tumor nodules between the primary tumor site and draining nodal basin formed by tumor deposits within the lymphatic channels
B. They are often subtle in appearance, lack pigmentation, and may only be appreciated as a palpable nodule
C. Limited in-transit disease need to be adequately treated with extensive excision with 2 cms margin
D. SLN biopsy in the setting of in-transit disease should be considered, as the results carry prognostic significance

76. The most common chemotherapy agent delivered into the circuit for hyperthermic isolated limb perfusion (HILP) is:

A. Methotrexate B. Melphalan
C. Cisplatin D. Carboplatin

77. False among the following is:

A. Talimogene laherparepvec (T-VEC) is a herpes simplex virus type 1–derived oncolytic immunotherapy that is serially injected into palpable target lesions to induce both a direct local effect and potentially a systemic response
B. In the OPTiM trial, the overall response rate was greater in the T-VEC group (26% vs. 6%) and median overall survival was marginally improved
C. On the basis of OPTiM trial, T-VEC received FDA approval for intralesional therapy of stage III or IV cutaneous melanoma
D. The addition of T-VEC to systemic immunotherapy doesn't appear to improve the response rate to immunotherapy in unresectable stage III/IV disease

78. Monoclonal anti–CTLA-4 antibody is:

A. Ipilimumab B. Vemurafenib
C. Pembrolizumab D. Nivolumab

79. PD-1 inhibitor is:

A. Ipilimumab B. Vemurafenib
C. Pembrolizumab D. Dabrafenib

80. The preferred first line agent for metastatic melanoma:

A. Ipilimumab B. Vemurafenib
C. Pembrolizumab D. Dabrafenib

81. The first agent used to target metastatic melanoma with the BRAF V600E mutation was:

A. Ipilimumab B. Vemurafenib
C. Pembrolizumab D. Dabrafenib

82. Drug active at the shown site is:

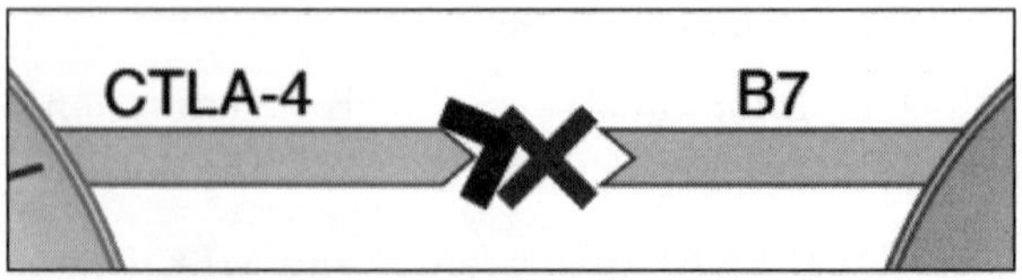

A. Ipilimumab B. Vemurafenib
C. Pembrolizumab D. Dabrafenib

83. **Drug active at the shown site is:**

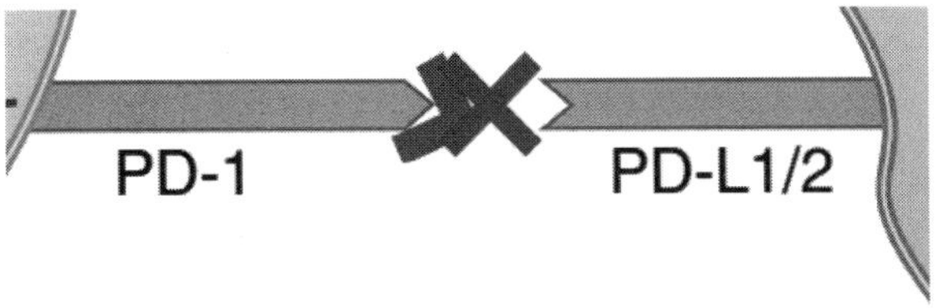

A. Ipilimumab
B. Vemurafenib
C. Pembrolizumab
D. Dabrafenib

84. **False about Unknown Primary Melanoma is:**

A. It occurs in < 2% of melanoma cases overall and in < 5% of all cases involving metastatic disease
B. A diagnosis of unknown primary melanoma should prompt a thorough skin examination, including the perianal area, external genitalia, nail beds, scalp and external auditory canal
C. PET/CT and MRI of the brain are warranted to assess the extent of disease
D. In the setting of lymph node metastasis without a primary lesion, the patient should be treated as a patient with stage II melanoma

85. **False about Melanoma and Pregnancy is:**

A. The placenta should be examined pathologically for evidence of melanoma in women who develop melanoma during pregnancy as a marker for metastasis as well as possible transmission to the child
B. There is therapeutic benefit to early termination of the pregnancy
C. SLN biopsy may be performed if indicated by the pathologic factors of the primary tumor, although vital blue dye should not be used
D. For patients who have tumors with poor prognostic factors, it may be advisable to wait 2 to 3 years before the next pregnancy as this represents the time during which recurrence is most likely

86. **False about ocular melanoma is:**

A. Ocular melanoma is the most common intraocular malignant neoplasm in adults
B. Primary treatment consists of enucleation or iodine-125 brachytherapy, although other options include photocoagulation and partial resection
C. Metastatic spread of ocular melanoma occurs hematogenously
D. Ocular melanoma is more responsive to immunotherapy compared to cutaneous melanoma

87. **The most common sites for mucosal melanoma is/are:**

A. Female genitalia
B. Head and neck
C. Anal canal
D. All of the above

88. **False about mucosal melanoma is:**

A. Given the high risk of metastatic disease, extensive local resections, such as abdomino-perineal resection or pelvic exenteration, improve overall survival
B. Patients tend to present with more advanced disease and have a poor prognosis
C. These tumors should be excised to negative margins when possible
D. Response rate to immunotherapy for mucosal melanoma is similar to that of cutaneous melanoma

NONMELANOMA SKIN CANCERS

89. **Most common skin cancer is:**

A. Squamous cell carcinoma
B. Basal cell carcinoma
C. Melanoma
D. Merkel cell carcinoma

90. **Of the total NMSCs' Basal cell carcinoma constitutes about:**

A. 20%
B. 40%
C. 60%
D. 80%

91. **False about Squamous Cell Carcinoma is:**

A. Most SCCs occur on sun-exposed surfaces, particularly the head and neck
B. Individuals with dark complexions have a lower risk of SCC, even with prolonged sun exposure
C. UV radiation, and UVA in particular, increases the risk of SCC
D. The amount of sun exposure is also proportional to the incidence of known precursor lesions for SCC, including actinic keratosis

92. **Risk factors for the development of SCC include:**

A. Compromised immunity
B. Susceptible skin types
C. Underlying genetic disorders
D. Intense intermittent sun exposure

93. **False about Squamous Cell Carcinoma is:**

A. Occupational and environmental carcinogens, including arsenic, organic hydrocarbons, ionizing radiation, and cigarette smoke are associated with an increased risk for SCC

B. SCC that develops in immunosuppressed patients are less aggressive and have an decreased risk of systemic metastases

C. A history of chronic inflammation from burn scars (Marjolin ulcer), draining sinuses, infections (including osteomyelitis), and non-healing ulcers can precede the development of SCCs

D. There is the direct carcinogenic effect of UV light on the frequently dividing keratinocytes within the basal layer of the epidermis

94. UVB induced silencing of the p53 tumor suppressor gene occurs in:

A. >60% B. >70%
C. >80% D. >90%

95. Compared to normal population, the incidence of SCC in posttransplant patients is:

A. 15 times B. 25 times
C. 45 times D. 65 times

96. Compared to normal population, the incidence of BCC in posttransplant patients is:

A. 5-fold B. 10-fold
C. 20-fold D. 40-fold

97. After 20 years of immunosuppression, malignant neoplasms develop in:

A. 40% to 60% B. 10% to 20%
C. 70% to 80% D. 5% to 10%

98. False about SCC is:

A. Most SCCs begin with a proliferation of keratin cells in the basal layer of the epidermis that appear as red or pink areas, clinically termed actinic keratoses (solar keratoses)

B. Lesions are scaling, with an even surface and an whitish base

C. Human papillomavirus, an infection associated with immunosuppression, is a proposed risk factor for the development of SCCs

D. The risk of malignant transformation of actinic keratosis to SCC is approximately 0.01%– 0.6% over 1 year and up to 2.5% over 4 years

99. Erythroplasia of Queyrat is sometimes referred to as bowen disease confined to the:

A. Vulva B. Glans penis
C. Both A and B D. Scrotum

100. False about the management of SCC is:

A. Curettage may be used for patients with superficial lesions <5 cm

B. Unlike melanoma, SCC T category is based on the diameter of the lesion

C. For higher-risk lesions, 20 mm margins are recommended

D. The typical margin of excision is a gross 5-mm resection, although MMS can be used when a cosmetically sensitive area demands skin conservation

101. High risk factors for local recurrence or metastases in squamous cell carcinoma of the skin includes all except:

A. Poorly defined border
B. Location: Area H
C. Adenosquamous subtype
D. Clark level III

102. Low risk factors for local recurrence or metastases in squamous cell carcinoma of the skin includes all except:

A. No prior radiation therapy
B. Area M ≥10 mm
C. No vascular involvement
D. Primary disease

103. Cryotherapy is best suited for small superficial lesions and can be expected to achieve local control rates:

A. >50% B. >60%
C. >70% D. >90%

104. True about the management of SCC is:

A. In precursor lesions of SCC, such as actinic keratosis, cryotherapy is a commonly performed therapy

B. Tissue biopsy is indicated when the actinic keratosis is raised or recurrent after topical therapy

C. Adjuvant radiation to the primary tumor is recommended by the NCCN for any SCC with extensive perineural or large nerve involvement

D. All of the above

105. FDA approved PD-1 inhibitor for refractory advanced cutaneous SCC is:

A. Nivolumab B. Cemiplimab
C. Pembrolizumab D. Ipilimumab

106. In SCC, SLN biopsy may have a role in high-risk lesions, as clinically occult lymph node metastases may be identified in:

A. 50% - 60%
B. 5% - 20%
C. 25% - 40%
D. 60% - 75%

107. False about Basal Cell Carcinoma is:

A. Basal cell lesions are more often associated with intense, intermittent exposure to UV radiation
B. BCC is the most common NMSC, and lesions are most commonly found on the sun-exposed areas of the head and neck
C. Both activating mutations in SMO and inactivating mutations in Patched have been linked to BCC
D. Actinic keratoses is a precursor skin lesion for BCCs

108. In BCC, hedgehog-signaling pathway is a key signaling pathway in embryonic development is mutated in up to:

A. 30%
B. 60%
C. 75%
D. 90%

109. False about Basal Cell Carcinoma is:

A. Lesions may have an appearance that varies from nodules in the skin to a large non-healing sore with drainage and crusting
B. In comparison to SCCs, they have a fast growth rate
C. BCCs commonly infiltrate locally but rarely metastasize
D. The nodular growth pattern is characterized by a well-defined, elevated lesion with a waxy appearance

110. In BCC, once metastatic disease develops, the median survival decreases to:

A. <6 months
B. <1 year
C. <2 years
D. <3 years

111. False about Basal Cell Carcinoma is:

A. In nodular growth pattern as the lesion grows, pearly opalescent nodules develop along the margins
B. In nodular growth pattern, distinct blood vessels (telangiectasia) may be seen across the surface or along the edges of the lesion
C. Cystic BCCs are very common and have a distinctive translucent appearance
D. Although most BCCs are pink or skin-coloured, they may also have shades of brown or black pigmentation, thereby mimicking a benign mole or melanoma.

112. False about the treatment of BCC is:

A. Similar to SCC, a gross 5-mm margin is usually adequate for local disease control
B. Field therapies can be used for BCC, including radiation therapy, cryosurgery, photodynamic therapy, electrodessication and curettage, and topical agents like imiquimod
C. Evaluation of the lymph nodes by SLN biopsy is necessary for BCC
D. All of the above are true

113. A small molecule inhibitor of the hedgehog pathway used in locally advanced BCC is:

A. Cemiplimab
B. Vismodegib
C. Nivolumab
D. Pembrolizumab

114. High risk factors for recurrence in basal cell carcinoma of the skin are all except:

A. Nodular growth pattern
B. Recurrent disease
C. Area M ≥10 mm
D. Presence of perineural invasion

115. Area H includes all except:

A. Forehead
B. Eyelids/eyebrows
C. Periorbital nose
D. Vermillion

116. Aggressive growth patterns of BCC includes all except:

A. Morpheaform
B. Superficial
C. Basosquamous
D. Sclerosing

117. Area M includes all except:

A. Trunk
B. Scalp
C. Forehead
D. Cheeks

118. False about Merkel cell carcinoma (MCC) is:

A. It is locally aggressive with high local recurrence rates and has the potential for regional and distant metastases
B. MCC usually appears as a painless, raised nodule, often red or purplish, but it can be of the same colour as the surrounding skin
C. SLN biopsy is generally not recommended for any T stages of MCC
D. The AJCC has a separate staging system for MCC, based on maximum tumor diameter, rather than depth of invasion

119. Occult regional lymphatic metastases in Merkel cell carcinoma may occur in up to:

A. 25%
B. 33%
C. 50%
D. 66%

120. False about Merkel cell carcinoma (MCC) is:

A. MCC is a relatively radiosensitive tumor, and adjuvant radiation has been shown to reduce the local recurrence rate at the primary tumor site
B. If the SLN is positive, adjuvant radiation to the nodal basin after CLND may decrease the rate of regional recurrence and improve overall survival
C. An approximately 80% response rate has been reported with the PD-1 inhibitor pembrolizumab
D. The primary treatment is WLE (1- to 2-cm margins), although MMS has been used for some lesions where tissue conservation is necessary

121. PD-L1 inhibitor approved for use in Merkel cell carcinoma is:

A. Pembrolizumab B. Avelumab
C. Nivolumab D. Ipilimumab

122. False about Cutaneous angiosarcoma is:

A. Cutaneous angiosarcoma is a rare, aggressive, soft tissue sarcoma derived from blood or lymphatic vessel endothelium
B. On histologic evaluation, angiosarcomas are low grade and often solitary, with skip areas of normal-appearing skin
C. Cutaneous angiosarcoma predominantly occurs in elderly whites and most commonly arises on the head and neck
D. The typical finding is a smooth, firm, or spongy subcutaneous growth that develops a violaceous erythema similar to a bruise

123. False about treatment of Cutaneous angiosarcoma is:

A. The principal route of metastatic spread is hematogenous
B. SLN biopsy is usually performed
C. Treatment consists of complete resection with histologically negative margins and radiotherapy of the involved field
D. A gross margin of approximately 2 cm is attempted at the time of operation to achieve the desired negative pathologic margin

124. False about Dermatofibrosarcoma protuberans (DFSP) is:

A. Dermatofibrosarcoma protuberans (DFSP) is a low-grade sarcoma arising from dermal fibroblasts
B. Lesions appear as smooth, flesh-coloured nodules in or immediately beneath the skin and generally occur in relatively young patients between 20 and 50 years of age
C. Treatment consists of WLE with a gross 1 margin
D. DFSP grows slowly, so the lesions are usually not grossly very large at the time of diagnosis unless they have been neglected for a long period of time

125. Most common site of Dermatofibrosarcoma protuberans (DFSP) is:

A. Trunk
B. Proximal extremities
C. Head/neck region
D. Scalp

126. False about Kaposi's sarcoma is:

A. HSV 1 has been identified as the causative agent of Kaposi sarcoma in patients infected with human immunodeficiency virus
B. Kaposi sarcoma is a low-grade soft tissue, malignant neoplasm that arises from lymphatic vascular endothelial cells in the skin
C. In AIDS patients, the most effective treatment is aggressive antiretroviral therapy
D. Symptomatic skin lesions can be treated with radiation therapy, intralesional injection of chemotherapeutic agents, cryotherapy, or excision

127. False about Extramammary Paget's disease (EMPD) is:

A. Extramammary Paget disease (EMPD) is a rare form of adenocarcinoma that arises from apocrine glands of the skin
B. The clinical appearance is that of an erythematous plaque, but white or depigmented areas with crusts and scaling may also be present
C. Because EMPD can have many clinical characteristics in common with eczema, bacterial and fungal infections, and nonspecific dermatitis, the diagnosis is often made by biopsy of lesions not responding to standard therapies
D. In most cases, EMPD is confined to the dermis

128. True about Extramammary Paget's disease (EMPD) is:

A. If invasion of the deeper structures is present, the disease becomes increasingly difficult to control, and the mortality rate approaches 50%
B. Standard treatment is surgical resection extending to histologically negative margins
C. Radiation therapy may reduce the incidence of local recurrence after excision
D. All of the above

ANSWERS

1. **Ans: B. Melanoma**

   Ref: Chapter No.31, Page No.705

2. **Ans: B. John Hunter**

   Ref: Chapter No.31, Page No.705

3. **Ans: D. Melanoma is slightly more common in women across most races/ethnicities**

   Ref: Chapter No.31, Page No.705

4. **Ans: C. Fitzpatrick type III**

   Ref: Chapter No.31, Page No.705

5. **Ans: A. Lower socioeconomic status**

   Ref: Chapter No.31, Page No.705

6. **Ans: A. Chronic sun exposure (UV radiation) exposure appears to be a strong causative factor for melanoma**

   Ref: Chapter No.31, Page No.705-706

7. **Ans: B. UVB**

   Ref: Chapter No.31, Page No.706

8. **Ans: B. 40%**

   Ref: Chapter No.31, Page No.706

9. **Ans: B. 5-10%**

   Ref: Chapter No.31, Page No.706

10. **Ans: D. Small- or medium-sized congenital nevi represent a moderate risk and therefore are observed**

    Ref: Chapter No.31, Page No.706

11. **Ans: C. >20 cm**

    Ref: Chapter No.31, Page No.706

12. **Ans: C. The melanin content of the skin is the single best intrinsic factor for protecting the skin from the harmful effects of UV radiation**

    Ref: Chapter No.31, Page No.706

13. **Ans: B. A Spitz nevus is a slow growing, pink or brown, benign skin lesion with risk for further progression to melanoma**

    Ref: Chapter No.31, Page No.706

14. **Ans: C. Symmetry**

    Ref: Chapter No.31, Page No.706-707

15. **Ans: B. Mutant BRAF**

    Ref: Chapter No.31, Page No.707

16. **Ans: B. V600E**

    Ref: Chapter No.31, Page No.707

17. **Ans: A. Mutant RAS**

    Ref: Chapter No.31, Page No.707

18. **Ans: B. An inactivating mutation in the gene CDKN2A occurs in 25% to 40% of familial melanomas**

    Ref: Chapter No.31, Page No.707

19. **Ans: B. 25% to 50%**

    Ref: Chapter No.31, Page No.707

20. **Ans: D. Diameter >10 mm (and Evolution or changes over time)**

    Ref: Chapter No.31, Page No.707-708

21. **Ans: D. 25% of patients will present with regional disease, while up to 50% may present with metastases**

    Ref: Chapter No.31, Page No.708-709

22. **Ans: C. Seborrheic keratoses**

    Ref: Chapter No.31, Page No.708

23. **Ans: D. All of the above**

    Ref: Chapter No.31, Page No.708

24. **Ans: A. Transverse orientation of incision on the extremities is best**

    Ref: Chapter No.31, Page No.709

25. **Ans: C. Multiple punch biopsies should not be performed to sample larger lesions**

    Ref: Chapter No.31, Page No.709

26. **Ans: A. Shave biopsy**

    Ref: Chapter No.31, Page No.709

27. **Ans: D. Deep shave or saucerization biopsies, completely remove the lesion down to dermis but not the subcutaneous fat**

    Ref: Chapter No.31, Page No.709

28. **Ans: D. Histologic subtype is a major factor in prognosis**

    Ref: Chapter No.31, Page No.709

29. **Ans: A. Superficial spreading melanoma**

    Ref: Chapter No.31, Page No.709

30. **Ans: D. It most commonly appears on the neck and distal extremities**

    Ref: Chapter No.31, Page No.709

31. **Ans: C. The prognosis of lentigo maligna melanoma is worse than for the other subtypes given the deep nature of these tumors**

    Ref: Chapter No.31, Page No.709-710

32. **Ans: C. The diagnosis is often made at an early stage**

    Ref: Chapter No.31, Page No.710

33. **Ans: C. Acral lentiginous melanoma**

Ref: Chapter No.31, Page No.710

34. **Ans: A. Nodular melanomas often have a good prognosis**

Ref: Chapter No.31, Page No.711

35. **Ans: C. Pure desmoplastic melanomas have a high risk of lymph node metastases**

Chapter No.31, Page No.711

36. **Ans: A. <1 mm Breslow thickness**

Ref: Chapter No.31, Page No.711

37. **Ans: C. >4 mm Breslow thickness**

Ref: Chapter No.31, Page No.711

38. **Ans: B. T3b**

Ref: Chapter No.31, Page No.712

39. **Ans: C. T4a**

Ref: Chapter No.31, Page No.712

40. **Ans: B. T0**

Ref: Chapter No.31, Page No.712

41. **Ans: B. T0**

Ref: Chapter No.31, Page No.712

42. **Ans: C. T1b**

Ref: Chapter No.31, Page No.712

43. **43. Ans: B. M1b**

Ref: Chapter No.31, Page No.712

44. **Ans: D. M1d**

Ref: Chapter No.31, Page No.713

45. **Ans: D. N3c**

Ref: Chapter No.31, Page No.712

46. **Ans: C. Men have a better prognosis than women**

Ref: Chapter No.31, Page No.713

47. **Ans: B. Patients with thick primary tumors (stage IIA) can be considered for imaging to detect metastatic disease**

Ref: Chapter No.31, Page No.713

48. **Ans: B. Excision of the fascia is necessary in most cases**

Ref: Chapter No.31, Page No.714

49. **Ans: D. 2 cm**

Ref: Chapter No.31, Page No.714

50. **Ans: A. 0.5 cm**

Ref: Chapter No.31, Page No.714

51. **Ans: C. It is necessary to reexcise the melanoma if the final pathology report indicates that the measured distance from the melanoma to the edge of the excised skin is less than the recommended margin**

Ref: Chapter No.31, Page No.714

52. **Ans: B. Donald Morton**

Ref: Chapter No.31, Page No.715

53. **Ans: D. SLN biopsy is recommended for thin melanomas**

Ref: Chapter No.31, Page No.715

54. **Ans: B. T2 or greater (>1.0 mm) melanomas**

Ref: Chapter No.31, Page No.715

55. **Ans: D. Interval nodes have the less risk of harbouring melanoma cells than sentinel nodes in traditional nodal basins; therefore, it is not recommended to be removed at the time of sentinel node biopsy**

Ref: Chapter No.31, Page No.715-716

56. **Ans: B. A sentinel node is defined as any lymph node that is the most radioactive node in the nodal basin, any node that is blue, any node that has a radioactive count of 50% or higher of the most radioactive node in that basin**

Ref: Chapter No.31, Page No.716-717

57. **Ans: A. Immediate frozen section histology should be done**

Ref: Chapter No.31, Page No.717

58. **Ans: B. S-100**

Ref: Chapter No.31, Page No.717

59. **Ans: C. No improvement in 10-year disease-free was observed with SLN biopsy in both intermediate and thick melanomas**

Ref: Chapter No.31, Page No.717

60. **Ans: D. Around 30% to 50% of patients with SLN-positive micrometastatic lymph node disease have additional micrometastatic nonsentinel nodes after CLND**

Ref: Chapter No.31, Page No.717-718

61. **Ans: D. All of the above**

Ref: Chapter No.31, Page No.718

62. **Ans: C. The 3-year disease-free survival rate was numerically and statistically greater in the CLND group compared to the observation group**

Ref: Chapter No.31, Page No.718

63. **Ans: D. All of the above**

Ref: Chapter No.31, Page No.718

64. **Ans: D. All of the above**

Ref: Chapter No.31, Page No.718

65. **Ans: B. Vemurafenib**

Ref: Chapter No.31, Page No.720

66. **Ans: C. COMBI-AD trail**

Ref: Chapter No.31, Page No.720

67. **Ans: B. CheckMate 238 trail**

Ref: Chapter No.31, Page No.720

68. **Ans: A. Ipilimumab**

Ref: Chapter No.31, Page No.721

69. **Ans: B. CheckMate 238 trail**

Ref: Chapter No.31, Page No.721

70. **Ans: D. All of the above**

Ref: Chapter No.31, Page No.721

71. **Ans: B. Adjuvant radiation therapy appears to offer some improvement in control of regional lymph node disease in high-risk patients after lymphadenectomy**

Ref: Chapter No.31, Page No.722

72. **Ans: C. 10-fold**

Ref: Chapter No.31, Page No.722

73. **Ans: B. 5%**

Ref: Chapter No.31, Page No.722

74. **Ans: C. Although WLE guidelines for primary tumors do not apply, at least a 5-cm margin should be attempted with complete resection of the prior WLE scar**

Ref: Chapter No.31, Page No.722

75. **Ans: C. Limited in-transit disease need to be adequately treated with extensive excision with 2 cms margin**

Ref: Chapter No.31, Page No.722

76. **Ans: B. Melphalan**

Ref: Chapter No.31, Page No.722

77. **Ans: D. The addition of T-VEC to systemic immunotherapy doesn't appear to improve the response rate to immunotherapy in unresectable stage III/IV disease**

Ref: Chapter No.31, Page No.723

78. **Ans: A. Ipilimumab**

Ref: Chapter No.31, Page No.724

79. **Ans: C. Pembrolizumab**

Ref: Chapter No.31, Page No.724

80. **Ans: C. Pembrolizumab (and Nivolumab)**

Ref: Chapter No.31, Page No.724

81. **Ans: B. Vemurafenib**

Ref: Chapter No.31, Page No.724

82. **Ans: A. Ipilimumab**

Ref: Chapter No.31, Page No.725

83. **Ans: C. Pembrolizumab**

Ref: Chapter No.31, Page No.725

84. **Ans: D. In the setting of lymph node metastasis without a primary lesion, the patient should be treated as a patient with stage II melanoma**

Ref: Chapter No.31, Page No.726

85. **Ans: B. There is therapeutic benefit to early termination of the pregnancy**

Ref: Chapter No.31, Page No.726

86. **Ans: D. Ocular melanoma is more responsive to immunotherapy compared to cutaneous melanoma**

Ref: Chapter No.31, Page No.726-727

87. **Ans: D. All of the above**

Ref: Chapter No.31, Page No.727

88. **Ans: A. Given the high risk of metastatic disease, extensive local resections, such as abdominoperineal resection or pelvic exenteration, improve overall survival**

Ref: Chapter No.31, Page No.727

89. **Ans: B. Basal cell carcinoma**

Ref: Chapter No.31, Page No.727

90. **Ans: D. 80%**

Ref: Chapter No.31, Page No.727

91. **Ans: C. UV radiation, and UVA in particular, increases the risk of SCC**

Ref: Chapter No.31, Page No.727

92. **Ans: D. Intense intermittent sun exposure**

Ref: Chapter No.31, Page No.727

93. **Ans: B. SCC that develops in immunosuppressed patients are less aggressive and have an decreased risk of systemic metastases**

Ref: Chapter No.31, Page No.727

94. **Ans: D. >90%**

Ref: Chapter No.31, Page No.727

95. **Ans: D. 65 times**

Ref: Chapter No.31, Page No.727

96. **Ans: B. 10-fold**

Ref: Chapter No.31, Page No.727

97. **Ans: A. 40% to 60%**

Ref: Chapter No.31, Page No.727

98. **Ans: B. Lesions are scaling, with an even surface and a whitish base**

Ref: Chapter No.31, Page No.727

99. **Ans: C. Both A and B**

Ref: Chapter No.31, Page No.727

100. **Ans: A. Curettage may be used for patients with superficial lesions <5 cm**

Ref: Chapter No.31, Page No.728

101. **Ans: D. Clark level III**

Ref: Chapter No.31, Page No.729

102. **Ans: B. Area M ≥10 mm**

Ref: Chapter No.31, Page No.728

103. Ans: D. >90%

Ref: Chapter No.31, Page No.728

104. Ans: D. All of the above

Ref: Chapter No.31, Page No.728

105. Ans: B. Cemiplimab

Ref: Chapter No.31, Page No.728

106. Ans: B. 5% - 20%

Ref: Chapter No.31, Page No.728

107. Ans: D. Actinic keratoses is a precursor skin lesion for BCCs

Ref: Chapter No.31, Page No.728

108. Ans: D. 90%

Ref: Chapter No.31, Page No.728

109. Ans: B. In comparison to SCCs, they have a fast growth rate

Ref: Chapter No.31, Page No.728-729

110. Ans: B. <1 year

Ref: Chapter No.31, Page No.728

111. Ans: C. Cystic BCCs are very common and have a distinctive translucent appearance

Ref: Chapter No.31, Page No.729

112. Ans: C. Evaluation of the lymph nodes by SLN biopsy is necessary for BCC

Ref: Chapter No.31, Page No.729-730

113. Ans: B. Vismodegib

Ref: Chapter No.31, Page No.730

114. Ans: A. Nodular growth pattern

Ref: Chapter No.31, Page No.730

115. Ans: A. Forehead

Ref: Chapter No.31, Page No.730

116. Ans: B. Superficial

Ref: Chapter No.31, Page No.730

117. Ans: A. Trunk

Ref: Chapter No.31, Page No.730

118. Ans: C. SLN biopsy is generally not recommended for any T stages of MCC

Ref: Chapter No.31, Page No.730

119. Ans: B. 33%

Ref: Chapter No.31, Page No.730

120. Ans: C. An approximately 80% response rate has been reported with the PD-1 inhibitor pembrolizumab

Ref: Chapter No.31, Page No.730

121. Ans: B. Avelumab

Ref: Chapter No.31, Page No.730

122. Ans: B. On histologic evaluation, angiosarcomas are low grade and often solitary, with skip areas of normal-appearing skin

Ref: Chapter No.31, Page No.730-731

123. Ans: B. SLN biopsy is usually performed

Ref: Chapter No.31, Page No.731

124. Ans: C. Treatment consists of WLE with a gross 1 margin

Ref: Chapter No.31, Page No.731

125. Ans: A. Trunk

Ref: Chapter No.31, Page No.731

126. Ans: A. HSV 1 has been identified as the causative agent of Kaposi sarcoma in patients infected with human immunodeficiency virus

Ref: Chapter No.31, Page No.731

127. Ans: D. In most cases, EMPD is confined to the dermis

Ref: Chapter No.31, Page No.731

128. Ans: D. All of the above

Ref: Chapter No.31, Page No.731

32

Soft Tissue Sarcoma

EPIDEMIOLOGY

1. **False statement among the following is:**
   A. Extremity and trunk STS is more common than intraperitoneal and retroperitoneal STS
   B. Soft tissue sarcoma (STS) has a common mesoderm origin
   C. Among extremity STS, the distal limb is more commonly affected than the proximal portion
   D. Most STS occurs sporadically, but other well-documented causes include germline mutations, radiation exposure, and environmental exposure

2. **Types of histological subtypes in soft tissue sarcoma is:**
   A. 50 B. 60
   C. 75 D. 120

3. **Most common site of STS is:**
   A. Extremity B. Head and neck
   C. Retroperitoneum D. Trunk

CORE CONCEPTS

4. **False about Neurofibromatosis type 1 (NF1) is:**
   A. NF1 codes for a protein called neurofibromin, which acts as a tumor suppressor of the ras oncogene signaling pathway
   B. These patients have a 10% risk for development of a malignant peripheral nerve sheath tumor
   C. An autosomal dominant condition
   D. Caused by mutations of the NF1 gene, which is located at chromosome 13q11.2

5. **False about Li-Fraumeni syndrome is:**
   A. Caused by mutations of the TP53 gene, which is located at chromosome 17p13.1
   B. Wild-type p53 functions to facilitate the clearance of damaged cellular DNA and to prevent the clonal propagation of these mutated sequences
   C. Annual whole-body magnetic resonance imaging (MRI) has been advocated for patients with the Li-Fraumeni syndrome, in addition to dedicated breast imaging and colonoscopy
   D. An autosomal recessive disorder

6. **Most common cancer in Li-Fraumeni syndrome is:**
   A. Rhabdomyosarcoma
   B. Breast cancer
   C. Adrenocortical carcinoma
   D. Osteosarcoma

7. **Entities that may mimic soft tissue sarcoma includes:**
   A. Myositis ossificans
   B. Retroperitoneal lymphadenopathy
   C. Cutaneous malignant neoplasms
   D. All of the above

8. **False about familial adenomatous polyposis (FAP) syndrome is:**
   A. The familial adenomatous polyposis (FAP) syndrome is an autosomal dominant disorder
   B. Caused by mutation of the APC gene, which is located at chromosome 5q21-q22
   C. Desmoid tumors, typically arise approximately 25 years after FAP-related prophylactic colectomy
   D. The cardinal clinical feature is innumerable colonic polyps, but some patients also develop extracolonic manifestations, such as epidermoid cysts, osteomas and desmoid tumors

9. **False about radiation and soft tissue sarcomas is:**
   A. An increased risk of STS is not only attributable to therapeutic doses of radiation but also

has been linked to lower doses encountered by pediatric patients undergoing routine computed tomography (CT) scan

B. Compared with sporadic forms of these same STS subtypes, those arising after radiation exposure tend to have a better disease-specific survival

C. The effects of radiation are thought to be dose dependent, radiation-related STS typically occurs at the periphery of the radiation field

D. The main STS subtypes thought to be associated with prior radiation exposure include unclassified pleomorphic sarcoma, angiosarcoma, leiomyosarcoma, fibrosarcoma, and MPNST

10. Hepatic angiosarcoma is related to several carcinogenic substances except:

A. Thorotrast B. Polyvinyl chloride
C. Silica D. Arsenic

11. To demonstrate and predict metastasis-free survival, Complex Index in SARComas (CINSARC) [molecular analysis] consists of a group of how many genes?

A. 25 genes B. 67 genes
C. 76 genes D. 21 genes

12. As per AJCC staging for soft tissue sarcomas, a tumor of 13 cms is:

A. T1 B. T2
C. T3 D. T4

13. The French Fédération Nationale des Centres de Lutte Contre le Cancer (FNCLCC) is a score based on the sum of all categories except:

A. Size of tumor B. Tumor necrosis
C. Tumor differentiation D. Rate of mitoses

14. False among the following is:

A. The FNCLCC and the NIH systems were compared and the FNCLCC was found to be superior in estimating the risk of distant metastasis and survival

B. The AJCC 8th edition stages tumors based on histologic sarcoma subtype

C. Regional lymph node involvement for STS is uncommon (2% to 10%)

D. Regional nodal involvement is an important prognosticator of survival, patients with a single lymph node, multiple positive nodes, and distant metastatic disease all have similar survival

15. The common STS subtypes undergoing lymphadenectomy for nodal metastases are all except:

A. Rhabdomyosarcoma
B. Angiosarcoma
C. Leiomyosarcoma
D. Clear cell sarcoma

16. The most common clinical presentation of soft tissue sarcomas is:

A. Painful mass B. Painless mass
C. Bleeding D. Ulceration

17. Indications for preoperative imaging and biopsy include the following:

A. Suspected neurovascular involvement
B. Inability to determine the extent of the mass on physical examination
C. Need for operation that would likely result in a significant functional deficit
D. All of the above

18. True among the following is:

A. An image-guided core needle biopsy is more likely to provide a reliable diagnosis, but when it is applied to large cystic lesions or lesions with a considerable myxoid component, a core needle biopsy may still be nondiagnostic

B. MRI is generally considered the most informative imaging modality for trunk and extremity STS

C. A chest CT scan should generally be obtained as this is the most frequent site of metastasis

D. All of the above

19. In patients with STS, CT scan of the abdomen and pelvis should be considered for patients with all except:

A. Epithelioid sarcoma
B. Pleomorphic liposarcoma
C. Angiosarcoma
D. Leiomyosarcoma

20. In patients with STS, brain imaging may be considered to exclude metastasis from:

A. Alveolar soft part sarcoma
B. Clear cell sarcoma
C. Angiosarcoma
D. All of the above

21. In patients with STS, preoperative chemotherapy should be given to:

A. Synovial sarcoma
B. Angiosarcoma
C. Leiomyosarcoma
D. Clear cell sarcoma

22. A 45-year-old male with right thigh mass came to cancer OPD. After examination and investigations patient had low grade soft tissue sarcoma. He underwent a function sparing complete excision with negative margins. Patient asks you regarding the need of adjuvant therapy. What should be done?

A. Consider postoperative BRT
B. No need of adjuvant therapy
C. Consider postoperative IMRT
D. Consider chemotherapy

23. A 52-year-old male with left thigh mass came to cancer OPD. After examination and investigations patient had an 8 cm high grade soft tissue sarcoma. He underwent a function sparing complete excision with microscopic positive margin. Patient asks you regarding the need of adjuvant therapy. What should be done?

A. Consider perioperative BRT or postoperative IMRT
B. Consider postoperative IMRT
C. No adjuvant therapy needed
D. Consider chemotherapy

24. The most frequent STS subtype is:

A. Rhabdomyosarcoma
B. Angiosarcoma
C. Liposarcoma
D. Clear cell sarcoma

25. Radiation contributes to an absolute increase in the risk of STS of:

A. 0.13% during 5 years
B. 0.13% during 10 years
C. 0.13% during 15 years
D. 0.13% during 20 years

26. Doege-Potter syndrome is a paraneoplastic non-islet cell tumor hypoglycemia, secondary to:

A. Undifferentiated pleomorphic sarcoma
B. Solitary fibrous tumor
C. Rhabdomyosarcoma
D. Liposarcoma

27. The CT and MRI features that have been demonstrated to be associated with liposarcoma over lipoma include all except:

A. Lesions that are < 50% adipose tissue
B. Presence of thick (more than 2 mm) septa
C. Tumor size > 10 cm
D. Presence of nonadipose areas

28. Most common retroperitoneal sarcoma is:

A. Undifferentiated pleomorphic sarcoma
B. Solitary fibrous tumor
C. Rhabdomyosarcoma
D. Liposarcoma

29. Histologic varieties of liposarcoma is/are:

A. Pleomorphic liposarcoma
B. Well-differentiated and dedifferentiated liposarcoma
C. Myxoid/round cell liposarcoma
D. All of the above

30. Least common histologic variety of liposarcoma is:

A. Well-differentiated liposarcoma
B. Dedifferentiated liposarcoma
C. Myxoid/round cell liposarcoma
D. Pleomorphic liposarcoma

31. False about liposarcoma is:

A. Both well differentiated and dedifferentiated retroperitoneal liposarcomas are often unifocal
B. Well-differentiated and dedifferentiated liposarcomas more typically arise from the retroperitoneum versus the extremities, whereas the inverse is true for pleomorphic and myxoid/round cell liposarcoma
C. Compared with well-differentiated liposarcoma, the dedifferentiated variety has a worse prognosis
D. Myxoid liposarcoma is unusual in its relative sensitivity to radiation and chemotherapy, resulting in a 10-year disease-specific survival of 87%

32. The malignant behavior of well-differentiated and dedifferentiated liposarcomas is attributable to the amplification of chromosome:

A. 12q13-15
B. 22q16-21
C. 22q13-15
D. 12q16-21

33. True about liposarcoma is:

A. The round cell variety has a worse outcome than myxoid liposarcoma, with metastasis developing upto 21% of patients
B. In the event of equivocal microscopic tumor morphology, well-differentiated liposarcoma

can be distinguished from benign lipoma and dedifferentiated liposarcoma can be distinguished from other poorly differentiated STS subtypes on the basis of MDM2 and CDK4 immunohistochemistry

C. Well-differentiated liposarcoma has an extremely low risk of distant metastasis and has a favorable overall survival

D. All of the above

34. False about the treatment of retroperitoneal liposarcoma is:

A. The principal goal is a gross complete resection as incomplete gross resection is associated with an increased risk of mortality

B. Patients who develop recurrence after initial resection are likely to develop multifocal disease

C. Out-of-field recurrences are likely to have been prevented with an aggressive complete compartmental resection strategy

D. Patients whose recurrence grows < 0.9 cm/month benefitted from complete resection of the recurrence

TRUNK AND EXTREMITY SARCOMA

35. False about Extremity STS is:

A. Metallic clips within the resection bed will assist with radiation planning, and careful drain placement reduces an otherwise unnecessary expansion of the radiation field

B. When radiation is delivered with the tumor in situ, a lower preoperative dose is required versus in the postoperative setting

C. When most of the resected tumor is nonviable after neoadjuvant radiation therapy or chemoradiotherapy, patients with STS have improvements in overall survival or local recurrence

D. Positive margins are associated with an increased risk for local recurrence, whereas overall survival is generally unchanged

36. False statement among the following is:

A. Treatment strategy that has been employed in patients with locally advanced extremity STS is regional chemotherapy, namely, limb perfusion

B. Adjuvant doxorubicin has statistically significant improvements in local, distant, and overall recurrence

C. Retrospectively, the local recurrence rate after resection of extremity STS with a microscopic margin of 1 cm or more is superior to when the margin is <1 cm

D. Overall, the published data is sufficient to conclusively establish the role of regional chemotherapy in the care of extremity STS

37. The common perfusion agents used in limb perfusion is/are:

A. Tumor necrosis factor-α

B. Melphalan

C. Interferon-γ

D. All of the above

38. True statement among the following is/are:

A. Resections that proceed along the pseudocapsule plane are generally enucleations with involved margins

B. Reresection has been associated with improvements in local recurrence, patients with positive margins should be offered re-resection to achieve margins of 1 cm

C. The pseudocapsule is a characteristic plane of thickened tissue that radiographically and during intraoperative palpation gives the impression of representing the interface between tumor and normal tissue

D. All of the above

39. False among the following is:

A. Typical agents for metastatic STS include doxorubicin, dacarbazine, ifosfamide, gemcitabine, docetaxel, eribulin, pazopanib, regorafenib and olaratumab

B. Neoadjuvant therapy may be associated with formation of a more robust tumor pseudocapsule populated by fewer tumor cells

C. Tumor size is the most important predictor of metastasis

D. Important predictors of metastasis include tumor size, bone or neurovascular involvement, and tumor depth

40. False about Malignant Peripheral Nerve Sheath Tumors (MPNSTs) is:

A. MPNSTs occur in roughly equal frequency sporadically and as part of NF1

B. 10-year disease-specific survival of < 40%

C. These tumors are the malignant form of the benign schwannoma

D. The most common age at presentation is 20 to 50 years

41. False about Malignant Peripheral Nerve Sheath Tumors (MPNSTs) is:

A. Local recurrence rate of about 50%

B. The key prognostic factors include tumor size at presentation and tumor grade
C. Treatment of these tumors is similar to that of other STS subtypes, with a focus on margin-negative resection
D. Most retrospective reports agree that adjuvant radiation therapy is indicated to decrease the rate of local recurrence in extremity and superficial trunk lesions

42. False about Desmoid tumors is:

A. Approximately 75% to 85% of cases are related to FAP
B. Desmoid tumors, also known as aggressive fibromatosis
C. Approximately 20% of FAP patients develop desmoid tumors
D. These tumors are 2 to 3 times more common in women than in men

43. False about Desmoid tumors is:

A. Desmoid tumors are usually preceded by colonic polyposis in FAP patients and represent the 2nd leading cause of death in FAP patients
B. Desmoid tumors are usually fast-growing but on occasion do grow slowly
C. In the setting of FAP, APC mutations also cause β-catenin stabilization, which also activates nuclear transcription and cellular proliferation
D. Clinically, the most common areas of origin include the extremity, intraperitoneal, abdominal wall and chest wall

44. False about Desmoid tumors is:

A. Core needle biopsy is indicated in situations in which treatment recommendations will be altered on the basis of tumor histology
B. When tumors are large or infiltrating crucial anatomic structures, surgical resection with widely negative margins may not be possible
C. Desmoid tumors show a low likelihood of local recurrence
D. Both CT scan and MRI are useful imaging modalities

45. False about Angiosarcoma is:

A. In decreasing order of frequency, the most important primary sites are the trunk, head, and neck (particularly the scalp) and the viscera
B. Angiosarcoma is a malignant tumor that arises from the endothelial lining of blood vessels
C. Angiosarcoma typically is diagnosed in the 5th and 6th decades
D. Although most angiosarcoma is sporadic, risk factors include previous therapeutic radiation exposure and lymphedema

46. Percentage of all angiosarcomas that are radiation associated is:

A. 25% B. 40%
C. 60% D. 75%

47. Percentage of all angiosarcoma patients that present with metastasis is:

A. 5% B. 20%
C. 40% D. 65%

48. On IHC examination the most consistent markers of angiosarcoma are:

A. CD25 and FLI-8 B. CD31 and FLI-1
C. CD21 and FLI-4 D. CD30 and FLI-2

49. False about Angiosarcoma is:

A. Metastatic angiosarcoma may be manifested with hemopneumothorax
B. Angiosarcoma that arises within the breast after breast-conserving therapy is managed with chemotherapy only
C. The median survival of stage IV angiosarcoma is 8 to 12 months
D. The most typical agents employed in the unresectable or metastatic setting include paclitaxel and doxorubicin, followed by radiation therapy, except perhaps in patients whose tumor was incited by previous radiation therapy

50. False about Dermatofibrosarcoma Protuberans (DFSP) is:

A. The tumor affects men and women equally and appears to be more common in African American patients than in whites
B. The typical range of presentation is between the 4th and 7th decades
C. On histologic evaluation, DFSP is a dermal or subdermal tumor with penetration into the epidermis
D. The trunk, upper extremity, and lower extremity are equally frequent sites of DFSP

51. Cytogenetically, the majority of DFSP displays the translocation:

A. t(17;22)(q22;q13) B. t(11;22)(q22;q13)
C. t(17;22)(q28;q11) D. t(11;22)(q28;q11)

52. False about Dermatofibrosarcoma Protuberans (DFSP) is:

A. Recurrence can be successfully treated with resection
B. The 5-year survival is 70%
C. DFSP rarely metastasizes, but when it does, it often implies degeneration to fibrosarcoma
D. Because of the platelet-derived growth factor B upregulation, patients with unresectable disease may be treated with neoadjuvant imatinib

53. The most common site of angiosarcoma is:

A. Head and neck
B. Trunk
C. Viscera
D. Extremity

54. Indicators of poor prognosis in angiosarcoma is:

A. Tumor size > 20 cm
B. Tumor size > 5 cm
C. Tumor size > 10 cm
D. Tumor size > 15 cm

RETROPERITONEAL AND VISCERAL SARCOMA

55. False about Retroperitoneal sarcoma is:

A. The average tumor size at presentation is 5 cm
B. Retroperitoneal sarcoma represents approximately 15% of all STS
C. The most frequent retroperitoneal sarcoma subtypes are liposarcoma, leiomyosarcoma, and MFH undifferentiated pleomorphic sarcoma
D. The predominant intraperitoneal STS subtypes are GIST and leiomyosarcoma

56. Even after optimal surgical resection, patients with retroperitoneal sarcomas will relapse in:

A. 30%
B. 50%
C. 70%
D. 90%

57. False about the diagnosis of retroperitoneal sarcomas is:

A. Preoperative biopsy is obtained from a homogenous mass, the specimen should be obtained from the most concerning region under image guidance
B. The advantages of MRI include a wider range of soft tissue differentiation
C. The advantages of CT scan include rapid image acquisition, nearly universal availability, and a concise image set that can be more intuitive for the nonradiologist to interpret
D. The preoperative CT scan often contains enough information to proceed with treatment without a preoperative biopsy as long as the other basic considerations in the differential diagnosis are considered excluded

58. Predictors of poor prognosis include:

A. Gross residual disease after resection
B. Unresectable disease (either metastatic or locally advanced)
C. High tumor grade
D. All of the above

59. False about radiation in soft tissue sarcoma is:

A. The 60- to 70-Gy dose that is considered sarcoma lethal and typically used for extremity STS is not feasible in the adjuvant setting for retroperitoneal sarcoma because of bowel toxicity
B. Dose reduction to 50 to 55 Gy results in significant enteritis
C. Neoadjuvant radiation approach delivers 55 Gy to the planned target volume, and the projected at-risk margins are boosted up to 65 Gy
D. Neoadjuvant radiation is that the in-situ tumor displaces the bowel anteriorly, thus facilitating the delivery of a higher radiation dose posteriorly, which is the most likely site of a positive histologic margin

60. True about chemotherapy in soft tissue sarcoma is:

A. For patients with metastatic retroperitoneal sarcoma, second-line regimen is gemcitabine and docetaxel
B. For patients with metastatic retroperitoneal sarcoma, single or combination therapy with anthracyclines can be used as first-line therapy
C. Undifferentiated pleomorphic sarcoma or dedifferentiated liposarcoma have a somewhat more promising objective response rate than those with other STS subtypes when treated with pembrolizumab, a programmed death-1 inhibitor
D. All of the above

61. False about Gastrointestinal Stromal Tumor is:

A. GIST is the most common variety of visceral STS
B. These tumors are believed to originate from the interstitial cells of Cajal within the gastrointestinal myenteric plexus
C. GIST is classically a spindle cell neoplasm of smooth muscle origin
D. Cajal cells and GIST share common markers for CD111 and a calcium-activated chloride channel called DOG1

62. The most prevalent GIST site is:

A. Small bowel
B. Stomach
C. Sigmoid
D. Rectum

63. GISTs are differentiated on the basis of:

A. CD34
B. CD117
C. DOG1 expression
D. All of the above

64. Percentage of GISTs that have KIT gene mutations is:

A. 30%
B. 50%
C. 70%
D. 90%

65. The GISTs are characterized by a number of mutations affecting all except:

A. KRAS
B. NF2
C. BRAF
D. SDH

66. False about Gastrointestinal Stromal Tumor is:

A. On endoscopic examination, GIST usually appears as a smooth submucosal tumor that extrinsically impinges on the visceral lumen as opposed to an ulcerated mucosal mass
B. Because these are submucosal tumors, endoscopic forceps biopsies are often nondiagnostic
C. Some GISTs are serosally pedunculated and do not contribute to intestinal obstruction
D. CT imaging shows that these tumors are poorly encapsulated and generally have heterogeneous contrast enhancement because of regions of necrosis within the tumor

67. Syndromic involvement of GIST includes all except:

A. Germline SDH mutations
B. von Hippel-Lindau disease
C. NF2
D. Carney-Stratakis syndrome

68. False about the management of GIST is:

A. Appropriate preoperative staging for GIST includes a contrast-enhanced CT scan of the chest, abdomen and pelvis
B. Localized lesions are taken to the operating room for resection with grossly negative surgical margins
C. Lymphadenectomy is mandatory for GIST
D. As long as the risk of tumor rupture is not elevated, consideration of minimally invasive surgical resection techniques is appropriate and may accelerate the recovery

69. According to 8th edition of AJCC, GIST of 8 cms is:

A. T1
B. T2
C. T3
D. T4

70. Entities that can mimic GIST microscopically include all except:

A. Lymphoma
B. Nerve sheath tumors
C. Neuroendocrine tumors
D. Melanoma

71. False among the following is:

A. SDH mutations: Patients with these mutations are generally younger, have multiple gastric GISTs, and have a good response to imatinib
B. A KIT mutation in exon 13 resides within the tyrosine kinase domain and confers susceptibility to imatinib therapy
C. Exon 9 mutations correspond to the extracellular domain of the c-kit receptor, are observed principally in small bowel or colon GIST, and are less sensitive to imatinib
D. Imatinib was demonstrated to be associated with a dramatic improvement in the median overall survival of metastatic GIST from 20 months to 57 months

72. The five-parameter risk stratification score includes all except:

A. Duration of imatinib therapy
B. Nuclear morphology
C. Mitotic count
D. Size

73. False about leiomyosarcoma is:

A. The most common sites affected are the retroperitoneum and the peritoneal cavity, namely, the uterus; about 25% rise from the trunk and extremities
B. Leiomyosarcoma is a malignant smooth muscle tumor that can originate from virtually any part of the body
C. Retroperitoneal and uterine leiomyosarcoma is more common in women, and there is a female predominance in other leiomyosarcoma sites as well
D. Predisposing risk factors for leiomyosarcoma include prior radiation exposure and immunosuppression combined with Epstein-Barr virus–related tumor promotion

74. False about leiomyosarcoma is:

A. Leiomyosarcoma is generally a heterogeneous, well-circumscribed tumor with an often cystic or necrotic central area

B. This tumor stains poorly for desmin and smooth muscle actin

C. It has a wide variety of cytogenetic aberrations but no reliable or pathognomonic markers

D. First-line therapy for leiomyosarcoma is surgical resection with negative margins

75. True about management of leiomyosarcoma is:

A. For uterine leiomyosarcoma, a total abdominal hysterectomy and bilateral oophorectomy is indicated

B. Resection of tumors that invade or are intimately associated with the inferior vena cava (IVC) require special planning

C. Regardless of the organ of origin, adjuvant therapy is not currently recommended

D. All of the above

76. A recombinant human monoclonal antibody that binds PDGFRα is:

A. Alemtuzumab
B. Olaratumab
C. Pembrolizumab
D. Aducanumab

ANSWERS

1. **Ans: C. Among extremity STS, the distal limb is more commonly affected than the proximal portion**
   - Overall, 5-year survival for all stages of STS is **50-60%**
   - Translocation associated sarcomas are **14**
   - Oncogenic mutation associated sarcoma – **GIST**

   Ref: Chapter No.32, Page No.734

2. **Ans: B. 60 (70 as per Devita/Schwartz and >60 as per Sabiston)**

   Ref: Chapter No.32, Page No.734

3. **Ans: A. Extremity**
   - Most common site of STS is **extremity > visceral > retroperitoneum > trunk > head and neck**
   - Most common STS of hand and foot is Epitheliod sarcoma, synovial sarcoma

   Ref: Chapter No.32, Page No.734

4. **Ans: D. Caused by mutations of the NF1 gene, which is located at chromosome 13q11.2**

   Ref: Chapter No.32, Page No.734

5. **Ans: D. An autosomal recessive disorder**

   Ref: Chapter No.32, Page No.734

6. **Ans: B. Breast cancer**
   - FAP- Desmoid
   - NF-1- MPNST
   - Li-Fraumeni syndrome-Breast cancer, STS (Rhabdomyosarcoma, undifferentiated pleomorphic sarcoma and pleomorphic sarcoma), Adrenocortical carcinoma, Brain cancer, Osteosarcoma and Hematologic malignant neoplasms

   Ref: Chapter No.32, Page No.734

7. **Ans: D. All of the above**

   Ref: Chapter No.32, Page No.738

8. **Ans: C. Desmoid tumors, typically arise approximately 25 years after FAP-related prophylactic colectomy**

   Ref: Chapter No.32, Page No.738

9. **Ans: B. Compared with sporadic forms of these same STS subtypes, those arising after radiation exposure tend to have a better disease-specific survival**

   Ref: Chapter No.32, Page No.738

10. **Ans: C. Silica**

    (Trauma has *no true causal relationship* with STS)

    Ref: Chapter No.32, Page No.738

11. **Ans: B. 67 genes**

    Ref: Chapter No.32, Page No.738-739

12. **Ans: C. T3**

    Ref: Chapter No.32, Page No.739

13. **Ans: A. Size of tumor**

    Ref: Chapter No.32, Page No.739

14. **Ans: B. The AJCC 8th edition stages tumors based on histologic sarcoma subtype**

    Ref: Chapter No.32, Page No.739-740

15. **Ans: C. Leiomyosarcoma (MARCEL: M**FH, **A**ngiosarcoma, **R**habdomyosarcoma, **C**lear cell sarcoma, **E**pithelioid sarcoma, **L**iposarcoma)

    Ref: Chapter No.32, Page No.740

16. **Ans: B. Painless mass**

    Ref: Chapter No.32, Page No.740

17. **Ans: D. All of the above**

    Ref: Chapter No.32, Page No.740

18. **Ans: D. All of the above**

    Ref: Chapter No.32, Page No.741

19. **Ans: B. Pleomorphic liposarcoma (MALE: M**yxoid or round cell liposarcoma, **A**ngiosarcoma **L**eiomyosarcoma, **E**pithelioid sarcoma)

    Ref: Chapter No.32, Page No.741

20. **Ans: D. All of the above (Angiosarcoma has lymphadenopathy and needs brain imaging and CT scan of abdomen and pelvis)**
    - CT scan of the abdomen and pelvis: **MALE: M**yxoid or round cell liposarcoma, **A**ngiosarcoma **L**eiomyosarcoma, **E**pithelioid sarcoma
    - Brain imaging: Alveolar soft part sarcoma, Clear cell sarcoma, Angiosarcoma
    - MRI whole spine: **MRi** - **M**yxoid/**R**ound cell liposarcoma

    Ref: Chapter No.32, Page No.741

21. **Ans: A. Synovial sarcoma**
    - STS sensitive to chemotherapy: **SERUM-S**ynovial sarcoma, **E**wings sarcoma, **R**habdomyosarcoma, **U**terine leiomyosarcoma, **M**yxoid/round cell sarcoma
    - STS resistant to chemotherapy: **ACE-A**lveolar softpart sarcoma, **C**lear cell sarcoma, **E**ndometrial stromal sarcoma, **E**xtraskeletal myxoid chondrosarcoma

    Ref: Chapter No.32, Page No.741

22. **Ans: B. No need of adjuvant therapy**

    Ref: Chapter No.32, Page No.741

23. **Ans: A. Consider perioperative BRT or postoperative IMRT**

    Ref: Chapter No.32, Page No.741

24. **Ans: C. Liposarcoma** (Most common sarcoma in **pediatric** age group is **Rhabdomyosarcoma**)

Ref: Chapter No.32, Page No.742

25. **Ans: B. 0.13% during 10 years**

Ref: Chapter No.32, Page No.738

26. **Ans: B. Solitary fibrous tumor**

Ref: https://www.ncbi.nlm.nih.gov/pmc/articles/PMC5502173/

27. **Ans: A. Lesions that are < 50% adipose tissue**

Ref: Chapter No.32, Page No.742

28. **Ans: D. Liposarcoma** (Most common STS in **viscera** is **Leiomyosarcoma**)

Ref: Chapter No.32, Page No.742

29. **Ans: D. All of the above**

Ref: Chapter No.32, Page No.742

30. **Ans: C. Myxoid/round cell liposarcoma**

Ref: Chapter No.32, Page No.742

31. **Ans: A. Both well differentiated and dedifferentiated retroperitoneal liposarcomas are often unifocal**

Ref: Chapter No.32, Page No.742

32. **Ans: A. 12q13-15**

Ref: Chapter No.32, Page No.742

33. **Ans: D. All of the above**

Ref: Chapter No.32, Page No.742

34. **Ans: C. Out-of-field recurrences are likely to have been prevented with an aggressive complete compartmental resection strategy**

Ref: Chapter No.32, Page No.742-743

35. **Ans: C. When most of the resected tumor is nonviable after neoadjuvant radiation therapy or chemoradiotherapy, patients with STS have improvements in overall survival or local recurrence**

Ref: Chapter No.32, Page No.743-744

36. **Ans: D. Overall, the published data is sufficient to conclusively establish the role of regional chemotherapy in the care of extremity STS**

Ref: Chapter No.32, Page No.744

37. **Ans: D. All of the above**

Ref: Chapter No.32, Page No.744

38. **Ans: D. All of the above**

Ref: Chapter No.32, Page No.744-745

39. **Ans: C. Tumor size is the most important predictor of metastasis**

PICASSO III trial

- **Palifosfamide** is the active metabolite of ifosfamide and *does not require prodrug activation*, thereby avoiding the generation of toxic metabolites
- The **PICASSO III trial** compared *doxorubicin plus palifosfamide* with *doxorubicin plus placebo* in patients who *had received no prior systemic therapy for metastatic soft tissue sarcoma*
- **Conclusion:** *No significant difference* in PFS was observed in patients receiving doxorubicin plus palifosfamide compared with those receiving doxorubicin plus placebo

Ref: Chapter No.32, Page No.745

https://pubmed.ncbi.nlm.nih.gov/27621408/

40. **Ans: B. 10-year disease-specific survival of < 40%**

Ref: Chapter No.32, Page No.745

41. **Ans: A. Local recurrence rate of about 50%**

Ref: Chapter No.32, Page No.745

42. **Ans: A. Approximately 75% to 85% of cases are related to FAP**

Ref: Chapter No.32, Page No.745

43. **Ans: B. Desmoid tumors are usually fast-growing but on occasion do grow slowly**

Ref: Chapter No.32, Page No.745

44. **Ans: C. Desmoid tumors show a low likelihood of local recurrence**

Ref: Chapter No.32, Page No.745

45. **Ans: C. Angiosarcoma typically is diagnosed in the 5th and 6th decades**

Ref: Chapter No.32, Page No.746

46. **Ans: B. 40%**

Ref: Chapter No.32, Page No.746

47. **Ans: B. 20%**

Ref: Chapter No.32, Page No.746

48. **Ans: B. CD31 and FLI-1**

Ref: Chapter No.32, Page No.746

49. **Ans: B. Angiosarcoma that arises within the breast after breast-conserving therapy is managed with chemotherapy only**

Ref: Chapter No.32, Page No.746

50. **Ans: C. On histologic evaluation, DFSP is a dermal or subdermal tumor with penetration into the epidermis**

Ref: Chapter No.32, Page No.746

51. **Ans: A. t(17;22)(q22;q13)**

Ref: Chapter No.32, Page No.746

52. **Ans: B. The 5-year survival is 70%**

Ref: Chapter No.32, Page No.746

53. **Ans: B. Trunk**

Ref: Chapter No.32, Page No.746

54. **Ans: B. Tumor size > 5 cm (and histologic evidence of an epithelioid component)**

Ref: Chapter No.32, Page No.746

55. Ans: A. The average tumor size at presentation is 5 cm

Ref: Chapter No.32, Page No.746

56. Ans: C. 70%

Ref: Chapter No.32, Page No.746

57. Ans: A. Preoperative biopsy is obtained from a homogenous mass; the specimen should be obtained from the most concerning region under image guidance

Ref: Chapter No.32, Page No.746-747

58. Ans: D. All of the above

Ref: Chapter No.32, Page No.747

59. Ans: C. Neoadjuvant radiation approach delivers 55 Gy to the planned target volume, and the projected at-risk margins are boosted up to 65 Gy

Ref: Chapter No.32, Page No.747

60. Ans: D. All of the above

Chemotherapy Regimens in STS:

1. The **MAID regimen** is a common combination and consists of **M**esna, doxorubicin (**A**driamycin), **I**fosfamide and **D**acarbazine
2. **AIM**, another common chemotherapy regimen, consists of doxorubicin (**A**driamycin), **I**fosfamide, and **M**esna

Ref: Chapter No.32, Page No.747

https://www.ncbi.nlm.nih.gov/pmc/articles/PMC2566912/

61. Ans: D. Cajal cells and GIST share common markers for CD111 and a calcium-activated chloride channel called DOG1

Ref: Chapter No.32, Page No.748

62. Ans: B. Stomach

Ref: Chapter No.32, Page No.748

63. Ans: D. All of the above (Also the lack of smooth muscle staining)

Ref: Chapter No.32, Page No.748

64. Ans: C. 70%

Ref: Chapter No.32, Page No.748

65. Ans: B. NF2

Ref: Chapter No.32, Page No.748

66. Ans: D. CT imaging shows that these tumors are poorly encapsulated and generally have heterogeneous contrast enhancement because of regions of necrosis within the tumor

Ref: Chapter No.32, Page No.748

67. Ans: C. NF2

Carney-Stratakis syndrome is a rare ***autosomal dominant*** condition comprising familial paraganglioma and gastric stromal sarcoma

- **Carney triad** is a rare syndrome defined by the coexistence of 3 tumors:
  1. *Extra-adrenal paraganglioma*
  2. *Gastric gastrointestinal stromal tumors (GIST)*
  3. *Pulmonary chondroma*
- In most cases, only 2 of the 3 tumors are present at the time of diagnosis, with the most common combination being ***GIST*** and ***pulmonary chondromas***

Carney complex has ***autosomal dominant*** inheritance with almost ***100% penetrance***, related to ***inactivating mutations*** or ***large deletions*** of the **PRKAR1A** tumor suppressor gene on chromosome **17q22-24**

- **Carney complex** (not to be confused with the Carney triad) is a rare multiple endocrine neoplasia syndrome characterized by:
  1. **Cardiac myxoma:** Often ***multiple***, seen in ***two-thirds*** of patients with Carney complex
  2. **Skin pigmentation *(blue nevi)*:** Especially of the face, trunk, lips and sclera

Ref: Chapter No.32, Page No.748

https://www.ncbi.nlm.nih.gov/pmc/articles/PMC7481509/

https://www.ncbi.nlm.nih.gov/books/NBK1286/

68. Ans: C. Lymphadenectomy is mandatory for GIST

Ref: Chapter No.32, Page No.748

69. Ans: C. T3

Ref: Chapter No.32, Page No.748

70. Ans: A. Lymphoma

Ref: Chapter No.32, Page No.748

71. Ans: A. SDH mutations: Patients with these mutations are generally younger, have multiple gastric GISTs, and have a good response to imatinib

Ref: Chapter No.32, Page No.749-750

72. Ans: B. Nuclear morphology

Postresection Evaluation of Recurrence-free Survival for Gastrointestinal Stromal Tumors with 5 Years of Adjuvant Imatinib **[PERSIST-5]** showed that all patients who completed 5 years of adjuvant imatinib, no patient with sensitive mutations experienced tumor recurrence

Ref: Chapter No.32, Page No.750

73. Ans: C. Retroperitoneal and uterine leiomyosarcoma is more common in women, and there is a female predominance in other leiomyosarcoma sites as well

Ref: Chapter No.32, Page No.750

74. Ans: B. This tumor stains poorly for desmin and smooth muscle actin

Ref: Chapter No.32, Page No.750

75. Ans: D. All of the above

Ref: Chapter No.32, Page No.750

76. Ans: B. Olaratumab

Ref: Chapter No.32, Page No.750

33

Bone Tumors

BONE MICROENVIRONMENT

1. **True among the following is:**
   A. Osteoclasts are multinucleated cells derived from a hematopoietic lineage (macrophages), which resorb bone
   B. Osteoblasts represent a terminal differentiation of a mesenchymal stem cell
   C. The active and ongoing homeostasis of bone and its intramedullary inhabitants generate a microenvironment rich in growth factors and signaling molecules, making it an ideal soil for osteophilic tumors
   D. All of the above

2. **True among the following is:**
   A. The concept of metastasis to bone neoplasms "seed and soil" theory was given by Dr. Stephen Paget
   B. Intramedullary mesenchymal stem cells secrete CXCL12, and circulating stem cells that express the correlating CXCR4 receptor are recruited to the marrow space
   C. In the setting of metastatic breast cancer, tumor cells express CXCR4 receptor and therefore can also be recruited to the marrow space via the chemokine CXCL12.2
   D. All of the above

3. **False among the following is:**
   A. Receptor activator of nuclear factor-κB ligand (RANKL) is generated by osteoblasts, and recognized by its osteoclast receptor (RANK)
   B. RANKL stimulates osteoclastogenesis
   C. Osteoprotegerin is a decoy receptor secreted by osteoclasts, which inhibits RANKL binding and therefore stimulates osteoclastogenesis
   D. Tumor cells can directly stimulate osteoblasts to generate RANKL, which is the most prominent cytokine inducer of osteoclastogenesis

4. **False about Bisphosphonates is:**
   A. Bisphosphonates are a class of drugs that inhibits bone resorption and can decrease the number of skeletally related events (SREs)
   B. Zoledronic acid (Zometa) is commonly used for oncology patients as a means of preventing SREs
   C. Nitrogen-containing bisphosphonates bind to and inhibit key enzymes of the intracellular mevalonate pathway
   D. Bisphosphonates are only taken up by active osteoblasts

5. **False about Denosumab is:**
   A. Denosumab (Xgeva) is a monoclonal antibody generated against RANKL
   B. It mimics the natural action of osteoprotegerin, which prevents RANKL binding to RANK, thereby preventing osteoclast maturation
   C. Less effective in preventing SREs than zoledronic acid
   D. Denosumab was found to be superior to zoledronic acid in delaying time to SRE in patients with metastatic breast cancer

BONE MACROENVIRONMENT

6. **The primary differential diagnosis of epiphyseal tumors includes all except:**
   A. Chondroblastoma
   B. Ewing sarcoma
   C. Giant cell tumor
   D. Intraosseous ganglion

7. **Diaphyseal lesions includes all except:**
   A. Ewing sarcoma
   B. Adamantinoma
   C. Osteosarcoma
   D. Fibrous dysplasia

8. **Acral metastases and intracortical metastases are typically:**
   A. Lung cancer B. Prostate cancer
   C. Renal cancer D. Breast cancer

9. **True about the biopsy of bony lesion is:**
   A. Depending upon the proximity of the lesion to the greater trochanter, perform an intramedullary biopsy through a greater trochanteric starting point, using pituitary rongeurs to grab intramedullary bone at a predetermined location
   B. If done as mentioned in "Option A" biopsy entrance site does not destabilize the bone, and it still can be resected as part of a wide tumor resection if needed
   C. Biopsy of an intraosseous, diaphyseal femoral lesion through a transcortical approach, even with a large bore needle (core biopsy), doesn't increase the risk of fracture at the site of biopsy
   D. Lesions at the metaphyseal flare can often be biopsied directly, because the biomechanical stress in that area places it at much lower risk for fracture, even if a small bone window is created to obtain tissue

10. **A 38-year-old male came with mild pain and had a lower limb bony tumor involving > 1/3rd of the cortex. Patient underwent biopsy which showed a blastic lesion. According to Mirels scoring system the score of the patient is:**
    A. 3 B. 4
    C. 5 D. 7

11. **A 58-year-old female came with mild pain and had a greater trochanteric bony tumor involving > 1/3rd of the cortex. Patient underwent biopsy which showed a lytic lesion. According to Mirels scoring system the score of the patient is:**
    A. 5 B. 7
    C. 8 D. 10

12. **A 52-year-old female came with moderate pain and had a greater trochanteric bony tumor involving > 2/3rd of the cortex. Patient underwent biopsy which showed a lytic lesion. According to Mirels scoring system, management of the patient involves:**
    A. Radiation therapy
    B. Prophylactic fixation
    C. Medical therapies
    D. Chemotherapy

13. **Variables used in Mirels scoring system are all except:**
    A. Site of lesion B. Size of lesion
    C. Type of pain D. Age of patient

BIOPSY

14. **False about biopsy of bony lesion is:**
    A. Fine-needle aspirate (FNA) is commonly used because of its ease to do
    B. Open biopsy allows for acquisition of the most tissue as compared to other techniques
    C. Core biopsy, often performed with computed tomography (CT) scan guidance, can be performed through intact cortices (with adjunct use of a combined biopsy/drill system) or through areas of soft tissue extension
    D. Incisional biopsy is a surgical procedure during which a carefully planned small incision is made in line with the tumor, with respect to neurovascular structures and bone biomechanics

STAGING

15. **False about the imaging studies done for bony lesion's staging is:**
    A. Whole-body bone scan identifies possible osseous sites/metastases
    B. Plain radiographs of the affected bone show where in the bone the tumor is located, show what the tumor is doing to the bone, show what the bone is doing to the tumor and show the matrix of the lesion
    C. CT with 2D reconstructions of the affected bone allows a poor 3D dimensional understanding of how the tumor has affected the bone
    D. Magnetic resonance imaging (MRI) of the entire affected bone with contrast identifies a soft tissue component of the tumor that, if present, may be easier to sample and also helps to identify skip metastasis

16. **False among the following is:**
    A. In the Enneking system, tumors are characterized as latent, active, or aggressive
    B. Aggressive benign tumors often have a higher risk of local recurrence
    C. Aggressive benign tumors can't be technically resected in an intralesional fashion
    D. The most important factor in preventing recurrence is likely to be adequacy of resection

ONCOLOGIC RESECTION

17. True about Intralesional resections of tumors is:

A. Intralesional resections involve an incision made into the substance of tumor

B. Intralesional resections in bone are typically exemplified by curettage or debulking

C. Intralesional resections are used in the setting of benign bone tumors and metastatic to bone tumors

D. All of the above

18. False about types of surgical resections in bony tumors is:

A. Radical resections include not only the tumor and a rim of normal tissue but also the entirety of the compartment in which the tumor resides

B. Marginal resections involves resection of the tumor around its capsule and by definition leave microscopic disease behind

C. Radical resections are more commonly utilized in the treatment of skeletal sarcomas, as opposed to wide resections

D. Wide resections involve resection of the tumor with a surrounding rim of normal tissue, designed to remove the entirety of a tumor

SKELETAL RECONSTRUCTION

19. True about skeletal stabilization utilized in intralesional resections is:

A. Plates and screws that span defects can be used following curettage of lesions

B. Intramedullary nail fixation is a common strategy for prophylaxis of diaphyseal lesions, especially in the femur

C. Bone strength can be augmented through the insertion of polymethylmethacrylate (bone cement) into skeletal defects along with plates and screws (rebar)

D. All of the above

20. False about Allograft is:

A. Allografts can be fortified with cement augmentation, if possible, and then secured to the native bone utilizing plates and screws

B. Intercalary allografts are essentially bony place holders and can often be secured in situ through the use of intramedullary stabilization

C. Allografts can't be harvested with soft tissue attachments

D. An allograft with soft tissue attachments allows the rotator cuff tendons to be sewn to the implant, thereby potentiating some overhead mobility

21. False about Arthroplasty is:

A. The metal replacements are either potted into the bone using bone cement or press fit into the long bone canal

B. The megaprosthesis is named as such because large modular metal implants are combined to restore length to the limb and replace large bone defects

C. In the case of the proximal humerus and proximal femur, additional resurfacing of the acetabulum or glenoid is typically done

D. Press fit stems require ingrowth or ongrowth of host bone over time around the stem periphery

BENIGN BONE TUMORS

22. False about Enchondromas is:

A. Enchondromas are benign proliferations of hyaline cartilage typically found in the appendicular skeleton

B. Isolated lesions can cause progressive deformity of the bone

C. They typically are incidental findings discovered during radiographic evaluations for other symptoms, except in the phalanges, where they can cause pathologic fracture

D. Malignant transformation is rare

23. False about the treatment of Enchondromas is:

A. An enchondroma biopsied from the finger will look hypercellular but, because of its location, will be called an enchondroma

B. Surgical intervention is always required

C. Entire lesion is often curetted and submitted to surgical pathology

D. Treatment of enchondromas remains conservative and serial radiographic evaluation is the primary means of punctuated surveillance

24. False about Osteochondroma is:

A. If a lesion continues to grow after skeletal maturity, or if radiographically a cartilage cap >2 cm in thickness after skeletal maturity, then there is concern for potential malignant transformation

B. It presents as a painless mass, or a mass associated with pain due to mechanical symptoms

C. The majority of osteochondromas are multiple, and in those cases, the chance of malignant transformation is > 10%

D. An osteochondroma is better described as a hamartoma of bone

25. False about Hereditary multiple osteochondral exostosis is:

A. Hereditary multiple osteochondral exostosis is an autosomal dominant condition

B. 3 separate loci are implicated in its development: EXT1 (8q24.1), EXT2 (11p11-12) and EXT3 (19p)

C. The risk over time of malignant transformation of an osteochondroma in this scenario ranges from 1% - 3%

D. Affected children present with mass lesions and skeletal growth anomalies, including short stature, limb length discrepancies, angular deformity of knees and ankles, radial bowing and wrist deviation, and subluxation of the radiocapitellar joint

26. False about Osteoid osteoma is:

A. Although self-limited, the symptoms generated by this less than 1 cm in diameter lesion can be debilitating

B. Radiographically, these lesions show a radiolucent nidus, surrounded by an area of thickened cortical bone and sclerosis

C. Osteoid osteoma can be treated with radiofrequency ablation using CT-guided percutaneous techniques

D. The patient's history elicited is classic, in that pain is worse in daytime and not relieved with nonsteroidal anti-inflammatory drugs

27. False about Giant cell tumors is:

A. It represents approximately 20% of benign bone tumors, is the most aggressive benign bone tumor

B. Giant cell tumor occurs in the epiphyseal portion of a long bone or flat bones like the pelvis or sacrum in individuals between 20 - 40 years of age

C. Surgical management requires exposure of the affected bone and creation of a large bony window allowing access to the entirety of the tumor cavity and resection must be meticulous and often includes the use of adjuvants

D. Despite its benign description, there are instances of giant cell tumor lung metastases, which occur in approximately 10% to 20% of cases

28. Local recurrence rates after treatment of giant cell tumor in a bone is:

A. ~ 10% B. ~ 25%

C. ~ 40% D. ~ 50%

SKELETAL SARCOMAS

29. In children, the most common primary bone cancer is:

A. Chondrosarcoma B. Osteosarcoma

C. Ewing sarcoma D. Chordomas

30. In adults, the most common primary bone cancer is:

A. Chondrosarcoma B. Osteosarcoma

C. Ewing sarcoma D. Chordomas

31. In children, the 2nd most common primary bone cancer is:

A. Chondrosarcoma B. Osteosarcoma

C. Ewing sarcoma D. Chordomas

32. False about Osteosarcoma is:

A. There is a bimodal age of tumor occurrence

B. Spontaneous osteosarcomas are most common, but some osteosarcomas occur in the genetic syndromes of Li-Fraumeni, hereditary retinoblastoma and in postradiation scenarios

C. Defined as a malignant tumor that produces neoplastic osteoid

D. Conventional osteosarcomas occur in the 5th decade of life

33. True about treatment of Osteosarcoma is:

A. Survival is best predicted by the degree of chemotherapy-induced necrosis

B. Nonmetastatic extremity osteosarcoma with greater than 90% chemotherapy-induced necrosis has survival rates of 80% at 5 years

C. Pelvic osteosarcoma with less than 90% chemotherapy-induced necrosis has a survival rate of approximately 30%

D. All of the above

34. False about Ewing sarcoma is:

A. Ewing sarcoma and primitive neuroectodermal tumor are small blue cell malignancies of bone

B. Tumor is not sensitive to chemotherapy and radiation treatment

C. Translocation, t(11;22) (q24; q12), is seen in 85% of cases

D. Surgical extirpation in conjunction with chemotherapy is the preferred treatment

35. False about Chondrosarcoma is:

A. Chondrosarcoma is a malignant skeletal neoplasm that produces hyaline cartilage

B. Histopathology predicts biologic behavior

C. A low-grade cartilage tumor of the phalanx may have the same microscopic appearance as a pelvic chondrosarcoma

D. Secondary chondrosarcomas occur after malignant transformation of benign cartilage tumors such as enchondroma or osteochondroma

BONE METASTASES

36. The most common osteophilic carcinomas include:

A. Breast carcinoma
B. Thyroid carcinoma
C. Prostate carcinoma
D. All of the above

37. False about the management of bone tumors is:

A. Palliative relief of pain and maximization of function are the goals of surgery

B. When considering surgical stabilization, often whole bone prophylaxis is performed utilizing metal implants and cement augmentation

C. Isolated metastases such as from renal cell carcinoma or melanoma can be treated aggressively if they are indeed isolated and occur after a long hiatus (several years) from initial diagnosis

D. A surgical goal of a local recurrence rate < 25% is preferred

ANSWERS

1. **Ans: D. All of the above**
Ref: Chapter No.33, Page No.754

2. **Ans: D. All of the above**
Ref: Chapter No.33, Page No.754

3. **Ans: C. Osteoprotegerin is a decoy receptor secreted by osteoclasts, which inhibits RANKL binding and therefore stimulates osteoclastogenesis**
Ref: Chapter No.33, Page No.755

4. **Ans: D. Bisphosphonates are only taken up by active osteoblasts**
Ref: Chapter No.33, Page No.755

5. **Ans: C. Less effective in preventing SREs than zoledronic acid**
Ref: Chapter No.33, Page No.755

6. **Ans: B. Ewing sarcoma**
Ref: Chapter No.33, Page No.755

7. **Ans: C. Osteosarcoma**
Ref: Chapter No.33, Page No.756

8. **Ans: A. Lung cancer**
Ref: Chapter No.33, Page No.756

9. **Ans: C. Biopsy of an intraosseous, diaphyseal femoral lesion through a transcortical approach, even with a large bore needle (core biopsy), doesn't increase the risk of fracture at the site of biopsy**
Ref: Chapter No.33, Page No.756-757

10. **Ans: C. 5**
Ref: Chapter No.33, Page No.758

11. **Ans: C. 8**
Ref: Chapter No.33, Page No.758

12. **Ans: B. Prophylactic fixation**
Ref: Chapter No.33, Page No.758

13. **Ans: D. Age of patient**
Ref: Chapter No.33, Page No.758

14. **Ans: A. Fine-needle aspirate (FNA) is commonly used because of its ease to do**
Ref: Chapter No.33, Page No.757

15. **Ans: C. CT with 2D reconstructions of the affected bone allows a poor 3D dimensional understanding of how the tumor has affected the bone**
Ref: Chapter No.33, Page No.759

16. **Ans: C. Aggressive benign tumors can't be technically resected in an intralesional fashion**
Ref: Chapter No.33, Page No.759

17. **Ans: D. All of the above**
Ref: Chapter No.33, Page No.759

18. **Ans: C. Radical resections are more commonly utilized in the treatment of skeletal sarcomas, as opposed to wide resections**
Ref: Chapter No.33, Page No.759-760

19. **Ans: D. All of the above**
Ref: Chapter No.33, Page No.760

20. **Ans: C. Allografts can't be harvested with soft tissue attachments**
Ref: Chapter No.33, Page No.760-761

21. **Ans: C. In the case of the proximal humerus and proximal femur, additional resurfacing of the acetabulum or glenoid is typically done**

Ref: Chapter No.33, Page No.761

22. **Ans: B. Isolated lesions can cause progressive deformity of the bone**

Ref: Chapter No.33, Page No.761-762

23. **Ans: B. Surgical intervention is always required**

Ref: Chapter No.33, Page No.762

24. **Ans: C. The majority of osteochondromas are multiple, and in those cases, the chance of malignant transformation is > 10%**

Ref: Chapter No.33, Page No.762

25. **Ans: C. The risk over time of malignant transformation of an osteochondroma in this scenario ranges from 1% - 3%**

Ref: Chapter No.33, Page No.762-763

26. **Ans: D. The patient's history elicited is classic, in that pain is worse in daytime and not relieved with nonsteroidal anti-inflammatory drugs**

Ref: Chapter No.33, Page No.763

27. **Ans: D. Despite its benign description, there are instances of giant cell tumor lung metastases, which occur in approximately 10% to 20% of cases**

Ref: Chapter No.33, Page No.763

28. **Ans: C. ~ 40%**

Ref: Chapter No.33, Page No.763

29. **Ans: B. Osteosarcoma**

Ref: Chapter No.33, Page No.765

30. **Ans: A. Chondrosarcoma**

Ref: Chapter No.33, Page No.765

31. **Ans: C. Ewing sarcoma**

Ref: Chapter No.33, Page No.765

32. **Ans: D. Conventional osteosarcomas occur in the 5th decade of life**

Ref: Chapter No.33, Page No.765

33. **Ans: D. All of the above**

Ref: Chapter No.33, Page No.765

34. **Ans: B. This tumor is not sensitive to chemotherapy and radiation treatment**

Ref: Chapter No.33, Page No.765-766

35. **Ans: B. Histopathology predicts biologic behavior**

Ref: Chapter No.33, Page No.766

36. **Ans: D. All of the above**

Ref: Chapter No.33, Page No.766

37. **Ans: D. A surgical goal of a local recurrence rate < 25% is preferred**

Ref: Chapter No.33, Page No.766-767

34

Head and Neck

HISTOLOGY

1. **Which of the following is a type of elastic cartilage?**
   - A. Thyroid
   - B. Epiglottis
   - C. Cricoid
   - D. Arytenoid

2. **All of the following structures lined by respiratory epithelium except:**
   - A. Paranasal sinus
   - B. Middle ear
   - C. False vocal folds
   - D. Epiglottis

3. **Which statement is correct regarding histology of the head and neck?**
   - A. The nasal cavity entirely lined by ciliated respiratory epithelium
   - B. The Waldeyer ring consists of only palatine tonsils and adenoids
   - C. The adenoids have crypts lined by stratified squamous and epithelium
   - D. Minor salivary glands are present throughout the submucosa of oral cavity

4. **Parakeratosis is characterized by:**
   - A. Thickening of epithelium
   - B. An abnormal keratinization of epithelium
   - C. An abnormal presence of nuclei in the keratin layers
   - D. Presence of normal keratinization at abnormal place

EPIDEMIOLOGY AND CARCINOGENESIS

5. **Most common type of malignancy in head and neck:**
   - A. Squamous cell carcinoma
   - B. Adenocarcinoma
   - C. Lymphoma
   - D. Rhabdomyosarcoma

6. **All are true concerning HPV-associated head and neck (HNSCC) cancers except:**
   - A. E7 oncogene of HPV targets retinoblastoma gene for proteasomal degradation
   - B. It has a 4:1 female preponderance
   - C. Higher levels of APOBEC mutations in HPV-associated HNSCCs
   - D. Loss of heterozygosity at 9p21 and 3p21 was among the earliest detectable events

7. **Synchronous cancers are second primary cancers detected within _____ of index cancer.**
   - A. 3 months
   - B. 6 months
   - C. 1 year
   - D. 2 years

8. **Metachronous cancers are defined as:**
   - A. The occurrence of a metastatic lesion more than 6 months after the initial lesion
   - B. The occurrence of a second primary lesion less than 1 year after the initial lesion
   - C. The occurrence of a second primary lesion more than 6 months after the initial lesion
   - D. The occurrence of a metastatic lesion more than 1 year after the initial lesion

9. **Which is incorrect about head and neck cancers?**
   - A. Oropharyngeal cancers are most common form of HPV-associated cancers
   - B. Amplification of cyclin D1 is unique to HPV-negative HNSCC
   - C. Tyrosine kinase receptor targeted therapy may be used in HPV-negative HNSCC
   - D. PD-L1 immunotherapy is approved for use in recurrent and metastatic HNSCC

10. **All of the following mutations are associated with HPV-associated head and neck cancers except:**
    - A. Loss of CDKN2A
    - B. Amplification of FGFR3

C. Inactivation of CYLD
D. Inactivation of TRAF3

11. **Which is false about HPV- associated cancers?**
    A. High levels of inactivating defects in TRAF3 or CYLD seen only with HPV–associated HNSCC
    B. HPV integration is not required for carcinogenesis of HNSCC
    C. Uterine cervical cancers are most common form of HPV-associated cancers
    D. Somatic mutations are largely not shared between HPV-associated HNSCC and uterine cervical cancer

STAGING AND EVALUATION

12. **Most common distant metastasis for head and neck SCC:**
    A. Bone B. Lung
    C. Liver D. Brain

13. **Which is the most important risk factor for distant metastases form Head and neck SCC?**
    A. Histologic grade B. Lymph nodal stage
    C. Tumor size D. Tumor location

14. **Stage IV HPV-associated HNSCCs comprise which of the following disease:**
    A. T4 B. N3
    C. M1 D. All of the above

15. **HNSCC with involvement of bilateral or contralateral lymph nodes, but none more than 6 cm in size, has clinical nodal stage:**
    A. N2b B. N2c
    C. N3a D. N3b

16. **HNSCC with involvement single ipsilateral lymph node more than 6 cm in size, has clinical nodal stage:**
    A. N2b B. N2c
    C. N3a D. N3b

17. **Which is false regarding diagnostic evaluation in cases of HNSCC?**
    A. MRI is excellent at evaluating parotid and parapharyngeal space tumors
    B. CT scanning is best at evaluating bony destruction
    C. HPV DNA is used as prognostic marker of HPV-associated head and neck cancers
    D. Pathologic confirmation of cancer is mandatory before initiating treatment

18. **All are correct statements about anatomy of neck lymph nodes except:**
    A. The cervical lymphatic nodal basins contain 50 to 70 lymph nodes per side
    B. Level IA and level IB lymph nodes are divided by posterior belly of digastric muscle
    C. Lateral border of anterior neck triangle is formed by posterior border of sternocleidomastoid muscle
    D. Level IIB, so-called submuscular triangle, is posterior to the spinal accessory nerve

19. **All of the following cancers show bilateral lymph node metastases except:**
    A. Lower lip cancer
    B. Base of tongue cancer
    C. Supraglottic laryngeal cancer
    D. Upper lip cancer

20. **Following are recommendation of neck treatment in case of HNSCC except:**
    A. Clinically positive nodes
    B. Risk for occult disease > 5%
    C. Location of tumor
    D. Depth of primary tumor

21. **Which is correct statement regarding use of chemoradiation therapy for head and neck cancers?**
    A. Chemotherapy can be used as a single modality therapy for early stage head and neck cancers
    B. Postoperative concurrent chemotherapy and radiotherapy improves overall survival compared with postoperative radiation alone in high risk head and neck cancers
    C. Chemotherapy has no role in the palliative therapy for metastatic head and neck cancers
    D. Induction chemoradiotherapy has superior survival rates compared to surgery plus radiotherapy for the treatment of advanced laryngeal cancers

22. **Which is false regarding irradiation therapy in cases of HNSCC?**
    A. Photon irradiation is effective for eradicating microscopic SCC only
    B. Primary tumors caused by oncogenic viruses are usually responsive to photon irradiation
    C. Proton irradiation is used for the treatment of skull base cancers
    D. Electron irradiation commonly used in the head and neck for noncutaneous tumor

23. Radiation therapy is effective in HNSCC with following features:

A. Large-volume tumors
B. High-grade neoplasms
C. Involving bone or cartilage
D. Close proximity to the mandible

24. EXTREME Trial was based on:

A. Concurrent chemotherapy and radiotherapy in unresectable HNSCC
B. Radiotherapy alone for HNSCC
C. Adjuvant immunotherapy in HNSCC
D. Cytotoxic chemotherapy in recurrent or metastatic HNSCC

NECK

25. Who described radical neck dissection technique?

A. Bocca B. Crile
C. Morton D. Kocher

26. Who described modified radical neck dissection method?

A. Bocca B. Crile
C. Morton D. Kocher

27. Which structures are preserved in modified radical neck dissection surgery?

A. External jugular vein, Sternocleidomastoid muscle, Submandibular gland
B. Internal jugular vein, Spinal accessory nerve, Submandibular gland
C. Internal jugular vein, sternocleidomastoid muscle, Spinal accessory nerve
D. External jugular vein, Cervical plexus, Spinal accessory nerve

28. Which is false regarding neck dissection procedures?

A. Lateral neck dissections remove lymphatic tissue from levels II to IV
B. Supraomohyoid neck dissection is limited to levels I to III
C. Selective neck dissections are frequently used for clinically negative (cN0) neck
D. Sentinel neck lymph node biopsy is currently recommended for all clinically node negative necks

ORAL CAVITY

29. All are correct regarding oral cavity lesions except:

A. Oral leukoplakia is a white patch in the oral cavity with clinically insignificant risk of malignancy
B. Erythroplakia has higher risk of being malignant lesion
C. Carcinoma in situ is premalignant lesion
D. The oral cavity is the most common site of head and neck malignancy

30. Following are the benign lesions that can look like carcinoma, except:

A. Lichen planus
B. Pseudoepitheliomatous hyperplasia
C. Leukoplakia
D. Necrotizing sialometaplasia

31. Most common site of head and neck malignancy:

A. Nasopharynx B. Base of tongue
C. Oral cavity D. Neck

32. Following are the specific risks factors for oral cavity cancers:

A. Alcohol B. Tobacco
C. Areca nut D. All of the above

33. Highest risk of HNSCC seen with which familial syndrome?

A. Osteogenesis imperfect
B. Fanconi anaemia
C. Xeroderma pigmentosa
D. Cowden syndrome

34. 60-year-old female with history of chronic tobacco use presents with newly diagnosed 3 cm ulcerated right sided oral cavity lesion. Biopsy demonstrates SCC. CT evaluation reveals an enlarged two Level II lymph nodes of 2 cm size each on the right side of the neck. Findings on chest radiography are clear. What is the stage of cancer?

A. T1 N1 M0 B. T2 N2a M1
C. T2 N2b M0 D. T3 N2a M0

35. Which of the following structure does not constitute T4b stage?

A. Masticator space B. Facial skin
C. Pterygoid plate D. Skull base

36. A 60-year-old male presents with ulcerative lesion of 1.5 cm on right lateral border of the tongue. An FNA is consistent with SCC. A CT neck shows depth of invasion of 4.5 mm. No evidence of any lymph node involvement in bilateral neck and no distant metastasis. What is the appropriate management?

A. Partial glossectomy with ipsilateral MRND
B. Hemiglossectomy only
C. Radiation only
D. Partial glossectomy with ipsilateral selective neck dissection

37. Which is incorrect regarding management of oral cavity cancers?

A. Upfront surgery remains the preferred initial treatment for oral cavity carcinoma
B. Reconstructive surgery should be an integral part of the treatment decision
C. For early-stage oral cavity SCC, when the DOI is larger than 3 mm, an elective neck dissection is indicated
D. Advanced-stage tumors are generally treated with adjuvant chemotherapy alone

38. Adjuvant chemotherapy is recommended in setting of HNSCC for following conditions except:

A. Any cancer above T1
B. Extranodal extension
C. Close or positive margins which cannot be resected
D. High nodal burden

39. Wharton duct arises from:

A. Sublingual salivary gland
B. Submandibular salivary gland
C. Parotid gland
D. Lacrimal gland

40. Which nerve is in close relation with Wharton duct (Submandibular gland duct)?

A. Hypoglossal nerve
B. Glossopharyngeal nerve
C. Lingual nerve
D. Ansa cervicalis

41. Stensen duct (Parotid duct) opens at:

A. Floor of mouth
B. Adjacent to lower second molar
C. Adjacent to upper second molar
D. Adjacent to upper third molar

42. Which is false regarding hard palate cancers?

A. Hard palate is formed by the palatine process of the maxillary bone and the vomer
B. Torus palatini is a benign bone growth in the center hard palate
C. Necrotizing sialometaplasia is a self-limited ulcerative inflammatory lesion of minor salivary glands
D. Hard palate malignancies always require removal of bone for adequate margin

43. Which is incorrect about alveolar malignancy?

A. Squamous cell carcinoma is the most common malignancy of the alveolus
B. Lower alveolus is more commonly involved
C. The periosteum of the mandible is a strong tumor barrier
D. Tumors adherent to the periosteum can be treated with excision of periosteum only

44. Which oral cavity tumors are at higher risk of bone invasion?

A. Palate
B. Alveolus
C. Floor of mouth
D. Retromolar trigone

OROPHARYNX

45. Most common HPV associated cancers:

A. Oropharyngeal
B. Uterine cervical
C. Penile
D. Vaginal

46. Which of the following structure does not constitute the borders of oropharynx?

A. Posterior faucial pillars
B. Medial aspect of mandible
C. Soft palate
D. Plane of hyoid bone

47. Which is incorrect about management of the oropharyngeal HNSCC?

A. HPV-positive cancers are more likely to be asymptomatic and present with a neck mass as the only sign
B. Lymph node metastases generally occur in levels II to IV of neck nodes
C. Cystic metastatic nodes are frequently seen with HPV-positive oropharyngeal cancers
D. Smoking does not affect the overall outcome of HPV-associated cancers treated with concurrent chemoradiation

48. On complete evaluation of a 55-year-old male, he was diagnosed with HPV-associated right sided floor of mouth malignancy of clinical stage T4a N1 M0. What is most appropriate management for this patient?

A. Concurrent chemotherapy and radiotherapy
B. Chemotherapy followed by surgical resection

C. Surgical resection plus MRND followed by chemoradiotherapy
D. Palliative therapy

49. A 50-year old patient presents with oropharyngeal cancer involving more than half of the base of tongue and mandible. What will be most appropriate initial approach?

A. Radiation therapy only
B. Surgical excision followed by chemoradiation
C. Concurrent chemotherapy and radiation therapy
D. Palliative therapy

50. All are true regarding transoral robotic surgery for oropharyngeal cancer except:

A. Advantages for cosmesis and complication rate
B. Division and repair of soft tissues and bone under high quality visualization
C. Identification of the site of unknown primaries
D. It can be used as single modality for early-stage disease

HYPOPHARYNX

51. Which is incorrect regarding postcricoid hypopharyngeal cancer?

A. They are more common worldwide in women
B. Plummer-Vinson syndrome is a risk factor
C. Occurs in middle aged women with iron deficiency anemia
D. Postcricoid carcinoma may develop just distal to the web

52. All are true about management of hypopharyngeal cancers except:

A. Over 95% of all cancers arising in the hypopharynx are SCCs
B. Hypopharyngeal cancers have early lymphatic metastasis and worst outcome of all HNSCC
C. Patients with hypopharyngeal cancer have the highest rate of synchronous malignancies and the highest rate of development of second HNSCC primaries
D. Surgical excision is preferred initial treatment for early stage hypopharyngeal cancers

53. Which is the most common area of lymphatic spread in cases of hypopharyngeal cancers?

A. Upper jugular lymph nodes
B. Retropharyngeal lymph nodes
C. Paratracheal lymph nodes
D. Supraclavicular lymph nodes

LARYNX

54. Incorrect statement about nerve supply of the larynx:

A. External branch of superior laryngeal nerve supplies the cricoarytenoid
B. Internal branch of superior laryngeal nerve carries afferent sensory fibers from the mucosa of the false vocal folds and piriform sinuses
C. The recurrent laryngeal nerve supplies motor innervation to all the intrinsic muscles of the larynx
D. The recurrent laryngeal nerve provide sensory supply to the mucosa of the true vocal folds, subglottic region, and adjacent esophageal mucosa

55. All are true regarding management of laryngeal cancer except:

A. Formal pulmonary function testing (PFT) mandatory for all patients undergoing surgery
B. Early-stage larynx cancer (T1–T2 N0) can be treated with radiation therapy alone
C. CO_2 laser is the most common approach for T1 glottic tumor
D. Involvement of an entire vocal cord is a contraindications to vertical partial laryngectomy

56. Following are the contraindications for vertical partial laryngectomy surgery in cases of glottic cancers except:

A. Subglottic extension greater than 10 mm anteriorly
B. Subglottic extension greater than 5 mm posteriorly
C. T3 glottic cancers
D. Involvement of anterior commissure

57. Which of the following modalities are used for speech rehabilitation after total laryngectomy?

A. Electrolarynx
B. Esophageal speech
C. Tracheoesophageal puncture with prosthesis
D. All of the above

SALIVARY GLANDS

58. Which is incorrect about salivary gland infections?

A. Bacterial sialadenitis is typically unilateral and painful
B. A major cause of salivary obstruction is salivary stone
C. Viral sialadenitis is typically bilateral

D. Multiple, large, bilateral cysts of the parotid glands are characteristics of EBV infection

59. Multiple, large, bilateral cysts of the parotid glands are characteristically seen in:

A. EBV infection
B. HIV infection
C. Coxsackie viral infection
D. Sarcoidosis

60. Which is incorrect regarding salivary gland tumors?

A. Most salivary neoplasms are found in the parotid gland
B. Surgical removal is recommended for almost all tumors regardless of pathology
C. Most of parotid salivary tumors are benign
D. Sensitivity of FNA for distinguishing benign from malignant tumors of salivary glands being 95%

61. Most common benign tumor of salivary gland:

A. Warthin tumor
B. Pleomorphic adenoma
C. Myoepithelioma
D. Cystadenoma

62. Which salivary gland tumor is FDG-avid by PET scan?

A. Pleomorphic adenoma
B. Warthin tumor
C. Acinic cell carcinoma
D. Adenoid cystic carcinoma

63. Which is incorrect about management of malignant parotid tumors?

A. For deep lobe parotid malignancy, a total parotidectomy is usually required
B. Radiation therapy is typically recommended following removal of adenoid cystic carcinomas
C. Division of the auriculotemporal nerve is often required during parotidectomy
D. The facial nerve is located approximately 1 cm anterior, inferior, deep to the tragal pointer

64. A 45-year-old male undergone parotidectomy for parotid tumor. Which of the following statement is correct?

A. The facial nerve is located approximately 1 cm anterior, inferior, deep to the tragal pointer
B. Frey's syndrome is the result of an abnormal innervations of cutaneous sweat glands by parasympathetic fibres
C. A common complication of parotidectomy is injury to greater auricular nerve, which causes perioral numbness
D. The parotid gland is divided into superficial and deep lobe by facial artery

NASAL CAVITY AND PARANASAL SINUSES

65. Which of the following structure drains into inferior meatus of nasal cavity?

A. Maxillary sinus
B. Nasolacrimal duct
C. Frontal sinus
D. Anterior ethmoid sinus

66. Which is incorrect regarding anatomy of the paranasal sinuses?

A. The lamina papyracea is the thin medial wall of the ethmoid sinus
B. The posterior ethmoids drain via the sphenoethmoidal recess into the posterior nasal cavity
C. The sella turcica and optic chiasm are immediately superior to sphenoid sinus
D. Pterygopalatine fossa forms posterior border of maxillary sinus

67. Schneiderian papilloma is found in:

A. Nasal cavity
B. Nasopharynx
C. Pyriform fossa
D. Larynx

68. All are true about inverted papilloma of nasal cavity except:

A. It is most common benign tumor of nasal cavity
B. Rise along the medial nasal wall
C. 10% to 15% malignant degeneration rate
D. Removal of bone at the base of the tumor is important to prevent recurrence

69. Which is incorrect regarding management of sinonasal malignancy?

A. Biopsy of the primary site is required to establish pathologic diagnosis
B. Both CT and MRI imaging is recommended in preoperative planning
C. Elective neck dissection for primary sinonasal carcinomas is recommended
D. Postoperative radiation is considered for high-stage disease or high-grade pathologies only

70. Most frequent mutation found in sinonasal undifferentiated carcinoma:

A. SMARCB1
B. IDH2
C. BRD2
D. NUT

NASOPHARYNX

71. Which is incorrect about nasopharyngeal tumors?

A. Angiofibroma is the most common benign tumor of the nasopharynx in children
B. Juvenile angiofibroma is associated with mutations in β-catenin and APC
C. Thornwaldt cyst is a midline mass originates from a remnant of the caudal notochord
D. WHO type I nasopharyngeal cancer is associated with EBV

72. A 50-year-old male has complaints of recurrent right sided serous otitis media and hearing loss for the past 4 weeks. He has no history of a recent URTI or chronic ear disease. His clinical history is unremarkable. A 2 cm level V lymph node is palpable in right side of the neck. What is the next step of management?

A. Treatment with antibiotic for 14 days
B. Otitopic antibiotic drops
C. Grommet insertion with antibiotic treatment
D. Flexible nasopharyngeal examination

73. Which is false regarding nasopharyngeal carcinoma?

A. Non-keratinizing SCC associated with EBV is most common subtype
B. The most common presenting sign of a primary nasopharyngeal cancer is cervical node metastasis
C. High-dose radiation therapy with concurrent chemotherapy to the primary tumor and bilateral necks including the retropharyngeal nodal basins is the primary treatment
D. Surgery is most commonly used for persistent neck disease

74. What is the most common sarcoma of the head and neck?

A. Hemangiosarcoma
B. Rhabdomyosarcoma
C. Liposarcoma
D. Pleomorphic sarcoma

75. Incorrect statement regarding head and neck reconstruction:

A. Major neurovascular structures exposed during dissection should always be covered
B. Prior radiation therapy to the recipient area limits the use of bony and cartilaginous grafts
C. Regional flaps are based on axial blood flow and are located adjacent to the donor site
D. Most versatile donor site for head and neck free flap reconstruction is the system of flaps from the subscapularis vascular system

76. Patient with scalp vascular tumor undergoes wide local excision creating full thickness defect of 8 cm diameter with exposed underling periosteum. What is appropriate reconstructive approach?

A. Rotational local flap
B. Trapezius pedicle flap
C. Latissimus dorsi muscle free flap
D. Split skin grafting

77. A patient with a SCC of right alveolus undergoes right segmental mandibulectomy of 5 cm segment. Which is most appropriate reconstructive option?

A. Radial forearm osteocutaneous free flap
B. Anterolateral thigh fasciocutaneous free flap
C. Latissimus dorsi myocutaneous free flap
D. Fibula osteocutaneous free flap

78. A patient with laryngeal cancer was treated with total laryngectomy. The pharyngeal defect is reconstructed using pectoral myocutaneous regional pedicled flap. What is the blood supply this regional flap?

A. Branch from thoracoacromial artery
B. Thoracodorsal artery
C. Perforating vessel from internal mammary artery
D. Second intercostal artery

ANSWERS

1. **Ans: B. Epiglottis**
Ref: Chapter No. 34, Page No. 771

2. **Ans: D. Epiglottis**
Ref: Chapter No. 34, Page No. 771

3. **Ans: D. Minor salivary glands are present throughout the submucosa of oral cavity**
Ref: Chapter No. 34, Page No. 771

4. **Ans: C. An abnormal presence of nuclei in the keratin layers**
Ref: Chapter No. 34, Page No. 772

5. **Ans: A. Squamous cell carcinoma**
Ref: Chapter No. 34, Page No. 772

6. **Ans: B. It has a 4:1 female preponderance**
Ref: Chapter No. 34, Page No. 772

7. **Ans: B. 6 months**
Ref: Chapter No. 34, Page No. 772

8. **Ans: C. The occurrence of a second primary lesion more than 6 months after the initial lesion**
Ref: Chapter No. 34, Page No. 772

9. **Ans: C. Tyrosine kinase receptor targeted therapy may be used in HPV-negative HNSCC**
Ref: Chapter No. 34, Page No. 772-773

10. **Ans: A. Loss of CDKN2A**
Ref: Chapter No. 34, Page No. 773

11. **Ans: C. Uterine cervical cancers are most common form of HPV-associated cancers**
Ref: Chapter No. 34, Page No. 773

12. **Ans: B. Lung**
Ref: Chapter No. 34, Page No. 773

13. **Ans. B. Lymph nodal stage**
Ref: Chapter No. 34, Page No. 773

14. **Ans: C. M1**
Ref: Chapter No. 34, Page No. 773

15. **Ans: B. N2c**
Ref: Chapter No. 34, Page No. 774

16. **Ans: C. N3a**
Ref: Chapter No. 34, Page No. 774

17. **Ans: C. HPV DNA is used as prognostic marker of HPV-associated head and neck cancers**
Ref: Chapter No. 34, Page No. 774-775

18. **Ans: B. Level IA and level IB lymph nodes are divided by posterior belly of digastric muscle**
Ref: Chapter No. 34, Page No. 775

19. **Ans: D. Upper lip cancer**
Ref: Chapter No. 34, Page No. 775

20. **Ans: B. Risk for occult disease > 5%**
Ref: Chapter No. 34, Page No. 776

21. **Ans: B. Postoperative concurrent chemotherapy and radiotherapy improves overall survival compared with postoperative radiation alone in high risk head and neck cancers**
Ref: Chapter No. 34, Page No. 776

22. **Ans: D. Electron irradiation commonly used in the head and neck for noncutaneous tumor**
Ref: Chapter No. 34, Page No. 776

23. **Ans: B. High-grade neoplasms**
Ref: Chapter No. 34, Page No. 776

24. **Ans: D. Cytotoxic chemotherapy in recurrent or metastatic HNSCC**
Ref: Chapter No. 34, Page No. 777

25. **Ans: B. Crile**
Ref: Chapter No. 34, Page No. 777

26. **Ans: A. Bocca**
Ref: Chapter No. 34, Page No. 777

27. **Ans: C. Internal jugular vein, sternocleidomastoid muscle, Spinal accessory nerve**
Ref: Chapter No. 34, Page No. 777

28. **Ans: D. Sentinel neck lymph node biopsy is currently recommended for all clinically node negative necks**
Ref: Chapter No. 34, Page No. 777-778

29. **Ans: A. Oral leukoplakia is a white patch in the oral cavity with clinically insignificant risk of malignancy**
Ref: Chapter No. 34, Page No. 778

30. **Ans: C. Leukoplakia**
Ref: Chapter No. 34, Page No. 778

31. **Ans: C. Oral cavity**
Ref: Chapter No. 34, Page No. 778

32. **Ans: D. All of the above**
Ref: Chapter No. 34, Page No. 778

33. **Ans: B. Fanconi anaemia**
Ref: Chapter No. 34, Page No. 778

34. **Ans: C. T2 N2b M0**

Ref: Chapter No. 34, Page No. 778

35. **Ans: B. Facial skin**

Ref: Chapter No. 34, Page No. 778

36. **Ans: D. Partial glossectomy with ipsilateral selective neck dissection**

Ref: Chapter No. 34, Page No. 778

37. **Ans: D. Advanced-stage tumors are generally treated with adjuvant chemotherapy alone**

Ref: Chapter No. 34, Page No. 779

38. **Ans: A. Any cancer above T1**

Ref: Chapter No. 34, Page No. 779

39. **Ans: B. Submandibular salivary gland**

Ref: Chapter No. 34, Page No. 780

40. **Ans: C. Lingual nerve**

Ref: Chapter No. 34, Page No. 780

41. **Ans: C. Adjacent to upper second molar**

Ref: Chapter No. 34, Page No. 780

42. **Ans: A. Hard palate is formed by the palatine process of the maxillary bone and the vomer**

Ref: Chapter No. 34, Page No. 780

43. **Ans: D. Tumors adherent to the periosteum can be treated with excision of periosteum only**

Ref: Chapter No. 34, Page No. 780

44. **Ans: D. Retromolar trigone**

Ref: Chapter No. 34, Page No. 781

45. **Ans: A. Oropharyngeal**

Ref: Chapter No. 34, Page No. 781

46. **Ans: A. Posterior faucial pillars**

Ref: Chapter No. 34, Page No. 781

47. **Ans: D. Smoking does not affect the overall outcome of HPV-associated cancers treated with concurrent chemoradiation**

Ref: Chapter No. 34, Page No. 782-783

48. **Ans: C. Surgical resection plus MRND followed by chemoradiotherapy**

Ref: Chapter No. 34, Page No. 783

49. **Ans: C. Concurrent chemotherapy and radiation therapy**

Ref: Chapter No. 34, Page No. 783

50. **Ans: B. Division and repair of soft tissues and bone under high quality visualization**

Ref: Chapter No. 34, Page No. 783

51. **Ans: D. Postcricoid carcinoma may develop just distal to the web**

Ref: Chapter No. 34, Page No. 783

52. **Ans: D. Surgical excision is preferred initial treatment for early stage hypopharyngeal cancers**

Ref: Chapter No. 34, Page No. 784-785

53. **Ans: A. Upper jugular lymph nodes**

Ref: Chapter No. 34, Page No. 784

54. **Ans: A. External branch of superior laryngeal nerve supplies the cricoarytenoid**

Ref: Chapter No. 34, Page No. 785

55. **Ans: A. Formal pulmonary function testing (PFT) mandatory for all patients undergoing surgery**

Ref: Chapter No. 34, Page No. 787

56. **Ans: D. Involvement of anterior commissure**

Ref: Chapter No. 34, Page No. 788

57. **Ans: D. All of the above**

Ref: Chapter No. 34, Page No. 788

58. **Ans: D. Multiple, large, bilateral cysts of the parotid glands are characteristics of EBV infection**

Ref: Chapter No. 34, Page No. 789

59. **Ans: B. HIV infection**

Ref: Chapter No. 34, Page No. 789

60. **Ans: D. Sensitivity of FNA for distinguishing benign from malignant tumors of salivary glands being 95%**

Ref: Chapter No. 34, Page No. 789

61. **Ans: B. Pleomorphic adenoma**

Ref: Chapter No. 34, Page No. 789

62. **Ans: B. Warthin tumor**

Ref: Chapter No. 34, Page No. 789

63. **Ans: C. Division of the auriculotemporal nerve is often required during parotidectomy**

Ref: Chapter No. 34, Page No. 791-793

64. **Ans: B. Frey's syndrome is the result of an abnormal innervations of cutaneous sweat glands by parasympathetic fibers**

Ref: Chapter No. 34, Page No. 793

65. **Ans: B. Nasolacrimal duct**

Ref: Chapter No. 34, Page No. 793

66. **Ans: A. The lamina papyracea is the thin medial wall of the ethmoid sinus**

Ref: Chapter No. 34, Page No. 793

67. **Ans: A. Nasal cavity**

Ref: Chapter No. 34, Page No. 794

68. **Ans: B. Rise along the medial nasal wall**

Ref: Chapter No. 34, Page No. 794

69. **Ans: C. Elective neck dissection for primary sinonasal carcinomas is recommended**

Ref: Chapter No. 34, Page No. 794-796

70. **Ans: B. IDH2**

Ref: Chapter No. 34, Page No. 797

71. **Ans: D. WHO type I nasopharyngeal cancer is associated with EBV**

Ref: Chapter No. 34, Page No. 797

72. **Ans: D. Flexible nasopharyngeal examination**

Ref: Chapter No. 34, Page No. 797

73. **Ans: A. Non-keratinizing SCC associated with EBV is most common subtype**

Ref: Chapter No. 34, Page No. 797-798

74. **Ans: B. Rhabdomyosarcoma**

Ref: Chapter No. 34, Page No. 798

75. **Ans: C. Regional flaps are based on axial blood flow and are located adjacent to the donor site**

Ref: Chapter No. 34, Page No. 800-802

76. **Ans: A. Rotational local flap**

Ref: Chapter No. 34, Page No. 801

77. **Ans: D. Fibula osteocutaneous free flap**

Ref: Chapter No. 34, Page No. 802

78. **Ans: A. Branch from thoracoacromial artery**

Ref: Chapter No. 34, Page No. 802

35

Diseases of the Breast

ANATOMY

1. All are true statement about anatomy of breast except:

A. Multiple fibrous bands termed the suspensory ligaments of Cooper run from the chest wall to the dermis
B. The retromammary fat pad is a relatively avascular space that lies between the breast and pectoralis major muscle
C. Pectoralis minor muscle is enclosed in the clavipectoral fascia
D. Axillary nodes levels are defined by their relationship to the pectoralis major muscle

2. Location of Rotter nodes is:

A. Retromammary fat
B. Interpectoral
C. Retrosternal
D. Posterior to the pectoralis minor muscle

3. Apex of axilla is defined by:

A. Lateral third of clavicle
B. Lateral border of 1st rib
C. Halsted ligament
D. Acromioclavicular joint

4. Which is false regarding lymphatic supply of the breast?

A. Specialized lymphatic channels collect under the nipple and areola and form Sappey plexus
B. Axillary lymph nodes receives 75% of lymphatic flow from the breast
C. The internal mammary lymph nodes as the predominant drainage in 20% of patients
D. A major route of breast cancer metastasis is through lymphatic channels

5. Nerve of Bell is also known as:

A. Nerve to latissimus dorsi
B. Thoracodorsal nerve
C. Long thoracic nerve
D. 2nd intercostal brachial nerve

6. Which is false about anatomic relations of nerves to the breast?

A. The long thoracic nerve runs deep and close to the chest wall on the medial side of the axilla
B. The thoracodorsal nerve enters the axillary space over the axillary vein and crosses to lateral surface of the latissimus dorsi muscle
C. The axillary vein is superior and posterior the pectoral neurovascular bundle
D. Intercostal brachial nerves supply sensation to the upper inner surface of the arm

7. Which is false regarding lobular anatomy of the breast?

A. Multiple branching ends of terminal ducts, each ending in acini forms a lobule
B. Intra-lobular stroma is denser and less cellular
C. Functional independence is exhibited by each ductal system
D. The basement membrane layer is an important boundary in differentiating in situ from invasive breast cancer

BREAST DEVELOPMENT AND PHYSIOLOGY

8. Which is false about the breast tissue development?

A. Mammary ridge extends from the axilla to the inguinal area

B. 90% of newborns will have a breast secretion, which referred to as "witches milk"
C. Witches milk resolve on its own in 1 week
D. Thelarche entails the first appearance of lobular units

9. Prepubertal gynecomastia refers to symmetrical enlargement and projection of the breast bud in a girl before the age of:

A. 9 years
B. 12 years
C. 16 years
D. 18 years

10. Which is false statement regarding conditions associated with breast pain?

A. Fibrocystic changes manifest usually as premenstrual cyclic mastalgia
B. Breast pain as only symptom occurs in 20% of patients with breast cancer
C. Women 30 years and older with noncyclic mastalgia should undergo breast imaging with mammography and ultrasonography
D. The most common source of referred pain to the breast is scapulothoracic bursitis

11. Pain is an only symptom of the breast cancer in __% of patients with breast cancer.

A. 7%
B. 14%
C. 21%
D. 33%

12. Which of the following is most likely associated with breast pain?

A. Breast cancer
B. LCIS
C. Sclerosing adenosis
D. Breast cyst

13. Which is incorrect statement regarding fibrocystic disease of the breast?

A. It is common during the fourth and fifth decades of life
B. It manifests usually as premenstrual cyclic mastalgia
C. Palpable cysts or multiple small cysts are typical of fibrocystic disease
D. Fibrocystic change is a risk factor for the development of breast malignancy

14. Which is false about developmental anomalies of breast tissue?

A. Poland syndrome presents as a unilateral variable loss of the breast tissue, pectoralis major and minor, and serratus anterior muscles as well as several rib
B. Accessory nipples are usually removed only for cosmetic reasons
C. Accessory breast tissue is commonly located above the breast in the axilla
D. Axillary lymph nodes need to be removed along with accessory breast tissue

15. 16-year-old girl has asymmetric breast development with hypoplastic right breast along with hypoplasia of right pectoralis muscle. What is the diagnosis?

A. Li-Fraumeni syndrome
B. Amazia
C. Fragile X syndrome
D. Poland syndrome

16. All are true regarding features of gynecomastia except:

A. Pubertal hypertrophy is generally treated by observation without surgery
B. The enlargement is frequently unilateral in older patients
C. The mass is smooth, firm, saucer shaped and symmetrically distributed beneath the areola
D. It is frequently non-tender

17. What is the most common cause of spontaneous single duct discharge from the nipple?

A. Intraductal papilloma
B. Duct ectasia
C. Breast malignancy
D. Fibrocystic disease

18. Following are the causes of multi-ductal discharge from nipple except:

A. Duct ectasia
B. Breast malignancy
C. Intraductal papilloma
D. Hypothyroidism

19. A 40-year-old female presented with breast pain has recent onset spontaneous, bilateral, greenish nipple discharge from multiple ducts. She has bilateral breast tenderness without any palpable mass on breast examination. USG and mammographic findings are unremarkable. What is the best management?

A. USG guided core needle biopsy
B. Reassure the patient
C. Excise retroareolar ducts
D. MRI of breast

20. 50-year-old female has spontaneous onset single duct bloody discharge from left nipple. USG and mammography findings are unremarkable. What is best management?

A. Review medication and measure prolactin
B. Reassure and continue screening
C. Duct excision
D. Send sample for cytology and excise only if atypical cells are present

21. Following are the characteristics of intraductal papilloma of breast except:

A. Spontaneous nipple discharge from a single duct
B. Papillomas that are located near the nipple-areolar complex are at higher risk of malignancy
C. A papilloma is the most common benign tumor to develop breast cancer
D. Papilloma may progress to DCIS

22. What is the cause of bilateral spontaneous bloody nipple discharge?

A. Duct ectasia B. Physiological
C. Hypothyroidism D. Fibrocystic disease

23. Which of the following statement is incorrect concerning features of breast diseases?

A. Galactocele is round, easily movable cyst which occurs during lactation period
B. Paget's disease of nipple shows malignant Paget cells invading the epidermis without traversing the basement membrane
C. Skin dimpling is caused by involvement of Cooper ligaments by a scirrhous tumor
D. Dermal lymphatic obstruction by malignant cells is the pathologic hallmark of inflammatory carcinoma of breast

DIAGNOSIS OF BREAST DISEASE

24. Following are the characteristic features of inflammatory carcinoma of breast except:

A. Peau d'orange appearance of breast skin
B. Edematous warm and tenderness over the breast
C. Obstruction of dermal lymphatic channels by emboli of carcinoma cells
D. Palpable mass or localized induration in all patients

25. Specific sign which signifies presence of underlying carcinoma of the breast?

A. Blood stained nipple discharge
B. Nipple retraction
C. Palpable breast mass
D. Peau d'orange appearance

26. Following are the characteristic features of Paget's disease of nipple except:

A. It is commonly associated with an underlying breast cancer
B. Carcinoma cells invade epidermal layer of the skin of the nipple
C. Dermatitis that resembles eczematoid or psoriatic rash
D. Paget's disease originates on the areola and spread to skin

27. All are true regarding use of FNAC in the diagnosis of breast carcinoma except:

A. Multiple areas of a mass could be sampled at a time
B. FNA is a definitive diagnostic procedure for breast carcinoma
C. It helps to confirm the diagnosis of multifocal breast cancer
D. Lymph node metastasis can be detected with a specificity of 100%

28. All are true regarding use of core needle biopsy (CNB) in the diagnosis of breast carcinoma except:

A. CNB is the method of choice to sample breast lesion
B. The size of a CNB needle ranges from 8 to 14 gauge
C. CNB provides definitive diagnosis of breast carcinoma
D. 70% of patients with a diagnosis of DCIS on CNB are found to have some invasive carcinoma at definitive surgery

29. A 50-year-old female detected with non-tender well defined 2 cm palpable mass in upper outer quadrant of right breast. USG findings are unremarkable and mammography shows only dense breast. What is next step?

A. Reassure patient as it is benign mass
B. Follow up mammography after 6 months
C. Core needle biopsy of the lesion
D. Excisional biopsy

30. Patients with diagnosis of DCIS on CNB have invasive carcinoma at definitive surgery in __% of cases.

A. 11% B. 33%
C. 44% D. 66%

BREAST IMAGING

31. **Primary imaging modality for screening asymptomatic breast lesions:**
   A. USG B. Mammography
   C. CT scan D. MRI

32. **Which of the following view of breast is obtained on screening mammography?**
   A. Mediolateral
   B. Mediolateral oblique
   C. Anteroposterior
   D. Posteroanterior

33. **____% of clinically evident breast cancer have no visible abnormality on mammography.**
   A. 5% B. 15%
   C. 25% D. 30%

34. **Which is false regarding mammography as a screening modality for breast cancer?**
   A. Screening mammography is performed in asymptomatic women with the goal of detecting occult breast cancer
   B. American Cancer Society recommends annual screening mammography for women older than 40 years
   C. Screening mammography is not offered for women > 74 years old
   D. Tomosynthesis has significantly higher detection of breast cancer but a slightly higher false positive rate

35. **All are true statement about use ultrasonography in diagnosis of breast cancer except:**
   A. It is useful for discriminating lesions in patients with dense breasts
   B. It is useful as a breast cancer screening tool
   C. Use of ultrasonography resulted in more false-positive events
   D. It is useful tool to aid FNA or core needle biopsy of breast lesions

36. **Which of the following lesion has less detection rate with MRI?**
   A. Axillary lymph node metastases with unknown primary tumor
   B. Paget's disease of the nipple
   C. Multifocal or multicentric cancer
   D. Detection of DCIS

37. **Following are the advantages of MRI as imaging tool in breast lesions except:**
   A. Detection of lesions in young women with dense breast tissue
   B. Improved local recurrence rates or survival when used as guide for pre-operative decision making
   C. Best diagnostic tool in cases of implant rupture
   D. Useful to detect the extent of residual disease after lumpectomy with positive margins

38. **Following are the disadvantages of MRI in breast imaging:**
   A. Low sensitivity for the detection of DCIS
   B. Higher false-positive finding
   C. Screening of invasive lobular carcinoma
   D. Screening in women with a lifetime risk of developing breast cancer of less than 15%

39. **According to ACS, which of the following is not a high-risk criteria of MRI screening?**
   A. Known BRCA1 or BRCA2 gene mutation
   B. Radiation therapy to the chest between the ages of 10 and 30
   C. Lifetime risk of breast cancer of 15%–20%
   D. Li-Fraumeni syndrome or Cowden syndrome

40. **According to ACS, women with following factors have moderate lifetime risk of breast cancer except:**
   A. Lifetime risk of breast cancer of 15%–20% according to risk assessment tool
   B. Personal history of breast cancer, DCIS or LCIS
   C. Unevenly dense breasts on mammography
   D. Radiation therapy to the chest between the ages of 10 and 30

41. **All are true about MRI as screening modality for breast cancer except:**
   A. Annual MRI screening is recommended beginning at age 30 years for women at high lifetime risk
   B. MRI is recommended for women with a lifetime risk of developing breast cancer of less than 15%
   C. When MRI is used for screening, it should be used in addition to screening mammography
   D. MRI may fail to detect malignancies that a mammogram would detect

42. **Excisional biopsy is considered in following conditions except:**
   A. Atypical ductal hyperplasia in field of micro-calcification

B. Epithelial metaplasia
C. Hypercellular fibroadenoma
D. Diagnosis not concordant with imaging findings

43. All are correct statements about non-palpable breast lesion management except:

A. Non-palpable BI-RADS 3 category lesions should undergo excisional biopsy
B. Specimen radiography is carried out after surgical excision to confirm complete removal of targeted lesion
C. Patients who have a diagnosis of benign findings on excision should undergo new baseline mammogram 4 to 6 months after the surgical procedure
D. Iodine-125 radioactive seed can be used to guide the breast resection of non-palpable lesions

44. Following are the radiographic features suggestive of malignancy except:

A. Density with spiculated borders
B. Pleomorphic and linear microcalcifications
C. Cyst with enhanced posterior echoes
D. Solid, taller than wide lesion

RISK FACTORS

45. Which is the most important risk factor for breast cancer development?

A. Age
B. Gender
C. Race
D. Family history

46. Which is incorrect regarding risk association of breast cancer development?

A. Breast cancer is rare in women younger than 20 years
B. Women have an average lifetime risk of 12.2% of being diagnosed with breast cancer
C. Incidence of breast cancer in men is less than 1% of the incidence in women
D. Likelihood of a second primary cancer in the contralateral breast varies from 0.2% per year in younger patients

47. About the risk of breast cancer development, false statement is:

A. Twofold to fourfold risk in patients receiving mantle irradiation before the age of 30 years
B. Likelihood of a second primary cancer in the contralateral breast varies from 0.5% to 1% per year in younger patients
C. Likelihood of a second primary cancer in the contralateral breast is 0.2% per year in older patients
D. Breast cancer risk in patients with LCIS is more than 5% per year

48. Total categories involved in BI-RADS scoring:

A. 4
B. 5
C. 6
D. 7

49. Wrongly matched BI-RADS category:

A. Category 1 – Negative finding
B. Category 2 – Probably benign finding
C. Category 5 – Suggestive of malignancy
D. Category 6 – Proven malignancy

50. What is appropriate management of BI-RADS 3 category?

A. Continue annual screening
B. Initial short-interval follow-up imaging
C. FNA or core needle biopsy
D. Excisional biopsy

51. Risk of malignancy associated with BI-RADS 5 category:

A. < 50%
B. 50% - 75%
C. >75% - 95%
D. >95%

52. Risk of malignancy associated with BI-RADS 3 category:

A. < 2%
B. 5 - 10%
C. 10 - 25%
D. 25 - 50%

53. Which of the following is an non-modifiable risk factor of breast cancer?

A. Obesity
B. Use of hormone replacement therapy
C. Nulliparity
D. Reproductive factors

54. Which of the following is a modifiable risk factor of breast cancer?

A. Menstrual factors
B. Parity
C. History of radiation exposure
D. Age at menopause

55. All are true regarding LCIS of breast except:

A. It is observed predominantly in younger premenopausal women
B. It does not manifest as a palpable mass or suspicious microcalcifications on mammography

C. Risk ratio for patients with LCIS that develop into invasive carcinoma is 7:1
D. The invasive carcinomas that develop in patients with LCIS are predominantly lobular

56. Which of the following is false regarding LCIS?

A. LCIS carries lifelong and equal risk of breast cancer for both breasts
B. Breast cancer risk in patients with LCIS is less than 1% per year
C. A 5-year course of tamoxifen provides a 90% reduction in breast cancer risk
D. Bilateral total nipple skin-sparing mastectomy is the surgical procedure of choice

57. All are included in proliferative disease of breast without atypia except:

A. Fibrocystic change with epithelial metaplasia
B. Papillomatosis
C. Radial scar
D. Sclerosing adenosis

58. Which of the following breast lesions have highest relative risk of developing cancer?

A. Lobular carcinoma in situ
B. Atypical ductal hyperplasia with family history
C. Atypical lobular hyperplasia
D. Papillomatosis

59. Proliferative disease of breast without atypia has ____ relative risk of developing breast cancer.

A. 1.0 B. 1.3–1.9
C. 3.7–4.2 D. 4–9

60. Lobular carcinoma in situ lesion of breast has ____ relative risk of developing breast cancer.

A. 1.3–1.9 B. 2.0 – 3.5
C. 3.7–4.2 D. 7 – 9

61. Which is false about prevalence of genetic factors for breast cancer development?

A. Genetic factors are estimated to be responsible for 5% to 10% of all breast cancer
B. Genetic factors may account for 25% of cases in women younger than 30 years
C. Mutations in BRCA1 account for up to 60% of familial breast cancers
D. Mutations in BRCA2 accounts for 30% of familial breast cancers

62. The BRCA1 gene is located on:

A. Chromosome 13p12 B. Chromosome 13q21
C. Chromosome 17p12 D. Chromosome 17q21

63. The BRCA2 gene is located on:

A. Chromosome 11
B. Chromosome 13
C. Chromosome 15
D. Chromosome 17

64. False about BRCA1 gene mutation:

A. Proto-oncogene mutation inherited in autosomal dominant pattern
B. Mutations are unique and limited to a given family
C. Triple-negative breast cancer has 20% risk of a BRCA1 mutation
D. 45% lifetime risk of ovarian cancer in BRCA1 carrier

65. False concerning BRCA2 gene mutation:

A. Accounts for 40% of familial breast cancer
B. 30% lifetime risk for ovarian cancer
C. Association with the hormone receptor positive breast cancer subtype
D. Associated with increased breast cancer risk in men

66. False statement regarding BRCA gene mutations and breast cancer?

A. Responsible for 25% of all breast cancer case
B. Penetrance of BRCA1 and BRCA2 mutations has been estimated to be 50 – 70%
C. BRCA1 mutation are highly likely to have basal-like breast cancer
D. For the carriers of a BRCA gene mutation, prophylactic surgery is considered to be the most rational approach

67. Following factors are associated with unfavorable outcome except:

A. Triple negative breast cancer
B. Increased S phase fraction
C. Hormone receptor–positive
D. BRCA1-associated breast cancer

68. Following reproductive factors are associated with breast cancer risk except:

A. First live childbirth after age 30 years
B. Induced abortion
C. Nulliparity
D. Menopause after age 55 years

69. Which is incorrect regarding hormonal effect on breast cancer development?

A. Breast cancer risk doubles with delay in menopause after age 55
B. Breastfeeding has been reported to reduce breast cancer risk
C. Women receiving combination HRT for 5 years have approximately a 20% increased risk for breast cancer
D. Progesterone-only formulations do not appear to be at significant increased risk for breast cancer

70. Gail model for risk assessment of breast cancer does not include which of the following risk factor?

A. Race
B. Age at first live birth
C. Number of previous breast biopsies
D. Genetic factors

71. Gail model includes following risk factors except:

A. Age at menarche
B. Presence of proliferative disease with atypia
C. Radiation history
D. Number of first-degree female relatives with breast cancer

72. Regarding application of Gail model for breast cancer risk assessment, false statement is:

A. The Gail model assesses population risk using non-genetic factors
B. The model should not be used in women with a diagnosis of LCIS or DCIS
C. It may overestimate the risk for non-carriers
D. Race does not affect the assessment using Gail model

73. Which of the following risk assessment model is not based on genetic factors?

A. Claus model
B. Gail model
C. Couch model
D. Tyrer-Cuzick model

74. Couch model was developed to assess the risk of:

A. Mutation in BRCA1
B. Mutation in BRCA2
C. Rare genetic mutations
D. Both A and B

75. Which breast cancer risk assessment model gives more comprehensive and individual risk assessment?

A. Claus model
B. BRCAPro model
C. Couch model
D. Tyrer-Cuzick model

76. What is the incidence of clinically significant BRCA mutations in the general population?

A. 1 in 50
B. 1 in 500
C. 1 in 5000
D. 1 in 50000

77. Following are indications for genetic testing in cases of breast cancer except:

A. Breast cancer in men
B. Bilateral breast cancer
C. Breast cancer diagnosed before age 50
D. Family history of one individual with breast and ovarian cancer

78. Following are indications for genetic testing in cases of breast cancer except:

A. Breast and ovarian cancer in the same individual
B. Relative with breast or ovarian cancer
C. Close male relative with breast cancer
D. Family history of two or more individuals with breast and ovarian cancer

79. Following syndrome are associated with breast cancer except:

A. Cowden syndrome
B. Neurofibromatosis 1
C. Li-Fraumeni syndrome
D. Lynch syndrome

80. Following are recommended surveillance guidelines for high risk breast cancer women:

A. Monthly breast self-examination beginning at age 21 years
B. 6 monthly clinical breast examination beginning at age 25 years
C. Annual mammography beginning at age 25 years
D. Annual mammography beginning 10 years before the earliest age at onset of breast cancer in a family member

81. Which is incorrect regarding use of tamoxifen in breast cancer treatment?

A. Tamoxifen selective ER modulator
B. Adjuvant tamoxifen reduces the risk for a second breast cancer in the unaffected breast by 47%

C. Its use increases the risk of endometrial cancer
D. Tamoxifen is most effective for cancers involving BRCA1 mutation

82. Following are side effects of Tamoxifen except:

A. Risk of endometrial cancer
B. Risk of ovarian cancer
C. Pulmonary embolism
D. Venous thromboembolism

83. Following trials are based on use of selective estrogen modulators for chemoprevention of breast cancer except:

A. IBIS-1 Trial
B. STAR Trial
C. MORE Trial
D. MAP.3 Trial

84. All are true about drugs used for chemoprevention of breast cancer except:

A. Tamoxifen is most effective at reducing the incidence of ER-positive breast cancers
B. Raloxifene has more favorable toxicity profile
C. Tamoxifen and raloxifene each reduces the risk for invasive breast cancer by approximately 50%
D. Exemestane has been approved by the FDA as a chemopreventive agent

85. Which of the following is incorrect about prophylactic mastectomy?

A. Prophylactic mastectomy has been shown to reduce the chance of breast cancer development in high-risk women by 100%
B. BRCA mutation carriers should be counseled to consider risk-reducing surgeries as a strategy to reduce cancer incidence and improve survival
C. American Society of Breast Surgeons does not recommend the routine use of contralateral mastectomy in the sporadic cancer patient
D. Women who undergo annual mammographic screening have an overall 80% chance of surviving breast cancer after it has been detected

BENIGN BREAST TUMORS

86. Following are the features of breast cyst except:

A. Most cysts occur in women younger than 35 years and the incidence steadily decreases until menopause
B. 50% of cysts are multiple or recurrent
C. Intracystic carcinoma is exceedingly rare
D. CNB should be performed, if the cyst recurs more than twice

87. A 40-year-old female presented with 3 cm simple cyst. Aspiration yields straw colored fluid and there is complete resolution of cyst on USG. What should be the next step?

A. Repeat USG after 3 months
B. Send fluid to laboratory for occult blood test, cytology, tumor markers
C. Excision of cavity
D. Continue routine clinical breast examination

88. Which is incorrect regarding fibroadenoma of breast?

A. Fibroadenomas are benign solid tumors composed of stromal and epithelial elements
B. Most commonly occur in women younger than 30 years
C. Rarely, if cancer is detected in fibroadenoma; DCIS is more common finding
D. Fibroadenoma > 5 cm in size is called as Giant fibroadenoma

89. False regarding juvenile fibroadenoma:

A. Large in size
B. More cellular
C. Slower growth
D. Surgery is curative

90. 15-year-old girl has history of rapidly growing mass in left breast. Breast cancer was diagnosed in mother at age of 36 years. USG findings suggestive of 7 cm hypoechoic solid mass with distinct round borders. What is most appropriate management?

A. Bilateral mastectomy
B. Excisional biopsy
C. Cyst aspiration
D. Simple mastectomy

91. 34-year-old lactating female presented with right breast tenderness, erythema and warmth. USG demonstrates a hypoechoic collection with acoustic enhancement. What is best management?

A. Surgical incision and drainage
B. Needle aspiration and antibiotics
C. IV antibiotics
D. Core needle biopsy to rule out malignancy

92. All are true regarding duct ectasia or periductal mastitis except:

A. Chronic relapsing infection develop in the subareolar ducts of the breast

B. Develops in non lactating women
C. Associated with smoking and diabetes
D. Surgical excision is treatment of choice

93. A 45-year-old female undergone core needle biopsy of 1.5 cm spiculated, complex sclerosing lesion. Pathology report shows benign breast parenchyma. What is the most appropriate management?

A. Routine screening mammography at 1 year
B. Short term follow up in 4 - 6 months
C. Excisional biopsy of the lesion
D. Imaging with MRI

94. Which of the following is false about benign lesions of breast?

A. Papillomas are most commonly associated with the development of invasive ductal carcinoma
B. Papillomatosis consists of hyperplastic epithelium without stalk of fibrovascular tissue
C. Sclerosing adenosis is the most common pathologic finding in needle-directed biopsy of microcalcifications
D. Fat necrosis can mimic cancer on mammography by producing density with calcifications

PATHOLOGY OF BREAST CANCER

95. Following are types of ductal carcinoma of breast except:

A. Papillary
B. Scirrhous
C. Cribriform
D. Comedo

96. Which is most common type of invasive breast carcinoma?

A. Invasive ductal carcinoma
B. Invasive lobular carcinoma
C. Mucinous or colloid carcinoma
D. Medullary carcinoma

97. Which of the following feature is suggestive of invasive lobular carcinoma?

A. Discrete bilateral masses
B. Partially cystic appearance
C. Asymmetric density on mammogram
D. Densities with microcalcifications

98. Which is incorrect about invasive carcinoma of breast?

A. Tiny, pleomorphic and linear forms of micro-calcifications are characteristic of infiltrating ductal carcinoma
B. Invasive ductal cancer tends to grow as a cohesive mass
C. Invasive lobular cancer tends to permeate the breast in a single-file nature
D. Invasive lobular cancer is often remains clinically occult and often escapes detection on mammography

99. Which is correct about tubular carcinoma of breast?

A. Lymph node involvement is seen in 15%
B. It is usually ER negative
C. Neoadjuvant therapy should be considered
D. Favorable prognosis than other forms of ductal carcinoma

100. All are true concerning medullary carcinoma of breast except:

A. It is characterized by bizarre invasive cells with high-grade nuclear feature
B. It forms sheets of cells in an almost syncytial fashion, surrounded by an infiltrate of small mononuclear lymphocyte
C. The borders of the tumor infiltrate the stroma
D. They are usually triple negative cancers

101. Which is false regarding metaplastic carcinoma of breast?

A. Typically high grade and aggressive
B. Negative for ER, PR and HER-2
C. Most metaplastic carcinomas are node positive
D. 50% experience local or distant relapse

102. Presence of mononuclear lymphocyte infiltrate surrounding syncytial pattern of malignant cells is a characteristic feature seen in:

A. Mucinous or colloid carcinoma
B. Medullary carcinoma
C. Metaplastic carcinoma
D. Adenoid cystic carcinoma

103. Which of the following test is used to define basal like cancers of breast?

A. Immunohistochemistry
B. Flow cytometry
C. Microarray assay
D. Fluorescence in situ hybridization

104. Which is incorrect regarding use of molecular markers for breast cancer management?

A. Estrogen receptor testing is now performed on all primary tumors

B. HER-2 is amplified in approximately 20% of human breast cancers
C. Fluorescence in situ hybridization, which directly detects the number of HER-2–gene copies
D. Basal-like cancers are defined using immunohistochemistry

105. About basal like breast cancer, false is:

A. Associated with BRCA1 mutation
B. Microarray assay for diagnosis
C. HER-2 positive and ER negative
D. Type of ductal carcinoma

106. All are true about Oncotype Dx assay except:

A. 21-gene recurrence score assay
B. Used on paraffin-embedded tumor material
C. Includes node-positive breast cancer treated with adjuvant endocrine therapy
D. It is used to determine the need of chemotherapy for high-risk ER-positive breast cancer

107. All are true about Mammaprint assay except:

A. 70 gene assay
B. ER positive or negative tumors
C. Node positive tumors
D. Guides clinical decision making

108. Following are characteristics of phyllodes tumor except:

A. Whorled stroma forms larger clefts lined by epithelium that resemble clusters of leaf-like structure
B. Usually occur in older patients
C. CNB differentiates benign and malignant phyllodes
D. Surgical excision of benign phyllodes is curative

109. All are true about management of malignant phyllodes tumors except:

A. Extent of tumor is main predictor of survival
B. Regional lymph node dissection is not required for staging or locoregional control
C. Metastases occur via hematogenous spread
D. Radiotherapy is not effective

110. Which is incorrect concerning angiosarcoma of breast?

A. Stewart-Treves syndrome develops after a latent period of 10 to 15 years post surgery
B. Mammography is the initial investigation in evaluation of angiosarcoma
C. Axillary dissection is not required.
D. Radiation therapy is beneficial in locoregional treatment of primary angiosarcoma

STAGING OF BREAST CANCER

111. According to AJCC, Paget's disease of nipple without presence of carcinoma in situ or underlying carcinoma has T stage:

A. Tx B. T0
C. Tis D. T1mi

112. Inflammatory carcinoma of breast has T stage:

A. T3 B. T4b
C. T4c D. T4d

113. According to AJCC, T3 stage involves tumor with size:

A. < 4 cm B. > 4 cm
C. > 5 cm D. > 7 cm

114. T1a stage of breast cancer includes tumor size:

A. < 1mm B. 1 to 2 mm
C. 1 to 5 mm D. < 2 cm

115. Tumor of 4 cm involving chest wall without any skin changes, 4 axillary lymph nodes, no evidence of metastasis is staged:

A. T3 N1 M0 B. T4a N2 M0
C. T4b N1 M0 D. T4c N2 M0

SURGICAL TREATMENT

116. Radical mastectomy does not involve which of the following step?

A. Removal of the whole breast tissue with overlying skin
B. Preservation of thoracodorsal and long thoracic nerve
C. Preservation of pectoralis muscles
D. Regional lymph nodes along the axillary vein up to the costoclavicular ligament

117. Oncotype Dx assay is recommended for breast cancers with:

A. ER-positive, node negative
B. ER-positive, node positive
C. ER-positive or negative, node negative
D. ER-positive or negative, node positive

118. Following are most common sites of metastasis from breast cancer except:

A. Bone
B. Liver
C. Lungs
D. Gonads

119. Which collagen vascular disease is contraindication for radiation therapy?

A. Marfan syndrome
B. Ankylosing spondylitis
C. Systemic scleroderma
D. Sjogren syndrome

120. Which is an absolute contraindication for radiation?

A. Systemic scleroderma
B. Active systemic lupus erythematosus
C. Pregnancy
D. p53 mutation

121. Which of the following is contraindication for breast conservative surgery?

A. High nuclear grade
B. Noncompliant to surveillance
C. Presence of lymphovascular invasion
D. Negative steroid hormone receptor status

122. 34-year-old female who is 27 weeks pregnant has palpable 2 cm mass in upper outer quadrant of right breast. CNB reports invasive ductal carcinoma, which is ER negative, HER-2 negative. She has palpable 1.5 cm lymph node in axilla that is positive on FNA. What is best management?

A. Immediate neoadjuvant chemotherapy followed by mastectomy
B. Modified radical mastectomy followed by chemotherapy
C. Lumpectomy, axillary dissection, chemotherapy and radiation therapy delayed until delivery
D. Simple mastectomy, SLND and radiation therapy

123. What is local recurrence rate for patients undergoing breast conservative surgery with irradiation?

A. 3 – 5%
B. 5 – 10%
C. 10 – 15%
D. 15 – 20%

124. Which of the following is incorrect concerning breast conservation surgery?

A. Mastectomy and breast-conserving therapy have been shown to be equivalent in terms of patient survival
B. The tumor, regardless of size, can be excised with clear margins and an acceptable cosmetic result
C. "No ink on tumor" should be used as the standard for an adequate margin in invasive breast cancer
D. Atypical hyperplasia and LCIS at resection margins increase local recurrence rates

125. 45-year-old female has CNB findings of atypical ductal hyperplasia. What is appropriate management?

A. Tamoxifen
B. Mammography after 6 months
C. Excisional biopsy of lesion
D. Bilateral prophylactic mastectomy

126. A 60-year-old female has undergone BCS for T1N0 invasive ductal carcinoma. Pathology report reveals close lateral margin of 1 mm. What is next step of management?

A. Re excision of lateral margin
B. Completion mastectomy
C. Radiation therapy
D. Re excision of all margin with radiation therapy

127. Following are correct statements regarding breast conservation therapy (BCS) except:

A. Local recurrence rates after BCS and radiation therapy are more than 5%
B. Local recurrence rates after BCS are higher for younger women
C. Shaved margins at the time of the BCS reduces the need for re-excision
D. Surgical staging of the axilla is performed through a separate incision in most patients undergoing breast conservation

128. Following factors are considered for oncoplastic breast surgery following tumor resection except:

A. Significant area of skin that to be resected with the tumor
B. Absolute breast volume that will be resected
C. Any tumor resection in the lower breast
D. Resection leading to nipple malposition

129. Which of the following technique of breast conservation surgery is used for lower pole lesions?

A. Round block technique
B. Crescent mastopexy
C. Hemi-batwing
D. J or V plasty

130. Which of the following technique of breast conservation surgery is used for upper pole lesions?

A. Triangle incision
B. Batwing resection
C. J or V plasty
D. Benelli technique

131. Benelli technique is used for breast lesions that are located in:

A. Upper outer quadrant
B. Lower outer quadrant
C. Lower inner quadrant
D. Upper inner quadrant

132. All are correct about oncoplastic procedures of breast except:

A. Oncoplastic procedures at the time of the initial surgical procedure are preferred to delayed approach
B. It has been associated with delay in delivery of adjuvant systemic therapy or radiation
C. Tissue expanders and implants are not recommended for patients undergoing radiation therapy
D. Reconstruction of the irradiated breast is generally not recommended for 1 to 2 years after radiation therapy has been completed

133. Mastectomy is always indicated for following conditions except:

A. Tumors that are large relative to breast size
B. Tumors with extensive calcifications
C. Any case of invasive carcinoma
D. Tumors in patients with contraindications to breast irradiation

134. Which is incorrect regarding modified radical mastectomy?

A. Removal of the mammary gland without pectoral fascia
B. Complete removal of axillary lymph nodes to level II
C. Removal of nipple areola complex
D. Preservation of pectoralis muscles

135. Which is false about surgical management of breast carcinoma?

A. Patients who desire to avoid radiation is an indication for mastectomy
B. Immediate reconstruction does not have a detrimental effect on long-term survival or local recurrence rates
C. Nipple-areola–sparing mastectomy has also been demonstrated to be safe in patients undergoing prophylactic mastectomy for risk reduction including BRCA mutations
D. In a modified radical mastectomy, level I to III axillary lymph nodes are taken with the axillary breast tissue

136. Which is incorrect regarding advantages of sentinel lymph node biopsy?

A. Patients with negative sentinel lymph nodes can avoid the morbidity of axillary dissection
B. SLND provides accurate staging information
C. An average of two or three sentinel nodes are present per patient
D. SLND considered to be less accurate in patients treated with preoperative chemotherapy

137. What is false negative rate of sentinel lymph node biopsy?

A. 1%
B. 11%
C. 18%
D. 21%

138. Which of the following does not include in the technique of SLND?

A. Subareolar or subdermal injection technique shows drainage of lymph to the axilla or the internal mammary nodal basin
B. A dose of 2.5 mCi of 99mTc-labeled sulfur colloid can be injected on the day before surgery without additional intraoperative dose
C. 0.5 to 1.0 mCi of 99mTc-labeled sulfur colloid used for intraoperative lymphatic mapping
D. 3 to 5 mL of blue dye can be injected peritumorally for intraoperative lymphatic mapping

139. All are true about sentinel lymph node biopsy for breast cancer except:

A. SLND false-negative rates are generally less than 5%
B. Axillary recurrence rates have been shown to be extremely low after a negative sentinel node biopsy without axillary dissection
C. If axillary metastasis is confirmed by FNAB, patient can proceed to sentinel node surgery for staging
D. ALND remains the standard for inflammatory breast cancer

140. Axillary lymph node surgery is standard of care for following conditions except:

A. Inflammatory breast cancer

B. Patients with clinically positive nodes
C. Positive sentinel node after neoadjuvant chemotherapy
D. Clinically negative sentinel lymph node micrometastasis

TREATMENT OF DCIS

141. Which of the following is not the indication for mastectomy?

A. Diffuse suspicious mammographic calcifications
B. Non-compliance with follow-up surveillance
C. Size of the tumor
D. Patient choice

142. 45-year-old female presented with extensive microcalcification in upper quadrant of right breast on mammography. CNB reports presence of high grade DCIS with solid pattern. What is appropriate management?

A. Wide local excision alone
B. Total mastectomy with SLND
C. Modified radical mastectomy
D. Wide local excision with Radiotherapy

143. What is local recurrence rate of DCIS after breast conservation surgery?

A. 1 – 2% per month B. 1 – 2% per year
C. 1 – 2% per 5 years D. 1 – 2% lifetime

144. Van Nuys criteria is used for:

A. Hormonal therapy in DCIS
B. Radiation therapy in DCIS
C. Chemotherapy in invasive carcinoma
D. Radiation therapy in invasive carcinoma

145. Van Nuys criteria is based on following factors except:

A. Size of lesion
B. Type of DCIS
C. Age of patient
D. Lymph node involvement

146. According Van Nuys criteria, radiotherapy can be omitted in patients with DCIS having following features, except:

A. Low DCIS nuclear grade
B. Small lesions < 2 cm
C. Older age of >60 years
D. Wide surgical margins of >1 cm

RADIATION THERAPY

147. Post mastectomy radiation for Stage II breast cancer is considered in patients with following risk factors except:

A. Lymphovascular invasion
B. Age 40 years or older
C. Nodal positivity ratio of 20% or greater
D. Close/positive surgical margins

148. Partial breast radiotherapy is recommended for:

A. Tumor size ≤4 cm
B. Age ≥ 60 years
C. Pure DCIS
D. ER status negative tumor

149. Following factors are in favor of considering partial breast radiotherapy except:

A. Tumor size ≤ 2 cm
B. Negative margins by at least 2 mm
C. Neoadjuvant chemotherapy has been given
D. ER positive tumor

150. Favorable factor for partial breast radiotherapy:

A. Age < 50 years
B. Multicentric tumor
C. Node positive disease
D. Invasive ductal carcinoma

SYSTEMIC THERAPY

151. Chemotherapy is not recommended in which of the following condition?

A. HER-2 positive
B. Node positive
C. Oncotype Dx recurrence scores of less than 16
D. ER/PR negative

152. Which of the following factor does not influence the choice of adjuvant chemotherapy for breast carcinoma?

A. Tumor size B. ER or HER-2 status
C. DNA ploidy D. Nodal status

153. In patients with age more than 50 years, chemotherapy is recommended if the Oncotype Dx score is:

A. < 16 B. < 25
C. > 16 D. > 25

154. Which is incorrect regarding anthracycline based chemotherapy?

A. Act as topoisomerase II inhibitors
B. Associated with the potential long-term toxic effect of cardiomyopathy
C. Cardiac dysfunction resulting from anthracyclines is dose independent
D. Associated with the risk of development of leukemia

155. Which is incorrect regarding taxane based chemotherapy?

A. Microtubule inhibitors
B. Treatment of metastatic breast cancer and anthracycline-resistant tumors
C. Permanent toxic effect of peripheral neuropathy
D. Long-term increased risk of second cancer

156. A 55-year-old female underwent lumpectomy with SLND. Pathology report shows invasive ductal carcinoma, low grade, 2 cm, node negative, ER positive and HER-2 negative. Which adjuvant treatment is recommended for this patient?

A. No adjuvant treatment required
B. Chemotherapy, radiation and anti hormonal therapy
C. Radiation and anti hormonal therapy
D. Chemotherapy and radiation

157. Which is false regarding trastuzumab therapy in case of breast cancers?

A. HER-2 gene amplification or protein overexpression occurs in approximately 20% to 25% of breast cancers
B. Trastuzumab and chemotherapy is indicated for all HER-2 positive patients
C. 3 years of treatment as standard of care
D. It increases the risk of cardiac dysfunction

158. Trastuzumab is recommended for ___ year/s of therapy as a standard of care.

A. 1 B. 2
C. 3 D. 4

159. 50-year-old female with 2 cm invasive ductal carcinoma without clinical nodal involvement is ER/PR negative and HER-2 positive. What will be the management for this patient?

A. Wide local excision and radiotherapy
B. Wide local excision, SLND, radiation and adjuvant chemotherapy with trastuzumab
C. Simple mastectomy, SLND, trastuzumab and tamoxifen
D. Modified radical mastectomy alone

160. Tamoxifen can be used for women who are:

A. Premenopausal B. Perimenopausal
C. Postmenopausal D. Any of the above

161. False regarding endocrine therapy in management of breast cancer:

A. Tamoxifen is a selective ER modulator
B. The most common side effect of tamoxifen use is hot flashes
C. Aromatase inhibitors are restricted for use in postmenopausal women
D. Endocrine therapy is recommended for 5 years

162. Total duration of endocrine therapy recommended for breast cancer treatment?

A. 2 years B. 5 years
C. 7 years D. 10 years

163. Which of the following is recommended endocrine therapy for breast cancer?

A. For premenopausal or perimenopausal women, tamoxifen for 5 years
B. After 5 years of tamoxifen, if the patient is still premenopausal, she should be offered an additional 5 years of tamoxifen therapy
C. If women are postmenopausal, choice is offered to continue tamoxifen or switch to an AI for 10-years total adjuvant therapy
D. Any of the above

164. Which of the following is incorrect concerning use of neoadjuvant therapy for breast cancer management?

A. Increased rates of breast conservation with the use of neoadjuvant systemic therapy
B. Neoadjuvant therapy significantly reduces the rate of in-breast recurrence
C. Decrease drug resistance by treating tumors before resistance has developed
D. Neoadjuvant chemotherapy does not alter the outcome of SLND

165. Which of the following is incorrect concerning use of neoadjuvant therapy for breast cancer management?

A. It is safe to omit ALND if the sentinel lymph node is negative
B. Pertuzumab, a HER-2 antagonist is approved by FDA for the neoadjuvant treatment of breast cancer
C. Some patients with HER-2–positive breast cancer could be treated with targeted therapy alone without chemotherapy

D. In postmenopausal women with ER-positive tumors, endocrine therapy provides more protection than standard chemotherapy

TREATMENT OF LOCALLY ADVANCED AND INFLAMMATORY BREAST CANCER

166. All of the following stages are considered locally advanced breast cancer except:

A. IIB
B. IIIA
C. IIIB
D. IVA

167. All are features of locally advanced breast cancer except:

A. Large primary tumors of size >5 cm
B. Ulceration or satellite skin nodules
C. Inflammatory carcinoma
D. Separately palpable axillary lymph nodes

168. Peau d'orange appearance of skin overlying breast is due to:

A. Involvement of ligaments of Cooper due to tumor
B. Edema of skin due to superficial thrombophlebitis
C. Edema of skin due to dermal lymphatic obstruction
D. Erythema due to secondary inflammation of skin

169. Following are characteristics of inflammatory carcinoma of breast except:

A. Accounting for approximately 1% to 5% of all breast tumors
B. The hallmark of inflammatory breast cancer is diffuse tumor involvement of the dermal lymphatic channels
C. Rapid onset of the disease, with progression over weeks to 3 months
D. SLND is recommended in all cases of inflammatory carcinoma

170. Incorrect regarding diagnosis of inflammatory carcinoma of breast except:

A. Pathologic hallmark of inflammatory cancer is the presence of tumor cells within dermal lymphatics is a prerequisite for diagnosis
B. Palpable mass is not required for the diagnosis
C. Axillary lymph node dissection should always be performed for all cases
D. Mammography may not be always diagnostic

TREATMENT OF SPECIAL CONDITIONS

171. All are true regarding Paget's disease except:

A. Accounts for 1% or less of breast malignancies
B. Nipple erythema and pruritus
C. Spread from the areola onto the nipple
D. Biopsy of the skin of the nipple for confirmation the diagnosis

172. Following are characteristics of Paget's disease except:

A. Paget cell is located between the normal keratinocytes of the nipple epidermis
B. Paget cells do not invade through the dermal basement membrane
C. Less than 50% of patients with Paget's disease have an underlying breast carcinoma
D. Invasive breast cancer is identified in more than 90% of patients with a palpable mass and Paget's disease

173. A 45-year-old female presented with chronic erythema, eczematoid rash involving right nipple and areola. No evidence of palpable breast mass and normal mammographic findings. What is appropriate management?

A. Oral vitamin E and topical emollient
B. Steroid therapy
C. Skin biopsy
D. Follow up mammography in 6 months

174. Paget's disease is associated with underlying carcinoma in ___ cases.

A. < 50%
B. 50 – 75%
C. 75 – 95%
D. > 95%

175. Nipple-areola reconstruction can be done after ___ months of post radiation therapy.

A. Immediately
B. 2 – 3 months
C. 4 – 6 months
D. 1 – 2 years

BREAST CANCER IN MEN

176. Incidence of breast cancer in men:

A. < 1%
B. 3%
C. 5%
D. 8%

177. Following are risk factors for breast cancer in men except:

A. Radiation exposure
B. Klinefelter syndrome
C. Gynecomastia
D. Cirrhosis

178. Which is the most common breast cancer type in men?

A. Ductal carcinoma in situ
B. Invasive ductal carcinoma
C. Invasive lobular carcinoma
D. Metaplastic carcinoma

179. All are true about male breast carcinoma except:

A. Gynecomastia is not a risk factor
B. Most men with breast cancer have a breast mass
C. Poor survival outcome in men with breast cancer as compared to women of same age and stage
D. Most breast cancers in men are hormone receptor positive

180. Which is true statement about male breast carcinoma?

A. Detected most commonly in age 60 to 70 years
B. Commonly associated with BRCA 1 mutation
C. SLND is contraindicated
D. Adjuvant endocrine therapy is not effective

ANSWERS

1. **Ans: D. Axillary nodes levels are defined by their relationship to the pectoralis major muscle**

Ref: Chapter No. 35, Page No. 809

2. **Ans: B. Interpectoral**

Ref: Chapter No. 35, Page No. 809

3. **Ans: C. Halsted ligament**

Ref: Chapter No. 35, Page No. 810

4. **Ans: C. The internal mammary lymph nodes as the predominant drainage in 20% of patients**

Ref: Chapter No. 35, Page No. 810

5. **Ans: C. Long thoracic nerve**

Ref: Chapter No. 35, Page No. 810

6. **Ans: B. The thoracodorsal nerve enters the axillary space over the axillary vein and crosses to lateral surface of the latissimus dorsi muscle**

Ref: Chapter No. 35, Page No. 811

7. **Ans: B. Intra-lobular stroma is denser and less cellular**

Ref: Chapter No. 35, Page No. 812

8. **Ans: C. Witches milk resolve on its own in 1 week**

Ref: Chapter No. 35, Page No. 813

9. **Ans: B. 12 years**

Ref: Chapter No. 35, Page No. 813

10. **Ans: B. Breast pain as only symptom occurs in 20% of patients with breast cancer**

Ref: Chapter No. 35, Page No. 813

11. **Ans: A. 7%**

Ref: Chapter No. 35, Page No. 813

12. **Ans: D. Breast cyst**

Ref: Chapter No. 35, Page No. 813

13. **Ans: D. Fibrocystic change is a risk factor for the development of breast malignancy**

Ref: Chapter No. 35, Page No. 813-814

14. **Ans: D. Axillary lymph nodes need to be removed along with accessory breast tissue**

Ref: Chapter No. 35, Page No. 814

15. **Ans: D. Poland syndrome**

Ref: Chapter No. 35, Page No. 814

16. **Ans: D. It is frequently non-tender**

Ref: Chapter No. 35, Page No. 814

17. **Ans: A. Intraductal papilloma**

Ref: Chapter No. 35, Page No. 814

18. **Ans: C. Intraductal papilloma**

Ref: Chapter No. 35, Page No. 814

19. **Ans: B. Reassure the patient**

Ref: Chapter No. 35, Page No. 814

20. **Ans: C. Duct excision**

Ref: Chapter No. 35, Page No. 814

21. **Ans: B. Papillomas that are located near the nipple-areolar complex are at higher risk of malignancy**

Ref: Chapter No. 35, Page No. 814

22. **Ans: C. Hypothyroidism**

Ref: Chapter No. 35, Page No. 815

23. **Ans: A. Galactocele is round, easily movable cyst which occurs during lactation period**

Ref: Chapter No. 35, Page No. 815

24. **Ans: D. Palpable mass or localized induration in all patients**

Ref: Chapter No. 35, Page No. 816

25. **Ans: B. Nipple retraction**

Ref: Chapter No. 35, Page No. 816

26. **Ans: D. Paget's disease originates on the areola and spread to skin**

Ref: Chapter No. 35, Page No. 816

27. **Ans: B. FNA is a definitive diagnostic procedure for breast carcinoma**

Ref: Chapter No. 35, Page No. 816-817

28. **Ans: D. 70% of patients with a diagnosis of DCIS on CNB are found to have some invasive carcinoma at definitive surgery**

Ref: Chapter No. 35, Page No. 817

29. **Ans: C. Core needle biopsy of the lesion**

Ref: Chapter No. 35, Page No. 817

30. **Ans: B. 33%**

Ref: Chapter No. 35, Page No. 817

31. **Ans: B. Mammography**

Ref: Chapter No. 35, Page No. 817

32. **Ans: B. Mediolateral oblique**

Ref: Chapter No. 35, Page No. 817

33. **Ans: B. 15%**

Ref: Chapter No. 35, Page No. 817

34. **Ans: C. Screening mammography is not offered for women > 74 years old**

Ref: Chapter No. 35, Page No. 818

35. **Ans: B. It is useful as a breast cancer screening tool**

Ref: Chapter No. 35, Page No. 818

36. **Ans: D. Detection of DCIS**

Ref: Chapter No. 35, Page No. 818

37. **Ans: B. Improved local recurrence rates or survival when used as guide for pre-operative decision making**

Ref: Chapter No. 35, Page No. 818

38. **Ans: C. Screening of invasive lobular carcinoma**

Ref: Chapter No. 35, Page No. 818-819

39. **Ans: C. Lifetime risk of breast cancer of 15%–20%**

Ref: Chapter No. 35, Page No. 819

40. **Ans: D. Radiation therapy to the chest between the ages of 10 and 30**

Ref: Chapter No. 35, Page No. 819

41. **Ans: B. MRI is recommended for women with a lifetime risk of developing breast cancer of less than 15%**

Ref: Chapter No. 35, Page No. 819

42. **Ans: B. Epithelial metaplasia**

Ref: Chapter No. 35, Page No. 819

43. **Ans: A. Non-palpable BI-RADS 3 category lesions should undergo excisional biopsy**

Ref: Chapter No. 35, Page No. 819

44. **Ans: C. Cyst with enhanced posterior echoes**

Ref: Chapter No. 35, Page No. 820

45. **Ans: A. Age**

Ref: Chapter No. 35, Page No. 820

46. **Ans: D. Likelihood of a second primary cancer in the contralateral breast varies from 0.2% per year in younger patients**

Ref: Chapter No. 35, Page No. 820-821

47. **Ans: D. Breast cancer risk in patients with LCIS is more than 5% per year**

Ref: Chapter No. 35, Page No. 821

48. **Ans: D. 7**

Ref: Chapter No. 35, Page No. 821

49. **Ans: B. Category 2 – Probably benign finding**

Ref: Chapter No. 35, Page No. 821

50. **Ans: B. Initial short-interval follow-up imaging**

Ref: Chapter No. 35, Page No. 821

51. **Ans: D. >95%**

Ref: Chapter No. 35, Page No. 821

52. **Ans: A. < 2%**

Ref: Chapter No. 35, Page No. 821

53. **Ans: C. Nulliparity**

Ref: Chapter No. 35, Page No. 821

54. **Ans: B. Parity**

Ref: Chapter No. 35, Page No. 821

55. **Ans: D. The invasive carcinomas that develop in patients with LCIS are predominantly lobular**

Ref: Chapter No. 35, Page No. 821

56. **Ans: C. A 5-year course of tamoxifen provides a 90% reduction in breast cancer risk**

Ref: Chapter No. 35, Page No. 821

57. **Ans: A. Fibrocystic change with epithelial metaplasia**

Ref: Chapter No. 35, Page No. 822

58. **Ans: B. Atypical ductal hyperplasia with family history**

Ref: Chapter No. 35, Page No. 822

59. **Ans: B. 1.3–1.9**

Ref: Chapter No. 35, Page No. 822

60. **Ans: D. 7 – 9**

Ref: Chapter No. 35, Page No. 822

61. **Ans: C. Mutations in BRCA1 account for up to 60% of familial breast cancers**

Ref: Chapter No. 35, Page No. 822

62. **Ans: D. Chromosome 17q21**

Ref: Chapter No. 35, Page No. 822

63. **Ans: B. Chromosome 13**

Ref: Chapter No. 35, Page No. 822

64. **Ans: A. Proto-oncogene mutation inherited in autosomal dominant pattern**

Ref: Chapter No. 35, Page No. 822

65. **Ans: A. Accounts for 40% of familial breast cancer**

Ref: Chapter No. 35, Page No. 822

66. **Ans: A. Responsible for 25% of all breast cancer case**

Ref: Chapter No. 35, Page No. 822

67. **Ans: C. Hormone receptor–positive**

Ref: Chapter No. 35, Page No. 822

68. **Ans: B. Induced abortion**

Ref: Chapter No. 35, Page No. 823

69. **Ans: D. Progesterone-only formulations do not appear to be at significant increased risk for breast cancer**

Ref: Chapter No. 35, Page No. 823

70. **Ans: D. Genetic factors**

Ref: Chapter No. 35, Page No. 823

71. **Ans: C. Radiation history**

Ref: Chapter No. 35, Page No. 823

72. **Ans: D. Race does not affect the assessment using Gail model**

Ref: Chapter No. 35, Page No. 823

73. **Ans: B. Gail model**

Ref: Chapter No. 35, Page No. 823

74. **Ans: A. Mutation in BRCA1**

Ref: Chapter No. 35, Page No. 823

75. **Ans: D. Tyrer-Cuzick model**

Ref: Chapter No. 35, Page No. 823

76. **Ans: B. 1 in 500**

Ref: Chapter No. 35, Page No. 823

77. **Ans: D. Family history of one individual with breast and ovarian cancer**

Ref: Chapter No. 35, Page No. 824

78. **Ans: B. Relative with breast or ovarian cancer**

Ref: Chapter No. 35, Page No. 824

79. **Ans: D. Lynch syndrome**

Ref: Chapter No. 35, Page No. 824

80. **Ans: A. Monthly breast self-examination beginning at age 21 years**

Ref: Chapter No. 35, Page No. 824

81. **Ans: D. Tamoxifen is most effective for cancers involving BRCA1 mutation**

Ref: Chapter No. 35, Page No. 824

82. **Ans: B. Risk of ovarian cancer**

Ref: Chapter No. 35, Page No. 824

83. **Ans: D. MAP.3 Trial**

Ref: Chapter No. 35, Page No. 825

84. **Ans: D. Exemestane has been approved by the FDA as a chemopreventive agent**

Ref: Chapter No. 35, Page No. 825

85. **Ans: A. Prophylactic mastectomy has been shown to reduce the chance of breast cancer development in high-risk women by 100%**

Ref: Chapter No. 35, Page No. 825

86. **Ans: A. Most cysts occur in women younger than 35 years and the incidence steadily decreases until menopause**

Ref: Chapter No. 35, Page No. 826

87. **Ans: D. Continue routine clinical breast examination**

Ref: Chapter No. 35, Page No. 826

88. **Ans: C. Rarely if cancer is detected in fibroadenoma; DCIS is more common finding**

Ref: Chapter No. 35, Page No. 826

89. **Ans: C. Slower growth**

Ref: Chapter No. 35, Page No. 826

90. **Ans: B. Excisional biopsy**

Ref: Chapter No. 35, Page No. 826

91. **Ans: B. Needle aspiration and antibiotics**

Ref: Chapter No. 35, Page No. 826

92. **Ans: D. Surgical excision is treatment of choice**

Ref: Chapter No. 35, Page No. 826

93. **Ans: C. Excisional biopsy of the lesion**

Ref: Chapter No. 35, Page No. 826

94. **Ans: A. Papillomas are most commonly associated with the development of invasive ductal carcinoma**

Ref: Chapter No. 35, Page No. 827

95. **Ans: B. Scirrhous**

Ref: Chapter No. 35, Page No. 828

96. **Ans: A. Invasive ductal carcinoma**

Ref: Chapter No. 35, Page No. 828

97. **Ans: C. Asymmetric density on mammogram**

Ref: Chapter No. 35, Page No. 828

98. **Ans: A. Tiny, pleomorphic and linear forms of microcalcifications are characteristic of infiltrating ductal carcinoma**

Ref: Chapter No. 35, Page No. 828

99. Ans: D. Favorable prognosis than other forms of ductal carcinoma

Ref: Chapter No. 35, Page No. 828

100. Ans: C. The borders of the tumor infiltrate the stroma

Ref: Chapter No. 35, Page No. 828

101. Ans: C. Most metaplastic carcinomas are node positive

Ref: Chapter No. 35, Page No. 828

102. Ans: B. Medullary carcinoma

Ref: Chapter No. 35, Page No. 828

103. Ans: C. Microarray assay

Ref: Chapter No. 35, Page No. 828

104. Ans: D. Basal-like cancers are defined using immunohistochemistry

Ref: Chapter No. 35, Page No. 828-829

105. Ans: C. HER-2 positive and ER negative

Ref: Chapter No. 35, Page No. 828

106. Ans: C. Includes node -positive breast cancer treated with adjuvant endocrine therapy

Ref: Chapter No. 35, Page No. 831

107. Ans: C. Node positive tumors

Ref: Chapter No. 35, Page No. 831

108. Ans: C. CNB differentiates benign and malignant phyllodes

Ref: Chapter No. 35, Page No. 832

109. Ans: D. Radiotherapy is not effective

Ref: Chapter No. 35, Page No. 832

110. Ans: B. Mammography is the initial investigation in evaluation of angiosarcoma

Ref: Chapter No. 35, Page No. 832

111. Ans: C. Tis

Ref: Chapter No. 35, Page No. 833

112. Ans: D. T4d

Ref: Chapter No. 35, Page No. 833

113. Ans: C. > 5 cm

Ref: Chapter No. 35, Page No. 833

114. Ans: C. 1 to 5 mm

Ref: Chapter No. 35, Page No. 833

115. Ans: B. T4a N2 M0

Ref: Chapter No. 35, Page No. 833

116. Ans: C. Preservation of pectoralis muscles

Ref: Chapter No. 35, Page No. 834

117. Ans: A. ER positive, node negative

Ref: Chapter No. 35, Page No. 835

118. Ans: D. Gonads

Ref: Chapter No. 35, Page No. 835

119. Ans: C. Systemic scleroderma

Ref: Chapter No. 35, Page No. 836

120. Ans: C. Pregnancy

Ref: Chapter No. 35, Page No. 836

121. Ans: B. Noncompliant to surveillance

Ref: Chapter No. 35, Page No. 836

122. Ans: C. Lumpectomy, axillary dissection, chemotherapy and radiation therapy delayed until delivery

Ref: Chapter No. 35, Page No. 836

123. Ans: A. 3 – 5%

Ref: Chapter No. 35, Page No. 836

124. Ans: D. Atypical hyperplasia and LCIS at resection margins increase local recurrence rates

Ref: Chapter No. 35, Page No. 836

125. Ans: C. Excisional biopsy of lesion

Ref: Chapter No. 35, Page No. 836

126. Ans: C. Radiation therapy

Ref: Chapter No. 35, Page No. 836

127. Ans: A. Local recurrence rates after BCS and radiation therapy are more than 5%

Ref: Chapter No. 35, Page No. 836-837

128. Ans: B. Absolute breast volume that will be resected

Ref: Chapter No. 35, Page No. 838

129. Ans: D. J or V plasty

Ref: Chapter No. 35, Page No. 838

130. Ans: B. Batwing resection

Ref: Chapter No. 35, Page No. 838

131. Ans: C. Lower inner quadrant

Ref: Chapter No. 35, Page No. 838

132. Ans: B. It has been associated with delay in delivery of adjuvant systemic therapy or radiation

Ref: Chapter No. 35, Page No. 838

133. Ans: C. Any case of invasive carcinoma

Ref: Chapter No. 35, Page No. 838

134. Ans: A. Removal of the mammary gland without pectoral fascia

Ref: Chapter No. 35, Page No. 838

135. Ans. D. In a modified radical mastectomy, level I to III axillary lymph nodes are taken with the axillary breast tissue

Ref: Chapter No. 35, Page No. 838-839

136. Ans: D. SLND considered to be less accurate in patients treated with preoperative chemotherapy

Ref: Chapter No. 35, Page No. 840-842

137. Ans: B. 11%

Ref: Chapter No. 35, Page No. 842

138. Ans: A. Subareolar or subdermal injection technique shows drainage of lymph to the axilla or the internal mammary nodal basin

Ref: Chapter No. 35, Page No. 842

139. Ans: C. If axillary metastasis is confirmed by FNAB, patient can proceed to sentinel node surgery for staging

Ref: Chapter No. 35, Page No. 842-843

140. Ans: D. Clinically negative sentinel lymph node micrometastasis

Ref: Chapter No. 35, Page No. 843

141. Ans: C. Size of the tumor

Ref: Chapter No. 35, Page No. 843

142. Ans: B. Total mastectomy with SLND

Ref: Chapter No. 35, Page No. 843

143. Ans: B. 1 – 2% per year

Ref: Chapter No. 35, Page No. 843

144. Ans: B. Radiation therapy in DCIS

Ref: Chapter No. 35, Page No. 844

145. Ans: D. Lymph node involvement

Ref: Chapter No. 35, Page No. 844

146. Ans: B. Small lesions < 2 cm

Ref: Chapter No. 35, Page No. 844

147. Ans: B. Age 40 years or older

Ref: Chapter No. 35, Page No. 845

148. Ans: B. Age ≥ 60 years

Ref: Chapter No. 35, Page No. 846

149. Ans: C. Neoadjuvant chemotherapy has been given

Ref: Chapter No. 35, Page No. 846

150. Ans: D. Invasive ductal carcinoma

Ref: Chapter No. 35, Page No. 846

151. Ans: C. Oncotype Dx recurrence scores of less than 16

Ref: Chapter No. 35, Page No. 847

152. Ans. C. DNA ploidy

Ref: Chapter No. 35, Page No. 847

153. Ans: D. > 25

Ref: Chapter No. 35, Page No. 847

154. Ans: C. Cardiac dysfunction resulting from anthracyclines is dose independent

Ref: Chapter No. 35, Page No. 847

155. Ans: D. Long-term increased risk of second cancer

Ref: Chapter No. 35, Page No. 847

156. Ans: C. Radiation and anti hormonal therapy

Ref: Chapter No. 35, Page No. 847

157. Ans: C. 3 years of treatment as standard of care

Ref: Chapter No. 35, Page No. 848-849

158. Ans: A. 1

Ref: Chapter No. 35, Page No. 848

159. Ans: B. Wide local excision, SLND, radiation and adjuvant chemotherapy with trastuzumab

Ref: Chapter No. 35, Page No. 848

160. Ans: D. Any of the above

Ref: Chapter No. 35, Page No. 849

161. Ans: D. Endocrine therapy is recommended for 5 years

Ref: Chapter No. 35, Page No. 849

162. Ans: D. 10 years

Ref: Chapter No. 35, Page No. 849

163. Ans: D. Any of the above

Ref: Chapter No. 35, Page No. 849

164. Ans: B. Neoadjuvant therapy significantly reduces the rate of in-breast recurrence

Ref: Chapter No. 35, Page No. 850

165. Ans: A. It is safe to omit ALND if the sentinel lymph node is negative

Ref: Chapter No. 35, Page No. 851

166. Ans: D. IVA

Ref: Chapter No. 35, Page No. 851

167. Ans: D. Separately palpable axillary lymph nodes

Ref: Chapter No. 35, Page No. 851

168. Ans: C. Edema of skin due to dermal lymphatic obstruction

Ref: Chapter No. 35, Page No. 851

169. Ans: D. SLND is recommended in all cases of inflammatory carcinoma

Ref: Chapter No. 35, Page No. 851

170. Ans: A. Pathologic hallmark of inflammatory cancer is the presence of tumor cells within dermal lymphatics is a prerequisite for diagnosis

Ref: Chapter No. 35, Page No. 851

171. Ans. C. Spread from the areola onto the nipple

Ref: Chapter No. 35, Page No. 852

172. Ans: C. Less than 50% of patients with Paget's disease have an underlying breast carcinoma

Ref: Chapter No. 35, Page No. 852

173. Ans: C. Skin biopsy

Ref: Chapter No. 35, Page No. 852

174. Ans: D. > 95%

Ref: Chapter No. 35, Page No. 852

175. Ans: C. 4 – 6 months

Ref: Chapter No. 35, Page No. 852

176. Ans: A. < 1%

Ref: Chapter No. 35, Page No. 852

177. Ans: C. Gynecomastia

Ref: Chapter No. 35, Page No. 852

178. Ans: B. Invasive ductal carcinoma

Ref: Chapter No. 35, Page No. 852

179. Ans: C. Poor survival outcome in men with breast cancer as compared to women of same age and stage

Ref: Chapter No. 35, Page No. 852

180. Ans: A. Detected most commonly in age 60 to 70 years

Ref: Chapter No. 35, Page No. 852

36

Breast Reconstruction

1. **Most common cancer in females:**
   A. Lung B. Breast
   C. Colorectal D. Uterine

2. **ACS guidelines for screening of breast cancer, recommends annual mammogram from age:**
   A. 30 years B. 35 years
   C. 40 years D. 45 years

3. **According to ACS guidelines of breast cancer screening, following are recommended except:**
   A. Annual mammograms from age 45 and older
   B. Women aged 40 to 44 should be given the opportunity to begin screening earlier according to the qualified recommendation
   C. Women 55 and older may switch to biennial screening but should be given the option to continue annual screening if they prefer
   D. Screening mammography should continue so long as a woman is healthy and life expectancy is 20 years or longer

ONCOPLASTIC TECHNIQUES

4. **Following are the goals of oncoplastic breast reconstruction techniques except:**
   A. Obliteration of dead space
   B. Vascular support of the nipple
   C. Aesthetically acceptable shape
   D. Prevention of disease recurrence

5. **Following are the oncoplastic breast reconstruction techniques except:**
   A. Mastopexy
   B. Breast augmentation
   C. Intrinsic tissue rearrangement
   D. Adjacent tissue transfer

6. **Which is false about fat grafting for breast reconstruction?**
   A. Low complications rate
   B. Readily available donor sites
   C. Can be performed in outpatient setting
   D. Cannot be used at radiated fields

POSTMASTECTOMY RECONSTRUCTION

7. **Following are relative contraindications for breast implants except:**
   A. Old age
   B. Very large breast
   C. Unwilling to follow-up
   D. Need for adjuvant radiation therapy

8. **Which of the following is not a contraindication for breast implants?**
   A. Young age
   B. Small breast
   C. Previous failed implants
   D. Very ptotic breast

9. **Most commonly done procedure for contralateral breast following unilateral breast reconstruction is:**
   A. Breast reduction B. Mastopexy
   C. Breast augmentation D. Locoregional flap

10. **What is the ideal method of reconstruction in a patient with prior chest wall irradiation?**
    A. Breast implant
    B. Mastopexy
    C. Autologous reconstruction
    D. Fat grafting

11. **Which autologous flap has most advantages in breast reconstruction?**

A. Transverse rectus abdominis muscle flap
B. Deep inferior epigastric perforator flap
C. Latissimus dorsi musculocutaneous flap
D. Thoracoepigastric flap

12. All are advantages of breast implants except:

A. Shorter recovery time
B. Usefulness in prior irradiated breast
C. Bilateral reconstruction
D. Shorter time for procedure

13. Direct-to-implant breast reconstruction may be considered in following conditions except:

A. Young age
B. Thin body habitus
C. Large breast
D. Non-smoker

14. Which of the following is disadvantage of prepectoral implant placement over subpectoral placement?

A. Capsular contracture
B. Surgical site infection
C. Hematoma formation
D. Reconstructive failure

15. Following are risk factors for post implant complications except:

A. Radiation
B. Small breast size
C. Smoking
D. Obesity

16. Following are the indications for latissimus dorsi pedicle based flap reconstruction except:

A. Previous abdominal surgery
B. Breast of all sizes
C. Salvage of previous breast reconstruction
D. Minor breast ptosis

17. Latissimus dorsi pedicle flap is preferred over TRAM in which of the following condition?

A. Breasts of all sizes
B. Significant breast ptosis
C. Bilateral reconstruction
D. Salvage of previous breast reconstruction

18. What is an absolute contraindication for TRAM pedicle flap?

A. Obesity
B. Previous abdominal surgery
C. Previous abdominoplasty
D. Abdominal liposuction

19. Which is false regarding TRAM pedicle flap breast reconstruction?

A. TRAM flap is based on the superior epigastric vessels
B. For unilateral breast reconstruction, usually the contralateral TRAM is used
C. Perfusion is most reliable over the TRAM on the side of the pedicle
D. The potential for complete flap loss

20. What is supercharged TRAM flap?

A. TRAM and latissimus dorsi composite flap
B. TRAM flap with two vascular pedicles
C. Deep inferior epigatric vessels anastomosed with the internal mammary in the chest
D. TRAM flap with implant placement

21. What is turbocharged TRAM flap?

A. TRAM and latissimus dorsi composite flap
B. TRAM flap with two vascular pedicles
C. Deep inferior epigastric vessels anastomosed with the internal mammary in the chest
D. TRAM flap with implant placement

22. Gracilis flap is based on which vessel?

A. Superficial femoral artery
B. Profunda femoris artery
C. External obturator artery
D. Inferior epigastric artery

23. Following findings are consistent with arterial insufficiency of flap except:

A. Pale flap
B. Edematous
C. Delayed capillary refill of more than 2 seconds
D. Cold flap

24. Following findings are consistent with venous congestion of flap except:

A. Hyperemic or purple
B. Edematous
C. Warm flap
D. Rapid capillary refill of more than 2 seconds

25. Which is the most reliable method of flap monitoring?

A. Physical examination
B. Doppler examination
C. Fluorescent angiography
D. Near-infrared spectroscopy

26. What are stacked flap?

A. Pedicle flap with two vascular pedicles
B. Pedicle flap with microvascular anastomosis to regional vessel
C. Two flaps anastomosed in continuity, performing intra-flap anastomosis
D. Free flap with two vascular pedicles

27. What should be the time interval for revision surgery post breast reconstruction procedure?

A. 3 months
B. 6 months
C. 9 months
D. 12 months

ANSWERS

1. **Ans: B. Breast**
Ref: Chapter No. 36, Page No. 856

2. **Ans: D. 45 years**
Ref: Chapter No. 36, Page No. 856

3. **Ans: D. Screening mammography should continue so long as a woman is healthy and life expectancy is 20 years or longer**
Ref: Chapter No. 36, Page No. 856

4. **Ans: D. Prevention of disease recurrence**
Ref: Chapter No. 36, Page No. 856

5. **Ans: B. Breast augmentation**
Ref: Chapter No. 36, Page No. 856

6. **Ans: D. Cannot be used at radiated fields**
Ref: Chapter No. 36, Page No. 857

7. **Ans: A. Old age**
Ref: Chapter No. 36, Page No. 858

8. **Ans: B. Small breast**
Ref: Chapter No. 36, Page No. 858

9. **Ans: A. Breast reduction**
Ref: Chapter No. 36, Page No. 858

10. **Ans: C. Autologous reconstruction**
Ref: Chapter No. 36, Page No. 858

11. **Ans: B. Deep inferior epigastric perforator flap**
Ref: Chapter No. 36, Page No. 858

12. **Ans: B. Usefulness in prior irradiated breast**
Ref: Chapter No. 36, Page No. 858

13. **Ans: C. Large breast**
Ref: Chapter No. 36, Page No. 859

14. **Ans: B. Surgical site infection**
Ref: Chapter No. 36, Page No. 859

15. **Ans: B. Small breast size**
Ref: Chapter No. 36, Page No. 860

16. **Ans: B. Breast of all sizes**
Ref: Chapter No. 36, Page No. 861

17. **Ans: D. Salvage of previous breast reconstruction**
Ref: Chapter No. 36, Page No. 861

18. **Ans: C. Previous abdominoplasty**
Ref: Chapter No. 36, Page No. 862

19. **Ans: D. The potential for complete flap loss**
Ref: Chapter No. 36, Page No. 861-862

20. **Ans: B. TRAM flap with two vascular pedicles**
Ref: Chapter No. 36, Page No. 862

21. **Ans: C. Deep inferior epigastric vessels anastomosed with the internal mammary in the chest**
Ref: Chapter No. 36, Page No. 862

22. **Ans: B. Profunda femoris artery**
Ref: Chapter No. 36, Page No. 865

23. **Ans: B. Edematous**
Ref: Chapter No. 36, Page No. 865

24. **Ans: D. Rapid capillary refill of more than 2 seconds**
Ref: Chapter No. 36, Page No. 866

25. **Ans: A. Physical examination**
Ref: Chapter No. 36, Page No. 866

26. **Ans: C. Two flaps anastomosed in continuity, performing intra-flap anastomosis**
Ref: Chapter No. 36, Page No. 867

27. **Ans: A. 3 months**
Ref: Chapter No. 36, Page No. 870

37

Thyroid

HISTORY

1. **Who coined the term thyroid?**
   A. Thomas Wharton B. Wilhelm Fabricius
   C. Pierre Dessault D. Johann Gudenus

2. **Who is the father of modern thyroid surgery?**
   A. Theodor Kocher B. Theodor Billroth
   C. William Halsted D. Charles Mayo

3. **Who is the father of modern surgery?**
   A. Theodor Kocher B. Theodor Billroth
   C. William Halsted D. Charles Mayo

4. **What is Dunhill procedure?**
   A. Thyroid lobectomy
   B. Total thyroidectomy
   C. Thyroid lobectomy with isthmectomy
   D. Unilateral thyroid lobectomy with contralateral subtotal lobectomy

EMBRYOLOGY AND ANATOMY

5. **Which statement is incorrect regarding thyroid gland development?**
   A. The thyroglossal duct becomes a solid structure in the fifth week
   B. Thyroid hormone produced by the twelfth week of gestation
   C. Median thyroid anlage becomes a bilobed diverticulum with a median tubal structure called the thyroglossal duct
   D. The lateral thyroid anlage comprises cells of the ultimobranchial bodies

6. **Thyroid hormone production begins by which week of gestation?**
   A. 8 B. 10
   C. 12 D. 14

7. **All are true about thyroglossal duct cyst except:**
   A. Hyoid bone forms starting at the seventh week of gestation
   B. Thyroglossal duct cyst typically presents as a painless lateral neck mass
   C. Sistrunk procedure is the surgical treatment of choice
   D. Central portion of the hyoid bone resection is carried out

8. **Which is wrong about ectopic thyroid tissue?**
   A. Aberrant thyroid tissue can be found from the base of tongue down to the posterior mediastinum
   B. Aberrant thyroid tissue is abnormal and often associated with inadequate thyroid hormone production
   C. Foci of normal thyroid tissue along the thyrothymic tract are typically referred to as thyroid rests
   D. These rests can occur in up to 50% of people and are typically not pathologic

9. **Ectopic thyroid tissue is found at following locations except:**
   A. Lingual
   B. Infrahyoid
   C. Isthmus
   D. Posterior mediastinum

10. **All are true about anatomy of thyroid gland except:**
    A. Adult gland typically weighing about 20g
    B. Isthmus is 2-3 mm thick and draped over the upper trachea just caudal to the cricoid cartilage

C. Ligament of Berry extends superiorly from the isthmus and represents the caudal remnant of the thyroglossal duct
D. Small posterolateral projection of lobe known as the tubercle of Zuckerkandl

11. The caudal remnant of the thyroglossal duct is:

A. Ligament of Berry
B. Pyramidal lobe
C. Tubercle of Zuckerkandl
D. Isthmus

12. Which is false about arterial supply of thyroid?

A. Superior thyroid arteries originate from the external carotid arteries and divide as they enter the superior poles
B. Inferior thyroid arteries are branches from the thyrocervical trunks of the subclavian arteries
C. In about 2% of people, a third artery called the thyroid ima artery arises directly from the aorta or innominate artery
D. RLN typically crosses the superior thyroid artery perpendicularly as it travels into the larynx is an important landmark

13. Thyroid ima artery is present in ___% of people.

A. 0.5% B. 2%
C. 4% D. 5%

14. All are true about vascular supply of thyroid except:

A. Branches of the inferior and superior arteries also supply the parathyroid glands
B. The superior thyroid veins drain into the internal jugular veins
C. The inferior thyroid veins drain into the innominate veins
D. The middle thyroid vein is constant and drain into the innominate vein

15. Which is false about level VI lymph nodes of thyroid?

A. Laterally bounded by sternocleidomastoid muscles
B. The hyoid bone superiorly
C. Sternal notch inferiorly
D. Skip metastases avoid Level VI and extend directly to the lateral neck in less than 15%

16. Injury to the external branch of superior laryngeal nerve results in:

A. High pitch
B. Low pitch
C. Vocal cord adduction
D. Vocal cord abduction

17. RLN supplies all of the muscles of larynx except:

A. Thyroarytenoid
B. Posterior cricoarytenoid
C. Cricothyroid
D. Vocalis

18. Which is incorrect regarding the course of RLN?

A. Right RLN travels in a slightly anterior plane and an oblique direction in the tracheoesophageal groove
B. Left RLN travels relatively deep and straight in the tracheoesophageal groove
C. The tubercle of Zuckerkandl typically lies just posterior and medial to the nerve
D. RLN may branch more proximally in up to 20%–30% and preservation of all of the branches is important

19. Which of the following condition is associated with right non recurrent laryngeal nerve?

A. Double aortic arch
B. Right pulmonary sling
C. Aberrant right subclavian artery
D. Right aortic arch

20. A right-sided non-RLN occurs in up to ___% of people.

A. 0.1% B. 1%
C. 5% D. 10%

HISTOLOGY AND PHYSIOLOGY

21. All are true about thyroid histology except:

A. Predominant type is the follicular cell, which is responsible for the production and secretion of thyroid hormone
B. Parafollicular C cell secretes calcitonin
C. Colloid is made up of thyroglobulin (Tg), which is the non-iodinated precursor to active thyroid hormone
D. Parafollicular C cell are mainly found in the medial aspect of the mid and upper thyroid lobes

22. False about thyroid hormone synthesis:

A. Follicular cells actively transport iodide anion via the Na/I symporter membrane protein
B. Colloid contains the enzyme thyroid peroxidase, which is required for iodination of tyrosine residues on thyroglobulin

C. T3 is the more potent form
D. The average daily iodine requirement for adult humans is 1 mg

23. What is daily requirement of iodine for an adult human?

A. 0.1 mg B. 0.7 mg
C. 1 mg D. 1.5 mg

24. All are true regarding calcitonin functions except:

A. It functions by increasing osteoblast and decreasing osteoclast activity
B. It decreases calcium absorption from the gut
C. It increases urinary calcium excretion
D. Absence of calcitonin cause significant change in calcium homeostasis

25. 5′-Deiodinase type II enzyme is present in all of the following tissue except:

A. Pituitary gland B. Brain
C. Liver D. Brown fat

26. Which tissue shows presence of 5′-Deiodinase type I enzyme?

A. Liver B. Kidney
C. Brain D. Both A and B

27. Which is incorrect concerning thyroid hormone function during pregnancy?

A. Thyroid hormone is required for neuronal and brain development of fetus
B. Transient gestational thyrotoxicosis occurring only in the first trimester
C. Free T4 levels are increased during first trimester
D. Hypothyroidism is the most common type of thyroid dysfunction in pregnancy

28. Most common cause of hyperthyroidism during pregnancy:

A. Trophoblastic disease
B. Graves' disease
C. Toxic multinodular goiter
D. Toxic adenoma

29. Most common cause of hypothyroidism during pregnancy in iodine-replete areas:

A. Hashimoto thyroiditis
B. De Quervain disease
C. Drug induced hypothyroidism
D. Multinodular goiter

30. Hypothyroidism in pregnancy, occurring in up to ___% of pregnant women.

A. 0.5% B. 1%
C. 3% D. 5%

31. All are characteristics of euthyroid sick syndrome except:

A. Low serum T3 concentrations with relatively normal to slightly elevated TSH concentrations
B. Signs of clinical thyroid dysfunction
C. Decreased activity of peripheral deiodinase type 2 enzyme
D. Treating the underlying condition resolves abnormal thyroid function tests

32. Euthyroid sick syndrome is seen in patients with:

A. Myocardial infarction
B. Thermal injury
C. Trauma
D. All of the above

THYROID BIOMARKERS

33. False regarding Thyroid stimulating hormone:

A. TSH is a peptide hormone secreted from the anterior pituitary gland
B. It is secreted in pulsatile fashion
C. Measurement of serum TSH is the most common and reliable test for screening for thyroid dysfunction
D. TSH secretion follows a log-linear relationship

34. What is normal range of serum TSH for adults?

A. 9 -23 pmol/L B. 3 -7 pmol/L
C. 0.4 – 5.5 mIU/L D. 11 – 21 ng/dL

35. Which of the following has most accurate interpretability in diagnosing and monitoring of thyroid dysfunction?

A. Free T3
B. Free T4
C. Serum TSH
D. Serum TSH and free T4

36. Which of the following is false regarding antibody assay in thyroid dysfunction?

A. Measurement of TgAb is the most accurate and commonly used screening test for autoimmune thyroiditis
B. The presence of TgAb interferes with the interpretation of Tg measurement for the surveillance of differentiated thyroid cancer

C. Measurement of TRAb is typically reserved for diagnostic confirmation of Graves disease
D. Thyroid-stimulating immunoglobulin (TSI) bioassay, which more specifically detects the stimulatory subtype of TRAb

37. Which is the most accurate and commonly used screening test for autoimmune thyroiditis?

A. Anti-TPO (TPOAb)
B. Anti-Tg (TgAb)
C. Anti-TSH receptor (TRAb)
D. Thyroid-stimulating immunoglobulin (TSI) bioassay

38. Which is false about thyroglobulin assay?

A. Thyroglobulin is a large 660-kDa glycosylated protein
B. Serum Tg measurement after total thyroidectomy is the most sensitive cancer biomarker for DTC
C. The accuracy of serum Tg testing is highly dependent upon the absence of TgAb
D. TgAb is present in 1% to 5% of the general population

39. Serum calcitonin is used as biomarker for the detection of which thyroid cancer?

A. Follicular thyroid cancer
B. Medullary thyroid cancer
C. Anaplastic thyroid cancer
D. Hurthle cell cancer

THYROID IMAGING

40. All are true regarding thyroid imaging except:

A. The normal sonographic appearance of the thyroid is homogeneously echogenic with a uniform echotexture
B. Nuclear scintigraphy is useful for the differential diagnosis of hypothyroidism
C. CT has important role in substernal (intrathoracic) goiter and advanced thyroid cancer
D. PET is mainly used for surveillance and staging of RAI-refractory DTC

41. Risk of malignancy associated with cold nodule on thyroid uptake scan is ___%.

A. 5% B. 10%
C. 15% D. 20%

HYPOTHYROIDISM

42. Most common cause of hypothyroidism:

A. Autoimmune B. Iodine-deficiency
C. Iatrogenic D. Idiopathic

43. Following are the symptoms of hypothyroidism except:

A. Heat intolerance B. Dry skin
C. Myxedema D. Lethargy

44. Which of the following is false about primary hypothyroidism?

A. Serum TSH is highly sensitive for screening for hypothyroidism
B. Decreased free T4 and T3 levels are diagnostic
C. Levothyroxine is recommended as the first-line therapy
D. Levothyroxine can be administered subcutaneously

45. Which is incorrect concerning Hashimoto's thyroiditis?

A. It is also known as acute lymphocytic thyroiditis
B. Female-to-male incidence is 10:1
C. First-degree relatives of Hashimoto's patients have a nine-fold risk of developing the disease
D. Presence of circulating autoantibodies to thyroid antigens which results in deposition of immune complexes and complement in the basement membrane of follicular cells

46. First-degree relatives of Hashimoto's patients have _____ risk of developing the disease.

A. 3-fold B. 6-fold
C. 9-fold D. 18-fold

47. Which is false regarding diagnosis of Hashimoto's thyroiditis?

A. Measurement of circulating TPOAb and TgAb autoantibodies
B. There is no role for imaging studies in the workup and diagnosis
C. Sonographic characteristics include hyperechoic parenchymal echotexture
D. Cytological features include a moderately cellular specimen with minimal colloid and infiltration of mature lymphocytes

48. Following are the sonographic features of Hashimoto's thyroiditis:

A. Coarse, heterogeneous and hypoechoic parenchymal echotexture
B. Increased vascularity
C. Fine echogenic septae producing a pseudonodular appearance
D. All of the above

49. **Hashimoto thyroiditis has an increased risk for development of which thyroid cancer?**

A. Follicular B. Papillary
C. Hurthle cell D. Anaplastic

50. **Which is incorrect regarding postpartum autoimmune thyroiditis?**

A. It occurs within the first 2 months of the postpartum period
B. It is often associated with the presence of circulating TPOAb
C. Postpartum thyroiditis is associated with a tenfold risk of ultimately developing Hashimoto thyroiditis
D. Postpartum thyroiditis is typically short-lived, with resolution in 2 to 4 months

51. **Postpartum autoimmune thyroiditis is seen in __% of women.**

A. 1% B. 5%
C. 10% D. 15%

52. **de Quervain disease is also known as:**

A. Acute suppurative thyroiditis
B. Subacute granulomatous thyroiditis
C. Acute lymphocytic thyroiditis
D. Chronic granulomatous thyroiditis

53. **All are true about de Quervain disease except:**

A. It is found primarily in the underdeveloped countries
B. Female-to-male incidence is 2:1
C. It often occurs after a viral prodrome of URTI
D. Elevated erythrocyte sedimentation rate is diagnostic

54. **All are true about de Quervain disease except:**

A. The hallmark of the clinical presentation is pain and swelling in the thyroid region
B. It is associated with transient hyperthyroidism followed by hypothyroidism
C. Surgery is not indicated due to its self-limited course
D. Corticosteroids are contraindicated for the treatment

55. **All are associated with de Quervain thyroiditis except:**

A. Pain
B. Fever
C. Increased RAI uptake
D. Increased ESR

56. **Histopathologic finding of de Quervain disease shows:**

A. Mononuclear infiltrate
B. Histiocyte infiltrate
C. Giant cell infiltrate
D. Lymphocytic infiltrate

57. **Which of the following statement is false about Riedel thyroiditis?**

A. It is known as chronic fibrous thyroiditis
B. An extremely firm and constricting gland
C. Fibrotic process limited to thyroid gland
D. Medical treatment consists of corticosteroids and tamoxifen

58. **Tamoxifen is used in the treatment of:**

A. de Quervain disease
B. Riedel's thyroiditis
C. Hashimoto's thyroiditis
D. Autoimmune thyroiditis

59. **Most common cause of acute pyogenic infection of thyroid:**

A. Infection of thyroglossal cyst
B. Infection of a congenital pyriform sinus fistula
C. Retropharyngeal abscess
D. Tracheobronchial fistula

60. **All of the following drugs inhibit thyroid hormone synthesis except:**

A. Lithium B. Amiodarone
C. Perchlorate D. Dopamine

61. **Which of the following drug inhibit peripheral conversion of T4 to T3?**

A. Propylthiouracil
B. Methimazole
C. Carbimazole
D. Both A and B

62. **Which is false about drugs causing iatrogenic hypothyroidism?**

A. RAI therapy leads to direct destruction of the thyroid follicular cells

B. Methimazole directly inhibit T4 and T3 synthesis
C. Lithium may act by directly inhibiting the cAMP-dependent pathway in thyroid hormone synthesis
D. Sorafenib causes direct destructive autoimmune thyroiditis

63. All of the following drugs causes hypothyroidism except:

A. Alemtuzumab B. Nivolumab
C. Pembrolizumab D. Certolizumab

64. All of the following drugs causes hypothyroidism except:

A. Interferon gamma B. Interleukin 2
C. Ipilimumab D. Interferon alpha

65. Which of the following drug causes TSH suppression?

A. Sunitinib B. Dopamine
C. Guaifenesin D. Potassium iodide

66. Which of the following drug causes destructive thyroiditis?

A. Sunitinib B. Sorafenib
C. Bexarotene D. Lithium

67. Sorafenib increases which enzyme activity?

A. Type 1 deiodinase B. Type 2 deiodinase
C. Type 3 deiodinase D. Thyroid peroxidase

68. Which drug causes TSH suppression and T4 clearance?

A. Sorafenib B. Bexarotene
C. Aminoglutethimide D. Nivolumab

HYPERTHYROIDISM

69. Subclinical hyperthyroidism is characterized by:

A. Suppressed TSH
B. Normal free T4 and T3
C. Clinically significant symptoms or signs
D. All of the above

70. Which is false regarding Graves' disease?

A. It is an autoimmune disease characterized by the constitutive activation of the TSH receptor by TRAb
B. Female-to-male incidence is 4:1
C. Typically presents between 20 and 40 years of age
D. The most common manifestation is Graves orbitopathy

71. Graves' disease characterized by following findings except:

A. Suppressed TSH, elevated free T4 and T3
B. Presence of TPOAb
C. Sonographic features may include a diffusely hypervascular gland, often with heterogeneous echogenicity
D. Nuclear scintigraphy shows diffuse uptake pattern

72. Patient presented with bilateral proptosis, palpitation and acropachy. What is probable diagnosis?

A. Hashimoto's thyroiditis
B. Riedel's thyroiditis
C. Graves' disease
D. Endemic goiter

73. Graves orbitopathy occurs in up to ____% of patients with Graves' disease.

A. 5 – 10% B. 15 – 20%
C. 25 – 30% D. 35 – 40%

74. Following are indications of thyroidectomy in Graves' disease except:

A. Presence of severe eye disease
B. Pregnancy or breastfeeding state
C. Presence of concomitant suspicious thyroid nodules
D. Lifelong requirement of medical therapy

75. What is recurrence of Graves' disease with subtotal thyroidectomy?

A. 1 – 5% B. 5 – 10%
C. 10 – 15% D. 15 – 20%

76. All of the following are the causes of hyperthyroidism associated with increased RAI uptake except:

A. Graves' disease
B. Toxic multinodular goiter
C. Subacute thyroiditis
D. TSH-producing pituitary adenoma

77. Which of the following is associated with increased RAI uptake?

A. Amiodarone-induced thyroiditis
B. Graves' disease
C. Struma ovarii
D. Iatrogenic thyrotoxicosis

78. Radioactive iodine therapy is contraindicated in all except:

A. Pregnancy
B. Patients with periodic paralysis
C. Active Graves ophthalmopathy
D. Confirmed or suspected thyroid malignancy

79. Radioactive iodine therapy is preferred treatment in all except:

A. Limited life expectancy
B. Liver disease
C. Previously operated or externally irradiated neck
D. One or more large thyroid nodules

80. What is the rate of permanent RLN injury during total thyroidectomy?

A. 2% B. 5%
C. 7% D. 10%

81. Which is false about preoperative preparation of thyroidectomy surgery?

A. Patients should ideally be rendered euthyroid prior to thyroidectomy
B. Methimazole was found to be associated with liver failure
C. Lugol solution can be given for 7 to 10 days prior to surgery, which rapidly achieve euthyroid state
D. Preoperative supplementation with calcitriol decreases the postoperative risk of transient hypocalcemia

82. Which of the following is known as Plummer disease?

A. Toxic adenoma
B. Toxic multinodular goiter
C. Chronic fibrous thyroiditis
D. Sporadic multinodular goiter

83. Which is incorrect regarding toxic multinodular goiter?

A. One or more autonomously functioning nodules in nodular thyroid gland
B. Female predominance, with an approximately 5:1 female-to-male ratio
C. Affects adults below the age of 50 years
D. These "warm" or "hot" nodules are rarely malignant and do not require biopsy

84. Which is the first line imaging modality in toxic multinodular goiter?

A. USG
B. FNAC
C. Nuclear scintigraphy
D. CT neck

85. Which is false about management of toxic multinodular goiter?

A. Antithyroid medication is generally not advocated as a long-term management strategy
B. Autonomous nodules undergo remission with medical therapy
C. RAI with 131-I is the most commonly used definitive treatment
D. Lugol solutions are not indicated preoperatively

86. All are true about solitary toxic adenoma except:

A. Single autonomously functioning nodule existing within an otherwise normal or non toxic nodular thyroid
B. Activating mutations in the TSH receptor gene
C. Female predominance
D. Near-total thyroidectomy as definitive treatment

87. All are true regarding amiodarone-induced thyrotoxicosis (AIT) except:

A. An iodine-rich compound with structural similarities to T4
B. Normal dosing schedule can deliver over 100 times the daily dietary iodine requirement
C. It occurs in up to 6% of patients taking this medication
D. Type 1 AIT is caused by the Wolff-Chaikoff phenomenon

88. Amiodarone contains ___% of iodine content by molecular weight.

A. 17% B. 27%
C. 37% D. 47%

89. Which is false about amiodarone-induced thyrotoxicosis (AIT)?

A. Type 1 AIT is caused by the Jod-Basedow phenomenon
B. Type 1 AIT is more common in patients with preexisting hypothyroid disease
C. Type 2 AIT usually occurs in patients with preexisting normal thyroid
D. Type 2 AIT caused by a destructive thyroiditis from direct drug toxicity leading to release of preformed thyroid hormone

NONTOXIC GOITER

90. Following are consistent with nontoxic goiter except:

A. Benign, non-inflammatory condition
B. Persistent TSH stimulation

C. Diffuse enlargement of thyroid gland
D. Elevated free T4 and T3

91. Which is incorrect about substernal goiter?

A. The incidence of substernal goiter is estimated at 0.02%
B. The most common subtype extends into the anterior mediastinum
C. Least common subtype is the isolated mediastinal goiter with unique blood supply from the chest
D. Vocal cord paralysis is more likely to occur due to RLN compression

92. All features are consistent with isolated mediastinal goiter except:

A. It is least common subtype of substernal goiter
B. Connection to the normal cervical orthotopic gland
C. Unique blood supply from the chest
D. Minor enlargement may cause significant tracheal compressive symptoms

93. Which of the following feature is not consistent with substernal goiter?

A. Shortness of breath
B. Dysphagia
C. Vocal cord paralysis
D. Thoracic outlet syndrome

94. Which of the following is incorrect about management of substernal goiter?

A. Every nodule of at least 1 cm should be evaluated for suspicious sonographic features and by FNAC
B. Cross-sectional imaging with either CT or MRI is essential for the preoperative assessment
C. Asymptomatic smaller goiters may need for lifelong suppression with levothyroxine
D. RAI is suitable for larger goiters

95. Absolute indication for thyroidectomy in nontoxic goiter are all except:

A. Local compressive symptoms
B. Substernal extension
C. Presence of suspicious nodules
D. RAI refractory goiter

96. What is most common approach used for thyroidectomy in case of substernal goiter?

A. Transcervical
B. Median sternotomy
C. Anterolateral thoracotomy
D. Axillary

THYROID NODULE

97. Following are indications for surgical intervention in case of thyroid nodule except:

A. Concern for malignancy
B. Hyperfunction
C. Local compressive symptoms
D. Multinodular gland

98. Following factors increases the risk of malignancy in case of thyroid nodule except:

A. Age younger than 20 years
B. Female sex
C. Hoarseness or dysphagia
D. History of neck irradiation

99. Following factors increases the risk of malignancy in case of thyroid nodule except:

A. Age older than 70 years
B. Nodules larger than 1.5 cm
C. Cervical lymphadenopathy
D. Male sex

100. Most common malignancy of thyroid gland:

A. Follicular thyroid cancer
B. Papillary thyroid cancer
C. Medullary thyroid cancer
D. Thyroid metastases

101. Patient presented with history of palpitation and anxiety. Serum TSH levels are undetectable. What is first investigation to be done for this patient?

A. USG
B. FNA
C. Radioisotope scan
D. Upfront thyroidectomy

102. Which is wrongly matched about sonographic pattern of nodule and its risk of malignancy according to ATA?

A. Benign nodule - < 1%
B. Nodule with low Suspicion - <3%
C. Nodule with intermediate Suspicion - 10%-20%
D. Nodule with high Suspicion - 70%-90%

103. Sonographic features of thyroid nodule with highest risk of malignancy includes following except:

A. The presence of microcalcifications

B. Hypoechogenicity
C. Irregular margins
D. Wider-than-tall nodule shape

104. Thyroid nodule characteristics are stratified into how many risk levels according to TI-RADS?

A. 4 B. 5
C. 6 D. 7

105. Following features of thyroid are considered in TI-RADS scoring except:

A. Nodule composition B. Echogenicity
C. Margin D. Size

106. Following features of thyroid are considered in TI-RADS scoring except:

A. Margin B. Vascularity
C. Shape D. Echogenic foci

107. ATA or TI-RADS does not recommend routine biopsy for thyroids nodules of size less than:

A. 0.5 cm B. 1 cm
C. 1.5 cm D. 2 cm

108. Which is false about FNA cytology?

A. Most accurate and cost-effective invasive procedure
B. Sensitivity of over 95%
C. Specificity of over 90%
D. FNA is performed with 23–27 gauge needle

109. Spongiform or partially cystic nodules without any microcalcification, irregular margin is classified according to ATA as:

A. Benign
B. Very low suspicion
C. Low suspicion
D. Intermediate suspicion

110. USG thyroid of 25 years old patient shows 1.5 cm nodule in left lobe of thyroid. It has spongiform appearance with regular margin and without any solid component. Serum TSH is elevated. What is the preferred management?

A. Observation with follow up USG
B. FNAC of the nodule
C. Radioisotope scan
D. Left thyroid lobectomy

111. Sonographic features of low suspicion thyroid nodule according to ATA includes all except:

A. Isoechoic or hyperechoic solid nodule
B. Partially cystic nodule with eccentric solid areas
C. Spongiform nodule
D. Absence of microcalcification

112. All are high risk characteristics of thyroid nodule except:

A. Solid hypoechoic component of a partially cystic nodule
B. Presence of microcalcifications
C. Taller than wide shape
D. Isoechoic solid nodule

113. Risk of malignancy associated with high suspicion sonographic features of thyroid nodule:

A. 40 – 50% B. 50 – 70%
C. 70 – 90% D. >95%

114. Wrongly matched FNA size cutoff according to ATA:

A. Very low suspicion features - FNA at ≥2 cm
B. Low suspicion features - FNA at ≥1 cm
C. High suspicion features - FNA at ≥1 cm
D. Benign features - No biopsy

115. Patient presented with palpable thyroid nodule on right side. Serum TSH levels are low. USG neck shows isoechoic solid nodule of 2 cm size with smooth margin and without any microcalcification in right lobe of thyroid. No evidence of any neck lymph node enlargement. What is appropriate next step in management?

A. Observation B. FNAC of nodule
C. Radioisotope scan D. CT neck

116. Wrongly matched about TI-RADS levels:

A. TR1 – 1 point B. TR3 – 3 points
C. TR4 – 4 to 6 points D. TR5 - ≥ 7 points

117. All of the following features have highest points according to TIRADS except:

A. Completely solid Composition
B. Taller-than-wide
C. Extrathyroidal extension
D. Punctate echogenic foci

118. Bethesda system is based on:

A. Breast imaging
B. Thyroid imaging
C. Breast FNA cytology
D. Thyroid FNA cytology

119. Bethesda system of FNA cytology includes ___ categories.

A. 4 B. 5
C. 6 D. 7

120. Hurthle cell neoplasm is included in which Bethesda category?

A. Category II B. Category III
C. Category IV D. Category V

121. Follicular cell neoplasm is included in which Bethesda category?

A. Category II B. Category III
C. Category IV D. Category V

122. Large sheet of neoplastic cells with enlarged oval "Orphan Annie eye" nuclei are classified into which Bethesda category?

A. Category III B. Category IV
C. Category V D. Category VI

123. "Orphan Annie eye" nuclei are characteristic of which thyroid cancer?

A. Papillary B. Follicular
C. Medullary D. Anaplastic

124. What is the recommended management of FNAC features suggestive of atypia of undetermined significance according to Bethesda system?

A. Repeat FNA B. Molecular testing
C. Lobectomy D. All of the above

125. Molecular testing is recommended by Bethesda system for which category?

A. Category I and II B. Category II and III
C. Category III and IV D. Category V and VI

126. Risk of malignancy associated with Bethesda category IV:

A. 5%–10% B. 6%–18%
C. 10%–40% D. 45%–60%

127. Risk of malignancy associated with Bethesda category III:

A. 5%–10% B. 6%–18%
C. 10%–40% D. 45%–60%

128. Benign cytological features are classified according to Bethesda system as:

A. Category 0 B. Category I
C. Category II D. Category III

129. Afirma product, molecular test for genetic sequencing, is based on:

A. 91-gene DNA microarray
B. 91-gene mRNA microarray
C. 167-gene DNA microarray
D. 167-gene mRNA microarray

130. Which of the following statement is false regarding molecular testing for thyroid nodules?

A. It is recommended for Bethesda category III and IV
B. Afirma product has relatively poor specificity and positive predictive value
C. Genomic Sequence Classifier correctly predict Hürthle cell adenoma and carcinoma
D. ThyroSeq product employs next-generation DNA sequencing to detect the presence or absence of known gene mutations and gene fusions for thyroid cancer

131. Which molecular test detects Hürthle cell carcinoma more accurately?

A. Afirma
B. Genomic Sequence Classifier
C. ThyroSeq
D. Any of the above

THYROID CANCER

132. Differentiated thyroid cancer includes all of the following except:

A. Papillary B. Follicular
C. Medullary D. Hurthle cell

133. Which is false regarding papillary thyroid cancer?

A. Female predominance with a 3:1 female-to-male ratio
B. Peak incidence is in the third to fifth decades of life
C. Disseminates primarily via the lymphatic route
D. Distant metastases do occur in up to 23% to 25% of patients

134. Psammoma bodies are histological feature of which thyroid cancer?

A. Papillary B. Follicular
C. Medullary D. Anaplastic

135. Following are histological characteristics of papillary thyroid cancer except:

A. Pseudoinclusions

B. Nuclear grooving
C. Psammoma bodies
D. Eosinophilic granular cytoplasm

136. Distant metastases with papillary thyroid cancer seen in ___% of patients.

A. 5% B. 10%
C. 15% D. 20%

137. Following are aggressive variants of papillary thyroid cancer except:

A. Hobnail B. Follicular variant
C. Tall cell D. Diffuse sclerosing

138. Which is incorrect regarding follicular thyroid cancer?

A. Peak incidence in the fourth and sixth decades
B. Female predominance, with a 3:1 female-to-male ratio
C. The pattern of spread of FTC is lymphatic route
D. FTC cannot be reliably diagnosed by FNAC

139. All are true regarding Hurthle cell cancer except:

A. More aggressive behavior
B. Peak incidence in the sixth and seventh decades
C. HCC is less RAI-avid
D. Presence of oxyphilic Hürthle cells abundant basophilic granular cytoplasm

140. Metastases from Hurthle cell cancer occurs through:

A. Lymphatics B. Hematogenous
C. Contiguous D. Both A and B

141. Which is wrong statement about follicular variant of papillary thyroid cancer?

A. It has neoplastic follicles without papillary structures but with nuclear features characteristic of PTC
B. Encapsulated fvPTC is also known as noninvasive follicular thyroid neoplasm with papillary-like nuclear features
C. It has a similar prognosis to classical PTC and more indolent nature
D. It is considered to be a malignancy

142. Following genetic mutations are related to MAPK pathway except:

A. BRAF B. RET
C. NTRK D. MET

143. Which is incorrect about Cowden syndrome?

A. It is caused by mutations in PTEN, an inhibitor of AKT activation
B. Multiple hamartomas of the skin and mucous membranes
C. Microcephaly
D. Increased risk of breast cancer and endometrial cancer

144. Cowden syndrome is associated with which thyroid cancer variant?

A. Papillary B. Follicular
C. Medullary D. Lymphoma

145. Following are newly detected genetic alterations associated with PTC:

A. CHEK2 B. ATM
C. TERT promoter D. All of the above

146. Ionizing radiation exposure is associated with which thyroid cancer variant?

A. Papillary B. Follicular
C. Medullary D. Hurthle cell

147. Following hereditary cancer syndromes are associated with thyroid cancer except:

A. Gardner syndrome B. Turcot syndrome
C. Carney complex D. Werner syndrome

148. Following hereditary cancer syndromes are associated with thyroid cancer except:

A. Gardner syndrome B. Cowden syndrome
C. Wermer syndrome D. Carney complex

149. Gardner syndrome is associated with which variant of thyroid cancer?

A. Papillary B. Follicular
C. Medullary D. Anaplastic

150. Following are characteristics of familial non-MTC tumor except:

A. Two or more first-degree relatives diagnosed with DTC
B. Absence of other hereditary cancer syndromes
C. Aggressive and portend a worse prognosis
D. Associated with BRAF mutation

151. Risk factors for thyroid cancer are:

A. Ionizing radiation B. Obesity
C. Volcanic regions D. All of the above

152. Following are example of ALK inhibitors except:

A. Crizotinib B. Ceritinib
C. Entrectinib D. Larotrectinib

153. Lenvatinib acts on which receptor?

A. EGFR B. VEGFR
C. FGFR D. Fusion RTK

154. Following targeted drug therapy acts on RET except:

A. Sorafenib B. Lenvatinib
C. Cabozantinib D. Crizotinib

155. Vemurafenib is targeted therapy against:

A. NTRK B. BRAF
C. MEK D. VEGR

156. Following are MEK inhibitors except:

A. Selumetinib B. Trametinib
C. Gefitinib D. Combimetinib

157. False regarding changes made in AJCC 8th edition for thyroid cancer:

A. The age cutoff for staging increased to 55 years at diagnosis
B. T3a is a new category for tumors of any size, demonstrating gross extrathyroidal extension
C. The presence of distant metastases in patients 55 years of age or older was reclassified from stage IVC to stage IVB
D. N1 disease no longer upstages a patient 55 years of age or older to stage III

158. According to AJCC 8th edition for thyroid cancer, T3a includes which of the following?

A. Tumor >2 cm confined to one thyroid lobe
B. Tumor 2 – 4 cm confined to thyroid gland
C. Tumor > 4 cm confined to thyroid gland
D. Tumor any size with microscopic extrathyroidal extension

159. Tumors with following characteristics require total thyroidectomy except:

A. Tumor at least 4 cm
B. Radiation-induced DTC
C. Microscopic extrathyroidal extension
D. Familial nonmedullary thyroid cancer

160. Which of the following is false regarding surgical treatment of DTC?

A. Surgery is the mainstay of therapy for DTC
B. Ipsilateral thyroid lobectomy recommended surgical option for DTCs that are less than1 cm
C. Therapeutic lymph node dissection should be performed in patients with radiographic or clinical evidence of metastatic disease
D. Total thyroidectomy is recommended for tumors of > 2 cm

161. Risk of recurrence for thyroid DTC with clinically positive lymph node is:

A. 5% B. 10%
C. 20% D. 40%

162. 45-year-old patient presented with palpable thyroid nodule without any symptoms. After appropriate investigations tumor was staged as T3a cN0 M0. What is best management for this patient?

A. Active surveillance
B. Ipsilateral lobectomy
C. Total thyroidectomy
D. Total thyroidectomy with central neck dissection

163. 50-year-old patient presented with right sided palpable nodule with sonographic evidence of 4 cm tumor, no evidence of extrathyroidal extension and presence of right lateral lymph node enlargement. What is the appropriate management of this patient?

A. Ipsilateral thyroidectomy with EBRT to neck
B. Ipsilateral thyroidectomy with right lateral neck dissection
C. Total thyroidectomy with EBRT to neck
D. Total thyroidectomy with central and lateral neck dissection and RAI therapy

164. Post thyroidectomy serum TSH levels recommended for high risk tumors are:

A. < 0.1 mU/L B. 0.1 to 0.5 mU/L
C. 0.5 to 1.0 mU/L D. 1.0 to 1.5 mU/L

165. Post thyroidectomy serum TSH levels recommended for intermediate risk tumors are:

A. < 0.1 mU/L B. 0.1 to 0.5 mU/L
C. 0.5 to 1.0 mU/L D. 1.0 to 1.5 mU/L

166. Post thyroidectomy serum TSH levels recommended for low risk tumors are:

A. < 0.1 mU/L B. 0.1 to 0.5 mU/L
C. 0.5 to 1.0 mU/L D. 1.0 to 1.5 mU/L

167. RAI therapy is useful in following thyroid cancers except:

A. Papillary B. Follicular
C. Hurthle D. Medullary

168. Which is incorrect about benefits of RAI therapy for DTC?

A. Increases the specificity of both postoperative serum Tg and subsequent 131I scanning for detection of recurrent disease
B. Prevents subsequent de novo thyroid cancer formation
C. Prevent clinical recurrences
D. Higher benefits in low risk DTC

169. Which is incorrect about RAI therapy for DTC?

A. In DTC, RAI is typically administered post-thyroidectomy
B. To treat clinically detectable disease that cannot be addressed by surgery
C. RAI is routinely recommended for low-risk cancers
D. RAI should be administered in patients in a low-iodine state and in a setting of high TSH levels

170. RAI therapy dosage used for treatment are:

A. 30 to 50 mCi
B. 50 to 100 mCi
C. 100 to 150 mCi
D. 150 to 200 mCi

MEDULLARY THYROID CANCER

171. Histological features of MTC are as follows except:

A. Plasmacytoid morphology with eccentric round nuclei
B. Salt-and-pepper chromatin
C. Amyloid infiltrate
D. Eosinophilic granular cytoplasm

172. Which of the following marker is secreted by MTC?

A. CA19-9
B. Alpha hCG
C. Chorioembryonic antigen
D. CA125

173. Location of RET proto-oncogene:

A. Chromosome 10p11.2
B. Chromosome 11p10.2
C. Chromosome 10q11.2
D. Chromosome 11q10.2

174. Most common RET mutation associated with MTC:

A. Codon 620
B. Codon 634
C. Codon 883
D. Codon 918

175. MTC is associated with following diseases as a syndromic manifestations except:

A. Primary hyperparathyroidism
B. Cutaneous lichen amyloidosis
C. Neuroendocrine tumors
D. Hirschsprung disease

176. Which of the following statement is false about MTC with RET mutation?

A. The highest-risk category includes patients with MEN2B and the codon 918 mutation
B. The high-risk category comprises patients with the codon 634 and 883 mutations in whom thyroidectomy is recommended by the age of 5 years
C. All patients with a diagnosis of MTC should undergo genetic testing to rule out hereditary disease
D. Sporadic MTC with somatic RET mutations has good prognosis

177. Age at which total thyroidectomy is recommended for patients with MEN2B or Codon 918 RET mutation:

A. Within first year of life
B. Within 3 years of age
C. Within 5 years of age
D. Within 7 years of age

178. What serum calcitonin levels are suggestive of metastatic MTC?

A. 200 pg/mL
B. 300 pg/mL
C. 400 pg/mL
D. 500 pg/mL

179. Elevated serum calcitonin may be seen with all except:

A. Age younger than 3 years
B. Autoimmune thyroiditis
C. Lung cancer
D. Hypoparathyroidism

180. Which is incorrect concerning management of MTC?

A. Clinically evident MTC is treated with at minimum total thyroidectomy and bilateral central neck dissection
B. The role of routine lateral neck dissection is not recommended
C. ATA guidelines recommend that in patient with ipsilateral neck metastasis, prophylactic

contralateral lateral neck dissection should be considered if the basal serum calcitonin level is at least 200 pg/mL

D. Patients with familial MTC, MEN2B require four gland exploration of parathyroid

181. All are correct regarding postoperative management of MTC except:

A. MTC is associated with an overall 50% rate of disease recurrence

B. The doubling time of calcitonin is a prognostic indicator

C. Systemic chemotherapy regimens are ineffective

D. EBRT to the neck for locoregional control improves overall survival

ANAPLASTIC THYROID CANCER

182. Which is false regarding anaplastic thyroid cancer?

A. The mean age at diagnosis is 65 years

B. 2:1 female-to-male incidence ratio

C. History multinodular goiter and previous thyroidectomy exists

D. Asymptomatic with painless neck mass

183. Which of the following is not a clinical symptom of ATC?

A. Dysphagia B. Palpable neck mass

C. Painless D. Hoarseness

184. All of the following statements are true about ATC except:

A. Anaplastic thyroid cancer avidly stain for thyroglobulin

B. Cross-sectional imaging of the neck and mediastinum to assess the extent of locoregional disease is essential component

C. PET scan is recommended for a metastatic survey in the initial evaluation of ATC

D. According to the AJCC TNM system, all ATCs are considered stage IV disease

185. Following are the FDA approved tyrosine kinase inhibitors for treatment of advanced thyroid cancer except:

A. Vandetanib B. Cabozantinib

C. Sunitinib D. Lenvatinib

186. RAI therapy is most useful in which thyroid cancer?

A. Anaplastic B. Papillary

C. Medullary D. Hurthle cell

187. Which tyrosine kinase inhibitor is FDA approved for the treatment of RAI refractory DTC?

A. Sunitinib B. Sorafenib

C. Vandetanib D. Pazopanib

188. Which tyrosine kinase inhibitor is FDA approved for the treatment of RAI refractory DTC?

A. Sunitinib B. Lenvatinib

C. Vandetanib D. Cabozantinib

189. Which tyrosine kinase inhibitor is FDA approved for the treatment of advanced MTC?

A. Sorafenib B. Vandetanib

C. Lenvatinib D. Sunitinib

190. Which tyrosine kinase inhibitor is FDA approved for the treatment of advanced MTC?

A. Sorafenib B. Lenvatinib

C. Cabozantinib D. Dabrafenib

191. Which targeted therapy is FDA approved for the treatment of advanced BRAF mutated ATC?

A. Sorafenib

B. Lenvatinib

C. Dabrafenib with trametinib

D. Everolimus

192. Only FDA approved cytotoxic chemotherapy for thyroid cancer:

A. Paclitaxel B. Cisplatin

C. Doxorubicin D. Epirubicin

THYROIDECTOMY

193. What is near total thyroidectomy?

A. 1 gm of remnant is left at parathyroid gland

B. 1 gm of remnant is left at ligament of Berry

C. 8 gm of remnant is left at parathyroid gland

D. 8 gm of remnant is left at ligament of Berry

194. Which is incorrect statement regarding transcutaneous laryngeal ultrasound?

A. It has sensitivity of 93%–100%

B. It has specificity of 97%–100%

C. It has slow learning curve and it is not cost effective

D. It is less reliable in older and male patients

195. Vocal cord paralysis can be associated with a normal voice in up to ___% of cases.

A. 5% B. 10%

C. 15% D. 20%

196. Space of Reeves is present between:

A. Avascular space between medial superior pole and cricothyroid muscle
B. Avascular space between RLN and ligament of Berry
C. Avascular space between medial inferior pole and cricothyroid muscle
D. Avascular space between isthmus and ligament of Berry

197. Which is false about technique of thyroidectomy?

A. The sternothyroid may be partially or completely divided near its inferior attachment to sternum
B. The superior pole vessels are divided individually close to the surface of the thyroid
C. Branches of the inferior thyroid vessels are ligated at the surface of the thyroid gland
D. The recurrent nerve is most vulnerable at ligament of Berry

198. Most vulnerable location to injure RLN during thyroidectomy is:

A. At point where RLN crosses inferior thyroid artery
B. Near tubercle of Zuckerkandl
C. At ligament of Berry
D. Tracheoesophageal groove near isthmus

199. Rate of permanent RLN injury during thyroidectomy is:

A. 2% B. 7%
C. 16% D. 21%

200. Most common complication of thyroidectomy:

A. Vocal cord paralysis
B. Neck hematoma
C. Hypoparathyroidism
D. Surgical site infection

201. Rate of permanent hypoparathyroidism following thyroidectomy is:

A. 3% B. 9%
C. 18% D. 21%

202. Risk factors for neck hematoma following thyroidectomy are all except:

A. Advanced age
B. Graves' disease
C. Bilateral neck exploration
D. Female gender

203. Patient complains of sudden onset of stridor with neck swelling on the evening of thyroidectomy surgery. What is most appropriate management for this patient?

A. Endotracheal intubation
B. Bedside opening of sutures
C. Transfer to operative theatre for revision surgery
D. Emergency tracheostomy

204. Wavelength used to detect parathyroid tissue autofluorescence:

A. 240 nm B. 285 nm
C. 340 nm D. 430 nm

205. Which of the following approach is not used for thyroidectomy through remote access surgery?

A. Transoral approach
B. Transaxillary approach
C. Anterior thoracotomy approach
D. Face lift approach

206. 45-year-old male patient presented with 4 cm right sided tumor confined to thyroid and central lymph node enlargement. No evidence of any distant metastases. This patient has which stage of thyroid cancer?

A. Stage I B. Stage II
C. Stage III D. Stage IVa

207. 36-year-old female has right sided palpable firm thyroid nodule with palpable left sided cervical lymph node. Patient also has lumbar spine pain which proven to be vertebral metastasis. What is the stage of the cancer?

A. Stage I B. Stage II
C. Stage III D. Stage IVb

208. 60-year-old male presented with enlarged thyroid, nodular and hard in consistency. USG neck findings suggestive 3 cm of hypoechoic nodule in left lobe with involvement of only strap muscles without any evident enlargement of neck lymph nodes. FNA shows anaplastic follicular cells. What is the stage of cancer?

A. Stage I B. Stage II
C. Stage III D. Stage IVa

209. According to AJCC 8th edition, thyroid malignancy with extrathyroidal extension involving RLN is:

A. T2 B. T3a
C. T3b D. T4a

210. According to AJCC 8th edition, category T4b includes:

A. Tumor < 4 cm with microscopic extrathyroidal extension
B. Tumor > 4 cm and intrathyroidal
C. Gross extrathyroidal extension into trachea, esophagus, larynx, RLN
D. Gross extrathyroidal extension to prevertebral fascia or encasing the carotid artery, mediastinal vessels

211. According to AJCC 8th edition, thyroid malignancy with gross extrathyroidal extension involving only strap muscles of neck is:

A. T2 B. T3a
C. T3b D. T4a

212. According to AJCC 8th edition, thyroid malignancy with level VI and VII lymph nodes positive has N stage:

A. N0 B. N1a
C. N1b D. N2

213. According to AJCC 8th edition, microcarcinoma of thyroid has T stage:

A. T0 B. Ta
C. T1a D. T1b

214. Level VI and VII neck lymph nodes involves:

A. Pretracheal
B. Delphian
C. Superior mediastinal
D. All of the above

215. According to AJCC 8th edition, tumor of > 4 cm completely confined to thyroid gland has T stage:

A. T2 B. T3a
C. T3b D. T4a

216. Thyroid malignancy of 3 cm with gross extension into only strap muscle, involvement of level VI lymph nodes without any distant metastases is staged as:

A. T2 N0 M0 B. T2 N1a M0
C. T3a N1a M0 D. T3b N1a M0

217. Thyroid malignancy of 6 cm with involvement of soft tissue and larynx and presence of contralateral level III cervical lymph node is stages as:

A. T3a N1a M0 B. T3b N1a M0
C. T4a N1b M0 D. T4a N2 M0

218. Thyroid tumor of 2 cm without any evidence of lymph node involvement is staged as:

A. T1a N0 M0 B. T1b N0 M0
C. T1b N1 M0 D. T2 N0 M0

219. In 60-year-old patient, thyroid malignancy of any size with involvement of larynx, ipsilateral lateral neck lymph node and no evidence of distant metastases are staged according to TNM as:

A. Stage I B. Stage II
C. Stage III D. Stage IVa

220. According to AJCC 8th edition, stage III thyroid malignancy in >55 years old includes:

A. T2 N1b M0 B. T3a N1a M0
C. T3b N1b M0 D. T4a any N M0

ANSWERS

1. **Ans: A. Thomas Wharton**

Ref: Chapter No. 37, Page No. 874

2. **Ans: A. Theodor Kocher**

Ref: Chapter No. 37, Page No. 874

3. **Ans: C. William Halsted**

Ref: Chapter No. 37, Page No. 874

4. **Ans: D. Unilateral thyroid lobectomy with contralateral subtotal lobectomy**

Ref: Chapter No. 37, Page No. 874

5. **Ans: B. Thyroid hormone by the twelfth week of gestation**

Ref: Chapter No. 37, Page No. 874

6. **Ans: B. 10**

Ref: Chapter No. 37, Page No. 874

7. **Ans: B. Thyroglossal duct cyst typically presents as a painless lateral neck mass**

Ref: Chapter No. 37, Page No. 875

8. **Ans: A. Aberrant thyroid tissue can be found from the base of tongue down to the posterior mediastinum**

Ref: Chapter No. 37, Page No. 875

9. **Ans: D. Posterior mediastinum**

Ref: Chapter No. 37, Page No. 875

10. **Ans: C. Ligament of Berry extends superiorly from the isthmus and represents the caudal remnant of the thyroglossal duct**

Ref: Chapter No. 37, Page No. 875-876

11. **Ans: B. Pyramidal lobe**

Ref: Chapter No. 37, Page No. 876

12. **Ans: D. RLN typically crosses the superior thyroid artery perpendicularly as it travels into the larynx is an important landmark**

Ref: Chapter No. 37, Page No. 876

13. **Ans: B. 2%**

Ref: Chapter No. 37, Page No. 876

14. **Ans: D. The middle thyroid vein is constant and drain into the innominate vein**

Ref: Chapter No. 37, Page No. 876

15. **Ans: A. Laterally bounded by sternocleidomastoid muscles**

Ref: Chapter No. 37, Page No. 876

16. **Ans: B. Low pitch**

Ref: Chapter No. 37, Page No. 876

17. **Ans: C. Cricothyroid**

Ref: Chapter No. 37, Page No. 876

18. **Ans: C. The tubercle of Zuckerkandl typically lies just posterior and medial to the nerve**

Ref: Chapter No. 37, Page No. 877

19. **Ans: C. Aberrant right subclavian artery**

Ref: Chapter No. 37, Page No. 877

20. **Ans: B. 1%**

Ref: Chapter No. 37, Page No. 877

21. **Ans: D. Parafollicular C cell are mainly found in the medial aspect of the mid and upper thyroid lobes**

Ref: Chapter No. 37, Page No. 879

22. **Ans: D. The average daily iodine requirement for adult humans is 1 mg**

Ref: Chapter No. 37, Page No. 879

23. **Ans: A. 0.1 mg**

Ref: Chapter No. 37, Page No. 879

24. **Ans: D. Absence of calcitonin cause significant change in calcium homeostasis**

Ref: Chapter No. 37, Page No. 879

25. **Ans: C. Liver**

Ref: Chapter No. 37, Page No. 880

26. **Ans: D. Both A and B**

Ref: Chapter No. 37, Page No. 880

27. **Ans: C. Free T4 levels are increased during first trimester**

Ref: Chapter No. 37, Page No. 880

28. **Ans: B. Graves' disease**

Ref: Chapter No. 37, Page No. 880

29. **Ans: A. Hashimoto thyroiditis**

Ref: Chapter No. 37, Page No. 880

30. **Ans: A. 0.5%**

Ref: Chapter No. 37, Page No. 880

31. **Ans: B. Signs of clinical thyroid dysfunction**

Ref: Chapter No. 37, Page No. 880-881

32. **Ans: D. All of the above**

Ref: Chapter No. 37, Page No. 881

33. **Ans: A. TSH is a peptide hormone secreted from the anterior pituitary gland**

Ref: Chapter No. 37, Page No. 881

34. **Ans: C. 0.4 – 5.5 mIU/L**

Ref: Chapter No. 37, Page No. 881

35. **Ans: D. Serum TSH and free T4**

Ref: Chapter No. 37, Page No. 881

36. **Ans: A. Measurement of TgAb is the most accurate and commonly used screening test for autoimmune thyroiditis**

Ref: Chapter No. 37, Page No. 881

37. **Ans: A. Anti-TPO (TPOAb)**

Ref: Chapter No. 37, Page No. 881

38. **Ans: D. TgAb is present in 1% to 5% of the general population**

Ref: Chapter No. 37, Page No. 882

39. **Ans: B. Medullary thyroid cancer**

Ref: Chapter No. 37, Page No. 882

40. **Ans: B. Nuclear scintigraphy is useful for the differential diagnosis of hypothyroidism**

Ref: Chapter No. 37, Page No. 882-883

41. **Ans: C. 15%**

Ref: Chapter No. 37, Page No. 882

42. **Ans: B. Iodine-deficiency**

Ref: Chapter No. 37, Page No. 884

43. **Ans: A. Heat intolerance**

Ref: Chapter No. 37, Page No. 884

44. **Ans: D. Levothyroxine can be administered sub-cutaneously**

Ref: Chapter No. 37, Page No. 884

45. **Ans: A. It is also known as acute lymphocytic thyroiditis**

Ref: Chapter No. 37, Page No. 884

46. **Ans: C. 9-fold**

Ref: Chapter No. 37, Page No. 884

47. **Ans: C. Sonographic characteristics include hyperechoic parenchymal echotexture**

Ref: Chapter No. 37, Page No. 884-885

48. **Ans: D. All of the above**

Ref: Chapter No. 37, Page No. 884

49. **Ans: B. Papillary**

Ref: Chapter No. 37, Page No. 884

50. **Ans: A. It occurs within the first 2 months of the postpartum period**

Ref: Chapter No. 37, Page No. 885

51. **Ans: C. 10%**

Ref: Chapter No. 37, Page No. 885

52. **Ans: B. Subacute granulomatous thyroiditis**

Ref: Chapter No. 37, Page No. 885

53. **Ans: A. It is found primarily in the underdeveloped countries**

Ref: Chapter No. 37, Page No. 885

54. **Ans: D. Corticosteroids are contraindicated for the treatment**

Ref: Chapter No. 37, Page No. 885

55. **Ans: C. Increased RAI uptake**

Ref: Chapter No. 37, Page No. 885

56. **Ans: C. Giant cell infiltrate**

Ref: Chapter No. 37, Page No. 885

57. **Ans: C. Fibrotic process limited to thyroid gland**

Ref: Chapter No. 37, Page No. 885

58. **Ans: B. Riedel's thyroiditis**

Ref: Chapter No. 37, Page No. 885

59. **Ans: B. Infection of a congenital pyriform sinus fistula**

Ref: Chapter No. 37, Page No. 885

60. **Ans: D. Dopamine**

Ref: Chapter No. 37, Page No. 886

61. **Ans: A. Propylthiouracil**

Ref: Chapter No. 37, Page No. 886

62. **Ans: D. Sorafenib causes direct destructive autoimmune thyroiditis**

Ref: Chapter No. 37, Page No. 886

63. **Ans: D. Certolizumab**

Ref: Chapter No. 37, Page No. 886

64. **Ans: A. Interferon gamma**

Ref: Chapter No. 37, Page No. 886

65. **Ans: B. Dopamine**

Ref: Chapter No. 37, Page No. 886

66. **Ans: A. Sunitinib**

Ref: Chapter No. 37, Page No. 886

67. **Ans: C. Type 3 deiodinase**

Ref: Chapter No. 37, Page No. 886

68. **Ans: B. Bexarotene**

Ref: Chapter No. 37, Page No. 886

69. **Ans: D. All of the above**

Ref: Chapter No. 37, Page No. 886

70. **Ans: B. Female-to-male incidence is 4:1**

Ref: Chapter No. 37, Page No. 886-887

71. **Ans: B. Presence of TPOAb**

Ref: Chapter No. 37, Page No. 887

72. **Ans: C. Graves' disease**

Ref: Chapter No. 37, Page No. 887

73. **Ans: C. 25 – 30%**

Ref: Chapter No. 37, Page No. 887

74. **Ans: D. Lifelong requirement of medical therapy**

Ref: Chapter No. 37, Page No. 887

75. **Ans: B. 5 – 10%**

Ref: Chapter No. 37, Page No. 887

76. **Ans: C. Subacute thyroiditis**

Ref: Chapter No. 37, Page No. 887

77. **Ans: B. Graves' disease**

Ref: Chapter No. 37, Page No. 887

78. **Ans: B. Patients with periodic paralysis**

Ref: Chapter No. 37, Page No. 888

79. **Ans: D. One or more large thyroid nodules**

Ref: Chapter No. 37, Page No. 888

80. **Ans: A. 2%**

Ref: Chapter No. 37, Page No. 888

81. **Ans: B. Methimazole was found to be associated with liver failure**

Ref: Chapter No. 37, Page No. 888

82. **Ans: B. Toxic multinodular goiter**

Ref: Chapter No. 37, Page No. 888

83. **Ans: C. Affects adults below the age of 50 years**

Ref: Chapter No. 37, Page No. 888

84. **Ans: C. Nuclear scintigraphy**

Ref: Chapter No. 37, Page No. 888

85. **Ans: B. Autonomous nodules undergo remission with medical therapy**

Ref: Chapter No. 37, Page No. 888-889

86. **Ans: D. Near-total thyroidectomy as definitive treatment**

Ref: Chapter No. 37, Page No. 889

87. **Ans: D. Type 1 AIT is caused by the Wolff-Chaikoff phenomenon**

Ref: Chapter No. 37, Page No. 889

88. **Ans: C. 37%**

Ref: Chapter No. 37, Page No. 889

89. **Ans: B. Type 1 AIT is more common in patients with preexisting hypothyroid disease**

Ref: Chapter No. 37, Page No. 889

90. **Ans: D. Elevated free T4 and T3**

Ref: Chapter No. 37, Page No. 889

91. **Ans: D. Vocal cord paralysis is more likely to occur due to RLN compression**

Ref: Chapter No. 37, Page No. 890

92. **Ans: B. Connection to the normal cervical orthotopic gland**

Ref: Chapter No. 37, Page No. 890

93. **Ans: C. Vocal cord paralysis**

Ref: Chapter No. 37, Page No. 890

94. **Ans: D. RAI is suitable for larger goiters**

Ref: Chapter No. 37, Page No. 890

95. **Ans: D. RAI refractory goiter**

Ref: Chapter No. 37, Page No. 890

96. **Ans: A. Transcervical**

Ref: Chapter No. 37, Page No. 890

97. **Ans: D. Multinodular gland**

Ref: Chapter No. 37, Page No. 890

98. **Ans: B. Female sex**

Ref: Chapter No. 37, Page No. 890

99. **Ans: B. Nodules larger than 1.5 cm**

Ref: Chapter No. 37, Page No. 890

100. **Ans: B. Papillary thyroid cancer**

Ref: Chapter No. 37, Page No. 890

101. **Ans: C. Radioisotope scan**

Ref: Chapter No. 37, Page No. 892

102. **Ans: B. Nodule with low Suspicion - <3%**

Ref: Chapter No. 37, Page No. 893

103. **Ans: D. Wider-than-tall nodule shape**

Ref: Chapter No. 37, Page No. 893

104. **Ans: B. 5**

Ref: Chapter No. 37, Page No. 893

105. **Ans: D. Size**

Ref: Chapter No. 37, Page No. 893

106. **Ans: B. Vascularity**

Ref: Chapter No. 37, Page No. 893

107. **Ans: B. 1 cm**

Ref: Chapter No. 37, Page No. 894

108. **Ans: B. Sensitivity of over 95%**

Ref: Chapter No. 37, Page No. 894

109. Ans: B. Very low suspicion

Ref: Chapter No. 37, Page No. 894

110. Ans: A. Observation with follow up USG

Ref: Chapter No. 37, Page No. 894

111. Ans: C. Spongiform nodule

Ref: Chapter No. 37, Page No. 894

112. Ans: D. Isoechoic solid nodule

Ref: Chapter No. 37, Page No. 894

113. Ans: C. 70 – 90%

Ref: Chapter No. 37, Page No. 894

114. Ans: B. Low suspicion features - FNA at $\geq$1 cm

Ref: Chapter No. 37, Page No. 894

115. Ans: C. Radioisotope scan

Ref: Chapter No. 37, Page No. 892-894

116. Ans: A. TR1 – 1 point

Ref: Chapter No. 37, Page No. 895

117. Ans: A. completely solid Composition

Ref: Chapter No. 37, Page No. 895

118. Ans: D. Thyroid FNA cytology

Ref: Chapter No. 37, Page No. 895

119. Ans: C. 6

Ref: Chapter No. 37, Page No. 895

120. Ans: C. Category IV

Ref: Chapter No. 37, Page No. 895

121. Ans: C. Category IV

Ref: Chapter No. 37, Page No. 895

122. Ans: D. Category VI

Ref: Chapter No. 37, Page No. 896

123. Ans: A. Papillary

Ref: Chapter No. 37, Page No. 896

124. Ans: D. All of the above

Ref: Chapter No. 37, Page No. 897

125. Ans: C. Category III and IV

Ref: Chapter No. 37, Page No. 897

126. Ans: C. 10%–40%

Ref: Chapter No. 37, Page No. 897

127. Ans: B. 6%–18%

Ref: Chapter No. 37, Page No. 897

128. Ans: C. Category II

Ref: Chapter No. 37, Page No. 897

129. Ans: D. 167-gene mRNA microarray

Ref: Chapter No. 37, Page No. 897

130. Ans: C. Genomic Sequence Classifier correctly predict Hürthle cell adenoma and carcinoma

Ref: Chapter No. 37, Page No. 897

131. Ans: C. ThyroSeq

Ref: Chapter No. 37, Page No. 898

132. Ans: C. Medullary

Ref: Chapter No. 37, Page No. 898

133. Ans: D. Distant metastases do occur in up to 23% to 25% of patients

Ref: Chapter No. 37, Page No. 898

134. Ans: A. Papillary

Ref: Chapter No. 37, Page No. 898

135. Ans: D. Eosinophilic granular cytoplasm

Ref: Chapter No. 37, Page No. 898

136. Ans: A. 5%

Ref: Chapter No. 37, Page No. 898

137. Ans: B. Follicular variant

Ref: Chapter No. 37, Page No. 898

138. Ans: C. The pattern of spread of FTC is lymphatic route

Ref: Chapter No. 37, Page No. 898

139. Ans: D. Presence of oxyphilic Hürthle cells abundant basophilic granular cytoplasm

Ref: Chapter No. 37, Page No. 898

140. Ans: D. Both A and B

Ref: Chapter No. 37, Page No. 898

141. Ans: D. It is considered to be a malignant

Ref: Chapter No. 37, Page No. 899

142. Ans: D. MET

Ref: Chapter No. 37, Page No. 899

143. Ans: C. Microcephaly

Ref: Chapter No. 37, Page No. 899

144. Ans: B. Follicular

Ref: Chapter No. 37, Page No. 899

145. Ans: D. All of the above

Ref: Chapter No. 37, Page No. 900

146. Ans: A. Papillary

Ref: Chapter No. 37, Page No. 900

147. Ans: D. Werner syndrome

Ref: Chapter No. 37, Page No. 900

148. Ans: C. Wermer syndrome

Ref: Chapter No. 37, Page No. 900

149. Ans: A. Papillary

Ref: Chapter No. 37, Page No. 900

150. Ans: D. Associated with BRAF mutation

Ref: Chapter No. 37, Page No. 900

151. Ans: D. All of the above

Ref: Chapter No. 37, Page No. 900-901

152. Ans: D. Larotrectinib

Ref: Chapter No. 37, Page No. 902

153. Ans: C. FGFR

Ref: Chapter No. 37, Page No. 902

154. Ans: D. Crizotinib

Ref: Chapter No. 37, Page No. 902

155. Ans: B. BRAF

Ref: Chapter No. 37, Page No. 902

156. Ans: C. Gefitinib

Ref: Chapter No. 37, Page No. 902

157. Ans: B. T3a is a new category for tumors of any size, demonstrating gross extrathyroidal extension

Ref: Chapter No. 37, Page No. 902

158. Ans: C. Tumor > 4 cm confined to thyroid gland

Ref: Chapter No. 37, Page No. 902

159. Ans: C. Microscopic extrathyroidal extension

Ref: Chapter No. 37, Page No. 903

160. Ans: D. Total thyroidectomy is recommended for tumors of > 2 cm

Ref: Chapter No. 37, Page No. 903

161. Ans: C. 20%

Ref: Chapter No. 37, Page No. 904

162. Ans: D. Total thyroidectomy with central neck dissection

Ref: Chapter No. 37, Page No. 904

163. Ans: D. Total thyroidectomy with central and lateral neck dissection and RAI therapy

Ref: Chapter No. 37, Page No. 904

164. Ans: A. < 0.1 mU/L

Ref: Chapter No. 37, Page No. 905

165. Ans: B. 0.1 to 0.5 mU/L

Ref: Chapter No. 37, Page No. 905

166. Ans: B. 0.1 to 0.5 mU/L

Ref: Chapter No. 37, Page No. 905

167. Ans: D. Medullary

Ref: Chapter No. 37, Page No. 905

168. Ans: D. Higher benefits in low risk DTC

Ref: Chapter No. 37, Page No. 905

169. Ans: C. RAI is routinely recommended for low-risk cancers

Ref: Chapter No. 37, Page No. 905

170. Ans: C. 100 to 150 mCi

Ref: Chapter No. 37, Page No. 905

171. Ans: D. Eosinophilic granular cytoplasm

Ref: Chapter No. 37, Page No. 906

172. Ans: C. Chorioembryonic antigen

Ref: Chapter No. 37, Page No. 906

173. Ans: C. Chromosome 10q11.2

Ref: Chapter No. 37, Page No. 906

174. Ans: B. Codon 634

Ref: Chapter No. 37, Page No. 906

175. Ans: C. Neuroendocrine tumors

Ref: Chapter No. 37, Page No. 906

176. Ans: D. Sporadic MTC with somatic RET mutations has good prognosis

Ref: Chapter No. 37, Page No. 906

177. Ans: A. Within first year of life

Ref: Chapter No. 37, Page No. 906

178. Ans: D. 500 pg/mL

Ref: Chapter No. 37, Page No. 907

179. Ans: D. Hypoparathyroidism

Ref: Chapter No. 37, Page No. 907

180. Ans: D. Patients with familial MTC, MEN2B require four gland exploration of parathyroid

Ref: Chapter No. 37, Page No. 907-908

181. Ans: D. EBRT to the neck for locoregional control improves overall survival

Ref: Chapter No. 37, Page No. 908

182. Ans: D. Asymptomatic with painless neck mass

Ref: Chapter No. 37, Page No. 908

183. Ans: C. Painless

Ref: Chapter No. 37, Page No. 908

184. Ans: A. Anaplastic thyroid cancer avidly stain for thyroglobulin

Ref: Chapter No. 37, Page No. 908

185. Ans: C. Sunitinib

Ref: Chapter No. 37, Page No. 909

186. Ans: B. Papillary

Ref: Chapter No. 37, Page No. 909

187. Ans: B. Sorafenib

Ref: Chapter No. 37, Page No. 909

188. Ans: B. Lenvatinib

Ref: Chapter No. 37, Page No. 909

189. Ans: B. Vandetanib

Ref: Chapter No. 37, Page No. 909

190. Ans: C. Cabozantinib

Ref: Chapter No. 37, Page No. 909

191. Ans: C. Dabrafenib with trametinib

Ref: Chapter No. 37, Page No. 909

192. Ans: C. Doxorubicin

Ref: Chapter No. 37, Page No. 909

193. Ans: B. 1 gm of remnant is left at ligament of Berry

Ref: Chapter No. 37, Page No. 910

194. Ans: C. It has slow learning curve and it is not cost effective

Ref: Chapter No. 37, Page No. 910

195. Ans: D. 20%

Ref: Chapter No. 37, Page No. 910

196. Ans: A. Avascular space between medial superior pole and cricothyroid muscle

Ref: Chapter No. 37, Page No. 911

197. Ans: A. The sternothyroid may be partially or completely divided near its inferior attachment to sternum

Ref: Chapter No. 37, Page No. 911

198. Ans: C. At ligament of Berry

Ref: Chapter No. 37, Page No. 913

199. Ans: A. 2%

Ref: Chapter No. 37, Page No. 914

200. Ans: C. Hypoparathyroidism

Ref: Chapter No. 37, Page No. 915

201. Ans: A. 3%

Ref: Chapter No. 37, Page No. 915

202. Ans: D. Female gender

Ref: Chapter No. 37, Page No. 916

203. Ans: B. Bedside opening of sutures

Ref: Chapter No. 37, Page No. 916

204. Ans: B. 285 nm

Ref: Chapter No. 37, Page No. 916

205. Ans: C. Anterior thoracotomy approach

Ref: Chapter No. 37, Page No. 917

206. Ans: A. Stage I

Ref: AJCC 8th edition, Thyroid cancer

207. Ans: B. Stage II

Ref: AJCC 8th edition, Thyroid cancer

208. Ans: B. Stage II

Ref: AJCC 8th edition, Thyroid cancer

209. Ans: D. T4a

Ref: AJCC 8th edition, Thyroid cancer

210. Ans: D. Gross extrathyroidal extension to prevertebral fascia or encasing the carotid artery, mediastinal vessels

Ref: AJCC 8th edition, Thyroid cancer

211. Ans: C. T3b

Ref: AJCC 8th edition, Thyroid cancer

212. Ans: B. N1a

Ref: AJCC 8th edition, Thyroid cancer

213. Ans: C. T1a

Ref: AJCC 8th edition, Thyroid cancer

214. Ans: D. All of the above

Ref: AJCC 8th edition, Thyroid cancer

215. Ans: B. T3a

Ref: AJCC 8th edition, Thyroid cancer

216. Ans: D. T3b N1a M0

Ref: AJCC 8th edition, Thyroid cancer

217. Ans: C. T4a N1b M0

Ref: AJCC 8th edition, Thyroid cancer

218. Ans: B. T1b N0 M0

Ref: AJCC 8th edition, Thyroid cancer

219. Ans: C. Stage III

Ref: AJCC 8th edition, Thyroid cancer

220. Ans: D. T4a any N M0

Staging guide for thyroid cancer (AJCC 8e)				
Age at diagnosis	T category	N category	M category	Stage
		Differentiated thyroid cancer		
<55 years	any T	any N	M0	**I**
	any T	any N	M1	**II**
≥ 55 years	T1	N0/NX	M0	**I**
	T1	N1	M0	**II**
	T2	N0/NX	M0	**I**
	T2	N1	M0	**II**
	T3a/T3b	any N	M0	**II**
	T4a	any N	M0	**III**
	T4b	any N	M0	**IVA**
	any T	any N	M1	**IVB**
		Medullary thyroid cancer		
any	T1	N0	M0	**I**
	T2	N0	M0	**II**
	T3	N0	M0	**II**
	T1-3	N1a	M0	**III**
	T4a	any N	M0	**IVA**
	T1-3	N1b	M0	**IVA**
	T4b	any N	M0	**IVB**
	any T	any N	M1	**IVC**
		Anaplastic thyroid cancer		
any	T1-T3a	N0/NX	M0	**IVA**
	T1-T3a	N1	M0	**IVB**
	T3b	any N	M0	**IVB**
	T4	any N	M0	**IVB**
	any T	any N	M1	**IVC**

TNM definitions (AJCC 8e) for papillary, follicular, poorly differentiated, Hürthle cell, medullary, and anaplastic thyroid carcinomas	
TX	Primary tumor cannot be assessed
T0	No evidence of primary tumor
T1	Tumor ≤ 2 cm in greatest dimension limited to the thyroid
T1a	Tumor ≤ 1 cm in greatest dimension limited to the thyroid
T1b	Tumor > 1 cm but ≤ 2 cm in greatest dimension limited to the thyroid
T2	Tumor > 2 cm but ≤ 4 cm in greatest dimension limited to the thyroid
T3*	Tumor > 4 cm limited to the thyroid or gross extrathyroidal extension invading only strap muscles
T3a*	Tumor > 4 cm limited to the thyroid
T3b*	Gross extrathyroidal extension invading only strap muscles (sternohyoid) from a tumor of any size
T4	Includes gross extrathyroidal extension into major neck structures
T4a	Gross extrathyroidal extension invading subcutaneous soft tissues, larynx, trachea, esophagus, or recurrent laryngeal nerve from a tumor of any size
T4b	Gross extrathyroidal extension invading prevertebral fascia or encasing carotid artery or mediastinal vessels from a tumor of any size
NX	Regional lymph nodes cannot be assessed
N0	No evidence of regional lymph nodes metastasis
N0a*	One or more cytologic or histologically confirmed benign lymph node
N0b*	No radiologic or clinical evidence of locoregional lymph node metastasis
N1*	Metastasis to regional nodes
N1a*	Metastasis to level VI or VII (pretracheal, paratracheal, or prelaryngeal/Delphian, or upper mediastinal) lymph nodes; this can be unilateral or bilateral disease
N1b*	Metastasis to unilateral, bilateral, or contralateral lateral neck lymph nodes (levels I, II, III, IV, or V) or retropharyngeal lymph nodes
M0	No distant metastasis
M1	Distant metastasis

*all categories may be subdivided as solitary tumor (s) and multifocal tumor (m) – the largest tumor determines the classification

Ref: AJCC 8th edition, Thyroid cancer

38

The Parathyroid Glands

1. **Who was the first person to discover parathyroid glands in human?**
   A. Richard Owen B. Ivar Sandstrom
   C. William MacCallum D. William Halstead

2. **Who described the association of tetany to the parathyroid function?**
   A. Richard Owen B. James Collip
   C. Eugene Gley D. Schlagenhaufer

3. **Osteitis fibrosa cystica includes all features except:**
   A. Multiple fractures of the long bones
   B. Sclerosis
   C. Cystic changes
   D. Brown tumor

4. **Who performed first parathyroidectomy?**
   A. Schlagenhaufer B. James B. Collip
   C. Felix Mandl D. Charles Martell

5. **Who developed radioimmunoassay?**
   A. Fuller Albright
   B. Rasmussen and Craig
   C. Nussbaum
   D. Rosalyn Yalow

6. **Who successfully sequenced and synthesized PTH?**
   A. Fuller Albright
   B. Rasmussen and Craig
   C. Potts
   D. Irvin

7. **What is half life of PTH?**
   A. 1 to 2 mins B. 3 to 5 mins
   C. 5 to 7 mins D. 7 to 10 mins

EMBRYOLOGY AND ANATOMY

8. **Which structure develops from third branchial pouch?**
   A. Superior parathyroid glands
   B. Inferior parathyroid glands
   C. Lateral lobes of thyroid gland
   D. Parafollicular cells

9. **Superior parathyroid glands develops from which structure?**
   A. Foramen caecum
   B. Third branchial pouch
   C. Fourth branchial pouch
   D. Ultimobranchial body

10. **Which of the following is false statement?**
    A. Thymus develop from the ventral aspects of third branchial pouch
    B. The dorsal aspect of the fourth pharyngeal pouch forms the superior parathyroid glands
    C. The fourth pharyngeal pouch is also give rise to the lateral lobes of the thyroid gland
    D. Superior parathyroid glands are more frequent in ectopic location

11. **Which gene is responsible for differentiation and development of parathyroid glands?**
    A. HRPT2 B. GCM2
    C. CDKN1B D. RET

12. **Which genetic mutation is associated with higher risk of parathyroid carcinoma?**
    A. MEN1 B. RET
    C. RB1 D. GCM2

13. **GCM2 gene mutation is associated with which condition?**

A. Parathyroid hyperplasia
B. Parathyroid carcinoma
C. Familial isolated HPT
D. Hyperparathyroidism-jaw tumor syndrome

14. Supernumerary parathyroid glands present in:

A. 3%
B. 13%
C. 21%
D. 33%

15. Which is wrong statement about parathyroid glands?

A. Parathyroid glands weigh 35 to 40 mg
B. The superior thyroid artery is the predominant vascular supply for all parathyroid glands
C. 80% of cases, the ipsilateral and contralateral parathyroid glands are located in symmetrical positions in the neck
D. The parathyroid glands are usually found within 5 mm of the superior and inferior margins of the tubercle of Zuckerkandl

16. Inferior thyroid artery is a branch of which vessel?

A. Common carotid artery
B. Thyrocervical trunk
C. External carotid artery
D. Internal carotid artery

17. Which is predominant vascular supply for all parathyroid glands?

A. Superior thyroid artery
B. Inferior thyroid artery
C. Superior parathyroid artery
D. Inferior parathyroid artery

18. ___% of patients with primary HPT will have ectopic parathyroid glands.

A. 4%
B. 16%
C. 24%
D. 33%

19. What is the landmark for the location of parathyroid glands?

A. Tracheoesophageal groove
B. Berry ligament
C. Tubercle of Zuckerkandl
D. Recurrent laryngeal nerve

20. Which is incorrect about location of superior parathyroid glands?

A. The superior parathyroid glands located posterior and superior to the recurrent laryngeal nerve
B. They have a more predictable anatomic location
C. Superior parathyroid glands lie outside the capsule of the thyroid gland
D. They are located 1 cm superior to the junction of the inferior thyroid artery and the recurrent laryngeal nerve at the level of the cricoid cartilage

21. All are ectopic locations of superior parathyroid glands except:

A. Tracheoesophageal groove
B. Behind the esophagus
C. Intrathyroidal
D. Anterior mediastinum

22. Which is incorrect about location of inferior parathyroid glands?

A. They are located anterior and medial to the recurrent laryngeal nerve
B. They are less often found in a subcapsular location
C. They are more commonly ectopic and can be found anywhere from the angle of the mandible to the pericardium
D. They are most commonly found 1 cm superior to the junction of the inferior thyroid artery and the recurrent laryngeal nerve

23. What is the most common location of inferior parathyroid glands?

A. Anterior superior mediastinum
B. Thymus
C. Aortopulmonary window
D. Intrathyroidal

24. All are ectopic locations of superior parathyroid glands except:

A. Carotid sheath
B. Aortopulmonary window
C. Submandibular location
D. Posterior mediastinum

HISTOLOGY AND PHYSIOLOGY

25. Which is false about parathyroid gland?

A. The parathyroid glands are darker with a reddish-brown color in young age
B. The percent of adipose cells within the parathyroid gland increases with age
C. Chief cells are responsible for synthesis and secretion of PTH
D. The number of oxyphil cells in the parathyroid gland decreases with age

26. Tc-99m-sestamibi imaging in identification of a parathyroid adenoma is depended on which cell type?

A. Chief cell
B. Oxyphil cell
C. Clear cell
D. Follicular cell

27. Which cell type synthesize and secrete PTH?

A. Chief cell
B. Oxyphil cell
C. Clear cell
D. Follicular cell

28. Which is false about regulation of PTH?

A. Calcium by acting on CaSR inhibits PTH secretion and PTH gene expression
B. The NH2 terminus is a biologically active part of the intact-PTH peptide
C. Vitamin D and Calcium receptors are present on chief cell
D. Sigmoidal relationship exists between extracellular calcium concentration and PTH secretion

29. Which of the following is not a regulator of PTH?

A. 25-hydroxyvitamin D
B. Lithium
C. FGF 23
D. Inorganic phosphate

30. The relationship of parathyroid hormone (PTH) to changes in extracellular calcium concentration is explained by:

A. Linear
B. Sigmoidal
C. Reverse sigmoidal
D. Exponential

31. Incorrect regarding action of PTH on renal tissue:

A. PTH acts on proximal convoluted tubule
B. Produces active metabolite 1,25[OH]2D
C. The PTH-mediated renal effects to maintain calcium homeostasis are rapid
D. Enhance calcium reabsorption and increase phosphate excretion

32. Which is wrong about effect of PTH on bones?

A. PTH binds to the PTHR1 receptor that is found on cells of the osteoclastic lineage
B. PTH has both anabolic and catabolic effects on bone remodeling
C. PTH increases osteoclast activity leading to increased bone resorption
D. Intermittent administration of recombinant human PTH has been shown to stimulate bone formation

33. Which of the following does not produce ectopic PTHrP?

A. SCC of lung
B. Bladder cancer
C. Renal cell cancer
D. Breast cancer

34. All are causes of hypercalcemia except:

A. Hyperthyroidism
B. Sarcoidosis
C. Lithium
D. DiGeorge's syndrome

PRIMARY HYPERPARATHYROIDISM

35. Which of the following is associated with low PTH levels?

A. Primary HPT
B. Prolonged lithium therapy
C. Familial hypocalciuric hypercalcemia
D. Vitamin D intoxication

36. Which is only known risk factor of PHPT?

A. Irradiation
B. Drug induced
C. Prior thyroid malignancy
D. Age

37. Which of the following is presented with hypocalcemia?

A. Primary HPT
B. Secondary HPT
C. Tertiary HPT
D. Hyperthyroidism

38. All are true about Familial hypocalciuric hypercalcemia except:

A. FHH is a rare autosomal dominant disorder
B. FHH develops after the age of 40
C. Asymptomatic hypercalcemia with elevated PTH
D. No treatment is required for FHH

39. Which defect is seen in Familial hypocalciuric hypercalcemia?

A. CaSR of parathyroid gland
B. Renal CaSR
C. Renal PTHR1
D. FGF 23

40. All are true about primary HPT except:

A. Primary HPT is more common in females
B. The parathyroid cells in a parathyroid adenoma have a increased sensitivity to calcium
C. In parathyroid hyperplasia, cells maintain their normal sensitivity to calcium

D. Parathyroid adenoma is most common cause of primary HPT

41. Which genetic mutation is not associated with parathyroid carcinoma?

A. MEN1 B. RB1
C. GCM2 D. RET

42. All are true concerning hyperparathyroidism-jaw tumor syndrome except:

A. CASR gene mutation
B. Autosomal dominant develops in second or third decade
C. Risk of parathyroid carcinoma
D. Ossifying fibromas of mandible and maxilla

43. All are associated with hyperparathyroidism-jaw tumor syndrome except:

A. Ossifying fibromas of mandible and maxilla
B. Wilms tumor
C. Uterine tumor
D. Adrenal tumor

44. Most common site of osteoporosis in case of PHPT is seen at:

A. Distal radius B. Lumbar spine
C. Femoral neck D. Pelvis

45. Following are symptoms of PHPT except:

A. Nephrocalcinosis
B. Fragility fractures
C. Distal muscle weakness
D. Emotional lability

46. Which test is used to screen familial hypocalciuric hypercalcemia syndrome?

A. Serum Ionized calcium
B. 24-hour urine calcium
C. Intact PTH
D. Calcium creatinine clearance ratio

47. All are indications for parathyroidectomy in case of PHPT except:

A. Serum calcium >1 mg/dL above the upper limit of normal
B. T score < -2.5 on DEXA scan
C. Impaired renal function with GFR < 60 ml/min
D. Urine calcium >200 mg/24 hours

48. All are indications for parathyroidectomy in case of PHPT except:

A. Age > 50 years
B. Vertebral compression fracture on spine imaging
C. Nephrolithiasis
D. Urine calcium >400 mg/24 hours

49. 30-year-old female is a known primary hyperparathyroidism patient, incidentally diagnosed with nephrolithiasis with asymptomatic hypercalcemia. What is the best management for this patient?

A. Observation
B. Medical management of hypercalcemia
C. Specific treatment of nephrolithiasis
D. Parathyroidectomy

50. Which is incorrect about localization of parathyroid glands?

A. Parathyroid imaging has no role in confirming or excluding the diagnosis of HPT
B. Negative imaging reduces the need of surgical exploration
C. On ultrasound, an abnormal parathyroid gland appears as a round or oval hypoechoic mass with a well-defined hypervascular echogenic capsule
D. Sestamibi is the dominant radioisotope used for parathyroid imaging

51. Which imaging modality has superior sensitivity to detect multigland parathyroid disease?

A. USG B. Sestamibi-SPECT
C. 4D-CT scan D. MRI

52. Which is best imaging modality to detect ectopic parathyroid glands?

A. USG B. Sestamibi-SPECT
C. 4D-CT scan D. MRI

53. Which parathyroid specific PET tracer is used for localization?

A. 18F- FDG B. 11C- Choline
C. 18F-Fluorocholine D. 123I-MIBG

54. All true about focused parathyroidectomy except:

A. Typically an outpatient procedure
B. Through a standard Kocher's incision
C. Focused dissection usually limited to only one gland
D. Performed under local or general anesthesia

55. Miami criteria is used for:

A. Thyroid excision
B. Parathyroid gland excision
C. Pituitary adenoma excision
D. Adrenal tumor excision

56. What is Miami criteria of parathyroidectomy?
A. More than 90% decline in PTH at 15 minutes following parathyroid gland removal
B. More than 75% decline in PTH at 15 minutes following parathyroid gland removal
C. More than 50% decline in PTH at 10 minutes following parathyroid gland removal
D. More than 25% decline in PTH at 10 minutes following parathyroid gland removal

57. What is Dual criteria used for parathyroidectomy?
A. More than 50% PTH decrease from the pre-incision level
B. Final PTH that is within the normal range
C. Both A and B
D. Either A or B

58. What is the most common ectopic location of superior parathyroid gland?
A. Retroesophageal
B. Tracheoesophageal groove
C. Posterior mediastinum
D. Intrathyroidal

59. What is the most common location of supernumerary parathyroid gland?
A. Tracheoesophageal groove
B. Intrathyroidal
C. Posterior mediastinum
D. Thymus

60. What is the best tool to confirm complete resection of abnormal parathyroid glands?
A. Intraoperative frozen section
B. Tissue aspiration and PTH measurement
C. Intraoperative USG
D. Intraoperative PTH measurement

61. Cure of primary HPT is defined as:
A. Eucalcemia at 3 months after surgery
B. Eucalcemia at 6 months after surgery
C. Normal PTH at 3 months after surgery
D. Normal PTH at 6 months after surgery

62. Which is incorrect statement regarding medical management of PHPT?
A. Cinacalcet is an allosteric activator of the CaSR
B. Cinacalcet improves bone mineralization
C. Surgery for PHPT is more cost-effective compared to medical therapy
D. Bisphosphonates improves bone mineralization but do not change calcium or PTH levels

63. Cinacalcet is approved for treating following conditions except:
A. Primary HPT
B. Hypercalcemic crisis
C. Secondary HPT
D. Metastatic parathyroid cancer

64. What is the most common complication following parathyroidectomy?
A. Hypocalcemia
B. Permanent hypoparathyroidism
C. Recurrent laryngeal nerve injury
D. Neck hematoma

65. What is the rate of recurrent laryngeal nerve injury in parathyroidectomy?
A. <1% B. 5%
C. 11% D. 18%

SECONDARY HYPERPARATHYROIDISM

66. All are true about secondary hyperparathyroidism except:
A. Elevated PTH levels with low or normal serum calcium levels
B. 90% of patients with chronic renal insufficiency develop secondary HPT
C. Cinacalcet is used to restore calcium-phosphate homeostasis
D. Maintaining intact-PTH levels below normal range are recommended in CKD patients

67. All are causes of secondary hyperparathyroidism except:
A. Chronic renal failure
B. Celiac disease
C. Hypomagnesemia
D. DiGeorge syndrome

68. All are surgical indications of secondary hyperparathyroidism except:
A. PTH greater than 400 pg/mL
B. Calcium-phosphorous product greater than 55 mg^2/dL
C. Calciphylaxis
D. Refractory hyperphosphatemia

69. PTH levels of ___ are considered to be a surgical indication in renal HPT.
A. >200 pg/mL B. >400 pg/mL
C. >600 pg/mL D. >800 pg/mL

70. While performing subtotal parathyroidectomy, _____ well-vascularized, parathyroid remnant is left in-situ.

A. 8 – 10 mg
B. 10 – 20 mg
C. 20 – 40 mg
D. 40 – 80 mg

TERTIARY HYPERPARATHYROIDISM

71. All are true about tertiary hyperparathyroidism except:

A. Autonomous overproduction of PTH
B. Persists or occurs after successful renal transplantation
C. Cinacalcet is mainstay of treatment
D. Hungry bone syndrome occurs due to the sudden decline in circulating PTH levels after surgery

72. Tertiary HPT is characterized by all except:

A. High serum Calcium
B. High PTH
C. Phosphaturia
D. High serum phosphate

73. Which of the following is cause of tertiary hyperparathyroidism?

A. Osteolytic bone metastasis
B. Tuberculosis
C. 25-Hydroxyvitamin D deficiency
D. Post renal transplant

CALCIPHYLAXIS

74. Which is false regarding calciphylaxis?

A. Microvascular calcification with signs of vasculitis of small subcutaneous vessels
B. Manifested by painful violaceous skin lesions with associated ulceration and eschar
C. Mortality rates of 50% to 80% are reported in patients with calciphylaxis
D. It predominantly affects patients with end-stage renal disease and secondary HPT

75. Which is correct regarding calciphylaxis?

A. Mortality rates of 10% to 20% are reported in patients with calciphylaxis
B. Debridement of dry eschar should be done regularly
C. Total parathyroidectomy with transcervical thymectomy is the preferred operation
D. Urgent parathyroidectomy is required for the management of calciphylaxis

HYPERCALCEMIC CRISIS

76. Which is incorrect concerning HPT-hypercalcemic crisis?

A. Albumin-corrected serum calcium level of 14 mg/dL or greater with associated organ dysfunction
B. They more likely to have a palpable neck mass
C. Acute pancreatitis is more common in patients with HIHC
D. They have elevated calcium and phosphorus levels

77. Which is false about management of HPT-hypercalcemic crisis?

A. It is an endocrine emergency requiring interventions to rapidly reduce serum calcium levels
B. Bisphosphonate drugs considered the first line therapy of HIHC in combination with intravenous volume expansion
C. They more likely to have parathyroid cancer
D. Parathyroidectomy should be performed expeditiously

78. Which of the following monoclonal antibody inhibits osteoclast function?

A. Abituzumab
B. Burosumab
C. Denosumab
D. Elotuzumab

PARATHYROID CANCER

79. Which is incorrect regarding parathyroid cancer?

A. It accounts for less than 1% of all patients with primary HPT
B. It affects men and women in an equal distribution
C. Parathyroid cancer most often occurs sporadically
D. Parathyroid cancer is almost non-functional tumor

80. Which genetic mutation is seen in HPT-Jaw tumor syndrome?

A. GCM2
B. HPRT2
C. CDKN1B
D. CASR

81. Which is incorrect concerning parathyroid cancer?

A. Most patients are symptomatic
B. 50% of patients with parathyroid cancer present with a palpable neck mass
C. Often present with serum calcium levels greater than 14 mg/dL

D. Non-functional parathyroid cancer patients have good prognosis

82. All are true about parathyroid cancer except:

A. Parathyroid cancer is identified as a solid mass with a firm consistency
B. It has grayish white appearance
C. Normal tissue planes between the parathyroid mass and the thyroid lobe are absent
D. Cervical lymph node metastases are common

83. All are true about parathyroid cancer except:

A. Parathyroid cancer is almost a uniformly functional tumor
B. Operative therapy consists of an en bloc resection, including the recurrent laryngeal nerve when it is invaded by cancer
C. Prophylactic central or lateral compartment neck dissection should be done
D. Parathyroid cancer is radioresistant and chemotherapy is ineffective

FAMILIAL PRIMARY HYPERPARATHYROIDISM

84. Genetic testing is recommended in primary HPT patient with all of the following except:

A. Family history of primary HPT
B. Male sex
C. Age younger than 25 years
D. Presence of multigland disease

85. All are true about familial primary hyperparathyroidism except:

A. Primary HPT is familial in 3% to 5% of patient
B. Familial PHPT requires lifelong follow up due higher recurrence rate
C. Genetic testing is recommended in patients with primary HPT younger than 40 years of age with multigland disease
D. CDC73 gene is most often associated with multi-gland disease

86. Which is incorrect about MEN1 association of PHPT?

A. MEN1 is the most common familial form of primary HPT
B. Somatic mutation in the MEN1tumor suppressor gene
C. MEN1 patients develop primary HPT by 50 years of age
D. Most likely to develop multi-gland disease

87. Which is incorrect about MEN2A association of PHPT?

A. MEN2A occurs due to a gain-of-function germline mutation in the RET proto-oncogene
B. Primary HPT in MEN2A has a penetrance of 15% to 35%
C. Specific RET mutations does not alter rate of primary HPT
D. Guidelines preferentially recommend resection of only visibly enlarged glands

88. Which is incorrect about HPT-Jaw tumor syndrome?

A. It is an autosomal recessive disorder
B. HPT-JT associated primary HPT occurs due to single gland disease
C. Parathyroid carcinoma develops in 15% to 20% of patients with HPT-JT
D. Genetic testing for the CDC73 gene are recommended for all patients with parathyroid carcinoma

89. All are correct about Familial isolated HPT except:

A. It is an autosomal dominant disorder
B. Lack of syndromic manifestations
C. Focused parathyroidectomy is recommended
D. Require lifelong follow-up

90. Persistent HPT is defined as failure to achieve normocalcemia within ____ of parathyroidectomy.

A. 4 weeks B. 3 months
C. 6 months D. 1 year

91. Recurrent hypercalcemia defined as elevate serum calcium levels after:

A. 8 weeks B. 6 months
C. 1 year D. 3 years

92. Which of the following is most sensitive modality for parathyroid localization?

A. PET/CT
B. Sestamibi SPECT
C. 4D-CT
D. Selective venous sampling

93. Which is incorrect regarding selective venous sampling?

A. It is reserved when noninvasive imaging localization is unsuccessful
B. It is done via a catheter placed in the jugular vein
C. Allows for cervical and mediastinal venous blood sampling
D. If there is failure of localization of abnormal glands, continued surveillance is recommended

ANSWERS

1. **Ans: B. Ivar Sandstrom**
Ref: Chapter No. 38, Page No. 921

2. **Ans: C. Eugene Gley**
Ref: Chapter No. 38, Page No. 921

3. **Ans: B. Sclerosis**
Ref: Chapter No. 38, Page No. 921

4. **Ans: C. Felix Mandl**
Ref: Chapter No. 38, Page No. 921

5. **Ans: D. Rosalyn Yalow**
Ref: Chapter No. 38, Page No. 922

6. **Ans: C. Potts**
Ref: Chapter No. 38, Page No. 922

7. **Ans: B. 3 to 5 mins**
Ref: Chapter No. 38, Page No. 922

8. **Ans: B. Inferior parathyroid glands**
Ref: Chapter No. 38, Page No. 922

9. **Ans: C. Fourth branchial pouch**
Ref: Chapter No. 38, Page No. 922

10. **Ans: D. Superior parathyroid glands are more frequent in ectopic location**
Ref: Chapter No. 38, Page No. 922

11. **Ans: B. GCM2**
Ref: Chapter No. 38, Page No. 922

12. **Ans: D. GCM2**
Ref: Chapter No. 38, Page No. 923

13. **Ans: C. Familial isolated HPT**
Ref: Chapter No. 38, Page No. 923

14. **Ans: B. 13%**
Ref: Chapter No. 38, Page No. 923

15. **Ans: B. The superior thyroid artery is the predominant vascular supply for all parathyroid glands**
Ref: Chapter No. 38, Page No. 923

16. **Ans: B. Thyrocervical trunk**
Ref: Chapter No. 38, Page No. 923

17. **Ans: B. Inferior thyroid artery**
Ref: Chapter No. 38, Page No. 923

18. **Ans: B. 16%**
Ref: Chapter No. 38, Page No. 923

19. **Ans: C. Tubercle of Zuckerkandl**
Ref: Chapter No. 38, Page No. 923

20. **Ans: C. Superior parathyroid glands lie outside the capsule of the thyroid gland**
Ref: Chapter No. 38, Page No. 923-924

21. **Ans: D. Anterior mediastinum**
Ref: Chapter No. 38, Page No. 924

22. **Ans: D. They are most commonly found 1 cm superior to the junction of the inferior thyroid artery and the recurrent laryngeal nerve**
Ref: Chapter No. 38, Page No. 924

23. **Ans: B. Thymus**
Ref: Chapter No. 38, Page No. 924

24. **Ans: D. Posterior mediastinum**
Ref: Chapter No. 38, Page No. 924

25. **Ans: D. The number of oxyphil cells in the parathyroid gland decreases with age**
Ref: Chapter No. 38, Page No. 924

26. **Ans: B. Oxyphil cell**
Ref: Chapter No. 38, Page No. 924

27. **Ans: A. Chief cell**
Ref: Chapter No. 38, Page No. 924

28. **Ans: D. Sigmoidal relationship exists between extracellular calcium concentration and PTH secretion**
Ref: Chapter No. 38, Page No. 924

29. **Ans: A. 25-hydroxyvitamin D**
Ref: Chapter No. 38, Page No. 924

30. **Ans: C. Reverse sigmoidal**
Ref: Chapter No. 38, Page No. 925

31. **Ans: A. PTH acts on proximal convoluted tubule**
Ref: Chapter No. 38, Page No. 925

32. **Ans: A. PTH binds to the PTHR1 receptor that is found on cells of the osteoclastic lineage**
Ref: Chapter No. 38, Page No. 925

33. **Ans: D. Breast cancer**
Ref: Chapter No. 38, Page No. 926

34. **Ans: D. DiGeorge's syndrome**
Ref: Chapter No. 38, Page No. 926

35. **Ans: D. Vitamin D intoxication**
Ref: Chapter No. 38, Page No. 926

36. **Ans: A. Irradiation**

Ref: Chapter No. 38, Page No. 926

37. **Ans: B. Secondary HPT**

Ref: Chapter No. 38, Page No. 926

38. **Ans: B. FHH develops after the age of 40**

Ref: Chapter No. 38, Page No. 926

39. **Ans: B. Renal CaSR**

Ref: Chapter No. 38, Page No. 926

40. **Ans: B. The parathyroid cells in a parathyroid adenoma have a increased sensitivity to calcium**

Ref: Chapter No. 38, Page No. 926

41. **Ans: D. RET**

Ref: Chapter No. 38, Page No. 927

42. **Ans: A. CASR gene mutation**

Ref: Chapter No. 38, Page No. 927

43. **Ans: D. Adrenal tumor**

Ref: Chapter No. 38, Page No. 927

44. **Ans: A. Distal radius**

Ref: Chapter No. 38, Page No. 928

45. **Ans: C. Distal muscle weakness**

Ref: Chapter No. 38, Page No. 928

46. **Ans: B. 24-hour urine calcium**

Ref: Chapter No. 38, Page No. 929

47. **Ans: D. Urine calcium >200 mg/24 hours**

Ref: Chapter No. 38, Page No. 929

48. **Ans: A. Age > 50 years**

Ref: Chapter No. 38, Page No. 929

49. **Ans: D. Parathyroidectomy**

Ref: Chapter No. 38, Page No. 929

50. **Ans: B. Negative imaging reduces the need of surgical exploration**

Ref: Chapter No. 38, Page No. 930

51. **Ans: C. 4D-CT scan**

Ref: Chapter No. 38, Page No. 930

52. **Ans: B. Sestamibi-SPECT**

Ref: Chapter No. 38, Page No. 931

53. **Ans: C. 18F-Fluorocholine**

Ref: Chapter No. 38, Page No. 931

54. **Ans: B. Through a standard Kocher's incision**

Ref: Chapter No. 38, Page No. 932

55. **Ans: B. Parathyroid gland excision**

Ref: Chapter No. 38, Page No. 932

56. **Ans: C. More than 50% decline in PTH at 10 minutes following parathyroid gland removal**

Ref: Chapter No. 38, Page No. 932

57. **Ans: C. Both A and B**

Ref: Chapter No. 38, Page No. 932

58. **Ans: B. Tracheoesophageal groove**

Ref: Chapter No. 38, Page No. 933

59. **Ans: D. Thymus**

Ref: Chapter No. 38, Page No. 933

60. **Ans: D. Intraoperative PTH measurement**

Ref: Chapter No. 38, Page No. 933

61. **Ans: B. Eucalcemia at 6 months after surgery**

Ref: Chapter No. 38, Page No. 933

62. **Ans: B. Cinacalcet improves bone mineralization**

Ref: Chapter No. 38, Page No. 933-34

63. **Ans: A. Primary HPT**

Ref: Chapter No. 38, Page No. 934

64. **Ans: A. Hypocalcemia**

Ref: Chapter No. 38, Page No. 934

65. **Ans: A. <1%**

Ref: Chapter No. 38, Page No. 934

66. **Ans: D. Maintaining intact-PTH levels below normal range are recommended in CKD patients**

Ref: Chapter No. 38, Page No. 934

67. **Ans: C. Hypomagnesemia**

Ref: Chapter No. 38, Page No. 934

68. **Ans: A. PTH greater than 400 pg/mL**

Ref: Chapter No. 38, Page No. 934

69. **Ans: D. >800 pg/mL**

Ref: Chapter No. 38, Page No. 934

70. **Ans: D. 40 – 80 mg**

Ref: Chapter No. 38, Page No. 935

71. **Ans: C. Cinacalcet is mainstay of treatment**

Ref: Chapter No. 38, Page No. 935

72. **Ans: D. High serum phosphate**

Ref: Chapter No. 38, Page No. 935

73. **Ans: D. Post renal transplant**

Ref: Chapter No. 38, Page No. 935

74. **Ans: A. Microvascular calcification with signs of vasculitis of small subcutaneous vessels**

Ref: Chapter No. 38, Page No. 935

75. **Ans: C. Total parathyroidectomy with transcervical thymectomy is the preferred**

Ref: Chapter No. 38, Page No. 936

76. Ans: D. They have elevated calcium and phosphorus levels

Ref: Chapter No. 38, Page No. 936

77. Ans: C. They more likely to have parathyroid cancer

Ref: Chapter No. 38, Page No. 936

78. Ans: C. Denosumab

Ref: Chapter No. 38, Page No. 936

79. Ans: D. Parathyroid cancer is almost non-functional tumor

Ref: Chapter No. 38, Page No. 937

80. Ans: B. HPRT2

Ref: Chapter No. 38, Page No. 937

81. Ans: D. Non-functional parathyroid cancer patients have good prognosis

Ref: Chapter No. 38, Page No. 937

82. Ans: D. Cervical lymph node metastases are common

Ref: Chapter No. 38, Page No. 937

83. Ans: C. Prophylactic central or lateral compartment neck dissection should be done

Ref: Chapter No. 38, Page No. 937

84. Ans: C. Age younger than 25 years

Ref: Chapter No. 38, Page No. 937

85. Ans: D. CDC73 gene is most often associated with multi-gland disease

Ref: Chapter No. 38, Page No. 937-38

86. Ans: B. Somatic mutation in the MEN1tumor suppressor gene

Ref: Chapter No. 38, Page No. 938

87. Ans: C. Specific RET mutations does not alter rate of primary HPT

Ref: Chapter No. 38, Page No. 938

88. Ans: A. It is an autosomal recessive disorder

Ref: Chapter No. 38, Page No. 938

89. Ans: C. Focused parathyroidectomy is recommended

Ref: Chapter No. 38, Page No. 938

90. Ans: C. 6 months

Ref: Chapter No. 38, Page No. 938

91. Ans: B. 6 months

Ref: Chapter No. 38, Page No. 938

92. Ans: C. 4D-CT

Ref: Chapter No. 38, Page No. 938

93. Ans: B. It is done via a catheter placed in the jugular vein

Ref: Chapter No. 38, Page No. 939

39

Endocrine Pancreas

EMBRYOLOGY AND PHYSIOLOGY

1. **Which of the following is false statement about development of pancreas?**
   A. Pancreatic formation begins during the third week of gestation
   B. First organized islets appear at approximately 10 weeks
   C. Acinar and islet cells differentiate from the endodermal cells
   D. B cell proliferate up to the first 2 years of life

2. **Wrongly matched of the following:**
   A. A cell – Glucagon
   B. F cell – VIP
   C. D cell – somatostatin
   D. B cell – Insulin

3. **Which is wrong about histology of pancreas?**
   A. Endocrine cells comprise less than 2% of the overall pancreatic mass
   B. All cell types are not evenly distributed within the islets or throughout the pancreas
   C. Islets largely (up to 70%) consist of B cells
   D. B cells are evenly distributed throughout the gland

4. **All are true statements except:**
   A. The center of the islet consists of B cells
   B. B cells to inhibit A cell secretion
   C. A cells to inhibit D cell secretion
   D. The B cells' insulin stimulates pancreatic exocrine secretion and synthesis of protein

5. **All are functions of insulin except:**
   A. Glucose transport into cell
   B. Inhibiting glycogenolysis
   C. Stimulate lipolysis
   D. Stimulating protein synthesis

6. **Insulin does not transport glucose into following cells:**
   A. B cells of pancreas B. Hepatocytes
   C. CNS cells D. All of the above

7. **All are inhibitors of insulin except:**
   A. Somatostatin B. Amylin
   C. Leptin D. GLP-1

8. **Wrongly matched of the following:**
   A. A cell – 10% B. B cell – 70%
   C. D cell – 5% D. F cell – 1%

9. **Which cell type is not present in normal physiologic state of pancreas?**
   A. D2 cells B. E cells
   C. F cells D. G cells

10. **Which is false about location of each cell type in islet of pancreas?**
    A. A cells present peripherally
    B. B cells are located centrally
    C. F cells are evenly distributed
    D. D cells are evenly distributed

11. **Wrongly matched about cell type and its location within pancreas:**
    A. A cells – Head and neck of pancreas
    B. B cells – Body and tail
    C. F cells – Head and uncinate process
    D. D cells – Evenly distributed

12. **All are secreted by alpha cells except:**
    A. Glucagon B. Endorphin
    C. Pancreastatin D. Substance P

13. **All are secreted by beta cells except:**
    A. Insulin B. Amylin
    C. Pancreastatin D. Cholecystokinin

14. Which hormone is secreted by D2 cells of pancreas?

A. Pancreatic polypeptide
B. Vasoactive intestinal peptide
C. Pancreastatin
D. Substance P

15. Which is wrongly matched regarding diagnostic values of endocrine pancreatic tumors?

A. Fasting glucagon >1000 pg/mL – Glucagonoma
B. Somatostatin >160 pg/mL – Somatostatinoma
C. With secretin test, an increase of >400 pg/mL Gastrin – Gastrinoma
D. Insulin >5 μU/mL in the face of hypoglycemia – Insulinoma

16. High volume secretary diarrhea with metabolic acidosis is presented in which pancreatic endocrine tumor?

A. Gastrinoma B. VIPoma
C. PPoma D. Glucagonoma

17. Necrolytic migratory erythema is seen in which pancreatic endocrine tumor?

A. Gastrinoma B. VIPoma
C. Somatostatinoma D. Glucagonoma

18. Which is not the function of incretin hormones?

A. Release of insulin
B. Maintain Beta cell mass
C. Gastric emptying
D. Inhibition of feeding

19. Which is incorrect regarding pancreatic hormonal function?

A. The B cell is highly sensitive to changes in glucose concentration and is maximally stimulated at concentrations of 400 to 500 mg/dL
B. Ghrelin primarily inhibits insulin release from the pancreas
C. Leptin functions as a feedback mechanism to inhibit food intake and to regulate body weight
D. Incretins are intestinal hormones which inhibits insulin release

20. Which is incorrect regarding pancreatic hormonal function?

A. Both insulin and glucagon secretions are under neuronal control
B. Somatostatin secreted by D cells has generalized inhibitory function
C. Pancreatic polypeptide is used as marker for other endocrine tumors of the pancreas
D. Amylin deposits in the pancreas of patients with type 1 diabetes

PANCREATIC NEUROENDOCRINE TUMORS

21. Which is incorrect about PNETs?

A. PNETs account for less than 3% of pancreatic neoplasms
B. PNETs comprised 7% of all gastroentero-pancreatic NET
C. Malignancy in PNETs can only definitely be determined by the presence of metastasis
D. WHO staging system based on site of origin and functional hormone secretion

22. WHO system classify NETs based on following variables except:

A. Histological Appearance
B. Mitotic rate
C. Ki-67 Index
D. Functional hormone

23. All are characteristics of low grade NET except:

A. Abundant neuroendocrine markers
B. < 2 mitoses/10 HPF
C. Ki-67 Index <10%
D. Indolent behavior

24. NET carcinoma (Grade 3) is characterized by all except:

A. Pleomorphic cells with necrosis
B. >20 mitoses/50 HPF
C. Ki-67 Index > 20%
D. Aggressive behavior

25. AJCC NET staging includes all except:

A. Size B. Lymph nodes
C. Grade D. Metastasis

26. Stage of a 5 cm PNET invading duodenal wall with 6 regional lymph nodes involvement, without any distant metastases:

A. T2N1M0 B. T2N2M0
C. T3N2M0 D. T4N1M0

27. Which is wrong about Menin gene?

A. Chromosome 11q13
B. Component of the histone methyltransferase complex

C. Control of G1 to S phase cell cycle progression
D. It is not involved in sporadic cases

28. Which is false about genetic causes of PNET?
A. Most PNETs occur sporadically
B. The most common genetic syndrome associated with PNETs is MEN1
C. Menin is involved in control of G2 to M phase cell cycle progression
D. Inactivating mutations in MEN1 were seen in 44% of sporadic tumors

29. All are true about VHL syndrome associated PNETs except:
A. PNETs are often multifocal and have syndromic association
B. PNETs associated with VHL generally behave in an indolent fashion
C. Specific germline mutations in exon 3 of the VHL gene may be associated with a good prognosis
D. Risk for the development of renal cell carcinoma and CNS tumors

30. Following tumors are associated with VHL syndrome except:
A. Pancreatic lesions B. Pheochromocytoma
C. Renal cell carcinoma D. Liver adenoma

31. Which mTOR inhibitor is FDA approved for advanced NETs?
A. Tacrolimus B. Everolimus
C. Sirolimus D. Temsirolimus

32. Which is most common genetic mutation is seen in PNETs?
A. MEN1
B. DAXX
C. ATRX
D. mTOR pathway gene

33. Which genetic mutation is not seen in PNETs?
A. mTOR pathway B. KRAS
C. DAXX D. ATRX

34. Which of the following mutation is seen in PNETs?
A. KRAS B. CDKN2A
C. DAXX D. SMAD4

35. Which mutation differentiate adenocarcinoma from PNETs?
A. mTOR pathway B. p53
C. KRAS D. DAXX

36. Which is false regarding chromogranin A?
A. Chromogranin A levels correlate with both functional and nonfunctional PNET
B. It is a biomarker for both confirmation and surveillance
C. Chromogranin A levels can also be elevated in patients on proton pump inhibitors (PPIs) or with atrophic gastritis
D. It has association with clinical syndromes

37. What is the first modality of choice to localize PNET?
A. USG B. MDCT
C. EUS D. SRS

38. Which is false about PNET localization?
A. MDCT is first step in suspected PNET
B. Capturing the vascular blush in the arterial phase is critical for identification
C. MRI has low sensitivity detecting lesions smaller than 2 cm
D. EUS has an overall sensitivity of approximately 90% for tumors of all sizes

39. All are true about SRS except:
A. Most PNETs have abundance of somatostatin receptors
B. The sensitivity for SRS is over 80%
C. SRS is also useful for detecting hepatic metastases
D. SRS gives anatomic precision in localization

40. Which PNET is not diagnosed with SRS study?
A. Glucagonoma
B. Insulinoma
C. Gastrinoma
D. Non-functional tumor

41. To detect PNETs, SPECT/CT has sensitivity and specificity of:
A. 95% and 90% B. 80% and 95%
C. 95% and 97% D. 98% and 80%

42. Which is most specific and sensitive modality for localization of PNET?
A. MDCT B. EUS
C. SRS D. SPECT/CT

43. What is used for hormonal stimulation in case of gastrinoma detection by angiography?
A. Calcium B. Secretin
C. Somatostatin D. CCK

44. Which is false regarding management of incidentally found non functional PNET?

A. Observation of low grade tumors less than 1 cm
B. ENETS recommends mandatory EUS and MRI repeated every 6 months
C. If an increase of ≥0.5 cm in the size of the lesion occurs, patients should be reevaluated for surgery
D. NCCN recommend CT or MRI of the abdomen 6 monthly and CT of the chest when indicated

45. Observation is recommended in which of the following PNET?

A. Functional tumor < 2 cm
B. Asymtomatic functional tumor < 1 cm
C. Nonfunctional tumor < 2 cm
D. Incidental tumor < 3 cm

46. Which is incorrect about intra-operative localization of PNET?

A. The entire pancreas needs to be mobilized
B. 7.5- to 10-MHz transducers are used for the pancreas
C. Islet tumors are detected as echogenic heterogeneous masses
D. Identification of the ductal system is necessary

47. Which is not considered a curative/palliative criteria in case of liver metastasis of PNET?

A. G1/G2 tumor
B. Absence of distant lymph node metastases
C. Absence of extrahepatic metastases
D. >50% resectable disease overall

48. Agent used for transarterial embolization of liver metastases:

A. Lipiodol
B. Gel foam particle
C. Polyvinyl alcohol foam
D. All of the above

49. Transarterial chemoembolization uses following agent:

A. Doxorubicin
B. Melphalan
C. Streptozocin
D. All of the above

50. PROMID Trial for treating PNET is based on:

A. Intra-arterial chemoembolization
B. Octreotide LAR
C. Systemic cytotoxic chemotherapy
D. Targeted therapy using everolimus

51. Pasireotide acts on which of the following receptors?

A. SSTR1
B. SSTR2
C. SSTR5
D. All of the above

52. Which of the following trial was done for use of Lanreotide in PNET?

A. PROMID
B. CLARINET
C. RADIANT
D. TELESTAR

53. Which is wrong regarding chemotherapy in case of PNET?

A. Somatostatin analog is recommended for G1/low G2 PNETs
B. Grade 3 PNET are aggressive and respond to cytotoxic chemotherapy
C. For high-grade tumors with poor differentiation, platinum-based regimens are preferred
D. Lenvatinib is FDA approved targeted therapy of advanced well-differentiated PNET

54. Which is the FDA approved tyrosine kinase inhibitor for PNET?

A. Sorafenib
B. Sunitinib
C. Vandetinib
D. Erlotinib

55. Which is false statement about transplant in PNET liver metastases?

A. Unresectable neuroendocrine metastases is the only metastatic indication for transplantation
B. Age younger than 45 years with well-differentiated tumor status
C. Less than 50% liver involvement by metastases
D. Completely resected primary tumor in absence of extrahepatic disease

56. Which is false about Milan criteria for liver transplant?

A. Age younger than 55 years
B. Ki-67 proliferative marker index less than 5%
C. Less than 75% liver involvement
D. Well-differentiated tumor status

INSULINOMA

57. Which is incorrect regarding insulinoma?

A. Insulinoma is the most common functioning PNET
B. The clinical syndrome defined by Whipple's triad
C. The average age at diagnosis is 45 years
D. Insulinomas are more common in body and tail the pancreas

58. About insulinoma, incorrect statement is:

A. Insulinomas are typically have an average size of 1.0 to 1.5 cm
B. Surgical resection of insulinoma is usually curative
C. They are usually benign and solitary
D. 25% are associated with MEN1

59. Which of the following is more commonly considered a benign tumor?

A. Insulinoma B. Glucagonoma
C. VIPoma D. Somatostatinoma

60. Which is the gold standard test for diagnosis of insulinoma?

A. C-peptide levels
B. Insulin: Glucose ratio
C. 72 hours monitored fast
D. EUS

61. What is characteristic of non-insulinoma pancreatogenous hypoglycemia syndrome?

A. Insulin receptor antibodies
B. Postprandial hypoglycemia
C. Insulin-glucose ratio >0.3
D. Pancreatic lesion

62. All findings are consistent with insulinoma except:

A. Insulin-glucose ratio <0.3
B. Fasting hypoglycemia
C. C-peptide levels higher than 1.2 µg/mL
D. Serum beta hydroxybutyrate levels < 2.7 mmol/L at the end of the fast

63. Which is correct regarding management of insulinoma?

A. SRS is indicated for localization
B. Pancreatic resection is usually preferred operative procedure
C. Surgical resection is the mainstay and is the only curative option for insulinoma
D. Enucleation should not be performed if the tumor is within 5 mm of the main pancreatic duct

64. Fasting hypoglycemia is seen with all conditions except:

A. Insulinoma
B. NIPHS
C. Insulin autoimmune hypoglycemia
D. IGF mediated hypoglycemia

65. Which drug can be used to prevent symptoms of hypoglycemia before surgical intervention?

A. Acetazolamide B. Diazoxide
C. Streptozotocin D. Temozolomide

GASTRINOMA

66. Which is false about gastrinoma incidence?

A. The mean age of patients at diagnosis is approximately 50 years
B. More common in women
C. Sporadic in 75% of patient
D. Associated with MEN1 in 25%

67. Most common location of ulcers in ZES:

A. Esophageal B. Gastric
C. Duodenal D. Jejunal

68. Which is the most common symptom of gastrinoma?

A. Abdominal pain B. Diarrhoea
C. GERD D. Vomiting

69. All are true about features of gastrinoma except:

A. It is suspected diagnosis in presence of jejunal ulcers
B. It causes acid-induced diarrhea which is stopped by nasogastric aspiration
C. Duodenal gastrinomas, most arising in the second part of duodenum
D. Ninety percent of gastrinomas are located within the gastrinoma triangle

70. Boundaries of gastrinoma triangle are formed by the lines connecting three of following except:

A. The cystic duct
B. The junction between the second and third portions of the duodenum
C. The junction between the neck and body of the pancreas
D. The junction between the head and neck of the pancreas

71. All are true about diagnosis of gastrinoma except:

A. Gastrin levels higher than 1000 pg/mL with increased acid secretion are highly suggestive of gastrinoma
B. All PPIs should be stopped 2 weeks prior to testing gastrin levels
C. A gastric pH higher than 3 without acid-suppressing medications or prior acid-reducing operations strongly exclude ZES
D. Gastrin levels greater than 400 pg/mL after administration of secretin is also diagnostic

72. Which is the cause of hypergastrinemia with normal or low acid secretion?

A. Gastrinoma
B. Gastric cancer
C. Gastric outlet obstruction
D. Retained gastric antrum

73. Which is false regarding gastrinoma?

A. Duodenotomy will detect 25% to 30% of tumors not seen on preoperative imaging
B. Total gastrectomy cures all symptoms produced by excessive acid but has no effect on disease progression or survival for metastatic disease
C. 90% of aggressive tumors are located in the pancreas
D. The best predictor of survival for patients with gastrinoma is the presence of lymph node metastases

74. Gastrinoma patient has increased risk for:

A. Gastric lymphoma
B. Esophageal adenocarcinoma
C. Gastric adenocarcinoma
D. Gastric carcinoid

75. Which is false regarding management of gastrinoma?

A. Exploration includes the entire pancreas and gastrinoma triangle for preoperatively non localized tumors
B. Most gastrinomas require pancreatic resection procedures
C. More than 50% of patients with gastrinomas have metastatic disease at the time of diagnosis
D. For patients with unresectable, symptomatic metastatic disease PPI therapy is the mainstay

VIPOMA

76. VIP is normally not found in:

A. Brain
B. G cells of antrum
C. Adrenal cortex
D. D2 cells of pancreas

77. VIPoma has following features except:

A. Watery diarrhea
B. Hypokalemia
C. Achlorhydria
D. Hypochlorhydria

78. Which is incorrect about VIPoma?

A. More than two thirds are benign
B. Most common location is the pancreas
C. 5% are associated with MEN1
D. Elevated VIP levels in children are most commonly caused by ganglioneuromas

79. Which is false regarding VIPoma?

A. Generally solitary
B. Larger than 3 cm at diagnosis
C. Commonly found in the pancreatic head
D. 95% are sporadic

80. Most common location of VIPoma:

A. Pancreatic head and neck
B. 2nd part of duodenum
C. Pancreatic body and tail
D. Mediastinal

81. All are true about feature of VIPoma except:

A. Profuse, watery, iso-osmotic secretory diarrhea is the most common presenting symptom
B. The diagnosis of VIPoma is unlikely if the stool volume is less than 700 mL/day
C. Normal VIP levels are lower than 100 pg/mL
D. The diarrhea persists despite fasting and nasogastric aspiration

GLUCAGONOMA

82. Which is incorrect about glucagonoma?

A. Incidence in male to female is 3:1
B. 5 to 10 cm in size at the time of diagnosis
C. Commonly located in the body or tail of pancreas
D. 5% to 17% are associated with MEN1

83. Classic presentation of glucagonoma includes all except:

A. Diabetes
B. Dermatitis
C. Deep vein thrombosis
D. Dementia

84. All are true regarding glucagonoma except:

A. Commonly a malignant tumor
B. The characteristic skin lesion, a necrolytic migrating erythema has serpiginous margins
C. A fasting glucagon level higher than 400 pg/mL is considered diagnostic
D. Prophylaxis against thromboembolism should be instituted early

85. What fasting levels of glucagon are diagnostic of glucagonoma?

A. > 200 pg/mL B. > 400 pg/mL
C. > 800 pg/mL D. > 1000 pg/mL

86. ____ % of malignant glucaganomas present with liver metastases at the time of diagnosis.

A. 45% B. 60%
C. 80% D. 95%

SOMATOSTATINOMA AND OTHER TUMOR

87. Somatostatioma has following features except:

A. Cholelithiasis B. Steatorrhea
C. Diabetes D. Achorhydria

88. Somatostatin levels more than ___ are considered diagnostic of somatostatinoma.

A. 100 ng/mL B. 160 pg/mL
C. 150 ng/mL D. 200 pg/mL

89. Which is false about somatostatinoma?

A. Usually found in head of pancreas
B. Larger than 2 cm
C. Metastases to the liver or lymph nodes common
D. They are commonly associated with MEN1

90. Somatostatinoma are commonly associated with:

A. MEN1 syndrome B. MEN2 syndrome
C. NF1 disease D. VHL syndrome

91. Following are features of malignant neurotensinoma except:

A. Diabetes B. Flushing
C. Hypotension D. Hyperkalemia

92. Which is incorrect about PPoma?

A. It is non functional tumor
B. Usually small and multiple
C. Most common PNET associated with MEN1
D. PP levels can be raised in other NETs

93. All are classified as non functional tumors except:

A. PPoma
B. VIPoma
C. Neurotensinoma
D. Calcitonin secreting tumor

94. What is the most common cause of tumor related death in MEN1?

A. Hyperparathyroidism
B. Pancreatic NETs
C. Metastases
D. Local invasion

95. Which is the most common PNET seen in MEN1?

A. Gastrinoma B. Insulinoma
C. PPoma D. Glucagonoma

96. Which is the most common pancreatic endocrine syndrome seen in MEN1?

A. Gastrinoma B. Insulinoma
C. PPoma D. Glucagonoma

97. Which is false regarding NIPHS (Nesidioblastosis)?

A. It is characterized by excessive pancreatic B cell function
B. Associated pancreatic islet hyperplasia and dysplasia
C. Postprandial hypoglycemia, within 4 hours of a meal, is the hallmark of NIPHS
D. Elevated insulin and beta hydroxybutyrate levels

SURGICAL THERAPY COMPLICATION

98. Which operative procedure is associated with NIPHS?

A. Sleeve gastrectomy
B. Roux en Y gastric bypass
C. Duodenal switch
D. Gastric banding

99. What % of pancreatic mass removal results in endocrine insufficiency?

A. 60% B. 75%
C. 85% D. 90%

100. Brittle diabetes is seen after:

A. Chronic pancreatitis
B. Whipple's procedure
C. Total pancreatectomy
D. Pancreatic fistula

ISLET TRANSPLANT

101. Islet cells are transplanted through:

A. Percutaneous directly into liver
B. Jugular vein
C. Portal vein
D. Hepatic artery

102. What is one year graft survival rate of pancreas only transplant?

A. 55% B. 65%
C. 75% D. 85%

103. Whole pancreatic transplant is gold standard for which condition?

A. Refractory type 1 diabetes
B. Refractory type 2 diabetes
C. Chronic calcific pancreatitis
D. Pancreatic NET

104. What is one year graft survival rate of simultaneous kidney-pancreas transplant?

A. 65%
B. 75%
C. 85%
D. 95%

105. Donor pancreas required for islet transplant per recipient:

A. 1
B. 2
C. 3
D. 4

ANSWERS

1. **Ans: A. Pancreatic formation begins during the third week of gestation**

   Ref: Chapter No. 39, Page No. 941

2. **Ans: B. F cell – VIP**

   Ref: Chapter No. 39, Page No. 941

3. **Ans: D. B cells are evenly distributed throughout the gland**

   Ref: Chapter No. 39, Page No. 941-942

4. **Ans: C. A cells to inhibit D cell secretion**

   Ref: Chapter No. 39, Page No. 942

5. **Ans: C. Stimulate lipolysis**

   Ref: Chapter No. 39, Page No. 942

6. **Ans: D. All of the above**

   Ref: Chapter No. 39, Page No. 942

7. **Ans: D. GLP-1**

   Ref: Chapter No. 39, Page No. 943

8. **Ans: D. F cell – 1%**

   Ref: Chapter No. 39, Page No. 943

9. **Ans: D. G cells**

   Ref: Chapter No. 39, Page No. 943

10. **Ans: C. F cells are evenly distributed**

    Ref: Chapter No. 39, Page No. 943

11. **Ans: A. A cells – Head and neck of pancreas**

    Ref: Chapter No. 39, Page No. 943

12. **Ans: D. Substance P**

    Ref: Chapter No. 39, Page No. 943

13. **Ans: D. Cholecystokinin**

    Ref: Chapter No. 39, Page No. 943

14. **Ans: B. Vasoactive intestinal peptide**

    Ref: Chapter No. 39, Page No. 943

15. **Ans: C. With secretin test, an increase of >400 pg/mL Gastrin – Gastrinoma**

    Ref: Chapter No. 39, Page No. 943

16. **Ans: B. VIPoma**

    Ref: Chapter No. 39, Page No. 943

17. **Ans: D. Glucagonoma**

    Ref: Chapter No. 39, Page No. 943

18. **Ans: C. Gastric emptying**

    Ref: Chapter No. 39, Page No. 943

19. **Ans: D. Incretins are intestinal hormones which inhibits insulin release**

    Ref: Chapter No. 39, Page No. 942-944

20. **Ans: D. Amylin deposits in the pancreas of patients with type 1 diabetes**

    Ref: Chapter No. 39, Page No. 944

21. **Ans: D. WHO staging system based on site of origin and functional hormone secretion**

    Ref: Chapter No. 39, Page No. 944

22. **Ans: D. Functional hormone**

    Ref: Chapter No. 39, Page No. 945

23. **Ans: C. Ki-67 Index <10%**

    Ref: Chapter No. 39, Page No. 945

24. **Ans: B. >20 mitoses/50 HPF**

    Ref: Chapter No. 39, Page No. 945

25. **Ans: C. Grade**

    Ref: Chapter No. 39, Page No. 945

26. **Ans: C. T3N2M0**

    Ref: Chapter No. 39, Page No. 945

27. **Ans: D. It is not involved in sporadic cases**

    Ref: Chapter No. 39, Page No. 945

28. **Ans: C. Menin is involved in control of G2 to M phase cell cycle progression**

    Ref: Chapter No. 39, Page No. 945-946

29. **Ans: C. Specific germline mutations in exon 3 of the VHL gene may be associated with a good prognosis**

    Ref: Chapter No. 39, Page No. 946

30. **Ans: D. Liver adenoma**

    Ref: Chapter No. 39, Page No. 946

31. **Ans: B. Everolimus**

    Ref: Chapter No. 39, Page No. 946

32. **Ans: A. MEN1**

    Ref: Chapter No. 39, Page No. 947

33. **Ans: B. KRAS**

    Ref: Chapter No. 39, Page No. 947

34. **Ans: C. DAXX**

    Ref: Chapter No. 39, Page No. 947

35. **Ans: C. KRAS**

    Ref: Chapter No. 39, Page No. 947

36. **Ans: D. It has association with clinical syndromes**

Ref: Chapter No. 39, Page No. 947

37. **Ans: B. MDCT**

Ref: Chapter No. 39, Page No. 947

38. **Ans: A. MDCT is first step in suspected PNET**

Ref: Chapter No. 39, Page No. 947

39. **Ans: D. SRS gives anatomic precision in localization**

Ref: Chapter No. 39, Page No. 947-948

40. **Ans: B. Insulinoma**

Ref: Chapter No. 39, Page No. 947-948

41. **Ans: C. 95% and 97%**

Ref: Chapter No. 39, Page No. 947-948

42. **Ans: D. SPECT/CT**

Ref: Chapter No. 39, Page No. 948

43. **Ans: B. Secretin**

Ref: Chapter No. 39, Page No. 949

44. **Ans: A. Observation of low grade tumors less than 1 cm**

Ref: Chapter No. 39, Page No. 951

45. **Ans: C. Nonfunctional tumor < 2 cm**

Ref: Chapter No. 39, Page No. 951

46. **Ans: C. Islet tumors are detected as echogenic heterogeneous masses**

Ref: Chapter No. 39, Page No. 951

47. **Ans: D. >50% resectable disease overall**

Ref: Chapter No. 39, Page No. 951

48. **Ans: D. All of the above**

Ref: Chapter No. 39, Page No. 952

49. **Ans: D. All of the above**

Ref: Chapter No. 39, Page No. 952

50. **Ans: B. Octreotide LAR**

Ref: Chapter No. 39, Page No. 952

51. **Ans: D.** All of the above

Ref: Chapter No. 39, Page No. 952

52. **Ans: B. CLARINET**

Ref: Chapter No. 39, Page No. 952

53. **Ans: D. Lenvatinib is FDA approved targeted therapy of advanced well-differentiated PNET**

Ref: Chapter No. 39, Page No. 952

54. **Ans: B. Sunitinib**

Ref: Chapter No. 39, Page No. 952

55. **Ans: B. Age younger than 45 years with well-differentiated tumor status**

Ref: Chapter No. 39, Page No. 952

56. **Ans: C. Less than 75% liver involvement**

Ref: Chapter No. 39, Page No. 952

57. **Ans: D. Insulinomas are more common in body and tail the pancreas**

Ref: Chapter No. 39, Page No. 953

58. **Ans: D. 25% are associated with MEN1**

Ref: Chapter No. 39, Page No. 953

59. **Ans: A. Insulinoma**

Ref: Chapter No. 39, Page No. 953

60. **Ans: C. 72 hours monitored fast**

Ref: Chapter No. 39, Page No. 953

61. **Ans: B. Postprandial hypoglycemia**

Ref: Chapter No. 39, Page No. 953

62. **Ans: A. Insulin-glucose ratio <0.3**

Ref: Chapter No. 39, Page No. 953

63. **Ans: C. Surgical resection is the mainstay and is the only curative option for insulinoma**

Ref: Chapter No. 39, Page No. 953

64. **Ans: B. NIPHS**

Ref: Chapter No. 39, Page No. 954

65. **Ans: B. Diazoxide**

Ref: Chapter No. 39, Page No. 955

66. **Ans: B. More common in women**

Ref: Chapter No. 39, Page No. 955

67. **Ans: C. Duodenal**

Ref: Chapter No. 39, Page No. 955

68. **Ans: A. Abdominal pain**

Ref: Chapter No. 39, Page No. 955

69. **Ans: C. Duodenal gastrinomas, most arising in the second part of duodenum**

Ref: Chapter No. 39, Page No. 955

70. **Ans: D. The junction between the head and neck of the pancreas**

Ref: Chapter No. 39, Page No. 955

71. **Ans: D. Gastrin levels greater than 400 pg/mL after administration of secretin is also diagnostic**

Ref: Chapter No. 39, Page No. 955

72. **Ans: B. Gastric cancer**

Ref: Chapter No. 39, Page No. 956

73. **Ans: D. The best predictor of survival for patients with gastrinoma is the presence of lymph node metastases**

Ref: Chapter No. 39, Page No. 957

74. **Ans: D. Gastric carcinoid**

Ref: Chapter No. 39, Page No. 957

75. **Ans: A. Exploration includes the entire pancreas and gastrinoma triangle for preoperatively non localized tumors**

Ref: Chapter No. 39, Page No. 957

76. **Ans: C. Adrenal cortex**

Ref: Chapter No. 39, Page No. 957

77. **Ans: D. Hypochlorhydria**

Ref: Chapter No. 39, Page No. 957

78. **Ans: A. More than two thirds are benign**

Ref: Chapter No. 39, Page No. 957

79. **Ans: C. Commonly found in the pancreatic head**

Ref: Chapter No. 39, Page No. 957

80. **Ans: C. Pancreatic body and tail**

Ref: Chapter No. 39, Page No. 957

81. **Ans: C. Normal VIP levels are lower than 100 pg/mL**

Ref: Chapter No. 39, Page No. 957

82. **Ans: A. Incidence in male to female is 3:1**

Ref: Chapter No. 39, Page No. 958

83. **Ans: D. Dementia**

Ref: Chapter No. 39, Page No. 958

84. **Ans: C. A fasting glucagon level higher than 400 pg/mL is considered diagnostic**

Ref: Chapter No. 39, Page No. 958

85. **Ans: D. > 1000 pg/mL**

Ref: Chapter No. 39, Page No. 958

86. **Ans: C. 80%**

Ref: Chapter No. 39, Page No. 958

87. **Ans: D. Achorhydria**

Ref: Chapter No. 39, Page No. 958

88. **Ans: B. 160 pg/mL**

Ref: Chapter No. 39, Page No. 958

89. **Ans: D. They are commonly associated with MEN1**

Ref: Chapter No. 39, Page No. 958

90. **Ans: C. NF1 disease**

Ref: Chapter No. 39, Page No. 958

91. **Ans: D. Hyperkalemia**

Ref: Chapter No. 39, Page No. 958

92. **Ans: B. Usually small and multiple**

Ref: Chapter No. 39, Page No. 958

93. **Ans: B. VIPoma**

Ref: Chapter No. 39, Page No. 958

94. **Ans: B. Pancreatic NETs**

Ref: Chapter No. 39, Page No. 959

95. **Ans: C. PPoma**

Ref: Chapter No. 39, Page No. 959

96. **Ans: A. Gastrinoma**

Ref: Chapter No. 39, Page No. 959

97. **Ans: D. Elevated insulin and beta hydroxybutyrate levels**

Ref: Chapter No. 39, Page No. 959

98. **Ans: B. Roux en Y gastric bypass**

Ref: Chapter No. 39, Page No. 959

99. **Ans: C.85%**

Ref: Chapter No. 39, Page No. 960

100. **Ans: C. Total pancreatectomy**

Ref: Chapter No. 39, Page No. 960

101. **Ans: C. Portal vein**

Ref: Chapter No. 39, Page No. 960

102. **Ans: C. 75%**

Ref: Chapter No. 39, Page No. 961

103. **Ans: A. Refractory type 1 diabetes**

Ref: Chapter No. 39, Page No. 961

104. **Ans: C. 85%**

Ref: Chapter No. 39, Page No. 961

105. **Ans: B. 2**

Ref: Chapter No. 39, Page No. 961

40

The Adrenal Glands

ANATOMY, EMBRYOLOGY AND HISTOLOGY

1. **The adrenal glands were first described by:**
   A. Kölliker B. Eustachi
   C. Thomas Addison D. Edward Kendall

2. **All are true about adrenal anatomy except:**
   A. Weighing approximately 4 g each
   B. Right adrenal is pyramidal in shape
   C. Left adrenal is crescent shaped
   D. Receiving 1 L/kg/min of blood

3. **Blood supply to the adrenals is:**
   A. 20 mL/g/min B. 2000 mL/kg/min
   C. 2 L/kg/Hr D. 200 mL/kg/Hr

4. **Which is false regarding adrenal development?**
   A. The primordial cortex arises from the endodermal tissue
   B. The adrenal medulla arises from the ectodermal tissues of the embryonic neural crest
   C. Cortical biosynthetic activity can be detected by the seventh week
   D. Pheochromocytomas may arise in extra-adrenal sites more commonly

5. **Primordial cortex of adrenal develops from:**
   A. Endoderm
   B. Ectoderm of neural crest tissue
   C. Coelomic mesoderm
   D. Mesonephros tissue

6. **Which is incorrect about relations to adrenal glands?**
   A. Bare area of the liver is anterosuperiorly to the right adrenal gland
   B. Inferior limb of left adrenal gland extends caudad toward the renal
   C. The tail of the pancreas and splenic hilum lie posterior to left adrenal gland
   D. Each adrenal gland is enveloped by its proper capsule

7. **All are true about vascular supply of adrenal glands except:**
   A. The arterial supply is diffuse, the venous drainage of each gland is usually solitary
   B. The left adrenal vein is approximately 2 cm long and drains into the left renal vein
   C. The right adrenal vein is typically as short as it is wide
   D. In up to 5% of individuals, the right adrenal vein has variant

8. **Arterial supply to the adrenals through all except:**
   A. Inferior phrenic B. Aorta
   C. Renal artery D. Lumbar artery

9. **Right adrenal vein may drain into all except:**
   A. Inferior phrenic vein B. Right hepatic vein
   C. Renal vein D. IVC

10. **Variant of right adrenal vein is seen __% of individuals.**
    A. 5% B. 10%
    C. 20% D. 25%

11. **All are true statements except:**
    A. The cortex is approximately 2 mm thick and composes more than 80% of the mass of the gland
    B. Most of the adrenal cortex is formed by the zona granulosa
    C. Chromaffin cells of adrenal medulla are large, polyhedral, and packed with basophilic secretory granules

D. The adrenal arteries before entering the capsule form a sub-capsular plexus

12. Wrongly matched of the following:

A. Zona glomerulosa – small cells, eosinophilic, lipid-poor cytoplasm
B. Zona fasciculata – large, clear, lipid-laden cells
C. Zona reticularis – small nests, basophilic cells
D. Adrenal medulla – large, polyhedral, basophilic

BIOCHEMISTRY AND PHYSIOLOGY

13. Which is false about steroid synthesis?

A. Cholesterol undergoes oxidative reactions catalyzed cytochrome P450 inside mitochondria
B. Pregnenolone is the immediate precursor to the adrenal steroid hormones
C. Cortisol is generated by the oxidation of corticosterone by CYP11B2 within the zona glomerulosa
D. CYP17 expression is confined to the zona fasciculata and zona reticularis

14. All are true about glucocorticoids except:

A. ACTH stimulates glucocorticoid secretion through G protein–coupled receptor
B. Continuous baseline secretion of ACTH is maintained
C. The highest levels of cortisol are generally detected on waking
D. Glucocorticoids are potent anti-inflammatory and immunosuppressive agents

15. Which is false regarding mineralocorticoids?

A. Aldosterone is released from the zona glomerulosa
B. The prohormone angiotensinogen is synthesized by the liver
C. Hyperkalemia reduces aldosterone release by suppressing renin secretion
D. Aldosterone promotes sodium and chloride retention by the distal tubule

16. All are true about catecholamine except:

A. Hydroxylation of tyrosine is first step in catecholamine synthesis
B. Dopamine synthesis is rate limiting step
C. Epinephrine synthesis, is localized to the chromaffin cells of the adrenal medulla and organ of Zuckerkandl
D. Metanephrine and nor-metanephrine are used for pheochromocytoma diagnosis

17. What is the precursor of catecholamines?

A. Tryptophan
B. Tyrosine
C. Phenylalanine
D. Threonine

18. Which enzyme of catecholamine pathway is specific to adrenal medulla?

A. DOPA decarboxylase
B. Phenylethanolamine N-methyltransferase
C. Catechol-O-methyl transferase
D. Monoamine oxidase

ADRENAL INSUFFICIENCY

19. All of the following are features of Addison's disease except:

A. It causes primary adrenal insufficiency
B. Hyperpigmentation due to ACTH induced melanogenesis
C. Adrenal destruction from autoimmune causes is the most common cause
D. It causes hypokalemia

20. Which is most common cause of primary adrenal insufficiency?

A. Autoimmune destruction
B. Tuberculosis
C. Adrenal hemorrhage
D. Metastatic tumor

21. About Waterhouse-Friderichsen syndrome, false statement is:

A. It causes tertiary adrenal insufficiency
B. More common in children and asplenia
C. It occurs in the setting of septicemia caused by meningococcal
D. It is caused due to adrenal hemorrhage

22. Causes of secondary adrenal insufficiency except:

A. Low supraphysiologic dose steroid therapy for > 3 weeks
B. ≥20 mg/day prednisone for > 5 days
C. Sheehan syndrome
D. Adrenal metastases

23. Sheehan syndrome is related to:

A. Meningococcal septicemia
B. Postpartum hemorrhage
C. Pituitary metastases
D. Miliary tuberculosis

24. Which is incorrect regarding acute adrenal insufficiency?

A. Sepsis or SIRS causes irreversible dysfunction of the HPA axis
B. It occurs in 30% of critically ill patients
C. Mineralocorticoid replacement is not an early priority in adrenal crisis
D. The treatment of adrenal crisis is large-volume intravenous resuscitation with isotonic saline and glucocorticoid administration

25. Hydrocortisone dosage in treatment of adrenal crisis:

A. 100 mg intravenous bolus followed by 75 mg every 8 hours
B. 200 mg intravenous bolus followed by 75 mg every 12 hours
C. 100 mg intravenous bolus followed by 100 mg every 8 hours
D. 200 mg intravenous bolus followed by 100 mg every 12 hours

26. Dexamethasone dosage used for acute adrenal insufficiency:

A. 4 mg intravenously every 24 hours
B. 6 mg intravenously every 12 hours
C. 8 mg intravenously every 24 hours
D. 12 mg intravenously every 24 hours

27. Which of the following does not require 17α-hydroxylase enzyme for synthesis?

A. Aldosterone B. Cortisol
C. DHEA D. Androstenedione

28. Which enzyme involved in synthesis of androgens from progesterone?

A. 3β- hydroxysteroid dehydrogenase
B. 11β- hydroxylase
C. 17α- hydroxylase
D. 21-hydroxylase

29. Aldosterone synthesis does not require which of the following enzyme?

A. 3β- hydroxysteroid dehydrogenase
B. 11β- hydroxylase
C. 17α- hydroxylase
D. 21-hydroxylase

30. All of the following enzyme deficiency causes increased androgen synthesis except:

A. 3β-hydroxysteroid dehydrogenase
B. 11β-hydroxylase
C. 17α-hydroxylase
D. 21-hydroxylase

31. Which enzyme is absent in zona glomerulosa?

A. 3β-hydroxysteroid dehydrogenase
B. 11β-hydroxylase
C. 17α-hydroxylase
D. 21-hydroxylase

32. What is the end product of catecholamine pathway?

A. 5-HIAA
B. Hydroxytryptamine
C. Vanillylmandelic acid
D. Metanephrine

33. Which is the first biochemical test to detect adrenal insufficiency?

A. Morning serum ACTH
B. Morning serum cortisol
C. 24-hour urine cortisol
D. Plasma-free metanephrines

34. Which of the following is consistent with diagnosis of adrenal insufficiency?

A. Morning serum cortisol concentration < 15 µg/dL
B. Morning salivary cortisol concentration < 5.8 ng/mL
C. Cosyntropin stimulated serum cortisol level < 30 µg/dL morning
D. ACTH level is determined to differentiate between primary and secondary adrenal insufficiency

35. What levels of serum cortisol with cosyntropin (250 µg) stimulation is suggestive of adrenal insufficiency?

A. <15 µg/dL B. < 5.8 µg/mL
C. < 18 µg/dL D. < 30 µg/dL

36. Which is most potent glucocorticoid?

A. Hydrocortisone B. Prednisolone
C. Methylprednisolone D. Dexamethasone

37. Potency of methylprednisolone is ___times the cortisol.

A. 0.8 B. 4
C. 5 D. 25

38. What is the dosage of fludrocortisones?

A. 0.1 mg/day B. 1 mg/day
C. 5 mg/day D. 10 mg/day

39. Patient having adrenal insufficiency on steroid therapy is planned for resection of ca colon. What is the recommended preoperative dosage of hydrocortisone?

A. Usual morning steroid dose
B. 25 mg before procedure
C. 50 mg before procedure
D. 100 mg before procedure

40. Patient on steroid therapy is undergoing inguinal hernia repair. What is the recommended dosage of hydrocortisone should be given?

A. Usual morning dose pre-operatively and continue same dose post-operatively
B. 50 mg before procedure and continue usual dose post-operatively
C. 50 mg before procedure and 25 mg every 8 hourly post-operatively
D. 100 mg before procedure and 50 mg every 8 hourly post-operatively

41. What is the dose of hydrocortisone is recommended for the patient on steroid therapy undergoing knee replacement?

A. Usual morning dose pre operatively
B. 25 mg before procedure
C. 50 mg before procedure
D. 100 mg before procedure

42. Hydrocortisone 50 mg before procedure is recommended in secondary adrenal insufficiency for following procedure except:

A. Peripheral vascular reconstruction
B. Orthopedic surgery
C. Cholecystectomy
D. Inguinal hernia repair

PRIMARY HYPERALDOSTERONISM

43. Which is false regarding Conn's disease?

A. Most patients may be normokalemic
B. Affect approximately 1% of hypertensives
C. Actual prevalence in unselected hypertensive patients is likely to be 7% or less
D. Most patients are symptomatic

44. All are true about Conn's disease except:

A. Causes resistant hypertension
B. The mean age at diagnosis is approximately 50 years
C. Female predilection
D. Aldesterone to renin ratio is used for screening

45. Aldosteronoma may have following mutation:

A. Somatic mutations in the potassium channel gene
B. Germline mutations in the potassium channel gene
C. Somatic mutations in the sodium channel gene
D. Germline mutations in the potassium channel gene

46. All are true about diagnosis of hyperaldosteronism except:

A. Screening should be performed in all patients with hypertension and unexplained hypokalemia
B. Ratio of plasma aldosterone concentration to plasma renin activity is used as screening method
C. An absolute aldosterone concentration should be higher than 15 mg/dL to improve specificity
D. Most commonly used cutoff values for the aldosterone-to-renin ratio is 20

47. Cut off values for the aldosterone-to-renin ratio used for screening of hyperaldosteronism is:

A. >10
B. >20
C. >30
D. >40

48. Which is most common cause of primary hyperaldosteronism with selective screening?

A. Bilateral adrenal hyperplasia
B. Aldosterone-producing adenoma
C. Adrenocortical carcinoma
D. Glucocorticoid-remediable aldosteronism

49. Which is most common cause of primary hyperaldosteronism with non-selective screening?

A. Bilateral adrenal hyperplasia
B. Aldosterone-producing adenoma
C. Adrenocortical carcinoma
D. Glucocorticoid-remediable aldosteronism

50. Which is wrong about familial hyperaldosteronism?

A. They have early onset younger than 30 years
B. Type I has glucocorticoid-remediable aldosteronism
C. This is rare autosomal recessive condition
D. It can be medically treated

51. Adrenal venous sampling is advised for patients with age more than:

A. 30 years
B. 40 years
C. 50 years
D. 60 years

52. Which is confirmatory biochemical test for primary hyperaldosteronism?

A. Serum aldosterone levels
B. Aldosterone to renin ratio
C. 24-hr urine free aldosterone
D. IV saline loading

53. Which is most preferred imaging modality used for aldosteronoma localization?

A. Thin cut CT
B. MRI
C. SPECT scan
D. Adrenal venous sampling

54. Successful cannulation of an adrenal vein is considered when cortisol concentration in a sample to peripheral blood is:

A. 2:1 B. 3:1
C. 4:1 D. 5:1

55. Lateralization is indicated by an unbalanced ratio of aldosterone to cortisol in the left and right adrenal veins, with the ratio on affected side being:

A. 2:1 B. 3:1
C. 4:1 D. 5:1

56. Which is most common reason for incomplete adrenal venous sampling?

A. Failure to cannulate the right adrenal vein
B. Failure to cannulate the left adrenal vein
C. Cannulation of renal vein
D. Bilateral adrenal adenoma

57. Partial success after adrenalectomy is considered as follows except:

A. Correction of hypokalemia
B. $\geq$50% decrease in plasma aldosterone
C. Persistently elevated aldosterone to renin ratio
D. Normalization of aldosterone to renin ratio

58. What is the outcome of adrenal venous sampling study with following values?

Right – Cortisol 40 μg/dL, Aldosterone 34 ng/dL

Left – Cortisol 190 μg/dL, Aldosterone 420 ng/dL

Peripheral blood – Cortisol 45 μg/dL, Aldosterone 32 ng/dL

A. Lateralization to right
B. Lateralization to left
C. Non-lateralizing
D. Failed study

59. What is the outcome of adrenal venous sampling study with following values?

Right – Cortisol 400 μg/dL, Aldosterone 3200 ng/dL, A/C ratio 8

Left – Cortisol 300 μg/dL, Aldosterone 60 ng/dL, A/C ratio 0.2

Peripheral blood – Cortisol 50 μg/dL, Aldosterone 60 ng/dL

A. Lateralization to right
B. Lateralization to left
C. Non-lateralizing
D. Failed study

60. Which is false regarding post adrenalectomy sequelae in hyperaldosteronism?

A. Patients with hyperaldosteronism have a higher incidence of chronic kidney disease
B. Hyperkalemia due to transient suppression of the contralateral adrenal gland may occur in 5%–10% of patients following adrenalectomy
C. Persistent hyperkalemia can be treated with renal replacement therapy
D. Pre-operative response to spironolactone predicts benefit from surgical treatment

61. Patients with following factors have reduced benefit from adrenalectomy for hyperaldosteronism except:

A. Men older than 45 years
B. Family history of hypertension
C. Requirement of more than two antihypertensive medications
D. Response to spironolactone

CUSHING'S SYNDROME

62. Which is not the feature of Cushing's syndrome?

A. Obesity
B. Hirsutism
C. Polymenorrhoea
D. Extreme muscle weakness

63. Cushing's syndrome is caused by:

A. Aldosterone excess
B. Cortisol excess
C. DHEA
D. Aldosterone deficiency

64. All are correct about Cushing's syndrome except:

A. Most common cause of Cushing's syndrome is pharmacologic glucocorticoid use

B. Cushing's disease is glucocorticoid excess caused by an adrenal adenoma
C. Specific mutation of protein kinase A is present in cortisol producing adenoma
D. Mortality is primarily because of cardiovascular complication

65. Ectopic ACTH production is seen with:

A. Mediastinal NET
B. Small cell carcinoma of lung
C. Thyroid cancer
D. Ganglioneuroma

66. Cushing's disease is caused by:

A. Excess ACTH production
B. Pituitary adenoma
C. Most common cause of endogenous Cushing's syndrome
D. All of the above

67. Primary adrenal Cushing's syndrome is seen in ___%.

A. 5% B. 15%
C. 25% D. 75%

68. All are true about diagnosis of Cushing's syndrome except:

A. 24-hour urine collection for urine-free cortisol used for initial screening
B. Early morning salivary cortisol measurement is confirmatory test
C. Dexamethasone suppression test has substantial number of false-positive tests
D. These tests should be performed at least twice

69. Which test is used as confirmatory for Cushing's syndrome diagnosis?

A. 24-hour urine free cortisol
B. Morning serum cortisol
C. Late evening salivary cortisol
D. Dexamethasone suppression test

70. Following are in favor of diagnosis of adrenal Cushing's syndrome except:

A. >3-fold elevation of 24-hr urine free cortisol
B. >550 ng/dL late evening salivary cortisol
C. Dexamethasone suppression test positive
D. Undetectable ACTH level < 5 pg/mL

71. Following tests are more likely to detect Cushing's disease except:

A. Late evening salivary cortisol
B. Dexamethasone suppression test
C. ACTH level
D. Inferior petrosal sinus sampling

72. Which is false regarding Cushing's disease diagnosis?

A. Elevated ACTH levels
B. Mass >4 mm on pituitary MRI requires surgery
C. Bilateral inferior petrosal sinus sampling to differentiate from ectopic source of ACTH
D. Bilateral adrenalectomy may be indicated

73. Which of the following is not evident on CT adrenal?

A. Solitary adrenal adenoma
B. Bilateral micronodular hyperplasia
C. Bilateral macronodular hyperplasia
D. Both B and C

74. What is most common cause of ACTH-independent Cushing's syndrome?

A. Solitary adrenal adenoma
B. Bilateral micronodular hyperplasia
C. Bilateral macronodular hyperplasia
D. Adrenocortical carcinoma

75. Which is false regarding management of hypercortisolism?

A. Hydrocortisone 100 mg intravenously every 12 hours for 48 hours are recommended perioperatively
B. Glucocorticoid supplementation for longer periods upto 1 year are required post operatively
C. A subnormal morning cortisol level on postoperative day 1 or 2 is indicative of cure in case of Cushing's disease
D. Laparoscopic bilateral adrenalectomy should be considered for failed pituitary surgery

76. Which is incorrect regarding subclinical Cushing's syndrome?

A. Absence of adrenal masses
B. Elevated cortisol levels
C. Without overt signs or symptoms of Cushing's syndrome
D. Improved outcome in surgically treated patients

77. Which of the following has best diagnostic accuracy for subclinical hypercortisolism?

A. Elevated evening salivary cortisol

B. Elevated ACTH levels
C. Low DHEA-S levels
D. Elevated morning serum cortisol

78. Which is wrong statement about sex steroid adrenal tumors?

A. Most of these tumors are feminizing
B. Almost all feminizing tumors are malignant
C. One third of virilizing tumors are malignant
D. Laparoscopic adrenalectomy remains the preferred procedure

ADRENOCORTICAL CARCINOMA

79. Which is false about incidence of adrenocortical carcinoma?

A. It is a rare tumor
B. Almost all cases occur in patients aged more than 60 years
C. Equal incidence among males and females
D. At the time of presentation, adrenocortical carcinomas tend to be very large

80. Which is most commonly seen with adrenocortical carcinoma?

A. Cushing's syndrome
B. Hyperaldosteronism
C. Virilization
D. Feminization

81. All are true about adrenocortical carcinoma except:

A. More than 50% of adrenocortical carcinomas are non-functional
B. 5-year survival is approximately 40%
C. CT shows a heterogeneous mass, irregular borders and central necrosis
D. The principal chemotherapeutic agent for the treatment of adrenocortical carcinoma is mitotane

82. FIRM-ACT Trial was carried out for which disease?

A. Breast cancer
B. Gastric cancer
C. Adrenocortical carcinoma
D. Neuroblastoma

PHEOCHROMOCYTOMA

83. Classic triad of pheochromocytoma includes all except:

A. Headache
B. Diaphoresis
C. Palpitations
D. Anxiety

84. All are true about pheochromocytoma except:

A. Affects approximately 0.2% of hypertensive individuals
B. Men and women are affected equally
C. Peak incidence in sporadic cases is between the ages of 30 to 40 years
D. Essential hypertension is common

85. All are true about pheochromocytoma diagnosed during pregnancy except:

A. It results in 12% fetal mortality in antenatal period
B. If diagnosis is made within the first 16 weeks of pregnancy adrenalectomy is recommended
C. Laparoscopic adrenalectomy performed in second trimester
D. Surgery should be postponed until after delivery if the diagnosis is made in the third trimester

86. Which screening test is used for pheochromocytoma?

A. 24-hr urine metanephrines
B. Serum catecholamines
C. Plasma-free metanephrines
D. Clonidine suppression test

87. Which confirmatory test is used for pheochromocytoma?

A. 24-hr urine metanephrines
B. Serum catecholamines
C. Plasma-free metanephrines
D. Clonidine suppression test

88. Which is false about pheochromocytoma diagnosis?

A. Plasma free metanephrine testing has low false positive rate
B. 24-hour urine testing of urinary total metanephrines and catecholamines is highly sensitive and highly specific, when it is performed twice
C. Localization with CT/MRI done after biochemical confirmation
D. MIBG scanning performed for younger patients < 50 years old

89. Highly specific to pheochromocytoma:

A. 131-I MIBG

B. 18F-DOPA
C. 68Ga-DOTATATE
D. 18F-Dopamine

90. Currently, the best PET/CT radiopharmaceutical for the localization of pheochromocytoma:

A. 131-I MIBG
B. 18F-DOPA
C. 68Ga-DOTATATE
D. 18F-Dopamine

91. All are true statements about peri-operative management of pheochromocytoma except:

A. Use of intraoperative α-adrenergic blockade followed by aggressive volume repletion is recommended
B. The administration of α-adrenergic agonists in the immediate postoperative period
C. The period of preoperative conditioning should last at least 2 week period to allow adequate reversal of α-adrenergic receptor downregulation
D. Phenoxybenzamine is a selective, reversible alpha antagonist

92. Which is wrong about phenoxybenzamine?

A. It is short-acting drug
B. Nonspecific, noncompetitive irreversible alpha antagonist
C. Provides the most complete alpha blockade among available agent
D. Nasal congestion can actually serve as a useful indicator of adequate blockade

93. Which is incorrect about surgical treatment of pheochromocytoma?

A. Surgery is curative in more than 90% cases
B. Laparoscopic approach contraindicated in local invasion
C. Open resection should be considered for size > 4 cm
D. Tumor rupture can lead to local recurrence even in benign cases

94. Laparoscopic approach can be successfully used for pheochromocytoma upto size:

A. 4 cm B. 5 cm
C. 6 cm D. 7 cm

95. All are associated with pheochromocytoma except:

A. Multiple endocrine neoplasia type 2 syndrome
B. Von Hippel-Lindau syndrome
C. Neurofibromatosis type 1
D. Li Fraumeni syndrome

96. Penetrance of pheochromocytoma in MEN2 syndrome:

A. 20 – 40% B. 40 – 50%
C. 60 – 70% D. 70 – 80%

97. Which is false regarding SDH associated pheochromocytomas?

A. Germline mutation of SDH inherited in an autosomal dominant fashion
B. Identified in 1% of apparently sporadic pheochromocytoma cases
C. SDH B mutation carriers have high rates of extra-adrenal pheochromocytomas and malignant disease
D. SDH D mutation present with multiple tumors and hormonally inactive paragangliomas of the head and neck

98. All are true about SDH D mutation associated pheochromocytoma except:

A. Autosomal dominant
B. Multiple tumors
C. Hormonally active paragangliomas
D. Paragangliomas of the head and neck

99. Which is false about management of familial pheochromocytoma?

A. Genetic counseling should be considered in all patients younger than 45 years
B. Germline mutation may influence prognosis and surveillance
C. Cortical-sparing adrenalectomy should be considered in familial cases
D. Preservation of at least two third of one adrenal gland is necessary

100. Following are the common site of metastases from pheochromocytoma except:

A. Axial skeleton B. Lung
C. Liver D. Brain

101. Which genetic mutation is not associated with pheochromocytoma?

A. RET B. Menin
C. NF1 D. VHL

102. Lisch nodules are seen in:

A. Multiple endocrine neoplasia type 2B

B. von Recklinghausen disease
C. von Hippel-Lindau syndrome
D. Neurofibromatosis 2

103. SDH mutation may be associated with:

A. GIST
B. Renal cell carcinoma
C. Pheochromocytoma
D. All of the above

104. von Hippel-Lindau is associated with:

A. CNS hemangioblastoma
B. Renal cell cancer
C. Neuroectodermal tumor
D. Breast cancer

105. Which genetic mutation is associated with Hereditary pheochromocytoma?

A. SDH B
B. HIF2A
C. RB
D. MET

ADRENAL INCIDENTALOMA

106. Which is most common adrenal incidentaloma?

A. Pheochromocytoma
B. Aldosteronoma
C. Nonfunctioning adenoma
D. Adrenal cyst

107. Surgery is indicated for incidentaloma in following conditions except:

A. Hormonally active tumors
B. High risk of malignancy
C. Growth on interval imaging
D. Old patient

108. Tumors larger than 6 cm carry a __% risk of malignancy.

A. 5%
B. 10%
C. 25%
D. 50%

109. All are characteristic of benign adrenal incidentaloma except:

A. Homogeneous appearance
B. High lipid content
C. Rapid washout of contrast material
D. Internal calcifications

110. Incidentaloma size upto ____ can be safely observed.

A. 2 cm
B. 3 cm
C. 4 cm
D. 5 cm

111. Which imaging modality has high sensitivity and specificity for distinguishing between benign and malignant adrenal lesions?

A. CT scan
B. MRI
C. SPECT/CT
D. 18F-FDG PET

112. Which is false about management of incidentaloma?

A. Tumor size correlates strongly with risk of malignancy
B. 18F-FDG PET cannot differentiate between a metastasis and primary adrenocortical carcinoma
C. The diagnosis of primary adrenal malignancy can be made on FNAC
D. Patients should undergo repeated imaging in 6 to 12 months during surveillance

METASTASES TO ADRENAL GLAND

113. All of the following primaries most often metastasize to adrenal except:

A. Melanoma
B. Breast carcinoma
C. Lung cancer
D. Gonadal cancer

114. Which is incorrect statement of the following concerning metastases to adrenal gland?

A. 25% of patients with carcinomas eventually develop adrenal involvement
B. In 80% of these cases, metastatic disease is bilateral
C. Adrenal insufficiency may occur in up to 30% of these patients
D. Most adrenal metastases are well encapsulated

ADRENALECTOMY

115. Following are indications for retroperitoneoscopic adrenaletomy except:

A. Tumors smaller than 6 cm
B. Body mass index >35
C. Bilateral tumors
D. History of extensive prior abdominal surgery

116. Which is correct regarding retroperitoneoscopic adrenalectomy?

A. Longer post operative recovery
B. Body mass index >35 is absolute contraindication
C. Patient operated in the prone position
D. Better approach for unilateral tumors

117. Open adrenalectomy is indicated for following conditions except:

A. Features suggestive of malignancy
B. Size > 6 cm
C. Clinical feminization
D. Hypersecretion of multiple steroid hormones

118. What size cut off is usually considered for open adrenalectomy in case of adrenal tumor?

A. 4 cm B. 6 cm
C. 8 cm D. 10 cm

119. Which position is used for laparoscopic adrenalectomy?

A. Supine
B. Semi-prone
C. Left or right lateral
D. 80 degree lateral decubitus

120. The left-hand page of the book in left laparoscopic adrenalectomy is composed of following structures except:

A. Spleen
B. Tail of the pancreas
C. Greater curvature of the stomach
D. Adrenal gland

121. Second right adrenal vein is seen in:

A. 2% B. 5%
C. 10% D. 15%

122. Which is incorrect about right laparoscopic adrenalectomy?

A. Left-hand page of the open book is made up by the kidney and adrenal gland
B. A significant second right adrenal vein may be found in up to 10% of patients
C. Right adrenalectomy centers on the avoidance of venous bleeding
D. Junction of the inferior vena cava and right renal vein used as an anatomic landmark for identification of the adrenal vein

123. Which is false about retroperitoneoscopic adrenalectomy approach?

A. Need for repositioning during bilateral adrenalectomy
B. Best suited for tumors smaller than 7 cm in diameter
C. High insufflation pressures of 20 to 28 mm Hg are used
D. Left adrenal vein is almost always encountered early in the procedure

124. Complication specific to the retroperitoneal approach:

A. Air embolism
B. Renal injury
C. Injury to subcostal nerve
D. IVC injury

125. Which is false regarding open technique of adrenalectomy?

A. Subcostal Chevron incision with or without a vertical upper midline extension
B. The left adrenal can be exposed by entering the lesser sac through the gastrocolic ligament
C. Open right adrenalectomy begins with complete mobilization of the left lobe of the liver
D. Kocher maneuver performed during right adrenalectomy

ANSWERS

1. **Ans: B. Eustachi**

Ref: Chapter No. 40, Page No. 964

2. **Ans: D. Receiving 1 L/kg/min of blood**

Ref: Chapter No. 40, Page No. 964

3. **Ans: B. 2000 mL/kg/min**

Ref: Chapter No. 40, Page No. 964

4. **Ans: A. The primordial cortex arises from the endodermal tissue**

Ref: Chapter No. 40, Page No. 964

5. **Ans: C. Coelomic mesoderm**

Ref: Chapter No. 40, Page No. 964

6. **Ans: C. The tail of the pancreas and splenic hilum lie posterior to left adrenal gland**

Ref: Chapter No. 40, Page No. 965

7. **Ans: D. In up to 5% of individuals, the right adrenal vein has variant**

Ref: Chapter No. 40, Page No. 965

8. **Ans: D. Lumbar artery**

Ref: Chapter No. 40, Page No. 965

9. **Ans: A. Inferior phrenic vein**

Ref: Chapter No. 40, Page No. 965

10. **Ans: C. 20%**

Ref: Chapter No. 40, Page No. 965

11. **Ans: B. Most of the adrenal cortex is formed by the zona granulosa**

Ref: Chapter No. 40, Page No. 965

12. **Ans: C. Zona reticularis - small nests, basophilic cells**

Ref: Chapter No. 40, Page No. 965

13. **Ans: C. Cortisol is generated by the oxidation of corticosterone by CYP11B2 within the zona glomerulosa**

Ref: Chapter No. 40, Page No. 966

14. **Ans: B. Continuous baseline secretion of ACTH is maintained**

Ref: Chapter No. 40, Page No. 967

15. **Ans: C. Hyperkalemia reduces aldosterone release by suppressing renin secretion**

Ref: Chapter No. 40, Page No. 967

16. **Ans: B. Dopamine synthesis is rate limiting step**

Ref: Chapter No. 40, Page No. 967-968

17. **Ans: B. Tyrosine**

Ref: Chapter No. 40, Page No. 967

18. **Ans: B. Phenylethanolamine N-methyltransferase**

Ref: Chapter No. 40, Page No. 967

19. **Ans: D. It causes hypokalemia**

Ref: Chapter No. 40, Page No. 969

20. **Ans: A. Autoimmune destruction**

Ref: Chapter No. 40, Page No. 970

21. **Ans: A. It causes tertiary adrenal insufficiency**

Ref: Chapter No. 40, Page No. 970

22. **Ans: D. Adrenal metastases**

Ref: Chapter No. 40, Page No. 970

23. **Ans: B. Postpartum hemorrhage**

Ref: Chapter No. 40, Page No. 970

24. **Ans: A. Sepsis or SIRS causes irreversible dysfunction of the HPA axis**

Ref: Chapter No. 40, Page No. 970

25. **Ans: A. 100 mg intravenous bolus followed by 75 mg every 8 hours**

Ref: Chapter No. 40, Page No. 970

26. **Ans: A. 4 mg intravenously every 24 hours**

Ref: Chapter No. 40, Page No. 970

27. **Ans: A. Aldosterone**

Ref: Chapter No. 40, Page No. 971

28. **Ans: C. 17α-hydroxylase**

Ref: Chapter No. 40, Page No. 971

29. **Ans: C. 17α-hydroxylase**

Ref: Chapter No. 40, Page No. 971

30. **Ans: C. 17α-hydroxylase**

Ref: Chapter No. 40, Page No. 971

31. **Ans: C. 17α-hydroxylase**

Ref: Chapter No. 40, Page No. 971

32. **Ans: C. Vanillylmandelic acid**

Ref: Chapter No. 40, Page No. 972

33. **Ans: B. Morning serum cortisol**

Ref: Chapter No. 40, Page No. 972

34. **Ans: C. Cosyntropin stimulated serum cortisol level < 30 μg/dL morning**

Ref: Chapter No. 40, Page No. 972

35. **Ans: C. < 18 μg/dL**

Ref: Chapter No. 40, Page No. 972

36. **Ans: D. Dexamethasone**

Ref: Chapter No. 40, Page No. 973

37. **Ans: C. 5**

Ref: Chapter No. 40, Page No. 973

38. **Ans: A. 0.1 mg/day**

Ref: Chapter No. 40, Page No. 973

39. **Ans: D. 100 mg before procedure**

Ref: Chapter No. 40, Page No. 974

40. **Ans: A. Usual morning dose pre-operatively and continue same dose post-operatively**

Ref: Chapter No. 40, Page No. 974

41. **Ans: C. 50 mg before procedure**

Ref: Chapter No. 40, Page No. 974

42. **Ans: D. Inguinal hernia repair**

Ref: Chapter No. 40, Page No. 974

43. **Ans: D. Most patients are symptomatic**

Ref: Chapter No. 40, Page No. 974

44. **Ans: C. Female predilection**

Ref: Chapter No. 40, Page No. 974

45. **Ans: A. Somatic mutations in the potassium channel gene**

Ref: Chapter No. 40, Page No. 974

46. **Ans: D. Most commonly used cutoff values for the aldosterone-to-renin ratio is 20**

Ref: Chapter No. 40, Page No. 974

47. **Ans: C. >30**

Ref: Chapter No. 40, Page No. 974

48. **Ans: B. Aldosterone-producing adenoma**

Ref: Chapter No. 40, Page No. 975

49. **Ans: A. Bilateral adrenal hyperplasia**

Ref: Chapter No. 40, Page No. 975

50. **Ans: C. This is rare autosomal recessive condition**

Ref: Chapter No. 40, Page No. 975

51. **Ans: B. 40 years**

Ref: Chapter No. 40, Page No. 975

52. **Ans: D. IV saline loading**

Ref: Chapter No. 40, Page No. 975

53. **Ans: A. Thin cut CT**

Ref: Chapter No. 40, Page No. 976

54. **Ans: D. 5:1**

Ref: Chapter No. 40, Page No. 976

55. **Ans: C. 4:1**

Ref: Chapter No. 40, Page No. 976

56. **Ans: A. Failure to cannulate the right adrenal vein**

Ref: Chapter No. 40, Page No. 976

57. **Ans: C. Persistently elevated aldosterone to renin ratio**

Ref: Chapter No. 40, Page No. 976

58. **Ans: D. Failed study**

Ref: Chapter No. 40, Page No. 977

59. **Ans: A. Lateralization to right**

Ref: Chapter No. 40, Page No. 977

60. **Ans: C. Persistent hyperkalemia can be treated with renal replacement therapy**

Ref: Chapter No. 40, Page No. 977

61. **Ans: D. Response to spironolactone**

Ref: Chapter No. 40, Page No. 977

62. **Ans: C. Polymenorrhoea**

Ref: Chapter No. 40, Page No. 977

63. **Ans: B. Cortisol excess**

Ref: Chapter No. 40, Page No. 977

64. **Ans: B. Cushing's disease is glucocorticoid excess caused by an adrenal adenoma**

Ref: Chapter No. 40, Page No. 978

65. **Ans: A. Mediastinal NET**

Ref: Chapter No. 40, Page No. 978

66. **Ans: D. All of the above**

Ref: Chapter No. 40, Page No. 978

67. **Ans: B. 15%**

Ref: Chapter No. 40, Page No. 978

68. **Ans: B. Early morning salivary cortisol measurement is confirmatory test**

Ref: Chapter No. 40, Page No. 979

69. **Ans: C. Late evening salivary cortisol**

Ref: Chapter No. 40, Page No. 979

70. **Ans: C. Dexamethasone suppression test positive**

Ref: Chapter No. 40, Page No. 979

71. **Ans: A. Late evening salivary cortisol**

Ref: Chapter No. 40, Page No. 979

72. **Ans: B. Mass >4 mm on pituitary MRI requires surgery**

Ref: Chapter No. 40, Page No. 979

73. **Ans: B. Bilateral micronodular hyperplasia**

Ref: Chapter No. 40, Page No. 979

74. **Ans: A. Solitary adrenal adenoma**

Ref: Chapter No. 40, Page No. 979

75. **Ans: A. Hydrocortisone 100 mg intravenously every 12 hours for 48 hours are recommended peri-operatively**

Ref: Chapter No. 40, Page No. 980

76. **Ans: A. Absence of adrenal masses**

Ref: Chapter No. 40, Page No. 980

77. **Ans: C. Low DHEA-S levels**

Ref: Chapter No. 40, Page No. 980

78. **Ans: A. Most of these tumors are feminizing**

Ref: Chapter No. 40, Page No. 980

79. **Ans: B. Almost all cases occur in patients aged more than 60 years**

Ref: Chapter No. 40, Page No. 980

80. **Ans: A. Cushing's syndrome**

Ref: Chapter No. 40, Page No. 981

81. **Ans: A. More than 50% of adrenocortical carcinomas are non-functional**

Ref: Chapter No. 40, Page No. 981

82. **Ans: C. Adrenocortical carcinoma**

Ref: Chapter No. 40, Page No. 981

83. **Ans: D. Anxiety**

Ref: Chapter No. 40, Page No. 981

84. **Ans: C. Peak incidence in sporadic cases is between the ages of 30 to 40 years**

Ref: Chapter No. 40, Page No. 981

85. **Ans: B. If diagnosis is made within the first 16 weeks of pregnancy adrenalectomy is recommended**

Ref: Chapter No. 40, Page No. 981

86. **Ans: C. Plasma-free metanephrines**

Ref: Chapter No. 40, Page No. 982

87. **Ans: A. 24-hr urine metanephrines**

Ref: Chapter No. 40, Page No. 982

88. **Ans: A. Plasma free metanephrine testing has low false positive rate**

Ref: Chapter No. 40, Page No. 982

89. **Ans: A. 131-I MIBG**

Ref: Chapter No. 40, Page No. 983

90. **Ans: C. 68Ga-DOTATATE**

Ref: Chapter No. 40, Page No. 983

91. **Ans: D. Phenoxybenzamine is a selective, reversible alpha antagonist**

Ref: Chapter No. 40, Page No. 983

92. **Ans: A. It is short-acting drug**

Ref: Chapter No. 40, Page No. 983

93. **Ans: C. Open resection should be considered for size > 4 cm**

Ref: Chapter No. 40, Page No. 986

94. **Ans: C. 6 cm**

Ref: Chapter No. 40, Page No. 986

95. **Ans: D. Li Fraumeni syndrome**

Ref: Chapter No. 40, Page No. 986

96. **Ans: B. 40 – 50%**

Ref: Chapter No. 40, Page No. 986

97. **Ans: B. Identified in 1% of apparently sporadic pheochromocytoma cases**

Ref: Chapter No. 40, Page No. 986

98. **Ans: C. Hormonally active paragangliomas**

Ref: Chapter No. 40, Page No. 986

99. **Ans: D. Preservation of at least two third of one adrenal gland is necessary**

Ref: Chapter No. 40, Page No. 986

100. **Ans: D. Brain**

Ref: Chapter No. 40, Page No. 986

101. **Ans: B. Menin**

Ref: Chapter No. 40, Page No. 987

102. **Ans: B. von Recklinghausen disease**

Ref: Chapter No. 40, Page No. 987

103. **Ans: D. All of the above**

Ref: Chapter No. 40, Page No. 987

104. **Ans: D. Breast cancer**

Ref: Chapter No. 40, Page No. 987

105. **Ans: B. HIF2A**

Ref: Chapter No. 40, Page No. 987

106. **Ans: C. Nonfunctioning adenoma**

Ref: Chapter No. 40, Page No. 987

107. **Ans: D. Old patient**

Ref: Chapter No. 40, Page No. 987

108. **Ans: C. 25%**

Ref: Chapter No. 40, Page No. 987

109. **Ans: D. Internal calcifications**

Ref: Chapter No. 40, Page No. 987-988

110. **Ans: B. 3 cm**

Ref: Chapter No. 40, Page No. 988

111. **Ans: D. 18F-FDG PET**

Ref: Chapter No. 40, Page No. 988

112. **Ans: C. The diagnosis of primary adrenal malignancy can be made on FNAC**

Ref: Chapter No. 40, Page No. 988

113. **Ans: D. Gonadal cancer**

Ref: Chapter No. 40, Page No. 988

114. **Ans: B. In 80% of these cases, metastatic disease is bilateral**

Ref: Chapter No. 40, Page No. 989

115. Ans: B. Body mass index >35

Ref: Chapter No. 40, Page No. 989

116. Ans: C. Patient operated in the prone position

Ref: Chapter No. 40, Page No. 989

117. Ans: B. Size > 6 cm

Ref: Chapter No. 40, Page No. 989

118. Ans: C. 8 cm

Ref: Chapter No. 40, Page No. 989

119. Ans: D. 80 degree lateral decubitus

Ref: Chapter No. 40, Page No. 989

120. Ans: D. Adrenal gland

Ref: Chapter No. 40, Page No. 990

121. Ans: C. 10%

Ref: Chapter No. 40, Page No. 991

122. Ans: D. Junction of the inferior vena cava and right renal vein used as an anatomic landmark for identification of the adrenal vein

Ref: Chapter No. 40, Page No. 991

123. Ans: A. Need for repositioning during bilateral adrenalectomy

Ref: Chapter No. 40, Page No. 991-992

124. Ans: C. Injury to subcostal nerve

Ref: Chapter No. 40, Page No. 992

125. Ans: C. Open right adrenalectomy begins with complete mobilization of the left lobe of the liver

Ref: Chapter No. 40, Page No. 993

41

The Multiple Endocrine Neoplasia Syndrome

1. **Which is associated with menin gene mutation?**
   A. MEN 1 B. MEN 2A
   C. MEN 2B D. MEN 4

2. **All are associated with MEN1 syndrome except:**
   A. Multigland parathyroid adenomas
   B. NETs of the gastrointestinal system
   C. Ganglioneuromatosis
   D. Thymus carcinoids

3. **MEN1 associated with all except:**
   A. Thymus carcinoids
   B. Facial angiofibromas
   C. Collagenomas
   D. Mucosal neuromas

4. **MEN2A associated with all except:**
   A. Medullary thyroid carcinoma
   B. Pheochromocytomas
   C. Parathyroid tumor
   D. NETs of the gastrointestinal system

5. **All are associated with MEN2B except:**
   A. Thyroid C- cell hyperplasia
   B. Pheochromocytoma
   C. Mucosal neuromas
   D. Collagenomas

6. **Which is false statement?**
   A. MEN type 2 occurs due to mutation of the RET proto-oncogenes
   B. Lifelong risk of development of benign and malignant tumor
   C. Prophylactic surgery is required in case of MEN1 syndrome
   D. MEN2B is characterized by marfanoid appearance

MEN1

7. **Wrong statement about MEN1 syndrome:**
   A. Incidence of MEN1 is 1 of 3,00,000 people
   B. Clinical manifestations of MEN1 will have developed by age 29
   C. 1 – 18% of primary hyperparathyroidism (PHPT) will have MEN1
   D. Mean age at death is 50 to 55 years

8. **Wermer's syndrome is associated with which genetic mutation?**
   A. Menin B. RET
   C. MET D. CDKN1B

9. **What is incorrect regarding MEN1?**
   A. Hereditary cancer syndrome inherited in an autosomal dominant
   B. It results due to germline mutation and loss of heterozygosity in MEN1 gene
   C. It is proto-oncogene on chromosome 11p
   D. MEN1 are at increased risk for the development of breast cancer

10. **What is the location of MEN1 gene?**
   A. Chromosome 11p13
   B. Chromosome 11p15
   C. Chromosome 11q13
   D. Chromosome 11q15

11. **Which of the following is associated with MEN1 syndrome?**
   A. Diffuse large cell lymphoma
   B. Chronic myeloid leukemia
   C. Non-Hodgkin's lymphoma
   D. Mixed lineage leukemia

12. **Which is most common mutation seen in MEN1 syndrome?**

A. Missense mutations
B. Nonsense mutations
C. Frameshift mutations
D. RNA splice mutations

13. Somatic MEN1 mutations most commonly associated with which tumors?
A. Glucagonoma
B. Gastrinoma
C. Insulinomas
D. Nonfunctioning PNET

14. Which of the following is wrong about genetic diagnosis of MEN1?
A. Clinical practice guidelines recommend genetic testing for index patients with MEN1 as well as their first-degree relatives
B. The chance of inheriting the mutation is 50%
C. No genotype-phenotype correlations have been established for MEN1
D. Genetic testing predicts the disease course or severity

15. Which is false regarding MEN1 diagnosis?
A. Diagnosis of MEN1 is made clinically in patients with one or more MEN1-associated tumors
B. Patient with one MEN1-associated tumor and a first-degree relative with MEN1
C. An individual with a known MEN1 mutation but no clinical manifestations
D. 10% to 20% will not have a mutation identifiable by conventional testing

16. MEN4 is associated with which genetic mutation?
A. RET mutation
B. MET mutation
C. Menin gene mutation
D. CDKN1B mutation

17. What is the first manifestation of MEN1 syndrome?
A. Zollinger Ellison syndrome
B. Prolactinoma
C. Primary hyperparathyroidism
D. Insulinoma

18. Which is incorrect about MEN1 syndrome screening?
A. Pituitary screening started at age 5
B. Parathyroid screening started at age 8
C. Pancreatic screening started at age 20
D. Screening is done every 3 yearly after the diagnosis of MEN1

19. Which is false about parathyroid involvement is MEN1?
A. PHPT is the most common feature, occurring in more than 90% of patients
B. PHPT occurs in the setting of MEN1 at age 20–25 years
C. Female: male ratio is 3:1 in patients with MEN1
D. Surgery is the treatment of choice for PHPT in MEN1

20. All are true about parathyroid adenoma in MEN1 except:
A. It is multiglandular disease
B. All glands are at equal risk
C. Symmetric hyperplasia
D. Benign involvement

21. Which is incorrect concerning PHPT management in MEN1?
A. The diagnosis of PHPT is made by imaging
B. Sestamibi parathyroid scintigraphy may be useful to screen for parathyroid glands that are ectopic
C. Bilateral neck exploration via a standard open approach with the goal of identifying all four parathyroid gland
D. Choice of operation is either subtotal or total parathyroidectomy

22. What is recurrence rate of PHPT post subtotal parathyroidectomy?
A. < 5%
B. 5 – 10%
C. 10 – 20%
D. 20 – 30%

23. Which is incorrect about imaging of PNETs in MEN1?
A. Endoscopic ultrasound (EUS) is useful for obtaining a tissue diagnosis, staging and follow up
B. SRS has the advantage of being whole-body imaging but cannot detect lesions less than 1 cm
C. EUS is most useful to detect duodenal gastrinomas
D. 68-GaSAPET/CT is better diagnostic modality for primary and metastatic lesions than SRS

24. Which is not the characteristic of PNET on CT imaging?
A. Isointense on precontrast study
B. Hyperintense in arterial phase
C. Contrast washout on portal venous phase
D. Rim enhancement

25. Most common functional PNET in MEN1:

A. Gastrinoma
B. Insulinoma
C. VIPoma
D. Somatostatinoma

26. All are true about gastrinoma except:

A. 50% of enteropancreatic NETs that develop in the setting of MEN1 are gastrin-secreting tumor
B. 20% of patients with gastrinomas will have MEN1
C. 90% of gastrinomas diagnosed within the setting of MEN1 are malignant
D. Liver metastases are common when tumor size is > 1 cm

27. Survival of the patient with gastrinoma is majorly affected by:

A. Size
B. Lymph node status
C. Liver metastases
D. Location

28. "Whipple Triad" is observed with which condition?

A. Gastrinoma
B. Glucagonoma
C. Somatostatinoma
D. Insulinoma

29. All are true about Whipple triad except:

A. Fasting glucose levels less than 40 mg/dL
B. Symptoms of hypoglycemia corresponds to low plasma glucose
C. Resolution of symptoms upon administration of glucose
D. It is characteristic of insulinoma

30. Which is incorrect regarding insulinoma?

A. Insulinoma represent up to 30% of PNETs in patients with MEN1
B. 4% of patients with an insulinoma have MEN1
C. 72-hour supervised fast is diagnostic test
D. Insulinomas may be multifocal and occur most commonly in tail of pancreas

31. Most common location of insulinoma in pancreas:

A. Tail
B. Head
C. Body
D. Equally distributed

32. What is the diagnostic test used for insulinoma?

A. Glucose – insulin ratio
B. Insulin – C-peptide ratio
C. 72 hours fast test
D. Plasma insulin levels

33. What percentage of insulinomas are malignant?

A. 10%
B. 25%
C. 50%
D. 90%

34. Necrolytic migratory erythema is characteristic of which condition?

A. Gastrinoma
B. Glucagonoma
C. VIPoma
D. Somatostatinoma

35. Which of the following is not seen with VIPoma?

A. Intermittent watery diarrhea
B. Hypokalemia
C. Achlorhydria
D. Metabolic alkalosis

36. Which is seen with somatostatinoma?

A. Cholelithiasis
B. Diabetes
C. Steatorrhea
D. All of the above

37. Most common PNET in MEN1:

A. Gastrinoma
B. Insulinoma
C. PPoma
D. Non-functional

38. What is the cut-off size for operative indication in case of PNETs?

A. 1 cm
B. 2 cm
C. 4 cm
D. 5 cm

39. Which is false concerning MEN1 with thymic carcinoids?

A. Thymic carcinoid tumors are most likely to be malignant and aggressive
B. They occur twice as often in men
C. It has an association with smoking
D. Preventative transcervical thymectomy is recommended

40. All are indications for operative procedure for adrenal tumors except:

A. Tumors that exhibit radiologic features suspicious for malignancy
B. Excess hormone production
C. Tumors 6 cm or greater in size
D. Significant growth over at least a 6-month imaging interval

41. What is cut-off size of adrenal tumors for operative intervention?

A. 2 cm
B. 4 cm
C. 6 cm
D. 7 cm

MEN2 SYNDROME

42. Which is incorrect about MEN2A syndrome?

A. Its prevalence is estimated at 1/35,000 persons

B. Medullary thyroid cancer occurs in 50% of patients
C. There is a distinct genotype-phenotype correlation based on the type of RET mutation
D. Prophylactic thyroidectomy in known carriers can prevent MTC and improve survival

43. What is the location of RET proto-oncogene?
A. Chromosome 10p11.2
B. Chromosome 10q11.2
C. Chromosome 11p10.2
D. Chromosome 11q10.2

44. Which is false about MEN2 syndrome?
A. MEN2 syndromes occurs as a result of a RET mutation, inherited in an autosomal dominant pattern
B. Mutations that result in the development of MTC are missense mutations
C. Gain of function mutations in RET were found to be associated with Hirschsprung disease
D. Presence or absence of specific RET mutations can predict disease course

45. Which is not associated with MEN2A syndrome?
A. Pituitary adenoma
B. Pheochromocytoma
C. Medullary thyroid cancer
D. Parathyroid adenoma

46. Which of the following is associated with MEN2A?
A. Neurofibromas of tongue
B. Meningioma
C. Cutaneous lichen amyloidosis
D. Facial angiofibromas

47. Hirschsprung disease is seen with which endocrine syndrome?
A. MEN1 B. MEN2A
C. MEN2B D. MEN4

48. Which codon mutation of RET oncogene is associated with cutaneous lichen amyloidosis?
A. 634 B. 918
C. 609 D. 620

49. Which codon mutations of RET oncogene are associated with Hirschsprung disease?
A. 634 B. 618
C. 883 D. 918

50. Hirschsprung disease affects ___ % of MEN2A patients.
A. 1% B. 7%
C. 14% D. 24%

51. What % of patients with Hirschsprung disease will have MEN2A?
A. 5% B. 10%
C. 20% D. 30%

MEN2B SYNDROME

52. What is hallmark characteristic of MEN2B?
A. Marfanoid body habitus
B. Medullary thyroid cancer
C. Pheochromocytoma
D. Elongated facies

53. Which is not associated with MEN2B?
A. Medullary thyroid cancer
B. Pheochromocytoma
C. Primary hyperparathyroidism
D. Ganglioneuromatosis of GIT

54. Which skeletal abnormalities associated with MEN2B?
A. Pectus excavatum B. Kyphosis
C. Vertebra plana D. Pectus carinatum

55. Which germline mutation of RET oncogene is associated with MEN2B?
A. Codon 620 B. Codon 634
C. Codon 804 D. Codon 918

MEDULLARY THYROID CANCER

56. All are predictors of poor outcome in case of MTC except:
A. Male sex
B. Age
C. Tumor size larger than 1 cm
D. Lateral neck lymph node metastases

57. Which is false about MTC?
A. Arises from the parafollicular C-cells
B. Radioactive iodine (RAI) avid
C. Relatively indolent malignancy
D. 25% of MTC is familial

58. Which of the following is a marker for MTC?
A. CEA B. CA 19-9
C. CA125 D. None of the above

59. Which is incorrect about diagnosis of MTC?
A. CEA is most useful surrogate marker for both diagnosis and recurrence

B. Ultrasound is the most sensitive method of imaging the neck in patients with primary, persistent, or recurrent MTC
C. CT is more useful in imaging of chest and abdominal metastases
D. MRI is helpful to determine the presence or absence of liver metastases

60. MTC metastases to all of the following sites except:

A. Liver B. Bone
C. Lungs D. Brain

61. What is cut-off levels of calcitonin to evaluate distant metastases in case of MTC?

A. 200 pg/ml B. 500 pg/ml
C. 800 pg/ml D. 1000 pg/ml

62. 20-year-old patient presented with neck swelling. USG suggestive of multifocal nodules and no enlarged lymph nodes. FNA report came to be MTC. What is best management of this patient?

A. Near total thyroidectomy
B. Total thyroidectomy with RAI irradiation
C. Total thyroidectomy with central lymph node dissection
D. Total thyroidectomy with MRND

63. All are boundaries of central (level VI) lymph node dissection except:

A. Hyoid bone superiorly
B. The arch of aorta inferiorly
C. The carotid sheaths laterally
D. Anterior to trachea and deepest layer of cervical fascia

64. Which RET mutation is classified as highest risk category?

A. Codon 609 B. Codon 634
C. Codon 883 D. Codon 918

65. Which of the following RET mutation is not included under moderate risk category?

A. Codon 611 B. Codon 618
C. Codon 620 D. Codon 634

66. Which RET mutation is classified as high risk category?

A. Codon 609 B. Codon 620
C. Codon 883 D. Codon 918

67. Prophylactic thyroidectomy is carried out at what age for patients with codon 918 mutation of RET?

A. Within a year of age B. Within 5 years of age
C. At 10 years of age D. At 16 years of age

68. Prophylactic thyroidectomy is carried out at what age for patients with high risk category of RET mutation?

A. Within a year of age
B. Within 5 years of age
C. At 10 years of age
D. At 16 years of age

69. What is recommended interval of calcitonin/CEA measurement post thyroidectomy in case of MTC?

A. Monthly B. 3 monthly
C. 6 monthly D. Yearly

70. Regional recurrences of MTC are best managed with:

A. Repeat operation B. EBRT
C. Chemotherapy D. RAI ablation

71. Which of the following drug is approved by FDA for metastatic MTC?

A. Sorafenib B. Sunitinib
C. Vandetanib D. Lenvatinib

PHEOCHROMOCYTOMA

72. Which is false regarding pheochromocytoma associated with MEN2?

A. MEN2-pheochromocytoma patients were more than 10 years younger on average and had bilateral tumors
B. Evaluation is done by measuring plasma or timed urinary metanephrines prior to surgery
C. Screening for pheochromocytoma prior to thyroidectomy is necessary
D. MEN2-pheochromocytoma tend to be malignant and require lifelong monitoring

73. Which is most common RET mutation identified in patients with MEN2-pheochromocytoma?

A. Codon 620 B. Codon 634
C. Codon 883 D. Codon 918

PRIMARY HYPERPARATHYROIDISM

74. Which RET mutation is associated with PHPT?

A. Codon 609 B. Codon 620
C. Codon 634 D. Codon 918

75. What is preferred choice of procedure for PHPT in MEN syndrome?

A. Subtotal parathyroidectomy
B. Total parathyroidectomy with autotransplantation
C. Removal of abnormal looking glands
D. External beam radiation

ANSWERS

1. **Ans: A. MEN 1**
Ref: Chapter No. 41, Page No. 998

2. **Ans: C. Ganglioneuromatosis**
Ref: Chapter No. 41, Page No. 998

3. **Ans: D. Mucosal neuromas**
Ref: Chapter No. 41, Page No. 998

4. **Ans: D. NETs of the gastrointestinal system**
Ref: Chapter No. 41, Page No. 998

5. **Ans: D. Collagenomas**
Ref: Chapter No. 41, Page No. 998

6. **Ans: C. Prophylactic surgery is required in case of MEN1 syndrome**
Ref: Chapter No. 41, Page No. 998

7. **Ans: A. Incidence of MEN1 is 1 of 3,00,000 people**
Ref: Chapter No. 41, Page No. 998

8. **Ans: A. Menin**
Ref: Chapter No. 41, Page No. 998

9. **Ans: C. It is pro-oncogene on chromosome 11p**
Ref: Chapter No. 41, Page No. 998-999

10. **Ans: C. Chromosome 11q13**
Ref: Chapter No. 41, Page No. 999

11. **Ans: D. Mixed lineage leukemia**
Ref: Chapter No. 41, Page No. 999

12. **Ans: C. Frameshift mutations**
Ref: Chapter No. 41, Page No. 999

13. **Ans: A. Glucagonoma**
Ref: Chapter No. 41, Page No. 999

14. **Ans: D. Genetic testing predicts the disease course or severity**
Ref: Chapter No. 41, Page No. 999

15. **Ans: A. Diagnosis of MEN1 is made clinically in patients with one or more MEN1-associated tumors**
Ref: Chapter No. 41, Page No. 999

16. **Ans: D. CDKN1B mutation**
Ref: Chapter No. 41, Page No. 999

17. **Ans: C. Primary hyperparathyroidism**
Ref: Chapter No. 41, Page No. 999

18. **Ans: D. Screening is done every 3 yearly after the diagnosis of MEN1**
Ref: Chapter No. 41, Page No. 1000

19. **Ans: C. Female: male ratio is 3:1 in patients with MEN1**
Ref: Chapter No. 41, Page No. 1000

20. **Ans: C. Symmetric hyperplasia**
Ref: Chapter No. 41, Page No. 1000

21. **Ans: A. The diagnosis of PHPT is made by imaging**
Ref: Chapter No. 41, Page No. 1000

22. **Ans: D. 20 – 30%**
Ref: Chapter No. 41, Page No. 1001

23. **Ans: C. EUS is most useful to detect duodenal gastrinomas**
Ref: Chapter No. 41, Page No. 1001-1002

24. **Ans: D. Rim enhancement**
Ref: Chapter No. 41, Page No. 1001

25. **Ans: A. Gastrinoma**
Ref: Chapter No. 41, Page No. 1002

26. **Ans: D. Liver metastases are common when tumor size is > 1 cm**
Ref: Chapter No. 41, Page No. 1002

27. **Ans: C. Liver metastases**
Ref: Chapter No. 41, Page No. 1002

28. **Ans: D. Insulinoma**
Ref: Chapter No. 41, Page No. 1002

29. **Ans: A. Fasting glucose levels less than 40 mg/dL**
Ref: Chapter No. 41, Page No. 1002

30. **Ans: D. Insulinomas may be multifocal and occur most commonly in tail of pancreas**
Ref: Chapter No. 41, Page No. 1002

31. **Ans: D. Equally distributed**
Ref: Chapter No. 41, Page No. 1002

32. **Ans: C. 72 hours fast test**
Ref: Chapter No. 41, Page No. 1002

33. **Ans: A. 10%**
Ref: Chapter No. 41, Page No. 1003

34. **Ans: B. Glucagonoma**
Ref: Chapter No. 41, Page No. 1003

35. **Ans: D. Metabolic alkalosis**
Ref: Chapter No. 41, Page No. 1003

36. **Ans: D. All of the above**
Ref: Chapter No. 41, Page No. 1003

37. **Ans: D. Non-functional**

Ref: Chapter No. 41, Page No. 1003

38. **Ans: B. 2 cm**

Ref: Chapter No. 41, Page No. 1003

39. **Ans: D. Preventative transcervical thymectomy is recommended**

Ref: Chapter No. 41, Page No. 1004

40. **Ans: C. Tumors 6 cm or greater in size**

Ref: Chapter No. 41, Page No. 1004

41. **Ans: B. 4 cm**

Ref: Chapter No. 41, Page No. 1004

42. **Ans: B. Medullary thyroid cancer occurs in 50% of patients**

Ref: Chapter No. 41, Page No. 1004

43. **Ans: B. Chromosome 10q11.2**

Ref: Chapter No. 41, Page No. 1004

44. **Ans: C. Gain of function mutations in RET were found to be associated with Hirschsprung disease**

Ref: Chapter No. 41, Page No. 1004

45. **Ans: A. Pituitary adenoma**

Ref: Chapter No. 41, Page No. 1005

46. **Ans: C. Cutaneous lichen amyloidosis**

Ref: Chapter No. 41, Page No. 1005

47. **Ans: B. MEN2A**

Ref: Chapter No. 41, Page No. 1005

48. **Ans: A. 634**

Ref: Chapter No. 41, Page No. 1005

49. **Ans: B. 618**

Ref: Chapter No. 41, Page No. 1005

50. **Ans: B. 7%**

Ref: Chapter No. 41, Page No. 1005

51. **Ans: A. 5%**

Ref: Chapter No. 41, Page No. 1005

52. **Ans: B. Medullary thyroid cancer**

Ref: Chapter No. 41, Page No. 1005

53. **Ans: C. Primary hyperparathyroidism**

Ref: Chapter No. 41, Page No. 1005

54. **Ans: A. Pectus excavatum**

Ref: Chapter No. 41, Page No. 1005

55. **Ans: D. Codon 918**

Ref: Chapter No. 41, Page No. 1006

56. **Ans: B. Age**

Ref: Chapter No. 41, Page No. 1006

57. **Ans: B. Radioactive iodine (RAI) avid**

Ref: Chapter No. 41, Page No. 1006

58. **Ans: A. CEA**

Ref: Chapter No. 41, Page No. 1006

59. **Ans: A. CEA is a useful surrogate marker for both diagnosis and recurrence**

Ref: Chapter No. 41, Page No. 1006

60. **Ans: D. Brain**

Ref: Chapter No. 41, Page No. 1006

61. **Ans: B. 500 pg/ml**

Ref: Chapter No. 41, Page No. 1006

62. **Ans: C. Total thyroidectomy with central lymph node dissection**

Ref: Chapter No. 41, Page No. 1007

63. **Ans: B. The arch of aorta inferiorly**

Ref: Chapter No. 41, Page No. 1007

64. **Ans: D. Codon 918**

Ref: Chapter No. 41, Page No. 1007

65. **Ans: D. Codon 634**

Ref: Chapter No. 41, Page No. 1007

66. **Ans: C. Codon 883**

Ref: Chapter No. 41, Page No. 1007

67. **Ans: A. Within a year of age**

Ref: Chapter No. 41, Page No. 1007

68. **Ans: B. Within 5 years of age**

Ref: Chapter No. 41, Page No. 1007

69. **Ans: B. 3 monthly**

Ref: Chapter No. 41, Page No. 1008

70. **Ans: A. Repeat operation**

Ref: Chapter No. 41, Page No. 1008

71. **Ans: C. Vandetanib**

Ref: Chapter No. 41, Page No. 1008

72. **Ans: D. MEN2-pheochromocytoma tend to be malignant and require lifelong monitoring**

Ref: Chapter No. 41, Page No. 1008

73. **Ans: B. Codon 634**

Ref: Chapter No. 41, Page No. 1008

74. **Ans: C. Codon 634**

Ref: Chapter No. 41, Page No. 1009

75. **Ans: C. Removal of abnormal looking glands**

Ref: Chapter No. 41, Page No. 1009

42

Esophagus

ANATOMY

1. **False about esophagus is:**
   A. At the level of the carina, it deviates to the right to accommodate the arch of the aorta
   B. At the level of the carina, the heart and pericardium lie directly anterior to the thoracic esophagus
   C. 25 to 30 cm long
   D. The cervical esophagus begins as a midline structure that deviates slightly to the right of the trachea as it passes through the neck into the thoracic inlet

2. **Esophagus commences at the base of the pharynx and terminates in the abdomen where it joins the cardia of the stomach at:**
   A. C5 to T12 B. C6 to T11
   C. C6 to L1 D. C5 to T11

3. **False about esophagus is:**
   A. Immediately before entering the abdomen, the esophagus is pushed anteriorly by the descending thoracic aorta
   B. The pharyngeal constrictor muscles are three consecutive muscles that begin at the base of the palate and end at the crest of the esophagus
   C. The cricopharyngeus muscle is responsible for generating a high-pressure zone that marks the position of the UES and esophageal introitus
   D. All of the above are true

4. **The inferior pharyngeal constrictor muscle is composed of:**
   A. Palatopharyngeus and salpingopharyngeus muscles
   B. Stylopharyngeus and cricopharyngeus muscles
   C. Thyropharyngeus and cricopharyngeus muscles
   D. Salpingopharyngeus and thyropharyngeus muscle

5. **Killian triangle is the transition between:**
   A. The oblique fibers of the salpingopharyngeus muscle and the horizontal fibers of the cricopharyngeus muscle which creates a point of potential weakness
   B. The oblique fibers of the stylopharyngeus muscle and the horizontal fibers of the cricopharyngeus muscle which creates a point of potential weakness
   C. The oblique fibers of the thyropharyngeus muscle and the horizontal fibers of the palatopharyngeus muscle which creates a point of potential weakness
   D. The oblique fibers of the thyropharyngeus muscle and the horizontal fibers of the cricopharyngeus muscle which creates a point of potential weakness

6. **V-shaped area of Laimer is a:**
   A. Point of transition is flanked by the circular esophageal muscles that extend superiorly to attach to the midportion of the anterior surface of the cricoid cartilage
   B. Point of transition is flanked by the longitudinal esophageal muscles that extend superiorly to attach to the midportion of the posterior surface of the cricoid cartilage
   C. Point of transition is flanked by the circular esophageal muscles that extend superiorly to attach to the midportion of the posterior surface of the cricoid cartilage
   D. Point of transition is flanked by the longitudinal esophageal muscles that extend superiorly to attach to the midportion of the anterior surface of the cricoid cartilage

7. **True about esophageal deviation is all except:**
   A. Thoracic - right B. Cervical - left
   C. Abdominal - left D. Thoracic - left

8. **Meissner neural plexus is in:**
   A. Muscularis propria B. Submucosa
   C. Mucosa D. Serosa

9. **The collar of Helvetius marks the transition of:**
   A. The circular muscles of the esophagus to longitudinal muscles of the stomach at the incisura (cardiac notch)
   B. The oblique muscles of the esophagus to circular muscles of the stomach at the incisura (cardiac notch)
   C. The circular muscles of the esophagus to oblique muscles of the stomach at the incisura (cardiac notch)
   D. The longitudinal muscles of the esophagus to oblique muscles of the stomach at the incisura (cardiac notch)

10. **Auerbach plexus is in:**
   A. Muscularis propria B. Submucosa
   C. Mucosa D. Serosa

11. **True about narrowings in esophagus is:**
   A. Bronchoaortic constriction -14 mm
   B. Cricopharyngeus muscle -16 mm
   C. Bronchoaortic constriction - 15 to 17 mm
   D. Diaphragmatic constriction - 14 to 17 mm

12. **The narrowest point of the gastrointestinal tract is:**
   A. Duodenum
   B. Diaphragmatic constriction
   C. Cricopharyngeus muscle
   D. Bronchoaortic constriction

13. **False about anatomic points that identify the gastroesophageal junction (GEJ) except:**
   A. The transition from the smooth esophageal lining to the rugal folds of the stomach-endoscopically
   B. The squamocolumnar epithelial junction (Z-line)-endoscopically
   C. The gastroesophageal fat pad are consistent identifiers of the GEJ-externally
   D. All of the above are true

14. **The cervical esophagus receives most of its blood supply from the:**
   A. Superior thyroid arteries
   B. Inferior thyroid arteries
   C. Bronchial arteries
   D. Aorta

15. **The thoracic esophagus receives its blood supply directly from all except:**
   A. Left bronchial arteries
   B. Inferior thyroid arteries
   C. 4 to 6 esophageal arteries coming off the aorta
   D. Light bronchial arteries

16. **The cricopharyngeus muscle is supplied by the:**
   A. Superior thyroid arteries
   B. Inferior thyroid arteries
   C. Bronchial arteries
   D. Descending aorta

17. **False about venous drainage of esophagus is:**
   A. The abdominal esophagus drains into the systemic and portal venous systems through right gastric vein
   B. In all parts of the esophagus, the rich sub-mucosal venous plexus is the first basin for venous drainage of the esophagus
   C. The submucosal venous plexus of the thoracic esophagus joins with the more superficial esophageal venous plexus and the venae comitantes that envelop the esophagus at this level
   D. In the cervical esophagus, the submucosal venous plexus drains into the inferior thyroid veins, which are tributaries of the left subclavian vein and right brachiocephalic vein

18. **True about lymphatic drainage of esophagus is:**
   A. In the upper two-thirds, flow tends to be downward
   B. In the upper one-thirds, lymphatic flow is upward
   C. In the distal third, flow tends to be downward
   D. In the two-thirds, flow tends to be upward

19. **False about nerve supply of esophagus is:**
   A. Inferiorly, the greater and lesser splanchnic nerves innervate the distal thoracic esophagus
   B. The cervical sympathetic trunk arises from the superior ganglion in the neck
   C. In the abdomen, the sympathetic fibers lay posteriorly alongside the right gastric artery
   D. The parasympathetic fibers arise from the vagus nerve, which gives rise to the superior and recurrent laryngeal nerves

20. **False about nerve supply of esophagus is:**
   A. The parasympathetic fibers coalesce 5 cm above the diaphragm into the left (anterior) and right (posterior) vagus nerves

B. Unilateral injury to the superior or recurrent laryngeal nerve results in hoarseness and aspiration from laryngeal and UES dysfunction
C. The sympathetic and parasympathetic fibers penetrate through the muscular wall, forming networks between the muscle layers to become Auerbach plexus and within the submucosal layer to become Meissner plexus
D. They provide an intrinsic autonomic nervous system within the esophageal wall that is responsible for peristalsis

PHYSIOLOGY

21. The tone of UES (Upper esophageal sphincter) is:

A. 60 mm Hg
B. 60 cm H_2O
C. 40 mm Hg
D. 40 cm H_2O

22. The tone of LES (Lower esophageal sphincter) is:

A. 34 cm H_2O
B. 24 mm Hg
C. 34 mm Hg
D. 24 cm H_2O

23. Which of the following is not seen during swallowing?

A. Elevation of the larynx
B. Elevation of the hyoid
C. Depression of the soft palate
D. Tilting of the epiglottis

24. Within 0.5 second of the initiation of swallowing, the UES closes and reaches close to:

A. 30 mm Hg
B. 60 mm Hg
C. 90 mm Hg
D. 120 mm Hg

25. Amplitude of esophageal body contractions is:

A. 10–20 mm Hg
B. 20–40 mm Hg
C. 30–50 mm Hg
D. 40–80 mm Hg

26. False about esophageal peristalsis is:

A. Secondary peristaltic contractions are also progressive but are generated from distention or irritation of the esophagus
B. Primary peristaltic contractions are progressive and voluntary
C. Tertiary contractions represent coordinated contractions of the smooth muscle
D. Tertiary contractions are nonprogressive, nonperistaltic, monophasic or multiphasic, simultaneous waves that can occur after voluntary swallowing or spontaneously between swallows throughout the esophagus

27. Primary peristaltic contractions are progressive and move down the esophagus at a rate of:

A. 1 to 2 cm/sec
B. 2 to 4 cm/sec
C. 4 to 8 cm/sec
D. 8 to 10 cm/sec

28. Vagal-mediated relaxation of the LES occurs after pharyngeal swallowing and lasts:

A. 1 to 2 seconds
B. 2 to 4 seconds
C. 4 to 6 seconds
D. 6 to 8 seconds

DIAGNOSIS AND MANAGEMENT OF ESOPHAGEAL MOTILITY DISORDERS

29. Chicago classification, which was derived from data obtained by:

A. High-resolution manometry (HRM) + Esophageal pressure topography
B. High-resolution manometry (HRM) + Esophageal ultrasound
C. Impedance monitoring + Esophageal pressure topography
D. Impedance monitoring + Esophageal ultrasound

30. No. of sensors in High-resolution manometry (HRM) is:

A. 36
B. 24
C. 12
D. 6

31. False about diffuse esophageal spasm is:

A. It is now called as distal esophageal spasm
B. Patients will complain of a squeezing pressure in the chest that may radiate to the jaw, arms and upper back
C. It is seen most often in men and is often found in patients with multiple medical complaints
D. DES esophageal contractions are repetitive, simultaneous and of high amplitude

32. False about diffuse esophageal spasm is:

A. Regurgitation of esophageal contents, saliva and acid reflux is common
B. The clinical presentation of DES is typically that of chest pain and dysphagia
C. The mainstay of treatment for DES is nonsurgical and pharmacologic or endoscopic intervention is preferred
D. The classic picture of the corkscrew esophagus or pseudo diverticulosis on an esophagram is caused by the presence of tertiary contractions and indicates advanced disease

33. HRM findings in DES are all except:

A. At least 20% premature contractions
B. DCI >450 mm Hg·s·cm
C. Normal median integrated relaxation pressure (IRP)
D. DCI >8000 mm Hg·s·cm

34. Following image of barium esophagram shows:

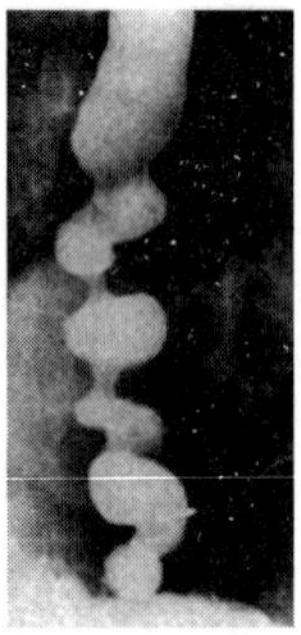

A. Type I achalasia
B. Diffuse esophageal spasm
C. Jackhammer esophagus
D. Nutcracker esophagus

35. Bougie dilatation of the esophagus up to 50 or 60 Fr provides relief for severe dysphagia in:

A. 30% to 50% B. 50% to 80%
C. 70% to 80% D. 20% to 30%

36. False about management of DES is:

A. Dor fundoplication is recommended to provide reflux protection
B. Results of a long esophagomyotomy for DES are poor, it is reported to provide relief of symptoms in up to only 20% of patients
C. Surgery is indicated for patients in the presence of a pulsion diverticulum of the thoracic esophagus
D. Surgery is indicated for patients with incapacitating chest pain or dysphagia who have failed to respond to medical and endoscopic therapy

37. Spastic achalasia is:

A. Type I achalasia
B. Type II achalasia
C. Type III achalasia
D. Esophagogastric junction outflow obstruction

38. The most painful of all esophageal motility disorders is:

A. Type I achalasia
B. Diffuse esophageal spasm
C. Type III achalasia
D. Nutcracker esophagus

39. The most common of all esophageal hypermotility disorders is:

A. Type I achalasia
B. Diffuse esophageal spasm
C. Type III achalasia
D. Nutcracker esophagus

40. Median IRP >15 mm Hg; no normal peristalsis, spastic contractions with DCI >450 mm Hg·s·cm with ≥20% of swallows is diagnostic of:

A. Type I achalasia
B. Type II achalasia
C. Type III achalasia
D. Esophagogastric junction outflow obstruction

41. False about nutcracker esophagus is:

A. Diagnosis of nutcracker esophagus as the subjective complaint of chest pain with at least 2 swallows showing a distal contractile integral >8000 mm Hg·s·cm with single or multipeaked contractions on HRM
B. The primary initial treatment of nutcracker esophagus is surgical
C. Patients with nutcracker esophagus may have triggers and are counselled to avoid caffeine, cold and hot foods
D. It is described as an esophagus with hypertensive peristalsis or high-amplitude peristaltic contractions

42. False about hypertensive lower esophageal sphincter is:

A. Defined on HRM as a median IRP greater than 15 mm Hg (ineffective EGJ relaxation with swallowing)
B. Hypertensive LES has been renamed in the Chicago classification as EGJ outflow obstruction
C. About 50% of the time, peristalsis in the esophageal body is normal
D. Motility of the esophageal body is always hyperperistaltic

43. False about achalasia cardia is:

A. It is the best understood of all esophageal motility disorders
B. Meaning of the term achalasia is "failure to relax"
C. The incidence is 6/100,000 persons/year with a predilection to affect elderly women
D. The muscles of the esophagus and LES are affected

44. The classic triad of presenting symptoms of achalasia consists of all except:

A. Regurgitation B. Dysphagia
C. Heartburn D. Weight loss

45. Long-standing achalasia leads to:

A. Lung abscess B. Pneumonia
C. Bronchiectasis D. All of the above

46. The most common type of cancer identified by achalasia cardia is:

A. Adenocarcinoma
B. Squamous cell carcinoma
C. Lymphoma
D. Carcinoid

47. Chance for development of carcinoma in a patient of achalasia cardia after 20 years is:

A. 8% B. 15%
C. 40% D. 25%

48. False about diagnosis of achalasia cardia is:

A. Manometry is the "gold standard" test for diagnosis
B. In type I (classic) achalasia, the median IRP greater than 15 mm Hg and there is 100% failed peristalsis with minimal esophageal pressurization
C. In type II achalasia, the median IRP greater than 15 mm Hg, 100% failed peristalsis, and panesophageal pressurization with at least 20% of swallows
D. In type III (spastic or vigorous) achalasia, the median IRP greater than 15 mm Hg without normal peristalsis and there are spastic contractions (distal contractile integral >4500 mm Hg·s·cm) with at least 50% of swallow

49. Pseudoachalasia is seen in all except:

A. Neuropathy
B. Strictures
C. GEJ tumors
D. DES

50. False about treatment of achalasia cardia is:

A. Pneumatic dilatation has been shown to provide poor relief of symptoms
B. Nonsurgical treatment options include medications and endoscopic interventions but usually are only a short-term solution to a lifelong problem
C. Surgical treatment - modified laparoscopic Heller myotomy is now the operation of choice
D. POEM-through the submucosal tunnel, the muscular layer of the distal esophagus, LES, and cardia is visualized and divided

51. Esophagectomy as treatment in achalasia cardia is considered in any symptomatic patient with a:

A. Sigmoid esophagus
B. Reflux stricture that is not amenable to dilatation
C. Tortuous dilated esophagus megaesophagus
D. Failure of more than 3 myotomies

52. False about ineffective esophageal motility is:

A. Patients usually present with symptoms of reflux and dysphagia
B. IEM is defined by greater than 50% of swallows being deemed ineffective (distal contractile integral <450 mm Hg·s·cm)
C. It is defined as a contraction abnormality of the distal esophagus and is usually associated with GERD
D. The best treatment of IEM is surgery

DIVERTICULAR DISORDERS

53. False about esophageal diverticular diseases is:

A. Traction, or true, diverticula are more common in the lower esophageal region
B. Most diverticula are a result of a primary motor disturbance or an abnormality of the UES or LES
C. True diverticula involve all layers of the esophageal wall, including mucosa, submucosa and muscularis
D. A false diverticulum consists of mucosa and submucosa

54. Most common esophageal diverticula is:

A. Epiphrenic Diverticula
B. Pharyngoesophageal Diverticulum
C. Midesophageal Diverticula
D. All of the above

55. False about pharyngoesophageal diverticulum is:

A. As the diverticulum enlarges, the mucosal and submucosal layers dissect down the right side of the esophagus into the superior mediastinum, posteriorly along the prevertebral space
B. Result of loss of tissue elasticity and muscle tone with age
C. It is specifically found herniating from Killian triangle, between the oblique fibers of the thyropharyngeus muscle and the horizontal fibers of the cricopharyngeus muscle
D. It is usually manifested in older patients

56. **False about pharyngoesophageal diverticulum is:**
   A. The most serious complication from an untreated Zenker diverticulum is aspiration pneumonia or lung abscess
   B. Halitosis, voice changes, retrosternal pain, and respiratory infections are especially common in older adults
   C. The gold standard of treatment surgical or endoscopic repair of a zenker diverticulum
   D. At the level of the cricothyroid cartilage, the diverticulum can be seen filled with barium resting anteriorly alongside the esophagus

57. **False about the treatment of zenker's diverticulum is:**
   A. When a diverticulopexy performed, it is important to suture the diverticulum to the prevertebral fascia
   B. Large sac (>5 cm), excision of the sac is indicated
   C. Small diverticulum (<2 cm) a myotomy alone is often sufficient
   D. Endoscopic division of the common wall between the esophagus and diverticulum using a laser, electrocautery, or stapler device

58. **False about midesophageal diverticula is:**
   A. Traction diverticula due to inflamed mediastinal nodes due to TB and Histoplasmosis
   B. Some may also be caused by a primary motility disorder, such as achalasia, DES, or other esophageal motility disorder
   C. Dysphagia, chest pain, and regurgitation can be present and are usually indicative of an underlying primary motility disorder
   D. Most patients with a midesophageal diverticulum have chest pain

59. **All are true about midesophageal diverticula except:**
   A. Manometric studies are undertaken in all patients, symptomatic or not, to identify a primary motor disorder
   B. Midesophageal diverticula typically are on the left
   C. Endoscopy is important to rule out mucosal abnormalities, including cancer
   D. CT scan is helpful to identify any mediastinal lymphadenopathy and may help lateralize the sac

60. **False about management of midesophageal diverticula is:**
   A. In patients with severe chest pain or dysphagia and a documented motor abnormality, a long esophagomyotomy is also indicated
   B. Diverticulopexy can be performed, whereby the diverticulum is suspended from the thoracic vertebral fascia
   C. If the diverticulum is smaller than 5 cm, it can be observed
   D. If the diverticulum is 2 cm or larger, surgical intervention is indicated

61. **Endoscopic Dohlman procedure is done in:**
   A. Epiphrenic Diverticula
   B. Pharyngoesophageal Diverticulum
   C. Midesophageal Diverticula
   D. None

62. **Epiphrenic diverticula is seen in:**
   A. Proximal esophagus
   B. Distal esophagus
   C. Mid esophagus
   D. Equal incidence in all the above

63. **False about epiphrenic diverticula is:**
   A. Epiphrenic diverticula are more common on the right side and tend to be wide-mouthed
   B. CT scan is the best diagnostic tool to detect an epiphrenic diverticulum
   C. They are pulsion, or false, diverticula that are often associated with DES, achalasia, or hypertensive LES disorders
   D. Most patients with epiphrenic diverticula present asymptomatically

64. **In the treatment of esophageal diverticulum all of the following are true except:**
   A. If a diverticulopexy is performed, a myotomy is begun at the neck of the diverticulum and extended onto the LES
   B. It is essential to relieve outflow obstruction in patients with diverticula; failure to do so can result in significant complications of leak or recurrence
   C. Small (<2 cm) diverticula should be excised
   D. If a large hiatal hernia is also present, the diverticulum is excised, a myotomy performed, and the hiatal hernia repaired

GASTROESOPHAGEAL REFLUX DISEASE

65. **The most common benign condition of the esophagus is:**
   A. Zeneker's diverticula B. GERD
   C. Achalasia cardia D. Hiatus hernia

66. Complications of GERD includes all except:

A. Carcinoma B. Diverticula
C. Metaplasia D. Strictures

67. False about medical management of GERD is:

A. Patients with the greatest likelihood of successful surgical therapy are those who have typical symptoms and good response to anti-secretory therapy
B. Patients for whom medical therapy never relieved symptoms or who demonstrate atypical symptoms
C. Medical therapy is usually maximal with twice-daily PPI therapy
D. Lifestyle modifications will eliminate GERD symptoms

68. Regarding diagnosis of GERD, all are true except:

A. Patients with severe dysmotility should be considered for surgery
B. Video esophagram shows both structure and function
C. Patient should be off of antisecretory and antacid medications at the time of 24 hrs pH testing (usually cease medications 5 days to 2 weeks prior)
D. A DeMeester score greater than 14.72 confirms pathologic GERD

69. Surgical therapy of GERD includes all except:

A. "Shoeshine maneuver" ensures adequate mobility and lack of tension in fundoplication
B. The passage of instruments easily through the hiatus ensures that fundoplication it is not too tight
C. Nissen fundoplication has become a standard in antireflux surgery
D. At least 5 to 7 cm of intraabdominal esophagus should be present to minimize the likelihood of postoperative hiatal hernia

70. Toupet fundoplication involves:

A. Anterior partial wrap of 270 degrees
B. Posterior complete wrap of 270 degrees
C. Posterior partial wrap of 270 degrees
D. Anterior complete wrap of 270 degrees

71. Dor fundoplication is:

A. Posterior 180 degree B. Anterior 180 degree
C. Anterior 270 degree D. Posterior 270 degree

72. Series of magnetic beads that are placed around the EGJ that will stretch with slight pressure in the esophagus is:

A. EsophyX B. LINX
C. Endoclinch D. Enteryx

73. The patient undergoing fundoplication in whom there is less than adequate intra-abdominal esophagus may require an esophageal lengthening procedure also called as:

A. Vertical gastroplasty
B. Nissen gastroplasty
C. Collis gastroplasty
D. Watson's gastroplasty

ACQUIRED BENIGN DISORDERS OF THE ESOPHAGUS

74. The most common cause of esophageal perforation is:

A. Boerhaave syndrome
B. Iatrogenic
C. Tumor perforation
D. Foreign body ingestion

75. False about esophageal perforation is:

A. Overall mortality is 50% - 60%
B. The key to management and patient survival is early recognition with timely diagnosis and therapy
C. A CT scan may show mediastinal air and periesophageal air or fluid
D. Barium esophagram is the standard for diagnosis

76. False about Pittsburgh esophageal perforation severity score is:

A. As per the criteria age >75 years has score of 1
B. Score ranges 0 to 18 with higher scores indicating greater morbidity with worse prognosis
C. Score has been correlated with morbidity, mortality and hospital stay
D. As per the criteria hypotension has score of 2

77. Not seen as a variable in Pittsburgh esophageal perforation severity score is:

A. Leukocytosis (>12,000 white blood cells/mL)
B. Presence of cancer
C. Respiratory rate >30
D. Tachycardia (>100 beats/min)

78. Pittsburgh esophageal perforation severity score of 4 has a mortality rate of:

A. 2
B. 6
C. 15
D. 27

79. The principles of management after diagnosis includes:

A. Wide local drainage
B. Treatment of contamination
C. Enteral feeding access
D. All of the above

80. False about treatment of esophageal perforation is:

A. Midesophageal are approached through a left thoracotomy
B. High perforations are approached through a left-sided neck incision
C. Gastrostomy and jejunostomy tubes at the first operation are important to provide decompression and drainage near the perforation as well as enteral access for nutrition
D. Distal esophageal are approached through a left thoracotomy or thoracoabdominal approach

81. Pittsburgh esophageal perforation severity score of <3 has a mortality rate of:

A. 2
B. 6
C. 15
D. 27

82. True about endoscopic vacuum therapy (EVT) is:

A. EVT has been described for both esophageal perforation and anastomotic leak after esophagectomy
B. This technique involves endoscopic placement of a sponge into the site of esophageal injury
C. Tubing from the sponge is connected externally to a vacuum device with continuous negative pressure applied to the site of perforation
D. All of the above

83. False about caustic injury is:

A. Majority of caustic ingestion is accidental small-volume drinking of household products by young children
B. Radiographic studies to guide the first procedure, ideally a CT scan of chest and abdomen with intravenous and oral administration of contrast material
C. Nasogastric and orogastric tubes should be inserted blindly initially
D. Endoscopic evaluation of the degree and extent of injury is recommended to be done early in the hospital course as the risk of perforation increases after 48 hours

84. Classification scheme for caustic ingestion is called:

A. Pittsburgh's classification
B. Zargar's classification
C. Seibert's classification
D. Southampton's classification

85. Endoscopic finding in caustic injury shows superficial edema/erythema, as per Zargar's classification it is:

A. Grade 1
B. Grade 2A
C. Grade 2B
D. Grade 3A

86. Endoscopic finding in caustic injury shows transmural ulcerations with focal necrosis, as per Zargar's classification it is:

A. Grade 1
B. Grade 2A
C. Grade 2B
D. Grade 3A

87. To assess for signs of worsening caustic injury, depending on the clinical course, patients may benefit from repeated endoscopy after the event at:

A. 12 to 24 hours
B. 24 to 48 hours
C. 48 to 72 hours
D. 72 to 96 hours

88. In the long term, patients after caustic injury may develop esophageal cancer the risk increases:

A. >10 times
B. >100 times
C. >500 times
D. >1000 times

89. False about Schatzki ring is:

A. Presence of a ring is pathologic
B. Concentric, non-malignant, fibrous thickening and narrowing of the GEJ with squamous epithelium above and columnar cells below
C. The area should always be biopsied to rule out malignancy
D. The majority of patients with a Schatzki ring have a concomitant finding of hiatal hernia

BENIGN AND RARE TUMORS OF THE ESOPHAGUS

90. False about benign tumors of esophagus is:

A. Barium esophagram characteristically demonstrates a smooth defect in the lumen
B. Benign tumors of the esophagus are more common than esophageal cancer

C. Tumors of the submucosa and muscularis propria occur more frequently than mucosal tumors
D. Most commonly these lesions are asymptomatic

91. The most common benign tumors of the esophagus is:

A. Granular cell tumor B. Leiomyoma
C. Fibrovascular polyp D. Lipomas

92. False about granular cell tumor is:

A. The proximal esophagus is the most common location
B. Derive from Schwann cells of nerve sheath origin
C. 11% of patients may have multiple tumors
D. Granular cell tumors may be found in a variety of locations, including the skin, respiratory tract, gastrointestinal tract, breast and tongue

93. False about the management of esophageal granular cell tumor is:

A. Endoscopic resection is a valuable tool for these lesions when diagnosis is in question and to rule out malignancy
B. Standard biopsies are diagnostic
C. Tunneled biopsies will reveal eosinophilic granules
D. On endoscopic ultrasound (EUS), lesions typically have regular borders and arise within the first and second sonographic layers

94. False about fibrovascular polyp is:

A. They appear cylindrical or elongated with a stalk
B. Large tumors may cause dysphagia and some may even prolapse into the hypopharynx, causing airway obstruction
C. Most often found in the cervical esophagus at or near the cricopharyngeus
D. Large tumors can't be resected endoscopically

95. Most common location of squamous papilloma is:

A. Distal esophagus
B. Proximal esophagus
C. Middle third of esophagus
D. GE junction

96. False about squamous papilloma is:

A. Complete excision is warranted to rule out carcinoma and can usually be performed endoscopically
B. There is evidence suggesting a link between squamous papillomas and human papillomavirus (HPV)
C. They appear as red, endophytic projections
D. Most common location is distal esophagus

97. Benign submucosal tumors, false statement is:

A. Benign submucosal tumors include lipomas, hemangiomas and neural tumors
B. Hemangiomas typically appear as a purple or reddish nodule; smooth, hyperchoic, submucosal mass on EUS
C. Lipomas have a characteristic, homogeneous, hyperechoic, smooth appearance on EUS
D. Neural tumors including neurofibromas and schwannomas and are rare in the esophagus

98. False about leiomyoma is:

A. The tumors arise in the muscularis propria and are usually found in the mid to distal esophagus
B. The endoscopic appearance is a round protrusion into the lumen of the esophagus with smooth, reddened mucosa
C. They have a 2:1 male predominance
D. Tumors with EUS characteristics suggestive of a leiomyoma should not be biopsied

99. False about management of leiomyoma is:

A. Large, symptomatic lesions with this appearance may be safely observed without biopsy
B. On EUS, leiomyomas are hypoechoic, have regular borders and arise from the fourth endosonographic
C. Symptomatic lesions may be enucleated and even large lesions can usually be removed with a VATS approach
D. Differential diagnosis of a large smooth esophageal tumor, including leiomyosarcoma, gastrointestinal stromal tumor (GIST) and leiomyomas.

100. False about small cell carcinomas of the esophagus is:

A. Stage at diagnosis is the most important prognostic factor
B. The tumors typically present with lymph node involvement
C. The overall prognosis is good
D. These tumors have the same aggressive phenotype and histologic appearance of other poorly differentiated neuroendocrine cancers

101. **True about leiomyosarcoma is:**

A. EUS may show more irregular borders or a heterogeneous appearance that is uncharacteristic for leiomyoma
B. In general, esophagectomy with radical lymphadenectomy is the treatment of choice for leiomyosarcomas
C. Although well-differentiated leiomyosarcomas may be difficult to distinguish from leiomyoma, these are rare tumors that often erode through the mucosa, appearing as an ulcerated or exophytic mass on endoscopy
D. All of the above

102. **False about GIST is:**

A. GISTs tend to be larger, with uptake of IV contrast on CT, and often have significant positron emission tomography (PET) avidity
B. Imatinib should be considered for any GIST larger than 3 cm or with other high-risk features
C. GISTs have similar appearance to leiomyomas but can be distinguished histologically by CD117 (c-kit) and CD34 stain positivity
D. Esophageal GISTs tend to have good disease-free and overall survival

ESOPHAGEAL CANCER

103. **Most common histology of esophageal cancer in westernized counties is:**

A. Squamous cell carcinoma
B. Adenocarcinoma
C. Leiomyosarcoma
D. GIST

104. **False about CA esophagus - SCC is:**

A. 3 to 4 times more prevalent in women
B. Tobacco and alcohol are strong risk factors for SCC and they have a synergistic effect on risk
C. Hereditary cancer syndromes associated with esophageal SCC include tylosis and Fanconi anemia
D. SCC is associated with certain intrinsic disorders of the esophagus, such as Plummer-Vinson syndrome and achalasia

105. **Most common site of SCC is:**

A. Middle and distal esophagus
B. Proximal and middle esophagus
C. Distal esophagus
D. GE junction

106. **Most common site of adenocarcinoma is:**

A. Middle and distal esophagus
B. Proximal and middle esophagus
C. Distal esophagus
D. GE junction

107. **Siewert III tumors are classified as:**

A. Esophageal cancers B. Gastric cancers
C. Both D. None

108. **GEJ adenocarcinomas are staged and classified as:**

A. Esophageal cancers B. Gastric cancers
C. Both D. None

109. **False about esophageal cancers is:**

A. Locally advanced tumors may be manifested with laryngeal nerve involvement causing hoarseness or with tracheoesophageal fistula
B. Many patients with adenocarcinoma will endorse a long history of reflux symptoms including heartburn and regurgitation
C. Majority of esophageal cancers are symptomatic at the time of diagnosis
D. Early-stage tumors are often symptomatic and are discovered during endoscopy done for Barrett's esophagus

110. **Most common symptom of esophageal cancer is:**

A. Reflux B. Chest pain
C. Heartburn D. Dysphagia

111. **False about diagnosis of esophageal cancer is:**

A. Tumor location affects pathologic stage for adenocarcinoma but not for SCC
B. Barium esophagram: "Apple-core" filling defect is seen only if there is symmetrical, circumferential narrowing
C. Diagnosis of esophageal cancer is almost always made by endoscopic biopsy
D. The most proximal extent and circumferential extent of any Barrett's esophagus should also be noted according to the Prague criteria

112. **True about esophageal cancer is:**

A. Lower tumors arise distal to the lower border of the inferior pulmonary vein to the GEJ; usually more than 30 cm from the incisors
B. Upper thoracic esophagus begins at the thoracic inlet and extends to the azygos vein; approximately 20 to 25 cm from the incisors

C. Midthoracic tumors arise from the lower border of the azygos vein to the inferior pulmonary vein; approximately 25 to 30 cm from the incisors

D. All of the above

113. Tumors that invade into the submucosa are:

A. T1a tumors B. T1b tumors
C. T2 tumors D. T3 tumors

114. Tumors that invade the adventitia but not surrounding structures are:

A. T1a tumors B. T1b tumors
C. T2 tumors D. T3 tumors

115. Esophageal tumors that invade into azygos vein are:

A. T3 tumors B. T2 tumors
C. T4a tumors D. T4b tumors

116. Esophageal lesions with high-grade dysplasia are:

A. Tis B. TX
C. T0 D. T1a

117. T2 N1 M0 is which clinical stage of esophageal cancer?

A. Stage I B. Stage IIA
C. Stage IIB D. Stage III

118. T2 N0 M0 is which clinical stage of esophageal cancer?

A. Stage I B. Stage IIA
C. Stage IIB D. Stage III

119. T4a N1 M0 is which clinical stage of esophageal cancer?

A. Stage IIB B. Stage III
C. Stage IVA D. Stage IVB

120. False about esophageal cancer is:

A. If there is no evidence of distant metastatic disease, EUS should be done to assess T-status and regional lymph nodes

B. For T1a tumors resected by EMR, the risk of lymph node metastasis is low and additional staging studies are required

C. EUS is superior to CT or PET for assessment of both T and N-status

D. EUS has less accuracy for superficial disease and will seldom obviate the need for EMR

121. False about esophageal cancer is:

A. Use of narrow-band imaging is associated with low accuracy is diagnosing dysplasia

B. Dysplasia arising in Barrett's esophagus is characterized by cytologic malignant changes including atypical nuclei, increased mitoses, and lack of surface maturation

C. The Seattle biopsy protocol is still widely accepted for mapping of Barrett's esophagus with high-grade dysplasia

D. Barrett's esophagus is a significant risk factor for the development of esophageal adenocarcinoma

122. The Seattle biopsy protocol is:

A. 4 quadrant biopsies at 0.5-cm intervals along the entire length of Barrett's esophagus in addition to targeted biopsies of all visible lesions

B. 4 quadrant biopsies at 1-cm intervals along the entire length of Barrett's esophagus in addition to targeted biopsies of all visible lesions

C. 4 quadrant biopsies at 2-cm intervals along the entire length of Barrett's esophagus in addition to targeted biopsies of all visible lesions

D. 4 quadrant biopsies at 3-cm intervals along the entire length of Barrett's esophagus in addition to targeted biopsies of all visible lesions

123. False about ablation used in esophageal cancer is:

A. RFA is much less effective than photodynamic therapy with a higher stricture (and overall complication) rate

B. The standard ablation program uses two double pulses of 12 J/cm^2

C. The most commonly used technology today is radiofrequency ablation (RFA)

D. RFA may be delivered with a circumferential balloon or an electrical plate using a bipolar electrode that transmits radiofrequency energy, which generates heat and destroys superficial tissue

124. False about cryotherapy used in esophageal cancer is:

A. Advantage of cryotherapy compared with RFA is that cryotherapy does not require a probe to be in contact with the tissue

B. Cryotherapy is not well tolerated with pain and high stricture rates

C. A decompression tube is typically required to prevent overdistention of the stomach and intestine with gas

D. Endoscopists typically use either an endoscopic spray catheter or in some cases, an endoscopic balloon, to deliver cold liquid nitrogen (–196°C)

125. **False about EMR: Endoscopic mucosal resection is:**

A. EMR can technically remove lesions involving the submucosa (T1b), but the risk of lymph node involvement increases with depth of submucosal invasion
B. EMR provides large specimens to accurately determine the depth of invasion
C. NCCN guidelines currently recommend use of EMR ± ablation in patients with Tis and T1a tumors as a preferred therapy over esophagectomy
D. T1b cancers with adenocarcinoma appear to have a higher risk of nodal metastasis compared with squamous cell histology

126. **Complications of EMR includes:**

A. Perforation B. Stricture
C. Bleeding D. All of the above

127. **Which variable for predicting lymph node metastases in early esophageal adenocarcinoma using a scoring system has maximum points?**

A. Moderate differentiation
B. Lymphovascular invasion
C. Poor differentiation
D. Size

128. **False about EMR for early esophageal cancer is:**

A. For superficial lesions treated endoscopically, radiologic imaging, such as fluorodeoxyglucose (FDG) PET, should be used for surveillance
B. Patients should receive high-dose acid suppression therapy with a PPI to help EMR and ablation sites to heal
C. Any residual Barrett epithelium may be focally ablated at that time
D. Short-interval follow-up endoscopy should be performed 3 months after endoscopic treatment is completed

129. **True about esophagectomy is:**

A. Esophagectomy with an adequate lymphadenectomy would be expected to confer an overall 5-year survival of anywhere between 40% and 65% for a pathologic T2N0 cancer, depending on histology, grade and location of tumor
B. The benefit of a transthoracic approach is the ability to perform an extensive lymphadenectomy
C. Hybrid Ivor Lewis esophagectomy was associated with almost half as many major complications as open surgery with differences in pulmonary events being a driving factor
D. All of the above

130. **Dysphagia, generally signifies transmural tumor involvement of:**

A. T1 lesion B. T2 lesion
C. T3 lesion D. T4a lesion

131. **Probability of lymph node metastases in T3 disease reaches:**

A. 80% B. 60%
C. 50% D. 30%

132. **Regarding use of radiation in locally advanced esophageal cancer false statement is:**

A. Adjuvant radiation: deliver lower doses (20–40 Gy) of radiation postoperatively
B. Postoperative radiation therapy for esophageal cancer appeared to be potentially beneficial in several trials
C. Radiation was employed as the first treatment modality for esophageal cancer
D. Radiation is a part of multimodality treatment for locally advanced esophageal cancer

133. **The main cause of death in patients with esophageal cancer:**

A. Bleeding B. Distant recurrence
C. Malnutrition D. Heart failure

134. **False about radiotherapy is:**

A. Radiotherapy and chemotherapy used have synergistic effect
B. Current chemotherapeutic regimens are based on platinum compounds (cisplatin and carboplatin) in combination with 5-fluorouracil or taxanes as a doublet
C. In the adjuvant setting, the results of chemotherapy have not been convincing
D. All of the above are true

135. **True among the following about the management of locally advanced esophageal cancer is:**

A. The synergistic effect of chemoradiation combined with surgical resection maximizes the chances of effectively treating both locoregional disease and potential undetectable metastases
B. Concomitant administration of chemotherapy and radiation has a synergistic effect with increased tumor cytotoxicity at low doses

C. Chemoradiation may be administered in a preoperative or postoperative setting, as definitive bimodality therapy, or as part of trimodality therapy when combined with surgery
D. All of the above

136. False about the CROSS trial is:

A. Compared chemoradiation followed by surgery with surgery alone for esophageal and EGJ cancer
B. The chemoradiation regimen consisted of a 4-week course of carboplatin and paclitaxel administered concurrently with radiation therapy at a dose of 41.4 Gy given in 23 fractions seven days a week
C. Esophagectomy was performed within 4 to 6 weeks in the treatment group and immediately after randomization in the control group
D. Established the standard of care as trimodality treatment for the treatment of locally advanced esophageal carcinoma

137. As per NCCN guidelines, Esophageal cancer patient surveillance includes that providers should consider observing patients every 3 to 6 months with:

A. Endoscopy studies
B. Clinical examination
C. CT chest/abdomen ± PET
D. All of the above

138. More than 98% of local recurrences after esophageal cancer treatment occur in the first:

A. 12 months
B. 24 months
C. 36 months
D. 48 months

ANSWERS

1. **Ans: D. The cervical esophagus begins as a midline structure that deviates slightly to the right of the trachea as it passes through the neck into the thoracic inlet**

   Ref: Chapter No.42, Page No.1014

2. **Ans: B. C6 to T11**

   Ref: Chapter No.42, Page No.1014

3. **Ans: D. All of the above are true**

   Ref: Chapter No.42, Page No.1014

4. **Ans: C. Thyropharyngeus and cricopharyngeus muscles**

   Ref: Chapter No.42, Page No.1015

5. **Ans: D. The transition between the oblique fibers of the thyropharyngeus muscle and the horizontal fibers of the cricopharyngeus muscle which creates a point of potential weakness**

   Ref: Chapter No.42, Page No.1015

6. **Ans: B. Point of transition is flanked by the longitudinal esophageal muscles that extend superiorly to attach to the midportion of the posterior surface of the cricoid cartilage**

   Ref: Chapter No.42, Page No.1015

7. **Ans: D. Thoracic - left**

   Ref: Chapter No.42, Page No.1014-1015

8. **Ans: B. Submucosa**

   Ref: Chapter No.42, Page No.1015-1016

9. **Ans: C. The circular muscles of the esophagus to oblique muscles of the stomach at the incisura (cardiac notch)**

   Ref: Chapter No.42, Page No.1016

10. **Ans: A. Muscularis propria**

    Ref: Chapter No.42, Page No.1016

11. **Ans: C. Bronchoaortic constriction - 15 to 17 mm**

    Ref: Chapter No.42, Page No.1016

12. **Ans: C. Cricopharyngeus muscle**

    Ref: Chapter No.42, Page No.1016

13. **Ans: D. All of the above are true**

    Ref: Chapter No.42, Page No.1016

14. **Ans: B. Inferior thyroid arteries**

    Ref: Chapter No.42, Page No.1016

15. **Ans: B. Inferior thyroid arteries**

    Ref: Chapter No.42, Page No.1016

16. **Ans: A. Superior thyroid arteries**

    Ref: Chapter No.42, Page No.1016

17. **Ans: A. The abdominal esophagus drains into the systemic and portal venous systems through right gastric vein**

    Ref: Chapter No.42, Page No.1017

18. **Ans: C. In the distal third, flow tends to be downward**

Ref: Chapter No.42, Page No.1017

19. **Ans: C. In the abdomen, the sympathetic fibers lay posteriorly alongside the right gastric artery**

Ref: Chapter No.42, Page No.1018

20. **Ans: A. The parasympathetic fibers coalesce 5 cm above the diaphragm into the left (anterior) and right (posterior) vagus nerves**

Ref: Chapter No.42, Page No.1018

21. **Ans: A. 60 mm Hg**

Ref: Chapter No.42, Page No.1019

22. **Ans: B. 24 mm Hg**

Ref: Chapter No.42, Page No.1019

23. **Ans: C. Depression of the soft palate**

Ref: Chapter No.42, Page No.1019

24. **Ans: C. 90 mm Hg**

Ref: Chapter No.42, Page No.1019

25. **Ans: D. 40–80 mm Hg**

Ref: Chapter No.42, Page No.1021

26. **Ans: C. Tertiary contractions represent coordinated contractions of the smooth muscle**

Ref: Chapter No.42, Page No.1021

27. **Ans: B. 2 to 4 cm/sec**

Ref: Chapter No.42, Page No.1021

28. **Ans: C. 4 to 6 seconds**

Ref: Chapter No.42, Page No.1021

29. **Ans: A. High-resolution manometry (HRM) + Esophageal pressure topography**

Ref: Chapter No.42, Page No.1022

30. **Ans: A. 36**

Ref: Chapter No.42, Page No.1022

31. **Ans: C. It is seen most often in men and is often found in patients with multiple medical complaints**

Ref: Chapter No.42, Page No.1022-1023

32. **Ans: A. Regurgitation of esophageal contents, saliva and acid reflux is common**

Ref: Chapter No.42, Page No.1023-1024

33. **Ans: D. DCI >8000 mm Hg·s·cm**

Ref: Chapter No.42, Page No.1024

34. **Ans: B. Diffuse esophageal spasm**

Ref: Chapter No.42, Page No.1024

35. **Ans: C. 70% to 80%**

Ref: Chapter No.42, Page No.1024

36. **Ans: B. Results of a long esophagomyotomy for DES are poor, it is reported to provide relief of symptoms in up to only 20% of patients**

Ref: Chapter No.42, Page No.1024-1025

37. **Ans: C. Type III achalasia**

Ref: Chapter No.42, Page No.1024

38. **Ans: D. Nutcracker esophagus**

Ref: Chapter No.42, Page No.1025

39. **Ans: D. Nutcracker esophagus**

Ref: Chapter No.42, Page No.1025

40. **Ans: C. Type III achalasia**

Ref: Chapter No.42, Page No.1024

41. **Ans: B. The primary initial treatment of nutcracker esophagus is surgical**

Ref: Chapter No.42, Page No.1025

42. **Ans: D. Motility of the esophageal body is always hyperperistaltic**

Ref: Chapter No.42, Page No.1025

43. **Ans: C. The incidence is 6/100,000 persons/year with a predilection to affect elderly women**

Ref: Chapter No.42, Page No.1025

44. **Ans: C. Heartburn**

Ref: Chapter No.42, Page No.1025

45. **Ans: D. All of the above**

Ref: Chapter No.42, Page No.1026

46. **Ans: B. Squamous cell carcinoma**

Ref: Chapter No.42, Page No.1026

47. **Ans: A. 8%**

Ref: Chapter No.42, Page No.1026

48. **Ans: D. In type III (spastic or vigorous) achalasia, the median IRP greater than 15 mm Hg without normal peristalsis and there are spastic contractions (distal contractile integral >4500 mm Hg·s·cm) with at least 50% of swallow**

Ref: Chapter No.42, Page No.1026

49. **Ans: D. DES**

Ref: Chapter No.42, Page No.1026-1027

50. **Ans: A. Pneumatic dilatation has been shown to provide poor relief of symptoms**

Ref: Chapter No.42, Page No.1027

51. **Ans: D. Failure of more than 3 myotomies**

Ref: Chapter No.42, Page No.1027

52. **Ans: D. The best treatment of IEM is surgery**

Ref: Chapter No.42, Page No.1028

53. **Ans: A. Traction, or true, diverticula are more common in the lower esophageal region**

Ref: Chapter No.42, Page No.1028

54. **Ans: B. Pharyngoesophageal Diverticulum**

Ref: Chapter No.42, Page No.1028

55. **Ans: A. As the diverticulum enlarges, the mucosal and submucosal layers dissect down the right side of the esophagus into the superior mediastinum, posteriorly along the prevertebral space**

Ref: Chapter No.42, Page No.1028

56. **Ans: D. At the level of the cricothyroid cartilage, the diverticulum can be seen filled with barium resting anteriorly alongside the esophagus**

Ref: Chapter No.42, Page No.1029

57. **Ans: A. When a diverticulopexy performed, it is important to suture the diverticulum to the prevertebral fascia**

Ref: Chapter No.42, Page No.1029

58. **Ans: D. Most patients with a midesophageal diverticulum have chest pain**

Ref: Chapter No.42, Page No.1029

59. **Ans: B. Midesophageal diverticula typically are on the left**

Ref: Chapter No.42, Page No.1029

60. **Ans: C. If the diverticulum is smaller than 5 cm, it can be observed**

Ref: Chapter No.42, Page No.1029

61. **Ans: B. Pharyngoesophageal Diverticulum**

Ref: Chapter No.42, Page No.1029

62. **Ans: B. Distal esophagus**

Ref: Chapter No.42, Page No.1029

63. **Ans: B. CT scan is the best diagnostic tool to detect an epiphrenic diverticulum**

Ref: Chapter No.42, Page No.1029

64. **Ans: C. Small (<2 cm) diverticula should be excised**

Ref: Chapter No.42, Page No.1030

65. **Ans: B. GERD**

Ref: Chapter No.42, Page No.1030

66. **Ans: B. Diverticula**

Ref: Chapter No.42, Page No.1031

67. **Ans: D. Lifestyle modifications will eliminate GERD symptoms**

Ref: Chapter No.42, Page No.1031

68. **Ans: A. Patients with severe dysmotility should be considered for surgery**

Ref: Chapter No.42, Page No.1031

69. **Ans: D. At least 5 to 7 cm of intraabdominal esophagus should be present to minimize the likelihood of postoperative hiatal hernia**

Ref: Chapter No.42, Page No.1031-1033

70. **Ans: C. Posterior partial wrap of 270 degrees**

Ref: Chapter No.42, Page No.1033

71. **Ans: B. Anterior 180 degree**

Ref: Chapter No.42, Page No.1033

72. **Ans: B. LINX**

Ref: Chapter No.42, Page No.1033

73. **Ans: C. Collis gastroplasty**

Ref: Chapter No.42, Page No.1033

74. **Ans: B. Iatrogenic**

Ref: Chapter No.42, Page No.1034

75. **Ans: A. Overall mortality is 50% - 60%**

Ref: Chapter No.42, Page No.1034

76. **Ans: D. As per the criteria hypotension has score of 2**

Ref: Chapter No.42, Page No.1034

77. **Ans: A. Leukocytosis (>12,000 white blood cells/mL)**

Ref: Chapter No.42, Page No.1034

78. **Ans: B. 6**

Ref: Chapter No.42, Page No.1035

79. **Ans: D. All of the above**

Ref: Chapter No.42, Page No.1034

80. **Ans: A. Midesophageal are approached through a left thoracotomy**

Ref: Chapter No.42, Page No.1035

81. **Ans: A. 2**

Ref: Chapter No.42, Page No.1035

82. **Ans: D. All of the above**

Ref: Chapter No.42, Page No.1035

83. **Ans: C. Nasogastric and orogastric tubes should be inserted blindly initially**

Ref: Chapter No.42, Page No.1035

84. **Ans: B. Zargar's classification**

Ref: Chapter No.42, Page No.1036

85. **Ans: A. Grade 1**

Ref: Chapter No.42, Page No.1036

86. **Ans: D. Grade 3A**

Ref: Chapter No.42, Page No.1036

87. **Ans: C. 48 to 72 hours**

Ref: Chapter No.42, Page No.1036

88. **Ans: D. >1000 times**

Ref: Chapter No.42, Page No.1036

89. **Ans: A. Presence of a ring is pathologic**

Ref: Chapter No.42, Page No.1036

90. **Ans: B. Benign tumors of the esophagus are more common than esophageal cancer**

Ref: Chapter No.42, Page No.1036

91. **Ans: B. Leiomyoma**

Ref: Chapter No.42, Page No.1037

92. **Ans: A. The proximal esophagus is the most common location**

Ref: Chapter No.42, Page No.1036

93. **Ans: B. Standard biopsies are diagnostic**

Ref: Chapter No.42, Page No.1036-1037

94. **Ans: D. Large tumors can't be resected endoscopically**

Ref: Chapter No.42, Page No.1037

95. **Ans: A. Distal esophagus**

Ref: Chapter No.42, Page No.1037

96. **Ans: C. They appear as red, endophytic projections**

Ref: Chapter No.42, Page No.1037

97. **Ans: B. Hemangiomas typically appear as a purple or reddish nodule; smooth, hyperchoic, submucosal mass on EUS**

Ref: Chapter No.42, Page No.1037

98. **Ans: B. The endoscopic appearance is a round protrusion into the lumen of the esophagus with smooth, reddened mucosa**

Ref: Chapter No.42, Page No.1037-1038

99. **Ans: A. Large, symptomatic lesions with this appearance may be safely observed without biopsy**

Ref: Chapter No.42, Page No.1038

100. **Ans: C. The overall prognosis is good**

Ref: Chapter No.42, Page No.1038

101. **Ans: D. All of the above**

Ref: Chapter No.42, Page No.1038

102. **Ans: D. Esophageal GISTs tend to have good disease-free and overall survival**

Ref: Chapter No.42, Page No.1038

103. **Ans: B. Adenocarcinoma**

Ref: Chapter No.42, Page No.1038

104. **Ans: A. 3 to 4 times more prevalent in women**

Ref: Chapter No.42, Page No.1038

105. **Ans: B. Proximal and middle esophagus**

Ref: Chapter No.42, Page No.1039

106. **Ans: C. Distal esophagus**

Ref: Chapter No.42, Page No.1039

107. **Ans: B. Gastric cancers**

Ref: Chapter No.42, Page No.1039

108. **Ans: A. Esophageal cancers**

Ref: Chapter No.42, Page No.1039

109. **Ans: D. Early-stage tumors are often symptomatic and are discovered during endoscopy done for Barrett's esophagus**

Ref: Chapter No.42, Page No.1039

110. **Ans: D. Dysphagia**

Ref: Chapter No.42, Page No.1039

111. **Ans: A. Tumor location affects pathologic stage for adenocarcinoma but not for SCC**

Ref: Chapter No.42, Page No.1039

112. **Ans: D. All of the above**

Ref: Chapter No.42, Page No.1039

113. **Ans: B. T1b tumors**

Ref: Chapter No.42, Page No.1039

114. **Ans: D. T3 tumors**

Ref: Chapter No.42, Page No.1039

115. **Ans: C. T4a tumors**

Ref: Chapter No.42, Page No.1040

116. **Ans: A. Tis**

Ref: Chapter No.42, Page No.1040

117. **Ans: D. Stage III**

Ref: Chapter No.42, Page No.1040

118. **Ans: C. Stage IIB**

Ref: Chapter No.42, Page No.1040

119. **Ans: B. Stage III**

Ref: Chapter No.42, Page No.1040

120. **Ans: B. For T1a tumors resected by EMR, the risk of lymph node metastasis is low, and additional staging studies are required**

Ref: Chapter No.42, Page No.1040-1041

121. **Ans: A. Use of narrow-band imaging is associated with low accuracy is diagnosing dysplasia**

Ref: Chapter No.42, Page No.1041-1042

122. **Ans: B. 4 quadrant biopsies at 1-cm intervals along the entire length of Barrett esophagus in addition to targeted biopsies of all visible lesions**

Ref: Chapter No.42, Page No.1042

123. **Ans: A. RFA is much less effective than photodynamic therapy with a higher stricture (and overall complication) rate**

Ref: Chapter No.42, Page No.1044

124. Ans: B. Cryotherapy is not well tolerated with pain and high stricture rates

Ref: Chapter No.42, Page No.1045

125. Ans: D. T1b cancers with adenocarcinoma appear to have a higher risk of nodal metastasis compared with squamous cell histology

Ref: Chapter No.42, Page No.1046

126. Ans: D. All of the above

Ref: Chapter No.42, Page No.1046

127. Ans: B. Lymphovascular invasion

Ref: Chapter No.42, Page No.1047

128. Ans: A. For superficial lesions treated endoscopically, radiologic imaging, such as fluorodeoxyglucose (FDG) PET, should be used for surveillance

Ref: Chapter No.42, Page No.1047

129. Ans: D. All of the above

Ref: Chapter No.42, Page No.1048

130. Ans: C. T3 lesion

Ref: Chapter No.42, Page No.1048

131. Ans: A. 80%

Ref: Chapter No.42, Page No.1048

132. Ans: A. Adjuvant radiation: deliver lower doses (20–40 Gy) of radiation postoperatively

Ref: Chapter No.42, Page No.1049

133. Ans: B. Distant recurrence

Ref: Chapter No.42, Page No.1049

134. Ans: D. All of the above are true

Ref: Chapter No.42, Page No.1049-1050

135. Ans: D. All of the above

Ref: Chapter No.42, Page No.1050

136. Ans: B. The chemoradiation regimen consisted of a 4-week course of carboplatin and paclitaxel administered concurrently with radiation therapy at a dose of 41.4 Gy given in 23 fractions seven days a week

Ref: Chapter No.42, Page No.1050-1051

137. Ans: D. All of the above

Ref: Chapter No.42, Page No.1051

138. Ans: C. 36 months

Ref: Chapter No.42, Page No.1052

43

Gastroesophageal Reflux Disease and Hiatal Hernia

1. **The most common benign medical condition of the stomach and esophagus:**
   A. Hiatus hernia
   B. Gastroesophageal reflux disease
   C. Barrett's esophagus
   D. Gastric ulcers

GASTROESOPHAGEAL REFLUX DISEASE

2. **LES is made up of:**
   A. Crura of the diaphragm
   B. Sling fibers of the gastric cardia
   C. The intrinsic musculature of the distal esophagus
   D. All of the above

3. **LES pressure is measured at:**
   A. Beginning of expiration
   B. Mid-expiration
   C. Mid-inspiration
   D. End-inspiration

4. **Sling fibers of the gastric cardia are located at the same anatomic depth as the:**
   A. Longitudinal fibers of the esophagus
   B. Circular muscle fibers of the esophagus
   C. Adventia of esophagus
   D. Oblique muscle fibers of the esophagus

5. **False about GER is:**
   A. Gastroesophageal reflux (GER) occurs when intragastric pressure is greater than the high-pressure zone of the distal esophagus
   B. The distinction between physiologic reflux (i.e., GER) and pathologic reflux (i.e., GERD) hinges on the total amount of esophageal acid exposure, the patient's symptoms, and the presence of mucosal damage of the esophagus
   C. Physiologic GER provides us the ability to rapidly evacuate swallowed air from the stomach
   D. Hypertensive LES is frequently associated with hiatal hernia because of displacement of the GEJ into the posterior mediastinum

6. **The most common type of hiatal hernia is:**
   A. Type I B. Type II
   C. Type III D. Type IV

7. **Sliding hiatal hernia is:**
   A. Type I B. Type II
   C. Type III D. Type IV

8. **When the GEJ migrates cephalad into the posterior mediastinum it is:**
   A. Type I hiatal hernia
   B. Type II hiatal hernia
   C. Type III hiatal hernia
   D. Type IV hiatal hernia

9. **Paraoesophageal hernias are:**
   A. Type II hiatal hernia
   B. Type III hiatal hernia
   C. Type IV hiatal hernia
   D. All of the above

10. **When both the GEJ and fundus located in the mediastinum it is:**
    A. Type I hiatal hernia
    B. Type II hiatal hernia
    C. Type III hiatal hernia
    D. Type IV hiatal hernia

11. **When small bowel migrates cephalad to the esophageal hiatus and into the mediastinum it is:**
    A. Type I hiatal hernia

B. Type II hiatal hernia
C. Type III hiatal hernia
D. Type IV hiatal hernia

12. When the GEJ is anchored in the abdomen and the gastric fundus migrates into the mediastinum through the hiatal defect it is:

A. Type I hiatal hernia
B. Type II hiatal hernia
C. Type III hiatal hernia
D. Type IV hiatal hernia

13. The most common presenting symptom of GERD is:

A. Dysphagia
B. Heartburn
C. Regurgitation
D. Cough

14. False about the symptoms of GERD is:

A. In severe cases, patients will be unable to bend over or lie supine without experiencing an episode of regurgitation
B. Water brash: Regurgitation of gastric contents to the oropharynx and mouth can produce a sour taste that patients will describe as either acid or bile
C. The presence of regurgitation often indicates progression of GERD
D. Regurgitation of undigested food is common in GERD

15. Which of the following is not an extraesophageal manifestation of GERD?

A. Wheezing
B. Rhinitis
C. Postnasal drip
D. Shortness of breath

16. False about extraoesophageal symptoms of GERD is:

A. A lack of response of extraoesophageal symptoms to proton pump inhibitor (PPI) therapy can reliably refute GERD as the cause of these symptoms
B. The most common mechanism is proximal esophageal reflux and microaspiration of gastroduodenal contents cause direct caustic injury to the larynx and lower respiratory tract
C. Extraesophageal symptoms of GERD arise from the respiratory tract and include both laryngeal and pulmonary symptoms
D. If a patient's laryngeal or pulmonary symptoms are not due to abnormal GER, an antireflux operation is not performed

17. True about asthma and GERD is:

A. Antireflux surgery is associated with improvement in respiratory symptoms in nearly 90% of children and 70% of adults with asthma and GERD
B. Compared with patients treated with antisecretory medications, patients treated with antireflux surgery were more likely to experience relief of asthma symptoms, to discontinue systemic steroid therapy, and to improve peak expiratory flow rate
C. In patients with asthma and GERD, antireflux surgery appears to be more effective than medical therapy at managing pulmonary symptoms
D. All of the above

18. False about idiopathic pulmonary fibrosis (IPF) and GERD is:

A. Proximal esophageal reflux with microaspiration of acid and non-acid gastric contents has been implicated as one possible cause of alveolar epithelial injury that can lead to IPF
B. The threshold for testing patients with IPF for GERD should be high
C. Medical treatment of GERD in patients with IPF is associated with longer survival and slower pulmonary decline
D. The incidence of GERD in patients with IPF has been reported to be as high as 94%

19. Patients who have severe proximal esophageal reflux and regurgitation of gastric contents into the mouth may develop:

A. Erosion of their dentition
B. Signs of chronic sinusitis
C. Injected oropharyngeal mucosa
D. All of the above

20. The "gold standard" test to diagnose GERD is:

A. Esophagogastroduodenoscopy
B. Ambulatory pH monitoring
C. Esophageal manometry
D. Barium Esophagram

21. The most effective way to assess function of the esophageal body and the LES is:

A. Esophagogastroduodenoscopy
B. Ambulatory pH monitoring
C. Esophageal manometry
D. Barium Esophagram

22. Abnormal distal esophageal acid exposure is defined by a DeMeester score of:

A. 4.7 or lower
B. 4.7 or higher
C. 14.7 or lower
D. 14.7 or higher

23. Ambulatory pH monitoring generates a large amount of data concerning esophageal acid exposure, including:

A. Number of episodes lasting longer than 5 minutes
B. Total number of reflux episodes (pH <4)
C. Longest episode of reflux
D. All of the above

24. During the interpretation of the pH study, symptom index and symptom-associated probability are calculated on the basis of the temporal relationship between the symptom event and episodes of distal esophageal acid exposure; Close temporal relationship is defined as symptom episode that occurs within:

A. 2 minutes of a reflux episode
B. 5 minutes of a reflux episode
C. 10 minutes of a reflux episode
D. 20 minutes of a reflux episode

25. Impedance catheters use electrodes placed at:

A. 0.5-cm intervals
B. 1-cm intervals
C. 2-cm intervals
D. 3-cm intervals

26. To ensure valid ambulatory esophageal pH study results, the distal electrode must be placed:

A. 5 cm distal to the LES
B. 5 cm proximal to the LES
C. 2 cm distal to the LES
D. 2 cm proximal to the LES

27. False about impedance-pH monitoring is:

A. Impedance decreases in the presence of air and increases in the presence of a liquid bolus
B. Esophageal impedance monitoring identifies episodes of non-acid reflux
C. Disadvantage of impedance technology, however, is that the automated analytic software is very sensitive and tends to overestimate the number of non-acid reflux episodes
D. When pH-impedance catheters are used, it is possible to determine the direction of movement of esophageal acid exposures and therefore to differentiate between an antegrade event (as in a swallow) and a retrograde event (as in GER)

28. High-resolution esophageal manometry gathers data using a 32-channel flexible catheter with pressure-sensing devices arranged at:

A. 0.5-cm intervals
B. 1-cm intervals
C. 2-cm intervals
D. 3-cm intervals

29. No of swallows and the time needed to perform esophageal manometry is:

A. 15 swallows, 10 mins
B. 15 swallows, 5 mins
C. 10 swallows, 15 mins
D. 10 swallows, 10 mins

30. Esophagitis can be reported according to:

A. Siewert classification
B. Chicago classification
C. Savary-Miller classification
D. Paris classification

31. False among he following is:

A. LA class A and B esophagitis should undergo pH testing to confirm abnormal distal esophageal acid exposure
B. Barium esophagram can confirm the diagnosis of GERD
C. Both peptic strictures and LA class C and D esophagitis can be considered pathognomonic for GERD & hence ambulatory pH monitoring is unnecessary in these patients
D. Endoscopic evaluation should also include an assessment of the GEJ flap valve

32. True among the following is:

A. Peptic strictures are pathognomonic for long-standing reflux and develop from the chronic mucosal inflammation that occurs with GERD
B. In patients with GERD, the most common cause of dysphagia is a reflux associated inflammatory process of the esophageal wall
C. Strictures can be associated with esophageal shortening
D. All of the above

33. False about peptic strictures in GERD is:

A. Refractory strictures can pose a significant challenge to surgeons and gastroenterologists and in these patients, LARS should not be considered
B. Steroid injections of the stricture have been shown to result in fewer dilations
C. The majority of peptic strictures are effectively treated with dilation and PPI therapy

D. Refractory peptic strictures are defined as strictures that recur despite dilation and PPI therapy

34. True about Schatzki's ring is:

A. Schatzki rings are pathognomonic for GERD
B. Schatzki rings are mucosal fibrotic bands
C. Schatzki rings develop in the submucosal space, so in the absence of other endoscopically identified mucosal abnormalities, biopsies do not need to be performed
D. Peptic strictures and Schatzki rings can't be differentiated on endoscopy

35. False about GERD and obesity is:

A. Fundoplication in patients with a body mass index (BMI) above 40 should be considered
B. GERD is a common comorbid condition with obesity
C. Severely obese patients with GERD, serious consideration should be given to performing a laparoscopic RYGB instead of a fundoplication
D. 45% of patients undergoing assessment for bariatric surgery have evidence of silent (asymptomatic) reflux

36. False about Barrett's esophagus and GERD is:

A. On endoscopic evaluation, Barrett's esophagus appears as velvety-red "tongues" of mucosa that extend cephalad from the GEJ
B. Because of the variability in regression in Barrett's esophagus following antireflux surgery, it should be considered an indication for antireflux surgery
C. Long-standing acid and alkaline reflux can result in histologic change of the distal esophageal mucosa from its normal squamous epithelium to a columnar configuration
D. Based on endoscopic measurements, it can be classified into long segment ($\geq$3 cm) and short segment (<3 cm)

37. The incidence of adenocarcinoma in patients with Barrett's esophagus is about ___ greater than that in the general population.

A. 20 times B. 30 times
C. 40 times D. 50 times

38. Recommended course of PPI therapy for patients who present with typical symptoms of GERD, is:

A. 6-week B. 8-week
C. 10-week D. 12-week

39. False about the medical management of GERD is:

A. Before empirically prescribing a PPI, it is necessary to ensure that the patient does not have symptoms that may indicate the presence of a gastroesophageal malignant neoplasm or other non-GERD diagnosis
B. Lifestyle modification has been advocated before or as an adjunct to medical therapy, the efficacy of such changes in the treatment of esophagitis has been proved
C. The maximal pharmacologic effect occurs approximately 4 days after initiation of therapy
D. LARS is cost-effective compared with prolonged PPI therapy

40. Before ambulatory pH monitoring, to avoid a false-negative test results, patients must stop PPI therapy for:

A. 1 week B. 2 weeks
C. 4 weeks D. 6 weeks

41. PPI use has been associated with the following except:

A. Interactions with antiplatelet medications
B. Loss of bone density and risk of fracture
C. Liver disease
D. Myocardial infarction

42. False about operative technique for treatment of GERD is:

A. The patient is placed in steep reverse Trendelenburg position
B. A Nathanson liver retractor does not require a trocar and is placed through a small epigastric incision
C. Laparoscopic antireflux operations with the patient in low lithotomy position
D. Preoperative antibiotics are not needed

43. False about operative technique of surgical treatment of GERD is:

A. The most common technical failure in performing a Nissen fundoplication is failure to create appropriate fundoplication anatomy
B. The esophagus is mobilized in the posterior mediastinum to obtain a minimum of 1 cm of intra-abdominal esophagus
C. With use of three or four interrupted permanent sutures, the fundoplication is created to a length of 2.5 to 3 cm

D. To maintain appropriate orientation of the fundus during the creation of the fundoplication, the posterior aspect of the fundus is marked with a suture 3 cm distal to the GEJ and 2 cm off the greater curvature

44. The most common partial fundoplication is:

A. Watson fundoplication
B. Dor fundoplication
C. Toupet fundoplication
D. Nissen fundoplication

45. False about short esophagus management in GERD is:

A. An option for achieving adequate intra-abdominal esophageal length is a stapled wedge gastroplasty
B. At the time of LARS, a minimum of 1 cm of intra-abdominal esophagus should be obtained
C. A unilateral vagotomy can result in an additional 1 to 2 cm of esophageal length
D. Division of both vagus nerves typically yields 3 to 4 cm of additional esophagus

46. Patients after LARS should expect to resume a diet without limitations in about:

A. 1 to 2 weeks   B. 2 to 4 weeks
C. 4 to 6 weeks   D. 6 to 10 weeks

47. Most common complication after laparoscopic antireflux procedures is:

A. Postoperative ileus   B. Pneumothorax
C. Urinary retention   D. Dysphagia

48. False about operative complications is:

A. Most commonly, splenic injury occurs during mobilization of the fundus and greater curvature of the stomach
B. Partial splenic infarction, which can occur during transection of the short gastric vessels and inadvertent coagulation of superior pole branch of the main splenic artery
C. Gastric and esophageal injuries have been reported to occur in approximately 1% of patients undergoing LARS
D. All of the above are true

49. Post operatively it is expected that patients will experience mild, temporary dysphagia during the first ___ postoperatively.

A. 1 to 2 weeks   B. 2 to 4 weeks
C. 4 to 6 weeks   D. 6 to 8 weeks

50. False about failed antireflux surgery is:

A. Anatomic problems after a fundoplication that can cause symptoms include persistent or recurrent hiatal hernia, slipped fundoplication, and incorrectly constructed fundoplication
B. Re operative antireflux surgery comes with higher stakes than first-time antireflux surgery as tissues are less pliable
C. The most common symptoms of failed LARS are typical symptoms of GERD and dysphagia
D. All of the above are true

51. False about GERD in the setting of previous bariatric surgery is:

A. Sleeve gastrectomy (SG) is a safe and effective alternative to RYGB for the control of obesity and its related conditions
B. Operative management strategies for GERD in patients following SG and RYGB are limited due to the lack of gastric fundus for creation of a fundoplication
C. In patients who have undergone bariatric surgery and have GERD that is unresponsive to maximal medical therapy, operative management strategies should not be considered
D. GERD following RYGB can result from an overly large gastric pouch, gastrogastric fistula, and development of hiatal hernia

52. Injection of inert biopolymers for GERD is called:

A. Enteryx   B. Endocinch
C. LINX   D. Esophyx

53. False about Transoral Incisionless Fundoplication is:

A. The procedure is performed under general anesthesia; the device is inserted over a gastroscope
B. TIF is performed with a flexible, multichannel endoluminal device that uses fasteners to construct a full-thickness gastric plication and to create an antireflux valve at the GEJ
C. TIF is associated with significant reduction in acid exposure and improvement in GERD symptoms, normalization of esophageal acid exposure and complete cessation of PPI use have not been demonstrated in these short-term studies
D. The endoluminal fundoplication can be created up to 3 cm in length and 360 degrees

54. False about MSAD is:

A. Postoperative rates of dysphagia appear similar between MSAD and Nissen fundoplication

B. Laparoscopic placement of the MSAD is harder to reproduce than creating a fundoplication

C. Patients with device erosion present most commonly years following device placement with new onset chest pain or dysphagia

D. Device erosion is a feared complication of MSAD implantation

PARAESOPHAGEAL HERNIA

55. False about paraoesophageal hernias is:

A. Gastric volvulus develops because of laxity in the stomach's peritoneal attachments and subsequent rotation of the gastric fundus on the organoaxial or mesenteric axis of the stomach

B. PEH is frequently associated with obstructive symptoms and, less frequently, typical symptoms of GERD

C. Key event that facilitates the formation of a PEH are the widening of the diaphragmatic crura at the esophageal hiatus and stretching of the phrenoesophageal membrane

D. All of the above are true

56. The most common structure to herniate through the esophageal hiatus is the:

A. Small intestine

B. Left lobe of liver

C. Fundus of the stomach

D. Transverse colon

57. False about paraesophageal hernias is:

A. Respiratory symptoms, primarily shortness of breath, can be explained by the mass effect of the hernia contents in the chest

B. The diagnosis of PEH is often made on the basis of symptoms

C. The most common symptoms attributed to PEH are gastroesophageal obstructive symptoms

D. Gastrointestinal bleeding can result from mucosal ischemia or mechanical ulceration of the gastric mucosa

58. False about the preoperative evaluation of paraesophageal hernia is:

A. Endoscopy evaluates the gastric and esophageal mucosa for mechanical gastric mucosal erosions

B. The results of ambulatory pH monitoring rarely change the decision for operative repair of PEH, preoperative documentation of GERD is particularly useful as a baseline for comparison

C. A barium esophagogram rarely provides the operating surgeon the an image of the gastroesophageal anatomy

D. Manometry is necessary to determine the motor function of the esophageal body, which can affect the type of antireflux operation performed at the time of PEH repair

59. True about the operative repair of paraesophageal hernias is:

A. Tension-free closure of the esophageal hiatus is a key step in the repair of PEH

B. After the hernia contents are returned to the peritoneal cavity, the hernia sac must be transected circumferentially at the hiatus

C. The most challenging aspect of the sac dissection is encountered during the mobilization of the posterior sac

D. All of the above

60. Key aspects of operative repair of paraesophageal hernia is:

A. Reduction of the hernia contents to the abdominal cavity

B. Complete excision of the hernia sac from the posterior mediastinum

C. Mobilization of the distal esophagus to achieve a minimum of 3 cm of intra-abdominal esophageal length

D. All of the above

61. False about gastric volvulus is:

A. Gastric volvulus is necessary but and sufficient for gastric ischemia to develop

B. Patients present with sudden onset of chest or epigastric pain associated with retching without the production of emesis

C. Initial management of acute gastric volvulus should include placement of a nasogastric tube for gastric decompression

D. The development of fever, tachycardia, and leukocytosis suggests gastric strangulation and impending perforation

ANSWERS

1. **Ans: B. Gastroesophageal reflux disease**

   Ref: Chapter No.43, Page No.1056

2. **Ans: D. All of the above**

   Ref: Chapter No.43, Page No.1056

3. **Ans: B. Mid-expiration**

   Ref: Chapter No.43, Page No.1056

4. **Ans: B. Circular muscle fibers of the esophagus**

   Ref: Chapter No.43, Page No.1056

5. **Ans: D. Hypertensive LES is frequently associated with hiatal hernia because of displacement of the GEJ into the posterior mediastinum**

   Ref: Chapter No.43, Page No.1057

6. **Ans: A. Type I**

   Ref: Chapter No.43, Page No.1057

7. **Ans: A. Type I**

   Ref: Chapter No.43, Page No.1057

8. **Ans: A. Type I hiatal hernia**

   Ref: Chapter No.43, Page No.1057

9. **Ans: D. All of the above**

   Ref: Chapter No.43, Page No.1057

10. **Ans: C. Type III hiatal hernia**

    Ref: Chapter No.43, Page No.1057

11. **Ans: D. Type IV hiatal hernia**

    Ref: Chapter No.43, Page No.1057

12. **Ans: B. Type II hiatal hernia**

    Ref: Chapter No.43, Page No.1057

13. **Ans: B. Heartburn**

    Ref: Chapter No.43, Page No.1058

14. **Ans: D. Regurgitation of undigested food is common in GERD**

    Ref: Chapter No.43, Page No.1058

15. **Ans: B. Rhinitis**

    Ref: Chapter No.43, Page No.1058

16. **Ans: A. Lack of response of extraoesophageal symptoms to proton pump inhibitor (PPI) therapy can reliably refute GERD as the cause of these symptoms**

    Ref: Chapter No.43, Page No.1058-1059

17. **Ans: D. All of the above**

    Ref: Chapter No.43, Page No.1059

18. **Ans: B. The threshold for testing patients with IPF for GERD should be high**

    Ref: Chapter No.43, Page No.1059

19. **Ans: D. All of the above**

    Ref: Chapter No.43, Page No.1059

20. **Ans: B. Ambulatory pH monitoring**

    Ref: Chapter No.43, Page No.1060

21. **Ans: C. Esophageal manometry**

    Ref: Chapter No.43, Page No.1060

22. **Ans: D. 14.7 or higher**

    Ref: Chapter No.43, Page No.1060

23. **Ans: D. All of the above**

    Ref: Chapter No.43, Page No.1060

24. **Ans: A. 2 minutes of a reflux episode**

    Ref: Chapter No.43, Page No.1060

25. **Ans: B. 1-cm intervals**

    Ref: Chapter No.43, Page No.1060

26. **Ans: B. 5 cm proximal to the LES**

    Ref: Chapter No.43, Page No.1060

27. **Ans: A. Impedance decreases in the presence of air and increases in the presence of a liquid bolus**

    Ref: Chapter No.43, Page No.1060

28. **Ans: B. 1-cm intervals**

    Ref: Chapter No.43, Page No.1060-1061

29. **Ans: C. 10 swallows, 15 mins**

    Ref: Chapter No.43, Page No.1061

30. **Ans: C. Savary-Miller classification**

    Ref: Chapter No.43, Page No.1061

31. **Ans: B. Barium esophagram can confirm the diagnosis of GERD**

    Ref: Chapter No.43, Page No.1061-1062

32. **Ans: D. All of the above**

    Ref: Chapter No.43, Page No.1062

33. **Ans: A. Refractory strictures can pose a significant challenge to surgeons and gastroenterologists and in these patients, LARS should not be considered**

    Ref: Chapter No.43, Page No.1062

34. **Ans: C. Schatzki rings develop in the submucosal space, so in the absence of other endoscopically identified mucosal abnormalities, biopsies do not need to be performed**

    Ref: Chapter No.43, Page No.1063

35. **Ans: A. Fundoplication in patients with a body mass index (BMI) above 40 should be considered**

Ref: Chapter No.43, Page No.1063

36. **Ans: B. Because of the variability in regression in Barrett esophagus following antireflux surgery, it should be considered an indication for antireflux surgery**

Ref: Chapter No.43, Page No.1063-1064

37. **Ans: C. 40 times**

Ref: Chapter No.43, Page No.1063

38. **Ans: B. 8-week**

Ref: Chapter No.43, Page No.1064

39. **Ans: B. Lifestyle modification has been advocated before or as an adjunct to medical therapy, the efficacy of such changes in the treatment of esophagitis has been proved**

Ref: Chapter No.43, Page No.1064

40. **Ans: A. 1 week**

Ref: Chapter No.43, Page No.1064

41. **Ans: C. Liver disease**

Ref: Chapter No.43, Page No.1064

42. **Ans: D. Preoperative antibiotics are not needed**

Ref: Chapter No.43, Page No.1064

43. **Ans: B. The esophagus is mobilized in the posterior mediastinum to obtain a minimum of 1 cm of intra-abdominal esophagus**

Ref: Chapter No.43, Page No.1064-1066

44. **Ans: C. Toupet fundoplication**

Ref: Chapter No.43, Page No.1066

45. **Ans: B. At the time of LARS, a minimum of 1 cm of intra-abdominal esophagus should be obtained**

Ref: Chapter No.43, Page No.1066-1067

46. **Ans: C. 4 to 6 weeks**

Ref: Chapter No.43, Page No.1067

47. **Ans: A. Postoperative ileus**

Ref: Chapter No.43, Page No.1069

48. **Ans: D. All of the above are true**

Ref: Chapter No.43, Page No.1069

49. **Ans: B. 2 to 4 weeks**

Ref: Chapter No.43, Page No.1069

50. **Ans: D. All of the above are true**

Ref: Chapter No.43, Page No.1070

51. **Ans: C. In patients who have undergone bariatric surgery and have GERD that is unresponsive to maximal medical therapy, operative management strategies should not be considered**

Ref: Chapter No.43, Page No.1071

52. **Ans: A. Enteryx**

Ref: Chapter No.43, Page No.1071

53. **Ans: D. The endoluminal fundoplication can be created up to 3 cm in length and 360 degrees**

Ref: Chapter No.43, Page No.1071

54. **Ans: B. Laparoscopic placement of the MSAD is harder to reproduce than creating a fundoplication**

Ref: Chapter No.43, Page No.1072

55. **Ans: D. All of the above are true**

Ref: Chapter No.43, Page No.1073

56. **Ans: C. Fundus of the stomach**

Ref: Chapter No.43, Page No.1073

57. **Ans: B. The diagnosis of PEH is often made on the basis of symptoms**

Ref: Chapter No.43, Page No.1073

58. **Ans: C. A barium esophagogram rarely provides the operating surgeon the an image of the gastroesophageal anatomy**

Ref: Chapter No.43, Page No.1073

59. **Ans: D. All of the above**

Ref: Chapter No.43, Page No.1074

60. **Ans: D. All of the above**

Ref: Chapter No.43, Page No.1074

61. **Ans: A. Gastric volvulus is necessary but and sufficient for gastric ischemia to develop**

Ref: Chapter No.43, Page No.1075

44

Abdominal Wall, Umbilicus, Peritoneum, Mesenteries, Omentum and Retroperitoneum

ABDOMINAL WALL AND UMBILICUS

1. **The abdominal wall begins to develop in the earliest stages of embryonic differentiation from:**
   A. Medial plate of the embryonic mesoderm
   B. Lateral plate of the embryonic mesoderm
   C. Paraxial mesoderm
   D. Intermediate mesoderm

2. **False among the embryology of abdominal wall and umbilicus is:**
   A. By the end of the third month of gestation, the body wall has closed, except at the umbilical ring
   B. After division of the umbilical cord, the umbilical ring heals rapidly by scarring
   C. The splanchnic layer of mesoderm contributes to the development of the abdominal wall
   D. As the embryo enlarges and the abdominal wall components grow toward one another, the ventral open area, bounded by the edge of the amnion, becomes smaller

3. **Superficial subcutaneous layer is called:**
   A. Scarpa fasciae
   B. Camper fasciae
   C. Both of the above
   D. None of the above

4. **Approximation of which fascia aids in the alignment of the skin after surgical incisions in the lower abdomen:**
   A. Scarpa fasciae B. Camper fasciae
   C. Both of the above D. None of the above

5. **The largest and thickest of the flat abdominal wall is:**
   A. Internal oblique muscle
   B. Transversalis fascia
   C. External oblique muscle
   D. Transversus abdominis muscle

6. **False about internal oblique muscle is:**
   A. The uppermost fibers insert into the lower five ribs and their cartilages
   B. Below the semi-circular line, the aponeurosis of the internal oblique muscle courses posteriorly to the rectus abdominis muscle as part of the rectus sheath
   C. Its fibers course in a direction opposite to those of the external oblique
   D. The internal oblique muscle originates from the iliopsoas fascia beneath the lateral half of the inguinal ligament

7. **The smallest of the muscles of the anterolateral abdominal wall is:**
   A. Internal oblique muscle
   B. Transversalis fascia
   C. External oblique muscle
   D. Transversus abdominis muscle

8. **The floor of Hesselbach triangle is the:**
   A. Internal oblique muscle
   B. Transversalis fascia
   C. External oblique muscle
   D. Transversus abdominis muscle

9. **False about rectus abdominis muscle is:**
   A. Each muscle is composed of long parallel fascicles interrupted by three to five tendinous inscriptions
   B. These muscles lie adjacent to each other, separated only by the linea alba
   C. The rectus abdominis muscles are contained within the rectus sheath, which is derived from

the aponeuroses of the three flat abdominal muscles

D. The rectus abdominis muscles are paired muscles that appear as long, flat, triangular ribbons wider at their origin on the anterior surfaces of the 4th costal cartilages

10. Below the semi-circular line, all the fascial layers pass anterior to the rectus abdominis muscle except:

A. Internal oblique muscle
B. Transversalis fascia
C. External oblique muscle
D. Transversus abdominis muscle

11. Coursing through the preperitoneal space are all of the following except:

A. Medial umbilical ligaments
B. Falciform ligament of the liver
C. Superior epigastric artery and vein
D. Median umbilical ligament

12. The anterolateral abdominal wall receives its arterial supply from all except:

A. Superficial circumflex iliac arteries
B. Superior epigastric arteries
C. Last six intercostal and four lumbar arteries
D. Inferior epigastric arteries

13. False about the vascular supply of abdominal wall is:

A. The superior epigastric artery, one of the terminal branches of the internal mammary artery
B. The inferior epigastric artery, derived from the internal iliac artery just proximal to the inguinal ligament
C. The deep circumflex iliac artery, arising from the lateral aspect of the external iliac artery near the origin of the inferior epigastric artery
D. All of the above are true

14. The trunks of the intercostal and lumbar arteries, together with the intercostal, iliohypogastric, and ilioinguinal nerves, course between the:

A. External oblique muscles and internal oblique muscles
B. Scarpa's fascia and external oblique muscles
C. Transversus abdominis and internal oblique muscles
D. Transversus abdominis and transversalis fascia

15. Carcinoma in the liver may spread to involve the anterior abdominal wall at the umbilicus and is called as:

A. Sister Mary Joseph node
B. Virchow's node
C. Callot's node
D. Irish node

16. False about innervation of abdominal wall is:

A. The anterior ramus of the 10th thoracic nerve reaches the skin at the level of the umbilicus, and the 12th thoracic nerve innervates the skin of the hypogastrium
B. The 7th and 8th nerves course slightly upward or horizontally to reach the epigastrium, whereas the lower nerves have an increasingly caudal trajectory
C. Thoracic nerves 7 to 12 pass behind the costal cartilages and lower ribs to enter a plane between the internal oblique muscle and the transversus abdominis
D. The ilioinguinal nerve runs parallel to the 12th thoracic nerve to pierce the transversus abdominis muscle near the iliac crest

17. Infants who are born with an omphalocele will have concomitant congenital anomalies of all except:

A. Branchial arches
B. Gastrointestinal (GI) tract
C. Cardiopulmonary system
D. Genitourinary (GU) system

18. False about omphalocele is:

A. Omphalocele is a funnel-shaped defect in the central abdomen through which the viscera protrude into the base of the umbilical cord
B. Of infants who are born with an omphalocele, 10% will have concomitant congenital anomalies
C. It is caused by failure of the abdominal wall musculature to unite in the midline during fetal development
D. The umbilical vessels may be splayed over the viscera or pushed to one side

19. The defect of gastrochisis is almost always to the:

A. Left of the umbilical cord
B. Right of the umbilical cord
C. Superior to the umbilical cord
D. Inferior to the umbilical cord

20. False about gastroschisis is:

A. Concomitant congenital anomalies occur in about 10% of these patients
B. The intestine is covered with skin or amnion
C. Gastroschisis is a congenital defect of the abdominal wall in which the umbilical membrane has ruptured in utero allowing the intestine to herniate outside the abdominal cavity
D. Typically, the intestine has not undergone complete mesenteric rotation and fixation

21. Most of infantile umbilical hernias resolve within the first:

A. 6 months of life B. 12 months of life
C. 24 months of life D. 48 months of life

22. False about Meckel diverticulum is:

A. False diverticula arise from the antimesenteric border of the small intestine
B. GI bleeding is caused by peptic ulceration of adjacent intestinal mucosa from hydrochloric acid secreted by ectopic parietal cells located within the diverticulum
C. Persistence of the intestinal end of the omphalomesenteric duct
D. Meckel diverticula may be complicated by inflammation, perforation, hemorrhage, or obstruction

23. These true diverticula arise from the antimesenteric border of the small intestine, most often the:

A. Jejunum
B. Ileum
C. Duodenum
D. Equal incidence in all

24. Following image represents:

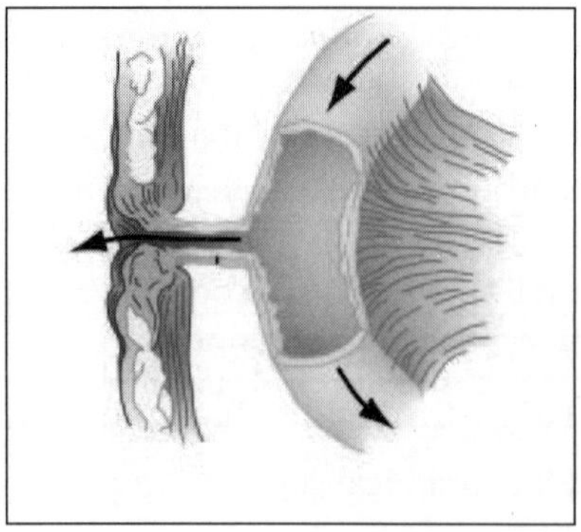

A. Omphalomesenteric duct cyst
B. Persistent omphalomesenteric duct with an enterocutaneous fistula
C. Omphalomesenteric duct cyst and sinus
D. Meckel diverticulum

25. Following image represents:

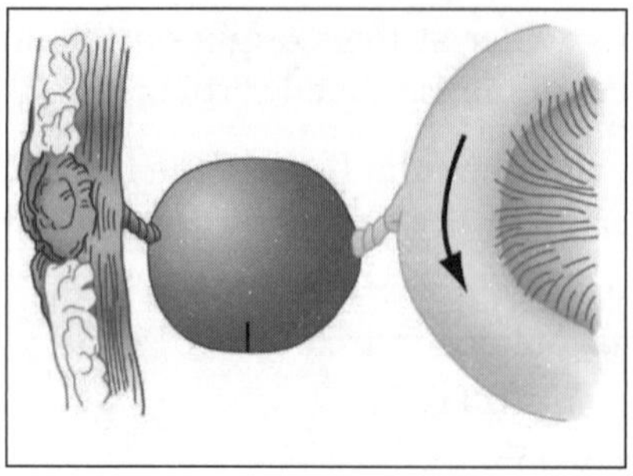

A. Omphalomesenteric duct cyst
B. Persistent omphalomesenteric duct with an enterocutaneous fistula
C. Omphalomesenteric duct cyst and sinus
D. Meckel diverticulum

26. Following image represents:

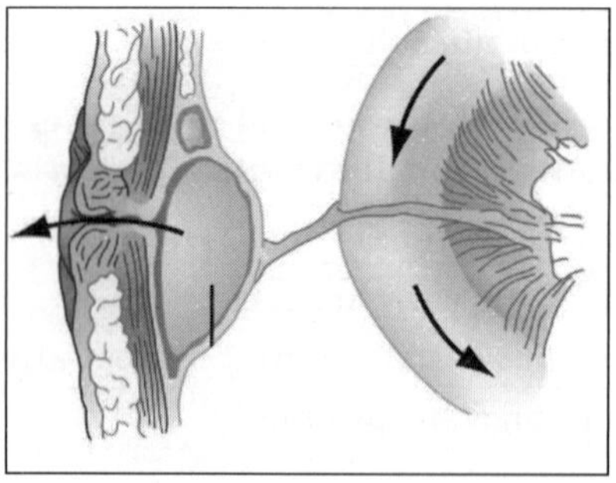

A. Omphalomesenteric duct cyst
B. Persistent omphalomesenteric duct with an enterocutaneous fistula
C. Omphalomesenteric duct cyst and sinus
D. Meckel diverticulum

27. False about persistence of the allantois is:

A. The allantois is the caudal-most component of the embryologic ventral cloaca
B. The intra-abdominal portion is termed the urachus and connects the urinary bladder with the umbilicus, whereas the extraabdominal allantois is contained within the umbilical cord
C. Because of the risk of complications, including transformation into malignancy, treatment is excision of the urachal remnant with closure of the bladder if necessary
D. All of the above are true

28. False about Diastasis recti is:

A. There is no risk for intestinal strangulation
B. The transversalis fascia has a defect

C. Appropriate treatment consists of reassurance of the patient
D. Diastasis recti refers to a thinning of the linea alba in the epigastrium and is manifested as a smooth midline protrusion of the anterior abdominal wall

29. False about anterior abdominal wall hernias is:

A. Treatment consists of operative closure of the fascial defect
B. Epigastric hernias occur at sites through which vessels and nerves perforate the linea alba to course into the subcutaneum
C. Ultrasonography of the abdominal wall or computed tomography (CT) with thin cuts through the abdomen should be diagnostic
D. All of the above are true

30. False about rectus sheath hematoma is:

A. The pain and tenderness associated with this process may be severe enough to suggest peritonitis
B. It is more common in men than in women and in younger than in older individuals
C. Physical examination demonstrates tenderness over the rectus sheath often with voluntary guarding
D. Patients with rectus sheath hematomas usually present with the sudden onset of abdominal pain, which may be severe and is often exacerbated by movements requiring contraction of the abdominal wall musculature

31. Periumbilical ecchymosis is called:

A. Cullen sign
B. Bryant sign
C. Fox's sign
D. Grey Turner sign

32. Blue discoloration in the flanks is called:

A. Fox's sign
B. Cullen sign
C. Grey Turner sign
D. Bryant sign

33. False about the management of rectus sheath hematoma is:

A. Ultrasonography or CT will confirm the presence of the hematoma and localize it to the abdominal wall
B. Progression of the hematoma may necessitate angiographic embolization of the bleeding vessel or uncommonly operative evacuation of the hematoma and hemostasis
C. Almost 50% of patients were managed successfully with rest and analgesics and, if necessary, blood transfusion
D. Patients may be managed successfully with rest and analgesics and, if necessary, blood transfusion

34. The most common primary neoplasms of the abdominal wall are:

A. Squamous cell carcinoma
B. Melanoma
C. Desmoid tumors
D. Basal cell carcinoma

35. False about desmoid tumors is:

A. These tumors occur in young or middle-age adults and are uncommon in children or elderly patients
B. Uncommon mesenchymal neoplasms that are locally aggressive and have high metastatic potential
C. 10% to 15% of cases occur in patients with familial adenomatous polyposis and males are affected as commonly as females in these instances
D. In sporadic cases, there is a female predominance of two to one

36. Gardner syndrome has all except:

A. Osteomas of the skull and mandible
B. Dermoid cysts
C. Desmoid tumor
D. Subcutaneous fibromas

37. Sporadic desmoid tumors are most commonly associated with:

A. Accumulation of β-catenin
B. Somatic mutations of the CTNNB1 gene
C. An abnormal stabilization of β-catenin
D. Activation of the Wnt signaling pathway

38. Desmoid tumors present as all except:

A. Painful
B. Firm
C. Non tender mass
D. All of the above

39. Percentage of patients with FAP who will develop a desmoid tumor is:

A. 5% to 10%
B. 10% to 15%
C. 20% to 30%
D. 30% to 50%

40. Investigation preferred imaging modality for diagnosis of desmoid is:

A. MRI
B. CT Scan
C. PET CT Scan
D. USG

41. Spontaneous regression of desmoid tumor occurs in ___ of cases.

A. 5% B. 10%
C. 30% D. 50%

42. Systemic treatment options for patients with desmoid tumors includes all except:

A. High-dose methotrexate
B. Tamoxifen
C. NSAIDs
D. Sorafenib

43. Patients of abdominal wall sarcoma present most commonly with all except:

A. Painless
B. Poorly circumscribed
C. Firm
D. Well circumscribed

44. False about abdominal wall sarcoma is:

A. Open biopsy of the tumor should be avoided because of the risk of compromising the curative resection by inappropriate orientation of the incision
B. Depth, size, positive margin status and high tumor grade are associated with increased risk of recurrence
C. Most surgeons attempt to obtain at least a 5-cm margin of normal tissue around the tumor
D. The diagnosis is best established by core needle biopsy

45. Malignancies most commonly associated with hematogenous metastasis to the abdominal wall includes all except:

A. Colon carcinoma
B. Pancreatic carcinoma
C. Renal carcinoma
D. Lung carcinoma

46. Stimulation of nociceptors in right colon causes the sensation of pain in:

A. Right iliac fossa B. Epigastric region
C. Peri umbilical region D. Hypogastrium

PERITONEUM AND PERITONEAL CAVITY

47. The surface area of peritoneum is:

A. 1.0 to 1.7 m^2 B. 1.7 to 2.0 m^2
C. 2.0 to 2.7 m^2 D. 2.7 to 3.7 m^2

48. Normally, the peritoneal cavity contains ___ of sterile serous fluid.

A. <50 mL B. <100 mL
C. >150 mL D. >100 mL

49. Perihepatitis of Fitz-Hugh Curtis syndrome is in patients with:

A. Acute hepatitis B. Acute appendicitis
C. Acute salpingitis D. Acute cervicitis

50. Most common complication of cirrhosis is:

A. Ascitis B. Hematemesis
C. Melena D. Malnutrition

51. False about ascitic fluid analysis is:

A. Paracentesis with ascitic fluid analysis is the most rapid and cost-effective method of determining the cause of ascites
B. It is usually performed in the lower abdomen with the right lower quadrant preferred
C. Ultrasound guidance may be useful in obese patients and in those with a history of laparotomy
D. Important indication for early paracentesis in a patient with ascites is the occurrence of signs and symptoms of infection

52. False about ascites is:

A. Renal sodium retention is driven by activation of the renin-angiotensin-aldosterone and sympathetic nervous systems, which cause proximal and distal renal tubule sodium reabsorption
B. The onset of ascites is an important prognostic factor in patients with cirrhosis
C. Increased hydrostatic pressure within the hepatic sinusoids and splanchnic vasculature drives the extravasation of fluid from the microvasculature into the extracellular compartment
D. Ascites is the most common complication of cirrhosis, with approximately 90% of compensated cirrhotic patients developing ascites within 20 years of diagnosis

53. Amount of fluid required to be present before dullness can be detected by percussion is:

A. 0.5 L of fluid B. 1.0 L of fluid
C. 1.5 L of fluid D. 2.0 L of fluid

54. False about ascitic fluid is:

A. The presence of more than 5000 leukocytes/ mm^3 will cause the fluid to be cloudy
B. Nontraumatic blood-tinged ascitic fluid clots
C. Normal ascitic fluid is slightly yellow and transparent

D. Ascitic fluid with fewer than 1000 cells/mm^3 is almost clear

55. Ascitic fluid from patients with uncomplicated cirrhosis will have a total leukocyte count:

A. > 250 cell/mm^3
B. < 250 cell/mm^3
C. < 50 cell/mm^3
D. > 50 cell/mm^3

56. False about SAAG is:

A. If the SAAG is <1.1 g/dL the patient has portal hypertension
B. The accuracy of this measurement in predicting the presence or absence of portal hypertension is approximately 97%
C. The SAAG is calculated by measuring the albumin concentration of serum and ascitic fluid specimens and subtracting the ascitic fluid value from the serum value
D. The serum-ascites albumin gradient (SAAG) is the most reliable method to differentiate causes of ascites due to portal hypertension from those due to other causes

57. A reasonable dietary sodium restriction for most cirrhotic patients with ascites is:

A. 0.5 g per day
B. 1 g per day
C. 2 g per day
D. 5 g per day

58. Dosing ratio of Spironolactone and furosemide, that will promote natriuresis while maintaining normokalemia is:

A. 100:50
B. 100:40
C. 80:40
D. 80:50

59. In large-volume paracentesis, ascites fluid removed from the peritoneal cavity is:

A. 2 L
B. 3 L
C. 5 L
D. 8 L

60. Which among the following doesn't have SAAG ≥1.1g/dL?

A. Cirrhosis
B. Alcoholic hepatitis
C. Cardiac failure
D. Nephrotic syndrome

61. Which among the following doesn't have SAAG <1.1g/dL?

A. Myxedema
B. Tuberculous peritonitis
C. Peritoneal carcinomatosis
D. Biliary ascites

62. The most common cause of chylous ascites in adults is an obstructing:

A. Congenital lymphatic abnormalities
B. Iatrogenic
C. Intra-abdominal malignancy
D. Blunt or penetrating trauma

63. The most common malignant neoplasm associated with chylous ascites is:

A. Gastric malignant neoplasms
B. Lymphoma
C. Ovarian malignant neoplasms
D. Pancreatic malignant neoplasms

64. False about chylous ascites is:

A. Paracentesis yields a characteristic milky fluid with a high protein and fat content
B. Patients with chylous ascites most often present with painless abdominal distention
C. The SAAG will be >1.1 mg/dL
D. Malnutrition and dyspnea occur in approximately 50% of cases

65. False about spontaneous bacterial peritonitis is:

A. SBP is defined as a bacterial infection of ascitic fluid in the presence of an intra-abdominal source of infection
B. Third-generation cephalosporin, are started immediately in patients suspected of having ascitic fluid infection
C. Bacterial translocation from the GI tract is thought to be an important step in the pathogenesis of SBP
D. It is extremely rare for patients with ascitic fluid containing a high protein concentration to develop SBP, such as patients with peritoneal carcinomatosis

66. The most common pathogens in adults with SBP are the aerobic enteric flora like:

A. Staphylococcus aureus
B. Pseudomonas
C. Streptococcus pneumoniae
D. Escherichia coli

67. In a clinical setting consistent with SBP diagnosis, the diagnosis of SBP is made initially by demonstrating ___ of ascitic fluid.

A. > 150 neutrophils/mm^3
B. > 250 neutrophils/mm^3

C. > 500 neutrophils/mm^3
D. > 1000 neutrophils/mm^3

68. False about tuberculous peritonitis is:

A. Abdominal pain caused by ascites formation is the most common symptom, occurring in more than 50% of cases
B. Its clinical presentation mimics inflammatory conditions such as Crohn's disease and malignant diseases, so obtaining a diagnosis can be problematic at times
C. Constitutional symptoms such as low-grade fever and night sweats, weight loss, anorexia and malaise are reported in approximately 60% of patients
D. Peritoneal tuberculosis is the sixth most common site of extrapulmonary tuberculosis, after lymphatic, GU, bone and joint, miliary and meningeal

69. In patients with peritoneal tuberculosis abdominal tenderness is present in approximately ___ of patients.

A. 30% B. 50%
C. 70% D. 80%

70. No of patients with tuberculous peritonitis will have an abnormal chest radiograph is:

A. 30% B. 50%
C. 70% D. 80%

71. False about tuberculous peritonitis is:

A. Ultrasound may demonstrate the ascitic fluid containing echogenic material, seen as fine mobile strands or particulate matter
B. The ascitic fluid SAAG is >1.1 g/dL, consistent with a high protein concentration in the ascitic fluid
C. The gross appearance of the peritoneal cavity is similar to that of peritoneal carcinomatosis
D. CT will document a thickened and nodular mesentery with mesenteric lymphadenopathy and omental thickening

72. The gross appearance of the peritoneal cavity is similar to that of:

A. Appendicitis
B. Sarcoidosis
C. Peritoneal carcinomatosis
D. Crohn's disease

73. False about peritonitis associated with chronic ambulatory peritoneal dialysis is:

A. 25% of infections are cured by culture directed antibiotic therapy
B. Refractory or recurrent peritonitis was the most common cause of technical failure
C. Peritonitis is one of the most common complications of CAPD, occurring with an incidence of approximately one episode every 1 to 3 years
D. Patients present with abdominal pain, fever, and cloudy peritoneal dialysate containing more than 100 leukocytes/mm more than 50% of the cells being neutrophils

74. False about Pseudomyxoma peritonei is:

A. The histology of appendiceal tumors is an important predictor of survival
B. Pseudomyxoma peritonei is a rare disease characterized by mucinous ascites
C. Peritoneal mucinous carcinomatosis has the best survival rate
D. The grading of these tumors is based upon the presence or absence of infiltrative invasion, high cytologic grade, high tumor cellularity, angiolymphatic invasion, perineural invasion and signet ring cells

75. Pseudomyxoma peritonei most often arises from a perforated mucinous tumor of the:

A. Appendix B. Ovary
C. Caecum D. Sigmoid

76. False about Pseudomyxoma peritonei is:

A. Patients are often asymptomatic until late in the course of their disease
B. Pseudomyxoma peritonei occurs most commonly in individuals 20 to 30 years of age
C. Similar frequency in men and women
D. Physical examination may reveal a new hernia, ascites, abdominal distention with nonshifting dullness, and on occasion a palpable abdominal mass

77. False about management of pseudomyxoma peritonei is:

A. Preoperative colonoscopy will differentiate a mucinous neoplasm of the appendix from that arising from the colon
B. The current treatment of patients with pseudomyxoma peritonei involves resection of as much of the tumor as possible (cytoreduction) and hyperthermic intraperitoneal chemotherapy (HIPEC)

C. Patients with low-grade tumors who undergo complete cytoreduction with HIPEC have 5-year survival rates of 20% to 30%
D. The goal is to leave no visible disease or, if this is not feasible, to leave no nodules larger than 2 mm in diameter

78. The most commonly used drugs for intraperitoneal chemotherapy are:

A. Methotrexate
B. Mitotane
C. Mitomycin C
D. Adriamycin

79. Most common complication of Cytoreduction and HIPEC is:

A. Pulmonary complications
B. Intra-abdominal infections
C. Hemorrhage
D. Enterocutaneous fistula

80. False about carcinomatosis from colorectal cancer is:

A. The use intraperitoneal chemotherapy did not have an additional benefit over cytoreduction alone
B. Untreated, metastatic disease is uniformly fatal
C. Cytoreductive surgery with HIPEC has been performed in all patients
D. About 8% of patients with colorectal cancer develop peritoneal metastases

81. False about peritoneal mesothelioma is:

A. Encasement of the small bowel may create a bowel obstruction and eventually death
B. The most common primary malignant neoplasm of the peritoneum is mesothelioma
C. It has male predominance
D. Peritoneal mesothelioma tends to involve all peritoneal surfaces, producing hard, white masses and plaques of tumor

82. False about peritoneal mesothelioma is:

A. Paracentesis has a high diagnostic yield
B. Peritoneal mesothelioma has a variable rate of progression and tends to remain confined to the abdominal cavity until very late in the course of the disease
C. Ascites is common and is often intractable
D. Most patients with peritoneal mesothelioma present with abdominal pain and weight loss

83. Factors associated with improved outcomes in peritoneal mesothelioma include all except:

A. High histologic tumor grade
B. Complete or near complete cytoreduction
C. Epithelioid histology
D. Use of cisplatin for HIPEC

MESENTERY AND OMENTUM

84. Between the layers of the lesser omentum, and at its right border is:

A. Hepatic artery
B. Hepatic vein
C. Common hepatic duct
D. Portal vein

85. The posterior line of attachment of the mesentery extends obliquely from the duodenojejunal junction at the:

A. Left side of the 4th lumbar vertebra toward the right iliac fossa to terminate anterior to the sacroiliac articulation
B. Left side of the 3rd lumbar vertebra toward the right iliac fossa to terminate anterior to the sacroiliac articulation
C. Left side of the 2nd lumbar vertebra toward the right iliac fossa to terminate anterior to the sacroiliac articulation
D. Left side of the 1st lumbar vertebra toward the right iliac fossa to terminate anterior to the sacroiliac articulation

86. False about omental cyst is:

A. Omental cysts contains cloudy fluid
B. Omental cysts are unilocular or multilocular cysts
C. These lesions are most common in children and young adults
D. They are lined by a lymphatic endothelium similar to that of cystic lymphangiomas

87. Complications of omental cysts are more common in children and include:

A. Infection
B. Torsion
C. Rupture
D. All of the above

88. All of the following are true about omental cysts except:

A. Diagnosis is made by excision of the cyst and histologic examination of the wall
B. Ultrasound or CT will show a fluid-filled, complex cystic mass with internal septations
C. Local excision, either laparoscopically or open, is curative
D. Uncomplicated cysts usually lie in the lower mid-abdomen and are freely movable, smooth and tender

89. False about Omental Torsion and Infarction is:

A. Secondary when the torsion occurs in association with a causative condition such as a hernia, tumor, or adhesion

B. Primary omental torsion usually involves the left side of the omentum

C. Omental torsion occurs twice as often in men as in women

D. Omental torsion is classified as primary when no coexisting causative condition is identified

90. False regarding management of Omental Torsion and Infarction is:

A. CT often demonstrates an omental mass without signs of inflammation

B. Palpation of the abdomen demonstrates localized abdominal tenderness with guarding suggesting peritonitis

C. Treatment consists of resection of the involved omentum and correction of any related condition

D. Patients often present with the acute onset of severe abdominal pain localized to the right side of the abdomen

91. The most common non-neoplastic mesenteric cysts are:

A. Urachal cyst

B. Endothelial cyst

C. Chylolymphatic cyst

D. Mesothelial cysts

92. False about Mesenteric Cysts is:

A. Enucleation of the cyst at laparotomy is curative

B. The cysts contain chyle or a clear serous fluid and occur in the mesentery of the small intestine (60%) or colon (40%)

C. Internal drainage of the cyst into the peritoneal cavity has also been successfully used in the treatment of very large cysts

D. These cysts usually occur in adults, with a mean age of 45 years, and are twice as common in men as in women

93. False about acute mesenteric lymphadenitis is:

A. Syndrome occurs most commonly in children and young adults with increased frequency in males

B. Physical examination demonstrates right lower quadrant tenderness with abdominal wall muscle rigidity and rebound tenderness

C. It is recommended that abdominal ultrasound be obtained for definitive diagnosis

D. Yersinia enterocolitica in particular has been associated with this syndrome in children

94. False about sclerosing mesenteritis is:

A. Sclerosing mesenteritis is twice as common in men as in women and usually occurs in the fifth decade of life

B. An abdominal mass is palpable in more than 80% of patients

C. Characterized histologically by sclerosing fibrosis, fat necrosis with lipid-laden macrophages, chronic inflammation with germinal centers and focal calcification

D. This condition is characterized grossly by marked thickening of the mesentery of the small intestine with irregular areas of discoloration suggesting fat necrosis

95. False about sclerosing mesenteritis is:

A. Laparotomy or laparoscopy with biopsy of the involved mesentery remains necessary for definitive diagnosis

B. Operative management is always indicated

C. Most patients are asymptomatic, and the diagnosis is discovered incidentally on imaging for an unrelated condition

D. Laboratory studies are usually normal except that the erythrocyte sedimentation rate and C.-reactive protein levels may be elevated

96. CT characteristics of sclerosing mesenteritis are all except:

A. A fatty mass arising from the base of the mesentery that has well-delineated margins separating it from normal mesentery, a feature described as a tumoral pseudocapsule

B. The presence of normal mesenteric vessels coursing through the fatty mass, without evidence of vascular involvement or deviation

C. The presence of inflamed adipose tissue surrounding mesenteric vessels

D. An intra-abdominal mass that displaces adjacent bowel loops without invading them

97. False about mesocolic hernia is:

A. Left mesocolic hernias are thought to be caused by in utero herniation of the small intestine between the inferior mesenteric vein and posterior parietal attachments of the descending mesocolon to the retroperitoneum

B. Approximately 75% of mesocolic hernias occur on the right side

C. The inferior mesenteric artery and vein are integral components of the hernia sac
D. A right mesocolic hernia occurs when the prearterial limb of the midgut loop fails to rotate around the superior mesenteric artery

98. Which vessel courses along the medial border of the neck of the right sided mesocolic hernia?

A. Inferior mesenteric artery
B. Superior mesenteric vein
C. Superior mesenteric artery
D. Inferior mesenteric vein

99. The most common location for mesenteric hernias is:

A. Near the transverse colon
B. Near the ileocolic junction
C. Near the duodenojejunal junction
D. Near the rectosigmoid junction

100. False about acquired internal hernias is:

A. Hernia rates after laparoscopic Roux-en-Y gastric bypass (i.e., Peterson hernia) are reported as high
B. Herniation after laparoscopic colectomy is very common
C. These usually result from inadequate closure (or dehiscence) of mesenteric defects created during the performance of gastrojejunostomy, colostomy, ileostomy, or bowel resection
D. Treatment of these patients is operative reduction of the hernia and closure of the peritoneal defect

101. The most common neoplasm affecting the mesentery is:

A. Sarcomas
B. Desmoid tumor
C. Metastatic disease
D. Hemangioma

102. The most common primary malignant tumor of the mesentery is:

A. Sarcomas
B. Desmoid tumor
C. Metastatic disease
D. Hemangioma

103. Overall the 10-year survival rate for patients with intra-abdominal desmoid tumors is:

A. 10% to 20%
B. 20% to 30%
C. 30% to 50%
D. 60% to 70%

RETROPERITONEUM

104. Most common cause of retroperitoneal abscesses is:

A. Mycobacterium tuberculosis
B. E. coli
C. Bacteroides
D. Proteus mirabilis

105. The most common symptoms of retroperitoneal abscesses is:

A. Flank pain
B. Fever and chills
C. Malaise
D. Weight loss

106. False about retroperitoneal abscess is:

A. CT will demonstrate a high-density mass in the retroperitoneum with surrounding inflammation and gas is present in as many as one third of these lesions
B. The mortality rate for patients with retroperitoneal abscesses is related in large part to the presence of significant medical comorbidities
C. Treatment of retroperitoneal abscesses includes appropriate antibiotics and adequate drainage
D. Operative drainage through a retroperitoneal approach is indicated for lesions not amenable to percutaneous drainage or those that fail percutaneous drainage

107. False about retroperitoneal hematoma is:

A. Patients who develop retroperitoneal hematomas as a result of anticoagulation are best managed by the restoration of circulating blood volume and correction of the underlying coagulopathy
B. CT establishes the diagnosis by demonstrating a high-density mass in the retroperitoneum
C. Patients present with abdominal or flank pain that may radiate into the groin, labia, or scrotum
D. As many as 50% to 60% of patients will develop signs of a femoral neuropathy

108. False about retroperitoneal fibrosis is:

A. The fibrosis is usually confined to the central and paravertebral spaces between the renal arteries and sacrum
B. 70% of cases are idiopathic
C. The process usually begins at the level of the aortic bifurcation and spreads cephalad
D. The mean age at presentation is 20 to 30 years

109. HLA-DRB1*03 is linked with all except:

A. Myasthenia gravis
B. Retroperitoneal fibrosis
C. Type 2 diabetes mellitus
D. Systemic lupus erythematosus

110. False about retroperitoneal fibrosis is:

A. Scrotal swelling is common as is the occurrence of a varicocele or hydrocele
B. Laboratory tests may demonstrate azotemia, and 80% to 100% of patients will have elevated concentrations of acute-phase reactants
C. The mainstay of treatment has been the administration of corticosteroids
D. Ureteral involvement is present in 50% to 60% of cases

111. False about retroperitoneal fibrosis is:

A. Operative management is generally performed to relieve ureteral obstruction by open ureterolysis with intraperitoneal transposition and omental wrapping of the ureters
B. MRI of early benign retroperitoneal fibrosis may show areas of high signal intensity on T2-weighted images
C. In the mature and quiescent stages of benign retroperitoneal fibrosis, there is a low signal intensity on T1- and T2-weighted images
D. Evaluation of patients thought to have retroperitoneal fibrosis often starts with a MRI

112. When retroperitoneal fibrosis is associated with an abdominal aortic aneurysm, repair of the aneurysm is warranted when the aortic diameter exceeds:

A. 3.5 to 4 cm
B. 4.5 to 5 cm
C. 4.0 to 4.5 cm
D. 5 to 5.5 cm

113. The most common primary malignant neoplasm of the retroperitoneum is:

A. Sarcomas
B. Desmoid tumor
C. Renal cancer
D. Haemangioendothelioma

114. False about retroperitoneal sarcomas is:

A. The most common histologic subtypes are liposarcoma and leiomyosarcoma
B. Treatment of choice is R0 resection with lymphadenectomy
C. Retroperitoneal sarcomas generally present as a large, well-circumscribed mass that displaces rather than invades intraabdominal organs
D. CT or MRI will provide important information about the size and precise location of the tumor and its relationship to major vascular structures

115. Abdominal pain is present in retroperitoneal sarcomas in about ___ of the patients.

A. 10%
B. 50%
C. 70%
D. 30%

ANSWERS

1. **Ans: B. Lateral plate of the embryonic mesoderm**

Ref: Chapter No.44, Page No.1080

2. **Ans: C. The splanchnic layer of mesoderm contributes to the development of the abdominal wall**

Ref: Chapter No.44, Page No.1080

3. **Ans: B. Camper fasciae**

Ref: Chapter No.44, Page No.1080

4. **Ans: A. Scarpa fasciae**

Ref: Chapter No.44, Page No.1080

5. **Ans: C. External oblique muscle**

Ref: Chapter No.44, Page No.1080

6. **Ans: B. Below the semi-circular line, the aponeurosis of the internal oblique muscle courses posteriorly to the rectus abdominis muscle as part of the rectus sheath**

Ref: Chapter No.44, Page No.1081

7. **Ans: D. Transversus abdominis muscle**

Ref: Chapter No.44, Page No.1082

8. **Ans: B. Transversalis fascia**

Ref: Chapter No.44, Page No.1082

9. **Ans: D. The rectus abdominis muscles are paired muscles that appear as long, flat, triangular ribbons wider at their origin on the anterior surfaces of the 4th costal cartilages**

Ref: Chapter No.44, Page No.1082

10. **Ans: B. Transversalis fascia**

Ref: Chapter No.44, Page No.1082

11. **Ans: C. Superior epigastric artery and vein**

Ref: Chapter No.44, Page No.1082

12. **Ans: A. Superficial circumflex iliac arteries**

Ref: Chapter No.44, Page No.1082

13. **Ans: B. The inferior epigastric artery, derived from the internal iliac artery just proximal to the inguinal ligament**

Ref: Chapter No.44, Page No.1082

14. **Ans: C. Transversus abdominis and internal oblique muscles**

Ref: Chapter No.44, Page No.1082

15. **Ans: A. Sister Mary Joseph node**

Ref: Chapter No.44, Page No.1083

16. **Ans: D. The ilioinguinal nerve runs parallel to the 12th thoracic nerve to pierce the transversus abdominis muscle near the iliac crest**

Ref: Chapter No.44, Page No.1083

17. **Ans: A. Branchial arches**

Ref: Chapter No.44, Page No.1083

18. **Ans: B. Of infants who are born with an omphalocele, 10% will have concomitant congenital anomalies**

Ref: Chapter No.44, Page No.1083

19. **Ans: B. Right of the umbilical cord**

Ref: Chapter No.44, Page No.1083

20. **Ans: B. The intestine is covered with skin or amnion**

Ref: Chapter No.44, Page No.1083

21. **Ans: C. 24 months of life**

Ref: Chapter No.44, Page No.1085

22. **Ans: A. False diverticula arise from the antimesenteric border of the small intestine**

Ref: Chapter No.44, Page No.1085

23. **Ans: B. Ileum**

Ref: Chapter No.44, Page No.1085

24. **Ans: B. Persistent omphalomesenteric duct with an enterocutaneous fistula**

Ref: Chapter No.44, Page No.1085

25. **Ans: A. Omphalomesenteric duct cyst**

Ref: Chapter No.44, Page No.1085.

26. **Ans: C. Omphalomesenteric duct cyst and sinus**

Ref: Chapter No.44, Page No.1085

27. **Ans: A. The allantois is the caudal-most component of the embryologic ventral cloaca**

Ref: Chapter No.44, Page No.1086

28. **Ans: B. The transversalis fascia has a defect**

Ref: Chapter No.44, Page No.1086

29. **Ans: D. All of the above are true**

Ref: Chapter No.44, Page No.1086

30. **Ans: B. It is more common in men than in women and in younger than in older individuals**

Ref: Chapter No.44, Page No.1086

31. **Ans: A. Cullen sign**

Ref: Chapter No.44, Page No.1086

32. **Ans: C. Grey Turner sign**

Ref: Chapter No.44, Page No.1086

33. **Ans: C. Almost 50% of patients were managed successfully with rest and analgesics and, if necessary, blood transfusion**

Ref: Chapter No.44, Page No.1086

34. **Ans: C. Desmoid tumors**

Ref: Chapter No.44, Page No.1086

35. **Ans: B. Uncommon mesenchymal neoplasms that are locally aggressive and have high metastatic potential**

Ref: Chapter No.44, Page No.1086-1087

36. **Ans: B. Dermoid cysts**

Ref: Chapter No.44, Page No.1086

37. **Ans: B. Somatic mutations of the CTNNB1 gene**

Ref: Chapter No.44, Page No.1087

38. **Ans: A. Painful**

Ref: Chapter No.44, Page No.1087

39. **Ans: B. 10% to 15%**

Ref: Chapter No.44, Page No.1087

40. **Ans: A. MRI**

Ref: Chapter No.44, Page No.1087

41. **Ans: C. 30%**

Ref: Chapter No.44, Page No.1087

42. **Ans: A. High-dose methotrexate**

Ref: Chapter No.44, Page No.1087

43. **Ans: D. Well circumscribed**

Ref: Chapter No.44, Page No.1088

44. **Ans: C. Most surgeons attempt to obtain at least a 5-cm margin of normal tissue around the tumor**

Ref: Chapter No.44, Page No.1088

45. **Ans: B. Pancreatic carcinoma**

Ref: Chapter No.44, Page No.1088

46. **Ans: C. Peri umbilical region**

Ref: Chapter No.44, Page No.1088

47. **Ans: A. 1.0 to 1.7 m^2**

Ref: Chapter No.44, Page No.1089

48. **Ans: B. <100 mL**

Ref: Chapter No.44, Page No.1089

49. **Ans: C. Acute salpingitis**

Ref: Chapter No.44, Page No.1089

50. **Ans: A. Ascitis**

Ref: Chapter No.44, Page No.1090

51. **Ans: B. It is usually performed in the lower abdomen with the right lower quadrant preferred**

Ref: Chapter No.44, Page No.1091

52. **Ans: D. Ascites is the most common complication of cirrhosis, with approximately 90% of compensated cirrhotic patients developing ascites within 20 years of diagnosis**

Ref: Chapter No.44, Page No.1090

53. **Ans: C. 1.5 L of fluid**

Ref: Chapter No.44, Page No.1090

54. **Ans: B. Nontraumatic blood-tinged ascitic fluid clots**

Ref: Chapter No.44, Page No.1091

55. **Ans: B. < 250 cell/mm^3**

Ref: Chapter No.44, Page No.1091

56. **Ans: A. If the SAAG is <1.1 g/dL the patient has portal hypertension**

Ref: Chapter No.44, Page No.1091

57. **Ans: C. 2 g per day**

Ref: Chapter No.44, Page No.1091

58. **Ans: B. 100:40**

Ref: Chapter No.44, Page No.1091

59. **Ans: C. 5 L**

Ref: Chapter No.44, Page No.1091

60. **Ans: D. Nephrotic syndrome**

Ref: Chapter No.44, Page No.1091

61. **Ans: A. Myxedema**

Ref: Chapter No.44, Page No.1091

62. **Ans: C. Intra-abdominal malignancy**

Ref: Chapter No.44, Page No.1091

63. **Ans: B. Lymphoma**

Ref: Chapter No.44, Page No.1091

64. **Ans: C. The SAAG will be >1.1 mg/dL**

Ref: Chapter No.44, Page No.1092

65. **Ans: A. SBP is defined as a bacterial infection of ascitic fluid in the presence of an intraabdominal source of infection**

Ref: Chapter No.44, Page No.1092

66. **Ans: D. Escherichia coli**

Ref: Chapter No.44, Page No.1092

67. **Ans: B. > 250 neutrophils/mm^3**

Ref: Chapter No.44, Page No.1092

68. **Ans: A. Abdominal pain caused by ascites formation is the most common symptom, occurring in more than 50% of cases**

Ref: Chapter No.44, Page No.1092-1093

69. **Ans: B. 50%**

Ref: Chapter No.44, Page No.1093

70. **Ans: B. 50%**

Ref: Chapter No.44, Page No.1093

71. **Ans: B. The ascitic fluid SAAG is >1.1 g/dL, consistent with a high protein concentration in the ascitic fluid**

Ref: Chapter No.44, Page No.1093

72. **Ans: A. Appendicitis**

Ref: Chapter No.44, Page No.1093

73. **Ans: A. 25% of infections are cured by culture directed antibiotic therapy**

Ref: Chapter No.44, Page No.1093

74. **Ans: C. Peritoneal mucinous carcinomatosis has the best survival rate**

Ref: Chapter No.44, Page No.1093

75. **Ans: A. Appendix**

Ref: Chapter No.44, Page No.1093

76. **Ans: B. Pseudomyxoma peritonei occurs most commonly in individuals 20 to 30 years of age**

Ref: Chapter No.44, Page No.1093

77. **Ans: C. Patients with low-grade tumors who undergo complete cytoreduction with HIPEC have 5-year survival rates of 20% to 30%**

Ref: Chapter No.44, Page No.1094

78. **Ans: C. Mitomycin C**

Ref: Chapter No.44, Page No.1094

79. **Ans: A. Pulmonary complications**

Ref: Chapter No.44, Page No.1094

80. **Ans: C. Cytoreductive surgery with HIPEC has been performed in all patients**

Ref: Chapter No.44, Page No.1094

81. **Ans: C. It has male predominance**

Ref: Chapter No.44, Page No.1094

82. **Ans: A. Paracentesis has a high diagnostic yield**

Ref: Chapter No.44, Page No.1094-1095

83. **Ans: A. High histologic tumor grade**

Ref: Chapter No.44, Page No.1095

84. **Ans: B. Hepatic vein**

Ref: Chapter No.44, Page No.1095

85. **Ans: C. Left side of the 2nd lumbar vertebra toward the right iliac fossa to terminate anterior to the sacroiliac articulation**

Ref: Chapter No.44, Page No.1095

86. **Ans: A. Omental cysts contains cloudy fluid**

Ref: Chapter No.44, Page No.1095

87. **Ans: D. All of the above**

Ref: Chapter No.44, Page No.1095

88. **Ans: D. Uncomplicated cysts usually lie in the lower mid-abdomen and are freely movable, smooth and tender**

Ref: Chapter No.44, Page No.1095

89. **Ans: B. Primary omental torsion usually involves the left side of the omentum**

Ref: Chapter No.44, Page No.1095

90. **Ans: A. CT often demonstrates an omental mass without signs of inflammation**

Ref: Chapter No.44, Page No.1095-1096

91. **Ans: D. Mesothelial cysts**

Ref: Chapter No.44, Page No.1096

92. **Ans: D. These cysts usually occur in adults, with a mean age of 45 years, and are twice as common in men as in women**

Ref: Chapter No.44, Page No.1096

93. **Ans: A. Syndrome occurs most commonly in children and young adults with increased frequency in males**

Ref: Chapter No.44, Page No.1096

94. **Ans: B. An abdominal mass is palpable in more than 80% of patients**

Ref: Chapter No.44, Page No.1096-1097

95. **Ans: B. Operative management is always indicated**

Ref: Chapter No.44, Page No.1097

96. **Ans: C. The presence of inflamed adipose tissue surrounding mesenteric vessels**

Ref: Chapter No.44, Page No.1097

97. **Ans: B. Approximately 75% of mesocolic hernias occur on the right side**

Ref: Chapter No.44, Page No.1097

98. **Ans: C. Superior mesenteric artery**

Ref: Chapter No.44, Page No.1097

99. **Ans: B. Near the ileocolic junction**

Ref: Chapter No.44, Page No.1097

100. **Ans: B. Herniation after laparoscopic colectomy is very common**

Ref: Chapter No.44, Page No.1097

101. **Ans: C. Metastatic disease**

Ref: Chapter No.44, Page No.1098

102. **Ans: B. Desmoid tumor**

Ref: Chapter No.44, Page No.1098

103. **Ans: D. 60% to 70%**

Ref: Chapter No.44, Page No.1099

104. **Ans: B. E. coli**

Ref: Chapter No.44, Page No.1100

105. **Ans: A. Flank pain**

Ref: Chapter No.44, Page No.1100

106. **Ans: A. CT will demonstrate a high-density mass in the retroperitoneum with surrounding inflammation & gas is present in as many as one third of these lesions**

Ref: Chapter No.44, Page No.1100

107. **Ans: D. As many as 50% to 60% of patients will develop signs of a femoral neuropathy**

Ref: Chapter No.44, Page No.1100

108. **Ans: D. The mean age at presentation is 20 to 30 years**

Ref: Chapter No.44, Page No.1100

109. **Ans: C. Type 2 diabetes mellitus**

Ref: Chapter No.44, Page No.1100

110. **Ans: D. Ureteral involvement is present in 50% to 60% of cases**

Ref: Chapter No.44, Page No.1100-1101

111. **Ans: D. Evaluation of patients thought to have retroperitoneal fibrosis often starts with a MRI**

Ref: Chapter No.44, Page No.1101

112. **Ans: B. 4.5 to 5 cm**

Ref: Chapter No.44, Page No.1101

113. **Ans: A. Sarcomas**

Ref: Chapter No.44, Page No.1101

114. **Ans: B. Treatment of choice is R0 resection with lymphadenectomy**

Ref: Chapter No.44, Page No.1101-1102

115. **Ans: B. 50%**

Ref: Chapter No.44, Page No.1101

45

Hernias

1. **False statement among the following is:**
   A. There is a consistent relationship between the area of a hernia defect and the size of a hernia sac
   B. Hernia is derived from the Latin word for rupture
   C. A hernia is defined as an abnormal protrusion of an organ or tissue through a defect in its surrounding walls
   D. The so-called neck or orifice of a hernia is located at the innermost musculoaponeurotic layer, whereas the hernia sac is lined by peritoneum and protrudes from the neck

2. **False statement among the following is:**
   A. Strangulated hernia has compromised blood supply to its contents, which is a serious and potentially fatal complication
   B. A hernia is reducible when its contents can be replaced within the surrounding musculature, and it is irreducible or incarcerated when it cannot be reduced
   C. An internal hernia protrudes through all layers of the abdominal wall
   D. Adhesions between the contents of the hernia and peritoneal lining of the sac can provide a tethering point that entraps the hernia contents and predisposes to intestinal obstruction and strangulation

3. **Anterior abdominal wall hernias include all except:**
   A. Lumbar B. Umbilical
   C. Epigastric D. Spigelian

4. **Pelvic hernias include all except:**
   A. Sciatic B. Obturator
   C. Lumbar D. Perineal

INGUINAL HERNIAS

5. **Grynfeltt's hernia is also called as:**
   A. Inferior lumbar hernia
   B. Superior lumbar hernia
   C. Esophageal hernia
   D. Obturator hernia

6. **Petit's hernia is also called as:**
   A. Inferior lumbar hernia
   B. Superior lumbar hernia
   C. Esophageal hernia
   D. Obturator hernia

7. **False about incidence of Inguinal hernias is:**
   A. It is estimated that 5% of the population will develop an abdominal wall hernia
   B. About 75% of all hernias occur in the inguinal region
   C. Two-thirds of these are direct and the remainder are indirect inguinal hernias
   D. Femoral hernias represent only 3% of all groin hernias

8. **False about incidence of Inguinal hernias is:**
   A. In men, indirect hernias predominate over direct hernias at a ratio of 2:1
   B. Indirect hernias are by far the most common type of hernia in women
   C. Femoral hernias are the most common hernia in women
   D. The female-to-male ratio for femoral and umbilical hernias is about 10:1 and 2:1 respectively

9. **As compared to women, groin hernias are more common in men upto:**
   A. 5 times B. 10 times
   C. 20 times D. 25 times

10. Percent of men who have a femoral hernia and who will develop an inguinal hernia is:

A. 10% B. 20%
C. 40% D. 50%

11. Which of the following statements is false regarding the incidence of abdominal wall hernias?

A. Two-thirds of all inguinal hernias are classified as indirect
B. Femoral hernias are more common in females than in males
C. Indirect hernias are common in females
D. Hernias generally occur with equal frequency in males and females

12. Percent of women who have a femoral hernia and who will develop an inguinal hernia is:

A. 10% B. 20%
C. 40% D. 50%

13. False about of Inguinal hernias is:

A. Indirect inguinal and femoral hernias occur more commonly on the left side
B. The predominance of right-sided femoral hernias is thought to be caused by the tamponading effect of the sigmoid colon on the left femoral canal
C. Strangulation, the most common serious complication of a hernia, occurs in only 1% - 3% of groin hernias and is more common at the extremes of life
D. The likelihood of strangulation and need for hospitalization increase with aging

14. False about of groin hernias is:

A. Most strangulated hernias are direct inguinal hernias
B. Femoral hernias have the highest rate of strangulation (15%–20%) of all hernias
C. The prevalence of hernias increases with age, particularly for inguinal, umbilical, and femoral hernias
D. Femoral hernias be repaired at the time of discovery

15. False about external oblique muscle and aponeurosis is:

A. The aponeurosis of the external oblique muscle is formed by a superficial and deep layer
B. Aponeurosis, along with the bilaminar aponeuroses of the internal oblique and transversus abdominis, forms the posterior rectus sheath
C. The external (superficial) inguinal ring is an ovoid opening of the external oblique aponeurosis that is positioned superiorly and slightly laterally to the pubic tubercle
D. The external oblique aponeurosis serves as the superficial boundary of the inguinal canal

16. The inguinal ligament is also called as:

A. Poupart ligament
B. Lacunar ligament
C. Cooper's ligament
D. Hesselbach's ligament

17. The letter A marked in the image is:

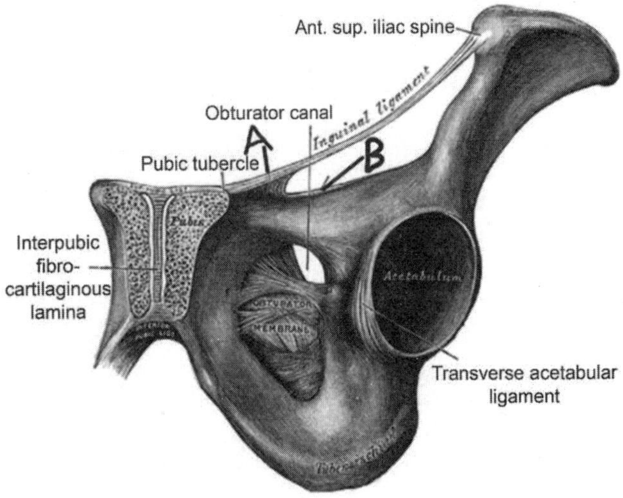

A. Pectineal ligament
B. Lacunar ligament
C. Cooper's ligament
D. Hesselbach's ligament

18. The letter B marked in the image is:

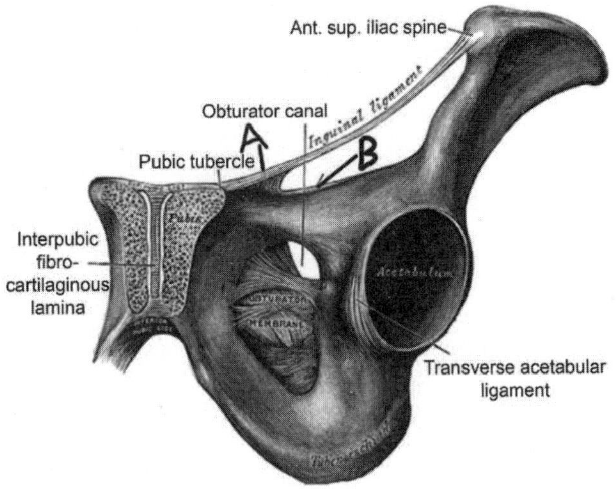

A. Poupart ligament
B. Lacunar ligament
C. Cooper's ligament
D. Hesselbach's ligament

19. False about internal oblique muscle and aponeurosis is:

A. The internal oblique muscle serves as the posterior border of the inguinal canal
B. The internal oblique muscle forms the middle layer of the lateral abdominal musculoaponeurotic complex
C. The cremaster muscle fibers should be minimally disrupted during open inguinal hernia repair to help reduce chronic groin pain
D. The cremaster muscle fibers arise from the internal oblique

20. Conjoined tendon is present in only:

A. 1% to 5% of patients
B. 5% to 10% of patients
C. 10% to 20% of patients
D. 20% to 40% of patients

21. False about transversus abdominis muscle and aponeurosis and transversalis fascia is:

A. The transversus abdominis muscle layer is oriented horizontally throughout most of its area; in the inguinal region, these fibers course in a slightly oblique downward direction
B. The strength and continuity of this muscle and aponeurosis are important for the prevention and treatment of inguinal hernia
C. The transversalis fascia, sometimes referred to as the endoabdominal fascia, is a component of the inguinal floor and tends to be thinner in this area
D. The inferior crus of the deep inguinal ring is composed of the iliopubic tract; the superior crus of the deep ring is formed by the transversus abdominis aponeurotic arch

22. False about iliopubic tract is:

A. It composes the inferior margin of most anterior repairs
B. The iliopubic tract is an aponeurotic band that is formed by the transversalis fascia and transversus abdominis aponeurosis and fascia
C. The iliopubic tract is located posterior to the inguinal ligament and crosses over the femoral vessels and inserts on the anterior superior iliac spine and inner lip of the wing of the ilium
D. The femoral, lateral femoral cutaneous, and genitofemoral nerves are located superior to the iliopubic tract

23. False about Cooper's ligament is:

A. This structure is anterior to the iliopubic tract and forms the anterior border of the femoral canal
B. The Cooper's ligament is formed by the periosteum and aponeurotic tissues along the superior ramus of the pubis
C. Also called as pectineal ligament
D. Cooper's ligament is an important landmark for open and laparoscopic repairs and is a useful anchoring structure, particularly in laparoscopic repairs

24. False about the inguinal canal and hernias is:

A. The inguinal canal is about 4 cm in length and is located just cephalad to the inguinal ligament
B. The posterior wall, or floor of the inguinal canal, is formed by the aponeurosis of the transversus abdominis muscle and transversalis fascia
C. Indirect hernias occur within Hesselbach triangle, whereas direct inguinal hernias arise lateral to the triangle
D. The inguinal canal contains the spermatic cord in men and the round ligament of the uterus in women

25. The spermatic cord is composed of all except:

A. Femoral branch of the genitofemoral nerve
B. Vas deferens
C. Cremaster muscle fibers
D. Testicular artery and accompanying veins

26. The cremasteric vessels are branches of the:

A. Superior epigastric vessels
B. Inferior epigastric vessels
C. Medial circumflex femoral vessels
D. Internal iliac artery

27. Boundaries of Hesselbach triangle are all except:

A. *Medially:* Rectus abdominis
B. *Laterally:* Inferior epigastric vessels
C. *Superiorly:* Superior epigastric vessels
D. *Inferiorly:* Inguinal ligament

28. The letter A marked in the image denotes:

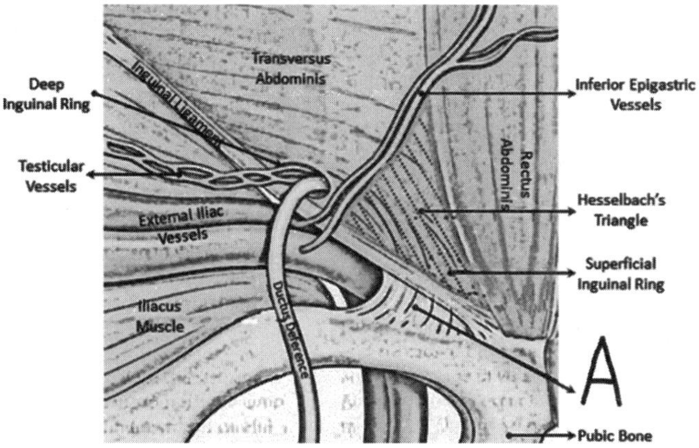

A. Poupart ligament
B. Lacunar ligament
C. Cooper's ligament
D. Hesselbach's ligament

29. False among the following is:

A. The iliohypogastric and ilioinguinal nerves and genital branch of the genitofemoral nerve are the important sensory nerves in the groin area
B. The iliohypogastric and ilioinguinal nerves lie beneath the internal oblique muscle to a point just medial and superior to the anterior superior iliac spine, where they penetrate the internal oblique muscle and course beneath the external oblique aponeurosis
C. The main trunk of the iliohypogastric nerve runs on the anterior surface of the internal oblique muscle and aponeurosis medial and superior to the internal ring
D. The femoral branch of the genitofemoral nerve innervates the cremaster muscle and skin on the lateral side of the scrotum and labia

30. False among the following is:

A. The nerves of the preperitoneal space of specific concern to the surgeon include the lateral femoral cutaneous nerve and genitofemoral nerve
B. The lateral femoral cutaneous nerve originates as a root of L4 – L5 and is occasionally a direct branch of the femoral nerve
C. The vas deferens courses through the preperitoneal space from caudad to cephalad and medial to lateral to join the spermatic cord at the deep inguinal ring
D. The genital branch enters the inguinal canal through the deep ring, whereas the femoral branch enters the femoral sheath lateral to the artery

31. Femoral canal boundaries are all except:

A. Iliopubic tract anteriorly
B. Cooper's ligament posteriorly
C. Femoral vein medially
D. Lacunar ligament medially

32. False about the diagnosis of groin hernias is:

A. The inguinal region is examined with the patient in the only supine position
B. A bulge identified below the inguinal ligament is consistent with a femoral hernia
C. Ultrasonography also can aid in the diagnosis
D. There is a high degree of sensitivity and specificity for ultrasound in the detection of occult direct, indirect and femoral hernias

33. Differential diagnosis of groin and scrotal masses includes all except:

A. Ectopic testis
B. Inguinal lymphadenopathy
C. Popliteal artery aneurysm
D. Femoral hernia

34. As per Nyhus classification of groin hernias, femoral hernia is:

A. Type I B. Type II
C. Type III D. Type IV

35. As per Nyhus classification of groin hernias, recurrent hernia is:

A. Type I B. Type II
C. Type III D. Type IV

36. As per Nyhus classification of groin hernias, pediatric hernias is/are:

A. Type I B. Type II
C. Type III D. Type IV

37. False about the non-operative management of inguinal hernias is:

A. Patients electing non-operative management can occasionally have symptomatic improvement with the use of a truss
B. Symptom control has been reported in about 70% of patients
C. Complications associated with the use of a truss include testicular atrophy, ilioinguinal or femoral neuritis and hernia incarceration
D. Fitzgibbons and colleagues reported a prospective randomized trial of a watchful waiting strategy for men with asymptomatic or minimally symptomatic inguinal hernias

38. False about anterior repair in inguinal hernia is:

A. The genital branch of the genitofemoral nerve and the ilioinguinal and iliohypogastric nerves are identified and transected

B. The cremaster muscle of the mobilized spermatic cord is separated parallel to its fibers from the underlying cord structures

C. The cremaster muscle of the mobilized spermatic cord is separated perpendicularly to its fibers from the underlying cord structures

D. A "lipoma" of the cord actually represents retroperitoneal fat that has herniated through the deep inguinal ring; this should be suture ligated and removed

39. The Bassini repair is performed by suturing:

A. The transversus abdominis and external oblique musculoaponeurotic arches to the inguinal ligament

B. The transversus abdominis and internal oblique musculoaponeurotic arches or conjoined tendon to the inguinal ligament

C. The transversus abdominis and external oblique musculoaponeurotic arches to the lacunar ligament

D. The transversus abdominis and external oblique musculoaponeurotic arches to the pectineal ligament

40. McVay repair is also called as:

A. Cooper's ligament repair

B. Lacunar ligament repair

C. Inguinal ligament repair

D. Femoral ligament repair

41. False about Shouldice repair is:

A. The Shouldice repair emphasizes a multilayer imbricated repair of the posterior wall of the inguinal canal with a continuous running suture technique

B. After completion of the dissection, the posterior wall of the inguinal canal is reconstructed by superimposing running suture lines progressing from deep to more superficial layers

C. The initial suture line secures the transversus abdominis aponeurotic arch to the iliopubic tract

D. The Shouldice repair is associated with a high recurrence rate and a low degree of patient satisfaction in patients

42. Following image shows which tissue repair of inguinal hernia:

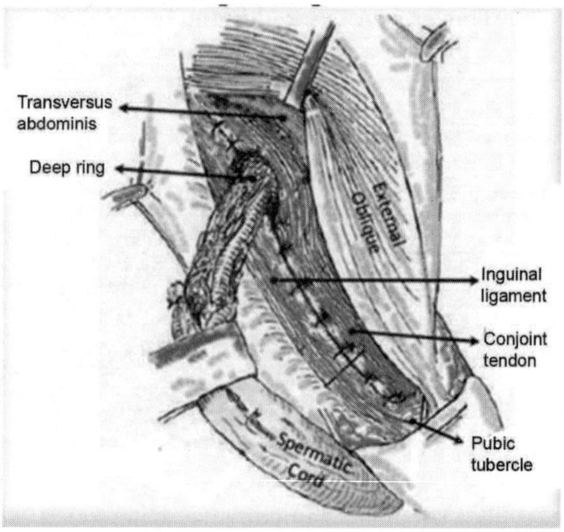

A. Bassini repair

B. McVay repair

C. Iliopubic tract repair

D. Shouldice repair

43. Following image shows which tissue repair of inguinal hernia:

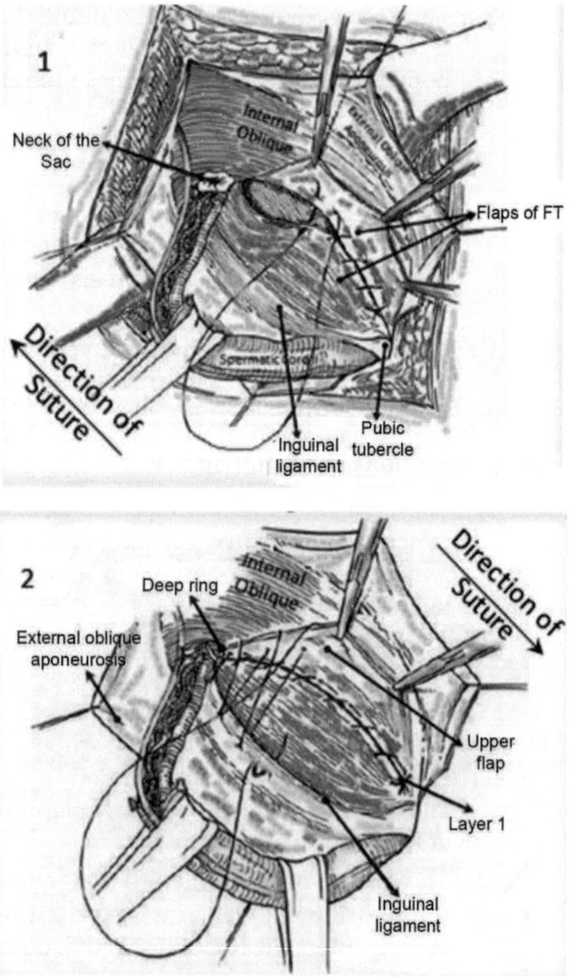

A. Bassini repair B. McVay repair
C. Iliopubic tract repair D. Shouldice repair

44. Following image shows which repair of inguinal hernia:

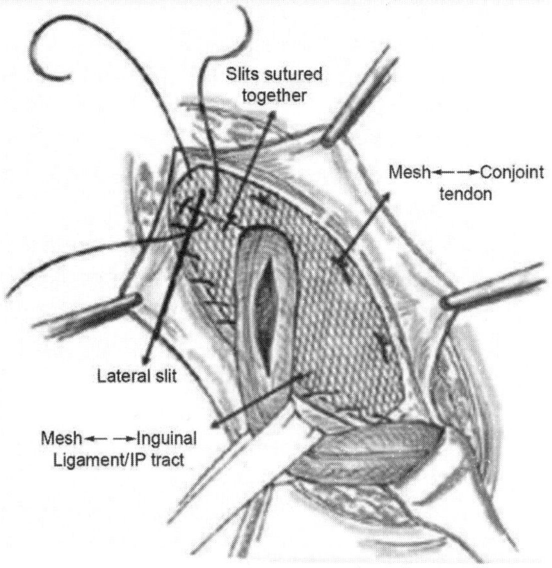

A. Iliopubic tract repair B. Lichtenstein repair
C. McVay repair D. Bassini repair

45. False about tension-free anterior inguinal hernia repair is:

A. Fixation of mesh to the pubic tubercle itself should be avoided to minimize the risk of chronic groin pain
B. The medial aspect of the mesh is allowed to generously overlap the pubic tubercle by at least 15 mm
C. This so-called plug and patch repair, an extension of the Lichtenstein original mesh repair, has now become the most commonly performed primary anterior inguinal hernia repair
D. The sandwich technique involves a bilayered device, with 2 polypropylene components

46. The Stoppa-Rives technique is particularly useful for all except:

A. Large hernia B. Recurrent hernias
C. Unilateral hernias D. All of the above

47. False about Lichtenstein tension-free hernia repair is:

A. The medial aspect of the mesh overlaps the pubic bone by approximately 1 cm
B. The external oblique aponeurosis is separated from the underlying internal oblique muscle high enough to accommodate a 6- to 8-cm-wide mesh patch
C. Overlap of the internal oblique muscle edge by 2 to 3 cm is necessary
D. The suture is continued laterally by suturing the inferior edge of the mesh to the shelving edge of the inguinal ligament to a point just lateral to the internal inguinal ring

48. False about preperitoneal repair is:

A. The open preperitoneal approach is useful for the repair of recurrent inguinal hernias, sliding hernias, femoral hernias, and some strangulated hernias
B. The inferior epigastric artery and veins are generally beneath the midportion of the posterior rectus sheath and usually need to be divided
C. The transversalis fascia and transversus abdominis aponeurosis are identified and sutured to the iliopubic tract with permanent sutures
D. Femoral hernias repaired by this approach require closure of the femoral canal by securing the repair to Cooper's ligament

49. False about laparoscopic inguinal hernia repair is:

A. Laparoscopic repair is associated with an approximately 3% risk of visceral or vascular injury
B. The most popular techniques are totally extraperitoneal (TEP) and transabdominal preperitoneal (TAPP) approaches
C. In the TEP approach, the dissection begins in the preperitoneal space using a balloon dissector
D. With the TAPP repair, the preperitoneal space is accessed after initially entering the peritoneal cavity

50. Boundaries of triangle of doom are all except:

A. Ductus deferens B. Testicular vessels
C. Peritoneal fold D. Iliopubic tract

51. Boundaries of triangle of pain are all except:

A. Ductus deferens B. Testicular vessels
C. Peritoneal fold D. Iliopubic tract

52. This triangle of pain has all except:

A. The femoral nerve
B. The genital branch of the genitofemoral nerve
C. The lateral femoral cutaneous nerve
D. The femoral branch of the genitofemoral nerve

53. Which of the following is not true regarding laparoscopic hernia repair?

A. Local anesthesia with sedation is the most common form of anesthesia used
B. It is best suited for recurrent and bilateral hernias
C. Transabdominal preperitoneal or total extra-peritoneal approaches are commonly used
D. Fixation devices for the mesh should not be placed below the iliopubic tract

54. False about the complications and results of inguinal hernia repair is:

A. There is a greater mortality associated with the repair of strangulated hernias
B. Large series, including multiple types of repairs, have suggested that recurrence ranges from 1.7% to 10%
C. Approximately 50% of recurrences are found within 3 years after primary repair
D. The Shouldice repair has a lower recurrence rate than mesh repairs

55. Most common complication after open inguinal hernia repair is:

A. Urinary retention B. Seroma
C. Chronic pain D. Recurrence

56. Most common complication after laparoscopic inguinal hernia repair is:

A. Urinary retention B. Seroma
C. Chronic pain D. Recurrence

57. Which of the following urologic complications does not occur with hernia repair?

A. Ischemic orchitis
B. Transection of the vas deferens
C. Prostatitis
D. Testicular atrophy

58. Which of the following statements is true regarding surgical technique?

A. Bassini repair can be used for femoral hernias
B. Shouldice repair approximates the transversus abdominis aponeurosis to Cooper's ligament medially and the iliopubic tract laterally. It requires a relaxing incision
C. Total extraperitoneal repair (TEP) is a laparoscopic approach that stays in the preperitoneal space by using a balloon dissector
D. Bassini repair uses a piece of mesh to reinforce the floor of the inguinal canal and recreate the internal ring in a tension-free manner

59. Which of the following statements are true regarding laparoscopic inguinal hernia anatomy?

A. The triangle of doom is bordered by the vas deferens, iliopubic tract, and gonadal vessels and contains the ilioinguinal and iliohypogastric nerves that must be avoided to prevent pain
B. The lateral-most border of the dissection is the anterior superior iliac spine
C. The femoral branch of the genitofemoral nerve and the lateral femoral cutaneous nerve are located medial and superior to the iliopubic tract
D. A transabdominal preperitoneal repair (TAPP) approach uses a dissecting balloon to stay in the preperitoneal space throughout the procedure and a TEP approach initially accesses the peritoneum before creating a peritoneal flap

FEMORAL HERNIAS

60. False among the following is:

A. Approximately 50% of men with a femoral hernia will have an associated direct inguinal hernia, whereas this relationship occurs in only 20% of women
B. The incidence of strangulation in femoral hernias is high; therefore, all femoral hernias should be repaired, and incarcerated femoral hernias should have the hernia sac contents examined for viability
C. In patients with a compromised bowel, the Cooper ligament approach is the preferred technique because mesh is contraindicated
D. The occurrence of a femoral hernia after repair of an inguinal hernia has been reported to be 15 times the normal expected rate

61. Which of the following statements is true regarding femoral hernias?

A. Femoral hernias should not be repaired through an infrainguinal approach
B. If an incarcerated femoral hernia cannot be reduced intraoperatively, the insertion of the inguinal ligament can be cut from the pubic tubercle to allow more space
C. Femoral hernias are more common than inguinal hernias in females
D. A laparoscopic repair is an inappropriate choice for a femoral hernia repair

SPECIAL PROBLEMS

62. False statement among the following is:

A. Recurrent hernias almost always require placement of prosthetic mesh for successful repair
B. Recurrences after anterior hernia repair using mesh are best managed by a laparoscopic or open posterior approach, without placement of a second prosthesis
C. Repair of a suspected strangulated hernia is most easily done using a intraperitoneal approach
D. The use of a giant prosthetic reinforcement of the visceral sac (Stoppa repair) or the laparoscopic repair is preferred for simultaneous repair of bilateral inguinal hernias

63. The most common viscus involved in sliding inguinal hernia is the:

A. Colon
B. Small intestine
C. Urinary bladder
D. Both A and C

64. False about Sliding inguinal hernia is:

A. Sliding hernia occurs when an internal organ composes a portion of the wall of the hernia sac
B. Most sliding hernias are a variant of direct inguinal hernias, although femoral and indirect sliding hernias can occur
C. The primary danger associated with a sliding hernia is the failure to recognize the visceral component of the hernia sac before injury to the bowel or bladder
D. Sliding hernia contents are reduced into the peritoneal cavity and any excess hernia sac is ligated and divided

COMPLICATIONS AND RESULTS

65. Overall complication rate from hernia repair has been estimated to be approximately:

A. 5% B. 10%
C. 20% D. 25%

66. False about surgical site infection in inguinal hernia repair is:

A. The risk for surgical site infection is estimated to be 5% to 10% after open inguinal hernia repair and slightly less with laparoscopic repairs
B. There is an increased risk for infection for patients who have had prior hernia incision infections, chronic skin infections, or infection at a distant site
C. Superficial surgical site infections are treated by opening the incision, local wound care, and healing by secondary intention
D. Deep surgical site infections usually involve the prosthetic mesh, which should be explanted

67. False statement about nerve injuries and chronic pain syndrome among the following is:

A. Nerve injury can occur from traction, electrocautery, transection and entrapment
B. The use of prosthetic mesh can result in dysesthesias, which are usually permanent
C. Persistent neuralgias usually result in pain and hyperesthesia in the area of distribution
D. Transient neuralgias involving sensory nerves can occur and are usually self-limited and resolve within a few weeks after surgery

68. The nerves most commonly affected during open hernia repair are all except:

A. Genital branch of the genitofemoral
B. The ilioinguinal
C. Iliohypogastric nerves
D. Lateral femoral cutaneous nerve

69. Chronic postherniorrhaphy pain, is defined as pain persisting:

A. > 1 month after operation
B. > 2 months after operation
C. > 3 months after operation
D. > 6 months after operation

70. False statement about nerve injuries and chronic pain syndrome among the following is:

A. Approximately 10% of patients will have chronic postherniorrhaphy pain
B. Strategies of routine nerve division in open surgery have not been associated with a reduction in chronic pain in mesh-based anterior repairs
C. Measures to reduce chronic groin pain during open repair include identification and preservation of all three major nerves leaving them in situ (ilioinguinal, iliohypogastric, genital branch of the genital nerve)
D. Early symptoms are treated with surgical removal of mesh

71. After surgery, ischemic orchitis results in venous congestion of the testis, which becomes swollen and tender in:

A. 1 to 2 days
B. 2 to 5 days
C. 5 to 10 days
D. 10 to 14 days

72. False statement among the following is:

A. Ischemic orchitis usually occurs from thrombosis of the small veins of the pampiniform plexus within the spermatic cord
B. Ischemic orchitis also can be caused by ligation of the testicular artery
C. Testicular atrophy is a consequence of ischemic orchitis and is more common after repair of recurrent hernias, particularly when an anterior approach is used
D. Orchiectomy is often necessary

73. With each subsequent hernia recurrence, the incidence of ischemic orchitis increases by a factor of:

A. 2-3
B. 3-4
C. 4-6
D. 6-10

74. Hernia recurrences are usually caused by:

A. Missed hernias
B. Less tension on the repair
C. Improper mesh size and placement
D. Failure to include an adequate musculoaponeurotic margin in the repair

75. False about Inguinal hernia recurrence is:

A. Recurrences are best managed by excision prosthesis and repair without mesh
B. Recurrences are more common in patients with direct hernias and usually involve the floor of the inguinal canal near the pubic tubercle, where suture line tension is greatest
C. The use of a relaxing incision when there is excessive tension at the time of primary hernia repair is helpful to reduce recurrence
D. Recurrences after initial prosthetic mesh repairs can be caused by displaced prostheses or the use of a prosthetic of inadequate size

76. Compared with more traditional repairs, tension-free and mesh-based repairs have the lowest rates of reoperation after recurrence and result in a reduction in recurrence of approximately:

A. 10%
B. 20%
C. 40%
D. 60%

VENTRAL HERNIAS

77. False statement among the following is:

A. Epigastric hernias occur from the xiphoid process to the umbilicus
B. Umbilical hernias occur at the umbilicus
C. Hypogastric hernias spontaneous hernias that occur below the umbilicus in the midline
D. Diastasis recti can present as a midline bulge with a hernia sac

78. False statement among the following is:

A. Incisional hernias account for 15% to 20% of all abdominal wall hernias
B. Umbilical and epigastric hernias constitute 10% of hernias
C. The use of a suture to wound length ratio of 4:1 has been shown to significantly reduce incisional hernia formation
D. Incisional hernias are twice as common in men as in women

79. Patient-related factors linked to ventral hernia formation includes all except:

A. Female gender
B. Obesity
C. Sleep apnea
D. Older age

80. False about the anatomy of the anterior abdominal wall is:

A. At the midline, 2 anterior rectus sheaths form the tendinous linea alba
B. An important anatomic structure of the anterior abdominal wall is the arcuate line, which is located 3 to 6 cm below the umbilicus
C. The posterior rectus sheath below the arcuate line is composed of the peritoneum only
D. The abdominal wall receives most of its innervation from intercostal nerves 7 through 12 and the 1st and 2nd lumbar nerves

81. The lateral abdominal muscles receive their blood supply from:

A. Deep circumflex iliac artery
B. Lower 3 or 4 intercostal arteries
C. Deep superior epigastric artery
D. Lumbar arteries

82. True about the diagnosis of abdominal wall hernias is:

A. As with the inguinal region, the anterior abdominal wall is evaluated with the patient in standing and supine positions, and a valsalva maneuver is also useful to demonstrate the site and size of a hernia
B. Imaging modalities may play a greater role in the diagnosis of more unusual hernias of the abdominal wall

C. Computed tomography (CT) evaluation and surgeon-performed ultrasound (dynamic abdominal sonography for hernia [DASH]) are the most useful adjuncts to physical examination
D. All of the above

83. False about umbilical hernia is:

A. Umbilical hernias in infants are congenital and are common
B. There is a strong predisposition toward the development of these hernias in individuals of African descent
C. The incidence of umbilical hernia is 8 times higher in African American than in white infants
D. Umbilical hernias in adults are largely congenital

84. Pediatric umbilical hernias close spontaneously in most cases by the age of:

A. 6 months B. 1 year
C. 2 years D. 5 years

85. Which of the following is a true statement regarding umbilical hernias?

A. They are the embryonic equivalent of a small omphalocele
B. Repair in infants is usually deferred until approximately 5 years of age
C. Repair in adults is generally indicated
D. They are most common in white infants

86. Pediatric umbilical hernias are frequently repaired surgically if they persist after the age of:

A. 6 months B. 1 year
C. 2 years D. 5 years

87. False about umbilical hernia is:

A. Adult umbilical hernias are more common in women and in patients with conditions that result in increased intra-abdominal pressure, such as pregnancy, obesity, ascites, or chronic abdominal distention
B. Umbilical hernia is more common in those who have only a single midline aponeurotic decussation compared with the normal decussation of fibers from all 3 lateral abdominal muscles
C. Spontaneous rupture of umbilical hernias in patients with ascites can result in peritonitis and death
D. Mayo's repair is the most common repair for umbilical hernia performed today

88. The technique of repair shown in the following image is:

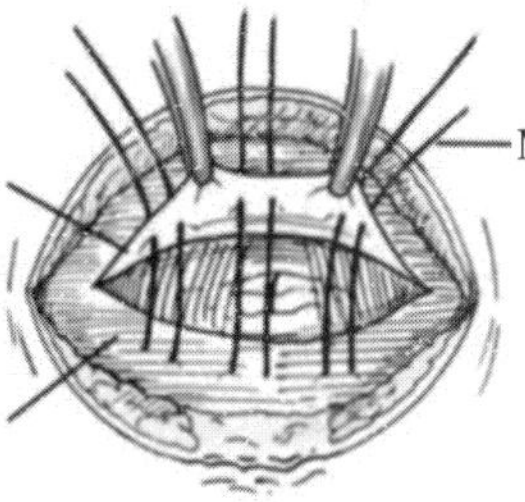

A. Lichtenstein's repair B. Mayo's repair
C. Bassini's repair D. Stoppa's repair

89. False about Epigastric hernias is:

A. Epigastric hernias are 2 to 3 times more common in women
B. Approximately 3% to 5% of the population has epigastric hernias
C. These hernias are located between the xiphoid process and umbilicus and are usually within 5 to 6 cm of the umbilicus
D. Umbilical hernias, epigastric hernias are more common in individuals with a single aponeurotic decussation

90. False about Epigastric hernias is:

A. The defects are small and often produce pain out of proportion to their size because of incarceration of preperitoneal fat
B. They are multiple in up to 20% of patients and approximately 80% are in the midline
C. Epigastric hernias are better repaired preperitoneally
D. Repair usually consists of excision of the incarcerated preperitoneal tissue and simple closure of the fascial defect, similar to that for umbilical hernias

91. False about incisional hernias is:

A. Incisional hernias occur as a result of excessive tension and inadequate healing of a previous incision, which may be associated with surgical site infection
B. Conditions that decrease intra-abdominal pressure are factors that predispose to the development of an incisional hernia
C. Obesity can cause an incisional hernia to occur because of increased tension on the abdominal wall from the excessive bulk of a thick pannus and large omental mass
D. Medications such as corticosteroids and chemotherapeutic agents and surgical site

infection can contribute to poor wound healing and increase the risk for development of an incisional hernia

92. True about incisional hernias is:

A. Two of the most popular ventral hernia classification tools to date have been generated from expert opinion: the Ventral Hernia Working Group grading scale and the European Hernia Society system

B. Respiratory dysfunction can occur because these large ventral defects cause paradoxic respiratory abdominal motion

C. With loss of domain, the natural rigidity of the abdominal wall becomes compromised and the abdominal musculature is often retracted

D. All of the above

93. A 55-year-old obese woman returns to the office 2 weeks after an open incisional hernia repair with mesh complaining of increasing pain and redness. On examination, the wound is red and fluctuant consistent with a postoperative wound infection. Which of the following is true regarding wound infections?

A. Laparoscopic hernia repairs have lower rates of wound infections than open repairs

B. Polytetrafluoroethylene (PTFE) mesh is an absorbable mesh that can be left in place even with a wound infection

C. Suture ventral hernia repair has higher infection rates and recurrence rates than mesh ventral hernia repair

D. Surgical site infections have no effect on the recurrence rate after a ventral hernia repair

94. Stage I Incisional hernia is:

A. <10 cm, clean

B. <10 cm, contaminated

C. 10–20 cm, clean

D. ≥10 cm, contaminated

95. Stage III Incisional hernia is:

A. <10 cm, clean

B. <10 cm, contaminated

C. 10–20 cm, clean

D. ≥10 cm, contaminated

96. Which of the following hernias is most likely to recur after a primary repair?

A. Epigastric hernia   B. Spigelian hernia

C. Incisional hernia   D. Femoral hernia

97. False about the treatment of incisional hernias is:

A. Primary repair of incisional hernias can be done when the defect is small (≤2–3 cm in diameter) and there is viable surrounding tissue

B. Larger defects (<3 cm in diameter) have a high recurrence rate if closed primarily and are repaired with a prosthesis

C. Incisional hernia is likely a chronic disease and an array of management options will need to be utilized to care for a patient throughout the course of their life

D. Prosthetic material may be placed as an onlay patch to buttress a tissue repair, interposed between the fascial defect, sandwiched between tissue planes, or put in a sublay position

98. Desirable characteristics of a synthetic mesh includes all except:

A. Carcinogenic

B. Chemically inert

C. Resistant to mechanical stress while maintaining compliance

D. Incite minimal inflammatory reaction

99. False about prosthetic materials for ventral hernia repair is:

A. Mesh constructs can be classified on the basis of weight of the material, pore size, water angle (hydrophobic or hydrophilic) and whether there is an antiadhesive barrier present

B. Polypropylene mesh is a hydrophilic macroporous mesh that allows the ingrowth of native fibroblasts and incorporation into the surrounding fascia

C. It is semirigid, somewhat flexible and porous

D. Lighter weight polypropylene mesh has been introduced to address some of the long-term complications of heavyweight polypropylene mesh

100. The definition of lightweight mesh was chosen at:

A. < 20 g/m^2 B. < 40 g/m^2

C. < 60 g/m^2 D. < 80 g/m^2

101. The definition of heavyweight mesh is a mesh weighing:

A. >25 g/m^2 B. >50 g/m^2

C. >75 g/m^2 D. >100 g/m^2

102. Which of the following is true regarding characteristics of mesh used in hernia repair?

A. Lightweight mesh, compared with heavyweight mesh, provokes an intense inflammatory reaction in the body causing scarring, pain, and shrinkage
B. Synthetic meshes can never be placed into a contaminated field
C. Polypropylene meshes have high adhesion risks, so they should not be placed directly next to bowel
D. Biologic meshes are processed human, bovine and porcine tissues composed of a collagen matrix and immune cells

103. The definition of intermediate weight mesh is a mesh weighing:

A. 30 to 45 g/m^2 B. 40 to 60 g/m^2
C. 60 to 75 g/m^2 D. 75 to 90 g/m^2

104. False among the following is:

A. In a randomized controlled trials, heavyweight mesh has been shown to exhibit less recurrence and chronic pain 2 years after laparoscopic TEP inguinal repair compared to lightweight mesh
B. Given the lightweight polypropylene mesh had less overall mesh-related issues compared to heavyweight mesh in this setting, lightweight mesh is favored
C. In a randomized controlled trial evaluating lightweight versus heavyweight polypropylene mesh for ventral hernia repair, the recurrence rate in the heavyweight group was more than twice that in the lightweight group
D. Large-pore lightweight mesh has an ability to resist bacterial contamination

105. True about Polyester mesh is:

A. Polyester mesh is composed of polyethylene terephthalate and is a hydrophilic, heavyweight, macroporous mesh
B. This mesh has several different weaves that can yield a 2-dimensional flat screen-like mesh and a 3-dimensional multifilament weave
C. When it is placed in the preperitoneal position in complex ventral hernia repairs, complication rates are comparable to other products
D. All of the above

106. False about PTFE mesh is:

A. Encapsulation occurs slowly and infection can occur during the encapsulation process
B. This prosthetic has a visceral side that is microporous (3 μm) and an abdominal wall side that is macroporous (17–22 μm) and promotes tissue ingrowth
C. Some fibroblast proliferation occurs through the pores, and PTFE is permeable to fluid
D. Encapsulation occurs slowly and infection can occur during the encapsulation process

107. False about biologic prostheses for ventral hernia is:

A. Biologic prostheses for ventral hernia repair are non synthetic, natural tissue mesh
B. These products are largely composed of cellular collagen
C. Biologic mesh has found increased use in very challenging contaminated situations where permanent prosthetic use would be ill advised and native tissue coverage is difficult or impossible
D. Biologic mesh used in a bridge configuration can be used to minimize evisceration and provide a barrier separating viscera from atmosphere

108. Which of the following is not derived from human dermis?

A. Permacol B. AlloDerm
C. AlloMax D. FlexHD

109. Which of the following is not derived from porcine dermis?

A. Veritas B. Strattice
C. XenMatrix D. Surgisis

110. False about absorbable synthetic materials is:

A. The original absorbable synthetic material used for repair, polyglactin, remains a mainstay of managing challenging situations in contaminated fields
B. Polyglactin is slowly absorbable and hydrolyzes completely in 8 to 9 months
C. Slowly resorbable polyglactin mesh was found to have an acceptable recurrence rate of 17% when placed in a retromuscular position during contaminated complex ventral hernia repair
D. Poly-4-hydroxybutyrate resorbs completely between 12 and 18 months

111. Following image shows which technique of abdominal wall reconstruction?

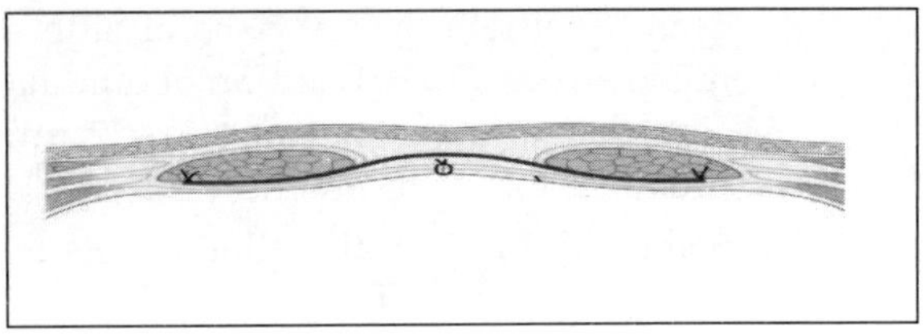

A. Sublay (Preperitoneal)
B. Sublay (Retromuscular)
C. Sublay (Intraperitoneal)
D. Inlay

112. Following image shows which technique of abdominal wall reconstruction?

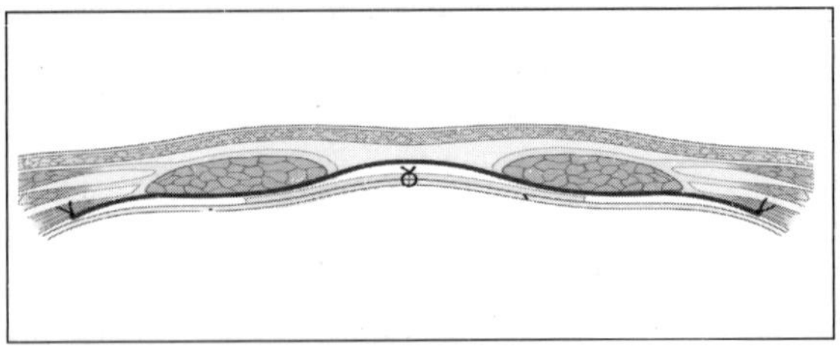

A. Sublay (Preperitoneal)
B. Sublay (Retromuscular)
C. Sublay (Intraperitoneal)
D. Inlay

113. Following image shows which technique of abdominal wall reconstruction?

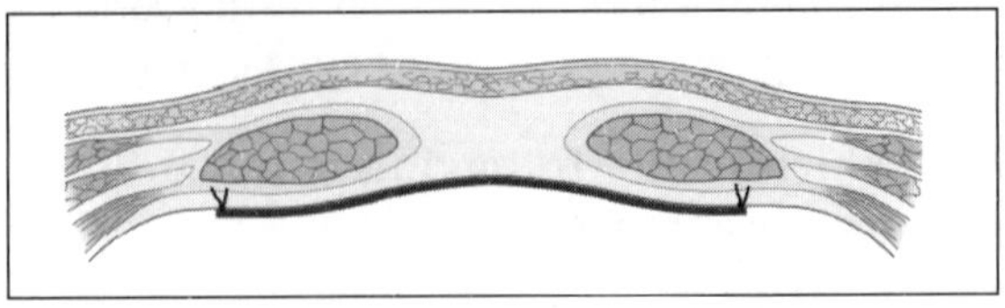

A. Sublay (Preperitoneal)
B. Sublay (Retromuscular)
C. Sublay (Intraperitoneal)
D. Inlay

114. False statement among the following is:

A. The onlay technique involves primary closure of the fascia defect and placement of a mesh over the anterior fascia
B. Modifications of the traditional onlay repair in highly selected patients using midweight polypropylene mesh and fibrin glue fixation have shown comparable infection rates compared to permanent synthetic mesh placed in the sublay position
C. Interposition prosthetic repairs involve securing the mesh to the fascial edge without overlap
D. It is highly desirable to have the mesh placed above the fascia

115. False about intraperitoneal mesh placement is:

A. Mesh can be placed in an intraperitoneal position at least 4 cm beyond the fascial margin and secured with interrupted mattress sutures
B. A minimum 5-cm overlap should be utilized beyond the edge of the fascial defect
C. The laparoscopic approach for ventral hernia repair relies on the same principles as the retrorectus repair; however, the mesh is placed within the peritoneal cavity
D. There are fewer wound complications with the laparoscopic approach because large incisions and subcutaneous undermining are avoided

116. False about posterior rectus sheath incision with retromuscular mesh placement is:

A. This technique involves placing prosthetic mesh in the extraperitoneal position in the preperitoneal space or retrorectus position
B. A large piece of mesh is placed in the retromuscular space behind the posterior rectus sheath
C. Retromuscular space must be dissected laterally on both sides of the linea alba to a distance of 8 to 10 cm beyond the defect
D. The prosthetic mesh extends 5 to 6 cm beyond the superior and inferior borders of the defect

117. In posterior component separation advancement can be obtained by incising the posterior rectus sheath approximately:

A. 1 cm medial to the linea semilunaris
B. 1 cm lateral to the linea semilunaris
C. 2 cm medial to the linea semilunaris
D. 2 cm lateral to the linea semilunaris

118. In anterior component separation, on the lateral external oblique aponeurosis from several centimeters above the costal margin to the pubis, a relaxing incision is made:

A. 5 cm medial to the linea semilunaris
B. 5 cm lateral to the linea semilunaris
C. 2 cm medial to the linea semilunaris
D. 2 cm lateral to the linea semilunaris

119. False about robotic intraperitoneal mesh placement is:

A. After identification of the entire hernia defect, it is closed with a continuous barbed suture
B. A tissue separating mesh is chosen and typically sized to overlap the size of the original hernia defect by 8 to 10 cm on each side

C. The "baseball" stitch alternates between the edge of the mesh and the adjacent peritoneum/posterior fascia

D. The "dolphin" stitch is a horizontal mattress-type suture placed just inside the edge of the mesh, where the suture passes through the mesh, through the tissue and back through the mesh

120. False about robotic retromuscular repair with TAR is:

A. Patients with risk factors for increased wound morbidity, such as smoking, diabetes, and obesity, appear to be well suited for robotic hernia repair

B. A robotic approach is ideal as the surgeon can replicate the steps of an open repair, with the benefit of decreased wound complications seen with laparoscopic surgery

C. An increased SSO rate was noted with the robotic approach, which were mostly seromas

D. Defects 20 to 25 cm in widest dimension seem to be best suited for the robotic TAR technique with good cosmetic results

121. Following image shows:

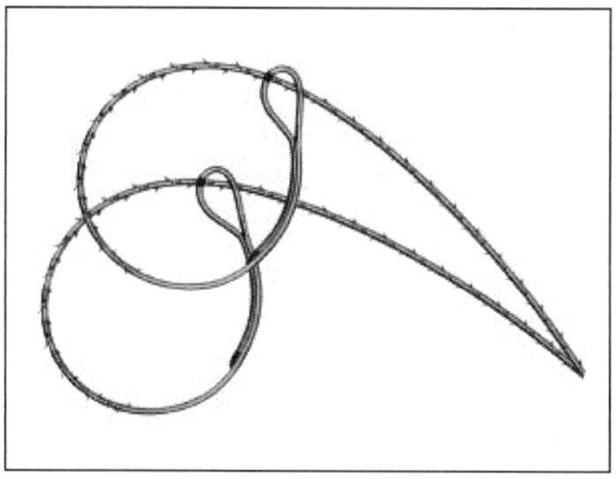

A. Barbed suture material

B. Force Fiber Fusion

C. Smart surgical suture

D. Zipstitch suture material

122. The following image shows:

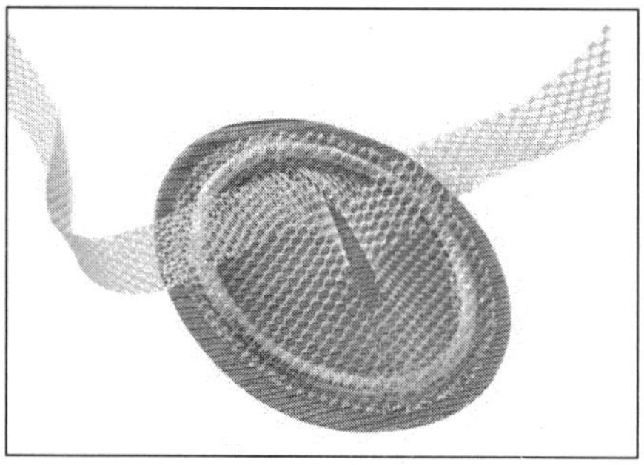

A. Ventralex™ hernia patch

B. Dextile™ anatomical mesh

C. Parietene™ DS Composite Mesh

D. ProGrip™ Laparoscopic Self-Fixating Mesh

123. The following image shows:

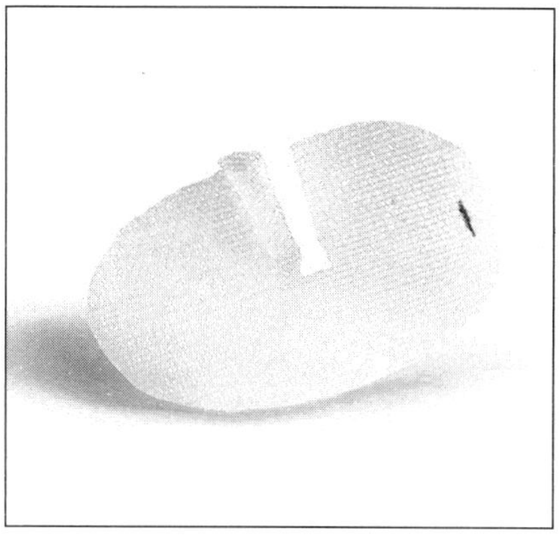

A. Ventralex™ hernia patch

B. Dextile™ anatomical mesh

C. Parietene™ DS Composite Mesh

D. Parietex ProGrip™ Self-Fixating Mesh

124. The following image shows:

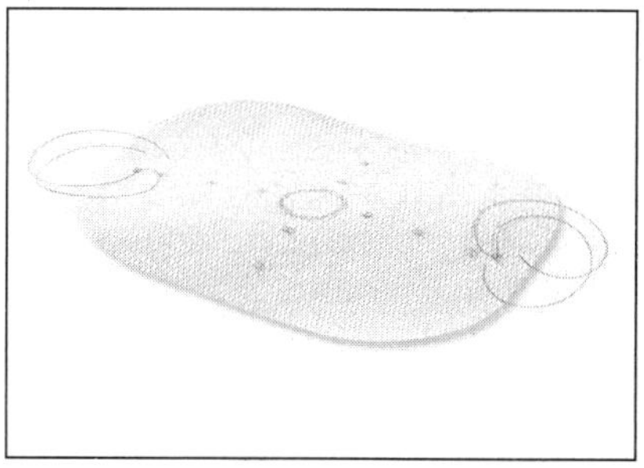

A. Ventralex™ hernia patch

B. Dextile™ anatomical mesh

C. Parietene™ DS Composite Mesh

D. Parietex ProGrip™ Self-Fixating Mesh

125. The following image shows:

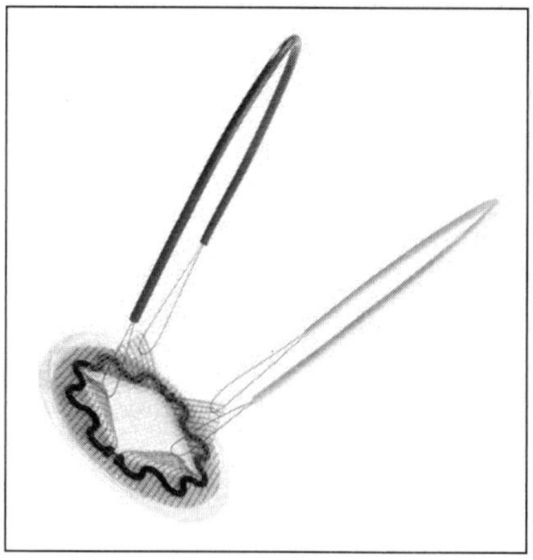

A. Parietex™ Plug and Patch System
B. Parietex™ Composite Ventral Patch
C. Parietex™ Composite (PCO) Parastomal Mesh
D. Parietex™ Composite Hiatal (PCO 2H) Mesh

126. The following image shows:

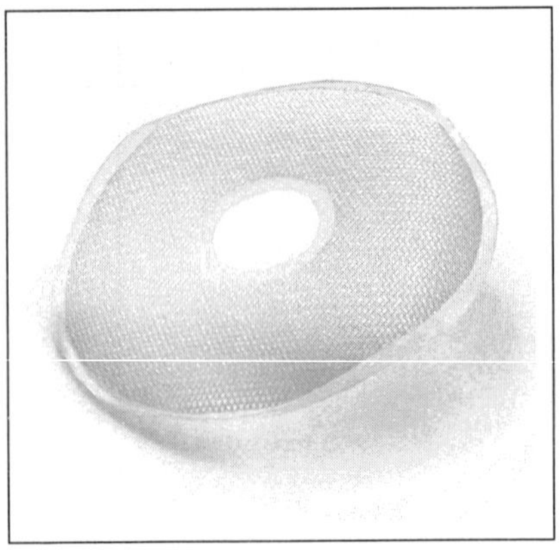

A. Parietex™ Plug and Patch System
B. Parietex™ Composite Ventral Patch
C. Parietex™ Composite (PCO) Parastomal Mesh
D. Parietex™ Composite Hiatal (PCO 2H) Mesh

UNUSUAL HERNIAS

127. False about spigelian hernia is:

A. A spigelian hernia occurs through the spigelian fascia, which is composed of the aponeurotic layer between the rectus muscle medially and semilunar line laterally
B. The absence of posterior rectus fascia may contribute to an inherent weakness in this area
C. Most spigelian hernias are small (1–2 cm in diameter) and develop during the 4th to 7th decades of life
D. A spigelian hernia is generally not repaired because of the risk for incarceration associated with it is very low

128. False about the treatment of spigelian hernia is:

A. A spigelian hernia is repaired because of the risk for incarceration associated with its relatively narrow neck
B. The hernia site is marked before operation; the DASH technique is very useful to localize the hernia prior to anesthetic induction and can minimize the size of open incision
C. The defect is closed transversely by simple suture repair of the transversus abdominis and internal oblique muscles, followed by closure of the external oblique aponeurosis
D. Recurrence is common

129. False about Obturator hernia is:

A. Weakening of the obturator membrane may result in enlargement of the canal and formation of a hernia sac, which can lead to intestinal incarceration and strangulation
B. The patient can present with evidence of compression of the obturator nerve, which causes pain in the anteromedial aspect of the thigh (Howship-Romberg sign) that is relieved by thigh flexion
C. The obturator foramen is repaired with prosthetic mesh, with care taken to avoid injury to the obturator nerve and vessels
D. A anterior approach, open or laparoscopic, is preferred

130. Percentage of patients with obturator hernia that present with complete or partial bowel obstruction is:

A. 20% B. 30%
C. 50% D. 70%

131. False about lumbar hernia is:

A. Lumbar hernias can be congenital or acquired after an operation on the flank and occur in the lumbar region of the posterior abdominal wall
B. Hernias through the inferior lumbar triangle (Petit triangle) are more common
C. Lumbar hernias are not prone to incarceration
D. Repair is best done by placement of prosthetic mesh, which is sutured beyond the margins of the hernia

132. The superior lumbar triangle is bounded all except:

A. Paraspinal muscles
B. 12th rib
C. Internal oblique muscle
D. External oblique muscle

133. Inferior lumbar triangle (Petit triangle), is bounded by all except:

A. External oblique muscle
B. Internal oblique muscle
C. The iliac crest
D. Latissimus dorsi muscle

134. False about Interparietal hernias is:

A. Interparietal hernias are very common and occur when the hernia sac lies between layers of the abdominal wall
B. Spigelian hernias are almost always interparietal

C. Large interparietal hernias usually require placement of prosthetic mesh for closure
D. These hernias most frequently occur in previous incisions

135. False about Sciatic hernia is:

A. The gluteus maximus muscle is opened, and the sac is visualized and muscle edges of the defect are reapproximated with interrupted sutures, or the defect is obliterated with mesh
B. These hernias are extremely unusual and difficult to diagnose and frequently are asymptomatic until intestinal obstruction occurs
C. In the absence of intestinal obstruction, the most common symptom is the presence of an uncomfortable or slowly enlarging mass in the gluteal or intragluteal area
D. Prosthetic mesh repair is usually not preferred

136. True about Perineal hernias is:

A. Perineal hernias are caused by congenital or acquired defects and may also occur after abdominoperineal resection or perineal prostatectomy
B. Symptoms are usually related to protrusion of a mass through the defect that is worsened by sitting or standing and a bulge is frequently detected on bimanual rectal-vaginal examination
C. Perineal hernias are generally repaired through a transabdominal approach or combined transabdominal and perineal approaches
D. All of the above

137. True about loss of domain hernia is:

A. Loss of domain implies a massive hernia in which the herniated contents have resided for so long outside the abdominal cavity that they cannot simply be replaced into the peritoneal cavity
B. A staged approach using ePTFE dual mesh for patients with loss of abdominal domain and lateral retraction of the abdominal wall musculature can be used
C. Repeated administrations of increasing volumes of air during 1 to 3 weeks allowed the muscles of the abdominal wall to become lax enough for primary closure of the defect & this technique is particularly suited for small defects and massive hernia sacs
D. All of the above

138. False about Parastomal hernia is:

A. The incidence of parastomal hernias is highest for colostomies and occurs in up to 50% of stomas
B. Most patients remain symptomatic, and life-threatening complications, such as bowel obstruction and strangulation, are common
C. Primary fascial repair involves hernia reduction and primary fascial reapproximation through a parastomal incision and this technique carries a predictably high recurrence rate
D. Prosthetic repairs of parastomal hernias can provide excellent long-term results with a lower rate of hernia recurrence, but a higher rate of prosthetic complications must be accepted

139. Surgical approaches for parastomal hernia repair includes:

A. Sugarbaker technique
B. Keyhole technique
C. Resisting with mesh reinforcement
D. All of the above

140. Identify the procedure for parastomal hernia shown in the image:

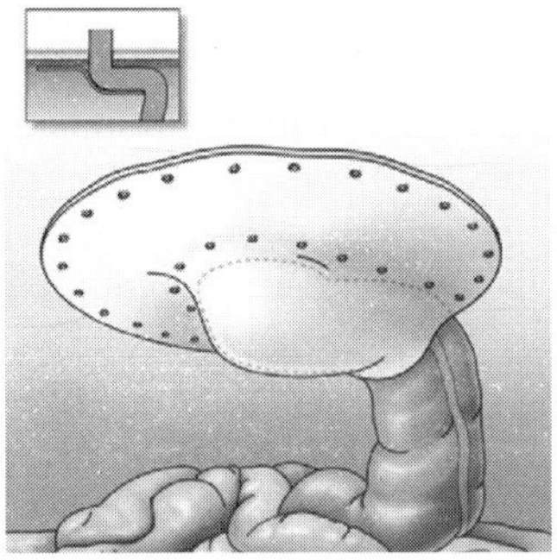

A. Sugarbaker technique
B. Keyhole technique
C. Resisting with mesh reinforcement
D. Bassini's technique

141. Identify the procedure for parastomal hernia shown in the image:

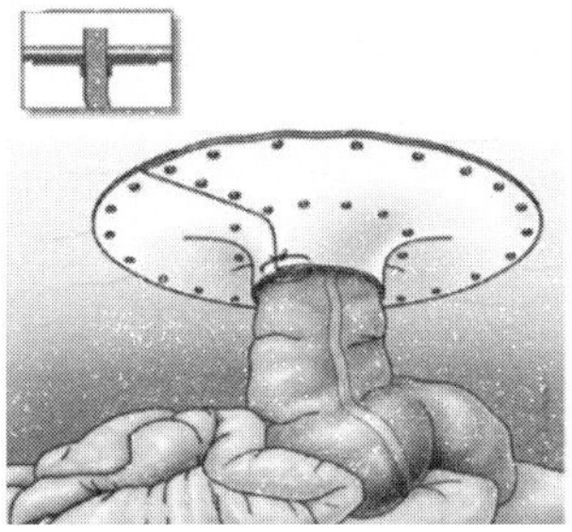

A. Sugarbaker technique
B. Keyhole technique
C. Resisting with mesh reinforcement
D. Bassini's technique

142. False about mesh infections is:

A. In acute infection with sepsis, the patients are emergently and aggressively treated including monitored admission to the hospital, intravenous antibiotics, and early debrided and mesh removal
B. If ePTFE becomes infected, it requires removal with the resultant morbidity of another defect, which often must be closed under tension, leading to inevitable recurrence
C. Infected polyester mesh often requires at least partial removal; areas of mesh that are still clearly well incorporated at the time of operation can usually be left in place taking into consideration the morbidity of complete removal
D. Polyester products tend to be the most successful in terms of mesh salvage

143. False about seroma formation is:

A. Seroma formation can occur after open ventral hernia repair and not after laparoscopic repair
B. Most of these seromas will resolve over time as the mesh becomes incorporated on the hernia sac
C. In open ventral hernia repair, drains are often placed in an attempt to obliterate the dead space caused by the hernia and tissue dissection
D. Aspiration is done for symptomatic or persistent seromas after 6 to 8 weeks

ANSWERS

1. **Ans: A. There is a consistent relationship between the area of a hernia defect and the size of a hernia sac**
Ref: Chapter No.45, Page No.1105

2. **Ans: C. An internal hernia protrudes through all layers of the abdominal wall**
Ref: Chapter No.45, Page No.1105-1106

3. **Ans: A. Lumbar**
Ref: Chapter No.45, Page No.1106

4. **Ans: C. Lumbar**
Ref: Chapter No.45, Page No.1106

5. **Ans: B. Superior lumbar hernia**
Ref: Chapter No.45, Page No.1106

6. **Ans: A. Inferior lumbar hernia**
Ref: Chapter No.45, Page No.1106

7. **Ans: C. Two-thirds of these are direct and the remainder are indirect inguinal hernias**
Ref: Chapter No.45, Page No.1107

8. **Ans: C. Femoral hernias are the most common hernia in women**
Ref: Chapter No.45, Page No.1107

9. **Ans: D. 25 times**
Ref: Chapter No.45, Page No.1107

10. **Ans: D. 50%**
Ref: Chapter No.45, Page No.1107

11. **Ans: D. Hernias generally occur with equal frequency in males and females**
Ref: Chapter No.45, Page No.1107

12. **Ans: A. 10%**
Ref: Chapter No.45, Page No.1107

13. **Ans: A. Indirect inguinal and femoral hernias occur more commonly on the left side**
Ref: Chapter No.45, Page No.1107

14. **Ans: A. Most strangulated hernias are direct inguinal hernias**
Ref: Chapter No.45, Page No.1107

15. **Ans: B. Aponeurosis, along with the bilaminar aponeuroses of the internal oblique and transversus abdominis, forms the posterior rectus sheath**
Ref: Chapter No.45, Page No.1107-1108

16. **Ans: A. Poupart ligament**
Ref: Chapter No.45, Page No.1108

17. **Ans: B. Lacunar ligament**
Ref: Chapter No.45, Page No.1108

18. **Ans: C. Cooper's ligament**
Ref: Chapter No.45, Page No.1108

19. **Ans: A. The internal oblique muscle serves as the posterior border of the inguinal canal**
Ref: Chapter No.45, Page No.1108

20. **Ans: B. 5% to 10% of patients**

Ref: Chapter No.45, Page No.1108

21. **Ans: C. The transversalis fascia, sometimes referred to as the endoabdominal fascia, is a component of the inguinal floor and tends to be thinner in this area**

Ref: Chapter No.45, Page No.1108-1109

22. **Ans: D. The femoral, lateral femoral cutaneous and genitofemoral nerves are located superior to the iliopubic tract**

Ref: Chapter No.45, Page No.1108-1109

23. **Ans: A. This structure is anterior to the iliopubic tract and forms the anterior border of the femoral canal**

Ref: Chapter No.45, Page No.1109

24. **Ans: C. Indirect hernias occur within Hesselbach triangle, whereas direct inguinal hernias arise lateral to the triangle**

Ref: Chapter No.45, Page No.1109

25. **Ans: A. Femoral branch of the genitofemoral nerve**

Ref: Chapter No.45, Page No.1109

26. **Ans: B. Inferior epigastric vessels**

Ref: Chapter No.45, Page No.1109

27. **Ans: C. Superiorly: Superior epigastric vessels**

Ref: Chapter No.45, Page No.1109

28. **Ans: B. Lacunar ligament**

Ref: Chapter No.45, Page No.1109

29. **Ans: D. The femoral branch of the genitofemoral nerve innervates the cremaster muscle and skin on the lateral side of the scrotum and labia**

Ref: Chapter No.45, Page No.1109

30. **Ans: B. The lateral femoral cutaneous nerve originates as a root of L4 – L5 and is occasionally a direct branch of the femoral nerve**

Ref: Chapter No.45, Page No.1109

31. **Ans: D. Lacunar ligament medially**

Femoral triangle: (SAIL)

Lateral border: **S**artorius muscle

Medial border: **A**dductor longus muscle

Base or superior border: **I**nguinal **L**igament

Contents of femoral triangle: (NAVEL)

Femoral **N**erve, Femoral **A**rtery, Femoral **V**ein, Femoral canal (**E**mpty space), **L**ymphatics

Ref: Chapter No.45, Page No.1109

32. **Ans: A. The inguinal region is examined with the patient in the only supine position**

Ref: Chapter No.45, Page No.1110

33. **Ans: C. Popliteal artery aneurysm**

Ref: Chapter No.45, Page No.1111

34. **Ans: C. Type III**

Ref: Chapter No.45, Page No.1111

35. **Ans: D. Type IV**

Ref: Chapter No.45, Page No.1111

36. **Ans: A. Type I**

Ref: Chapter No.45, Page No.1111

37. **Ans: B. Symptom control has been reported in about 70% of patients**

Ref: Chapter No.45, Page No.1111

38. **Ans: C. The cremaster muscle of the mobilized spermatic cord is separated perpendicularly to its fibers from the underlying cord structures**

Ref: Chapter No.45, Page No.1111-1112

39. **Ans: B. The transversus abdominis and internal oblique musculoaponeurotic arches or conjoined tendon to the inguinal ligament**

Ref: Chapter No.45, Page No.1112

40. **Ans: A. Cooper's ligament repair**

Ref: Chapter No.45, Page No.1112

41. **Ans: D. The Shouldice repair is associated with a high recurrence rate and a low degree of patient satisfaction in patients**

Ref: Chapter No.45, Page No.1112

42. **Ans: A. Bassini repair**

Ref: Chapter No.45, Page No.1112

43. **Ans: D. Shouldice repair**

Ref: Chapter No.45, Page No.1112

44. **Ans: B. Lichtenstein repair**

Ref: Chapter No.45, Page No.1112

45. **Ans: D. The sandwich technique involves a bilayered device with 2 polypropylene components**

Ref: Chapter No.45, Page No.1112-1113

46. **Ans: C. Unilateral hernias**

Ref: Chapter No.45, Page No.1114

47. **Ans: A. The medial aspect of the mesh overlaps the pubic bone by approximately 1 cm**

Ref: Chapter No.45, Page No.1114

48. **Ans: B. The inferior epigastric artery and veins are generally beneath the midportion of the posterior rectus sheath and usually need to be divided**

Ref: Chapter No.45, Page No.1114

49. **Ans: A. Laparoscopic repair is associated with an approximately 3% risk of visceral or vascular injury**

Ref: Chapter No.45, Page No.1115

50. **Ans: D. Iliopubic tract (The importance of this triangle is in this area you can find the *external iliac artery and vein*)**

Ref: Chapter No.45, Page No.1115

51. **Ans: A. Ductus deferens (Nerve injury can result in *chronic pain*)**

Ref: Chapter No.45, Page No.1115

52. **Ans: B. The genital branch of the genitofemoral nerve**

SYSTEMIZATION OF LAPAROSCOPIC INGUINAL HERNIA REPAIR (TAPP) BASED ON A. NEW ANATOMICAL CONCEPT: INVERTED Y AND 5 TRIANGLES

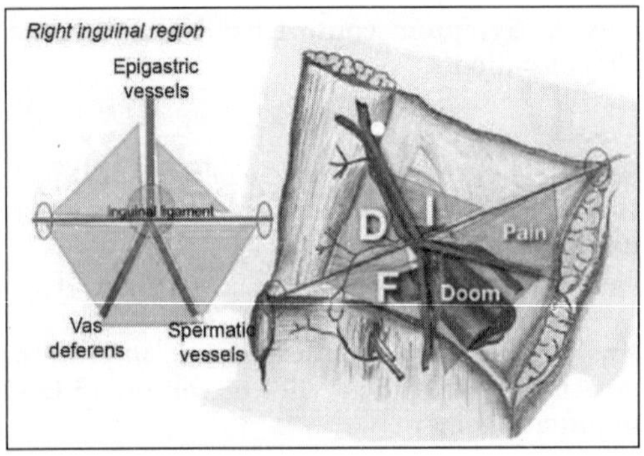

Illustration of **"5 triangles"**:

(A) Illustration of the iliopubic tract crossing the ***inverted Y*** and formation of the 5 triangles.

(B) Anatomical scheme of the inverted Y formed by inferior epigastric vessels, vas deferens and spermatic vessels.

The figure also illustrates in a didactic way the representation of 5 triangles, clockwise: indirect hernias (I), pain (P), doom (D), femoral (F) and direct (D) hernias

Ref: Chapter No.45, Page No.1115

https://doi.org/10.1590/0102-672020180001e1426

53. **Ans: A. Local anesthesia with sedation is the most common form of anesthesia used**

Ref: Chapter No.45, Page No.1115

54. **Ans: D. The Shouldice repair has a lower recurrence rate than mesh repairs**

Ref: Chapter No.45, Page No.1115-1117

55. **Ans: C. Chronic pain**

Ref: Chapter No.45, Page No.1118

56. **Ans: D. Recurrence**

Ref: Chapter No.45, Page No.1118

57. **Ans: C. Prostatitis**

Ref: Chapter No.45, Page No.1118

58. **Ans: C. Total extraperitoneal repair (TEP) is a laparoscopic approach that stays in the preperitoneal space by using a balloon dissector**

Ref: Chapter No.45, Page No.1111-1117

59. **Ans: B. The lateral-most border of the dissection is the anterior superior iliac spine**

Ref: Chapter No.45, Page No.1111-1117

60. **Ans: A. Approximately 50% of men with a femoral hernia will have an associated direct inguinal hernia, whereas this relationship occurs in only 20% of women**

Some unusual femoral hernias:

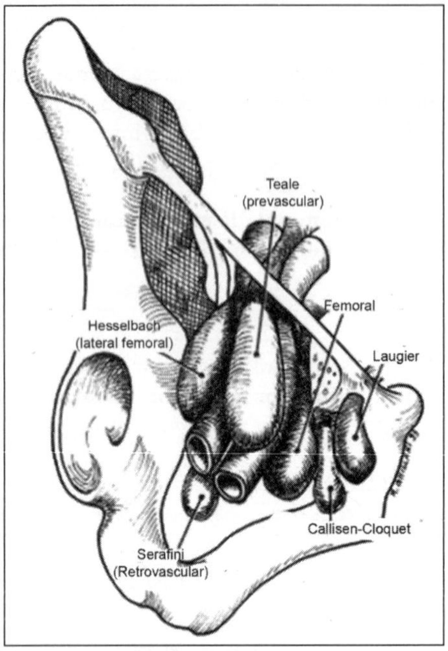

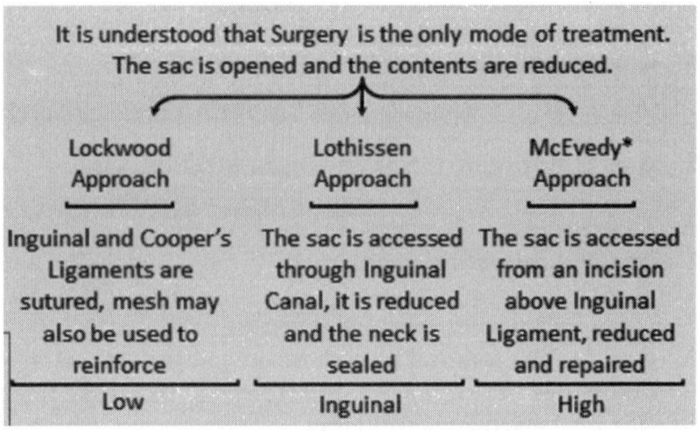

Ref: Chapter No.45, Page No.1117

https://link.springer.com/chapter/10.1007/978-1-4419-8574-3_68

61. **Ans: B. If an incarcerated femoral hernia cannot be reduced intraoperatively, the insertion of the inguinal ligament can be cut from the pubic tubercle to allow more space**

Ref: Chapter No.45, Page No.1117

62. **Ans: B. Recurrences after anterior hernia repair using mesh are best managed by a laparoscopic or open posterior approach, without placement of a second prosthesis**

Ref: Chapter No.45, Page No.1118

63. **Ans: D. Both A and C**

Ref: Chapter No.45, Page No.1118

64. **Ans: B. Most sliding hernias are a variant of direct inguinal hernias, although femoral and indirect sliding hernias can occur**

Ref: Chapter No.45, Page No.1118

65. **Ans: B. 10%**

Ref: Chapter No.45, Page No.1118

66. Ans: A. The risk for surgical site infection is estimated to be 5% to 10% after open inguinal hernia repair and slightly less with laparoscopic repairs

Ref: Chapter No.45, Page No.1118-1119

67. Ans: B. The use of prosthetic mesh can result in dysesthesias, which are usually permanent

Ref: Chapter No.45, Page No.1119

68. Ans: D. Lateral femoral cutaneous nerve (Affected in laparoscopic repair)

Ref: Chapter No.45, Page No.1119

69. Ans: C. > 3 months after operation

Ref: Chapter No.45, Page No.1119

70. Ans: D. Early symptoms are treated with surgical removal of mesh

Ref: Chapter No.45, Page No.1119

71. Ans: B. 2 to 5 days

Ref: Chapter No.45, Page No.1119

72. Ans: D. Orchiectomy is often necessary

Ref: Chapter No.45, Page No.1119

73. Ans: B. 3-4

Ref: Chapter No.45, Page No.1119

74. Ans: B. Less tension on the repair

Ref: Chapter No.45, Page No.1119

75. Ans: A. Recurrences are best managed by excision prosthesis and repair without mesh

Ref: Chapter No.45, Page No.1119

76. Ans: D. 60%

Ref: Chapter No.45, Page No.1120

77. Ans: D. Diastasis recti can present as a midline bulge with a hernia sac

Ref: Chapter No.45, Page No.1120

78. Ans: D. Incisional hernias are twice as common in men as in women

Ref: Chapter No.45, Page No.1120

79. Ans: A. Female gender

Ref: Chapter No.45, Page No.1120

80. Ans: C. The posterior rectus sheath below the arcuate line is composed of the peritoneum only

Ref: Chapter No.45, Page No.1120-1121

81. Ans: C. Deep superior epigastric artery

Ref: Chapter No.45, Page No.1121

82. Ans: D. All of the above

Ref: Chapter No.45, Page No.1121

83. Ans: D. Umbilical hernias in adults are largely congenital

Ref: Chapter No.45, Page No.1121-1122

84. Ans: C. 2 years

Ref: Chapter No.45, Page No.1121

85. Ans: C. Repair in adults is generally indicated

Ref: Chapter No.45, Page No.1121

86. Ans: D. 5 years

Ref: Chapter No.45, Page No.1121

87. Ans: D. Mayo's repair is the most common repair for umbilical hernia performed today

Ref: Chapter No.45, Page No.1122

88. Ans: B. Mayo's repair

Ref: Chapter No.45, Page No.1122

89. Ans: A. Epigastric hernias are 2 to 3 times more common in women

Ref: Chapter No.45, Page No.1122

90. Ans: C. Epigastric hernias are better repaired preperitoneally

Ref: Chapter No.45, Page No.1122

91. Ans: B. Conditions that decrease intra-abdominal pressure are factors that predispose to the development of an incisional hernia

Ref: Chapter No.45, Page No.1122

92. Ans: D. All of the above

Ref: Chapter No.45, Page No.1122

93. Ans: A. Laparoscopic hernia repairs have lower rates of wound infections than open repairs

Ref: Chapter No.45, Page No.1115-1124

94. Ans: A. <10 cm, clean

Ref: Chapter No.45, Page No.1123

95. Ans: D. $\geq$10 cm, contaminated

Ref: Chapter No.45, Page No.1123

96. Ans: C. Incisional hernia

Ref: Chapter No.45, Page No.1123

97. Ans: B. Larger defects (<3 cm in diameter) have a high recurrence rate if closed primarily and are repaired with a prosthesis

Ref: Chapter No.45, Page No.1123

98. Ans: A. Carcinogenic

Ref: Chapter No.45, Page No.1123

99. Ans: B. Polypropylene mesh is a hydrophilic macroporous mesh that allows the ingrowth of native fibroblasts and incorporation into the surrounding fascia

Ref: Chapter No.45, Page No.1123

100. Ans: B. < 40 g/m^2

Ref: Chapter No.45, Page No.1123

101. Ans: C. >75 g/m^2

Ref: Chapter No.45, Page No.1123

102. Ans: C. Polypropylene meshes have high adhesion risks, so they should not be placed directly next to bowel

Ref: Chapter No.45, Page No.1123-1124

103. Ans: C. 60 to 75 g/m^2

Ref: Chapter No.45, Page No.1123

104. Ans: C. In a randomized controlled trial evaluating lightweight versus heavyweight polypropylene mesh for ventral hernia repair, the recurrence rate in the heavyweight group was more than twice that in the lightweight group

Ref: Chapter No.45, Page No.1123

105. Ans: D. All of the above

Ref: Chapter No.45, Page No.1124

106. Ans: C. Some fibroblast proliferation occurs through the pores and PTFE is permeable to fluid

Ref: Chapter No.45, Page No.1124

107. Ans: B. These products are largely composed of cellular collagen

Ref: Chapter No.45, Page No.1124

108. Ans: A. Permacol

Ref: Chapter No.45, Page No.1124

109. Ans: D. Surgisis

Ref: Chapter No.45, Page No.1124

110. Ans: B. Polyglactin is slowly absorbable and hydrolyzes completely in 8 to 9 months

Ref: Chapter No.45, Page No.1124-1125

111. Ans: B. Sublay (Retromuscular)

Ref: Chapter No.45, Page No.1125

112. Ans: A. Sublay (Preperitoneal)

Ref: Chapter No.45, Page No.1125

113. Ans: C. Sublay (Intraperitoneal)

Ref: Chapter No.45, Page No.1125

114. Ans: D. It is highly desirable to have the mesh placed above the fascia

Ref: Chapter No.45, Page No.1125

115. Ans: B. A minimum 5-cm overlap should be utilized beyond the edge of the fascial defect

Ref: Chapter No.45, Page No.1125

116. Ans: B. A large piece of mesh is placed in the retromuscular space behind the posterior rectus sheath

Ref: Chapter No.45, Page No.1125-1126

117. Ans: A. 1 cm medial to the linea semilunaris

Ref: Chapter No.45, Page No.1126

118. Ans: D. 2 cm lateral to the linea semilunaris

Ref: Chapter No.45, Page No.1126

119. Ans: B. A tissue separating mesh is chosen and typically sized to overlap the size of the original hernia defect by 8 to 10 cm on each side

Ref: Chapter No.45, Page No.1127

120. Ans: D. Defects 20 to 25 cm in widest dimension seem to be best suited for the robotic TAR technique with good cosmetic results

Ref: Chapter No.45, Page No.1127

121. Ans: A. Barbed suture material (V-loc)

Ref: Chapter No.45, Page No.1127
https://www.sciencedirect.com/topics/medicine-and-dentistry/barbed-suture

122. Ans: A. Ventralex™ hernia patch

Ref: https://www.medtronic.com/covidien/en-us/products/hernia-repair/mesh-products

123. Ans: D. Parietex ProGrip™ Self-Fixating Mesh

Parietex ProGrip™ self-fixating mesh: Delivers security, patient comfort and ease of use.

- Its advanced ***micro grip*** technology provides ***immediate fixation*** of the entire mesh surface for a secure repair and ***even distribution of tension*** for patient comfort
- Designed for ease of use, the ***resorbable polylactic acid (PLA) micrograps*** enable surgeons to position and place the mesh in ***under 60 seconds***, without the use of additional fixation
- Surgeons and patients can depend on a secure repair with the potential for greater patient comfort

Ref: https://www.medtronic.com/covidien/en-us/products/hernia-repair/mesh-products

124. Ans: C. Parietene™ DS Composite Mesh

Parietene™ DS Composite Mesh:

- A strong, easy-to-use mesh for open and laparoscopic ventral hernia repairs
- On one side, a ***macroporous mesh*** to repair ventral hernia defects
- On the other, an ***absorbable synthetic film*** to minimize unwanted tissue attachment
- Two unique sides. One unique mesh.

Ref: https://www.medtronic.com/covidien/en-us/products/hernia-repair/mesh-products

125. Ans: B. Parietex™ Composite Ventral Patch

Parietex™ Composite Ventral Patch:

- Parietex™ Composite ventral patch is a mesh specifically designed for ***small ventral hernia repair.***
- The shape, size and the specific fixation and deployment system have been designed for ***optimal abdominal wall conformability and easy deployment and fixation***

Ref: https://www.medtronic.com/covidien/en-us/products/hernia-repair/mesh-products

126. Ans: C. Parietex™ Composite (PCO) Parastomal Mesh

Parietex™ Composite (PCO) parastomal mesh: Is a

monofilament mesh providing a custom design for parastomal hernia repair

- While ordinary meshes carry the risk of in-growth into the bowel, Parietex™ Composite is ***coated with a protective collagen-based film*** to help prevent tissue attachment
- Its unique design provides for ***easy placement of the mesh*** for parastomal hernia repair

Ref: https://www.medtronic.com/covidien/en-us/products/hernia-repair/mesh-products

127. Ans: D. A spigelian hernia is generally not repaired because of the risk for incarceration associated with it is very low

Ref: Chapter No.45, Page No.1128

128. Ans: D. Recurrence is common

Ref: Chapter No.45, Page No.1128

129. Ans: D. An anterior approach, open or laparoscopic, is preferred

Ref: Chapter No.45, Page No.1129

130. Ans: C. 50%

Ref: Chapter No.45, Page No.1129

131. Ans: B. Hernias through the inferior lumbar triangle (Petit triangle) are more common

Ref: Chapter No.45, Page No.1129

132. Ans: D. External oblique muscle

Ref: Chapter No.45, Page No.1129

133. Ans: B. Internal oblique muscle

Ref: Chapter No.45, Page No.1129

134. Ans: A. Interparietal hernias are very common and occur when the hernia sac lies between layers of the abdominal wall

Ref: Chapter No.45, Page No.1129

135. Ans: D. Prosthetic mesh repair is usually not preferred

Ref: Chapter No.45, Page No.1129

136. Ans: D. All of the above

Ref: Chapter No.45, Page No.1129

137. Ans: D. All of the above

Ref: Chapter No.45, Page No.1129

138. Ans: B. Most patients remain symptomatic, and life-threatening complications, such as bowel obstruction and strangulation, are common

Ref: Chapter No.45, Page No.1130

139. Ans: D. All of the above

Ref: Chapter No.45, Page No.1130

140. Ans: A. Sugarbaker technique

Ref: Chapter No.45, Page No.1130

141. Ans: B. Keyhole technique

Ref: Chapter No.45, Page No.1130

142. Ans: D. Polyester products tend to be the most successful in terms of mesh salvage

Ref: Chapter No.45, Page No.1130

143. Ans: A. Seroma formation can occur after open ventral hernia repair and not after laparoscopic repair

Ref: Chapter No.45, Page No.1130

46

Acute Abdomen

1. **True among the following is/are:**
   A. Diseases like appendicitis and mesenteric adenitis are more common in the young
   B. Toxins and drugs that can cause acute abdominal pain are lead and other heavy metal intoxications, narcotic withdrawal and black widow spider bites
   C. Biliary tract disease, diverticulitis and intestinal ischemia are more common in older populations
   D. All of the above

ANATOMY AND PHYSIOLOGY

2. **False about abdominal pain is:**
   A. Parietal pain is sharper and better localized than visceral pain
   B. Parietal pain is usually due to the distention of a hollow viscus
   C. Visceral pain is vague
   D. Referred pain is perceived at a site distant from the source of the pain

3. **Which among the following is not a nonsurgical cause of the acute abdomen?**
   A. Hemorrhagic pancreatitis
   B. Sickle cell crisis
   C. Acute leukemia
   D. Uremia

4. **Which among the following is not a surgical cause of the acute abdomen?**
   A. Ischemic colitis
   B. Buerger's disease
   C. Acute intermittent porphyria
   D. Gastrointestinal malignancy

5. **Which among the following is not a nonsurgical cause of the acute abdomen?**
   A. Mediterranean fever
   B. Addisonian crisis Hereditary
   C. Diabetic crisis
   D. All of the above are nonsurgical cause of the acute abdomen

6. **All of the following are referred to left shoulder except:**
   A. Heart
   B. Left hemidiaphragm
   C. Spleen
   D. Ureter

7. **All of the following are referred to right shoulder except:**
   A. Gallbladder
   B. Duodenum
   C. Liver
   D. Right hemidiaphragm

HISTORY

8. **False about vomiting is:**
   A. With an underlying surgical cause, vomiting precedes the pain
   B. Vomiting is more likely to precede the onset of significant abdominal pain in many nonsurgical conditions
   C. Vomiting may occur because of severe abdominal pain of any cause or as a result of either mechanical bowel obstruction or ileus
   D. All of the above true

9. **False about medications and acute abdominal conditions is:**
   A. NSAIDs drugs are associated with upper gastrointestinal inflammation and perforation

B. High dose narcotics can interfere with bowel motility and lead to obstipation and obstruction
C. Cocaine and methamphetamine use can create an intense vasodilatation
D. Narcotics can also contribute to spasm of the sphincter of Oddi and exacerbate biliary or pancreatic pain

PHYSICAL EXAMINATION

10. Ileus is associated with hearing fewer than:

A. 1 bowel sounds every 15 seconds per quadrant
B. 1 bowel sounds every 30 seconds per quadrant
C. 2 bowel sounds every 60 seconds per quadrant
D. 1 bowel sounds every 60 seconds per quadrant

11. Shoulder pain on inspiration is called:

A. Aaron sign
B. Danforth sign
C. Blumberg sign
D. Ten Horn sign

12. Yellow discoloration of umbilical region is seen in:

A. Hemoperitoneum
B. Portal hypertension
C. Ruptured common bile duct
D. Acute pancreatitis

13. Yellow discoloration of umbilical region is called as:

A. Cullen sign
B. Grey Turner sign
C. Cruveilhier sign
D. Ransohoff sign

14. Varicose veins at umbilicus is called as:

A. Cullen sign
B. Grey Turner sign
C. Cruveilhier sign
D. Ransohoff sign

15. Sharp pain created by compressing appendix between abdominal wall and iliacus is called:

A. Aaron sign
B. Bassler sign
C. Carnett sign
D. Murphy sign

16. Transient abdominal wall rebound tenderness is called:

A. Rovsing sign
B. Chandelier sign
C. Blumberg sign
D. Bassler sign

17. Loss of abdominal tenderness when abdominal wall muscles contracted is called:

A. Chandelier sign
B. Bassler sign
C. Carnett sign
D. Murphy sign

18. Extreme pelvic pain with movement of the cervix is called:

A. Chandelier sign
B. Fothergill sign
C. Obturator sign
D. Ten Horn sign

19. Pain caused by gentle traction of right testicle is called:

A. Chandelier sign
B. Fothergill sign
C. Obturator sign
D. Ten Horn sign

20. Which of the following is not seen in acute appendicitis?

A. Aaron sign
B. Rovsing sign
C. Ten Horn sign
D. Fothergill sign

21. Fothergill sign is seen in:

A. Pelvic inflammatory disease
B. Rectus muscle hematoma
C. Chronic appendicitis
D. Pelvic abscess

22. Which of the following is seen in pelvic inflammatory disease?

A. Chandelier sign
B. Fothergill sign
C. Obturator sign
D. Ten Horn sign

LABORATORY STUDIES

23. Laboratory tests for abdominal pain includes:

A. Clostridium difficile culture and toxin assay
B. Serum lactate levels
C. Urine human chorionic gonadotropin
D. All of the above

24. False about USG is:

A. Ultrasound is a relatively cheap and expedient imaging modality that can be very useful in evaluating the acute abdomen
B. Ultrasonography can have limitations with visualization due to abdominal wall thickness, bowel gas contents and operator experience
C. It remains the best modality for evaluating right upper quadrant pain, especially pain that is suspected to emanate from the gallbladder
D. USG can provide more information regarding location of perforation and specific cause

INTRA-ABDOMINAL PRESSURE MONITORING

25. Abdominal compartment syndrome (ACS) has intra-abdominal pressure is sustained above:

A. 12 mm Hg
B. 15 mm Hg
C. 20 mm Hg
D. 25 mm Hg

26. **Normal intra-abdominal pressure should be:**

A. 2 - 5 mm Hg B. 5 - 7 mm Hg
C. 7 - 9 mm Hg D. 10 - 12 mm Hg

27. **Grade 3 hypertension has intra-abdominal pressure of:**

A. 16–20 mm Hg B. >25 mm Hg
C. 12–15 mm Hg D. 21–25 mm Hg

SPECIAL PATIENT POPULATIONS

28. **False about surgery in pregnancy is:**

A. Ultrasound is the initial imaging study of choice in the pregnant patient
B. Maternal hemorrhage is often compensated by increased uterine flow, and marked fetal distress is often the last manifestation of an acute surgical pathology, even before maternal hypotension or tachycardia is identified
C. Laboratory studies such as white blood cell counts and other chemistries are also altered in pregnancy, making recognition of disease processes more difficult
D. Pregnancy can alter the presentation of some disease processes and make the physical examination more challenging because of the enlarging uterus, and fear of exposure of a fetus to radiation or unnecessary procedures

29. **Studies have shown that up to ___ of ionizing radiation, results in no significant increase in teratogenic effects of radiation.**

A. 10 mGy B. 25 mGy
C. 50 mGy D. 60 mGy

30. **The most common nonobstetric abdominal emergency requiring surgery is:**

A. Acute cholecystitis
B. Acute appendicitis
C. Acute salpingitis
D. Acute intestinal obstruction

31. **For perforated appendicitis, percentage of patients who will have peritonitis or established intra-abdominal abscess at presentation:**

A. 5% B. 10%
C. 20% D. 40%

32. **In pregnancy recommended imaging study for Diverticulitis is:**

A. CT scan B. MRI
C. USG D. Plain films

33. **In pregnancy recommended imaging study for Perforated ulcer is:**

A. CT scan B. MRI
C. USG D. Plain films

34. **In pregnancy recommended imaging study for inflammatory bowel disease is:**

A. CT scan B. MRI
C. USG D. Plain films

35. **In pregnancy recommended imaging study for Pancreatitis is:**

A. CT scan B. MRI
C. USG D. Plain films

36. **In pregnancy recommended imaging study for trauma is:**

A. CT scan B. MRI
C. USG D. Plain films

37. **Gallstone pancreatitis has been associated with a fetal loss of:**

A. 10% B. 30%
C. 45% D. 60%

38. **The most common cause of acute surgical abdomen in the pediatric population is:**

A. Acute cholecystitis
B. Acute appendicitis
C. Acute salpingitis
D. Acute intestinal obstruction

39. **Differential diagnosis of acute abdomen in hematopoietic stem cell transplantation is all except:**

A. Pancreatitis
B. Pneumatosis
C. Cholangitis
D. Neutropenic enterocolitis

40. **Risk factors for the development of gastrointestinal complications after cardiothoracic surgery includes all except:**

A. Low cardiac output
B. Cardiopulmonary bypass time >250 minutes
C. Liver failure
D. Peripheral vascular disease

41. Risk factors for the development of gastrointestinal complications after cardiothoracic surgery includes all except:

A. Active smoker

B. Age >50

C. Prolonged ventilation

D. Chronic obstructive pulmonary disease

42. Concerning CT imaging findings in the post bariatric surgery patient includes all except:

A. Transition between dilated and nondilated bowel

B. Cluster of small bowel loops

C. Vertical position of the superior mesenteric artery

D. Mesenteric swirl sign

43. False about abdominal emergencies in cardiac patients is:

A. The highest mortality is seen in patients with intestinal ischemia and in those patients who required a valve repair

B. The pathophysiology of gastrointestinal complications is thought to be associated with disturbances in the inferior mesenteric artery blood flow during cardiopulmonary bypass

C. Abdominal emergencies in the cardiac patient can be easily masked by their postoperative recovery, ongoing management of their cardiac dysfunction, mechanical ventilation, arrhythmias, hemodynamic instability and sedation

D. Patients undergoing an open abdominal aortic aneurysm repair have the highest incidence, especially those repaired through a transabdominal approach

ANSWERS

1. **Ans: D. All of the above**

Ref: Chapter No.46, Page No.1134

2. **Ans: B. Parietal pain is usually due to the distention of a hollow viscus**

Ref: Chapter No.46, Page No.1134

3. **Ans: A. Hemorrhagic pancreatitis**

Ref: Chapter No.46, Page No.1135

4. **Ans: C. Acute intermittent porphyria**

Ref: Chapter No.46, Page No.1135

5. **Ans: D. All of the above are nonsurgical cause of the acute abdomen**

Ref: Chapter No.46, Page No.1135

6. **Ans: D. Ureter**

Ref: Chapter No.46, Page No.1136

7. **Ans: B. Duodenum**

Ref: Chapter No.46, Page No.1136

8. **Ans: A. With an underlying surgical cause, vomiting precedes the pain**

Ref: Chapter No.46, Page No.1136-1137

9. **Ans: C. Cocaine and methamphetamine use can create an intense vasodilatation**

Ref: Chapter No.46, Page No.1137

10. **Ans: A. 1 bowel sounds every 15 seconds per quadrant**

Ref: Chapter No.46, Page No.1137

11. **Ans: B. Danforth sign**

Ref: Chapter No.46, Page No.1139

12. **Ans: C. Ruptured common bile duct**

Ref: Chapter No.46, Page No.1139

13. **Ans: D. Ransohoff sign**

Ref: Chapter No.46, Page No.1139

14. **Ans: C. Cruveilhier sign**

Ref: Chapter No.46, Page No.1139

15. **Ans: B. Bassler sign**

Ref: Chapter No.46, Page No.1139

16. **Ans: C. Blumberg sign**

Ref: Chapter No.46, Page No.1139

17. **Ans: C. Carnett sign**

Ref: Chapter No.46, Page No.1139

18. **Ans: A. Chandelier sign**

Ref: Chapter No.46, Page No.1139

19. **Ans: D. Ten Horn sign**

Ref: Chapter No.46, Page No.1139

20. **Ans: D. Fothergill sign**

Ref: Chapter No.46, Page No.1139

21. **Ans: B. Rectus muscle hematoma**

Ref: Chapter No.46, Page No.1139

22. **Ans: A. Chandelier sign**

Ref: Chapter No.46, Page No.1139

23. **Ans: D. All of the above**

Ref: Chapter No.46, Page No.1139

24. **Ans: D. USG can provide more information regarding location of perforation and specific cause**

Ref: Chapter No.46, Page No.1140

25. **Ans: C. 20 mm Hg**

Ref: Chapter No.46, Page No.1141

26. **Ans: B. 5 - 7 mm Hg**

Ref: Chapter No.46, Page No.1141

27. **Ans: D. 21–25 mm Hg**

Ref: Chapter No.46, Page No.1142

28. **Ans: B. Maternal hemorrhage is often compensated by increased uterine flow, and marked fetal distress is often the last manifestation of an acute surgical pathology, even before maternal hypotension or tachycardia is identified**

Ref: Chapter No.46, Page No.1143

29. **Ans: C. 50 mGy**

Ref: Chapter No.46, Page No.1143

30. **Ans: B. Acute appendicitis**

Ref: Chapter No.46, Page No.1143

31. **Ans: C. 20%**

Ref: Chapter No.46, Page No.1143

32. **Ans: B. MRI**

Ref: Chapter No.46, Page No.1144

33. **Ans: D. Plain films**

Ref: Chapter No.46, Page No.1144

34. **Ans: B. MRI**

Ref: Chapter No.46, Page No.1144

35. **Ans: C. USG**

Ref: Chapter No.46, Page No.1144

36. **Ans: C. USG**

Ref: Chapter No.46, Page No.1144

37. **Ans: D. 60%**

Ref: Chapter No.46, Page No.1144

38. **Ans: B. Acute appendicitis**

Ref: Chapter No.46, Page No.1144

39. **Ans: A. Pancreatitis**

Ref: Chapter No.46, Page No.1145

40. **Ans: B. Cardiopulmonary bypass time >250 minutes**

Ref: Chapter No.46, Page No.1146

41. **Ans: B. Age >50**

Ref: Chapter No.46, Page No.1146

42. **Ans: C. Vertical position of the superior mesenteric artery**

Ref: Chapter No.46, Page No.1146

43. **Ans: B. The pathophysiology of gastrointestinal complications is thought to be associated with disturbances in the inferior mesenteric artery blood flow during cardiopulmonary bypass**

Ref: Chapter No.46, Page No.1146

47

Acute Gastrointestinal Hemorrhage

1. **False about gastrointestinal bleeding is:**
   A. Upper GIB (UGIB) is defined as being proximal to the ligament of Treitz
   B. Lower GIB (LGIB) accounts for 60% to 70% of all bleeds and is defined as distal to the ligament of Treitz
   C. The term massive GIB refers to intestinal blood loss leading to hemodynamic instability or transfusion requirement
   D. Occult GIB refers to anemia that persists or recurs after negative endoscopic evaluation and imaging workup

ACUTE MANAGEMENT OF PATIENTS WITH GASTROINTESTINAL HEMORRHAGE

2. **False about management of acute hemorrhagic exsanguination is:**
   A. Intravenous (IV) access with two large-bore (14 or 16 gauge) catheters should be obtained
   B. Tachypnea, tachycardia, hypotension, agitation and mental status changes are all indicators of a severe degree of hemorrhage
   C. Systolic blood pressures under 90 mm Hg do not typically manifest until a patient has experienced a 15% to 20% blood loss
   D. The clinical response may be blunted in patients taking beta blockers or those patients who are at the extremes of age

3. **False about management of acute hemorrhagic exsanguination is:**
   A. In acute severe blood loss, the serum hematocrit is not a reliable marker of the amount of blood loss
   B. Rapid blood loss can be complicated by pre-existing or hemorrhage-related coagulopathy with deficiencies in both pro- and antithrombotic factors
   C. A role for viscoelastic tests such as thromboelastography or thromboelastometry has been well studied in GIB
   D. With large volume blood loss, the utilization of massive transfusion protocols can make universal donor blood products rapidly available in prespecified ratios

4. **A landmark study by Villanueva compared a restrictive transfusion threshold of a hemoglobin level to a liberal threshold and this randomized controlled trial found lower rates of mortality, rebleeding and other adverse outcomes with the restrictive strategy of:**
   A. 9 g/dL	B. 8 g/dL
   C. 7 g/dL	D. 6 g/dL

5. **False among the following is:**
   A. Hematemesis is the emesis of blood or coffee ground gastric secretions, most commonly from a UGIB
   B. Melena, a malodorous, black stool with a tar-like quality, is indicative of a proximal source of bleeding
   C. Hematochezia, the passage of bright red blood from the anus, is most commonly from fissure in ano
   D. Over 90% of melena arises from a UGIB, though it can originate from anywhere in the GI tract if intestinal transit is slow

6. **True about differentiating a UGIB from a LGIB is:**
   A. The first steps in differentiating a UGIB from a LGIB is aided by a nasogastric tube (NGT) lavage
   B. It can detect the presence of blood above the ligament of Treitz
   C. An aspiration, which is bilious and nonbloody, can effectively rule out an active UGIB
   D. All of the above

7. CT angiogram can detect bleeding rates as low as:

A. 0.04 mL/min B. 0.3 mL/min
C. 0.05 mL/min D. 0.5 mL/min

8. The sensitivity and specificity of CT angiogram approaches:

A. 100% and > 90% B. 90% and > 85%
C. 95% and > 80% D. 80% and > 85%

9. Technetium-99-m-labeled RBC scintigraphy can detect bleeding as low as:

A. 0.04 mL/min B. 0.3 mL/min
C. 0.05 mL/min D. 0.5 mL/min

10. Patients with bleeding localized to the UGI tract should proceed to upper endoscopy within:

A. 12 hours B. 24 hours
C. 36 hours D. 48 hours

11. The most common source of LGIB is:

A. Malignancy
B. Diverticular disease
C. Inflammatory bowel disease
D. Angiodysplasia

12. Rapid prep in colonoscopy preparation is:

A. Minimum of 2 L of polyethylene glycol solution given within a period of approximately 8 hours, followed by colonoscopy within 4 to 6 hours
B. Minimum of 2 L of polyethylene glycol solution given within a period of approximately 4 hours, followed by colonoscopy within 1 to 2 hours
C. Minimum of 4 L of polyethylene glycol solution given within a period of approximately 8 hours, followed by colonoscopy within 4 to 6 hours
D. Minimum of 4 L of polyethylene glycol solution given within a period of approximately 4 hours, followed by colonoscopy within 1 to 2 hours

13. In acute GIBs, middle GIB accounts for:

A. 2% B. 5%
C. 10% D. 18%

14. False about video capsule endoscopy is:

A. Bleeding is the most common indication for capsule endoscopy
B. The diagnostic rates are reported to be between about 35% and 67% and highest in acute GIB rather than obscure blood loss
C. These higher-risk patients may be better served by the alternative diagnostic strategies of computed tomography (CT) enterography or magnetic resonance (MR) enterography
D. The main risk of capsule endoscopy is capsule retention that can occur in up to 25% of patients when used for overt GIB

15. Factors that are associated with a positive capsule study are all except:

A. Male sex
B. Hospitalization at the time of test performance
C. Age >60 years
D. Female sex

16. Patients at high risk for capsule retention are those with:

A. Prior small bowel radiation
B. Hemorrhoids
C. Tumors
D. Heavy NSAID use

17. When upper and lower sources have been ruled out, the modality of choice for overt GIB in a stable patient is:

A. CT enterography B. MR enterography
C. Capsule endoscopy D. CT angiography

18. False about CT enterography is:

A. Multiphase CT enterography can be superior to capsule endoscopy in detecting bleeding from tumors
B. It is performed with a neutral or low-density oral contrast to distend the small bowel and includes IV contrast
C. If a patient is stable and can tolerate capsule endoscopy and CT enterography, these studies are complementary to each other
D. Scans are performed in only the arterial phase

19. Push enteroscopy using a small-caliber colonoscope can reach about:

A. 20 to 30 cm past the ligament of Treitz
B. 30 to 50 cm past the ligament of Treitz
C. 50 to 70 cm past the ligament of Treitz
D. 70 to 100 cm past the ligament of Treitz

20. In patients with obscure small bowel bleeding, push enteroscopy using a small-caliber colonoscope can lead to successful diagnosis in:

A. 20% B. 40%
C. 60% D. 80%

21. In patients with obscure small bowel bleeding, double-balloon endoscopy can lead to successful diagnosis in approximately:

A. 20% B. 40%
C. 60% D. 80%

22. In patients with obscure-overt bleeding, repeated upper endoscopy and lower endoscopy should be performed and may identify lesions in up to:

A. 15% B. 20%
C. 35% D. 50%

SPECIFIC CAUSES OF UGIB

23. True about peptic ulcer disease is:

A. PUD is responsible for up to two-thirds of UGIBs and can develop in the stomach or duodenum
B. The major etiologic factors in PUD are H. pylori and NSAIDs
C. It is estimated that up to 77% of duodenal ulcers are associated with H. pylori infection
D. All of the above

24. As part of the disease course, patients with PUD will develop bleeding in:

A. 2% - 5% B. 5% - 10%
C. 10% - 15% D. 20% - 25%

25. In patients with regular NSAID use, PUD has a prevalence of:

A. 2% - 5% B. 5% - 10%
C. 10% - 15% D. 15% to 20%

26. The most significant hemorrhage in PUD occurs when gastric ulcers penetrate branches of:

A. Left gastric artery
B. Gastroduodenal artery
C. Left gastroepiploic artery
D. Common hepatic artery

27. The most significant hemorrhage in PUD occurs when duodenal ulcers penetrate branches of:

A. Left gastric artery
B. Common hepatic artery
C. Left gastroepiploic artery
D. Gastroduodenal artery

28. pH required for healing of PUD is:

A. pH > 2 for 24 hours
B. pH > 3 for 24 hours
C. pH > 2 for 18 hours
D. pH > 3 for 18 hours

29. True about the management of PUD is:

A. Those with high clinical risk may benefit from EGD intervention within 12 hours of presentation
B. Erythromycin prior to endoscopy is proven to reduce the need for 2nd endoscopy, amount of blood transfusion and hospital length of stay
C. While awaiting EGD, patients should be treated with a PPI
D. All of the above

30. A 32-year-old female with known PUD came to emergency with an episode of hematemesis. After initial resuscitation patient underwent endoscopy and showed an adherent clot. According to Forrest classification, the grade is:

A. Grade IIa B. Grade IIb
C. Grade IIc D. Grade III

31. A 52-year-old male with known PUD came to emergency with 3 episodes of hematemesis. After initial resuscitation patient underwent endoscopy and showed active, nonpulsatile bleeding. According to Forrest classification, the grade is:

A. Grade Ia B. Grade Ib
C. Grade IIa D. Grade IIb

32. A 40-year-old male with known PUD came to emergency with 2 episodes of hematemesis. After initial resuscitation patient underwent endoscopy and showed nonbleeding visible vessel. According to Forrest classification, the grade is:

A. Grade IIa B. Grade IIb
C. Grade IIc D. Grade III

33. False about the medical management of PUD is:

A. All patients with confirmed peptic ulcer bleed should receive PPI therapy
B. If PPI has not been started prior to endoscopy; a bolus of 80 mg should be given, followed by an infusion at 8 mg an hour for 72 hours
C. Continuing PPI therapy post endoscopy also has been associated with reduced risk of further bleeding need for surgery and mortality
D. Once H. pylori has been eradicated, there is need for long-term acid suppression as it does decrease the rebleed risk

34. False about the medical management in PUD is:

A. Rebleeding rates with COX-2 inhibitors alone versus traditional NSAIDs plus a PPI are similar at 4% to 9%
B. COX-2 inhibitors plus PPI has a much lower

rebleed risk as compared to COX-2 selective NSAIDs alone

C. ASA for secondary risk should be restarted in combination with a PPI within 14 days after bleeding cessation

D. All of the above are true

35. False about the endoscopic management of PUD is:

A. The recommended endoscopic approach is to use thermal coagulation or clips, with or without epinephrine injection

B. Epinephrine monotherapy has a higher risk of rebleed compared to clipping or thermal coagulation

C. Epinephrine is diluted 1:1000 or 1:2000 and is injected into all four quadrants of a bleeding lesion

D. The rate of initial hemostasis with epinephrine monotherapy is as high as 100%

36. False about the endoscopic management of PUD is:

A. Large volume injection of epinephrine (>13 mL) is associated with improved hemostasis, suggesting that part of the mechanism is by tamponade and compression of the bleeding vessel

B. All heat modalities have similar efficacy and are effective in achieving initial hemostasis, reducing recurrent bleeding, surgery and mortality

C. Limitations of hemoclips are the difficulty in applying to fibrotic lesions and prolonged procedure time

D. Hemoclips are more effective than thermal therapy

37. In addition to epinephrine injection, heat or mechanical therapy is usually added and together can achieve initial hemostasis in gastric ulcer bleeding in up to:

A. 80% B. 85%

C. 90% D. 100%

38. With rebleeding after endoscopic management of PUD bleeding, a second attempt at endoscopic control is recommended and is successful in:

A. 45% B. 60%

C. 75% D. 90%

39. False about angiographic management of PUD bleeding is:

A. For suspected UGIB, the superior mesenteric artery and its branches are interrogated first

B. The superior mesenteric artery and inferior mesenteric artery can also be evaluated if no bleeding is identified

C. Transcatheter arterial embolization is effective at hemorrhage control when a bleeding source is found

D. Vasopressin infusion can be useful if there is diffuse bleeding or as a bridge to surgical intervention if super selective cannulation cannot be achieved

40. Various angiographic embolic agents are:

A. Polyvinyl alcohol particles

B. Gelfoam

C. Glue

D. All of the above

41. Which of the following is a temporary agent used in angiographic intervention for embolization and will recanalize over weeks to months is?

A. Polyvinyl alcohol particles

B. Gelfoam

C. Glue

D. Coils

42. Despite effective endoscopic management of PUD bleeding, surgical intervention is needed in:

A. 2% B. 5%

C. 10% D. 15%

43. Factors associated with increased risk of rebleeding are:

A. Large ulcer size >2 cm

B. Anterior duodenal wall ulcer

C. Active bleeding at time of endoscopy

D. Lesser gastric curve ulcer

44. Indications for surgery in gastrointestinal hemorrhage are all except:

A. Hemodynamic instability despite vigorous resuscitation (>6-unit transfusion)

B. Continued slow bleeding with a transfusion requirement exceeding 2 units/day

C. Recurrent hemorrhage after initial stabilization (with up to 2 attempts at obtaining endoscopic hemostasis)

D. Failure of endoscopic techniques to arrest hemorrhage

45. False about surgical management of duodenal ulcers is:

A. Most of the lesions are in the duodenal bulb

B. Hemorrhage typically can be controlled initially with pressure and then direct suture ligation with nonabsorbable suture
C. Suture ligature of the vessel proximal and distally, typically in a superior and inferior orientation, as placement of medial-stitch to control the pancreatic branches typically arrests the bleed
D. The duodenotomy is closed longitudinally with an NGT above and a nasojejunal tube placed beyond the repair for distal enteral access

46. False about surgical management of gastric ulcers is:
A. Surgical control of a bleeding gastric ulcer begins with a gastrotomy and suture ligation
B. Gastric ulcer resection is generally indicated due to the 40% incidence of malignancy
C. Proximal or near-total gastrectomies are associated with a particularly high mortality in the setting of acute hemorrhage
D. Simple excision alone is associated with rebleeding in as many as 20% of patients, so distal gastrectomy is generally preferred

47. False about esophagitis is:
A. Esophageal inflammation secondary to repeated exposure of the esophageal mucosa to the acidic gastric secretions in gastroesophageal reflux disease
B. The superficial mucosal ulcerations generally bleed acutely and are more commonly manifested as hematemesis
C. With infection, hemorrhage can occasionally be massive
D. Treatment typically includes acid suppressive therapy

48. False about gastritis is:
A. When stress ulceration is associated with major burns, these lesions are referred to as Cushing's ulcer
B. In those who develop bleeding, acid suppressive therapy is often successful in controlling the hemorrhage
C. Stress-related gastritis is characterized by the appearance of multiple superficial erosions of the entire stomach
D. Classically, gastritis commonly afflicted the critically ill

49. Stress-related gastritis is characterized by the appearance of multiple superficial erosions of the entire stomach, most commonly in:
A. Fundus B. Body
C. Antrum D. Cardia

50. False about Mallory-Weiss Tears is:
A. Classically, these lesions develop in alcoholic patients after a period of intense retching and vomiting following binge drinking
B. Mallory-Weiss tears are partial-thickness tears of the mucosa and submucosa that occur near the gastroesophageal junction
C. Recurrent bleeding from a Mallory-Weiss tear is common
D. Supportive therapy with acid suppression therapy is successful in 90% of bleeding episodes, the mucosa often healing within 72 hours

51. In the cases of UGIB, Mallory-Weiss tears account for:
A. 2% to 5% B. 5% to 10%
C. 10% to 20% D. 25% to 30%

52. False about gastric antral vascular ectasia is:
A. Gastric antral vascular ectasia is characterized by a collection of dilated arterioles
B. The success rate is upward of 90% with argon plasma coagulation
C. On endoscopy it appears as a linear red streak converging on the antrum, giving the appearance of a watermelon
D. Endoscopic therapy is indicated for persistent anemia or transfusion-dependent bleeding

53. False about Dieulafoy lesions is:
A. Erosion of the gastric mucosa overlying the sizable vessels (1 to 3 mm) found in the gastric submucosa leads to bleeding
B. The mucosal defect is usually small (2 to 5 mm), with an associated ulcer
C. Given the large size of the underlying artery, bleeding from a Dieulafoy lesion can be massive
D. Application of thermal or sclerosant therapy is effective in 80% to 100% of cases

54. Dieulafoy lesions are vascular malformations found primarily along:
A. The lesser curve of the stomach within 4 cm of the gastroesophageal junction
B. The lesser curve of the stomach within 6 cm of the gastroesophageal junction
C. The greater curve of the stomach within 4 cm of the gastroesophageal junction

D. The greater curve of the stomach within 6 cm of the gastroesophageal junction

55. False about Hemobilia is:

A. Endoscopy remains the gold standard for diagnosis and intervention

B. It is typically associated with trauma, recent instrumentation of the biliary tree or hepatic neoplasms

C. If angiographic embolization is performed, the portal vein must be verified to be patent

D. Endoscopy can be helpful by demonstrating blood at the ampulla or other biliary abnormalities suggestive of hemobilia

56. False about Malignancy and GI bleeding is:

A. Endoscopic therapy is often successful in controlling these bleeds and the rebleeding rate is low

B. Malignant neoplasms of the UGI tract are usually associated with chronic anemia or hemoccult-positive stool rather than episodes of significant hemorrhage

C. Palliative resections for control of bleeding usually entail wedge resections

D. Malignant neoplasms will be manifested as ulcerative lesions that bleed persistently and is most characteristic of the GI stromal tumor (GIST)

57. False about aortoenteric fistulas and GI bleeding is:

A. These are usually fatal as they represent free rupture of the aorta into the bowel

B. The interval between surgery and hemorrhage can be days to years with the median interval about 10 years

C. Secondary fistulas are much more common and are the result of an aortic graft-enteric erosion and may develop in up to 0.4% to 4% of aortic graft cases

D. Typically, patients with bleeding from an aortoenteric fistula will present first with a "sentinel bleed"

58. Aortoenteric fistulas most often involves the:

A. Duodenum B. Jejunum

C. Ileum D. Transverse colon

59. False about the management of aortoenteric fistulas and GI bleeding is:

A. This diagnosis of an aortoenteric fistula should be considered in all bleeding patients with a known abdominal aortic aneurysm or any prior aortic reconstruction

B. In stable patients, EGD is always the first-line test for UGIB

C. If the suspicion for an aortoenteric fistula is high, EGD should be the first-line study

D. A CT with IV contrast will often show air around the graft, which is suggestive of infection, possible pseudoaneurysm

60. False about Hemosuccus pancreaticus is:

A. Hemosuccus pancreaticus is bleeding from the pancreatic duct through the ampulla of Vater

B. ERCP is the diagnostic gold standard and first therapeutic line of action due to high efficacy

C. Bleeding is most typically from a pancreatic source such as a malformation, ductal wall ulceration, or a pancreatic pseudocyst that erodes into a pseudoaneurysm

D. Operative interventions may occasionally be required to treat the pseudocyst and should be aided by intraoperative ultrasonography or pancreatoscopy to diagnose the site of hemorrhage to guide operative planning

61. False about the procedure related GI bleeding is:

A. Bleeding from percutaneous endoscopic gastrostomy placement is from a punctured gastric vessel or mucosa is easily controlled by compression from traction on the bumper (temporary)

B. In bleeding from percutaneous endoscopic gastrostomy placement, if compression maneuvers are ineffective, then the tube may need to be removed and hemostasis achieved endoscopically

C. Bleeding after endoscopic sphincterotomy is often mild and self-limited

D. Most surgical anastomotic bleeding doesn't resolve with nonoperative management

62. Bleeding from percutaneous endoscopic gastrostomy placement is estimated to be:

A. 3% B. 5%

C. 10% D. 15%

63. Endoscopic sphincterotomy has bleeding rates of approximately:

A. 0.5% B. 2%

C. 5% D. 8%

64. False about variceal hemorrhage is:

A. The most common clinical scenario leading to variceal hemorrhage is portal hypertension from the sinusoidal fibrosis associated with cirrhosis

B. Portal hypertension is defined as a hepatic venous pressure gradient of more than 5 cm of H_2O
C. Due to the large capacitance of the venous system, veins may pathologically dilate to diameters upward of 1 to 2 cm with increased wall tension stressing the overlying mucosa
D. Catastrophic bleeding can occur with disruption of the overlying mucosa, which, despite medical advancement in the field, still has an associated 6-week mortality of 10% to 20%

65. The hepatic venous pressure gradient required for varices to form is:

A. >10 mm Hg
B. >12 cm of H_2O
C. >12 mm Hg
D. >10 cm of H_2O

66. False about the management of variceal hemorrhage is:

A. Vasoactive drugs such as terlipressin, somatostatin, octreotide and vapreotide should be used prior to endoscopic evaluation and continued for up to 5 days
B. Current recommendations are for oral fluoroquinolones or IV Ceftriaxone (1 g every 24 hours) for patients with advanced disease or nil per os status
C. Endoscopy is the first recommended step in any patient with cirrhosis and UGIB
D. Sclerotherapy is preferred over endoscopic venous ligation for acute esophageal bleeding

67. For high-risk variceal bleeding, definitive long-term management with early transjugular intrahepatic portosystemic shunt (TIPS) should be performed within:

A. 12 hours
B. 24 hours
C. 48 hours
D. 72 hours

68. TIPS effectively decreases the venous pressure and achieves definitive hemostasis in greater than:

A. 70%
B. 80%
C. 90%
D. 100%

69. In variceal bleeding, failure of hemorrhage control is predicted by all except:

A. Model for End-Stage Liver Disease (MELD) score > 20
B. Active bleeding at the time of intervention
C. Venous pressures > 25 mm Hg
D. Child-Pugh class C cirrhosis

70. Surgical intervention in variceal bleeding is associated with mortality of:

A. > 30%
B. > 50%
C. > 70%
D. > 90%

ACUTE LOWER GASTROINTESTINAL HEMORRHAGE

71. Most common cause of lower GI bleeding is:

A. Angiodysplasia
B. Anorectal disease
C. Diverticular disease
D. Neoplasia

72. Prevalence of lower GI bleeding due to neoplasia is:

A. 5%–10%
B. 10%–25%
C. 3%–4%
D. 1%–5%

73. False about acute lower GI bleeding is:

A. Melena, a common presentation of UGIB, can occasionally be a sign of LGIB
B. The most common presentation is painless hematochezia, defined as bright red blood, clots, or burgundy stools
C. In patients with LGIB, more than 50% will have a source in the small intestine
D. Altered bowel habits, iron-deficiency anemia, or unexplained weight loss may suggest malignancy

74. False about the diagnosis of acute lower GI bleeding is:

A. Hemorrhage from the lower GI tract tends to be less severe and intermittent
B. > 40% of patients with LGIB have multiple lesions identified as the potential source of bleeding
C. In up to 25% of patients with LGIB, the source of bleeding is never accurately identified
D. Up to 5% of patients with hematochezia had a UGI source to account for the bleed

75. Major LGIB can be defined as:

A. Need for 2 or more unit of blood
B. Hemorrhage associated with hemodynamic instability
C. Altered mental status
D. All of the above

76. True about colonoscopy in acute lower GI bleeding is:

A. The most common source of bleeding is diverticular, and even though an actively bleeding diverticulum may not be seen during endoscopy, certain features are predictive of high risk of rebleeding
B. Overall endoscopic success is good with one review showing a hemostasis rate of 92% and early and late rebleed rates of 8% and 12%, respectively
C. Colonoscopy is almost always the initial examination of choice for LGIB
D. All of the above

77. Angiography, when in lower GI bleeding is used to treat diverticular bleeding, the rate of successful hemostasis approaches:

A. 50% B. 80%
C. 90% D. 100%

78. Indications for surgery in acute lower GI bleeding is/are:

A. Administering > 4 units of blood in 24 hours
B. >10 units of blood during the hospital stay are considered
C. Persistent hemodynamic instability despite resuscitation attempts
D. All of the above

79. False about colonic diverticula is:

A. The incidence of diverticula increases with age, with 20% at age 40 and increasing to 60% and beyond at age 60
B. Among all with colonic diverticula, 3% to 15% will experience bleeding
C. In western countries, right-sided disease is far more common than left-sided disease; however, left-sided disease is responsible for over 50% of significant diverticular bleeding
D. The patients that bleed, > 75% stop spontaneously, although approximately 10% will rebleed within a year and almost 50% within 10 years

80. False about the management of colonic diverticula is:

A. If colonoscopy is unable to isolate or visualize bleeding or there is recurrent bleeding, angiography with superselective cannulation and embolization can be considered
B. Colonoscopy is the best modality for diagnosis and therapy
C. Blind total abdominal colectomy for GI hemorrhage carries with it high morbidity and mortality and does not entirely remove the risk for rebleed, which is approximately 40%
D. With recurrent bleeding, colonoscopy can be repeated, or mesenteric angiography can be performed

81. False about colitis is:

A. Ulcerative colitis (UC) is much more likely than Crohn's disease to manifest with GIB
B. Bleeding with ulcerative colitis (UC) will almost always be from a diffuse colitis with no discrete lesions amenable to endoscopic treatment
C. Crohn's disease is more typically associated with guaiac-positive diarrhea
D. Crohn's disease is less likely to have discrete lesions that can undergo endoscopic or angiographic intervention, usually in the form of an ulcer that has eroded into a vessel

82. False about Angiodysplasias is:

A. Angiodysplasias of the intestine are also referred to as arteriovenous malformations, angiectasias and vascular ectasia
B. More common in males
C. Unlike diverticular bleeding, this tends to be venous bleeding, so it is less brisk and often occult and will present more often as chronic bleeding
D. Their prevalence increases with age and they are associated with aortic stenosis and renal failure

83. Angiodysplasias can be found anywhere in the GI tract, typically they occur in the:

A. Ascending colon B. Caecum
C. Transverse colon D. Sigmoid colon

84. In angiodysplasias, significant bleeding can occur in up to:

A. 5% B. 10%
C. 15% D. 25%

85. False about the management of angiodysplasias is:

A. If the bleeding has been localized and these attempts at hemostasis fail or bleeding recurs, segmental colon resection, most commonly right colectomy, is also effective
B. Angiography demonstrates dilated, slowly emptying veins and sometimes early venous filling
C. When treated endoscopically, noncontact thermal therapy with argon plasma coagulation is the preferred method

D. On colonoscopy, these lesions appear as elevated, bright-red, stellate lesions with a surrounding rim of pale mucosa

86. GISTs are the most common soft tissue sarcoma in the digestive tract, with bleeding evident in:

A. 5% - 10%
B. 10% - 20%
C. 20% - 30%
D. 30% - 50%

87. False about ischemia and lower GI bleeding is:

A. Mesenteric ischemia should be considered in any patient with bleeding with a past medical history of cardiovascular disease, peripheral vascular disease or vasculitis
B. CT may show thickened bowel wall, pneumatosis, or more subtle signs of vascular disease such as calcification of the take-off of the mesenteric vasculature
C. Patients present with a characteristic "pain out of proportion to exam" and diarrhea that is often guaiac positive or bloody from mucosal degradation
D. Chronic colonic ischemia is the most common form of mesenteric ischemia

88. False about C difficile colitis and lower GI bleeding is:

A. C difficile colitis represents the overgrowth of a pathogenic clostridial bacterium that thrives after disruption of the normal gut microflora after antibiotic use
B. Treatment consists of stopping antibiotics, supportive care, and taking oral or IV metronidazole, oral vancomycin, or fidaxomicin
C. Explosive, voluminous, and, at times, bloody bowel movements can result from severe cases with associated mucosal sloughing
D. Profound leukocytosis is rarely observed

89. False about Meckel's diverticulum and Lower GI bleeding is:

A. Bleeding results from ulceration of the neighbouring ileal tissue from irritation from an active focus of gastric mucosa
B. Definitive treatment is surgical resection of the segment with care to incorporate the ulcerated ileal tissue, typically on the intestinal wall opposite the diverticulum
C. Bleeding is typically painful LGIB
D. A Meckel diverticulum scan, performed by administration of 99mTc-pertechnetate, can demonstrate ectopic gastric mucosa that can be localized with scintigraphy

90. False about radiation and lower GI bleeding is:

A. Endoscopic therapy with argon coagulation is recommended as an effective treatment as it is not associated with fistula and stricture formation
B. Bleeding from enteritis and, more commonly, proctitis complicates 1% to 5% of treated patients
C. The American Society of Colon and Rectal Surgeons has published guidelines for therapy, which include strong recommendations for treatment with formalin 4% to 10%, sucralfate enemas, and hyperbaric oxygen
D. Bleeding results from mucosal changes that, on endoscopy, reveal friability, angioectasias, and ulcerations

ANSWERS

1. **Ans: B. Lower GIB (LGIB) accounts for 60% to 70% of all bleeds and is defined as distal to the ligament of Treitz**
Ref: Chapter No.47, Page No.1150

2. **Ans: C. Systolic blood pressures under 90 mm Hg do not typically manifest until a patient has experienced a 15% to 20% blood loss**
Ref: Chapter No.47, Page No.1150

3. **Ans: C. A role for viscoelastic tests such as thromboelastography or thromboelastometry has been well studied in GIB**
Ref: Chapter No.47, Page No.1151

4. **Ans: C. 7 g/ dL**
Ref: Chapter No.47, Page No.1151

5. **Ans: C. Hematochezia, the passage of bright red blood from the anus, is most commonly from fissure in ano**
Ref: Chapter No.47, Page No.1151-1152

6. **Ans: D. All of the above**
Ref: Chapter No.47, Page No.1152

7. **Ans: B. 0.3 mL/min**
Ref: Chapter No.47, Page No.1152

8. **Ans: A. 100% and > 90%**
Ref: Chapter No.47, Page No.1152

9. **Ans: A. 0.04 mL/min**
Ref: Chapter No.47, Page No.1152

10. **Ans: B. 24 hours**
Ref: Chapter No.47, Page No.1152

11. **Ans: B. Diverticular disease**
Ref: Chapter No.47, Page No.1152

12. **Ans: D. Minimum of 4 L of polyethylene glycol solution given within a period of approximately 4 hours, followed by colonoscopy within 1 to 2 hours**
Ref: Chapter No.47, Page No.1152

13. **Ans: B. 5%**
Ref: Chapter No.47, Page No.1152

14. **Ans: D. The main risk of capsule endoscopy is capsule retention that can occur in up to 25% of patients when used for overt GIB**
Ref: Chapter No.47, Page No.1152

15. **Ans: D. Female sex**
Ref: Chapter No.47, Page No.1152

16. **Ans: B. Hemorrhoids**
Ref: Chapter No.47, Page No.1152

17. **Ans: C. Capsule endoscopy**
Ref: Chapter No.47, Page No.1152

18. **Ans: D. Scans are performed in only the arterial phase**
Ref: Chapter No.47, Page No.1152

19. **Ans: C. 50 to 70 cm past the ligament of Treitz**
Ref: Chapter No.47, Page No.1153

20. **Ans: B. 40%**
Ref: Chapter No.47, Page No.1153

21. **Ans: D. 80%**
Ref: Chapter No.47, Page No.1153

22. **Ans: C. 35%**
Ref: Chapter No.47, Page No.1153

23. **Ans: D. All of the above**
Ref: Chapter No.47, Page No.1153

24. **Ans: C. 10% - 15%**
Ref: Chapter No.47, Page No.1153

25. **Ans: D. 15% to 20%**
Ref: Chapter No.47, Page No.1153

26. **Ans: A. Left gastric artery**
Ref: Chapter No.47, Page No.1153

27. **Ans: D. Gastroduodenal artery**
Ref: Chapter No.47, Page No.1153

28. **Ans: D. pH > 3 for 18 hours**
Ref: Chapter No.47, Page No.1153

29. **Ans: D. All of the above**
Ref: Chapter No.47, Page No.1153

30. **Ans: B. Grade IIb**
Ref: Chapter No.47, Page No.1154

31. **Ans: B. Grade Ib**
Ref: Chapter No.47, Page No.1154

32. **Ans: A. Grade IIa**
Ref: Chapter No.47, Page No.1154

33. **Ans: D. Once H. pylori has been eradicated, there is need for long-term acid suppression as it does decrease the rebleed risk**
Ref: Chapter No.47, Page No.1154

34. **Ans: C. ASA for secondary risk should be restarted in combination with a PPI within 14 days after bleeding cessation**
Ref: Chapter No.47, Page No.1154

35. **Ans: C. Epinephrine is diluted 1:1000 or 1:2000 and is injected into all four quadrants of a bleeding lesion**

Ref: Chapter No.47, Page No.1154

36. **Ans: D. Hemoclips are more effective than thermal therapy**

Ref: Chapter No.47, Page No.1154

37. **Ans: C. 90%**

Ref: Chapter No.47, Page No.1154

38. **Ans: C. 75%**

Ref: Chapter No.47, Page No.1155

39. **Ans: A. For suspected UGIB, the superior mesenteric artery and its branches are interrogated first**

Ref: Chapter No.47, Page No.1155

40. **Ans: D. All of the above**

Ref: Chapter No.47, Page No.1155

41. **Ans: B. Gelfoam**

Ref: Chapter No.47, Page No.1155

42. **Ans: C. 10%**

Ref: Chapter No.47, Page No.1155

43. **Ans: B. Anterior duodenal wall ulcer**

Ref: Chapter No.47, Page No.1155

44. **Ans: B. Continued slow bleeding with a transfusion requirement exceeding 2 units/day**

Ref: Chapter No.47, Page No.1155

45. **Ans: D. The duodenotomy is closed longitudinally with an NGT above and a nasojejunal tube placed beyond the repair for distal enteral access**

Ref: Chapter No.47, Page No.1155

46. **Ans: B. Gastric ulcer resection is generally indicated due to the 40% incidence of malignancy**

Ref: Chapter No.47, Page No.1156

47. **Ans: B. The superficial mucosal ulcerations generally bleed acutely and are more commonly manifested as hematemesis**

Ref: Chapter No.47, Page No.1156

48. **Ans: A. When stress ulceration is associated with major burns, these lesions are referred to as Cushing's ulcer**

Ref: Chapter No.47, Page No.1156

49. **Ans: B. Body**

Ref: Chapter No.47, Page No.1156

50. **Ans: C. Recurrent bleeding from a Mallory-Weiss tear is common**

Ref: Chapter No.47, Page No.1156

51. **Ans: B. 5% to 10%**

Ref: Chapter No.47, Page No.1156

52. **Ans: A. Gastric antral vascular ectasia is characterized by a collection of dilated arterioles**

Ref: Chapter No.47, Page No.1156

53. **Ans: B. The mucosal defect is usually small (2 to 5 mm) with an associated ulcer**

Ref: Chapter No.47, Page No.1156-1157

54. **Ans: B. The lesser curve of the stomach within 6 cm of the gastroesophageal junction**

Ref: Chapter No.47, Page No.1156

55. **Ans: A. Endoscopy remains the gold standard for diagnosis and intervention**

Ref: Chapter No.47, Page No.1157-1158

56. **Ans: A. Endoscopic therapy is often successful in controlling these bleeds and the rebleeding rate is low**

Ref: Chapter No.47, Page No.1158

57. **Ans: B. The interval between surgery and hemorrhage can be days to years with the median interval about 10 years**

Ref: Chapter No.47, Page No.1158

58. **Ans: A. Duodenum**

Ref: Chapter No.47, Page No.1158

59. **Ans: C. If the suspicion for an aortoenteric fistula is high, EGD should be the first-line study**

Ref: Chapter No.47, Page No.1158

60. **Ans: B. ERCP is the diagnostic gold standard and first therapeutic line of action due to high efficacy**

Ref: Chapter No.47, Page No.1158

61. **Ans: D. Most surgical anastomotic bleeding doesn't resolve with nonoperative management**

Ref: Chapter No.47, Page No.1159

62. **Ans: A. 3%**

Ref: Chapter No.47, Page No.1159

63. **Ans: B. 2%**

Ref: Chapter No.47, Page No.1159

64. **Ans: B. Portal hypertension is defined as a hepatic venous pressure gradient of more than 5 cm of H_2O**

Ref: Chapter No.47, Page No.1159

65. **Ans: C. >12 mm Hg**

Ref: Chapter No.47, Page No.1159

66. **Ans: D. Sclerotherapy is preferred over endoscopic venous ligation for acute esophageal bleeding**

Ref: Chapter No.47, Page No.1159

67. **Ans: B. 24 hours**

Ref: Chapter No.47, Page No.1159

68. **Ans: C. 90%**

Ref: Chapter No.47, Page No.1159

69. **Ans: C. Venous pressures > 25 mm Hg**

Ref: Chapter No.47, Page No.1160

70. **Ans: B. > 50%**

Ref: Chapter No.47, Page No.1160

71. **Ans: C. Diverticular disease**

Ref: Chapter No.47, Page No.1160

72. **Ans: A. 5%–10%**

Ref: Chapter No.47, Page No.1160

73. **Ans: C. In patients with LGIB, more than 50% will have a source in the small intestine**

Ref: Chapter No.47, Page No.1160

74. **Ans: D. Up to 5% of patients with hematochezia had a UGI source to account for the bleed**

Ref: Chapter No.47, Page No.1160

75. **Ans: D. All of the above**

Ref: Chapter No.47, Page No.1160-1161

76. **Ans: D. All of the above**

Ref: Chapter No.47, Page No.1161

77. **Ans: D. 100%**

Ref: Chapter No.47, Page No.1162

78. **Ans: D. All of the above**

Ref: Chapter No.47, Page No.1162

79. **Ans: C. In western countries, right-sided disease is far more common than left-sided disease; however, left-sided disease is responsible for over 50% of significant diverticular bleeding**

Ref: Chapter No.47, Page No.1162

80. **Ans: C. Blind total abdominal colectomy for GI hemorrhage carries with it high morbidity and mortality and does not entirely remove the risk for rebleed, which is approximately 40%**

Ref: Chapter No.47, Page No.1162

81. **Ans: D. Crohn's disease is less likely to have discrete lesions that can undergo endoscopic or angiographic intervention, usually in the form of an ulcer that has eroded into a vessel**

Ref: Chapter No.47, Page No.1162

82. **Ans: B. More common in males**

Ref: Chapter No.47, Page No.1163

83. **Ans: B. Caecum**

Ref: Chapter No.47, Page No.1163

84. **Ans: C. 15%**

Ref: Chapter No.47, Page No.1163

85. **Ans: D. On colonoscopy, these lesions appear as elevated, bright-red, stellate lesions with a surrounding rim of pale mucosa**

Ref: Chapter No.47, Page No.1163

86. **Ans: C. 20% - 30%**

Ref: Chapter No.47, Page No.1163

87. **Ans: D. Chronic colonic ischemia is the most common form of mesenteric ischemia**

Ref: Chapter No.47, Page No.1163

88. **Ans: D. Profound leukocytosis is rarely observed**

Ref: Chapter No.47, Page No.1163

89. **Ans: C. Bleeding is typically painful LGIB**

Ref: Chapter No.47, Page No.1163

90. **Ans: A. Endoscopic therapy with argon coagulation is recommended as an effective treatment as it is not associated with fistula and stricture formation**

Ref: Chapter No.47, Page No.1164

48

Morbid Obesity

OBESITY: THE MAGNITUDE OF THE PROBLEM

1. **Mortality also increases significantly even for individuals with minimal increases in BMI greater than:**

   A. 25.0 B. 30.0
   C. 35.0 D. 40.0

PATHOPHYSIOLOGY AND ASSOCIATED MEDICAL PROBLEMS

2. **The most common single gene etiology of severe obesity is the:**

   A. FTO gene
   B. Ghrelin receptor
   C. MC4R
   D. Proopiomelanocortin (POMC)

3. **Which of the following gene mutations associated with obesity has autosomal dominant trait?**

   A. Ghrelin receptor
   B. Neuropeptide Y (NPY)
   C. Leptin/leptin receptor
   D. Melanocortin 4 receptor

4. **Severe childhood obesity is linked with:**

   A. Ghrelin receptor
   B. Neuropeptide Y (NPY)
   C. Leptin/leptin receptor
   D. Melanocortin 4 receptor

5. **Short stature and obesity is linked with:**

   A. Ghrelin receptor
   B. Neuropeptide Y (NPY)
   C. Leptin/leptin receptor
   D. Melanocortin 4 receptor

6. **Severe early onset obesity is linked with:**

   A. Ghrelin receptor
   B. Neuropeptide Y (NPY)
   C. Leptin/leptin receptor
   D. Proopiomelanocortin (POMC)

7. **Which of the following is appetite inhibitor?**

   A. Ghrelin receptor
   B. Neuropeptide Y (NPY)
   C. Leptin/leptin receptor
   D. Proopiomelanocortin (POMC)

8. **False about ghrelin among the following is:**

   A. Increased levels of ghrelin produce increased food intake, and decreased levels of ghrelin develop in individuals after low-calorie diets
   B. Ghrelin, the only known orexigenic gut hormone, is also known as the hunger hormone and is secreted by P/D1 cells of the gastric fundus
   C. Ghrelin receptor is linked with short stature and obesity
   D. Ghrelin stimulates release of various neuropeptides, such as neuropeptide Y (NPY) and growth hormone, from the hypothalamus, which creates an orexigenic or increased appetite state

9. **Most common medical conditions associated with severe obesity is:**

   A. Arthritis
   B. Asthma
   C. Gastroesophageal reflux
   D. Hypertension

10. **The metabolic syndrome includes all except:**

    A. Dyslipidemia

B. Type 2 diabetes mellitus
C. Stroke
D. Hypertension

11. Obesity has been shown to increase the risk of developing cancer of all except:

A. Liver B. Gallbladder
C. Endometrium D. Pancreas

12. Central body obesity, a primary essential feature the waist circumference in women is:

A. >30 inches B. >35 inches
C. >38 inches D. >40 inches

13. Musculoskeletal conditions associated with severe obesity includes all except:

A. Lumbar disk disease
B. Degenerative joint disease
C. Inguinal hernias
D. Osteoarthritis

14. Neurologic/Psychiatric conditions associated with severe obesity includes all except:

A. Anxiety
B. Low self-esteem
C. Pseudotumor cerebri
D. Stroke

15. Pulmonary conditions associated with severe obesity includes all except:

A. Obstructive sleep apnea
B. Hypoventilation syndrome of obesity
C. Interstitial lung disease
D. Asthma

MEDICAL VERSUS SURGICAL THERAPY

16. Once severely obese, the likelihood that a person will lose enough weight by dietary means alone and remain at a BMI below 35 kg/m² is estimated at:

A. 1% or less B. 3% or less
C. 5% or less D. 7% or less

17. The most common cause of death in the Swedish Obese Subjects (SOS) study was:

A. Heart failure B. Cancer
C. Cardiac arrest D. Stroke

18. False about SOS trial among the following is:

A. SOS trial showed an 80% decrease in the annual mortality of diabetic individuals in the surgical weight loss group versus the matched control patients
B. The majority of procedures performed in SOS study were Roux-en-Y gastric bypass (RYGB)
C. SOS study found improvement in all-cause mortality after 10 years of follow-up
D. The SOS study suicide and nonfatal health self-harm events were greater in the surgery group than in the matched controls

19. False among the following about is:

A. It is remarkable that the medically treated patients require intensive medical therapy while the metabolic surgery patients had reduced or eliminated diabetic medications
B. The reduced incidence rate of microvascular disease was largest in the reduction of nephropathy (59% reduction)
C. Metabolic surgery reduced hemoglobin A1c (HgbA1c) by 2% to 3.5% while medical therapy was only able to reduce HgbA1c by 1% to 1.5%
D. Diabetic patients who undergo bariatric surgery have a similar rate of incident of microvascular disease

BARIATRIC SURGERY MECHANISM OF ACTION

20. False among the following is:

A. RYGB and LSG are known to decrease satiety and reduce hunger
B. Release of NPY is modulated by hormones secreted into the circulation by gastrointestinal cells, such as ghrelin and peptide YY (PYY)
C. NPY is the dominant hormonal signal regulating energy intake
D. Most studies show that ghrelin levels fall significantly following LSG

21. False among the following is:

A. GLP-1 has been found to be consistently elevated (peak and postprandial AUC) in response to both RYGB and LSG, with significant higher magnitude in RYGB than LSG
B. In obese subjects, there is a delay in the postprandial release of GLP-1 and overall significantly reduced circulating levels of the peptide
C. The effect of both RYGB and LSG on postprandial GLP-1 secretion is also observed in subjects with an equivalent degree of weight loss achieved only by caloric restriction

D. GLP-1 is known to exert anorexigenic effects in obese subjects secondary to a reduction in gastric emptying

PREOPERATIVE EVALUATION AND SELECTION

22. Selection of patients for bariatric surgery based on currently accepted NIH and American Heart Association/American College of Cardiology/The Obesity Society guidelines is:

A. BMI greater than 30 kg/m^2 with an associated comorbid medical problem
B. BMI greater than 40 kg/m^2 without associated comorbid medical conditions
C. BMI greater than 40 kg/m^2 with an associated comorbid medical problem
D. BMI greater than 35 kg/m^2 without associated comorbid medical conditions

23. Indications for bariatric surgery includes all except:

A. Psychiatrically stable without alcohol dependence or illegal drug use
B. Medical problems precluding probable survival from surgery
C. Failed dietary therapy
D. Motivated individual

24. False among the following is:

A. For adolescents, most pediatric and bariatric surgeons recommend that the operation be performed after the major growth spurt
B. Surgery is contraindicated in patients who are unable to ambulate
C. Patients who weigh more than 300 lbs are at increased risk for mortality and have more complications
D. The duration and degree of obesity are the most important factors in evaluating an older patient

25. Contraindications to LAGB include:

A. Need for chronic administration of steroids
B. Autoimmune connective tissue disorders
C. Inflammatory bowel disease
D. All of the above

26. Absolute contraindication of bariatric surgery is:

A. Edwards syndrome
B. Prader-Willi syndrome
C. Down syndrome
D. Congenital hypothyroidism

27. False about bariatric surgery preparation is:

A. Bariatric surgery patients are at moderate to high risk for venous thromboembolism (VTE), and they should receive mechanical prophylaxis such as early ambulation and use of SCDs
B. A first-generation cephalosporin, in a dose appropriate for weight, is given preoperatively
C. Antibiotics are continued for >24 hours
D. High-risk patients are given low-molecular-weight heparin administered twice daily for a full 2-week course

28. False among the following is:

A. The prevalence of obstructive sleep apnea diagnosed using sleep studies in the morbidly obese ranges between 35% and 94%
B. Reactive asthma requires more preoperative preparation in terms of testing than sleep apnea does and it is more dangerous
C. Reactive asthma is a common problem of the severely obese and one that is underrecognized
D. In patients with obstructive sleep apnea, use of a continuous or bilevel positive airway pressure apparatus postoperatively while sleeping can eliminate the stressful periods of hypoxia

29. False about Pickwickian syndrome is:

A. These patients have significantly increased high cardiopulmonary morbidity and mortality and require significant preoperative weight loss and optimization
B. Arterial blood gas analysis reveals PaO_2 higher than $PaCO_2$ and an elevated hematocrit
C. Individuals with this diagnosis have plethoric faces, may appear clinically cyanotic, and clearly exhibit difficulty in normal respiratory efforts at baseline or with mild exertion
D. Pulmonary artery pressure is greatly elevated

30. Hypoventilation syndrome of obesity is a diagnosis that should be suspected in the superobese with BMI:

A. >60
B. >50
C. >40
D. >35

31. The most prevalent of the gastrointestinal condition in patients with obesity is:

A. Acute appendicitis
B. Renal stones
C. Acute hepatitis
D. Gallstones

32. The incidence of gallstone or sludge formation after gastric bypass is approximately:

A. 10%
B. 20%
C. 30%
D. 50%

33. Current recommendation for patients undergoing laparoscopic bariatric surgery if the gallbladder is normal:

A. Simultaneous cholecystectomy
B. Ursodiol therapy for 6 months after surgery
C. Interval cholecystectomy after 6 weeks of bariatric surgery
D. Ursodiol therapy for 12 months after surgery

34. False among the following is:

A. Bariatric surgery is beneficial for NASH and weight loss improves the prognosis
B. Preoperative upper endoscopy is indicated in all patients who have GERD symptoms to detect Barrett esophagus and the presence of hiatal hernias
C. Liver biopsy should be performed at the time of bariatric surgery in any patient whose liver appears abnormal
D. Patients with known enlarged fatty livers may benefit from calorie restriction, especially carbohydrate restriction, for a period of 15 to 20 days preoperatively

OPERATIVE PROCEDURES

35. False about Laparoscopic Adjustable Gastric Banding is:

A. Suturing is carried as far anterolaterally as possible because this region has been the most frequent area of fundus herniation through the band
B. The pars flaccid technique has become the approach of choice for placing the adjustable band
C. The anterior branch of the vagus nerve is spared and any aberrant left hepatic artery is preserved
D. Advantage over other bariatric procedures is individualized adjustability and a markedly lower initial operative morbidity and mortality

36. The Laparoscopic Adjustable Gastric band is ideally secured about:

A. 1 cm below the gastroesophageal junction
B. 2 cm below the gastroesophageal junction
C. 1 cm above the gastroesophageal junction
D. 2 cm above the gastroesophageal junction

37. False about Roux-en-Y Gastric Bypass is:

A. The lesser sac is entered through the gastrohepatic ligament, 3 to 4 cm below the gastroesophageal junction
B. Create a 20- to 50-mL proximal gastric pouch based on the upper lesser curvature of the stomach
C. A location approximately 30 to 40 cm distal to the ligament is chosen for division of the jejunum with an endoscopic stapler
D. The mesenteric defect in the jejunojejunostomy is closed with a purse-string suture of 2-0 polypropylene

38. Patients with a BMI in the 40s and undergoing Roux-en-Y Gastric Bypass will be served with a Roux limb of:

A. 150 cms
B. 120 cms
C. 200 cms
D. 250 cms

39. Patients with a BMI in the 50s and undergoing Roux-en-Y Gastric Bypass will be served with a Roux limb of:

A. 150 cms
B. 120 cms
C. 200 cms
D. 250 cms

40. Pouch size in RYGB is:

A. 150 to 200 ml
B. 15–20 ml
C. 30-50 ml
D. 100 to 120 ml

41. True about RYGB is:

A. The antecolic, antegastric approach is preferred
B. The retrocolic, postgastric approach is preferred
C. The antecolic, postgastric approach is preferred
D. The retrocolic, antegastric approach is preferred

42. In Biliopancreatic diversion (BPD) the intestinal tract is reconstructed to allow only a short, so-called common channel of the distal:

A. 100 cm of terminal ileum
B. 50 cm of terminal ileum
C. 150 cm of terminal ileum
D. 70 cm of terminal ileum

43. In the DS procedure, the common channel is:

A. 50 cm
B. 75 cm
C. 100 cm
D. 150 cm

44. In duodenal switch (DS) the goal is to produce a lesser curvature gastric sleeve with a volume of:

A. 150 to 200 ml
B. 15–20 ml
C. 30-50 ml
D. 100 to 120 ml

45. In duodenal switch (DS) the duodenoileostomy is an:

A. Retrocolic end-to-side anastomosis
B. Retrocolic end-to-end anastomosis
C. Antecolic end-to-end anastomosis
D. Antecolic end-to-side anastomosis

46. False about the technical considerations during laparoscopic sleeve gastrectomy is:

A. Staple line reinforcement is recommended
B. Bougie size used is 34–40 French as smaller bougie size associated with GERD and larger is associated with weight regain
C. Staple line extent extends into antrum
D. All of the above are true

POSTOPERATIVE CARE AND FOLLOW-UP

47. False about LAGB is:

A. Saline is added in 1.0- to 1.5-mL increments to produce a desired weight loss
B. The band is initially placed without adding any saline to distend it
C. Plain abdominal radiographs show the normally located 10 to 4 o'clock band position is either vertical or horizontal
D. Desired weight loss is 1 to 2 kg/week

48. Patients undergoing laparoscopic bariatric surgery usually have much less third space and operative blood loss than do patients undergoing open surgery and can be managed with:

A. 1 mL/kg/hour of intravenous fluids
B. 2 mL/kg/hour of intravenous fluids
C. 3 mL/kg/hour of intravenous fluids
D. 4 mL/kg/hour of intravenous fluids

49. False about LSG is:

A. Achilles heel of LSG is a leak along the long gastric staple line
B. The leaks are most likely to be located in the distal third of the stomach
C. Leaks after LSG appear between 1 - 4 weeks postoperative
D. Management of the leak includes adequate drainage, by either CT-guided percutaneous catheter placement or operative approaches, with institution of total parenteral nutrition, no oral intake and antibiotics

50. The cause of leaks after LSG appears to be multifactorial, with early leaks (≤2 days postoperatively) related to:

A. Ischemia
B. High intragastric pressure
C. Stapler misfires
D. All of the above

51. The cause of leaks after LSG appears to be multifactorial, with late leaks are related to:

A. Tissue trauma
B. High intragastric pressure
C. Stapler misfires
D. Both A and B

BARIATRIC SURGERY RESULTS

52. Post Roux-en-Y Gastric Bypass there is immediate resolution of symptoms of GERD in:

A. >50% of cases
B. >60% of cases
C. >80% of cases
D. >90% of cases

53. Highest estimated weight loss after bariatric operations is after:

A. Laparoscopic Adjustable Gastric Banding
B. Laparoscopic Sleeve Gastrectomy
C. Biliopancreatic Diversion and Duodenal Switch
D. Roux-en-Y Gastric Bypass

54. After undergoing BPD/DS most common deficiency is:

A. Vitamin K
B. Vitamin D
C. Zinc
D. Vitamin A

55. False about BPD/DS:

A. Excessive flatulence and foul-smelling stools are the rule
B. Malabsorption of starch and fat provides the major mechanism of weight loss
C. Supplements include multivitamins as well as at least 2 g of oral calcium per day
D. After BPD/DS, patients typically have between 5 and 8 bowel movements per day

COMPLICATIONS OF BARIATRIC SURGERY

56. The most common cause of death after RYGB was:

A. Sepsis
B. Pulmonary embolism
C. Cardiac causes
D. Renal failure

57. Post RYGB leaks are most common from:

A. Jejunojejunostomy
B. Gastrojejunostomy

C. Stapled end of proximal jejunum
D. Same at all sites

58. Post bariatric surgery, false statement is:

A. One specific problem that may arise with persistent vomiting after any of the bariatric operations and that is imperative for the surgeon to treat is Wernicke's encephalopathy
B. If the neurologic symptoms become significant after Wernicke's encephalopathy, they may often not be fully reversed despite thiamine therapy
C. Pulmonary embolism is one of the most feared complications after any form of bariatric surgery
D. Severe postoperative depression may develop after LSG only

59. After RYGB, false statement is:

A. The incidence of marginal ulcers can't be decreased by preoperative treatment of patients for Helicobacter pylori colonization of the stomach
B. After RYGB, postoperative anastomotic stenosis is usually manifested at 4 to 6 weeks postoperatively as progressive intolerance to solids and then liquids
C. Unless a marginal ulcer is associated with the stenosis, the problem does not require a reoperation
D. A marginal ulcer occurs after 2% to 10% of RYGB procedures

60. Each additional 1 cm added in the vertical stapling height in RYGB, increased the risk of marginal ulcer by:

A. 7% B. 14%
C. 21% D. 35%

61. False about marginal ulcers after RYGB is:

A. Treatment of marginal ulcer consists of medical therapy with proton pump inhibitors and avoidance of nonsteroidal anti inflammatory drugs
B. Medical treatment resolves most of the marginal ulcers
C. Surgery to divide the fistula is necessary when present to effect healing of the ulcer
D. All of the above are true

62. False about vitamin B_{12} deficiency after RYGB is:

A. Vitamin B_{12} deficiency is due to inefficient absorption because of delayed mixing with intrinsic factor
B. B_{12} deficiency can't develop with plentiful oral administration
C. The incidence of vitamin B_{12} deficiency after RYGB is reported as being 15% to 20%, it causes anemia
D. Routes of vitamin B_{12} administration include sublingual medication, nasal spray and parenteral injections

63. The most significant and specific long-term complication seen after BPD/DS is:

A. Vitamin D deficiency
B. Vitamin B_{12} deficiency
C. Iron deficiency
D. Protein malnutrition

64. RYGB is contraindicated in all except:

A. Iron deficiency anemia
B. Patients with pre existing vitamin deficiencies
C. Autoimmune connective tissue disorder
D. Crohn small bowel disease

65. In cardiac failure patients, which of the following procedure is not contraindicated?

A. DS B. LSG
C. RYGB D. BPD

REOPERATIVE SURGERY

66. True about revisional surgery for bariatric surgery is/are:

A. All bariatric operations have some incidence of failure, which includes inadequate weight loss and inadequate resolution of medical comorbid conditions
B. Stenosis causing gastric outlet obstruction after vertical banded gastroplasty is an indication of revisional surgery
C. The incidence of infection, organ ischemia, anastomotic leakage, blood transfusion, and other severe intra-abdominal complications is increased in revisional surgery
D. All of the above

ENDOSCOPIC PROCEDURES IN BARIATRIC SURGERY

67. False about endoscopic management of complications after bariatric surgery is:

A. One of the most commonly used interventions for a leak is the use of a fully covered stent
B. The endoscopically placed stent traverses the perforation, thereby decreasing ongoing contamination

C. Migration of the stent was noted in 8/20 patients, which appears to be a major issue with these stents and the Achilles heel of this management approach

D. Use of stents noted a healing period of 4 weeks and a 50% success rate

68. True about endoscopic vacuum-assisted closure is:

A. Endoscopic vacuum-assisted closure technique involves placing the vacuum sponge on the end of an orogastric tube into the cavity external to the leak

B. Endoscopic vacuum-assisted closure is now being used for the closure of large leaks

C. Patients will require 8 to 12 procedures over a period of weeks

D. All of the above

69. False about strictures after bariatric surgery is:

A. Strictures may require multiple dilations as one should not try to dilate the stricture more than 3 to 5 mm at any one sitting

B. After a gastric bypass, the anastomotic strictures can often be managed with through-the-scope balloons

C. Strictures after LSG are most often at the fundus

D. If the scope cannot traverse the stricture, the balloon can be placed over a wire or with fluoroscopic guidance to avoid perforation

70. True about primary endoscopic weight loss procedures is:

A. Most patients lose 30 to 50 lbs

B. The original gastric balloon was the Garren-Edwards balloon

C. Orbera balloon is placed endoscopically, remains in place for 6 months and then is removed endoscopically

D. All of the above

ANSWERS

1. **Ans: B. 30.0**

Ref: Chapter No.48, Page No.1168

2. **Ans: C. MC4R**

Ref: Chapter No.48, Page No.1168

3. **Ans: D. Melanocortin 4 receptor**

Ref: Chapter No.48, Page No.1168

4. **Ans: C. Leptin/leptin receptor**

Ref: Chapter No.48, Page No.1168

5. **Ans: A. Ghrelin receptor**

Ref: Chapter No.48, Page No.1168

6. **Ans: D. Proopiomelanocortin (POMC)**

Ref: Chapter No.48, Page No.1168

7. **Ans: D. Proopiomelanocortin (POMC)**

Ref: Chapter No.48, Page No.1168

8. **Ans: A. Increased levels of ghrelin produce increased food intake and decreased levels of ghrelin develop in individuals after low-calorie diets**

Ref: Chapter No.48, Page No.1168

9. **Ans: A. Arthritis**

Ref: Chapter No.48, Page No.1168

10. **Ans: C. Stroke**

Ref: Chapter No.48, Page No.1168

11. **Ans: A. Liver**

Ref: Chapter No.48, Page No.1169

12. **Ans: B. >35 inches**

Ref: Chapter No.48, Page No.1168

13. **Ans: C. Inguinal hernias**

Ref: Chapter No.48, Page No.1169

14. **Ans: A. Anxiety**

Ref: Chapter No.48, Page No.1169

15. **Ans: C. Interstitial lung disease**

Ref: Chapter No.48, Page No.1169

16. **Ans: B. 3% or less**

Ref: Chapter No.48, Page No.1169

17. **Ans: B. Cancer**

Ref: Chapter No.48, Page No.1169

18. **Ans: B. The majority of procedures performed in SOS study were Roux-en-Y gastric bypass (RYGB)**

Ref: Chapter No.48, Page No.1170-1171

19. **Ans: D. Diabetic patients who undergo bariatric surgery have a similar rate of incident of microvascular disease**

Ref: Chapter No.48, Page No.1171

20. **Ans: A. RYGB and LSG are known to decrease satiety and reduce hunger**

Ref: Chapter No.48, Page No.1172

21. **Ans: C. The effect of both RYGB and LSG on postprandial GLP-1 secretion is also observed in subjects with an equivalent degree of weight loss achieved only by caloric restriction**

Ref: Chapter No.48, Page No.1173

22. **Ans: B. BMI greater than 40 kg/m2 without associated comorbid medical conditions**

Ref: Chapter No.48, Page No.1173

23. **Ans: B. Medical problems precluding probable survival from surgery**

Ref: Chapter No.48, Page No.1174

24. **Ans: C. Patients who weigh more than 300 lbs are at increased risk for mortality and have more complications**

Ref: Chapter No.48, Page No.1174-1175

25. **Ans: D. All of the above**

Ref: Chapter No.48, Page No.1174

26. **Ans: B. Prader-Willi syndrome**

Ref: Chapter No.48, Page No.1174

27. **Ans: C. Antibiotics are continued for >24 hours**

Ref: Chapter No.48, Page No.1175

28. **Ans: B. Reactive asthma requires more preoperative preparation in terms of testing than sleep apnea does and it is more dangerous**

Ref: Chapter No.48, Page No.1175-1176

29. **Ans: B. Arterial blood gas analysis reveals PaO_2 higher than $PaCO_2$ and an elevated hematocrit**

Ref: Chapter No.48, Page No.1176

30. **Ans: A. >60**

Ref: Chapter No.48, Page No.1176

31. **Ans: D. Gallstones**

Ref: Chapter No.48, Page No.1176

32. **Ans: C. 30%**

Ref: Chapter No.48, Page No.1176

33. **Ans: B. Ursodiol therapy for 6 months after surgery**

Ref: Chapter No.48, Page No.1176

34. **Ans: D. Patients with known enlarged fatty livers may benefit from calorie restriction, especially carbohydrate restriction, for a period of 15 to 20 days preoperatively**

Ref: Chapter No.48, Page No.1176

35. **Ans: A. Suturing is carried as far anterolaterally as possible because this region has been the most frequent area of fundus herniation through the band**

Ref: Chapter No.48, Page No.1177

36. **Ans: A. 1 cm below the gastroesophageal junction**

Ref: Chapter No.48, Page No.1177

37. **Ans: B. Create a 20- to 50-mL proximal gastric pouch based on the upper lesser curvature of the stomach**

Ref: Chapter No.48, Page No.1177-1179

38. **Ans: B. 120 cms**

Ref: Chapter No.48, Page No.1177

39. **Ans: A. 150 cms**

Ref: Chapter No.48, Page No.1177

40. **Ans: B. 15–20 ml**

Ref: Chapter No.48, Page No.1180

41. **Ans: A. The antecolic, antegastric approach is preferred**

Ref: Chapter No.48, Page No.1179

42. **Ans: B. 50 cm of terminal ileum**

Ref: Chapter No.48, Page No.1179

43. **Ans: C. 100 cm**

Ref: Chapter No.48, Page No.1179-1181

44. **Ans: A. 150 to 200 ml**

Ref: Chapter No.48, Page No.1181

45. **Ans: D. Antecolic end-to-side anastomosis**

Ref: Chapter No.48, Page No.1181

46. **Ans: A. Staple line reinforcement is recommended**

Ref: Chapter No.48, Page No.1184

47. **Ans: C. Plain abdominal radiographs show the normally located 10 to 4 o'clock band position is either vertical or horizontal**

Ref: Chapter No.48, Page No.1183

48. **Ans: D. 4 mL/kg/hour of intravenous fluids**

Ref: Chapter No.48, Page No.1183

49. **Ans: B. The leaks are most likely to be located in the distal third of the stomach**

Ref: Chapter No.48, Page No.1184

50. **Ans: C. Stapler misfires**

Ref: Chapter No.48, Page No.1184

51. **Ans: B. High intragastric pressure**

Ref: Chapter No.48, Page No.1184

52. **Ans: D. >90% of cases**

Ref: Chapter No.48, Page No.1185

53. **Ans: C. Biliopancreatic Diversion and Duodenal Switch**

Ref: Chapter No.48, Page No.1185

54. **Ans: B. Vitamin D.**

Ref: Chapter No.48, Page No.1185

55. **Ans: D. After BPD/DS, patients typically have between 5 and 8 bowel movements per day**

Ref: Chapter No.48, Page No.1186

56. **Ans: A. Sepsis**

Ref: Chapter No.48, Page No.1187

57. **Ans: B. Gastrojejunostomy**

Ref: Chapter No.48, Page No.1187

58. **Ans: D. Severe postoperative depression may develop after LSG only**

Ref: Chapter No.48, Page No.1188

59. **Ans: A. The incidence of marginal ulcers can't be decreased by preoperative treatment of patients for Helicobacter pylori colonization of the stomach**

Ref: Chapter No.48, Page No.1188

60. **Ans: B. 14%**

Ref: Chapter No.48, Page No.1188

61. **Ans: D. All of the above are true**

Ref: Chapter No.48, Page No.1188

62. **Ans: B. B_{12} deficiency can't develop with plentiful oral administration**

Ref: Chapter No.48, Page No.1188

63. **Ans: D. Protein malnutrition**

Ref: Chapter No.48, Page No.1188

64. **Ans: C. Autoimmune connective tissue disorder**

Ref: Chapter No.48, Page No.1190

65. **Ans: B. LSG**

Ref: Chapter No.48, Page No.1190

66. **Ans: D. All of the above**

Ref: Chapter No.48, Page No.1189

67. **Ans: D. Use of stents noted a healing period of 4 weeks and a 50% success rate**

Ref: Chapter No.48, Page No.1190

68. **Ans: D. All of the above**

Ref: Chapter No.48, Page No.1190

69. **Ans: C. Strictures after LSG are most often at the fundus**

Ref: Chapter No.48, Page No.1191

70. **Ans: D. All of the above**

Ref: Chapter No.48, Page No.1191

49

Stomach

ANATOMY

1. **Stomach is derived from the tubular embryonic foregut and begins as a dilation during:**
   A. 5th week of gestation in the cranial portion
   B. 7th week of gestation in the caudal portion
   C. 5th week of gestation in the caudal portion
   D. 7th week of gestation in the cranial portion

2. **The stomach descends, rotates and further dilates with a disproportionate elongation of the greater curvature into its normal anatomic shape and position by which week?**
   A. 5th week B. 7th week
   C. 8th week D. 10th week

3. **Angle of His is formed by:**
   A. Fundus and left margin of oesophagus
   B. Fundus and cardia
   C. Cardia and left margin of oesophagus
   D. Fundus and body

4. **False statement regarding blood supply off stomach:**
   A. Left gastric artery-splenic artery
   B. Right gastric artery-hepatic artery
   C. Right gastroepiploic artery-superior mesenteric artery
   D. Left gastroepiploic artery-splenic artery

5. **Largest artery to stomach:**
   A. Right gastric artery
   B. Left gastric artery
   C. Left gastroepiploic artery
   D. Right gastroepiploic artery

6. **All of the following are false regarding nerve supply of stomach except:**
   A. Left vagus - anterior
   B. Hepatic branch - branch of posterior vagus
   C. Celiac branch - branch of anterior vagus
   D. First branch of anterior vagus - nerve of Latarjet

7. **Criminal nerve of Grassi is:**
   A. First branch of posterior vagus
   B. First branch of anterior vagus
   C. Last branch of posterior vagus
   D. Last branch of anterior vagus

8. **False statement about vagus nerve:**
   A. The vagus nerve originates in the vagal nucleus in the floor of the fourth ventricle
   B. Most (90%) of the vagal fibres are afferent, carrying stimuli to the brain
   C. Efferent vagal fibres originate in the dorsal nucleus of the medulla and synapse with neurons in the myenteric and submucosal plexuses
   D. The so-called criminal nerve of Grassi is the first branch of the left vagus nerve

9. **Layer of the stomach, which is responsible for gastric rugae?**
   A. Mucosa B. Muscularis mucosa
   C. Lamina propria D. Submucosa

10. **Only complete muscle layer of the stomach is:**
    A. Muscularis mucosae
    B. Oblique muscle fibres
    C. Circular muscle fibres
    D. Longitudinal muscle fibres

11. **Percentage of patients who have an aberrant left hepatic artery originating from the left gastric artery?**

A. 10 B. 20
C. 50 D. 30

12. False statement about the venous drainage of stomach:

A. Veins of the stomach parallel the arteries
B. Left gastric and right gastric veins usually drain into the portal vein
C. The left gastroepiploic vein drains into the splenic vein
D. The right gastroepiploic vein drains into the IVC

13. True statement about the lymphatic drainage of stomach:

A. The superior gastric group drains lymph from the upper lesser curvature into the left gastric and paracardial nodes
B. The supra pyloric group of nodes drains the antral segment on the lesser curvature of the stomach into the right suprapancreatic nodes
C. The pancreaticolienal group of nodes drains lymph high on the greater curvature into the left gastroepiploic and splenic nodes
D. All of the above are true statements

14. Strongest layer of the gastric wall is:

A. Submucosa B. Serosa
C. Muscularis Propria D. MuscularisMucosae

15. Sympathetic nerve supply to stomach comes from:

A. T10-T12 B. T1-T4
C. T5-T10 D. Vagus Nerve

16. All of the following are present in gastric body except:

A. Parietal cells B. Chief cell
C. G cells D. D cells

17. The endocrine G cells are present in greatest quantity at:

A. Body B. Antrum
C. Fundus D. Diffuse

18. Parietal cells are present at all except:

A. Body B. Proximal Antrum
C. Fundus D. Cardia

19. Which of the following is largest artery to stomach?

A. Left gastroepiploic artery
B. Right gastroepiploic artery
C. Right gastric artery
D. Left gastric artery

20. Criminal nerve of grassi is:

A. First branch of posterior vagus
B. First branch of anterior vagus
C. Last branch of right vagus
D. Last branch of left vagus

PHYSIOLOGY

21. Which of the following undergoes post translational modification?

A. Ghrelin B. CCK
C. Secretin D. Gastrin

22. Most common form of released antral gastrin:

A. Big gastrin B. Little gastrin
C. Mini gastrin D. Micro gastrin

23. Which is the biologically active component of gastrin?

A. Pentapeptide component at carboxyl terminus of gastrin
B. Octapeptide component at carboxyl terminus of gastrin
C. Pentapeptide component at N terminus of gastrin
D. Octapeptide component at N terminus of gastrin

24. Active component of the 2 following peptides are same .... is.

A. Gastrin and ghrelin
B. Ghrelin and CCK
C. Gastrin and CCK
D. Gastrin and somatostatin

25. Release of gastrin in the stomach is mainly stimulated by:

A. Protein meal B. Carbohydrates meal
C. Fatty meal D. All of the above

26. Major hormonal regulator of gastric phase of gastric acid secretion:

A. Histamine B. Acetylcholine
C. Gastrin D. Ghrelin

27. Gastrin has trophic effect on:

A. Parietal cells B. Zygomen cells
C. ECL cells D. Both option A + C

28. All are non-ulcerogenic causes of hypergastrinemia except:

A. Pernicious anemia

B. Short gut syndrome
C. H Pylori infection
D. Chronic renal failure

29. All are ulcerogenic causes of hypergastrinemia except:

A. Gastric Outlet Obstruction
B. Pernicious Anemia
C. Retained excluded Antrum
D. Zollinger-Ellison Syndrome

30. All are ulcerogenic causes of hypergastrinemia except:

A. Gastric Outlet Obstruction
B. H Pylori Infection
C. ZE Syndrome
D. Short Gut Syndrome

31. Majority of gastrin released as:

A. G34 B. G17
C. G14 D. G11

32. True Statement about Gastrin are all except:

A. Gastrin initiates its biologic actions by activation of surface membrane receptors
B. These surface receptors are members of the classic G protein–coupled receptor family
C. The gastrin or CCK-B receptor has high affinity for both gastrin and CCK
D. Type A CCK receptors have an affinity for sulphated CCK analogues and Gastrin

33. Major hormonal regulator of the gastric phase of acid secretion:

A. Secretin B. Gastrin
C. CCK D. Histamine

34. Predominant form of somatostatin in stomach:

A. Somatostatin 28 B. Somatostatin 20
C. Somatostatin 14 D. Somatostatin 12

35. The principal stimulus for somatostatin release is:

A. Antral acidification
B. Gastrin-releasing peptide
C. Acetylcholine
D. Both A and B

36. The stimulus for somatostatin inhibition is:

A. Acetylcholine B. GRP
C. Antral Acidification D. None of the above

37. All are true statements about Ghrelin except:

A. Under both endocrine and metabolic control
B. Has a diurnal rhythm
C. Plays a major role in the neuroendocrine and metabolic responses to changes in nutritional status
D. Increased ghrelin levels have been associated with gastritis

38. Gastric acid hypersecretion is regulated by:

A. Gastrin B. Histamine
C. Acetylcholine D. All of the Above

39. Basal acid output of acid secretion in absence of food:

A. 10% of the maximal acid output
B. 20% of the maximal acid output
C. 35% of the maximal acid output
D. 50% of the maximal acid output

40. Basal acid output of acid secretion in absence of food:

A. 1 to 5 mmol/hr B. 10 to 15 mmol/hr
C. 20 to 25 mmol/hr D. 10 to 50 mmol/hr

41. Which of the following is False?

A. Cephalic phase - 20-30% of the maximal acid output
B. Gastric phase - 60-70% of the maximal acid output
C. Gastric phase - 90% of the maximal acid output
D. Intestinal phase - 10% of the maximal acid output

42. False about gastric acid secretion is:

A. The intensity of the acid secretory response in the cephalic phase surpasses that of the other phases
B. Gastric distention activates stretch receptors in the stomach to elicit the vasovagal reflex arc
C. Intestinal phase of gastric secretion is initiated by entry of chyme into the stomach
D. Gastric phase of acid secretion begins when food enters the gastric lumen

43. The most potent of the H2-receptor antagonists:

A. Famotidine B. Ranitidine
C. Nizatidine D. Cimetidine

44. True about PPI are all except:

A. Because of the covalent nature of the bond, PPIs have more prolonged inhibition of gastric acid secretion than H2 blockers

B. For recovery of acid secretion after PPI, new protein pumps must be synthesized
C. H2 blockers have more prolonged inhibition of gastric acid secretion than PPI
D. Sucralfate is a sucrose octasulfate complexed with aluminum hydroxide

45. True statement amongst the following:

A. There is a non-linear relationship between maximal acid output and parietal cell number
B. There is a linear relationship between maximal acid output and parietal cell number
C. Patients with proximal gastric ulcers have higher secretory rates
D. All of the above are true

46. The lowest intraluminal pH commonly measured in the stomach:

A. 1
B. 2
C. 3
D. 4

47. Which of the following is not correct for intrinsic factor?

A. Essential for absorption of vitamin B_{12}
B. PPI don't block intrinsic factor secretion
C. Secreted in equal amounts to amount necessary for vitamin B_{12} secretion
D. Secretion if intrinsic factor parallel gastric acid secretion

48. Each cycle of MMC last for:

A. 60-90 mins
B. 90-120 mins
C. 80-120 mins
D. 100-120 mins

49. pH observed at the surface epithelial cell:

A. 2
B. 4
C. 7
D. 3

50. All are true except:

A. Gastric mucin is a large glycoprotein and the mucus is a viscoelastic gel containing approximately 65% water and 35% mucin
B. It provides a mechanical barrier to injury
C. Mucus is in a constant state of flux
D. Mucus production is stimulated by vagal stimulation, cholinergic agonists, prostaglandins and some bacterial toxins

51. All are true except:

A. Group 1 pepsinogens are secreted by chief cells and by mucous neck cells
B. Group 2 pepsinogens are produced by surface epithelial cells throughout the acid-secreting portion of the stomach, antrum and proximal duodenum
C. Pepsins have optimal function at a pH of 1.5 to 2.0 and become inactive at higher pH
D. Pepsin is an endopeptidase that preferentially hydrolyses peptide linkages where one of the amino acids is aromatic and accounts for approximately 50% of the protein digestion in the GI tract

52. All are true except:

A. Hot and cold liquids tend to empty at a slower rate than ambient temperature fluids
B. Hot and cold liquids tend to empty at a faster rate than ambient temperature fluids
C. Ingestion of a meal results in a decrease in the resting tone of the proximal stomach and fundus, referred to as receptive relaxation and gastric accommodation
D. None of the above

53. All are true about Fasting gastric motility except:

A. Gastric motility starts from pace maker cells greater curvature of mid body of stomach
B. Pace maker cells produce slow waves which travel circumferential and antegrade fashion
C. The cyclical activity of slow waves and action potential happening during fasting is called myoelectric migrating complex
D. The MMC is lost after vagal denervation

54. The number of smooth waves produced from gastric greater curvature:

A. 2 cycle/min
B. 3 cycle/min
C. 4 cycle/min
D. 5 cycle/min

55. Abnormal gastric motility symptoms:

A. Nausea
B. Fullness
C. Early satiety
D. All of the above

56. The most common cause of gastroparesis:

A. Diabetes mellitus
B. Viral infections
C. Stroke
D. Idiopathic

57. Evaluation of abnormal gastric motility is done by all except:

A. Endoscopy
B. Gamma scintigraphy
C. Real-time USG
D. MRI

58. Effects of hyperglycaemia in gastric motility are:

A. Decrease contractility of antrum
B. Increase contractility of pylorus
C. Suppression of MMC
D. All

59. Regarding radionuclide scintigraphy after 4 hours of ingestion, moderate gastroparesis is:

A. 10-15% B. 15-35%
C. >35% D. <10%

60. Regarding radionuclide scintigraphy after 4 hours of ingestion, severe gastroparesis is:

A. 10-15% B. 15-35%
C. >35% D. <10%

61. All are true regarding treatment of gastroparesis except:

A. Initial treatment is diet modification and environmental factors
B. Medication that affects gastric motility should be stopped
C. Gastric electrostimulators for refractory idiopathic and diabetic gastroparesis
D. Gastrojejunostomy gives very good results

62. Drugs that cause gastroparesis are all except:

A. Tricyclic anti antidepressants
B. Opioids
C. Calcium channel blockers
D. Dopamine antagonists

63. False about surgical management about gastroparesis:

A. Surgery for gastroparesis is rarely required and only indicated for refractory symptoms despite maximal medical therapy
B. Pyloromyotomy and pyloroplasty are options for the surgical management of gastroparesis
C. Surgical implantation of gastric electro stimulators use electrical leads that are placed onto the body laparoscopically and connected to a subcutaneously positioned simulator that delivers low-frequency, high-energy current
D. Endoscopic therapies, such as the gastric peroral endoscopic myotomy, are also being explored

64. Marked mucosal injury occurs when blood supply is reduced by:

A. 50% B. 65%
C. 55% D. 75%

65. Decreased gastric mucosal blood flow has minimal effects of ulcer formation till it approaches:

A. 50% B. 65%
C. 55% D. 75%

66. In normal gastric mucosa, potential difference across the mucosa is:

A. -30 to -50mV B. 30 to 50 mV
C. -30 to 150 mV D. 30 to -150 mV

PEPTIC ULCER DISEASE

67. Which of the following gastric ulcers behave more like duodenal ulcer?

A. Type 1 B. Type 2
C. Type 4 D. Type 5

68. Which of the following statement is false regarding abdominal pain in duodenal ulcer?

A. It is most common symptom
B. Relieved by food intake
C. Pain is episodic, seasonal in spring and fall
D. Improves in time of stress

69. Which of the following is true regarding abdominal pain in duodenal ulcer?

A. If pain becomes constant, it suggests deeper penetration of ulcer
B. Referral of pain to back usually a sign of penetration of ulcer into pancreas
C. Diffuse peritoneal irritation is usually a sign of free perforation
D. All are true

70. What is the prevalence in peptic ulcers in developed countries?

A. 50 to 75% B. 80 to 90%
C. 90 to 95% D. 60 to 90%

71. All are true statements about H pylori except:

A. Infection with H pylori has been shown to temporally precede ulcer formation
B. When the organism is eradicated as part of ulcer treatment, ulcer recurrence is still common
C. Observations have secured the place of H pylori as a primary causative factor in the pathogenesis of PUD
D. The interplay between bacterial and host factors determines the clinical outcome of H pylori infection

72. Which of the following is not a mechanism of H pylori pathogenesis?

A. Production of toxic products that cause local tissue injury
B. Induction of a local mucosal immune response
C. Decreased gastrin levels and changes in acid secretion
D. Gastric metaplasia occurring in the duodenum

73. For their pioneering work in H. pylori, who were jointly awarded the Nobel Prize in Medicine?

A. Louis Pasteur
B. Marshall and Warren
C. Lister and Koch
D. None of the above

74. True statements about urease assay:

A. Sensitivity in diagnosing infection is greater than 90% and specificity is 95% to 100%
B. Rapid urease test kits can detect urease in gastric biopsy specimens within 30 mins
C. Gold standard
D. All are true

75. Which test is used for checking antibiotic sensitivity?

A. Culture B. Histology
C. Urea breath test D. Serology

76. In patients taking PPIs or H_2-receptor antagonists, which is the most accurate test available?

A. Culture B. Histology
C. Urea breath test D. Serology

77. How long is it recommended for patients to discontinue antibiotics and PPIs to ensure optimal test accuracy?

A. 2 weeks and PPIs for 4 weeks for Antibiotics
B. 4 weeks and PPIs for 2 weeks for Antibiotics
C. 4 weeks and PPIs for 6 weeks for Antibiotics
D. 6 weeks and PPIs for 4 weeks for Antibiotics

78. Antibody titres can remain high for:

A. 1 year or longer after eradication
B. 2 years or longer after eradication
C. 1/2 years or longer after eradication
D. 3 years or longer after eradication

79. What is the accuracy of stool antigen testing in detecting eradication of infection after treatment?

A. 70% B. 80%
C. 90% D. 85%

80. Most cost-effective method for assessing treatment efficacy:

A. Culture B. Stool Antigen
C. Urea breath test D. Serology

81. Regarding Gastric Ulcers all are true except:

A. Most occur within 1.5 cm of the histologic transition zone
B. They usually manifest on the lesser curvature near the incisura
C. Modified Johnson anatomic classification system is used
D. Gastric ulcers are more likely to occur in individuals in a higher socio-economic class

82. Regarding Gastric Ulcers all are true except:

A. Patients who develop significant bleeding from gastric ulcers usually are older
B. Have higher morbidity and mortality rates than patients with bleeding from a duodenal ulcer
C. The most frequent complication of gastric ulceration is perforation
D. Most perforations occur along the Posterior aspect of the lesser curvature

83. _____% of ulcers that appear radiographically benign are malignant.

A. 1% B. 5%
C. 10% D. 7%

84. Most reliable method for diagnosing gastric and duodenal ulcers:

A. USG B. CECT scan
C. X-ray D. Endoscopy

85. True regarding Upper GI endoscopy:

A. Endoscopic biopsy showed that the first biopsy sample taken of an ulcer had only a 70% sensitivity in detecting gastric cancer
B. Taking four biopsy specimens increased this yield to 95%
C. Taking seven specimens increased it to 98%
D. All are true

86. All are true statements regarding:

A. The gold standard for diagnosis of H pylori is mucosal biopsy performed during upper endoscopy
B. Evaluation of serum antibodies is the test of choice for initial diagnosis when endoscopy is not required but has the drawback of remaining positive after treatment and eradication of infection

C. For monitoring treatment efficacy, stool antigen and urea breath testing are both adequate choices
D. All are true

87. Sensitivity and specificity of following tests in relation to H. pylori are true except:

A. Urease assay – 90%, 95-100
B. Histology – 95%, 99%
C. Culture – 80%, 100%
D. All of the above

88. Which of the following statements is false regarding urea breath test?

A. Antibiotics should be stopped 4 weeks before test
B. PPI should be stopped 4 weeks before test
C. In checking efficacy of treatment, it should be done after 4 weeks of treatment
D. It is done by carbon labelled

89. Which of the following is false regarding antacids?

A. Reduces acidity by reacting with HCL and forming salt
B Magnesium antacids cause diarrhoea
C. Phosphorus causes constipation
D. Magnesium antacids cause hypophosphatemia

90. Which of following is false regarding sucralfate?

A. It is an aluminium salt of sulfated sucrose
B. It can last for 6 hours in stomach
C. Treatment of 4-6 weeks is needed for healing
D. It is structurally related to warfarin have anticoagulant effects

91. Which of the following is false regarding H_2 receptor antagonist?

A. Similar to histamine
B. Most potent is famotidine
C. Ranitidine is weakest
D. Undergoes hepatic metabolism and excretion by kidney

92. Which of the following is false regarding PPIs?

A. The most potent antisecretory agents are PPIs
B. These agents irreversibly bind and inhibit the hydrogen potassium ATPase on the parietal cell
C. PPIs have a healing rate of 75% at 4 weeks and 90% at 8 weeks and produce more rapid healing of ulcers than standard H2-receptor antagonists
D. PPIs require an acidic environment within the gastric lumen to become activated maintenance PPI therapy is considered in patients with large (>2 cm) ulcers

93. Which of the following is not a triple therapy regimen?

A. Metronidazole + Clarithromycin + PPI
B. Amoxicillin + Clarithromycin + PPI
C. Amoxicillin + Tetracycline + PPI
D. None

94. Quadruple therapy is adding of?

A. 2nd PPI
B. H_2 antagonist
C. Tetracycline
D. Bismuth

95. Clinical guidelines generally recommend treatment with a:

A. 7-day course of triple therapy
B. 10-day course of triple therapy
C. 14-day course of triple therapy
D. 21-day course of triple therapy

96. Regarding surgical treatment recommendations for complications related: to peptic ulcer disease, all are true except:

A. Intractable: Parietal cell vagotomy ± antrectomy
B. Bleeding: Oversewing of bleeding vessel with treatment of H. pylori
C. Perforation: Patch closure with treatment of H pylori
D. Obstruction: Only gastrojejunostomy

97. Risk factors for complicated PUD:

A. NSAIDs
B. H. pylori
C. Size of ulcer >1 cm
D. All of the above

98. Which test is the best initial procedure for diagnosis of the source of upper GI bleeding and for therapeutic intervention, including in the setting of bleeding ulcers?

A. CT scan
B. Upper flexible endoscopy
C. USG
D. MRI

99. Which of the following is false regarding Forrest classification?

A. Type 1a – Active spurting
B. Type 1b – Diffuse bleeding
C. Type 2a – Adherent clot
D. Type 2c – Flat pigmented spot

100. Risk of rebleeding is least in which of the following?

A. Type 1a B. Type 1b
C. Type 2a D. Type 2b

101. PUD haemorrhage is associated with an approximately _____ % mortality rate.

A. 1% to 5% B. 6% to 10%
C. 10% to 20% D. 25% to 30%

102. Almost all patients with a potentially substantial acute upper GI bleed should undergo endoscopy within:

A. 48 hrs B. 24 hrs
C. 72 hrs D. 96 hrs

103. All are true except:

A. For high-risk patients requiring intervention, the best initial approach is endoscopic control
B. Patients with recurrent bleeding can be considered for interventional angiography with transarterial embolization
C. Epinephrine injection monotherapy is not recommended given the high rebleeding rates
D. Patients who have a second episode of bleeding after initially successful endoscopic therapy are typically treated with surgery

104. ________ % of patients with persistent bleeding that requires surgical intervention.

A. 1% to 5% B. 5% to 10%
C. 10% to 15% D. 15% to 20%

105. Indications for surgical intervention persistent bleeding are all except:

A. Failed endoscopic treatment hemodynamic
B. Instability, or continued slow bleeding with transfusion requirement
C. After 1 try of endoscopic treatment
D. Recurrent hemorrhage after multiple endoscopic treatments

106. In 3-point U stitch for UGI bleed, the medial stitch is for stopping the bleeding from:

A. Splenic artery
B. Gastroduodenal artery
C. Transverse pancreatic artery
D. Retropancreatic artery

107. Which of the following complication had highest mortality rate?

A. Bleeding
B. Gastric Outlet Obstruction
C. Perforation
D. Scarring

108. Which of the following is false regarding perforation?

A. < 1cm – Primary closure
B. > 1cm – Graham's patch
C. An elective upper endoscopy should be performed 6 to 8 weeks after surgery to assess for evidence of malignancy
D. A routine contrast radiograph is required before initiating eating

109. Which of the following is not seen in GOO?

A. Hypochloremia alkalosis
B. Hypokalemic alkalosis
C. Metabolic alkalosis
D. Metabolic acidosis

110. Which of the following statement is false?

A. GOO is mostly due to benign disease
B. Refractory GOO is treated by Antrectomy + Vagotomy
C. Intractable ulcer is treated by Antrectomy + TV
D. Intractability is failure of ulcer to heal after trial of 8-12 weeks

111. All are true regarding Gastric outlet obstruction except:

A. Gastric outlet obstruction from PUD is a surgical emergency and should undergo immediate surgical intervention
B. Upper endoscopy should be performed to rule out a malignancy and assess for H pylori infection
C. Endoscopic dilation (with or without stenting) and H pylori eradication are the mainstays of initial therapy
D. Patients with refractory obstruction are best managed with primary antrectomy and reconstruction along with vagotomy

112. All are true regarding Intractability except:

A. Failure of an ulcer to heal after an initial trial of 8 to 12 weeks of therapy
B. For any intractable ulcer, adequate duration of antisecretory therapy, H pylori eradication and elimination of NSAID use must be confirmed
C. It is estimated to occur in 15% to 20% of patients
D. All the above are true

113. Perforation complicates 2% to 10% of PUD and has the highest mortality rate of any complication of ulcer disease, reported as high ______ %.

A. 20% B. 30%
C. 40% D. 50%

114. Vagotomy decreases peak acid output by approximately ______ %.

A. 70% B. 60%
C. 50% D. 85%

115. Vagotomy plus antrectomy decreases peak acid output by approximately ______%.

A. 70% B. 60%
C. 50% D. 85%

116. All are true regarding Truncal vagotomy except:

A. Truncal vagotomy is performed by division of the left and right vagus nerves above the hepatic and celiac branches, just above the GE junction
B. Vagotomy with a drainage procedure can cause delayed gastric emptying
C. When the duodenal bulb is scarred, a Finney pyloroplasty or Jaboulay gastroduodenostomy may be a useful alternative
D. Significant scarring or inflammation may necessitate a gastrojejunostomy

117. In general side effects associated with the type of drainage procedure performed with truncal vagotomy, true statement is:

A. Bile reflux may be more common after gastroenterostomy
B. Diarrhoea is more common after pyloroplasty
C. The incidence of dumping syndrome is similar for both gastroduodenostomy and pyloroplasty
D. All of the above

118. Parietal cell vagotomy or Proximal gastric vagotomy is also known as:

A. Truncal vagotomy
B. Highly selective vagotomy
C. Truncal vagotomy and antrectomy
D. Selective vagotomy

119. In highly selective vagotomy, nerves are divided up until a point:

A. 5 cm proximal to the pylorus and point at least 7 cm proximal to the GE junction on the esophagus
B. 7 cm proximal to the pylorus and point at least 5 cm proximal to the GE junction on the esophagus
C. 7 cm proximal to the pylorus and point at least 7 cm proximal to the GE junction on the esophagus
D. 5 cm proximal to the pylorus and point at least 5 cm proximal to the GE junction on the esophagus

120. All the following nerves are divided in highly selective vagotomy except:

A. Nerve of Latarjet B. Crow feet
C. Nerve of Grassi D. None

121. Acid level increased in which types of gastric ulcers?

A. Type 1 and 2 B. Type 2 and 3
C. Type 3 and 4 D. Type 4 and 5

122. NSAID associated with which type of gastric ulcer?

A. Type 2 B. Type 3
C. Type 4 D. Type 5

123. All are true regarding diagnosis of ZES except:

A. Serum Gastrin levels more than 400 pg/ml are diagnostic
B. Gastrin values higher than 1000 pg/ml are diagnostic
C. Renal failure all can cause an elevation of fasting serum gastrin levels
D. All above are true

124. Boundaries of the Gastrinoma triangle are all except:

A. Cystic-common bile duct junction
B. The pancreas Body-neck junction
C. The pancreas Head-neck junction
D. The junction between the second and third portions of the duodenum

125. The best initial imaging study to localize the gastrin secreting tumor is:

A. Triple-phase CT B. USG
C. PET CT D. EUS

126. Modified Johnson classification is used for:

A. Esophageal carcinoma
B. Gastric ulcers
C. Gastric carcinoma
D. Gastric GIST

127. Which of the following types of gastric ulcers are associated with low acid levels?

A. Type I B. Type II
C. Type III D. Type IV

128. Gold standard for diagnosis of H. pylori is:

A. Urease assay on endoscopic biopsies
B. Culture of biopsies
C. Serology
D. Stool antigen

129. Location of Gastric pacemaker is situated at:

A. Cardia
B. Antrum along the lesser curvature
C. Mid body of stomach along the greater curvature
D. Pylorus

STRESS GASTRITIS

130. Stress gastritis (Curling's ulcer) occurs in the setting of thermal burns, when the burnt BSA is more than > _____%.

A. 30% B. 50%
C. 40% D. 60%

131. All are true regarding diagnosis of Stress Gastritis except:

A. Stress is considered present when hypoxia, sepsis, or organ failure occurs
B. When stress is present, mucosal ischemia is thought to be the main factor responsible for the breakdown of these normal defense mechanisms
C. Presence of luminal acid is not a prerequisite for this form of gastritis to evolve
D. Stress gastritis is characterized by multiple superficial (nonulcerating) erosions that typically begin in the proximal portion of the stomach and progress distally

132. All are true regarding diagnosis of Stress Gastritis except:

A. Stress gastritis develops within 1 to 2 weeks after a traumatic event in more than 50% to 75% of patients
B. Endoscopy is required to confirm the diagnosis and differentiate stress gastritis from other sources of GI hemorrhage
C. Painless upper GI bleeding
D. Prophylaxis should be limited only to high-risk patients, as gastric acid suppression has been associated with increased rates of nosocomial pneumonia and C difficile infection

133. Strongest risk factor for developing clinically significant bleeding from gastric stress ulcers:

A. Cardiac Failure
B. Prolonged mechanical ventilation (>48 hours)
C. Stroke
D. Diabetes mellitus

134. Stress Gastritis is most commonly located at:

A. Distal stomach
B. Body of stomach
C. Fundus of the stomach
D. Greater curvature

135. All are true about stress gastritis except:

A. Bleeding that results in hemodynamic instability or requires persistent transfusions is an indication for surgery
B. All bleeding areas are oversewn with figure-of-eight stitches taken deep within the gastric wall
C. Most superficial erosions are not actively bleeding and do not require ligation unless a blood vessel is seen at its base
D. The bleeding from stress ulcers is usually focal and the rebleeding rate is low

POST GASTRECTOMY SYNDROMES

136. _____ % patients who undergo surgery for PUD subsequently develop some degree of post gastrectomy syndrome.

A. 10% to 15% B. 5% to 10%
C. 20% to 25% D. 30% to 40%

137. Following is true regarding Dumping syndrome:

A. Early Dumping is 20-30 mins after meal and Late dumping is 2-3 hours after meal
B. More common after partial gastrectomy with the Billroth II reconstruction than Billroth I
C. Early dumping is more common than late dumping
D. All of the above

138. Most common metabolic defect after gastrectomy:

A. Anemia B. Jaundice
C. Diarrhoea D. Malignancy

139. Anemia in post gastrectomy syndromes, all are true except:

A. Iron deficiency (more common) or impairment in vitamin B_{12} metabolism
B. More than 30% of patients undergoing gastrectomy have iron deficiency anemia
C. In general, the addition of iron supplements to the patient's diet doesn't correct this problem

D. Megaloblastic anemia from vitamin B_{12} deficiency, rarely develops after partial gastrectomy but is dependent on the amount of stomach removed

140. All statements about afferent loop syndrome are true except:

A. The afferent loop is the duodenojejunal loop proximal to the gastrojejunal anastomosis

B. After obstruction of the afferent limb, pancreatic and hepatobiliary secretions accumulate within the limb, resulting in its distention, which causes epigastric discomfort and cramping

C. Failure to visualize the afferent limb on upper endoscopy is suggestive of the diagnosis

D. None

141. All statements about afferent loop syndrome are true except:

A. Surgical correction is indicated for this mechanical problem to prevent bowel necrosis or duodenal stump blowout

B. The intraluminal pressure increases enough to empty the contents of the afferent loop forcefully into the stomach, resulting in projectile bilious vomiting that offers immediate relief of symptoms

C. Remedies include conversion of the Billroth II construction into a Billroth I anastomosis, enteroenterostomy below the afferent and efferent loops, and conversion to a Roux-en-Y reconstruction

D. All are true

142. Alkaline Reflux Gastritis, false statement is:

A. Upper endoscopy demonstrates friable, beefy red mucosa

B. There is no clear correlation between the volume or composition of bile and the subsequent development of alkaline reflux gastritis

C. Medical therapies that have been tried to treat alkaline reflux gastritis have shown consistent benefits

D. In general, a Roux-en-Y procedure should be preferred over a Billroth II for reconstruction at the time of partial or subtotal distal gastrectomy to decrease the likelihood of alkaline reflux

143. Gastric Atony, false statement is:

A. The agents most commonly used are prokinetic agents such as metoclopramide and erythromycin

B. Mechanical cause of gastric outlet obstruction, such as postoperative adhesions, afferent or efferent loop obstruction, and internal herniation, must be ruled out

C. Erythromycin markedly accelerates gastric emptying by binding to motilin receptors on GI smooth muscle cells, where it acts as a motilin antagonist

D. Metoclopramide exerts its prokinetic effects by acting as a dopamine antagonist and has cholinergic-enhancing effects because of facilitation of acetylcholine release from enteric cholinergic neurons

144. Mechanism of action of erythromycin is:

A. Motilin antagonist

B. Motilin agonist

C. Dopamine agonist

D. Dopamine antagonist

145. For patients with intractable symptoms, the surgical procedure of choice is conversion of the Billroth II anastomosis into a Roux-en-Y gastrojejunostomy, in which the Roux limb has been lengthened to:

A. >25 cms B. >30 cms

C. >40 cms D. >75 cms

GASTRIC CANCER

146. Which of the following is not a risk factor for gastric carcinoma?

A. High protein

B. Salted meat/fish

C. Male sex

D. High complex carbohydrates

147. Which of the following molecular altercation is not involved in gastric carcinoma?

A. Over expression of cyclooxygenase-2

B. P53 mutation

C. Decreased p27 expression

D. Microsatellite stability

148. Which of the following is not a hereditary risk factor in gastric cancer?

A. FAP

B. HNPCC

C. Li Fraumeni syndrome

D. RET

149. Which of the following is not involved in gastric carcinoma?

A. C-met proto oncogene

B. K-sam oncogene

C. C-erb b2 oncogene
D. CDK1

150. **E. Catherin is involved in:**
A. Intestinal type gastric ca
B. Diffuse type gastric ca
C. Rectal cancer
D. Renal ca

151. **Which of the following is not a risk factor for gastric carcinoma?**
A. PPI
B. Adenomatous polyp
C. Pernicious anaemia
D. Cooked fish

152. **Which interleukin is involved as a risk factor in gastric cancer?**
A. IL-1 beta B. IL-2 alpha
C. IL-1 alpha D. IL-4

153. **Number of lymph nodes required in staging evaluation of gastric cancer surgery:**
A. 10 B. 13
C. 16 D. 18

154. **False statement regarding gastric cancer is:**
A. The disease affects men disproportionately, with more than 60% of new cases and deaths occurring in men
B. The second leading cause of cancer death
C. Among developed countries, Japan and Korea have the highest rates of the disease
D. Among racial groups, the disease is more common and has a higher mortality Whites

155. **True about CA stomach is all except:**
A. Intestinal metaplasia is a risk factor for the development of gastric carcinoma; however, not every patient with intestinal metaplasia develops invasive cancer
B. Higher levels of interleukin-1β and tumor necrosis factor-α expression lead to an increased risk of gastric cancer development
C. The presence of the cytotoxin associated gene A leads to decreased virulence and risk of gastric cancer
D. H. pylori can inhibit the secretion of ascorbic acid, preventing effective scavenging of oxygen free radicals and N-nitroso compounds

156. **Gene mutation for the cell adhesion molecule E-cadherin (CDH1); what is the lifetime incidence of developing gastric cancer?**
A. 30% to 50% B. 50% to 80%
C. 60% to 70% D. 80% to 90%

157. **Prophylactic total gastrectomy should be considered for patients with CDH1 mutation at what age?**
A. 30 years B. 25 years
C. 15 years D. 40 years

158. **Patients with an isolated polyp greater than _____ cm in size should have a complete polypectomy.**
A. 5 mm B. 1 cm
C. 2 cm D. 4 cm

159. **Regarding fundic gland polyps true is all except:**
A. Benign lesions
B. They are strongly associated with PPI use and occur in one third of patients by 1 year
C. Dysplasia, although common in patients whose polyps result from familial adenomatous polyposis
D. Hyperplastic polyps are associated with H pylori infection and chronic gastritis, with an associated malignancy rate of over 10%

160. **Which is not a risk factor for stomach cancer?**
A. Obesity B. Epstein-Barr virus
C. Smoking D. All of the above

161. **Which of the following is not associated with gastric cancer?**
A. Borrmann classification
B. Japanese and Paris classification systems
C. Lauren classification
D. Montreal classification

162. **Which type of Borrmann classification is called Ulcerating type?**
A. Type I B. Type II
C. Type III D. Type IV

163. **Which type of Borrmann classification is called fungating type?**
A. Type I B. Type II
C. Type III D. Type IV

164. **Which type of Borrmann classification is called linitis plastica?**
A. Type I B. Type II
C. Type III D. Type IV

165. As per Lauren's Classification, all are true about intestinal type of gastric cancer except:

A. Men > women
B. Hematogenous spread
C. APC gene mutations
D. Familial

166. As per Lauren's Classification, all are true about diffuse of gastric cancer except:

A. Blood type A
B. Decreased E-cadherin
C. Increasing incidence with age
D. Transmural, lymphatic spread

167. p53, p16 inactivation is seen in which type of gastric cancer?

A. Diffuse type
B. Intestinal type
C. Both
D. None

168. Siewert classification is for:

A. SCC of GE junction
B. Adenocarcinoma of GE junction
C. Adenocarcinoma of proximal stomach
D. SCC of distal esophagus

169. Siewert type 2 is:

A. 2 cm above GE junction and 2 cm below GE junction
B. 1cm above GE junction and 2 cm below GE junction
C. 5 cm above GE junction and 5 cm below GE junction
D. 3 cm above GE junction and 5 cm below GE junction

170. Type 3 Siewert with extension to GE junction treated as:

A. Gastric adenocarcinoma
B. Esophageal adenocarcinoma
C. Esophageal achalasia
D. Wide excision

171. A minimum of _____ nodes must be evaluated for accurate staging.

A. 15
B. 16
C. 20
D. 10

172. Current National Comprehensive Cancer Network (NCCN) guidelines recommend harvesting biopsies from different areas of the lesion in order to maximize the diagnostic yield:

A. 4-6 biopsy specimens
B. 6-8 biopsy specimens
C. 8-12 biopsy specimens
D. 2-4 biopsy specimens

173. Which statement about EUS in gastric cancer evaluation is wrong?

A. EUS provides the most accurate evaluation of the depth of tumor invasion, assessment of perigastric lymph node involvement
B. EUS is performed using a flexible endoscope with a 7.5- to 12-MHz ultrasound transducer
C. The stomach is filled with water to provide an acoustic window, and the stomach wall is visualized as five alternating hypoechoic and hyperechoic layers
D. Ascitis cannot be identified by EUS

174. Which statement about EUS in gastric cancer evaluation is wrong?

A. The mucosa and submucosa represent the first three layers (T1)
B. FNA cannot be performed if ascites is present to evaluate for peritoneal spread
C. Expansion of the tumor beyond the muscularis propria causing an irregular border correlates with expansion into the subserosa, or a T3 tumor
D. Direct invasion of surrounding structures, including named vessels, indicates a T4b tumor

175. Which statement about PET/CT in gastric cancer evaluation is wrong?

A. Combined PET/CT is more accurate in preoperative staging than either PET or CT
B. The utility of PET/CT for initial staging of diffuse and mucinous cancers is limited due to low tracer accumulation
C. NCCN guidelines recommend considering PET/CT as part of staging for patients with greater than T4 disease without evidence of metastatic disease on initial CT
D. In patients with locally advanced disease and patients being considered for neoadjuvant therapy, there may be a role for PET/CT

176. PET/CT in gastric cancer evaluation is recommended in all cases with T stage greater than:

A. T1
B. T2
C. T3
D. T4

177. Tumor penetrates subserosal connective tissue without invasion of visceral peritoneum or adjacent structures; which T stage does it belong?

A. T1
B. T2
C. T3
D. T4

178. Intraepithelial tumor without invasion of the lamina propria; which T stage does it belong?

A. T1
B. T2
C. Tis
D. T0

179. Which statement about Diagnostic Laproscopy in gastric cancer evaluation is wrong?

A. Staging laparoscopy is an integral part of the standard workup for gastric cancer
B. 20% to 30% of patients with no prior evidence of metastases will be found to have peritoneal disease on staging laparoscopy
C. The NCCN recommends staging laparoscopic in T4 or greater gastric cancer and prior evidence of metastases will be found to have peritoneal disease
D. The overall sensitivity of laparoscopy for detecting metastatic disease is greater than 95%

180. The NCCN recommends staging laparoscopic in which gastric cancer stage?

A. T1 or greater gastric cancer and no prior evidence of metastases will be found to have peritoneal disease
B. T2 or greater gastric cancer and prior evidence of metastases will be found to have peritoneal disease
C. T1 or greater gastric cancer and prior evidence of metastases will be found to have peritoneal disease
D. T2 or greater gastric cancer and no prior evidence of metastases will be found to have peritoneal disease

181. For cancers of the distal stomach, including the body and antrum, a distal gastrectomy is the appropriate operation; all statements are wrong except:

A. The proximal stomach is transected at the level of the incisura at a margin of at least 2 to 3 cm for early cancers and at least 4 to 6 cm for advanced cancers
B. The proximal stomach is transected at the level of the incisura at a margin of at least 5 cm for early cancers and at least 4 to 6 cm for advanced cancers
C. The distal margin is the proximal duodenum just distal to the pylorus
D. Roux-en-Y reconstruction has been shown to result in less alkaline reflux gastritis and improved quality of life at 1 year compared to Billroth reconstruction

182. Standard criteria for endoscopic resection of gastric adenocarcinoma includes all except:

A. Intestinal-type adenocarcinoma
B. Tumor confined to the mucosa
C. Absence of lymphovascular invasion
D. Ulcerated tumor

183. Standard criteria for endoscopic resection of gastric adenocarcinoma includes:

A. Intestinal-type adenocarcinoma
B. Tumor confined to the submucosa
C. Less than 4 cm in diameter
D. Ulcerated tumor

184. Expanded criteria for endoscopic resection of gastric adenocarcinoma includes:

A. Any differentiated mucosal tumor without ulceration
B. Mucosal tumors up to 3 cm without ulceration
C. Undifferentiated mucosal tumors up to 2 cm
D. Slight submucosal invasion

185. All are indications for surgery for gastric carcinoma without metastatic disease or invasion of unresectable vascular structures are candidates for curative resection; these structures include all except:

A. Aorta
B. Celiac trunk
C. Proximal common hepatic
D. Distal splenic arteries

186. False regarding gastric cancer:

A. ARTIST trial - No difference chemo radiotherapy Vs chemotherapy alone
B. MAGIC trial - compare perioperative chemotherapy with surgery alone
C. CROSS trial - compared surgery alone vs neoadjuvant chemoradiotherapy
D. DUTCH trial - advocates D1 lymph node dissection with splenic preservation

187. NCCN and European Society for Medical Oncology have recommended:

A. D1 dissection in patients undergoing surgery for curative intent

B. D2 dissection in patients undergoing surgery for curative intent
C. D3 dissection in patients undergoing surgery for curative intent
D. Extended D2 dissection in patients undergoing surgery for curative intent

188. Which statements in the following is false regarding gastric cancer surgery?

A. D1- Perigastric Nodes
B. D2- Nodes along left gastric, common hepatic artery, celiac, Splenic artery
C. D3- Nodes along SMA, middle colic and periaortic nodes
D. Number of positive lymph nodes doesn't correlate with survival in gastric cancer

189. Regarding D3 dissection, false statement is:

A. For more advanced disease, it has not been shown to offer a survival benefit
B. It increases morbidity and should not be considered standard
C. For more advanced disease, it has been shown to offer a survival benefit
D. None of the above

190. Which trial is associated with Neoadjuvant + Radiotherapy?

A. Southwest Oncology Group (9008/INT-0116) trial
B. CLASSIC trial
C. MAGIC trial
D. ARTIST trial

191. Common first-line regimens for gastric cancer includes:

A. ECF (Epirubicin, cisplatin and 5-FU)
B. CAPOX (Capecitabine and oxaliplatin)
C. FOLFOX (5-FU, leucovorin and oxaliplatin)
D. All of the above

192. Patients with unresectable or metastatic gastric cancer account for:

A. 20% B. 30%
C. 50% D. 60%

193. Patients presenting with bleeding in gastric cancer; which procedure can the patient undergo?

A. Endoscopic control
B. Angiographic embolization
C. External beam radiation therapy
D. All of the Above

194. Obstructing gastric cancers; which procedure can be done?

A. Endoscopic enteral stent
B. Radiation therapy
C. Gastrojejunostomy
D. All of the Above

195. Which statement about HER2 neu overexpression is false?

A. HER2 testing is now recommended by the NCCN guidelines for all patients with metastatic disease at time of initial diagnosis
B. HER2 positivity has been reported about 20% of gastric cancers
C. ToGA trial: Capecitabine or 5-FU with cisplatin and trastuzumab or cisplatin alone
D. The trastuzumab group had a better median survival and rates of severe complications differed between the groups

196. The common sites of locoregional recurrence are all except:

A. Gastric remnant at the anastomosis
B. The gastric bed
C. Regional nodal basins
D. Liver

197. Lymph node station for Celiac artery:

A. 8 B. 9
C. 10 D. 11

198. Lymph node station for Left Gastric Artery:

A. 6 B. 7
C. 8 D. 9

199. Match the following:

1. 10 a. Proximal splenic
2. 11p b. Splenic hilum
3. 13 c. Anterior common hepatic
4. 8a d. Retropancreatic

A. 1-b, 2-a, 3-c, 4-d
B. 1-b, 2-d, 3-a, 4-c
C. 1-b, 2-a, 3-d, 4-c
D. 1-a, 2-b, 3-c, 4-d

OTHER GASTRIC CANCERS

200. Most common site of extra nodal lymphoma is:

A. Small intestine B. Colon
C. Stomach D. Kidney

201. Most common site of gastric lymphoma is:

A. Gastric body B. Cardia
C. Antrum D. Fundus

202. Constitutional B symptoms (i.e., fever, night sweats) occur in about ______% of patients.

A. 10% B. 20%
C. 30% D. 40%

203. Conditions have been shown to be associated with gastric lymphoma, all except:

A. Celiac disease
B. Rheumatoid arthritis
C. Inflammatory bowel disease
D. Systemic lupus erythematous

204. The most common gastric lymphoma is:

A. MALT lymphoma
B. Diffuse large B cell lymphoma
C. Peripheral T-cell lymphoma
D. Follicular lymphomas

205. Which of the following is not a gastrointestinal lymphoma classification?

A. Real
B. Lukes-Collins
C. Who classification
D. All of the above

206. Classification used for evaluation and staging of gastric lymphoma?

A. WHO Staging B. Real Staging
C. Lugano Staging D. Siewert Staging

207. As per Lugano's staging, serosa penetration to involve adjacent organs/tissues is:

A. Stage II B. Stage IE
C. Stage IIE D. Stage II2

208. False regarding gastric lymphoma treatment is all except:

A. The most common chemotherapeutic combination is R-CHOP
B. The primary role of surgery is currently limited to patients with symptomatic recurrence after treatment failure and patients who develop complications, such as bleeding, gastric outlet obstruction, or perforation
C. Chemotherapy for gastric lymphoma is associated with a 5% rate of gastric perforation and GI bleeding
D. All of the above are true

209. Genetically, MALT lymphoma is characterized by all translocations except:

A. t(1;14) B. t(3;14)
C. t(11;14) D. t(14;18)

210. Increased FOXP1 transcription factor levels, which have been shown to expand marginal zone B cells are due to:

A. t(1;14) B. t(3;14)
C. t(11;18) D. t(14;18)

211. False statement regarding MALT Lymphoma is:

A. All patients should be evaluated for active infection with H pylori
B. Successful eradication of H pylori results in remission in more than 75% of cases
C. Some patients with MALT lymphoma are H pylori–negative, in these patients consideration should be given to surgical resection
D. The presence of transmural tumor extension, nodal involvement, transformation into a large cell phenotype, and nuclear BCL-10 expression all predict failure after H. pylori eradication alone

212. MALT lymphoma prognostic index includes all except:

A. Age of 70 or above
B. Stage IV disease
C. Elevated lactate dehydrogenase (LDH) level
D. Presence of t(3;14)

213. KIT is a receptor tyrosine kinase and approximately ______% of GISTs overexpress KIT.

A. 80% B. 90%
C. 95% D. 100%

214. Most GISTs that lack a KIT mutation will have a mutation in:

A. PDGFA B. PDGFB
C. PDGFRA D. PDGFRB

215. GISTs can appear anywhere within the GI tract, their most common site is:

A. Small intestine B. Stomach
C. Appendix D. Pancreas

216. 5% of GISTs are associated with an underlying heritable mutation; all of the following are involved except:

A. Familial GIST syndrome
B. Neurofibromatosis 2

C. Carney-Stratakis syndrome
D. All of the above are involved

217. Carney-Stratakis syndrome involves all except:

A. GIST
B. Paraganglioma with pulmonary chondroma
C. Paraganglioma without pulmonary chondroma
D. Autosomal Recessive syndrome

218. Regarding evaluation of gastric lymphoma, false statement is:

A. EUS is useful for the assessment of depth of gastric wall invasion
B. Endoscopy often reveals non-specific gastritis or gastric ulceration
C. Biopsy should be performed for any enlarged lymph nodes
D. Serological H pylori testing should be done if negative confirm with biopsy

219. Risk of perforation in patients of gastric lymphoma treated with chemotherapy is:

A. 1% B. 5%
C. 10% D. 12%

220. CHOP regimen for gastric lymphoma includes all except:

A. Cyclophosphamide B. Doxorubicin
C. Vinblastine D. Prednisone

221. To document clearance of H pylori infection in gastric MALTOMA endoscopy should be done at:

A. 1 month B. 2 months
C. 6 months D. 12 months

222. To document regression of the gastric MALTOMA endoscopy should be done:

A. Biannually for 3 years
B. Annually for 3 years
C. Biannually for 5 years
D. Annually for 5 years

223. 100% specificity in the diagnosis of GIST is:

A. Endoscopy B. EUS guided FNA
C. CT scan D. Tumor markers

224. False statement regarding GIST evaluation is:

A. Preoperative biopsy is recommended if there is a high suspicion for GIST and the patient is otherwise operable
B. Biopsy is preferred to confirm presence of metastatic disease or if the patient is being considered for neoadjuvant imatinib therapy
C. CT of the abdomen and pelvis with oral and IV contrast is used to assess for metastatic disease
D. Immunohistochemical staining for CD117, CD34 and PDGFRA are used to confirm the diagnosis

225. Main stay of treatment for GIST is:

A. Gastric resection B. Chemotherapy
C. Radiotherapy D. Endoscopic

226. Surgical resection should be done for GIST for tumor size more than:

A. 1 cm B. 2 cm
C. 5 cm D. 10 cm

227. High risk features on endoscopy for GIST are:

A. Irregular borders B. Ulceration
C. Heterogeneity D. All of the above

228. Most common site of recurrence in GIST is:

A. Stomach B. Lung
C. Liver D. Intestine

229. Which of the following statement is false about GIST?

A. The two primary prognostic factors for gastric GISTs are tumor size and mitotic rate
B. Most patients who experience recurrence demonstrate metastasis to the liver, with one-third having only isolated local recurrence
C. Recurrence doesn't occur over 2 years after resection; thus, long-term follow-up is not warranted
D. Patients presenting with recurrent or metastatic disease are primarily treated with imatinib or a second-line tyrosine kinase inhibitor

230. The results of which trial have established a 3-year course as the standard of care after surgical resection of high-risk GIST?

A. Scandinavian Sarcoma Group XVIII trial
B. The ACOSOG Z9001 phase III
C. Scandinavian Sarcoma Group XVI trial
D. All of the above

231. Malignant potential of tumor t >10 cm; no more than 5 mitoses/HPF is:

A. High malignant potential
B. Low to moderate malignant potential
C. Uncertain or low malignant potential
D. Probably benign

232. Imatinib in the treatment of GIST is used in following conditions except:

A. Metastatic GIST

B. Unresectable GIST

C. GIST with high risk of recurrence

D. Early GIST

233. Dosage and duration of imatinib in the treatment of high-risk gastric GIST after surgical resection is:

A. 400 mg and 3 years

B. 400 mg and 18 months

C. 800 mg and 1 year

D. 800 mg and 2 years

234. Which of the following type of gastric carcinoid is associated with Zollinger-Ellison syndrome?

A. Type 1　B. Type 2

C. Type 3　D. Type 4

235. Type of gastric carcinoid associated with chronic atrophic gastritis?

A. Type 1　B. Type 2

C. Type 3　D. Type 4

236. Gastric carcinoid is associated with all of the following except:

A. MEN 1

B. ZES

C. Chronic atrophic gastritis

D. MEN 2 B

237. Gastric Carcinoid with highest rate of metastatic spread is:

A. Type 1　B. Type 2

C. Type 3　D. Type 4

238. All of the following are true about GIST except:

A. The most common sites in the GI tract are the small intestine, rectum and appendix

B. The stomach is becoming an increasing common site of NETs

C. There are three distinct subtypes of gastric NETs

D. Gastric NETs are typically functioning and cause carcinoid syndrome

239. Determine whether these statements are correct:

(A) Assertion: The stomach is becoming an increasing common site of NETs

(R) Reason: This increasing incidence is thought to be due to a combination of improved surveillance and the widespread use of PPIs

A. Both Assertion (A) and Reason (R) are the true and Reason (R) is a correct explanation of Assertion (A)

B. Both Assertion (A) and Reason (R) are the true but Reason (R) is not a correct explanation of Assertion (A)

C. Assertion (A) is true and Reason (R) is false

D. Assertion (A) is false and Reason (R) is true

240. Neuroendocrine carcinoma has been referred to as:

A. Type 1　B. Type 2

C. Type 3　D. Type 4

241. All of the following are true about GIST evaluation except:

A. Diagnosis of gastric NET is established on esophagogastroduodenoscopy (EGD) with biopsy of the lesion

B. EUS can be performed to assess for depth of invasion subsequently

C. Either CT or MRI can be useful to evaluate for metastatic disease

D. Chromogranin B is often elevated and can serve as a biomarker for these tumors

242. All of the following are true about GIST treatment except:

A. The treatment for localized NETs is complete removal

B. For small pedunculated lesions that do not invade beyond the submucosa, complete removal can be accomplished endoscopically

C. Smaller (<2 cm) lesions may require wedge resection or partial gastrectomy

D. Patients with numerous gastric NETs may require total gastrectomy

243. True statement about GIST treatment:

A. In patients with type II NETs: Gastrinoma resection should be performed as well, if possible

B. Patients with localized type III NETs: Should undergo oncologic resection with lymphadenectomy

C. For patients with recurrent or metastatic disease: somatostatin analogues or chemotherapy can be used to decrease the burden of disease and treat carcinoid syndrome
D. All the above are true

244. What is the most common location of heterotopic pancreas within the stomach?

A. Antral greater curvature
B. Antral lesser curvature
C. Fundus of stomach
D. Cardia of stomach

OTHER GASTRIC LESIONS

245. Cobblestone/cerebriform appearance is seen in:

A. Mallory Weiss disease
B. Menetrier's disease
C. Dieulafoy lesion
D. Gastric volvulus

246. All are true about Menetrier's disease except:

A. Acquired premalignant condition
B. Characterized by massive gastric folds in fundus and corpus
C. Foveolar hyperplasia with absent parietal cells
D. Reduced mucus production

247. Menetrier's disease in children is usually associated with:

A. CMV
B. H Pylori
C. Campylobacter
D. HSV

248. Which of the following is increased in Menetrier's disease?

A. IL 2
B. IL12
C. TGF Alpha
D. TGF Beta

249. Given the increased risk of gastric neoplasms in patients with Menetrier's disease, patients should undergo endoscopic surveillance every:

A. 1 to 2 years
B. 3 to 4 years
C. 5 to 10 years
D. 10 to 20 years

250. All are true about Menetrier's disease except:

A. Total gastrectomy should be performed in patients who continue to have massive protein loss despite optimal medical therapy and high-protein diet or if dysplasia or carcinoma develops
B. Typical gastric mucosal changes can be detected by radiographic or endoscopic examination
C. Biopsy should be performed to establish the diagnosis and to rule out gastric carcinoma or lymphoma
D. Medical treatment yields consistent results

251. Mallory Weiss tear account for _____ % of acute upper GI haemorrhage.

A. 5%
B. 10%
C. 15%
D. 20%

252. Mallory Weiss tear usually has greater risk when associated with:

A. Alcoholics
B. Pre-existing portal hypertension
C. Smoking
D. Both A and B

253. False statement regarding Mallory Weiss syndrome:

A. Most patients with active bleeding cannot be managed by endoscopic methods
B. Angiographic transarterial embolization may be useful in patients who have persistent or recurrent bleeding after endoscopy
C. If surgery is required, the lesion at the GE junction is approached through an anterior gastrotomy, and the bleeding site is oversewn with several deep 2-0 silk ligatures to reapproximate the gastric mucosa in an anatomic fashion
D. All of the above are true

254. False regarding Dieulafoy lesion is:

A. Lesion 6 to 10 cm from GE Junction
B. Generally occurs at fundus
C. Women are usually involved
D. All of the above are true

255. The Dieulafoy lesion's most common site is:

A. Near the GE junction along the lesser curvature
B. Near the GE junction along the greater curvature
C. Near the GE junction along the lower Esophagus
D. Near the GE junction along the Fundus

256. False regarding Dieulafoy lesion:

A. The classic presentation of a patient with a Dieulafoy lesion is sudden onset of massive, painless hematemesis

B. The diagnostic modality of choice is upper endoscopy, which correctly identifies the lesion in 80% of patients
C. Surgical management consists of gastric wedge resection to include the offending vessel
D. Angiography is generally not useful

257. Angiographic findings in Dieulafoy's lesion may include a tortuous ectatic artery along which artery?

A. Right gastric artery
B. Left gastric artery
C. Short gastric artery
D. Left gastroepiploic artery

258. The classic presentation of a patient with a Dieulafoy lesion includes all except:

A. Sudden onset
B. Painless hematemesis
C. Painful hematemesis
D. Massive bleeding

259. Diagnostic modality of choice in Dieulafoy lesion is:

A. Biopsy
B. Angiography
C. Esophagoduodenoscopy
D. Barium swallow

260. False regarding Dieulafoy lesion is:

A. Bleeding from a gastric Dieulafoy lesion is caused by an abnormally large (1–3 mm)
B. Tortuous artery coursing through the submucosa with a primary ulcer
C. Erosion of the superficial mucosa overlying the artery occurs secondary to the pulsations of the large submucosal vessel
D. The mucosal defect is 2 to 5 mm and is surrounded by normal-appearing gastric mucosa

261. More prone to bleeding in gastric varices:

A. Isolated gastric varices
B. Type 1
C. Type 2
D. Type 3

262. True about gastric varices:

A. Type 1 varices are located in fundus of stomach
B. Type 2 varices occur anywhere in stomach
C. Develops secondary to portal hypertension
D. All of the above

263. True about gastric varices treatment is all except:

A. An emerging treatment modality is EUS-guided cyanoacrylate-lipiodol injection or coil embolization of perforating veins
B. Temporary tamponade can be attempted with a Sengstaken-Blakemore tube
C. A major problem with gastric varices after endoscopic treatment is rebleeding, occurring in more than 50% of patients
D. TIPS can be effective in controlling gastric variceal hemorrhage that does not respond to endoscopic treatments, with initial haemostasis rates over 90% and rebleeding rates of approximately 10% to 30%.

264. Regarding gastrorenal shunt between gastric varices and the left renal vein, false statement is:

A. A gastrorenal shunt between gastric varices and the left renal vein is present in 60% to 85% of patients with gastric varices
B. This spontaneous shunt decompresses the portal system and improves the efficacy of transjugular intrahepatic portosystemic shunting
C. A balloon catheter can be inserted into the gastrorenal shunt through the left renal vein, and the shunt can be occluded by inflating the balloon
D. Balloon-occluded retrograde transvenous obliteration can be done (BORTO)

265. Major complication of BORTO:

A. Death
B. Aggravation of Esophageal varices
C. Pulmonary Embolus
D. Failure of TIPS

266. Most common form of gastric volvulus is:

A. Organoaxial
B. Mesenterical
C. Both have equal incidence
D. None of the above

267. Characteristics of mesenterico axial volvulus include all except:

A. Partial (<180)
B. Recurrent
C. Associated with diaphragmatic defect
D. All of the above

268. Borchardt triad include all except:

A. Sudden onset of severe upper abdominal pain
B. Recurrent Retching
C. Inability to pass NG Tube
D. Hematemesis

269. True about gastric volvulus management is all except:

A. Acute volvulus is a surgical emergency
B. NG decompression should not be performed immediately
C. Patients should proceed with surgical intervention
D. The stomach is reduced and uncoiled through a transabdominal approach

270. True about gastric volvulus management is all except:

A. Percutaneous endoscopic gastrostomy tube placement can also be used as a temporizing measure in a hemodynamically unstable patient prior to definitive surgical repair
B. The diaphragmatic defect is repaired, with consideration given to a fundoplication in the setting of a paraesophageal hernia
C. If strangulation has occurred, the compromised segment of stomach is resected
D. Spontaneous volvulus, without an associated diaphragmatic defect, is treated by gastric resection

271. True about Phytobezoars:

A. Collections of nondigestible materials
B. Impaired gastric emptying
C. Risk of diabetes
D. All of the above

272. Complications of Trichobezoars include:

A. Gastric outlet obstruction
B. Gastric perforation
C. Small bowel obstruction
D. All of the above

273. True about gastric volvulus management is all except:

A. Initial management of symptomatic bezoars is attempted chemical dissolution
B. There are a wide array of options, including soda, cellulose, papain and acetylcysteine
C. Trichobezoars are typically effectively managed with chemical dissolution
D. Pharmacobezoars may require decontamination depending on the medication involved

274. True about gastric volvulus is all except:

A. The impaired grinding mechanism of the stomach and migrating motor complexes have been implicated as pathogenic causes of bezoars
B. The sodium concentration in Adolph's Meat Tenderizer is low, so hyponatremia may result if large quantities are administered
C. Physical exam is usually unremarkable, although sometimes a large mass may be palpable
D. Papain, found in Adolph's Meat Tenderizer, is given in a dose of 1 tsp in 150 to 300 mL water several times daily

ANSWERS

1. **Ans: C. 5th week of gestation in the caudal portion**

   Ref: Chapter No.49, Page No.1196

2. **Ans: B. 7th week**

   Ref: Chapter No.49, Page No. 1196

3. **Ans: A. Fundus and left margin of oesophagus**

   Ref: Chapter No.49, Page No. 1196

4. **Ans: C. Right gastroepiploic artery-superior mesenteric artery**

   Ref: Chapter No.49, Page No.1197

5. **Ans: B. Left gastric artery**

   Ref: Chapter No.49, Page No.1197

6. **Ans: B. Hepatic branch - branch of posterior vagus**

   Ref: Chapter No.49, Page No.1197

7. **Ans: A. First branch of posterior vagus**

   Ref: Chapter No.49, Page No.1198

8. **Ans: D. The so-called criminal nerve of Grassi is the first branch of the left vagus nerve**

   Ref: Chapter No.49, Page No.1198

9. **Ans: B. Muscularis mucosa**

   Ref: Chapter No.49, Page No.1198

10. **Ans: C. Circular muscle fibres**

    Ref: Chapter No.49, Page No.1198

11. **Ans: C. B. 20**

    Ref: Chapter No.49, Page No.1197

12. **Ans: D. The right gastroepiploic vein drains into the IVC**

    Ref: Chapter No.49, Page No.1197

13. **Ans: D. All of the above are true statements**

    Ref: Chapter No.49, Page No.1198

14. **Ans: A. Submucosa**

    Ref: Chapter No.49, Page No.1198

15. **Ans: C. T5-T10**

    Ref: Chapter No.49, Page No.1198

16. **Ans: C. G cells**

    Ref: Chapter No.49, Page No.1199

17. **Ans: B. Antrum**

    Ref: Chapter No.49, Page No.1199

18. **Ans: D. Cardia**

    Ref: Chapter No.49, Page No.1199

19. **Ans: D. Left gastric artery**

    Ref: Chapter No.49, Page No.1197

20. **Ans: A. First branch of posterior vagus**

    Ref: Ref: Chapter No.49, Page No.1198

21. **Ans: D. Gastrin**

    Ref: Chapter No.49, Page No.1199

22. **Ans: B. Little gastrin**

    Ref: Chapter No.49, Page No.1199

23. **Ans: A. Pentapeptide component at carboxyl terminus of gastrin**

    Ref: Chapter No.49, Page No.1199

24. **Ans: C. Gastrin and CCK**

    Ref: Chapter No.49, Page No.1199

25. **Ans: A. Protein meal**

    Ref: Chapter No.49, Page No.1199

26. **Ans: C. Gastrin**

    Ref: Chapter No.49, Page No.1199

27. **Ans: D. Both option A + C**

    Ref: Chapter No.49, Page No.1199

28. **Ans: B. Short gut syndrome**

    Ref: Chapter No.49, Page No.1200

29. **Ans: B. Pernicious Anemia**

    Ref: Chapter No.49, Page No.1200

30. **Ans: B. H pylori Infection**

    Ref: Chapter No.49, Page No.1200

31. **Ans: B. G17**

    Ref: Chapter No.49, Page No.1199

32. **Ans: D. Type A CCK receptors have an affinity for sulphated CCK analogues and Gastrin**

    Ref: Chapter No.49, Page No.1199

33. **Ans: B. Gastrin**

    Ref: Chapter No.49, Page No.1199

34. **Ans: C. Somatostatin 14**

    Ref: Chapter No.49, Page No.1200

35. **Ans: D. Both A and B**

    Ref: Chapter No.49, Page No.1200

36. **Ans: A. Acetylcholine**

    Ref: Chapter No.49, Page No.1200

37. **Ans: D. Increased ghrelin levels have been associated with gastritis**

Ref: Chapter No.49, Page No.1200

38. **Ans: D. All of the Above**

Ref: Chapter No.49, Page No.1200

39. **Ans: A. 10% of the maximal acid output**

Ref: Chapter No.49, Page No.1200

40. **Ans: A. 1 to 5 mmol/hr**

Ref: Chapter No.49, Page No.1200

41. **Ans: C. Gastric phase -90% of the maximal acid output**

Ref: Chapter No.49, Page No.1201

42. **Ans: C. Intestinal phase of gastric secretion is initiated by entry of chyme into the stomach (Entry into the duodenum not stomach)**

Ref: Chapter No.49, Page No.1201

43. **Ans: A. Famotidine**

Ref: Chapter No.49, Page No.1202

44. **Ans: C. H2 blockers have more prolonged inhibition of gastric acid secretion than PPI**

Ref: Chapter No.49, Page No.1202

45. **Ans: B. There is a linear relationship between maximal acid output and parietal cell number**

Ref: Chapter No.49, Page No.1202

46. **Ans: B. 2**

Ref: Chapter No.49, Page No.1203

47. **Ans: C. Secreted in equal amounts to amount necessary for vitamin B_{12} secretion. (It is secreted in amounts that far exceed the amounts necessary for vitamin B_{12} absorption)**

Ref: Chapter No.49, Page No.1203

48. **Ans: B. 90-120 mins**

Ref: Chapter No.49, Page No.1203

49. **Ans: C. 7**

Ref: Chapter No.49, Page No.1203

50. **Ans: A. Gastric mucin is a large glycoprotein and the mucus is a viscoelastic gel containing approximately 65% water and 35% mucin**

Ref: Chapter No.49, Page No.1203

51. **Ans: D. Pepsin is an endopeptidase that preferentially hydrolyses peptide linkages where one of the amino acids is aromatic and accounts for approximately 50% of the protein digestion in the GI tract**

Ref: Chapter No.49, Page No.1203

52. **Ans: B. Hot and cold liquids tend to empty at a faster rate than ambient temperature fluids**

Ref: Chapter No.49, Page No.1203

53. **Ans: D. The MMC is lost after vagal denervation**

Ref: Chapter No.49, Page No.1203

54. **Ans: B. 3 cycle/min**

Ref: Chapter No.49, Page No.1203

55. **Ans: D. All of the above**

Ref: Chapter No.49, Page No.1203

56. **Ans: D. Idiopathic**

Ref: Chapter No.49, Page No.1204

57. **Ans: A. Endoscopy**

Ref: Chapter No.49, Page No.1204

58. **Ans: D. All**

Ref: Chapter No.49, Page No.1204

59. **Ans: B. 15-35%**

Ref: Chapter No.49, Page No.1204

60. **Ans: C. >35%**

Ref: Chapter No.49, Page No.1204

61. **Ans: D. Gastrojejunostomy gives very good results**

Ref: Chapter No.49, Page No.1204

62. **Ans: D. Dopamine antagonists**

Ref: Chapter No.49, Page No.1204

63. **Ans: C. Surgical implantation of gastric electro stimulators use electrical leads that are placed onto the body laparoscopically and connected to a subcutaneously positioned simulator that delivers low-frequency, high-energy current**

Ref: Chapter No.49, Page No.1204

64. **Ans: D. 75%**

Ref: Chapter No.49, Page No.1204

65. **Ans: A. 50%**

Ref: Chapter No.49, Page No.1204

66. **Ans: A. -30 to -50mV**

Ref: Chapter No.49, Page No.1204

67. **Ans: B. Type 2**

Ref: Chapter No.49, Page No.1207

68. **Ans: D. Improves in time of stress**

Ref: Chapter No.49, Page No.1207-1208

69. **Ans: D. All are true**

Ref: Chapter No.49, Page No.1207-1208

70. **Ans: A. 50 to 75%**

Ref: Chapter No.49, Page No.1205

71. **Ans: B. When the organism is eradicated as part of ulcer treatment, ulcer recurrence is still common**

Ref: Chapter No.49, Page No.1205

72. **Ans: C. Decreased gastrin levels and changes in acid secretion**

Ref: Chapter No.49, Page No.1205

73. **Ans: B. Marshall and Warren**

Ref: Chapter No.49, Page No.1206

74. **Ans: A. Sensitivity in diagnosing infection is greater than 90%, and specificity is 95% to 100%**

Ref: Chapter No.49, Page No.1206

75. **Ans: A. Culture**

Ref: Chapter No.49, Page No.1206

76. **Ans: B. Histology**

Ref: Chapter No.49, Page No.1206

77. **Ans: A. 2 weeks and PPIs for 4 weeks for Antibiotics**

Ref: Chapter No.49, Page No.1206

78. **Ans: A. 1 year or longer after eradication**

Ref: Chapter No.49, Page No.1206

79. **Ans: C. 90%**

Ref: Chapter No.49, Page No.1206

80. **Ans: B. Stool Antigen**

Ref: Chapter No.49, Page No.1206

81. **Ans: D. Gastric ulcers are more likely to occur in individuals in a higher socio-economic class**

Ref: Chapter No.49, Page No.1207

82. **Ans: D. Most perforations occur along the posterior aspect of the lesser curvature**

Ref: Chapter No.49, Page No.1207

83. **Ans: B. 5%**

Ref: Chapter No.49, Page No.1209

84. **Ans: D. Endoscopy**

Ref: Chapter No.49, Page No.1209

85. **Ans: D. All are true**

Ref: Chapter No.49, Page No.1209

86. **Ans: D. All are true**

Ref: Chapter No.49, Page No.1209

87. **Ans: D. All of the above**

Ref: Chapter No.49, Page No.1206

88. **Ans: B. PPI should be stopped 4 weeks before test**

Ref: Chapter No.49, Page No.1206

89. **Ans: D. Magnesium antacids cause hypophosphatemia**

Ref: Chapter No.49, Page No.1209

90. **Ans: D. It is structurally related to warfarin, have anticoagulant effects**

Ref: Chapter No.49, Page No.1209

91. **Ans: C. Ranitidine is weakest**

Ref: Chapter No.49, Page No.1209

92. **Ans: C. PPIs have a healing rate of 75% at 4 weeks and 90% at 8 weeks and produce more rapid healing of ulcers than standard H2-receptor antagonists**

Ref: Chapter No.49, Page No.1209-1210

93. **Ans: D. None**

Ref: Chapter No.49, Page No.1210

94. **Ans: D. Bismuth**

Ref: Chapter No.49, Page No.1210

95. **Ans: C. 14-day course of triple therapy**

Ref: Chapter No.49, Page No.1210

96. **Ans: D. Obstruction: Only gastrojejunostomy**

Ref: Chapter No.49, Page No.1210

97. **Ans: D. All of the above**

Ref: Chapter No.49, Page No.1210

98. **Ans: B. Upper flexible endoscopy**

Ref: Chapter No.49, Page No.1210

99. **Ans: C. Type 2a – Adherent clot**

Ref: Chapter No.49, Page No.1211

100. **Ans: B. Type 1b**

Ref: Chapter No.49, Page No.1211

101. **Ans: B. 6% to 10%**

Ref: Chapter No.49, Page No.1211

102. **Ans: B. 24 hrs**

Ref: Chapter No.49, Page No.1211

103. **Ans: D. Patients who have a second episode of bleeding after initially successful endoscopic therapy are typically treated with surgery**

Ref: Chapter No.49, Page No.1211

104. **Ans: B. 5% to 10%**

Ref: Chapter No.49, Page No.1211

105. **Ans: C. After 1 try of endoscopic treatment**

Ref: Chapter No.49, Page No.1211

106. **Ans: C. Transverse pancreatic artery**

Ref: Chapter No.49, Page No.1212

107. **Ans: C. Perforation**

Ref: Chapter No.49, Page No.1212

108. **Ans: D. A routine contrast radiograph is required before initiating eating**

Ref: Chapter No.49, Page No.1213

109. **Ans: D. Metabolic acidosis**

Ref: Chapter No.49, Page No.1213

110. Ans: A. GOO is mostly due to benign disease

Ref: Chapter No.49, Page No.1213

111. Ans: A. Gastric outlet obstruction from PUD is a surgical emergency

Ref: Chapter No.49, Page No.1213

112. Ans: C. It is estimated to occur in 15% to 20% of patients

Ref: Chapter No.49, Page No.1213

113. Ans: B. 30%

Ref: Chapter No.49, Page No.1212

114. Ans: C. 50%

Ref: Chapter No.49, Page No.1213

115. Ans: D. 85%

Ref: Chapter No.49, Page No.1213

116. Ans: B. Vagotomy with a drainage procedure can cause delayed gastric emptying

Ref: Chapter No.49, Page No.1213

117. Ans: D. All of the above

Ref: Chapter No.49, Page No.1213

118. Ans: B. Highly selective vagotomy

Ref: Chapter No.49, Page No.1213

119. Ans: B. 7 cm proximal to the pylorus and point at least 5 cm proximal to the GE junction on the esophagus

Ref: Chapter No.49, Page No.1214

120. Ans: D. None

Ref: Chapter No.49, Page No.1214

121. Ans: B. Type 2 and 3

Ref: Chapter No.49, Page No.1207

122. Ans: D. Type 5

Ref: Chapter No.49, Page No.1207

123. Ans: A. Serum Gastrin levels more than 400 pg/ml are diagnostic

Ref: Chapter No.49, Page No.1215

124. Ans: C. The pancreas Head-neck junction

Ref: Chapter No.49, Page No.1215

125. Ans: A. Triple-phase CT

Ref: Chapter No.49, Page No.1215

126. Ans: B. Gastric ulcers

Ref: Chapter No.49, Page No.1207

127. Ans: A. Type I

Ref: Chapter No.49, Page No.1207

128. Ans: A. Urease assay on endoscopic biopsies

Ref: Chapter No.49, Page No.1207

129. Ans: C. Mid body of stomach along the greater curvature

Ref: Chapter No.49, Page No.1203

130. Ans: A. 30%

Ref: Chapter No.49, Page No.1216

131. Ans: C. Presence of luminal acid is not a prerequisite for this form of gastritis to evolve

Ref: Chapter No.49, Page No.1216

132. Ans: A. Stress gastritis develops within 1 to 2 weeks after a traumatic event in more than 50% to 75% of patients

Ref: Chapter No.49, Page No.1216

133. Ans: B. Prolonged mechanical ventilation (>48 hours)

Ref: Chapter No.49, Page No.1216

134. Ans: C. Fundus of the stomach

Ref: Chapter No.49, Page No.1216

135. Ans: D. The bleeding from stress ulcers is usually focal and the rebleeding rate is low

Ref: Chapter No.49, Page No.1217

136. Ans: C. 20% to 25%

Ref: Chapter No.49, Page No.1216

137. Ans: D. All of the above

Ref: Chapter No.49, Page No.1217

138. Ans: A. Anemia

Ref: Chapter No.49, Page No.1218

139. Ans: C. In general, the addition of iron supplements to the patient's diet doesn't correct this problem

Ref: Chapter No.49, Page No.1218

140. Ans: D. None

Ref: Chapter No.49, Page No.1218

141. Ans: D. All are true

Ref: Chapter No.49, Page No.1218

142. Ans: C. Medical therapies that have been tried to treat alkaline reflux gastritis have shown consistent benefits

Ref: Chapter No.49, Page No.1218

143. Ans: C. Erythromycin markedly accelerates gastric emptying by binding to motilin receptors on GI smooth muscle cells, where it acts as a motilin antagonist

Ref: Chapter No.49, Page No.1218-1219

144. Ans: B. Motilin agonist

Ref: Chapter No.49, Page No.1219

145. Ans: C. >40 cms

Ref: Chapter No.49, Page No.1218

146. Ans: A. High protein

Ref: Chapter No.49, Page No.1219

147. Ans: D. Microsatellite stability

Ref: Chapter No.49, Page No.1219

148. Ans: D. RET

Ref: Chapter No.49, Page No.1220

149. Ans: D. CDK1

Ref: Chapter No.49, Page No.1220

150. Ans: B. Diffuse type gastric ca

Ref: Chapter No.49, Page No.1220

151. Ans: D. Cooked fish

Ref: Chapter No.49, Page No.1219

152. Ans: A. IL-1beta

Ref: Chapter No.49, Page No.1219

153. Ans: C. 16

Ref: Chapter No.49, Page No.1222

154. Ans: D. Among racial groups, the disease is more common and has a higher mortality in Whites

Ref: Chapter No.49, Page No.1219

155. Ans: C. The presence of the cytotoxin associated gene A leads to decreased virulence and risk of gastric cancer

Ref: Chapter No.49, Page No.1219-1220

156. Ans: C. 60% to 70%

Ref: Chapter No.49, Page No.1220

157. Ans: A. 30 years

Ref: Chapter No.49, Page No.1220

158. Ans: B. 1 cm

Ref: Chapter No.49, Page No.1220

159. Ans: D. Hyperplastic polyps are associated with H. pylori infection and chronic gastritis with an associated malignancy rate of over 10%

Ref: Chapter No.49, Page No.1220

160. Ans: D. All of the above

Ref: Chapter No.49, Page No.1221

161. Ans: D. Montreal classification

Ref: Chapter No.49, Page No.1221

162. Ans: C. Type III

Ref: Chapter No.49, Page No.1221

163. Ans: B. Type II

Ref: Chapter No.49, Page No.1221

164. Ans: D. Type IV

Ref: Chapter No.49, Page No.1221

165. Ans: D. Familial

Ref: Chapter No.49, Page No.1221

166. Ans: C. Increasing incidence with age

Ref: Chapter No.49, Page No.1221

167. Ans: C. Both

Ref: Chapter No.49, Page No.1221

168. Ans: B. Adenocarcinoma of GE junction

Ref: Chapter No.49, Page No.1222

169. Ans: B. 1 cm above and 2 cm below

Ref: Chapter No.49, Page No.1222

170. Ans: B. Esophageal adenocarcinoma

Ref: Chapter No.49, Page No.1222

171. Ans: B. 16

Ref: Chapter No.49, Page No.1222

172. Ans: B. 6-8 biopsy specimens

Ref: Chapter No.49, Page No.1222

173. Ans: D. Ascitis cannot be identified by EUS

Ref: Chapter No.49, Page No.1224

174. Ans: B. FNA cannot be performed if ascites is present to evaluate for peritoneal spread

Ref: Chapter No.49, Page No.1224

175. Ans: C. NCCN guidelines recommend considering PET/CT as part of staging for patients with greater than T4 disease without evidence of metastatic disease on initial CT

Ref: Chapter No.49, Page No.1225

176. Ans: A. T1

Ref: Chapter No.49, Page No.1225

177. Ans: C. T3

Ref: Chapter No.49, Page No.1223

178. Ans: C. Tis

Ref: Chapter No.49, Page No.1223

179. Ans: C. The NCCN recommends staging laparoscopic in T4 or greater gastric cancer and no prior evidence of metastases will be found to have peritoneal disease

Ref: Chapter No.49, Page No.1225

180. Ans: D. T2 or greater gastric cancer and no prior evidence of metastases will be found to have peritoneal disease

Ref: Chapter No.49, Page No.1225

181. Ans: B. The proximal stomach is transected at the level of the incisura at a margin of at least 5 cm for early cancers and at least 4 to 6 cm for advanced cancers

Ref: Chapter No.49, Page No.1225

182. Ans: D. Ulcerated tumor

Ref: Chapter No.49, Page No.1226

183. Ans: A. Intestinal-type adenocarcinoma

Ref: Chapter No.49, Page No.1226

184. Ans: B. Mucosal tumors up to 3 cm without ulceration

Ref: Chapter No.49, Page No.1226

185. Ans: D. Distal splenic arteries

Ref: Chapter No.49, Page No.1225

186. Ans: D. DUTCH trial - advocates D1 lymph node dissection with splenic preservation

Ref: Chapter No.49, Page No.1229

187. Ans: B. D2 dissection in patients undergoing surgery for curative intent

Ref: Chapter No.49, Page No.1228

188. Ans: D. Number of positive lymph nodes doesn't correlate with survival in gastric cancer

Ref: Chapter No.49, Page No.1227-1228

189. Ans: C. For more advanced disease, it has been shown to offer a survival benefit

Ref: Chapter No.49, Page No.1228

190. Ans: D. ARTIST trial

Ref: Chapter No.49, Page No.1229-1230

191. Ans: D. All of the above

Ref: Chapter No.49, Page No.1229

192. Ans: C. 50%

Ref: Chapter No.49, Page No.1230

193. Ans: D. All of the Above

Ref: Chapter No.49, Page No.1230

194. Ans: D. All of the Above

Ref: Chapter No.49, Page No.1230

195. Ans: D. The trastuzumab group had a better median survival and rates of severe complications differed between the groups

Ref: Chapter No.49, Page No.1230

196. Ans: D. Liver

Ref: Chapter No.49, Page No.1230

197. Ans: B. 9

Ref: Chapter No.49, Page No.1228

198. Ans: B. 7

Ref: Chapter No.49, Page No.1228

199. Ans: C. 1-b, 2-a, 3-d, 4-c

Ref: Chapter No.49, Page No.1228

200. Ans: C. Stomach

Ref: Chapter No.49, Page No.1231

201. Ans: C Antrum

Ref: Chapter No.49, Page No.1231

202. Ans: A. 10%

Ref: Chapter No.49, Page No.1231

203. Ans: C. Inflammatory bowel disease

Ref: Chapter No.49, Page No.1231

204. Ans: B. Diffuse large B cell lymphoma

Ref: Chapter No.49, Page No.1231

205. Ans: D. All of the above

Ref: Chapter No.49, Page No.1231

206. Ans: C. Lugano Staging

Ref: Chapter No.49, Page No.1231

207. Ans: C. Stage IIE

Ref: Chapter No.49, Page No.1232

208. Ans: D. All of the above are true.

Ref: Chapter No.49, Page No.1232

209. Ans: C. t(11;14)

Ref: Chapter No.49, Page No.1232

210. Ans: B. t(3;14)

Ref: Chapter No.49, Page No.1232

211. Ans: C. Some patients with MALT lymphoma are H pylori–negative, in these patients, consideration should be given to surgical resection

Ref: Chapter No.49, Page No.1232

212. Ans: D. Presence of t(3;14)

Ref: Chapter No.49, Page No.1232

213. Ans: C. 95%

Ref: Chapter No.49, Page No.1232

214. Ans: C. PDGFRA

Ref: Chapter No.49, Page No.1232

215. Ans: B. Stomach

Ref: Chapter No.49, Page No.1232

216. Ans: B. Neurofibromatosis 2

Ref: Chapter No.49, Page No.1232

217. Ans: D. Autosomal Recessive syndrome (It is a rare Autosomal Dominant Disorder)

Ref: Chapter No.49, Page No.1232

218. Ans: D. Serological H pylori testing should be done if negative confirm with biopsy

Ref: Chapter No.49, Page No.1231-1232

219. Ans: B. 5%

Ref: Chapter No.49, Page No.1232

220. Ans: C. Vinblastine

Ref: Chapter No.49, Page No.1232

221. Ans: B. 2 months

Ref: Chapter No.49, Page No.1232

222. Ans: A. Biannually for 3 years

Ref: Chapter No.49, Page No.1232

223. Ans: B. EUS guided FNA

Ref: Chapter No.49, Page No.1232

224. Ans: A. Preoperative biopsy is recommended if there is a high suspicion for GIST and the patient is otherwise operable

Ref: Chapter No.49, Page No.1233

225. Ans: A. Gastric resection

Ref: Chapter No.49, Page No.1233

226. Ans: B. 2 cm

Ref: Chapter No.49, Page No.1233

227. Ans: D. All of the above

Ref: Chapter No.49, Page No.1233

228. Ans: C. Liver

Ref: Chapter No.49, Page No.1233

229. Ans: C. Recurrence doesn't occur over 2 years after resection; thus, long-term follow-up is not warranted

Ref: Chapter No.49, Page No.1233

230. Ans: A. Scandinavian sarcoma Group XVIII trial

Ref: Chapter No.49, Page No.1233

231. Ans: B. Low to moderate malignant potential

Ref: Chapter No.49, Page No.1233

232. Ans: D. Early GIST

Ref: Chapter No.49, Page No.1233-1234

233. Ans: A. 400 mg and 3 years

Ref: Chapter No.49, Page No.1233

234. Ans: B. Type 2

Ref: Chapter No.49, Page No.1234

235. Ans: A. Type 1

Ref: Chapter No.49, Page No.1234

236. Ans: D. MEN 2 B

Ref: Chapter No.49, Page No.1234

237. Ans: C. Type 3

Ref: Chapter No.49, Page No.1234

238. Ans: D. Gastric NETs are typically functioning and cause carcinoid syndrome

Ref: Chapter No.49, Page No.1234

239. Ans: A. Both Assertion (A) and Reason (R) are the true and Reason (R) is a correct explanation of Assertion (A)

Ref: Chapter No. 49, Page No.1234

240. Ans: D. Type 4

Ref: Chapter No. 49, Page No.1234

241. Ans: D. Chromogranin B is often elevated and can serve as a biomarker for these tumors

Ref: Chapter No.49, Page No.1234

242. Ans: C. Smaller (<2 cm) lesions may require wedge resection or partial gastrectomy

Ref: Chapter No.49, Page No.1234

243. Ans: D. All the above are true

Ref: Chapter No.49, Page No.1234

244. Ans: A. Antral greater curvature

Ref: Chapter No.49, Page No.1234

245. Ans: B. Menetrier's disease

Ref: Chapter No.49, Page No.1235

246. Ans: D. Reduced mucus production

Ref: Chapter No.49, Page No.1235

247. Ans: C. Campylobacter

Ref: Chapter No.49, Page No.1235

248. Ans: C. TGF Alpha

Ref: Chapter No.49, Page No.1235

249. Ans: A. 1 to 2 years

Ref: Chapter No.49, Page No.1235

250. Ans: D. Medical treatment yields consistent results

Ref: Chapter No.49, Page No.1235

251. Ans: C. 15%

Ref: Chapter No.49, Page No.1235

252. Ans: D. Both A and B

Ref: Chapter No.49, Page No.1235

253. Ans: D. All of the above are true

Ref: Chapter No.49, Page No.1235

254. Ans: C. Women are usually involved

Ref: Chapter No.49, Page No.1235

255. Ans: A. Near the GE junction along the lesser curvature

Ref: Chapter No.49, Page No.1235

256. Ans: D. Angiography is generally not useful

Ref: Chapter No.49, Page No.1235

257. Ans: B. Left gastric artery

Ref: Chapter No.49, Page No.1235

258. Ans: C. Painful hematemesis

Ref: Chapter No.49, Page No.1235

259. Ans: C. Esophagoduodenoscopy

Ref: Chapter No.49, Page No.1235

260. Ans: B. Tortuous artery coursing through the submucosa with a primary ulcer (without a primary ulcer)

Ref: Chapter No.49, Page No.1235

261. Ans: A. Isolated gastric varices

Ref: Chapter No.49, Page No.1235

262. Ans: D. All of the above

Ref: Chapter No.49, Page No.1235

263. Ans: C. A major problem with gastric varices after endoscopic treatment is rebleeding, occurring in more than 50% of patients

Ref: Chapter No.49, Page No.1236

264. Ans: B. This spontaneous shunt decompresses the portal system and improves the efficacy of transjugular intrahepatic portosystemic shunting

Ref: Chapter No.49, Page No.1236

265. Ans: B. Aggravation of Esophageal varices

Ref: Chapter No.49, Page No.1236

266. Ans: A. Organoaxial

Ref: Chapter No.49, Page No.1236

267. Ans: C. Associated with diaphragmatic defect

Ref: Chapter No.49, Page No.1236

268. Ans: D. Hematemesis

Ref: Chapter No.49, Page No.1236

269. Ans: B. NG decompression should not be performed immediately

Ref: Chapter No.49, Page No.1236

270. Ans: D. Spontaneous volvulus, without an associated diaphragmatic defect, is treated by gastric resection

Ref: Chapter No.49, Page No.1236

271. Ans: D. All of the above

Ref: Chapter No.49, Page No.1236

272. Ans: D. All of the above

Ref: Chapter No.49, Page No.1236-1237

273. Ans: C. Trichobezoars are typically effectively managed with chemical dissolution

Ref: Chapter No.49, Page No.1237

274. Ans: B. The sodium concentration in Adolph's Meat Tenderizer is low, so hyponatremia may result if large quantities are administered

Ref: Chapter No.49, Page No.1237

50

Small Intestine

1. **The largest endocrine organ in the body is:**
   A. Pituitary gland B. Pancreas
   C. Small bowel D. Adrenal gland

EMBRYOLOGY

2. **False about the development of small intestine is:**
   A. Splanchnic mesoderm surrounding the endoderm gives rise to the muscular connective tissue and all the other layers of the intestine
   B. Nerves and neurons found in the wall are derived from the neuroectoderm
   C. The endodermal layer gives rise to the epithelial lining of the digestive tract
   D. Except for the duodenum, which is a primitive foregut structure, the small intestine is derived from the midgut

3. **Meckel diverticulum is present in approximately:**
   A. 1% of the population
   B. 2% of the population
   C. 5% of the population
   D. 10% of the population

4. **False about small intestine is:**
   A. Epithelial cell turnover occurs rapidly, with a life span of 7 to 10 days in humans
   B. The primitive small bowel is lined by a sheet of cuboidal cells until about the 9th week of gestation
   C. 4 types of cells are present: Absorptive enterocytes, goblet cells, paneth cells and enteroendocrine cells
   D. Crypt formation begins in the 10th to 12th weeks of gestation

5. **Most common type of small intestinal cell is:**
   A. Absorptive enterocytes
   B. Paneth cells
   C. Enteroendocrine cells
   D. Goblet cells

6. **Which of the following cells doesn't have rapid turnover?**
   A. Absorptive enterocytes
   B. Paneth cells
   C. Enteroendocrine cells
   D. Goblet cells

ANATOMY

7. **Jejunal length is around:**
   A. 20 cms B. 50 cms
   C. 100 cms D. 150 cms

8. **Duodenal length is:**
   A. 20 cms B. 50 cms
   C. 100 cms D. 150 cms

9. **False about small bowel is:**
   A. In the jejunum, only one or two arcades send out long, straight vasa recta to the mesenteric border
   B. The ileum has a somewhat larger circumference, is thicker than the jejunum
   C. The mucosa of the small bowel is characterized by transverse folds (plicae circulares)
   D. The blood supply to the ileum may have 4 or 5 separate arcades with shorter vasa recta

10. **Ligament of Treitz is present at:**
    A. Gastroduodenal junction
    B. Duodenojejunal junction
    C. Jejunoileal junction
    D. Ileocolic junction

11. **Ileal length is:**
    A. 20 cms B. 50 cms
    C. 100 cms D. 150 cms

12. **The base of the mesentery of small intestine attaches to the posterior abdominal wall to:**

A. Right of the T12 vertebra and passes obliquely to the right and inferiorly to the right sacroiliac joint
B. Left of the L2 vertebra and passes obliquely to the right and inferiorly to the right sacroiliac joint
C. Right of the L2 vertebra and passes obliquely to the right and inferiorly to the right sacroiliac joint
D. Left of the T12 vertebra and passes obliquely to the right and inferiorly to the right sacroiliac joint

13. **False about nervous supply of small intestine is:**

A. The sympathetic fibers come from 3 sets of splanchnic nerves
B. Pain from the intestine is transmitted through general visceral afferent fibers of the parasympathetic system
C. The parasympathetic fibers derive from the vagus nerve
D. Motor impulses affect blood vessel motility and probably gut secretion and motility

14. **False about the lymphatic drainage of small intestine is:**

A. Lymphatic drainage proceeds from the mucosa through the wall of the bowel to a set of nodes adjacent to the bowel in the mesentery
B. The lymphatic drainage of the small intestine plays a major role in immune defense
C. Small intestine lymphatics are noted as major deposits of lymphatic tissue, particularly in the Peyer patches of the proximal small bowel
D. Lymph flows into the cisterna chyli and then up the thoracic duct, ultimately to empty into the venous system at the confluence of the left internal jugular and subclavian veins

15. **The strongest component of the intestinal wall is:**

A. Mucosa B. Submucosa
C. Serosa D. Muscularis propria

16. **False about the microanatomy of small intestine is:**

A. Villi are tallest in the distal duodenum and proximal jejunum and shortest in the distal ileum
B. The serosa is the outermost layer of the small intestine and consists of visceral peritoneum
C. The submucosa consists of a layer of fibroelastic connective tissue containing blood vessels and nerves
D. The muscularis propria consists of two muscle layers, a thick outer longitudinal layer and a thin inner circular layer of smooth muscle

17. **Meissner plexus is present in:**

A. Mucosa B. Submucosa
C. Serosa D. Muscularis propria

18. **Auerbach plexus is present in:**

A. Mucosa B. Submucosa
C. Serosa D. Muscularis propria

19. **False about the function of small intestinal cells is:**

A. The main functions of the villous epithelium are digestion and absorption
B. The microvilli increase the absorptive capacity by 10-fold
C. The main functions of the crypt epithelium are cell renewal as well as exocrine, endocrine, water and ion secretion
D. Paneth cells, which secrete lysozyme, tumor necrosis factor (TNF) and cryptdins, which are homologues of leukocyte defensin peptides thought to be related to the host mucosal defense system

PHYSIOLOGY

20. **The stomach initiates the process of digestion with the breakdown of solids to particles:**

A. 10 mm or smaller B. 5 mm or smaller
C. 3 mm or smaller D. 1 mm or smaller

21. **True about the following is:**

A. Maltase hydrolyzes maltose to produce glucose monomers
B. Amylose is broken down at the α-1,4 bonds by salivary and pancreatic amylases that convert amylose to maltotriose and maltose
C. Lactase hydrolyzes lactose into glucose and galactose
D. All of the above

22. **False about protein digestion is:**

A. Protein digestion is initiated in the stomach, where gastric acid denatures proteins
B. In normal humans, digestion and absorption of protein are usually 80% to 90% completed in the ileum

C. The endopeptidases, which include trypsin, chymotrypsin and elastase, act on peptide bonds at the interior of the protein molecule

D. All of the above are true

23. **False about pancreatic proteases is:**

A. Elastase: Attacks peptide bonds involving neutral aliphatic amino acids; yields products with neutral amino acids at carboxyl-terminal end

B. Trypsin: Attacks peptide bonds involving basic amino acids; yields products with basic amino acids at carboxyl-terminal end

C. Endopeptidases: Hydrolyze interior peptide bonds of polypeptides and proteins

D. Carboxypeptidase B: Attacks peptides with aromatic and neutral aliphatic amino acids at carboxyl-terminal end

24. **False about enterohepatic circulation is:**

A. Although unconjugated bile acids are absorbed into the jejunum by passive diffusion

B. The proximal intestine absorbs most of the dietary fat

C. The total bile acid pool (approximately 2–3 g) recirculates about 3 times every 24 hours through the enterohepatic circulation

D. Almost all the bile salts are reabsorbed, with only about 0.5 g lost in the stool every day

25. **False about absorption through small intestine is:**

A. Vitamin C is absorbed by an active transport process that incorporates a sodium-coupled mechanism as well as a specific carrier system

B. Calcium is absorbed, particularly in the proximal intestine

C. Iron is absorbed as a heme or nonheme component in the duodenum by a passive process

D. Potassium, magnesium, phosphate and other ions also can be actively absorbed throughout the mucosa

26. **False about the absorption of vitamin B is:**

A. Vitamin B_2 is absorbed in the upper intestine by facilitated transport

B. Vitamin B_6 appears to be rapidly absorbed by simple diffusion into the distal intestine

C. In the ileal enterocyte, free vitamin B_{12} is bound to an ileal pool of transcobalamin II, which transports it into the portal circulation

D. Vitamin B_1 is rapidly absorbed in the jejunum by an active process similar to the sodium-coupled transport system for vitamin C

27. **Which of the following is not absorbed through duodenum?**

A. Iron

B. Amino acids

C. Electrolytes, water

D. Monosaccharides

28. **Which of the following is not absorbed through jejunum?**

A. Free fatty acids

B. Folate, vitamins A, D, E, K

C. Monoglycerides

D. Bile acids

MOTILITY

29. **Peristalsis of small intestine consists of intestinal contractions passing aborally abnormally at a rate of:**

A. 0.5–1 cm/sec B. 1–2 cm/sec

C. 2–5 cm/sec D. 5–9 cm/sec

30. **Pacesetter potentials in intestinal motility is thought to originate in:**

A. Proximal jejunum B. Distal stomach

C. Duodenum D. Distal jejunum

31. **During the fasting period between meals, the bowel is regularly swept by cyclical contractions that move aborally along the intestine every:**

A. 15 to 30 minutes B. 30 to 60 minutes

C. 60 to 75 minutes D. 75 to 90 minutes

ENDOCRINE FUNCTION

32. **False about gastrin is:**

A. Produced by G cells in antrum

B. Bombesin is the major stimulant of gastrin secretion

C. Stimulates gastric acid and pepsinogen secretion

D. Relaxes sphincter of Oddi

33. **False about secretin is:**

A. Stimulates gastric acid secretion and motility

B. Stimulates release of water and bicarbonate from pancreatic ductal cells

C. Stimulates flow and alkalinity of bile

D. Produced by S cells in duodenum and jejunum

34. **Universal "off" switch peptide is:**
A. Cholecystokinin
B. Somatostatin
C. Gastrin-releasing peptide
D. Gastric inhibitory polypeptide

35. **Universal "on" switch peptide is:**
A. Cholecystokinin
B. Somatostatin
C. Gastrin-releasing peptide
D. Gastric inhibitory polypeptide

36. **False about cholecystokinin is:**
A. Produced by C cells in duodenum and jejunum
B. Stimulates gallbladder contraction
C. Inhibits gastric emptying
D. Relaxes sphincter of Oddi

37. **Gastric inhibitory polypeptide is secreted by:**
A. G cells B. K cells
C. I cells D. L cells

38. **L cells secretes:**
A. Enteroglucagon B. Peptide YY
C. Motilin D. Neurotensin

39. **False about Vasoactive intestinal peptide is:**
A. Primarily functions as a neuropeptide
B. Inhibits gastric acid secretion
C. Stimulates pancreatic and intestinal secretion
D. Potent vasoconstrictor

40. **False about Neurotensin is:**
A. Stimulates growth of small and large bowel mucosa
B. Stimulates growth of cancer with neurotensin receptors
C. Stimulates insulin release
D. Facilitates absorption of fats in the intestine

41. **False about Peptide YY is:**
A. Inhibits gallbladder contraction
B. Inhibits pancreatic glucagon release
C. Inhibits gastric and pancreatic secretion
D. Secreted by distal small bowel and colon

42. **False about diagnostic and therapeutic uses of gastrointestinal hormone is:**
A. Glucagon: Relieves sphincter of Oddi spasm
B. Secretin: Decrease secretion from pancreatic and intestinal fistulas
C. Cholecystokinin: Biliary imaging of gallbladder contraction
D. Gastrin: Pentagastrin (gastrin analogue) used to measure maximal gastric acid secretion

IMMUNE FUNCTION

43. **The gut-associated lymphoid tissue is localized in areas as:**
A. Lamina propria lymphoid cells
B. Intraepithelial lymphocytes
C. Peyer patches
D. All of the above

44. **False among the following is:**
A. The B lymphocytes become surface immunoglobulin A (IgA)
B. Peyer patches are unencapsulated lymphoid nodules that constitute an afferent limb of the gut-associated lymphoid tissue
C. Approximately 40% of the lymphoid cells in the lamina propria are B cells
D. Approximately 60% of the lymphoid cells are B cells

OBSTRUCTION

45. **Extraluminal causes of intestinal obstruction are all except:**
A. Adhesions B. Hernias
C. Carcinomas D. Bezoars

46. **Most common cause of intestinal obstruction is:**
A. Neoplasms B. Crohn's disease
C. Adhesions D. Hernias

47. **In the cases of small bowel obstruction, malignant tumors account for approximately of:**
A. 10% B. 20%
C. 40% D. 60%

48. **In the cases of small bowel obstruction, adhesions account for approximately of:**
A. 10% B. 20%
C. 40% D. 60%

49. **False about intestinal obstruction is:**
A. Primary small bowel tumors can cause obstruction but are exceedingly rare
B. Crohn's disease is the third leading cause of small bowel obstruction and accounts for approximately 10% of all cases

C. Most of these tumors are metastatic lesions that obstruct the intestine secondary to peritoneal implants that have spread from an intraabdominal primary tumor
D. Internal hernias, generally related to prior abdominal surgery, can also result in small bowel obstruction

50. Intraluminal cause of intestinal obstruction is all except:

A. Gallstone
B. Abscess
C. Bezoar
D. Enterolith

51. False about the pathophysiology of intestinal obstruction is:

A. Massive third-space fluid loss accounts for the dehydration and hypovolemia
B. The increase in peristalsis that occurs early in the course of bowel obstruction is present above and below the point of obstruction; this process can account for the finding of diarrhea
C. In distal obstruction of the small bowel, abnormalities in serum electrolyte levels are usually more dramatic
D. Later in the course of obstruction, the intestine becomes fatigued and dilates, with contractions becoming less frequent and less intense

52. With a proximal obstruction, increased vomiting associated with dehydration may be accompanied by all except:

A. Metabolic alkalosis
B. Hypokalemia
C. Hypochloremia
D. Hyperkalemia

53. With obstruction, the quantity of organisms reaches concentrations of:

A. 10^5 to 10^7 CFU/mL
B. 10^7 to 10^9 CFU/mL
C. 10^9 to 10^{10} CFU/mL
D. 10^{10} to 10^{12} CFU/mL

54. False about clinical manifestations of intestinal obstruction is:

A. The typical crampy abdominal pain associated with intestinal obstruction occurs in paroxysms at 4- to 5-minute intervals and occurs more frequently with distal obstruction
B. Complete bowel obstruction cannot be ruled out on the basis of a history of loose bowel movements
C. The cardinal symptoms of intestinal obstruction include colicky abdominal pain, nausea, vomiting, abdominal distention and obstipation
D. The typical crampy abdominal pain associated with intestinal obstruction occurs in paroxysms at 4- to 5-minute intervals and occurs more frequently with distal obstruction

55. True about physical examination in small bowel obstruction is:

A. Early in the course of bowel obstruction, the abdomen may demonstrate hyperactive bowel sounds with audible rushes associated with vigorous peristalsis (borborygmi)
B. A rectal examination should always be performed to rule out a distal colonic obstruction by intraluminal masses and to examine the stool for occult blood, which may be an indication of malignant disease, intussusception, or infarction
C. Late in the obstructive course, minimal or no bowel sounds are noted
D. All of the above

56. Plain abdominal film signs of small bowel obstruction in left lateral decubitus position are all except:

A. Air fluid levels longer than 2.5 cm
B. Multiple air fluid levels
C. String of beads sign
D. Pseudotumor sign

57. Plain abdominal film signs of small bowel obstruction in supine position are all except:

A. Stretch sign
B. Dilated gas or fluid filled small bowel >3 cm
C. Air fluid levels in same loop of small bowel of unequal lengths
D. Absence of rectal gas

58. False about diagnosis of small bowel obstruction is:

A. The absence of leukocytosis eliminates strangulation as a possibility
B. CT scan is less sensitive in patients with partial small bowel obstruction
C. The accuracy of diagnosis of the small intestinal obstruction on plain abdominal radiographs is estimated to be approximately 86%
D. Elevated lactic acid levels suggest intestinal ischemia or necrosis

59. **True about CT scan in small bowel obstruction is:**

A. CT is helpful to identify a transition zone in approximately 93% of cases
B. CT is particularly sensitive and specific (95% for both) for diagnosing complete or high-grade obstruction of the small bowel
C. CT findings associated with strangulation are those of irreversible ischemia and necrosis
D. All of the above

60. **False about enteroclysis in small bowel obstruction is:**

A. The suspension is then viewed continuously with use of either fluoroscopy or standard radiographs taken at frequent intervals
B. This technique is a single-contrast procedure that allows detailed imaging of the entire small intestine
C. Barium studies may be helpful for patients with a history of recurring obstruction or low-grade mechanical obstruction to precisely define the obstructed segment and degree of obstruction
D. The main disadvantages of enteroclysis are the need for nasoenteric intubation, slow transit of contrast material in patients with a fluid-filled hypotonic small bowel and enhanced expertise required by the radiologist

61. **Barium study procedure involves the continued infusion of:**

A. 100 to 300 mL of thin barium phosphate and methylcellulose suspension
B. 500 to 1000 mL of thin barium sulfate and methylcellulose suspension
C. 100 to 300 mL of thin barium sulfate and ethylcellulose suspension
D. 500 to 1000 mL of thin barium sulfate and ethylcellulose suspension

62. **True about small bowel obstruction is:**

A. Classic signs of strangulation include tachycardia, fever, leukocytosis and a constant, noncramping abdominal pain
B. In a strangulated obstruction, usually involves a closed loop obstruction with a compromised vascular supply to a segment of intestine, can lead to intestinal infarction
C. Noninvasive determinations of mesenteric ischemia have been described using a superconducting quantum interference device (SQUID) magnetometer to detect mesenteric ischemia noninvasively
D. All of the above

63. **CT scans demonstrates evidence of ischemia such as all except:**

A. Decreased bowel wall enhancement
B. Bowel wall thickening (>1 mm)
C. Mesenteric edema
D. Mesenteric or portovenous gas

64. **False about the management of small bowel obstruction is:**

A. Suction with a nasogastric tube empties the stomach, reducing the hazard of pulmonary aspiration of vomitus and minimizing further intestinal distention from swallowed air
B. Retrospective studies report that a 48- to 72-hour delay is safe but that the incidence of strangulation and other complications increases significantly after this time period
C. Resolution of symptoms and discharge without the need for surgery have been reported in up to 85% of patients with a partial obstruction
D. Patients with a partial intestinal obstruction may be treated conservatively with resuscitation and tube decompression alone

65. **The contrast challenge requires 100 mL of water-soluble contrast given through the nasogastric tube and follow-up radiographs obtained after:**

A. 4 and 6 hours
B. 6 and 18 hours
C. 8 and 24 hours
D. 12 and 36 hours

66. **False about operative management of small bowel obstruction is:**

A. Patients with intestinal obstruction secondary to an adhesive band may be treated with lysis of adhesions
B. Percutaneous drainage of the abscess may be sufficient to relieve the obstruction, but laparotomy and abdominal washout may be required for large and established abscesses
C. If a chronic fibrotic stricture is the cause of the obstruction, a bowel resection or strictureplasty may be required
D. Radiation enteropathy may cause bowel obstruction and can be treated nonoperatively with tube decompression and the potential addition of corticosteroids, particularly during the chronic setting

67. **During exploratory laparotomy if intestinal viability is questionable, the bowel segment should be completely released and placed in a warm, saline-moistened sponge for:**

A. 5 to 10 minutes
B. 10 to 12 minutes
C. 15 to 20 minutes
D. 25 to 30 minutes

68. The most effective means of limiting the number of adhesions is a:

A. Heparin
B. Use of corticosteroids
C. Good surgical technique
D. Dextran solutions

69. Given ample time, early postoperative obstructions will resolve spontaneously in:

A. >30%
B. >50%
C. >70%
D. >90%

70. Causes of ileus are all except:

A. Systemic sepsis
B. Retroperitoneal hemorrhage or inflammation
C. Intra-abdominal obstruction
D. Intra-abdominal inflammation

71. Metabolic and electrolyte derangements causing ileus includes all except:

A. Uremia
B. Hypoglycemia
C. Hypomagnesemia
D. Hypokalemia

72. False about ileus is:

A. The treatment of an ileus is entirely supportive, with nasogastric decompression and IV fluid
B. An ileus is defined as intestinal distention and the slowing or absence of passage of luminal contents without a demonstrable mechanical obstruction
C. Erythromycin has been effective and cisapride is beneficial in stimulating gastric motility and appears to alter intestinal ileus
D. Abdominal distention, usually without the colicky abdominal pain, is the typical and most notable finding

INFLAMMATORY AND INFECTIOUS DISEASES

73. The most common primary surgical disease of the small bowel is:

A. Crohn's disease
B. Tuberculosis
C. Ulcerative colitis
D. Pseudomembranous colitis

74. False about epidemiology of Crohn's disease is:

A. Two genders are affected equally
B. Crohn's disease primarily attacks middle aged adults in the 4th and 5th decades of life
C. Ashkenazi Jews, have a 2-4 fold higher incidence of Crohn's disease than age and gender matched control subjects
D. Crohn's disease have shown a concordance rate of only 4% in dizygotic twins but a 20% to 50% rate in monozygotic twins

75. As compared to non-smokers, in smokers the risk for development of Crohn's disease is:

A. 6 x
B. 5 x
C. 3 x
D. 2 x

76. There is a strong familial association in Crohn's disease, in siblings the risk for development of Crohn's disease is increased about:

A. 10-fold
B. 20-fold
C. 30-fold
D. 50-fold

77. The most important gene in Crohn's disease development is:

A. MST1 3p21
B. NOD2
C. MHC
D. CARD15

78. Homozygosity NOD2 variant confers increase in risk of:

A. 3- to 8-fold
B. 7- to 15-fold
C. 17- to 40-fold
D. 30- to 50-fold

79. False about genetic factors of Crohn's disease is:

A. NOD2 has been identified as a genetic predictor of ileal disease, ileal stenosis, fistula and Crohn-related surgery
B. CARD15 is also helpful in distinguishing Crohn's disease from ulcerative colitis as it is more strongly associated with ulcerative colitis
C. The genes with the strongest and most frequently replicated associations with Crohn's disease are NOD2, MHC and MST1 3p21
D. The FHIT gene located on 3p14.2 has been identified as a tumor suppressor gene and is suggested to play a role in the pathogenesis of Crohn's disease

80. True about environmental factors of Crohn's disease is:

A. Smoking is the single largest environment factor, with a 2 fold increase in risk of Crohn's disease
B. Dysbiosis with a decrease in intraluminal Bacteroides and Firmicutes and an increase in Gammaproteobacteria and Actinobacteria are associated with higher risk
C. Other factors that increase the risk of Crohn's disease include medications (oral contraceptives, aspirin, nonsteroidal antiinflammatory drugs [NSAIDs]), decreased dietary fiber and increase fat intake
D. All of the above

81. **True about Crohn's disease pathology is:**
   A. 30% percent of patients present with small bowel disease alone, and in 15%, the disease appears limited to the large intestine
   B. In patients with colonic disease, rectal sparing is characteristic of Crohn's disease and helps distinguish it from ulcerative colitis
   C. The involvement of the large and small intestine has been noted in about 55% of patients
   D. All of the above

82. **The earliest gross pathologic lesion is a:**
   A. Skip areas
   B. Superficial aphthous ulcer
   C. Transmural inflammation
   D. Noncaseating granulomas

83. **False about gross pathological features of Crohn's disease is:**
   A. The mesentery of the involved segment is usually thickened, with enlarged lymph nodes often noted
   B. The ulcers are characteristically transverse
   C. Areas of diseased bowel separated by areas of grossly appearing normal bowel, called skip areas, are commonly encountered
   D. A striking finding of Crohn's disease is the presence of extensive fat wrapping caused by the circumferential growth of the mesenteric fat around the bowel wall, also known as creeping fat

84. **Characteristic histologic lesions of Crohn's disease are:**
   A. Lymphocytes
   B. Noncaseating granulomas
   C. Caseating granulomas
   D. Plasma infiltration

85. **In Crohn's disease, granulomas appear later in the course and are found in the wall of the bowel or in regional lymph nodes in:**
   A. 10% to 20% of patients
   B. 30% to 50% of patients
   C. 60% to 70% of patients
   D. 80% to 90% of patients

86. **The most common symptom of Crohn's disease is:**
   A. Per rectal bleeding
   B. Chronic diarrhea
   C. Intermittent and colicky abdominal pain
   D. Bloody diarrhea

87. **The Montreal Classification divides all Crohn's disease patients into distinct categories based on all except:**
   A. Disease behaviour
   B. Disease site
   C. Symptom onset
   D. Disease etiology

88. **False about clinical manifestation of Crohn's disease is:**
   A. The main intestinal complications of Crohn's disease include obstruction and perforation
   B. Bleeding is typically indolent and chronic, but massive gastrointestinal bleeding can occasionally occur, particularly in duodenal Crohn's disease associated with chronic ulcer formation
   C. Localized abscesses can occur everywhere in peritoneum
   D. Free perforations into the peritoneal cavity leading to a generalized peritonitis can occur in patients with Crohn's disease

89. **False about Crohn's disease associated cancer is:**
   A. The relative risk for small bowel cancer in Crohn's disease is approximately 10-fold, the absolute risk is large
   B. Small bowel adenocarcinoma associated with Crohn's disease has an aggressive behavior and a strong probability of extracellular mucin
   C. Carcinomas typically arise at sites of chronic disease and more commonly occur in the ileum as a result of the chronic inflammation of the mucosa
   D. Extraintestinal cancer, such as squamous cell carcinoma of the vulva and anal canal and Hodgkin and non-Hodgkin lymphomas, may be more frequent in patients with Crohn's disease

90. **False about perianal disease in Crohn's disease is:**
   A. Crohn's disease should be suspected in any patient with multiple, chronic perianal fistulas
   B. Perianal disease (fissure, fistula, stricture, or abscess) is common and occurs in 25% of patients with Crohn's disease limited to the small intestine
   C. Perianal disease occurs in 80% of patients with colonic involvement alone
   D. Perianal disease may be the sole presenting feature in 5% of patients

91. The most common extraintestinal manifestation of Crohn's disease is:

A. Arthritis and arthralgias
B. Erythema nodosum
C. Uveitis and iritis
D. Aphthous stomatitis

92. Extraintestinal manifestations of Crohn's disease may be present in:

A. 10% of patients B. 30% of patients
C. 50% of patients D. 70% of patients

93. False about laboratory findings in Crohn's disease is:

A. Fecal calprotectin levels greater than 140 ng/mL, predicted small bowel inflammation with a sensitivity of 69% and a specificity of 82%
B. Fecal calprotectin is associated with elevated CRP and ESR levels
C. ASCA is also useful in differentiating Crohn's disease from ulcerative colitis as well as playing a role in determining patients who will require surgery in the future
D. Fecal lactoferrin is only associated with elevated ESR levels

94. As per Montreal classification of Crohn's disease, a 35-year-old male presenting with a colonic penetrating lesion is:

A. A2 B3 L1 B. A3 B2 L1
C. A2 B3 L2 D. A3 B2 L2

95. As per Montreal classification of Crohn's disease, a 52-year-old female presenting with a ileocolonic stricture is:

A. A2 B3 L3 B. A3 B2 L3
C. A2 B3 L2 D. A3 B2 L2

96. As per Montreal classification of Crohn's disease, an 18-year-old female presenting with an ileal perforation is:

A. A2 B3 L1 B. A1 B2 L2
C. A2 B1 L1 D. A1 B3 L2

97. False about the radiological features of Crohn's disease is:

A. Magnetic resonance enterography (MRE) is a useful adjunct to determine intestinal strictures as well as fistulas and sinus tracks
B. On barium enema, long lengths of narrowed terminal ileum (Kantor string sign) may be present with long-standing disease
C. Both MRE and CTE are equally accurate in assessing disease activity and bowel damage; however, MRE may be superior to CTE in detecting intestinal strictures and ileal wall enhancement
D. Ultrasonography has limited value in the evaluation of patients with Crohn's disease and has an especially high accuracy for detecting the disease proximal to the terminal ileum

98. False about endoscopy in Crohn's disease is:

A. The most commonly used criterion for an abnormal finding is the presence of three or more ulcers in the absence of NSAID use
B. Ileocolonoscopy with biopsies of the terminal ileum are the gold standard for the diagnosis of Crohn's disease
C. Capsule endoscopy has been found to be inferior to any endoscopy in the identification of intestinal ulceration
D. When the colon is involved, sigmoidoscopy or colonoscopy may reveal characteristic aphthous ulcers with granularity and a normal appearing surrounding mucosa

99. As compared to ulcerative colitis, Crohn's disease has all except:

A. More rectal bleeding
B. More anal complaints
C. Ileal disease
D. Rectal sparing

100. As compared to ulcerative colitis, Crohn's disease has all except:

A. Superficial ulcers on proctoscopy
B. Anal fissure, fistula or abscess
C. Linear, cobblestone ulcers on radiologic findings
D. Palpable mass

101. Clinical remission is achieved when Crohn's disease activity index (CDAI) is below:

A. 100 B. 150
C. 200 D. 300

102. False about Crohn's disease activity index (CDAI) is:

A. Score >450 is considered severe fulminant disease with failed medical therapy and complications of obstruction, peritonitis and abscess
B. Clinical response to therapy occurs with a drop of 150 points

C. A score between 150 - 220 is considered mild to moderate disease

D. Clinical remission is achieved when CDAI is <150

103. Crohn's disease activity index (CDAI) uses all of the following variables except:

A. Age

B. Number of liquid or soft stools

C. Number of listed complications

D. Hematocrit

104. True about aminosalicylates used in Crohn's disease is:

A. Mesalamine, which is also an aminosalicylate, provides a slow release of 5-aminosalicylic acid with passage through the small bowel and colon

B. Sulfasalazine is an aminosalicylate with 5-aminosalicylic acid as the active moiety

C. Clinical trials have demonstrated efficacy of mesalamine at a dosage of 4 g/day without an increase in side effects

D. All of the above

105. False about corticosteroids used in Crohn's disease is:

A. Patients with moderate to severe disease should be treated with high-dose (40–60 mg daily) prednisone until resolution of symptoms and resumption of weight gain

B. Budesonide is recommended as the preferred primary treatment to mesalamine for patients with mild to moderately active Crohn's disease with localized ileal disease

C. Prednisone is not ideal for maintenance therapy as more than 50% of patients, particularly smokers, treated with corticosteroids become "steroid dependent"

D. Steroids are fast acting and effective at inducing remission and are ideal as maintenance therapy

106. False about immunosuppressive agents used in Crohn's disease is:

A. AZT and 6-MP are effective for maintaining steroid-induced remission, and weekly IV MTX is effective for both induction and maintenance therapy

B. Low-dose cyclosporine was found to be efficacious

C. The most common side effects are pancreatitis, hepatitis, fever and rash

D. Patients with decreased TPMT activity have a significantly increased risk of fatal bone marrow suppression

107. True about anti-TNF therapy used in Crohn's disease is:

A. FDA-approved TNF antagonists include adalimumab and certolizumab

B. Infliximab is efficacious and safe as a monotherapy in the treatment of moderate to severe Crohn's disease and effective both an induction and maintenance agent

C. The first anti-TNF agent introduced was infliximab, a chimeric monoclonal antibody to TNF-α

D. All of the above

108. After anti-TNF therapy used in Crohn's disease, there is an increased risk for all except:

A. Invasive fungal infections

B. Tuberculosis reactivation

C. Increased risk of BCC

D. Activation of latent multiple sclerosis

109. Humanized IgG1 monoclonal antibody among the following is:

A. Adalimumab B. Certolizumab

C. Infliximab D. All of the above

110. Which of the following is ideal in pregnant and nursing women?

A. Adalimumab B. Certolizumab

C. Infliximab D. All of the above

111. True about the novel therapies in Crohn's disease is:

A. Ustekinumab is a humanized monoclonal antibody that specifically binds to α4β7 integrin and blocks its interaction with MadCAM-1

B. Natalizumab, a recombinant humanized monoclonal antibody against α4 integrin, showed effectiveness in the induction and maintenance of remission in patients with active Crohn's disease

C. Vedolizumab is a humanized IgG1 monoclonal antibody that inhibits IL-12/23 through targeting of a shared p40 subunit

D. All of the above

112. True about the nutritional therapy in Crohn's disease is:

A. Total parenteral nutrition (TPN) was also useful in patients with active Crohn's disease

B. Liquid polymeric diets may be as effective as elemental feedings and are more acceptable to patient

C. The use of chemically defined elemental diets has been shown in some studies to reduce disease activity, particularly in patients with disease localized to the small bowel, and they can reduce corticosteroid-induced toxicities

D. All of the above

113. False about smoking and treatment of Crohn's disease is:

A. Smoking is associated with the late bimodal onset of disease and has been shown to increase the incidence of relapse and failure of maintenance therapy

B. It appears to be associated with the severity of disease in a nonlinear dose-response relationship

C. Tobacco exposure is an independent predictor of the need for maintenance treatment, specifically biologic therapy

D. Smoking cessation therapy is an important component of medical therapy

114. False about surgical management of Crohn's disease is:

A. The goals are to preserve bowel length while minimizing postoperative complications and disease recurrence

B. Creating a wider anastomosis with a stapled functional side to side anastomosis may decrease fecal stasis and subsequent bacterial overgrowth

C. The extraintestinal complications of Crohn's disease, although not primary indications for operation, often subside after resection of the involved bowel

D. Often after removal of a diseased segment, endoscopic recurrence can occur up to 70% to 90% within 1 year after surgery in patients with Crohn's disease

115. No. of patients that will require surgical resection within 15 years after diagnosis of Crohn's disease is:

A. 30% B. 50%

C. 70% D. 90%

116. Indications for surgery in Crohn's disease includes:

A. Steroid dependence

B. Failure of medical treatment

C. Bowel obstruction

D. All of the above

117. The extraintestinal complications of Crohn's disease often subside after resection of the involved bowel except:

A. Erythema nodosum

B. Ankylosing spondylitis

C. Aphthous stomatitis

D. Uveitis and iritis

118. 25 years old male patient, known case of Crohn's disease came to emergency with complains of pain in abdomen. An exploratory laparotomy was performed. At exploration, the appendix is found to be normal. In the absence of acute inflammatory involvement of the appendix or the cecum, next step of management should be:

A. Biopsy of small bowel and closure of abdomen

B. Saline wash and closure of abdomen

C. Perform appendectomy

D. Closure of abdomen and do a second look laparotomy

119. The most common indication for surgical therapy in patients with Crohn's disease is:

A. Acute ileitis

B. Intestinal obstruction

C. Perforation

D. Fistula

120. False about Stricturing Crohn's disease:

A. Given the concerns for development of carcinoma at chronically strictured segments, full-thickness biopsy with frozen section of the stricture site has been advocated at the time of surgery to rule out malignant disease before strictureplasty is performed

B. In case of a chronic strictured segment, medical therapy is generally effective

C. For longer diseased segments (>10 cm), the strictureplasty can be performed similar to a Finney pyloroplasty or a side-to-side isoperistaltic strictureplasty

D. The treatment of choice for intestinal obstruction in patients with Crohn's disease is segmental resection of the involved segment with primary reanastomosis

121. Following image shows:

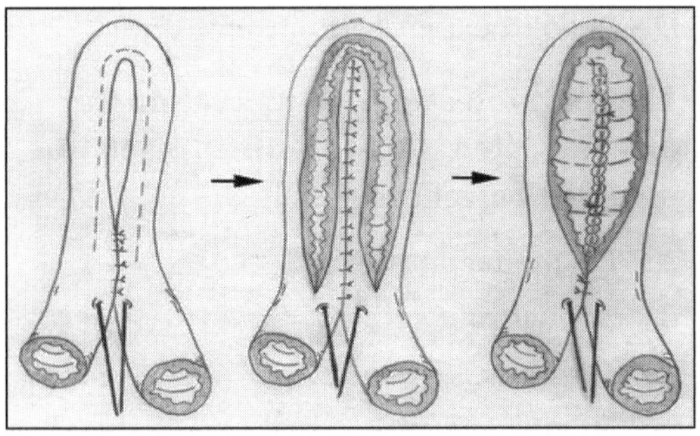

A. Finney strictureplasty
B. Heineke Mikulicz strictureplasty
C. Jaboulay strictureplasty
D. Ramstedt strictureplasty

122. Contraindications to strictureplasty includes all except:

A. Perforation of the intestine
B. Hemorrhagic strictures
C. Hypoalbuminemia (<3.0 g/dl)
D. Fistula or abscess formation at the intended strictureplasty site

123. False about penetrating Crohn's disease is:

A. Most patients with ileosigmoid fistulas require resection of the sigmoid
B. Enterocutaneous fistulas may develop but are rarely spontaneous and are more likely to follow resection or drainage of intraabdominal abscesses
C. Crohn's patients with penetrating disease tend to have longer operative times, higher reoperation rates, increased length of stay and postoperative complications
D. The presence of a radiographically demonstrable enteroenteral fistula with no signs of sepsis or other complications is not in itself an indication for surgery

124. True about treatment of perforation in Crohn's disease is:

A. Regardless of percutaneous or surgical drainage, in terms of time to resolution, early treatment of an abscess is key
B. Patients who have an abscess smaller than 3 cm and have not been on biologics or have an associated fistula can be treated with antibiotics alone
C. Penetration is manifested with a localized abscess densely adherent to the diseased segment of bowel
D. All of the above

125. True about urologic complications in Crohn's disease is:

A. Genitourinary complications occur in up to one third of patients with Crohn's disease
B. In long-standing inflammatory disease, periureteric fibrosis may be present and require ureterolysis with or without ureteral stenting
C. Surgical treatment of the primary intestinal disease is adequate in most patients
D. All of the above

126. The most common urologic complication is:

A. Renal stone
B. Ureteral obstruction
C. Acute epididymitis
D. Renal abscess

127. True about Colorectal Crohn's disease is:

A. More than half of perineal wounds are open 6 months after surgery in patients with Crohn's disease
B. Indications for surgery include a lack of response to medical management and complications of Crohn's colitis, which include obstruction, hemorrhage, perforation and toxic megacolon
C. Strictureplasty has limited usefulness in colonic Crohn's disease
D. All of the above

128. False about Perianal Crohn's disease is:

A. The treatment of perianal disease should be nonoperative unless an abscess or complex fistula develops
B. Fissures are usually lateral, painless, small and indolent and often respond to conservative management
C. Wide excision of abscesses or fistulas is not indicated, but more conservative interventions, including the liberal placement of drainage catheters and noncutting setons, are preferable
D. High transsphincteric, suprasphincteric and extrasphincteric fistulas are usually treated with noncutting setons

129. False about Duodenal Crohn's disease is:

A. Gastrojejunostomy to bypass the disease rather than duodenal resection is the procedure of choice
B. Strictureplasties have been performed with success in selected patients and may avoid the marginal ulceration and diarrhea associated with gastrojejunostomy
C. Operative intervention is common

D. Crohn's disease of the duodenum occurs in less than 5% of patients with Crohn's disease and occurs most commonly in the duodenal bulb

130. The leading cause of disease related deaths in patients with Crohn's disease is:

A. Sepsis
B. Electrolyte disorders
C. Gastrointestinal cancer
D. Thromboembolic complications

131. False about Typhoid Enteritis is:

A. Typhoid enteritis is an acute systemic infection caused primarily by Salmonella paratyphi
B. Children and young adults are most often affected
C. Peyer patches in the small bowel become hyperplastic and may subsequently ulcerate, complicated by hemorrhage or perforation
D. Hyperplasia of the reticuloendothelial system, including lymph nodes, liver and spleen, is characteristic of typhoid fever

132. During the first week of the illness, the diagnosis of typhoid fever in patients is confirmed by isolating the organism from blood in:

A. 40% B. 50%
C. 70% D. 90%

133. True about typhoid perforation is:

A. Multiple perforations, which occur in about 25% of patients, may require resection with primary anastomosis or exteriorization of the intestinal loop
B. Typically, there is a single perforation in the terminal ileum, and simple closure of the perforation is the treatment of choice
C. Intestinal perforation through an ulcerated Peyer patch occurs in approximately 2% of cases
D. All of the above

134. True about protozoal infection in immunocompromised patients is:

A. Symptoms are most commonly related to diarrhea, which may be at times intractable
B. The small bowel is the most common site of infection
C. Prophylactic cotrimoxazole and a highly active antiretroviral therapy appear to elicit a response to human immunodeficiency virus (HIV) related diarrheal illnesses
D. All of the above

135. True about bacterial infection in immunocompromised patients is:

A. Diarrhea caused by Clostridium difficile is more common in patients with AIDS because of the increased antibiotic use in this population compared with healthy hosts
B. Salmonella, Shigella and Campylobacter are associated with higher rates of bacteremia and antibiotic resistance in the immunocompromised patient
C. The incidence of Campylobacter infection among patients with AIDS who were treated with rifabutin prophylaxis was reported to be decreased compared with untreated controls
D. All of the above

136. True about Mycobacterial infection in immunocompromised patients is:

A. The usual route of infection is by swallowed organisms that directly penetrate the intestinal mucosa
B. Obstruction and fistula formation are the leading indications for surgery
C. The most frequent site of intestinal involvement of M. tuberculosis is the distal ileum and cecum, with approximately 90% of patients demonstrating disease at this site
D. All of the above

137. The most common viral cause of diarrhea in immunocompromised patients:

A. Adenovirus B. CMV
C. Rotavirus D. Astrovirus

138. A 40-year-old male with Crohn's disease underwent surgery for stricture. Patient had a low risk of clinical recurrence and was given metronidazole as a postoperative prophylaxis for 3 months. During the endoscopic surveillance, recurrence was observed. What should be the next line of management?

A. Continue metronidazole for 3 more months
B. Continue endoscopic surveillance
C. Intensify medical therapy
D. Start Anti-TNF or AZT/6MP

NEOPLASMS

139. False about small intestinal neoplasm is:

A. Most benign neoplasms are asymptomatic and often identified as an incidental finding
B. The small bowel develops relatively few primary neoplasms and less than 2% of gastrointestinal malignant neoplasms

C. The malignant neoplasms account for 25% of symptomatic lesions that lead to surgery
D. The 5-year survival for localized small bowel cancer is approximately 85%

140. Most common type of small intestinal malignancy is:

A. Carcinoid tumor B. Adenocarcinoma
C. GIST D. Lymphoma

141. Among small intestine malignant neoplasms, Neuroendocrine tumors (NETs) account for:

A. 5% - 10% B. 10% - 20%
C. 25% - 30% D. 45% - 50%

142. True about small intestinal neoplasm is:

A. Adenocarcinoma is the most common malignant neoplasm, accounting for 30% to 50% of malignant neoplasms of the small intestine
B. Adenocarcinomas are more prevalent in the proximal small bowel, whereas the other malignant lesions are more common in the distal small bowel
C. Neuroendocrine tumors (NETs) account for 25% to 30% of small intestine malignant neoplasms
D. All of the above

143. The risk factors and associated conditions related to small bowel neoplasms are all except:

A. Crohn's disease
B. Prior peptic ulcer disease
C. Heavy alcohol consumption (>20 g/day of ethanol)
D. Gluten-sensitive enteropathy

144. Small bowel carcinomas associated with celiac disease typically have:

A. 17q (p53 gene)
B. Microsatellite instability (MSI-H)
C. 5q (APC gene)
D. 18q (DCC)

145. False about clinical manifestations of small bowel neoplasia is:

A. Hemorrhage is the most common symptom
B. Most patients with benign neoplasms remain asymptomatic
C. Bleeding is usually occult; hematochezia or hematemesis may occur, although life-threatening hemorrhage is uncommon
D. Obstruction is the result of intussusception, and benign small tumors are the most common cause of this condition in adults

146. When symptoms are present the most frequent complaint of small bowel neoplasm is:

A. Hemorrhage
B. Vomiting
C. Pain
D. Electrolyte abnormalities

147. False about the diagnosis of small bowel neoplasia is:

A. A correct preoperative diagnosis is made in only 80% of symptomatic patients
B. CT of the abdomen can prove particularly useful in detecting extraluminal tumors, such as malignant gastrointestinal stromal tumors (GISTs), and can provide helpful information about the staging of malignant cancers
C. Ultrasonography has not proved effective for preoperative diagnosis of small bowel neoplasms
D. MRI enteroclysis has a sensitivity and specificity of 98% and 97%

148. False about the diagnosis of small bowel neoplasia is:

A. Despite these sophisticated imaging and diagnostic modalities, diagnosis of a small bowel tumor is often achieved only at the time of surgical exploration
B. The sensitivity and specificity for diagnosis of a small bowel tumor by capsule endoscopy in the setting of obscure bleeding are between 89% and 95% and between 75% and 95%, respectively
C. Flexible endoscopy may be useful, particularly in diagnosing duodenal lesions, and the colonoscope can be advanced into the terminal ileum for visualization and biopsy of ileal neoplasms
D. Push enteroscopy has been used routinely to evaluate lesions in the small bowel

149. The most common benign small bowel lesions that produce symptom is:

A. Adenomas B. Lipomas
C. Stromal tumors D. Carcinoids

150. The most common benign tumors reported in autopsy series is:

A. Adenomas B. Lipomas
C. Stromal tumors D. Carcinoids

151. Most common site of GIST is:

A. Jejunum and ileum
B. Stomach
C. Duodenum
D. Esophagus

152. False about GIST in small bowel is:

A. Median age of diagnosis is 65 years of age
B. Symptoms of GIST include abdominal pain, fullness, bowel obstruction, or tumor hemorrhage resulting in anemia, melena, or hematemesis
C. Incidence rates in M:F is 3:1
D. Stromal tumors arise from the interstitial cell of Cajal

153. GISTs can be malignant tumors in nearly _______ of patients.

A. 5%
B. 10%
C. 20%
D. 40%

154. False about the diagnosis of GIST is:

A. These tumors infrequently stain positive for actin (20%–30%), S100 (2%–4%) and desmin (2%–4%)
B. 50% to 60% express CD34
C. Surgical resection is necessary for appropriate treatment
D. Endoscopic core biopsy with immuno-histochemical staining for KIT (95%) and anoctamin-1 (98%) confirms the diagnosis

155. CD117 is expressed in of _____ patients of GIST.

A. 60%
B. 75%
C. 80%
D. 95%

156. False about the treatment of GIST is:

A. Tumors smaller than 5 cm, regardless of mitotic index, have higher rates of metastasis and recurrence
B. Surgical resection is necessary for appropriate treatment
C. The mitotic index is classified as low (5 mitoses/50 hpf) or high (>5 mitoses/50 hpf
D. GIST malignancy risk and prognosis is stratified based on the number of mitoses per high-power field and tumor size

157. Most common site of adenoma is:

A. Jejunum
B. Ileum
C. Duodenum
D. Ileocolic junction

158. True about adenoma is:

A. The most common presenting symptoms are bleeding and obstruction
B. Villous adenomas have a particular propensity for malignant degeneration and may be relatively large (>5 cm) in diameter
C. Endoscopic mucosal resection is gaining acceptance as a useful technique for the treatment of duodenal adenomas and Brunner gland tumors
D. All of the above

159. Villous adenomas of the small bowel are most commonly found in:

A. Jejunum
B. Ileum
C. Duodenum
D. Ileocolic junction

160. False about Familial adenomas is:

A. FAP patients carry a 5% lifetime risk for development of duodenal adenocarcinoma
B. Screening endoscopy with a forward- and side-viewing endoscope is performed at regular intervals with biopsy of all suspicious, villous, or large (>3 cm) adenomas in addition to random duodenal biopsy specimen
C. Familial adenomas typically occur in the presence of FAP syndrome
D. Adenomas in the ileum can be found in 50% to 90% of cases

161. As per Spigelman's classification, a patient with 9 points is:

A. Stage I
B. Stage II
C. Stage III
D. Stage IV

162. A 50-year-old patient with pain in abdomen was found to have, 6 villous polyps around 8 mm in size showing moderate degree dysplasia in ileum. As per Spigelman's classification, a patient's stage and management is:

A. Stage III and surveillance every 1 year
B. Stage II and surveillance every 2 years
C. Stage IV and consider surgery
D. Stage III and surveillance every 2 years

163. A 68-year-old patient with pain in abdomen was found to have, 3 tubulovillous polyps around 12 mm in size showing mild degree dysplasia in ileum. As per Spigelman's classification, a patient's stage and management is:

A. Stage II and surveillance every 2 years
B. Stage II and surveillance every 1 year
C. Stage III and surveillance every 1 year
D. Stage III and surveillance every 2 years

164. A 59-year-old patient with pain in abdomen was found to have, 14 tubular polyps around 9 mm in size showing mild degree dysplasia in ileum. As per Spigelman's classification, a patient's stage and management is:

A. Stage I and surveillance every 5 years
B. Stage II and surveillance every 2 years
C. Stage I and surveillance every 2 years
D. Stage II and surveillance every 4 years

165. False about Brunner gland adenomas is:

A. Brunner gland adenomas represent benign hyperplastic lesions arising from the Brunner glands of the proximal duodenum
B. Diagnosis can usually be accomplished by endoscopy and biopsy
C. There is malignant potential for Brunner gland adenomas and a radical resection should be considered
D. Adenomas may produce symptoms mimicking those of peptic ulcer disease

166. The most common site of lipoma is:

A. Jejunum B. Ileum
C. Duodenum D. Ileocolic junction

167. False about lipoma is:

A. Lipomas do not have malignant potential
B. Most common in the ileum and are manifested as single intramural lesions located in the submucosa
C. The treatment of choice for symptomatic lesions is excision
D. They usually occur in the sixth and seventh decades of life and are more frequent in women

168. False about Peutz-Jeghers syndrome is:

A. Hamartomas are most commonly found in the jejunum and ileum
B. Because of the widespread nature of intestinal involvement extensive resection is indicated
C. The most common symptom is recurrent colicky abdominal pain, usually the result of intermittent intussusception
D. The pattern of inheritance is autosomal dominant with a high degree of penetrance

169. The classic pigmented lesions in Peutz-Jeghers syndrome are small, 1 to 2 mm, as brown or black spots located in all except:

A. Buccal mucosa
B. Legs
C. Circumoral region of the face
D. Perianal area

170. False about Hemangiomas is:

A. Patients with Turner syndrome are likely also to have cavernous hemangiomas of the intestine
B. Hemangiomas of the small bowel may occur as part of an inherited disorder known as Osler-Weber-Rendu disease
C. If a hemangioma is localized preoperatively, resection of the involved intestinal segment is warranted
D. Hemangiomas account for 3% to 4% of all benign tumors of the small bowel and are multifocal in 10% of patients

171. False about malignant neoplasms in small intestine is:

A. Diarrhea with tenesmus and passage of large amounts of mucus may occur
B. Gastrointestinal bleeding, manifested by anemia and guaiac-positive stools or occasionally by melena or hematochezia is more common with adenocarcinoma
C. Malignant neoplasms almost always produce symptoms, the most common of which are pain and weight loss
D. A palpable mass may be felt in 10% to 20% of patients, and perforations develop in approximately 10%, usually secondary to lymphomas and sarcoma

172. True about Neuroendocrine Neoplasms is:

A. Intestinal NENs arise from enterochromaffin cells (Kulchitsky cells)
B. The classification of NENs is based predominately on tumor grade and differentiation
C. Most patients with small bowel NENs are in their 7th decade of life
D. All of the above

173. True about gastrointestinal NETs is:

A. Foregut NETs are characterized by having high serotonin production
B. Hindgut NETs rarely produce serotonin but may produce other hormones, such as somatostatin and peptide YY
C. Midgut NETs characteristically produce low levels of serotonin (5-hydroxytryptamine) but may secrete 5-hydroxytryptophan or adrenocorticotropic hormone
D. All of the above

174. The most common site for NETs is:

A. Respiratory tract
B. Appendix
C. Gastrointestinal tract
D. Thymus

175. The most common site for NETs is:

A. Appendix B. Ileum
C. Jejunum D. Duodenum

176. True about NETs is:

A. Primary tumors that secrete directly into the venous system, bypassing the portal system (e.g., ovary, lung), give rise to carcinoid syndrome without metastasis
B. Carcinoid syndrome, secondary to serotonin or tachykinin production, is characterized by episodic attacks of cutaneous flushing, bronchospasm, diarrhea, and vasomotor collapse and is mostly in those patients with hepatic metastases
C. NETs almost always occur within the last 2 feet of the ileum
D. All of the above

177. False about pathology of NETs is:

A. The malignant potential (ability to metastasize) is related to location, size, depth of invasion and growth pattern
B. They are associated with a larger mesenteric mass caused by nodal disease and desmoplastic invasion of the mesentery, which is often mistaken for the primary tumor
C. Small bowel NETs are multicentric in 50% to 60% of patients
D. In gross appearance, these tumors are small, firm, submucosal nodules that are usually yellow on the cut surface

178. NETs larger than 2 cm in diameter and are associated with metastasis in:

A. 20% of cases B. 40% of cases
C. 60% of cases D. 80% of cases

179. In NETs, a synchronous adenocarcinoma can occur in:

A. 5% to 10% B. 10% to 20%
C. 25% to 30% D. 40% to 50%

180. In NETs, the most common site of a synchronous adenocarcinoma is:

A. Ileum B. Large intestine
C. Duodenum D. Anus

181. Which of the following tachykinins are not secreted in neuroendocrine tumors?

A. Kallikrein B. Substance P
C. Neurotensin D. Neuropeptide K

182. Most common peptide secreted in neuroendocrine tumors is:

A. Pancreatic polypeptide
B. HCG-β
C. Neurotensin
D. Chromogranin

183. Most common amine secreted in neuroendocrine tumors is:

A. 5-HT B. 5-HIAA
C. 5-HTP D. Histamine

184. The most common symptom in NETs is:

A. Diarrhea
B. Abdominal pain
C. Cuatneous flushes
D. Weight loss

185. False about NETs of the small bowel is:

A. Diarrhea and weight loss may occur
B. Ischemia of the affected segment of intestine contribute to most symptoms and complications related to the tumor
C. Obstructive symptoms can be caused by intussusception but usually occur secondary to a local desmoplastic reaction
D. The diarrhea is a result of secretory diarrhea as noted in patients with the malignant carcinoid syndrome

186. The most common symptom in malignant carcinoid syndrome is:

A. Cutaneous flushing B. Diarrhea
C. Hepatomegaly D. Cardiac lesions

187. False about malignant carcinoid syndrome is:

A. The classic description of the carcinoid syndrome includes vasomotor, cardiac and gastrointestinal manifestations
B. Due to first-pass metabolism of the vasoactive peptides responsible for carcinoid syndrome, hepatic metastasis or extraabdominal disease is necessary to elicit the syndrome
C. Diarrhea is the most common symptom in malignant carcinoid syndrome
D. Tumors that bypass the liver, specifically ovarian and retroperitoneal NETs, may

produce the syndrome in the absence of liver metastasis

188. In patients with NETs, malignant carcinoid syndrome occurs in:

A. <5%
B. <10%
C. <20%
D. <25%

189. The most common cardiac lesions in malignant carcinoid syndrome is:

A. Tricuspid insufficiency
B. Pulmonary stenosis
C. Tricuspid stenosis
D. Aortic insufficiency

190. Cutaneous flushing seen in the gastric NETs is:

A. Violaceous
B. Bright-red patchy flushing
C. Prolonged flushes
D. Diffuse erythematous

191. Which type of cutaneous flushing may show permanent cyanotic flush?

A. Violaceous
B. Bright-red patchy flushing
C. Prolonged flushes
D. Diffuse erythematous

192. The diarrhea associated with carcinoid syndrome is controlled by:

A. Ondansetron
B. Methysergide
C. Erythromycin
D. Opioids

193. Cause of diarrhea in carcinoid syndrome is:

A. Dopamine
B. Histamine
C. Serotonin
D. Motilin

194. False about diagnosis of NETs is:

A. Elevated urinary levels of 5-HIAA measured during 24 hours with high-performance liquid chromatography are highly specific and sensitive
B. Chromogranin A (CgA) alone may be used for the diagnosis of NETs, given its specificity of 95%
C. In terms of surveillance after resection or as a prognostic marker to monitor response to therapy, CgA levels have proven efficacy over urine 5-HIAA levels
D. Provocative tests using pentagastrin, calcium, or epinephrine may be used to reproduce the symptoms of NETs

195. False about diagnostic imaging of NETs is:

A. Liver metastases are well demonstrated with MRI and usually have high signal intensity on T1-weighted images and low signal intensity on T2-weighted images
B. CT scan findings depend on the size, the degree of mesenteric invasion and desmoplastic reaction, and the presence of regional lymph node invasion
C. MRI is not used in the diagnosis of gastrointestinal NETs but can be helpful in diagnosing metastatic disease, especially in the liver
D. CT angiography may be useful in cases associated with a large mesenteric process to identify encasement and pseudoaneurysm formation, typical of a malignant process in the mesentery

196. False about diagnostic imaging of NETs is:

A. ^{68}Ga-DOTATATE imaging include better true positive lesion detection, longer shelf life and scanning window when compared with ^{64}Cu-DOTATATE
B. ^{68}Ga-DOTATATE PET/CT is a clinically useful imaging technique to localize primary tumors in patients with neuroendocrine metastases of unknown origin
C. Scintigraphic localization has a higher sensitivity than CT for delineating and localizing NETs
D. ^{64}Cu-DOTATATE, was FDA approved for diagnostic use in NETs

197. False about surgical therapy of NETs is:

A. For patients with lesions > 1 cm, with multiple tumors, or with regional lymph node metastasis, regardless of the size of the primary tumor, wide excision of bowel and mesentery is required
B. Extensive duodenal tumors require pancreaticoduodenectomy
C. For primary tumors <1 cm in diameter with evidence of regional lymph node metastasis, a segmental intestinal resection is adequate
D. Lesions of the terminal ileum are best treated by right hemicolectomy

198. Carcinoid crisis during anaesthesia is treated with:

A. IV octreotide given as a bolus of 10 to 20 µg, which may be continued as an infusion at 10 µg/hr

B. IV octreotide given as a bolus of 50 to 100 µg, which may be continued as an infusion at 50 µg/hr
C. IV octreotide given as a bolus of 100 to 200 µg, which may be continued as an infusion at 100 µg/hr
D. IV octreotide given as a bolus of 200 to 300 µg, which may be continued as an infusion at 200 µg/hr

199. Medical therapies for neuroendocrine tumor treatment include:

A. Lanreotide B. Streptozotocin
C. Sunitinib D. All of the above

200. False about the medical therapy for neuroendocrine tumor is:

A. Lanreotide relieves symptoms of the carcinoid syndrome in most patients and but doesn't delay cancer progression
B. Octreotide LAR is recommended for Grade 1 and 2 NETs and not recommended in grade 3 disease
C. Somatostatin analogs (SSAs) are the standard of care for controlling symptoms of patients with functional gastrointestinal NETs, and they control symptoms in more than 70% of patients with carcinoid syndrome
D. Serotonin synthesis inhibitor telotristat etiprate is a approved therapy

201. Which trial found that Lanreotide, an SSA, was associated with prolonged progression-free survival among patients with metastatic grade 1 or 2 enteropancreatic NETs?

A. PROMID trial B. CLARINET trial
C. RADIANT-4 trial D. NETTER-1 trial

202. Which trial demonstrated that treatment with radionuclide ^{177}LuDOTATATE had an improvement in progression-free survival when compared to high-dose octreotide?

A. PROMID trial B. CLARINET trial
C. RADIANT-4 trial D. NETTER-1 trial

203. False about the medical therapy for neuroendocrine tumor is:

A. Methysergide is no longer used because of the increased incidence of retroperitoneal fibrosis
B. In the TELESTAR trial, telotristat treatment reduced daily bowel movements by 35%
C. Currently, the role of chemotherapy is confined predominantly to patients with G1 metastatic disease who are symptomatic, are unresponsive to other therapies, or have high tumor proliferation rates
D. Temozolomide as monotherapy has acceptable toxicity and provides antitumoral effects in a small series of patients with advanced NETs

204. JS001 is:

A. Somatostatin drug conjugate
B. Checkpoint inhibitor
C. Peptide receptor radiotherapy
D. Dopamine agonists

205. PEN-221 is:

A. Somatostatin drug conjugate
B. Checkpoint inhibitor
C. Peptide receptor radiotherapy
D. Dopamine agonists

206. Medical therapy for neuroendocrine tumor treatment approved as an indication for Cushing's disease is:

A. Sunitinib B. 5-Fluorouracil
C. Capecitabine D. Pasireotide

207. Telotristat etiprate is:

A. Tyrosine kinase inhibitor
B. mTOR inhibitor
C. Cytotoxic therapy
D. Serotonin synthesis inhibitors

208. False about the prognosis of NETs is:

A. Resection of a NET localized to its primary site approaches a 100% survival rate
B. Metastatic disease at the time of diagnosis is approximately 10% to 20% and tumors recur in 70% to 90% of patients
C. 5-year survival rates are approximately 65% in patients with regional disease and 25% to 35% in those with distant metastasis
D. An elevated level of CgA, which is an independent predictor of an adverse prognosis, is probably the most useful factor identified

209. False about adenocarcinoma of small bowel is:

A. Most of these tumors are located in the duodenum and proximal jejunum
B. Adenocarcinomas constitute approximately 40% of the malignant tumors of the small bowel
C. The median age at diagnosis is in the sixth decade of life
D. Those arising in association with Crohn's disease tend to occur at a somewhat younger age and more than 70% arise in the duodenum

210. False about adenocarcinoma of small bowel is:

A. Perforation is uncommon

B. Tumors of the duodenum tend to manifest somewhat earlier than those in the jejunum and ileum because of the earlier presentation of symptoms

C. Intestinal obstruction and chronic bleeding may also occur

D. Adenocarcinomas of the jejunum and ileum usually produce more nonspecific symptoms that include vague abdominal pain and weight loss

211. True about the management of adenocarcinoma of small bowel is:

A. Lymph node invasion is the main prognostic factor for local small bowel adenocarcinoma

B. An R0 resection of the primary tumor with locoregional lymph node resection is the only curative treatment

C. In patients with metastatic disease, studies have determined that using FOLFOX and FOLFIRI as first-line therapy significantly improves the performance status and progression-free survival

D. All of the above

212. True about small intestinal lymphomas is:

A. An increased risk for development of primary small bowel lymphomas was reported in patients with celiac disease and immuno-deficient states

B. Approximately one-third of gastrointestinal lymphomas occur in the small bowel and these account for 5% of all lymphomas

C. Symptoms of small bowel lymphoma include pain, weight loss, nausea, vomiting and change in bowel habits

D. All of the above

213. The most common intestinal neoplasm in children younger than 10 years is:

A. Adenocarcinoma B. NETs

C. Lymphoma D. GIST

214. Small intestinal lymphomas are most commonly found in the:

A. 1st part of duodenum

B. Ileum

C. 2nd part of duodenum

D. Jejunum

215. In small intestinal lymphomas, perforation may occur in up to _______ of patients.

A. 25% B. 45%

C. 55% D. 75%

216. False about treatment of small intestinal lymphomas is:

A. T-cell lymphomas are more chemosensitive than B-cell lymphomas and have high remission rates with or without surgery

B. T-cell lymphomas are traditionally more resistant to therapy and will progress to symptoms of obstruction or perforation if not resected

C. In the absence of symptoms, small bowel lymphomas are often chemoresponsive and do not require surgery

D. Five-year survival of 50% to 60% can be expected and is dictated by response to systemic therapy rather than by the success of surgical resection

217. False about small bowel GIST is:

A. These tumors are more common in the jejunum and ileum, typically are diagnosed in the 5th and 6th decades of life

B. A laparoscopic approach in patients with large tumors is strongly encouraged

C. Malignant GISTs arise from mesenchymal tissue and constitute about 20% of malignant neoplasms of the small bowel

D. Surgical management includes complete resection for localized GISTs, with extreme care to avoid rupture of the tumor capsule

218. Malignant small bowel GISTs are larger than 5 cm at the time of diagnosis in ______ of patients.

A. 20% B. 40%

C. 60% D. 80%

219. GISTs mostly arise from the:

A. Muscularis mucosae

B. Submucosa

C. Muscularis propria

D. Serosa

220. Most common indication for surgery in small bowel GISTs is:

A. Bleeding B. Obstruction

C. Perforation D. Both A and B

221. The most useful indicator of survival and the risk for metastasis in small bowel GISTs includes:

A. Mitotic index
B. Evidence of tumor invasion into the lamina propria
C. Size of the tumor at presentation
D. All of the above

222. Rupture of the GIST tumor capsule results in relapse in _______ of patients.

A. 50% B. 70%
C. 85% D. 100%

223. False about the treatment of small bowel GISTs is:

A. Neoadjuvant imatinib should be considered for patients requiring extensive surgery to allow for tumor shrinkage prior to resection
B. Small GISTs (< 2 cm) found incidentally in surgical specimens do not require further treatment
C. Relapse-risk assessment for a primary GIST is critical as it provides prognostic information as well as estimates the potential benefits of medical therapy
D. Current guidelines suggest that patients with high-risk disease should receive 1 year of adjuvant treatment with imatinib

224. False about the treatment of small bowel GISTs is:

A. Imatinib is a first-line treatment for unresectable and metastatic GISTs with characteristic tumor biology
B. Adjuvant imatinib therapy is recommended in patients with D842V PDGFRα mutations
C. Exon 9 mutations exhibited a dose-dependent decrease in risk of progression and in this select group of patients, imatinib 400 mg twice per day should be given
D. Standard-dose therapy (400 mg daily) is recommended as no survival advantage is offered by increasing the dose unless the patient has an exon 9 mutation

225. A 30-year-old male with localised small intestinal GIST underwent R0 resection. Patient had a c-KIT mutation. Patient had a low risk of recurrence. What should be the next line of management?

A. Start imatinib for 12 months
B. Start regorafinib
C. Continue disease surveillance
D. Start imatinib for 36 months

226. A 40-year-old female with metastatic small intestinal GIST. Patient had a c-KIT mutation with exon 11 deletion. What should be the next line of management?

A. Imatinib 800 mg B. Imatinib 400 mg
C. Sunitinib D. Regorafenib

227. The most common extraabdominal source to involve the small intestine via metastasis is:

A. Adenocarcinoma of the breast
B. CA ovary
C. Cutaneous melanoma
D. CA lung

DIVERTICULAR DISEASE

228. The most common acquired diverticula of the small bowel is:

A. Ileal diverticula
B. Duodenal diverticula
C. Jejunal diverticula
D. Meckel diverticulum

229. The most common true congenital diverticulum of the small bowel is:

A. Ileal diverticula
B. Duodenal diverticula
C. Jejunal diverticula
D. Meckel diverticulum

230. False about duodenal diverticula is:

A. Duodenal diverticula occur twice as often in women as in men and are rare in patients younger than 40 years
B. Most common site for diverticulum formation
C. Extraluminal duodenal diverticula are considerably more common than intraluminal diverticula
D. Upper gastrointestinal radiographic studies identify duodenal diverticula in 1% to 5% of all studies

231. Extraluminal duodenal diverticula usually occur within the:

A. 1st portion of the duodenum
B. 2nd portion of the duodenum
C. 3rd portion of the duodenum
D. 4th portion of the duodenum

232. Extraluminal duodenal diverticula usually occur within the 2nd portion of duodenum along the:

A. Anterior wall
B. Lateral wall
C. Medial wall
D. Posterior wall

233. False about diagnosis of duodenal diverticula is:

A. CT can identify large diverticula by the presence of a mass-like structure interposed between the duodenum and pancreatic head containing air, air-fluid levels, fluid contrast material, or debris
B. Upper gastrointestinal endoscopy identifies approximately 25% of duodenal diverticula
C. Hemorrhage in diverticula is best diagnosed by a combination of angiography and 99mTc-labeled red blood cell scan
D. Majority of duodenal diverticula are asymptomatic

234. True about clinical manifestations of duodenal diverticula is/are:

A. <5% of duodenal diverticula will require surgery
B. Stasis of intestinal contents within a distended diverticulum can result in bacterial overgrowth, malabsorption, steatorrhea, and megaloblastic anemia, essentially producing a blind loop syndrome
C. Iatrogenic injuries, most commonly acquired during endoscopic instrumentation of an asymptomatic diverticulum, can result in perforation or hemorrhage
D. All of the above

235. True about treatment of extraluminal duodenal diverticula is:

A. An endoscopic stapler is most commonly used to traverse and to resect the diverticulum at its base, and an omental patch reinforcement can be placed over the staple line
B. The most common and effective treatment is diverticulectomy
C. Extraluminal duodenal diverticula should be resected in the setting of symptomatic disease or need for urgent surgery, such as free perforation or hemorrhage
D. All of the above

236. False about the treatment of a perforated duodenal diverticulum is:

A. If the diverticulum is posterior and perforates into the substance of the pancreas, wide drainage with duodenal diversion may be all that is feasible
B. The perforated diverticulum should be excised and the duodenum closed with a serosal patch from a jejunal loop
C. Surgical jejunostomy should also be considered for a few patients with acute perforation to ensure nutrition repletion
D. If the surrounding inflammation is severe, it may be necessary to divert the enteric flow away from the site of the perforation with a gastrojejunostomy or duodenojejunostomy

237. False about Jejunal and Ileal Diverticula is/are:

A. Jejunal diverticula are more common and are smaller than those in the ileum
B. Diverticula of the small bowel are much less common than duodenal diverticula
C. The cause of jejunoileal diverticulosis is thought to be a motor dysfunction of the smooth muscle or the myenteric plexus
D. All of the above are true

238. True about treatment of Jejunal and Ileal Diverticula is/are:

A. Patients presenting with malabsorption secondary to the blind loop syndrome and bacterial overgrowth in the diverticulum can usually be given antibiotics
B. Treatment of complications of obstruction, bleeding and perforation is usually by intestinal resection and end-to-end anastomosis
C. When the enterolith causes obstruction at the level of the diverticulum, bowel resection is necessary
D. All of the above

239. False about Meckel diverticulum is:

A. Pancreatic mucosa is encountered in about 5% of diverticula
B. Meckel diverticulum is located on the antimesenteric border of the ileum 45 to 60 cm proximal to the ileocecal valve
C. The usual manifestation is a relatively wide-mouthed diverticulum measuring about 5 cm in length, with a diameter of up to 2 cm
D. Incidence is more common in men as compared to women

240. Most common heterotopic tissue within the Meckel diverticulum is:

A. Colonic mucosa
B. Pancreatic tissue
C. Gastric mucosa
D. Neuroendocrine cells

241. False about clinical manifestation of Meckel diverticulum is:

A. Diverticulitis accounts for 10% to 20% of symptomatic presentations
B. Hemorrhage is the most common symptomatic presentation in children 2 years of age or younger
C. In intussusception, a broad-based diverticulum invaginates and then is carried forward by peristalsis
D. The usual source of the bleeding is a acute acid-induced ulcer in the diverticulum

242. The most common clinical presentation of Meckel diverticulum is:

A. Diverticulitis
B. Obstruction
C. Gastrointestinal bleeding
D. Volvulus

243. Most common malignant neoplasm in Meckel's diverticulum is:

A. Lymphoma B. NET
C. GIST D. Adenocarcinoma

244. In children, the single most accurate diagnostic test for Meckel diverticula is with:

A. Sodium ^{99m}Tc-pertechnetate scintigraphy
B. CT scan
C. USG
D. MRI

245. Drug used to increase the sensitivity of scintigraphy is:

A. Secretin
B. Somatostatin
C. Calcium channel blockers
D. Cimetidine

246. True about the treatment of Meckel diverticula is:

A. The treatment of a symptomatic Meckel diverticulum requires prompt surgical intervention with diverticulectomy or segmental resection of ileum containing the diverticulum
B. Segmental small bowel resection is required for treatment of patients with hemorrhage as the bleeding site is usually adjacent to the diverticulum
C. It is recommended that asymptomatic diverticula found in children during laparotomy should be resected
D. All of the above

247. The factors associated with a higher risk of complications in Meckel's diverticulum and warranting consideration of resection is all except:

A. Age < 50 years
B. Male sex
C. Diverticulum length >2 cm
D. Age > 50 years

MISCELLANEOUS PROBLEMS

248. NSAID-induced ulcers occur more commonly in the:

A. Duodenum B. Jejunum
C. Ileum D. Colon

249. True about Ingested foreign bodies is:

A. For most patients, treatment is observation, to permit safe passage of these objects through the intestinal tract
B. If abdominal pain, tenderness, fever, or leukocytosis occurs, immediate laparotomy and surgical removal of the offending object(s) is indicated
C. If the object is radiopaque, progress can be followed by serial abdominal films
D. All of the above

250. Most common cause of enterocutaneous fistulas is:

A. Malignant disease B. Iatrogenic
C. Diverticulitis D. Crohn's disease

251. High-output fistulas are those that discharge ____ per 24 hours.

A. 200 mL or more B. 300 mL or more
C. 500 mL or more D. 1000 mL or more

252. Favorable factors predictive of non-operative fistula closure are all except:

A. Transferrin >200 mg/dL
B. Length >2 cm, end fistula
C. Output >500 mL/24 hours
D. Appendicitis or diverticulitis

253. Non-favorable factors predictive of non-operative fistula closure are all except:

A. Inflammatory bowel disease
B. Surgical etiology
C. Sepsis, electrolyte disturbances
D. Distal small bowel obstruction

254. True about the stabilization phase of treatment of enterocutaneous fistulas is:

A. TPN is particularly valuable in the stabilization period to help minimize high-output fistula losses and for immediate nutritional repletion while the fistula is being delineated

B. All infections should be adequately drained percutaneously or operatively, if necessary, along with appropriate antibiotic administration

C. Protection of the skin around the fistulous opening is important to prevent excoriation with stomahesive product with applications of zinc oxide, aluminium paste, or karaya powder

D. All of the above

255. The most common cause of death in enterocutaneous fistula patient is:

A. Electrolyte abnormalities

B. Renal failure

C. Sepsis

D. Respiratory infection

256. Fistula output is best controlled by:

A. Prescribed anti diarrhoea medication

B. Restricting the total amount of oral hypotonic solutions

C. Intubation of the fistula tract with a drain

D. Addition of high fibrous food

257. No. of small intestinal fistulas that closed within 1 month is:

A. 50% B. 60%

C. 75% D. 90%

258. If closure has not been obtained after 6-week period of convalescence, surgical management should be considered if the preoperative albumin level is:

A. > 20 g/L B. > 25 g/L

C. > 30 g/L D. > 35 g/L

259. False about the staging and supportive care phase of treatment of enterocutaneous fistulas is:

A. Dysmotility agents such as loperamide and codeine can't assist with attempts at enteral therapy

B. Bowel rest with TPN therapy improves fistula closure rates and time to closure in patients with high-output fistulas

C. Vacuum devices are valuable in the setting of enteroatmospheric fistulas to help contract the open abdominal wound around the associated fistula

D. A period of 3 to 6 months is beneficial to allow the profound inflammatory response associated with intraabdominal sepsis to subside completely and for the adhesion formation to stabilize

260. All of the following is done in wound care of enterocutaneous fistulas except:

A. Drainage of excessive ECF fluid with sump suction

B. Collect ECF fluids with bag (wound manager, fistula bag)

C. Allow 500 mL/day clear liquids orally

D. Gauzes for low-output ECF paste to protect the skin

261. All of the following is done in surgical strategy of enterocutaneous fistulas except:

A. Wedge excision of intestinal resection

B. Increase the number of anastomoses

C. Careful adhesiolysis

D. Cover sutures with healthy, viable tissue

262. All of the following is done in Optimization of Nutritional Status of enterocutaneous fistulas except:

A. Rehydration and electrolyte supplementation

B. Parenteral nutrition to meet calorie requirements, small bowel ECF

C. Allow 1000 mL/day clear liquids orally

D. Enteral nutrition is preferred

263. False about Pneumatosis intestinalis is:

A. Pneumatosis in neonates is usually associated with necrotizing enterocolitis

B. They can occur anywhere along the gastrointestinal tract, from the esophagus to the rectum

C. The cysts may be located in the subserosa, submucosa, and, rarely, muscularis layer and vary in size from microscopic to several centimeters in diameter

D. There is an increased incidence in men, and the condition usually occurs in the fourth to seventh decades of life

264. Pneumatosis intestinalis are most common in:

A. Duodenum B. Jejunum

C. Ileum D. Colon

265. The majority of pneumatosis intestinalis (85%) are associated with:

A. Diabetes
B. Small bowel ischemia
C. COPD
D. Inflammatory bowel disease

266. False about Pneumatosis intestinalis is:

A. On histologic section, the involved portion has a honeycomb appearance
B. Treatment is always necessary
C. Upon gross inspection, the cysts resemble cystic lymphangiomas or hydatid cysts
D. Pneumatosis intestinalis is a radiographic finding and not a diagnosis

267. Complications associated with pneumatosis intestinalis includes:

A. Hemorrhage
B. Intestinal obstruction
C. Intestinal perforation
D. All of the above

268. False about blind loop syndrome is:

A. The bacteria compete for dietary vitamin B_{12}, producing a systemic deficiency of vitamin B_{12} and megaloblastic anemia
B. Bacterial overgrowth can be diagnosed with cultures obtained through an intestinal tube or by indirect tests such as the ^{14}C-xylose or ^{14}C-cholylglycine breath tests
C. Excessive bacterial use of ^{14}C substrate leads to an decrease in ^{14}C-labeled CO_2
D. Tetracyclines have been the mainstay of treatment, but studies have shown that rifaximin and metronidazole demonstrate less resistance and are also effective

269. True about acute radiation-induced small bowel disease is:

A. Acute radiation-induced small bowel disease usually is manifested with colicky abdominal pain, bloating, loss of appetite, nausea, diarrhea, and fecal urgency during or shortly after a course of radiotherapy
B. Most patients notice symptoms during the third week of treatment and these resolve 2 to 6 weeks after completion of radiation
C. The amount of radiation appears to correlate with the probability for the development of radiation enteritis
D. All of the above

270. Serious late complications are unusual if the total radiation dosage is:

A. < 2000 cGy B. < 3000 cGy
C. < 4000 cGy D. < 5000 cGy

271. Radiation induced morbidity risk increases with dosages exceeding:

A. 4000 cGy B. 5000 cGy
C. 6000 cGy D. 7000 cGy

272. After a completed course of radiotherapy, chronic radiation injury typically develops between:

A. 6 months and 1 year
B. 12 months and 2 years
C. 15 months and 4 years
D. 18 months and 6 years

273. The late effects of radiation injury are the result of:

A. Progressive obliterative arteritis and submucosal fibrosis
B. Damage to small submucosal blood vessels
C. Thrombosis and vascular insufficiency
D. All of the above

274. For prevention of radiation-induced small bowel disease all of the following are done except:

A. Use of modern imaging and radiotherapy techniques to minimize radiation exposure to normal tissues
B. Consideration of circadian rhythm effects and use of evening radiotherapy sessions
C. Continuation of angiotensin-converting enzyme inhibitors and statins and consideration of their introduction if appropriate
D. Consideration of the use of antibiotics

275. Pharmacological interventions used to reduce side effects of radiation enteritis is:

A. Sucralfate
B. Histamine agonists
C. ACE inhibitors
D. Superoxide dismutase

276. The most effective radioprotectant agent appears to be:

A. Amifostine B. Glutamine
C. Vitamin E D. Beta-carotene

277. False about treatment of acute radiation enteritis is:

A. The use of corticosteroids for acute radiation enteritis has proven value
B. Antispasmodics and analgesics may alleviate abdominal pain and cramping, and diarrhea

usually responds to opiates or other antidiarrheal agent
C. Bile acid malabsorption responds well to cholestyramine
D. Antibiotics are frequently used in the setting of bacterial overgrowth

278. False about operative intervention in radiation enteritis is:

A. Indications for operation include obstruction, fistula formation, perforation, and bleeding
B. Frozen section and laser doppler flowmetry techniques have been used to assist resection and anastomosis
C. Obstruction caused by rigid, fixed intestinal loops in the pelvis is best bypassed
D. In patients presenting with obstruction, extensive lysis of adhesions should be done

279. Most common presentation of radiation enteritis requiring operative intervention is:

A. Fistula formation B. Obstruction
C. Perforation D. Bleeding

280. False about short bowel resection is:

A. In cases of short bowel syndrome, 75% occur from massive intestinal resection
B. In the adult, mesenteric occlusion, midgut volvulus, and traumatic disruption of the superior mesenteric vessels are the most frequent causes
C. Multiple sequential resections, usually associated with recurrent Crohn's disease, account for 50% of patients
D. All of the above are true

281. In neonates, the most common cause of short bowel syndrome is bowel resection secondary to:

A. Portal vein thrombosis
B. Necrotizing enterocolitis
C. Mesenteric occlusion
D. Midgut volvulus

282. False about short bowel resection is:

A. Complications include an increased incidence of gallstones caused by disruption of the enterohepatic circulation and of nephrolithiasis from hyperoxaluria
B. The clinical hallmarks of short bowel syndrome include diarrhea, fluid and electrolyte deficiency, and malnutrition
C. Resection of up to 90% of the small bowel usually can be tolerated if the terminal ileum and ileocecal valve are preserved
D. In patients with short bowel syndrome, postabsorptive levels of plasma citrulline, a nonprotein amino acid produced by intestinal mucosa, may provide an indicator to differentiate transient from permanent intestinal failure

283. False about the treatment of short bowel resection is:

A. In its early phase, treatment is primarily directed at the control of diarrhea, replacement of fluid and electrolytes, and prompt institution of TPN in patients who cannot safely tolerate enteral feedings
B. The long-acting SSA octreotide also appears to reduce the amount of diarrhea during the early phase of short bowel syndrome
C. Volume losses may exceed 1 L/day, and vigorous monitoring of intake and output with adequate replacement must be carried out
D. Acid hypersecretion can be managed by H_2 receptor antagonists or proton pump blockers, such as omeprazole

284. False about the dietary management of short bowel resection is:

A. Milk products should be provided, and the diet should begin at hypo-osmolar concentrations and with small amounts
B. Vitamins, especially fat-soluble vitamins, as well as calcium, magnesium and zinc supplementation should be provided
C. Initially, a high-carbohydrate, high-protein diet is appropriate to maximize absorption
D. Reduction in dietary fat has long been considered important in the treatment of patients with short bowel syndrome

285. False about the management of short bowel resection is:

A. Intestinal transplantation remains the standard of care for patients for whom intestinal rehabilitation attempts have failed and who are at risk of life-threatening complications of TPN
B. Somatropin, a recombinant human growth hormone that elicits anabolic and anticatabolic influence on various cells, either as a direct effect or indirectly through IGF-I, is currently indicated to treat short bowel syndrome in conjunction with nutritional support
C. The first step in terms of surgical intervention is to restore digestive continuity, which can be accomplished by the reversal of a proximal stoma to reduce rates of dehydration
D. All of the above

286. Following image shows:

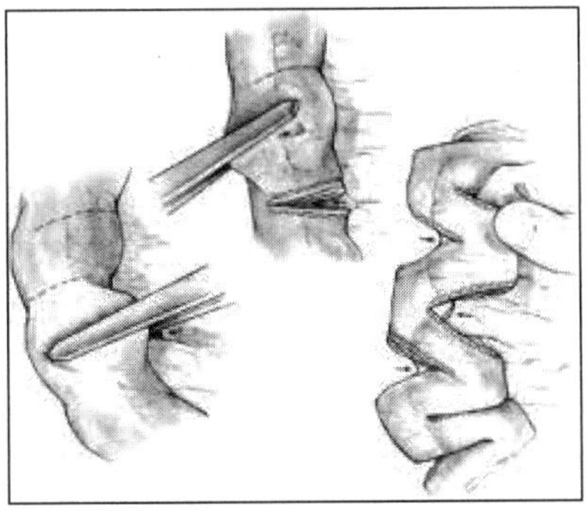

A. LILT (Longitudinal intestinal lengthening and tapering procedure)
B. STEP (Serial transverse enteroplasty procedure)
C. Bianchi procedure
D. Strong procedure

287. Following image shows:

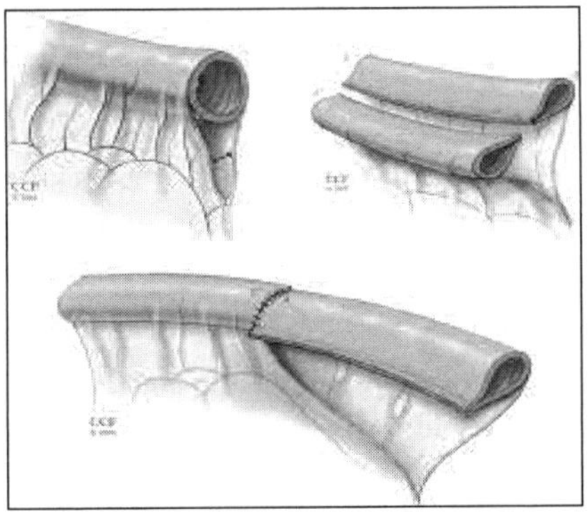

A. LILT (Longitudinal intestinal lengthening and tapering procedure)
B. STEP (Serial transverse enteroplasty procedure)
C. Bianchi procedure
D. Both A and C

288. Vascular compression of the duodenum, also known as:

A. Superior mesenteric artery syndrome
B. Wilkie syndrome
C. Nutcracker syndrome
D. Both A and B

289. False about Wilkie syndrome is:

A. Weight loss usually occurs after the onset of symptoms and contributes to the syndrome
B. Operative management may include duodeno-jejunostomy, gastrojejunostomy to bypass the obstructing segment, or duodenal derotation (*Strong procedure*)
C. This syndrome is most commonly seen in young asthenic individuals, with women more commonly affected than men
D. Diagnosis of this condition is made by a barium upper gastrointestinal series or hypotonic duodenography, which demonstrates abrupt or near-total cessation of flow of barium from the duodenum to the jejunum

290. Predisposing factors for vascular compression of the duodenum is all except:

A. Immobilization
B. Cast syndrome
C. Weight gain
D. Scoliosis

ANSWERS

1. **Ans: C. Small bowel**

Ref: Chapter No.50, Page No.1240

2. **Ans: B. Nerves and neurons found in the wall are derived from the neuroectoderm**

Ref: Chapter No.50, Page No.1240

3. **Ans: B. 2% of the population**

Ref: Chapter No.50, Page No.1240

4. **Ans: A. Epithelial cell turnover occurs rapidly, with a life span of 7 to 10 days in humans**

Ref: Chapter No.50, Page No.1241

5. **Ans: A. Absorptive enterocytes**

Ref: Chapter No.50, Page No.1241

6. **Ans: B. Paneth cells**

Ref: Chapter No.50, Page No.1241

7. **Ans: C. 100 cms**

Ref: Chapter No.50, Page No.1241

8. **Ans: A. 20 cms**

Ref: Chapter No.50, Page No.1241

9. **Ans: B. The ileum has a somewhat larger circumference, is thicker than the jejunum**

Ref: Chapter No.50, Page No.1242

10. **Ans: B. Duodenojejunal junction**

Ref: Chapter No.50, Page No.1242

11. **Ans: D. 150 cms**

Ref: Chapter No.50, Page No.1242

12. **Ans: B. Left of the L2 vertebra and passes obliquely to the right and inferiorly to the right sacroiliac joint**

Ref: Chapter No.50, Page No.1242

13. **Ans: B. Pain from the intestine is transmitted through general visceral afferent fibers of the parasympathetic system**

Ref: Chapter No.50, Page No.1242

14. **Ans: C. Small intestine lymphatics are noted as major deposits of lymphatic tissue, particularly in the Peyer patches of the proximal small bowel**

Ref: Chapter No.50, Page No.1243

15. **Ans: B. Submucosa**

Ref: Chapter No.50, Page No.1243

16. **Ans: D. The muscularis propria consists of two muscle layers, a thick outer longitudinal layer and a thin inner circular layer of smooth muscle**

Ref: Chapter No.50, Page No.1243

17. **Ans: B. Submucosa**

Ref: Chapter No.50, Page No.1243

18. **Ans: D. Muscularis propria**

Ref: Chapter No.50, Page No.1243

19. **Ans: B. The microvilli increase the absorptive capacity by 10-fold**

Ref: Chapter No.50, Page No.1243-1244

20. **Ans: D. 1 mm or smaller**

Ref: Chapter No.50, Page No.1244

21. **Ans: D. All of the above**

Ref: Chapter No.50, Page No.1244

22. **Ans: B. In normal humans, digestion and absorption of protein are usually 80% to 90% completed in the ileum**

Ref: Chapter No.50, Page No.1245

23. **Ans: D. Carboxypeptidase B: Attacks peptides with aromatic and neutral aliphatic amino acids at carboxyl-terminal end**

Ref: Chapter No.50, Page No.1246

24. **Ans: C. The total bile acid pool (approximately 2–3 g) recirculates about 3 times every 24 hours through the enterohepatic circulation**

Ref: Chapter No.50, Page No.1246

25. **Ans: C. Iron is absorbed as a heme or nonheme component in the duodenum by a passive process**

Ref: Chapter No.50, Page No.1247

26. **Ans: B. Vitamin B_6 appears to be rapidly absorbed by simple diffusion into the distal intestine**

Ref: Chapter No.50, Page No.1247

27. **Ans: D. Monosaccharides**

Ref: Chapter No.50, Page No.1247

28. **Ans: D. Bile acids**

Ref: Chapter No.50, Page No.1247

29. **Ans: B. 1–2 cm/sec**

Ref: Chapter No.50, Page No.1247

30. **Ans: C. Duodenum**

Ref: Chapter No.50, Page No.1247

31. **Ans: D. 75 to 90 minutes**

Ref: Chapter No.50, Page No.1248

32. **Ans: D. Relaxes sphincter of Oddi**

Ref: Chapter No.50, Page No.1249

33. **Ans: A. Stimulates gastric acid secretion and motility**
Ref: Chapter No.50, Page No.1249

34. **Ans: B. Somatostatin**
Ref: Chapter No.50, Page No.1249

35. **Ans: C. Gastrin-releasing peptide**
Ref: Chapter No.50, Page No.1249

36. **Ans: A. Produced by C cells in duodenum and jejunum**
Ref: Chapter No.50, Page No.1249

37. **Ans: B. K cells**
Ref: Chapter No.50, Page No.1249

38. **Ans: A. Enteroglucagon**
Ref: Chapter No.50, Page No.1249

39. **Ans: D. Potent vasoconstrictor**
Ref: Chapter No.50, Page No.1249

40. **Ans: C. Stimulates insulin release**
Ref: Chapter No.50, Page No.1249

41. **Ans: B. Inhibits pancreatic glucagon release**
Ref: Chapter No.50, Page No.1249

42. **Ans: B. Secretin: Decrease secretion from pancreatic and intestinal fistulas**
Ref: Chapter No.50, Page No.1249

43. **Ans: D. All of the above**
Ref: Chapter No.50, Page No.1250

44. **Ans: C. Approximately 40% of the lymphoid cells in the lamina propria are B cells**
Ref: Chapter No.50, Page No.1250

45. **Ans: D. Bezoars**
Ref: Chapter No.50, Page No.1250

46. **Ans: C. Adhesions**
Ref: Chapter No.50, Page No.1250

47. **Ans: B. 20%**
Ref: Chapter No.50, Page No.1250

48. **Ans: D. 60%**
Ref: Chapter No.50, Page No.1250

49. **Ans: B. Crohn's disease is the third leading cause of small bowel obstruction and accounts for approximately 10% of all cases**
Ref: Chapter No.50, Page No.1251

50. **Ans: B. Abscess**
Ref: Chapter No.50, Page No.1252

51. **Ans: C. In distal obstruction of the small bowel, abnormalities in serum electrolyte levels are usually more dramatic**
Ref: Chapter No.50, Page No.1252

52. **Ans: D. Hyperkalemia**
Ref: Chapter No.50, Page No.1252

53. **Ans: C. 10^9 to 10^{10} CFU/mL**
Ref: Chapter No.50, Page No.1252

54. **Ans: A. The typical crampy abdominal pain associated with intestinal obstruction occurs in paroxysms at 4- to 5-minute intervals and occurs more frequently with distal obstruction**
Ref: Chapter No.50, Page No.1253

55. **Ans: D. All of the above**
Ref: Chapter No.50, Page No.1253

56. **Ans: D. Pseudotumor sign**
Ref: Chapter No.50, Page No.1253

57. **Ans: C. Air fluid levels in same loop of small bowel of unequal lengths**
Ref: Chapter No.50, Page No.1253

58. **Ans: A. The absence of leukocytosis eliminates strangulation as a possibility**
Ref: Chapter No.50, Page No.1253

59. **Ans: D. All of the above**
Ref: Chapter No.50, Page No.1254-1255

60. **Ans: B. This technique is a single-contrast procedure that allows detailed imaging of the entire small intestine**
Ref: Chapter No.50, Page No.1255

61. **Ans: B. 500 to 1000 mL of thin barium sulfate and methylcellulose suspension**
Ref: Chapter No.50, Page No.1255

62. **Ans: D. All of the above**
Ref: Chapter No.50, Page No.1255-1256

63. **Ans: B. Bowel wall thickening (>1 mm)**
Ref: Chapter No.50, Page No.1255

64. **Ans: B. Retrospective studies report that a 48- to 72-hour delay is safe but that the incidence of strangulation and other complications increases significantly after this time period**
Ref: Chapter No.50, Page No.1256

65. **Ans: C. 8 and 24 hours**
Ref: Chapter No.50, Page No.1256

66. **Ans: D. Radiation enteropathy may cause bowel obstruction and can be treated nonoperatively with tube decompression and the potential addition of corticosteroids, particularly during the chronic setting**
Ref: Chapter No.50, Page No.1256-1257

67. **Ans: C. 15 to 20 minutes**
Ref: Chapter No.50, Page No.1257

68. **Ans: C. Good surgical technique**
Ref: Chapter No.50, Page No.1257

69. **Ans: D. >90%**

Ref: Chapter No.50, Page No.1258

70. **Ans: C. Intraabdominal obstruction**

Ref: Chapter No.50, Page No.1258

71. **Ans: B. Hypoglycemia**

Ref: Chapter No.50, Page No.1258

72. **Ans: C. Erythromycin has been effective and cisapride is beneficial in stimulating gastric motility and appears to alter intestinal ileus**

Ref: Chapter No.50, Page No.1258

73. **Ans: A. Crohn's disease**

Ref: Chapter No.50, Page No.1258

74. **Ans: B. Crohn's disease primarily attacks middle aged adults in the 4th and 5th decades of life**

Ref: Chapter No.50, Page No.1259

75. **Ans: D. 2x**

Ref: Chapter No.50, Page No.1259

76. **Ans: C. 30-fold**

Ref: Chapter No.50, Page No.1259

77. **Ans: B. NOD2**

Ref: Chapter No.50, Page No.1259

78. **Ans: C. 17- to 40-fold**

Ref: Chapter No.50, Page No.1259

79. **Ans: B. CARD15 is also helpful in distinguishing Crohn disease from ulcerative colitis as it is more strongly associated with ulcerative colitis**

Ref: Chapter No.50, Page No.1259

80. **Ans: D. All of the above**

Ref: Chapter No.50, Page No.1259-1260

81. **Ans: D. All of the above**

Ref: Chapter No.50, Page No.1260

82. **Ans: B. Superficial aphthous ulcer**

Ref: Chapter No.50, Page No.1260

83. **Ans: B. The ulcers are characteristically transverse**

Ref: Chapter No.50, Page No.1260-1261

84. **Ans: B. Noncaseating granulomas**

Ref: Chapter No.50, Page No.1261

85. **Ans: C. 60% to 70% of patients**

Ref: Chapter No.50, Page No.1261

86. **Ans: B. Chronic diarrhea**

Ref: Chapter No.50, Page No.1261

87. **Ans: D. Disease etiology**

Ref: Chapter No.50, Page No.1261

88. **Ans: C. Localized abscesses can occur everywhere in peritoneum**

Ref: Chapter No.50, Page No.1261

89. **Ans: A. The relative risk for small bowel cancer in Crohn's disease is approximately 10-fold, the absolute risk is large**

Ref: Chapter No.50, Page No.1261

90. **Ans: C. Perianal disease occurs in 80% of patients with colonic involvement alone**

Ref: Chapter No.50, Page No.1261

91. **Ans: B. Erythema nodosum**

Ref: Chapter No.50, Page No.1261

92. **Ans: B. 30% of patients**

Ref: Chapter No.50, Page No.1261

93. **Ans: D. Fecal lactoferrin is only associated with elevated ESR levels**

Ref: Chapter No.50, Page No.1262-1263

94. **Ans: C. A2 B3 L2**

Ref: Chapter No.50, Page No.1263

95. **Ans: B. A3 B2 L3**

Ref: Chapter No.50, Page No.1263

96. **Ans: A. A2 B3 L1**

Ref: Chapter No.50, Page No.1263

97. **Ans: D. Ultrasonography has limited value in the evaluation of patients with Crohn disease and has an especially high accuracy for detecting the disease proximal to the terminal ileum**

Ref: Chapter No.50, Page No.1263

98. **Ans: C. Capsule endoscopy has been found to be inferior to any endoscopy in the identification of intestinal ulceration**

Ref: Chapter No.50, Page No.1264

99. **Ans: A. More rectal bleeding**

Ref: Chapter No.50, Page No.1265

100. **Ans: A. Superficial ulcers on proctoscopy**

Ref: Chapter No.50, Page No.1265

101. **Ans: B. 150**

Ref: Chapter No.50, Page No.1265

102. **Ans: B. Clinical response to therapy occurs with a drop of 150 points**

Ref: Chapter No.50, Page No.1265

103. **Ans: A. Age**

Ref: Chapter No.50, Page No.1265

104. **Ans: D. All of the above**

Ref: Chapter No.50, Page No.1266

105. Ans: D. Steroids are fast acting and effective at inducing remission and are ideal as maintenance therapy

Ref: Chapter No.50, Page No.1266

106. Ans: B. Low-dose cyclosporine was found to be efficacious

Ref: Chapter No.50, Page No.1266

107. Ans: D. All of the above

Ref: Chapter No.50, Page No.1266

108. Ans: C. Increased risk of BCC

Ref: Chapter No.50, Page No.1266

109. Ans: A. Adalimumab

Ref: Chapter No.50, Page No.1266

110. Ans: B. Certolizumab

Ref: Chapter No.50, Page No.1266

111. Ans: B. Natalizumab, a recombinant humanized monoclonal antibody against α4 integrin, showed effectiveness in the induction and maintenance of remission in patients with active Crohn's disease

Ref: Chapter No.50, Page No.1267

112. Ans: D. All of the above

Ref: Chapter No.50, Page No.1267

113. Ans: B. It appears to be associated with the severity of disease in a nonlinear dose-response relationship

Ref: Chapter No.50, Page No.1267

114. Ans: B. Creating a wider anastomosis with a stapled functional side to side anastomosis may decrease fecal stasis and subsequent bacterial overgrowth

Ref: Chapter No.50, Page No.1267

115. Ans: C. 70%

Ref: Chapter No.50, Page No.1267

116. Ans: D. All of the above

Ref: Chapter No.50, Page No.1267

117. Ans: B. Ankylosing spondylitis

Ref: Chapter No.50, Page No.1267

118. Ans: C. Perform appendectomy

Ref: Chapter No.50, Page No.1268

119. Ans: B. Intestinal obstruction

Ref: Chapter No.50, Page No.1268

120. Ans: B. In case of a chronic strictured segment, medical therapy is generally effective

Ref: Chapter No.50, Page No.1268

121. Ans: A. Finney strictureplasty

Ref: Chapter No.50, Page No.1269

122. Ans: C. Hypoalbuminemia (<3.0g/dl)

Ref: Chapter No.50, Page No.1269

123. Ans: A. Most patients with ileosigmoid fistulas require resection of the sigmoid

Ref: Chapter No.50, Page No.1269

124. Ans: D. All of the above

Ref: Chapter No.50, Page No.1270

125. Ans: D. All of the above

Ref: Chapter No.50, Page No.1270

126. Ans: B. Ureteral obstruction

Ref: Chapter No.50, Page No.1270

127. Ans: D. All of the above

Ref: Chapter No.50, Page No.1270

128. Ans: B. Fissures are usually lateral, painless, small, and indolent and often respond to conservative management

Ref: Chapter No.50, Page No.1270

129. Ans: C. Operative intervention is common

Ref: Chapter No.50, Page No.1270

130. Ans: C. Gastrointestinal cancer

Ref: Chapter No.50, Page No.1271

131. Ans: A. Typhoid enteritis is an acute systemic infection caused primarily by Salmonella paratyphi

Ref: Chapter No.50, Page No.1271

132. Ans: D. 90%

Ref: Chapter No.50, Page No.1271

133. Ans: D. All of the above

Ref: Chapter No.50, Page No.1271-1272

134. Ans: D. All of the above

Ref: Chapter No.50, Page No.1272

135. Ans: D. All of the above

Ref: Chapter No.50, Page No.1272

136. Ans: D. All of the above

Ref: Chapter No.50, Page No.1272-1273

137. Ans: B. CMV

Ref: Chapter No.50, Page No.1273

138. Ans: D. Start Anti-TNF or AZT/6MP

Ref: Chapter No.50, Page No.1271

139. Ans: C. The malignant neoplasms account for 25% of symptomatic lesions that lead to surgery

Ref: Chapter No.50, Page No.1273

140. Ans: B. Adenocarcinoma

Ref: Chapter No.50, Page No.1273

141. Ans: C. 25% - 30%

Ref: Chapter No.50, Page No.1273

142. Ans: D. All of the above

Ref: Chapter No.50, Page No.1273

143. Ans: C. Heavy alcohol consumption (>20 g/day of ethanol)

Ref: Chapter No.50, Page No.1273

144. Ans: B. Microsatellite instability (MSI-H)

Ref: Chapter No.50, Page No.1274

145. Ans: A. Hemorrhage is the most common symptom

Ref: Chapter No.50, Page No.1274

146. Ans: C. Pain

Ref: Chapter No.50, Page No.1274

147. Ans: A. A correct preoperative diagnosis is made in only 80% of symptomatic patients

Ref: Chapter No.50, Page No.1274

148. Ans: D. Push enteroscopy has been used routinely to evaluate lesions in the small bowel

Ref: Chapter No.50, Page No.1274

149. Ans: C. Stromal tumors

Ref: Chapter No.50, Page No.1274-1275

150 Ans: A. Adenomas

Ref: Chapter No.50, Page No.1274

151. Ans: B. Stomach

Ref: Chapter No.50, Page No.1275

152. Ans: C. Incidence rates in M:F is 3:1

Ref: Chapter No.50, Page No.1275

153. Ans: C. 20%

Ref: Chapter No.50, Page No.1275

154. Ans: B. 50% to 60% express CD34

Ref: Chapter No.50, Page No.1275

155. Ans: D. 95%

Ref: Chapter No.50, Page No.1275

156. Ans: A. Tumors smaller than 5 cm, regardless of mitotic index, have higher rates of metastasis and recurrence

Ref: Chapter No.50, Page No.1275

157. Ans: B. Ileum

Ref: Chapter No.50, Page No.1275

158. Ans: D. All of the above

Ref: Chapter No.50, Page No.1275

159. Ans: C. Duodenum

Ref: Chapter No.50, Page No.1275

160. Ans: D. Adenomas in the ileum can be found in 50% to 90% of cases

Ref: Chapter No.50, Page No.1275

161. Ans: D. Stage IV

Ref: Chapter No.50, Page No.1276

162. Ans: C. Stage IV and consider surgery

Ref: Chapter No.50, Page No.1276

163. Ans: C. Stage III and surveillance every 1 year

Ref: Chapter No.50, Page No.1276

164. Ans: B. Stage II and surveillance every 2 years

Ref: Chapter No.50, Page No.1276

165. Ans: C. There is malignant potential for Brunner gland adenomas and a radical resection should be considered

Ref: Chapter No.50, Page No.1275

166. Ans: B. Ileum

Ref: Chapter No.50, Page No.1276

167. Ans: D. They usually occur in the sixth and seventh decades of life and are more frequent in women

Ref: Chapter No.50, Page No.1276

168. Ans: B. Because of the widespread nature of intestinal involvement extensive resection is indicated

Ref: Chapter No.50, Page No.1276

169. Ans: B. Legs

Ref: Chapter No.50, Page No.1276

170. Ans: D. Hemangiomas account for 3% to 4% of all benign tumors of the small bowel and are multifocal in 10% of patients

Ref: Chapter No.50, Page No.1276

171. Ans: B. Gastrointestinal bleeding, manifested by anemia and guaiac-positive stools or occasionally by melena or hematochezia is more common with adenocarcinoma

Ref: Chapter No.50, Page No.1276-1277

172. Ans: D. All of the above

Ref: Chapter No.50, Page No.1277

173. Ans: B. Hindgut NETs rarely produce serotonin but may produce other hormones, such as somatostatin and peptide YY

Ref: Chapter No.50, Page No.1277

174. Ans: C. Gastrointestinal tract

Ref: Chapter No.50, Page No.1277

175. Ans: A. Appendix

Ref: Chapter No.50, Page No.1277

176. Ans: D. All of the above

Ref: Chapter No.50, Page No.1277

177. Ans: C. Small bowel NETs are multicentric in 50% to 60% of patients

Ref: Chapter No.50, Page No.1277

178. Ans: D. 80% of cases

Ref: Chapter No.50, Page No.1277

179. Ans: B. 10% to 20%

Ref: Chapter No.50, Page No.1277

180. Ans: B. Large intestine

Ref: Chapter No.50, Page No.1277

181. Ans: C. Neurotensin

Ref: Chapter No.50, Page No.1277

182. Ans: D. Chromogranin

Ref: Chapter No.50, Page No.1277

183. Ans: B. 5-HIAA

Ref: Chapter No.50, Page No.1277

184. Ans: B. Abdominal pain

Ref: Chapter No.50, Page No.1278

185. Ans: D. The diarrhea is secretory diarrhea as noted in patients with the malignant carcinoid syndrome

Ref: Chapter No.50, Page No.1278

186. Ans: A. Cutaneous flushing

Ref: Chapter No.50, Page No.1278

187. Ans: C. Diarrhea is the most common symptom in malignant carcinoid syndrome

Ref: Chapter No.50, Page No.1278

188. Ans: B. <10%

Ref: Chapter No.50, Page No.1278

189. Ans: B. Pulmonary stenosis

Ref: Chapter No.50, Page No.1278

190. Ans: B. Bright-red patchy flushing

Ref: Chapter No.50, Page No.1278

191. Ans: A. Violaceous

Ref: Chapter No.50, Page No.1278

192. Ans: B. Methysergide

Ref: Chapter No.50, Page No.1278

193. Ans: C. Serotonin

Ref: Chapter No.50, Page No.1278

194. Ans: A. Elevated urinary levels of 5-HIAA measured during 24 hours with high-performance liquid chromatography are highly specific and sensitive

Ref: Chapter No.50, Page No.1279

195. Ans: A. Liver metastases are well demonstrated with MRI and usually have high signal intensity on T1-weighted images and low signal intensity on T2-weighted images

Ref: Chapter No.50, Page No.1279

196. Ans: A. ^{68}Ga-DOTATATE imaging include better true positive lesion detection, longer shelf life and scanning window when compared with ^{64}Cu-DOTATATE

Ref: Chapter No.50, Page No.1279-1280

197. Ans: C. For primary tumors <1 cm in diameter with evidence of regional lymph node metastasis, a segmental intestinal resection is adequate

Ref: Chapter No.50, Page No.1280

198. Ans: B. IV octreotide given as a bolus of 50 to 100 µg, which may be continued as an infusion at 50 µg/hr

Ref: Chapter No.50, Page No.1280

199. Ans: D. All of the above

Ref: Chapter No.50, Page No.1280-1281

200. Ans: A. Lanreotide relieves symptoms of the carcinoid syndrome in most patients and but doesn't delay cancer progression

Ref: Chapter No.50, Page No.1280-1281

201. Ans: B. CLARINET trial

Ref: Chapter No.50, Page No.1280

202. Ans: D. NETTER-1 trial

Ref: Chapter No.50, Page No.1281

203. Ans: C. Currently, the role of chemotherapy is confined predominantly to patients with G1 metastatic disease who are symptomatic, are unresponsive to other therapies, or have high tumor proliferation rates

Ref: Chapter No.50, Page No.1281

204. Ans: B. Checkpoint inhibitor

Ref: Chapter No.50, Page No.1281

205. Ans: A. Somatostatin drug conjugate

Ref: Chapter No.50, Page No.1281

206. Ans: D. Pasireotide

Ref: Chapter No.50, Page No.1281

207. Ans: D. Serotonin synthesis inhibitors

Ref: Chapter No.50, Page No.1281

208. Ans: B. Metastatic disease at the time of diagnosis is approximately 10% to 20% and tumors recur in 70% to 90% of patients

Ref: Chapter No.50, Page No.1282

209. Ans: D. Those arising in association with Crohn's disease tend to occur at a somewhat younger age and more than 70% arise in the duodenum

Ref: Chapter No.50, Page No.1282

210. Ans: A. Perforation is uncommon

Ref: Chapter No.50, Page No.1282

211. Ans: D. All of the above

Ref: Chapter No.50, Page No.1282-1283

212. Ans: D. All of the above

Ref: Chapter No.50, Page No.1283

213. Ans: C. Lymphoma

Ref: Chapter No.50, Page No.1283

214. Ans: B. Ileum

Ref: Chapter No.50, Page No.1283

215. Ans: A. 25%

Ref: Chapter No.50, Page No.1283

216. Ans: A. T-cell lymphomas are more chemosensitive than B.-cell lymphomas and have high remission rates with or without surgery

Ref: Chapter No.50, Page No.1283

217. Ans: B. A laparoscopic approach in patients with large tumors is strongly encouraged

Ref: Chapter No.50, Page No.1284

218. Ans: D. 80%

Ref: Chapter No.50, Page No.1284

219. Ans: C. Muscularis propria

Ref: Chapter No.50, Page No.1284

220. Ans: D. Both A and B

Ref: Chapter No.50, Page No.1284

221. Ans: D. All of the above

Ref: Chapter No.50, Page No.1284

222. Ans: D. 100%

Ref: Chapter No.50, Page No.1284

223. Ans: D. Current guidelines suggest that patients with high-risk disease should receive 1 year of adjuvant treatment with imatinib

Ref: Chapter No.50, Page No.1284

224. Ans: B. Adjuvant imatinib therapy is recommended in patients with D842V PDGFRα mutations

Ref: Chapter No.50, Page No.1285

225. Ans: C. Continue disease surveillance

Ref: Chapter No.50, Page No.1284

226. Ans: B. Imatinib 400 mg

Ref: Chapter No.50, Page No.1284

227. Ans: C. Cutaneous melanoma

Ref: Chapter No.50, Page No.1285

228. Ans: B. Duodenal diverticula

Ref: Chapter No.50, Page No.1286

229. Ans: D. Meckel diverticulum

Ref: Chapter No.50, Page No.1286

230. Ans: B. Most common site for diverticulum formation

Ref: Chapter No.50, Page No.1286

231. Ans: B. 2nd portion of the duodenum

Ref: Chapter No.50, Page No.1286

232. Ans: C. Medial wall

Ref: Chapter No.50, Page No.1286

233. Ans: B. Upper gastrointestinal endoscopy identifies approximately 25% of duodenal diverticula

Ref: Chapter No.50, Page No.1286

234. Ans: D. All of the above

Ref: Chapter No.50, Page No.1286

235. Ans: D. All of the above

Ref: Chapter No.50, Page No.1287

236. Ans: C. Surgical jejunostomy should also be considered for a few patients with acute perforation to ensure nutrition repletion

Ref: Chapter No.50, Page No.1287-1288

237. Ans: A. Jejunal diverticula are more common and are smaller than those in the ileum

Ref: Chapter No.50, Page No.1288

238. Ans: D. All of the above

Ref: Chapter No.50, Page No.1288

239. Ans: D. Incidence is more common in men as compared to women

Ref: Chapter No.50, Page No.1288-1289

240. Ans: C. Gastric mucosa

Ref: Chapter No.50, Page No.1289

241. Ans: D. The usual source of the bleeding is a acute acid-induced ulcer in the diverticulum

Ref: Chapter No.50, Page No.1289

242. Ans: C. Gastrointestinal bleeding

Ref: Chapter No.50, Page No.1289

243. Ans: B. NET

Ref: Chapter No.50, Page No.1289

244. Ans: A. Sodium ^{99m}Tc-pertechnetate scintigraphy

Ref: Chapter No.50, Page No.1289

245. Ans: D. Cimetidine

Ref: Chapter No.50, Page No.1289

246. Ans: D. All of the above

Ref: Chapter No.50, Page No.1290

247. Ans: D. Age > 50 years

Ref: Chapter No.50, Page No.1290

248. Ans: C. Ileum

Ref: Chapter No.50, Page No.1290

249. Ans: D. All of the above

Ref: Chapter No.50, Page No.1291

250. Ans: B. Iatrogenic

Ref: Chapter No.50, Page No.1291

251. Ans: C. 500 mL or more

Ref: Chapter No.50, Page No.1292

252. Ans: C. Output >500 mL/24 hours

Ref: Chapter No.50, Page No.1292

253. Ans: B. Surgical etiology

Ref: Chapter No.50, Page No.1292

254. Ans: D. All of the above

Ref: Chapter No.50, Page No.1292

255. Ans: C. Sepsis

Ref: Chapter No.50, Page No.1292

256. Ans: C. Intubation of the fistula tract with a drain

Ref: Chapter No.50, Page No.1292

257. Ans: D. 90%

Ref: Chapter No.50, Page No.1292

258. Ans: B. > 25 g/L

Ref: Chapter No.50, Page No.1292

259. Ans: A. Dysmotility agents such as loperamide and codeine can't assist with attempts at enteral therapy

Ref: Chapter No.50, Page No.1292-1293

260. Ans: C. Allow 500 mL/day clear liquids orally

Ref: Chapter No.50, Page No.1293

261. Ans: B. Increase the number of anastomoses

Ref: Chapter No.50, Page No.1293

262. Ans: C. Allow 1000 mL/day clear liquids orally

Ref: Chapter No.50, Page No.1293

263. Ans: D. There is an increased incidence in men, and the condition usually occurs in the fourth to seventh decades of life

Ref: Chapter No.50, Page No.1293

264. Ans: B. Jejunum

Ref: Chapter No.50, Page No.1293

265. Ans: C. COPD

Ref: Chapter No.50, Page No.1293

266. Ans: B. Treatment is always necessary

Ref: Chapter No.50, Page No.1293-1294

267. Ans: D. All of the above

Ref: Chapter No.50, Page No.1294

268. Ans: C. Excessive bacterial use of ^{14}C substrate leads to an decrease in ^{14}C-labeled CO_2

Ref: Chapter No.50, Page No.1294

269. Ans: D. All of the above

Ref: Chapter No.50, Page No.1294

270. Ans: C. < 4000 cGy

Ref: Chapter No.50, Page No.1295

271. Ans: B. 5000 cGy

Ref: Chapter No.50, Page No.1295

272. Ans: D. 18 months and 6 years

Ref: Chapter No.50, Page No.1295

273. Ans: D. All of the above

Ref: Chapter No.50, Page No.1295

274. Ans: D. Consideration of the use of antibiotics

Ref: Chapter No.50, Page No.1295

275. Ans: B. Histamine agonists

Ref: Chapter No.50, Page No.1295

276. Ans: A. Amifostine

Ref: Chapter No.50, Page No.1295

277. Ans: A. The use of corticosteroids for acute radiation enteritis has proven value

Ref: Chapter No.50, Page No.1295

278. Ans: D. In patients presenting with obstruction, extensive lysis of adhesions should be done

Ref: Chapter No.50, Page No.1295

279. Ans: B. Obstruction

Ref: Chapter No.50, Page No.1295

280. Ans: C. Multiple sequential resections, usually associated with recurrent Crohn disease, account for 50% of patients

Ref: Chapter No.50, Page No.1296

281. Ans: B. Necrotizing enterocolitis

Ref: Chapter No.50, Page No.1296

282. Ans: C. Resection of up to 90% of the small bowel usually can be tolerated if the terminal ileum and ileocecal valve are preserved

Ref: Chapter No.50, Page No.1296

283. Ans: C. Volume losses may exceed 1 L/day, and vigorous monitoring of intake and output with adequate replacement must be carried out

Ref: Chapter No.50, Page No.1296

284. Ans: A. Milk products should be provided, and the diet should begin at hypo-osmolar concentrations and with small amounts

Ref: Chapter No.50, Page No.1296

285. Ans: D. All of the above

Ref: Chapter No.50, Page No.1296-1297

286. Ans: B. STEP (Serial transverse enteroplasty procedure)

Ref: Chapter No.50, Page No.1297

287. Ans: D. Both A and C

Ref: Chapter No.50, Page No.1297

288. Ans: D. Both A and B

Ref: Chapter No.50, Page No.1297

289. Ans: A. Weight loss usually occurs after the onset of symptoms and contributes to the syndrome

Ref: Chapter No.50, Page No.1297

290. Ans: C. Weight gain

Ref: Chapter No.50, Page No.1297

51

The Appendix

1. **True about appendicitis is:**
   A. It is estimated that as much as 6% to 7% of the general population will develop appendicitis during their lifetime
   B. Low-fiber, high-fat intake, may play a role in the development of the disease process
   C. It is the most common urgent or emergent general surgical operation performed
   D. All of the above

ANATOMY AND EMBRYOLOGY

2. **The appendix is first identified at ___ of gestation.**
   A. 2 weeks B. 6 weeks
   C. 8 weeks D. 12 weeks

3. **False about appendix is:**
   A. Appendix is a midgut organ
   B. The appendiceal mucosa is of the colonic type, with columnar epithelium, neuroendocrine cells, and mucin-producing goblet cells lining its tubular structure
   C. Patients who have had previous appendectomy have been demonstrated to have a more difficult clinical course and overall poorer outcomes in recurrent cases of Clostridium difficile infection when compared with patients who have not undergone appendectomy
   D. Lymphoid tissue is found in the Muscularis mucosae of the appendix

4. **False about appendix is:**
   A. Appendix is pelvic in 30% cases
   B. The appendix is of variable size (5–35 cm in length) but averages 8 to 9 cm in length in adults
   C. Patients with the appendiceal tip in the midline pelvis may present with back or flank pain
   D. Agenesis of the appendix has been reported, as has duplication and even triplication

5. **The most common location of appendix is:**
   A. Retrocecal B. Pre ileal
   C. Pelvic D. Retroperitoneal

APPENDICITIS

6. **The first appendectomy was reported by:**
   A. Reginald Heber Fitz B. McBurney
   C. Claudius Amyand D. Kurt Semm

7. **True about appendicitis is:**
   A. The first formal description of the disease process, including the common clinical features and a recommendation for prompt surgical removal was done by Reginald Heber Fitz
   B. Laparoscopic appendectomy has become the preferred method for management of acute appendicitis
   C. The first laparoscopic appendectomy was done by Kurt Semm
   D. All of the above

8. **False about pathophysiology is:**
   A. With progressive distention of the appendix, the venous drainage becomes impaired, resulting in mucosal ischemia
   B. Infections associated with appendicitis should be considered monomicrobial
   C. Appendicitis is caused by luminal obstruction
   D. Bacterial overgrowth within the appendix results from bacterial stasis distal to the obstruction

9. **False about pain in appendicitis is:**
   A. Distention of the appendix is responsible for the initial vague abdominal pain (visceral) often experienced by the affected patient
   B. Pain associated with appendicitis has both visceral and somatic components

C. The pain typically does not localize to the right lower quadrant until the tip becomes inflamed and irritates the adjacent parietal peritoneum (somatic) or perforation occurs
D. All of the above

10. Differential diagnosis of appendicitis in children is all except:

A. Acute gastroenteritis
B. Intussusception
C. Mesenteric adenitis
D. All of the above

11. In the neutropenic patient, differential diagnosis specific for appendicitis is:

A. Mittelschmerz
B. Typhlitis
C. Nephrolithiasis
D. Meckel diverticulitis

12. False about the presentation of appendicitis is:

A. Patients with a retroperitoneal appendix may present in a more subacute manner with flank or back pain
B. Anorexia is often present, as is nausea with or without associated vomiting
C. Diarrhea may be present but constipation is not seen
D. All of the above are true

13. False about physical examination of appendicitis is:

A. Fever is frequently present, ranging from low-grade temperature elevations (<38.5°C)
B. Absence of fever excludes a diagnosis of appendicitis
C. Diffuse peritonitis or abdominal wall rigidity due to involuntary spasm of the overlying abdominal wall musculature is strongly suggestive of perforation
D. Tachycardia and mild dehydration are often present to varying degrees

14. The presence of right lower quadrant pain on palpation of the left lower quadrant in acute appendicitis is called:

A. Psoas sign
B. Obturator sign
C. Rovsing sign
D. McBurney's sign

15. Right lower quadrant pain on internal rotation of the hip in acute appendicitis is called:

A. Psoas sign
B. Obturator sign
C. Rovsing sign
D. McBurney's sign

16. Psoas sign in acute appendicitis is:

A. Pain with flexion of the ipsilateral hip
B. Pain with extension of the ipsilateral hip
C. Pain with flexion of the contralateral hip
D. Pain with extension of the contralateral hip

17. False about physical examination of appendicitis is:

A. The location of the tenderness is classically over McBurney point, which is located one third the distance between the anterior superior iliac spine and the umbilicus
B. Cervical motion tenderness may be present in appendicitis
C. Rectal examination findings show tenderness
D. The pain and tenderness are typically accompanied by localized peritonitis as evidenced by the presence of rebound tenderness

18. False about the laboratory studies in acute appendicitis is:

A. C-reactive protein appears to provide the most sensitive of the biomarkers, and provides sufficient specificity to definitively diagnose appendicitis
B. A leukocytosis, often with a "left shift" (a predominance of neutrophils and sometimes an increase in bands), is present in 90% of cases
C. Pregnancy testing is mandatory in women of childbearing age
D. A normal white blood cell count is found in 10% of cases

19. False about the Alvarado score in appendicitis is:

A. Alvarado score includes 8 clinical and laboratory variables used to assign a numerical score and remains the most widely used
B. Score of 7–8: Probable appendicitis
C. Alvarado score of <4 was most useful in excluding a diagnosis of appendicitis (96% sensitive) and a higher score have high specificity in diagnosing appendicitis as the cause of the patient's abdominal pain
D. All of the above are true

20. Imaging studies in patients suspected to have acute appendicitis can reduce the negative appendectomy rate, which can be as high as:

A. 5%
B. 15%
C. 25%
D. 40%

21. Most common anaerobe isolated in perforated appendicitis is:

A. Escherichia coli
B. Pseudomonas aeruginosa
C. Klebsiella pneumoniae
D. Citrobacter species

22. **Cause of luminal obstruction in acute appendicitis is:**

A. Intravenous barium
B. Fecolith
C. Vegetable material
D. All of the above

23. **Delayed presentation of appendicitis is defined as presentation delayed by more than:**

A. 24 hours
B. 48 hours
C. 72 hours
D. 96 hours

24. **Calcified fecalith in the right lower quadrant is typically present in only:**

A. 5%
B. 15%
C. 25%
D. 40%

25. **False about CT scan and acute appendicitis is:**

A. CT scanning is the most common imaging study used to diagnose appendicitis and is highly effective and accurate
B. CT has been shown to have a sensitivity ranging from 76% to 100% and a specificity of 83% to 100%
C. The recommended CT imaging technique involves the administration of intravenous contrast and oral contrast
D. The diagnosis of appendicitis on CT is based on the appearance of a thickened, inflamed appendix with surrounding "stranding" indicative of inflammation

26. **True about the diagnosis of acute appendicitis is:**

A. Periappendiceal fluid or air is also highly suggestive of appendicitis and suggests perforation
B. The inflamed appendix is typically enlarged, immobile and noncompressible on US
C. The appendix is typically more than 7 mm in diameter with a thickened, inflamed wall and mural enhancement or "target sign"
D. All of the above

27. **False about MRI and appendicitis is:**

A. MRI is typically reserved for use in the pregnant patient
B. MRI offers excellent resolution and is accurate in diagnosing appendicitis
C. The sensitivity of MRI to be 97% with a specificity of 95%
D. If it is obtained in a pregnant woman, the study should be contrast MRI

28. **Criteria for MRI diagnosis of acute appendicitis includes all except:**

A. Appendiceal enlargement (>7 mm)
B. Thickening (>5 mm)
C. The presence of inflammation
D. All of the above are true

29. **A 40-year-old man is suspected of having acute appendicitis. On physical examination his abdomen is soft and nondistended. He does not have pain with coughing or reproduction of tenderness in the right lower quadrant when palpated in the left lower quadrant. He experiences abdominal pain during extension of the right thigh while lying on his left side. He does not have pain with passive rotation of his right hip in a flexed position. Where do you suspect the location of the tip of his appendix to be?**

A. Extraperitoneal and lying anterior to the cecum
B. In the pelvis
C. In the left lower quadrant
D. Retrocecal over the psoas muscle

30. **A 25-year-old, 28-week pregnant female presents to the emergency department with a 24-hour history of right upper quadrant abdominal pain. The white blood cell (WBC) count is 16,000. An ultrasound was done showing a normal gallbladder and viable fetus. The appendix was not visualized. What is the next best step?**

A. Admit the patient for serial abdominal examinations and repeat lab tests in the morning
B. Treat with antibiotics in an attempt to avoid an operation
C. Proceed with laparoscopy after delivery
D. Obtain a magnetic resonance imaging (MRI) and proceed with an appendectomy if positive

TREATMENT OF APPENDICITIS

31. **McArthur-McBurney incision is:**

A. Midline incision
B. Oblique muscle-splitting incision
C. Transverse incision
D. Paramedian incision

32. **Rockey-Davis incision is:**

A. Midline incision
B. Oblique muscle-splitting incision
C. Transverse incision
D. Paramedian incision

33. **Post appendicectomy antibiotic administration is not continued beyond a:**

A. 1 preoperative dose
B. 1 post operative dose
C. 2 post operative doses
D. 3 post operative doses

34. **False about perforated appendicitis is:**

A. Once the appendix is successfully removed, careful attention should be given to the clearance of infectious material, including spilled fecal material or fecaliths from the abdomen
B. If an open technique was used, the skin and subcutaneous tissues are left open for 3 or 4 days to prevent development of wound infection
C. Cultures are not mandatory unless the patient has had exposure to a health care environment or has had recent exposure to antibiotic therapy because these factors increase the likelihood of encountering resistant bacteria
D. Drains are routinely placed

35. **In perforated appendicitis, postoperatively broad-spectrum antibiotics are continued for:**

A. 1 - 3 days
B. 4 - 7 days
C. 7 - 10 days
D. 10 - 14 days

36. **Abscess complicates perforated appendicitis in _____ of cases.**

A. 5% to 10%
B. 10% to 20%
C. 20% to 40%
D. 50% to 60%

37. **72-year-old female presents with a 6-day history of right lower quadrant abdominal pain and nausea. A computed tomography (CT) of the abdomen and pelvis shows perforated appendicitis with a 7-cm abscess. She was started on broad-spectrum antibiotics and underwent percutaneous drainage of the abscess. In 72 hours she was afebrile, and her leukocytosis and symptoms had resolved. What should the next treatment step be?**

A. Appendectomy prior to discharge
B. Continue broad-spectrum antibiotics until drain removal
C. Schedule a colonoscopy and consider an interval appendectomy in 4-6 weeks
D. Interval appendectomy in 4 weeks

38. **False about delayed presentation of appendicitis is:**

A. In general, treatment for these patients is initially accomplished operatively
B. If a localized abscess is identified, CT-guided percutaneous drainage is performed for source control
C. The drainage catheter is typically left in place for 4 to 7 days, during which the patient is treated with antibiotic therapy and after which time it is removed
D. If CT-guided drainage is not technically feasible, operative drainage may be accomplished through transrectal or transvaginal approaches

39. **28 years old male with pain in right iliac fossa was clinically diagnosed to have acute appendicitis and was taken up for emergency appendectomy. During the surgery the patient's appendix was found to be normal. All of the following should be done except:**

A. The abdominal and pelvic organs should be assessed for any abnormalities
B. The terminal 100 cm of ileum should be examined for a Meckel diverticulum and the serosa of the small bowel for any stigmata of Crohn's disease
C. The sigmoid colon should be examined for evidence of acute diverticulitis
D. Inspection of the ileal mesentery may reveal enlarged lymph nodes suggestive of mesenteric adenitis

40. **A 20-year-old woman is operated on through a right lower quadrant incision for presumed appendicitis, but the appendix is normal. At this point, which of the following would be an appropriate treatment?**

A. Exploration and appendectomy if no other pathology is found
B. Exploration, treatment of any associated pathologic condition, as indicated, and avoiding removal of a healthy appearing appendix
C. Exploration and diverticulectomy if a Meckel's diverticulum is present and is normal by inspection and palpation
D. Exploration and ileal resection if the terminal ileum appears acutely inflamed

APPENDICITIS IN SPECIAL POPULATIONS

41. False about appendicitis in the pregnant patients is:

A. Appendicitis remains the most common non-obstetric emergency in pregnancy
B. 50% of cases of appendicitis occur in the 1st trimester
C. When based on clinical presentation alone, high rate of negative appendectomy in pregnant patients, as high as 25% to 50%
D. Laparoscopic appendectomy is the most common approach currently used in pregnant patients

42. In pregnancy, appendicitis has a typical clinical presentation in only ______ of cases.

A. 10% to 20% B. 20% to 25%
C. 30% to 45% D. 50% to 60%

43. With complicated appendicitis the risk of preterm labor has been shown to be around:

A. 5% B. 10%
C. 20% D. 40%

44. With complicated appendicitis in a pregnant patient, fetal loss is seen in:

A. 2% B. 6%
C. 11% D. 20%

45. In the elderly population, perforation rate in acute appendicitis is:

A. 10% to 15% B. 20% to 30%
C. 40% to 70% D. 60% to 90%

46. With regard to appendicitis in immunocompromised patients, which of the following statements is false?

A. Immunocompromised patients with appendicitis often have a fever, a normal WBC count and nonspecific abdominal pain
B. Unusual infections such as those caused by mycobacteria protozoa and fungi do not usually mimic appendicitis
C. CT is particularly useful in immunocompromised patients
D. Typhlitis often mimics acute appendicitis

NEOPLASMS OF THE APPENDIX

47. True about appendiceal neoplasm is:

A. It is estimated that as many as 50% of appendiceal neoplasms present as appendicitis and are diagnosed on pathologic examination of the surgical specimen
B. Neoplasms arising from neuroendocrine cells from within the appendix and are detected in 0.2% to 0.7% of appendectomy specimens
C. Appendiceal neoplasms are thought to account for 0.4% to 1% of all gastrointestinal malignant neoplasms
D. All of the above

48. The most common primary tumor identified in the appendix is:

A. Carcinoids B. Adenocarcinoma
C. Mucinous tumors D. Small cell tumor

49. False about appendiceal neuroendocrine neoplasms (ANENs) is:

A. They are most commonly diagnosed in the 2nd or 3rd decade of life
B. The biologic behavior of ANENs is highly variable, and the prognosis subsequently depends greatly on the histologic type, malignant potential grade and stage at diagnosis
C. Size appears to be the best initial predictor of malignant behavior and metastatic potential
D. ANENs 3 cm or smaller are typically thought to behave in a benign manner and are most commonly treated with appendectomy with excision of the mesoappendix

50. True about treatment of appendiceal neuroendocrine neoplasms (ANENs) is/are:

A. For lesions between 1 and 2 cm in size, recommendations should be made after careful consideration of the individual tumor characteristics, as metastases have been reported in this subgroup of patients
B. ANENs larger than 2 cm are treated more aggressively, requiring right hemicolectomy and regional lymphadenectomy for adequate treatment
C. Attention should be given to the Ki-67 index (>3%), as a high proliferative index portends a worse prognosis and also warrants right hemicolectomy for proper staging and treatment
D. All of the above

51. True about Adenocarcinoma of appendix is/are:

A. Adenocarcinoma of the appendix is rare and occurs at a frequency of 0.08% to 0.1% of all appendectomies

B. Treatment is identical to that of cecal adenocarcinoma and consists of right hemicolectomy with regional lymphadenectomy
C. FOLFOX has also been used in the neoadjuvant setting in patients with mucinous adenocarcinoma before the implementation of cytoreductive (debulking) surgery
D. All of the above

52. **In staging of adenocarcinoma of the colon, the number of lymph nodes retrieved that may be associated with improved staging and subsequently improved survival is more than:**

A. 8
B. 10
C. 12
D. 16

53. **False about Mucinous tumors of the appendix is:**

A. Low-grade appendiceal mucinous neoplasms (AMNs) are often diagnosed incidentally at appendectomy
B. Mucinous appendiceal tumors, if ruptured, can result in intraperitoneal spread and the development of pseudomyxoma peritonei (PMP)
C. Patients with disseminated peritoneal adenomucinosis (DPAM) have an indolent course without distant extraperitoneal spread
D. Patients with peritoneal mucinous carcinomatosis (PMCA) are less likely to develop metastasis to lymph nodes and extraperitoneal organs, thus a good prognosis

54. **The most commonly used agent in HIPEC is:**

A. Cisplatin
B. Mitomycin C
C. Oxaliplatin
D. Methotrexate

55. **Which of the following is true regarding appendiceal carcinoid tumors?**

A. Carcinoid tumor is the second most common tumor of the appendix
B. For tumors greater than 2 cm, a formal right hemicolectomy is indicated
C. Carcinoid tumors arise from the smooth muscle within the appendiceal wall
D. All of the above

56. **A 25-year-old female underwent a laparoscopic appendectomy. On final pathology, he was found to have a 1.6-cm carcinoid tumor in the mid-appendix with direct extension to the mesoappendix, negative margins, and with lymphovascular invasion. What is the best treatment plan?**

A. No further treatment needed
B. Ileocecectomy
C. Right hemicolectomy
D. Medical treatment with octreotide

57. **A 35-year-old male undergoing appendicectomy was found to have a 3.4 cm mucocele. There was no involvement of the appendiceal base, no perforation. What is the appropriate line of treatment?**

A. Incisional biopsy with subsequent appendectomy if malignancy is confirmed by frozen section
B. Routine right hemicolectomy
C. Needle aspiration of cystic fluid for cytologic examination
D. Appendectomy

58. **During an exploratory laparotomy on a 46-year-old male with a small bowel obstruction, mucinous ascites is found throughout the abdomen along with a large cystic-appearing appendiceal mass. What is the most likely diagnosis?**

A. Malignant peritoneal mesothelioma
B. Appendiceal carcinoid tumor
C. Perforated acute appendicitis
D. Pseudomyxoma peritonei

ANSWERS

1. **Ans: D. All of the above**

   Ref: Chapter No.51, Page No.1301

2. **Ans: C. 8 weeks**

   Ref: Chapter No.51, Page No.1301

3. **Ans: D. Lymphoid tissue is found in the Muscularis mucosae of the appendix**

   Ref: Chapter No.51, Page No.1301

4. **Ans: C. Patients with the appendiceal tip in the midline pelvis may present with back or flank pain**

   Ref: Chapter No.51, Page No.1301-1302

5. **Ans: A. Retrocecal**

   Ref: Chapter No.51, Page No.1301

6. **Ans: C. Claudius Amyand**

   Ref: Chapter No.51, Page No.1302

7. **Ans: D All of the above**

   Ref: Chapter No.51, Page No.1302

8. **Ans: B. Infections associated with appendicitis should be considered monomicrobial**

   Ref: Chapter No.51, Page No.1302

9. **Ans: D. All of the above**

   Ref: Chapter No.51, Page No.1302

10. **Ans: D. All of the above**

    Ref: Chapter No.51, Page No.1302

11. **Ans: B. Typhlitis**

    Ref: Chapter No.51, Page No.1303

12. **Ans: C. Diarrhea may be present but constipation is not seen**

    Ref: Chapter No.51, Page No.1303

13. **Ans: B. Absence of fever excludes a diagnosis of appendicitis**

    Ref: Chapter No.51, Page No.1303

14. **Ans: C. Rovsing sign**

    Ref: Chapter No.51, Page No.1303

15. **Ans: B. Obturator sign**

    Ref: Chapter No.51, Page No.1303

16. **Ans: B. Pain with extension of the ipsilateral hip**

    Ref: Chapter No.51, Page No.1303

17. **Ans: C. Rectal examination findings show tenderness**

    Ref: Chapter No.51, Page No.1303

18. **Ans: A. C-reactive protein appears to provide the most sensitive of the biomarkers, and provides sufficient specificity to definitively diagnose appendicitis**

    Ref: Chapter No.51, Page No.1303

19. **Ans: C. Alvarado score of <4 was most useful in excluding a diagnosis of appendicitis (96% sensitive) and a higher score have high specificity in diagnosing appendicitis as the cause of the patient's abdominal pain**

    Ref: Chapter No.51, Page No.1303

20. **Ans: B. 15%**

    Ref: Chapter No.51, Page No.1303

21. **Ans: A. Escherichia coli**

    Ref: Chapter No.51, Page No.1302

22. **Ans: D. All of the above**

    Ref: Chapter No.51, Page No.1302

23. **Ans: B. 48 hours**

    Ref: Chapter No.51, Page No.1304

24. **Ans: A. 5%**

    Ref: Chapter No.51, Page No.1305

25. **Ans: C. The recommended CT imaging technique involves the administration of intravenous contrast and oral contrast**

    Ref: Chapter No.51, Page No.1305

26. **Ans: D. All of the above**

    Ref: Chapter No.51, Page No.1305

27. **Ans: D. If it is obtained in a pregnant woman, the study should be contrast MRI**

    Ref: Chapter No.51, Page No.1306

28. **Ans: B. Thickening (>5 mm)**

    Ref: Chapter No.51, Page No.1306

29. **Ans: D. Retrocecal over the psoas muscle**

    Ref: Chapter No.51, Page No.1303

30. **Ans: D. Obtain a magnetic resonance imaging (MRI) and proceed with an appendectomy if positive**

    Ref: Chapter No.51, Page No.1306

31. **Ans: B. Oblique muscle-splitting incision**

    Ref: Chapter No.51, Page No.1306

32. **Ans: C. Transverse incision**

    Ref: Chapter No.51, Page No.1306

33. **Ans: A. 1 preoperative dose**

Ref: Chapter No.51, Page No.1306

34. **Ans: D. Drains are routinely placed**

Ref: Chapter No.51, Page No.1306-1308

35. **Ans: B. 4 - 7 days**

Ref: Chapter No.51, Page No.1308

36. **Ans: B. 10% to 20%**

Ref: Chapter No.51, Page No.1308

37. **Ans: C. Schedule a colonoscopy and consider an interval appendectomy in 4-6 weeks (Rule out perforated tumors of the cecum in adults)**

Ref: Chapter No.51, Page No.1309

38. **Ans: A. In general, treatment for these patients is initially accomplished operatively**

Ref: Chapter No.51, Page No.1309

39. **Ans: B. The terminal 100 cm of ileum should be examined for a Meckel diverticulum and the serosa of the small bowel for any stigmata of Crohn's disease**

Ref: Chapter No.51, Page No.1309

40. **Ans: A. Exploration and appendectomy if no other pathology is found**

Ref: Chapter No.51, Page No.1309

41. **Ans: B. 50% of cases of appendicitis occur in the 1st trimester**

Ref: Chapter No.51, Page No.1313

42. **Ans: D. 50% to 60%**

Ref: Chapter No.51, Page No.1313

43. **Ans: B. 10%**

Ref: Chapter No.51, Page No.1314

44. **Ans: B. 6%**

Ref: Chapter No.51, Page No.1314

45. **Ans: C. 40% to 70%**

Ref: Chapter No.51, Page No.1314-1315

46. **Ans: B. Unusual infections such as those caused by mycobacteria, protozoa and fungi do not usually mimic appendicitis**

Ref: Chapter No.51, Page No.1315

47. **Ans: D. All of the above**

Ref: Chapter No.51, Page No.1315

48. **Ans: A. Carcinoids**

Ref: Chapter No.51, Page No.1315

49. **Ans: D. ANENs 3 cm or smaller are typically thought to behave in a benign manner and are most commonly treated with appendectomy with excision of the meso-appendix**

Ref: Chapter No.51, Page No.1315

50. **Ans: D. All of the above**

Ref: Chapter No.51, Page No.1315

51. **Ans: D. All of the above**

Ref: Chapter No.51, Page No.1315-1316

52. **Ans: C. 12**

Ref: Chapter No.51, Page No.1315

53. **Ans: D. Patients with peritoneal mucinous carcinomatosis (PMCA) are less likely to develop metastasis to lymph nodes and extraperitoneal organs, thus a good prognosis**

Ref: Chapter No.51, Page No.1316

54. **Ans: B. Mitomycin C**

Ref: Chapter No.51, Page No.1316

55. **Ans: B. For tumors greater than 2 cm, a formal right hemicolectomy is indicated**

Ref: Chapter No.51, Page No.1316

56. **Ans: C. Right hemicolectomy**

Ref: Chapter No.51, Page No.1317

57. **Ans: B. Routine right hemicolectomy**

Ref: Chapter No.51, Page No.1317

58. **Ans: D. Pseudomyxoma peritonei**

Ref: Chapter No.51, Page No.1316

52

Colon and Rectum

EMBRYOLOGY OF THE COLON AND RECTUM

1. **False about the embryology of colon is:**
   A. The dentate line marks the fusion of endodermal (hindgut) and ectodermal depression (proctodeum)
   B. The primitive gut tube is formed from the endodermal roof of the yolk sac
   C. Internal anal sphincter is formed by the posterior part of the cloacal sphincter
   D. Early in the development process, beginning in the 3rd week of gestation, the gut tube divides into three sections: the foregut, midgut and hindgut

2. **The foregut forms all except:**
   A. Distal duodenum
   B. Oral (buccopharyngeal) membrane
   C. Stomach
   D. Esophagus

3. **The midgut forms all except:**
   A. Right colon
   B. Proximal one third of the transverse colon
   C. Small intestine
   D. Distal part of the duodenum

4. **The foregut is supplied by:**
   A. Superior mesenteric artery (SMA)
   B. Celiac artery
   C. Inferior mesenteric artery (IMA)
   D. Gastroduodenal artery

5. **The midgut is supplied by:**
   A. Superior mesenteric artery (SMA)
   B. Celiac artery
   C. Inferior mesenteric artery (IMA)
   D. Gastroduodenal artery

6. **The hindgut part of the anal canal is supplied by:**
   A. Superior mesenteric artery (SMA)
   B. Celiac artery
   C. Inferior mesenteric artery (IMA)
   D. Gastroduodenal artery

7. **The lower third of anal canal is supplied by the:**
   A. External pudendal artery
   B. Internal pudendal artery
   C. Superior mesenteric artery (SMA)
   D. Inferior mesenteric artery (IMA)

ANATOMY OF THE COLON, RECTUM AND PELVIC FLOOR

8. **The cecum is the saccular beginning of the colon, with an average diameter of:**
   A. 2.5 cm B. 5 cm
   C. 7.5 cm D. 12.5 cm

9. **False about the anatomy of colon is:**
   A. The cecum has no mesentery and is completely covered with peritoneum and is therefore considered an intraperitoneal structure
   B. The cecum has a thick wall compared to the rest of the colon and considering its large diameter
   C. Patients with an abnormally mobile cecum and ascending colon, found in a small proportion of patients, can be predisposed to volvulus (torsion) or cecal bascule (intermittent anterior and superior folding of the cecum associated with obstructive symptoms)
   D. Although it is distensible, acute dilation of the cecum to a diameter of >12 cm, which can be measured on a plain abdominal radiograph, is associated with risk of ischemic necrosis and perforation of the bowel wall and should be treated promptly, usually with surgery

10. The site most likely to perforate in the presence of large bowel obstructions is:

A. Ileum B. Caecum
C. Sigmoid colon D. Descending colon

11. Length of vermiform appendix is:

A. 2 to 8 cm B. 4 to 6 cm
C. 8 to 10 cm D. 14 to 16 cm

12. The 2nd most common location of appendix is:

A. Pelvic position B. Retrocecal position
C. Subcecal position D. Preileal position

13. The most common location of appendix is:

A. Pelvic position B. Retrocecal position
C. Subcecal position D. Preileal position

14. True about the fold of Treves is:

A. The fold of Treves contains no sizable blood vessels
B. The bloodless fold of Treves extends from the antimesenteric border of the terminal ileum to the base of the appendix or the anterior surface of the mesoappendix, or to both areas
C. It is the only part of the ileum that has a fold on the antimesenteric side of the bowel, it can help in the recognition of the ileocecal region and the base of the appendix
D. All of the above

15. The ascending colon begins at the ileocecal junction and extends upward toward the hepatic flexure on the right side and is approximately:

A. 10 cm B. 15 cm
C. 20 cm D. 25 cm

16. The length of transverse colon is approximately:

A. 15 cm B. 30 cm
C. 45 cm D. 60 cm

17. The letter A in the image is:

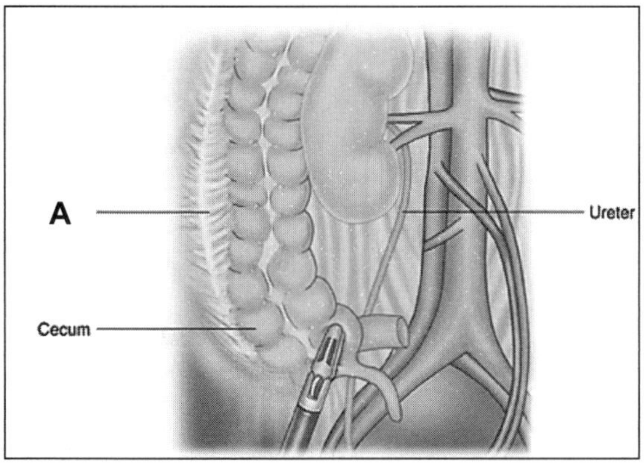

A. Avascular plane of Treves
B. Avascular plane of Toldt
C. Avascular plane of Reeve
D. Avascular plane of Brodel

18. False statement among the following is:

A. The greater omentum has 2 parts, the superior gastrocolic ligament composed of 4 serous layers, and the inferior portion, which is composed of 8 serous layers draping over the anterior abdominal cavity like an apron
B. The greater omentum's size and volume are highly variable, although in most cases correlated with body weight
C. Omentum provides a good patch, or reinforcement, in cases when closure of inflamed and friable tissues is not possible or likely to fail, such as in the treatment of perforated duodenal ulcer
D. Omental pedicle can be positioned between the rectum and vagina to buttress a colo- or rectovaginal fistula repair or used to fill the pelvic and perineal spaces after rectal excision

19. The splenic flexure is suspended by all of the following avascular ligaments except:

A. Splenocolic ligament to the lower pole of the spleen
B. Phrenicocolic ligament to the diaphragm
C. Gastrocolic ligament to the body of stomach
D. Renocolic ligament to the Gerota fascia

20. False statement among the following is:

A. The descending colon begins at the splenic flexure where the intestine loses its mesentery and extends downward on the left side of the abdomen approximately 25 cm until it transitions into the sigmoid colon
B. The descending colon is similar to the ascending colon with regard to its peritoneal coverage and approach to dissection
C. The sigmoid is thinner and more mobile compared to the descending colon varying in length from 15 to 50 cm
D. The mobile portion of the sigmoid colon is attached by the sigmoid mesocolon to the posterior abdominal wall and pelvis in the pattern of an inverted V creating the intersigmoid fossa

21. SMA is the 2nd unpaired anterior branch of the aorta, arising at the level of the:

A. Upper border of the L1 vertebra

B. Lower border of the L1 vertebra
C. Lower border of the L2 vertebra
D. Upper border of the L3 vertebra

22. The right colic artery is absent in up to:

A. 10% B. 20%
C. 40% D. 60%

23. The IMA is the 3rd unpaired anterior artery arising from the aorta at the level of the:

A. L1–2 vertebrae B. L2–3 vertebrae
C. L3–4 vertebrae D. L4–5 vertebrae

24. The letter A in the image shown below denotes:

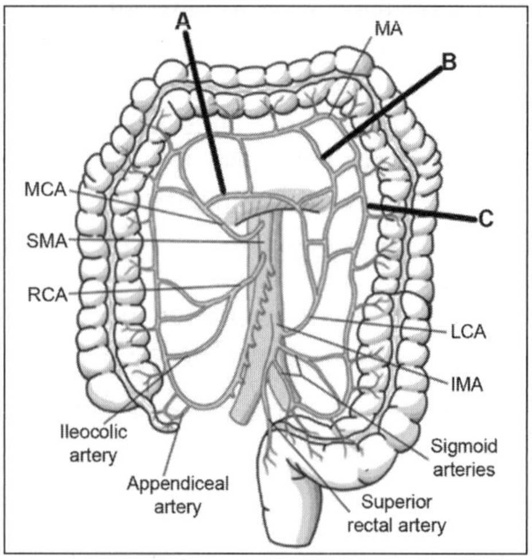

A. Marginal artery of Drummond
B. The artery of Percheron
C. The Moskowitz artery
D. The artery of Adamkiewicz

25. The letter C in the image shown below denotes:

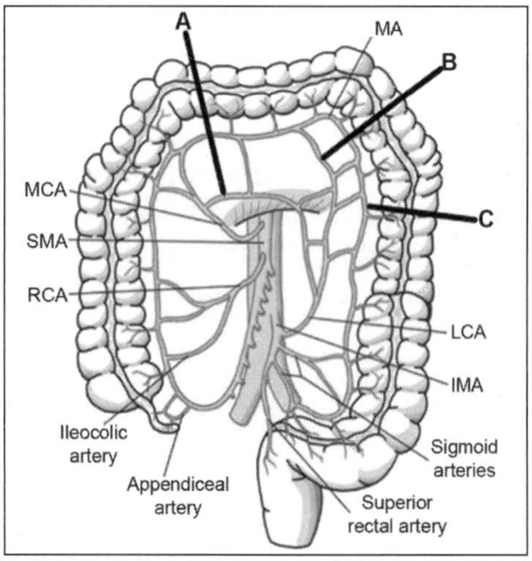

A. Marginal artery of Drummond
B. The recurrent artery of Heubner
C. The artery of Percheron
D. The artery of Adamkiewicz

26. False about rectal anatomy is:

A. The rectum with a total length of around 15 to 20 cm is divided into thirds based on its peritoneal relationships
B. The middle third of the rectum is totally extraperitoneal, extending from 1 to 5 cm above the dentate line
C. The anterior peritoneal reflection between the rectum and anterior structures, the rectovesical pouch in males and rectouterine or Douglas pouch in females, is 7 to 9 cm from the anal verge in men and 5 to 7.5 cm in women
D. The rectum has three lateral curves or valves of Houston, the proximal and distal valves fold to the right and the middle to the left

27. The 3 lateral curves or valves of Houston are lost after full surgical mobilization of the rectum, providing an additional length approximately:

A. 2 cm B. 5 cm
C. 8 cm D. 12 cm

28. The letter B in the image denotes:

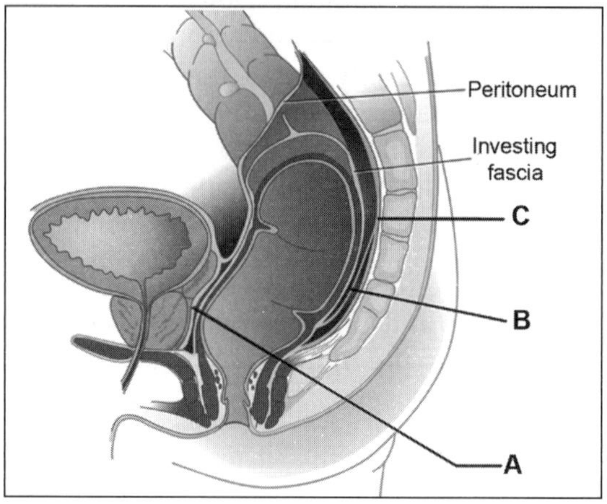

A. Presacral fascia B. Denonvilliers fascia
C. Waldeyer fascia D. Pouch of Douglas

29. The letter C in the image denotes:

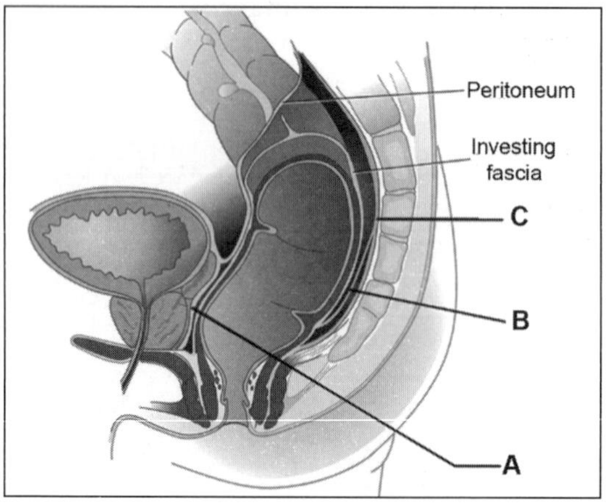

A. Presacral fascia
B. Denonvilliers fascia
C. Rectosacral fascia
D. Pouch of Douglas

30. False about the arterial supply of rectum is:

A. The blood supply to the rectum is derived from the superior, middle and inferior rectal (hemorrhoidal) arteries
B. The superior rectal artery is the end branch of the IMA
C. The middle rectal arteries are paired vessels derived from the internal iliac arteries to the lower rectum through the lateral columns
D. The inferior rectal arteries are branches of the external pudendal arteries

31. True about the lymphatic drainage of rectum is:

A. The lymph from the upper two thirds of the rectum drains upward toward the inferior mesenteric and paraaortic nodes
B. Below the dentate line, lymph drains toward the inguinal lymph nodes
C. The lower part of the rectum drains in 2 directions, cephalad toward the inferior mesenteric nodes and laterally and inferiorly toward the internal iliac nodes
D. All of the above

32. False about the nerve supply of rectum is:

A. A high IMA ligation injuring the superior hypogastric plexus or severing the hypogastric nerves near the sacral promontory may result in sympathetic dysfunction characterized by retrograde ejaculation in men
B. The sympathetic innervation of the rectum is derived from sympathetic nerves exiting at the level of L4–5, forming the superior hypogastric plexus
C. Division of the lateral stalks too close to the pelvic sidewall may injure the pelvic plexus and nervi erigentes and cause erectile dysfunction, impotence and atonic bladder
D. Left and right hypogastric nerves supply the rectum and send branches to supply the genitourinary system anteriorly

33. With regard to the anatomy of the colon and rectum, which of the following statements is true?

A. The colon has a complete outer longitudinal and an incomplete inner circular muscle layer
B. The haustra are separated by plicae circulares
C. The ascending colon and descending colon are usually fixed to the retroperitoneum
D. The rectum is totally invested by three complete muscle layers

PHYSIOLOGY OF THE COLON

34. Which of the following statements is true regarding colon physiology?

A. Transit time through the colon is independent of the fermentability of nonstarch polysaccharides such as lignin, cellulose and pectins
B. The left colon is the segment of colon where bacteria are the most metabolically active in the fermentation process. The right colon is the site of storage and dehydration of stool
C. Fifty percent of the daily energy expenditure is obtained from the absorption of short-chain fatty acids by the colon; this energy is used to stimulate blood flow, regulate the pH of the colonic environment and renew colonic mucosal cells
D. Butyrate, an SCFA, is the principal source of nutrition for the colonocyte

35. False about the physiology of colon is:

A. The body has the ability to adapt and sustain life without a colon
B. Succus in the ileum has a sodium concentration of 200 mEq/L that is reduced to approximately 30 mEq/L in rectal stool
C. Colon has the ability to absorb up to 2 L of fluid per day
D. By surface area, the colon is the most efficient site of absorption in the GI tract

36. Percentage of the fluid in succus that is reabsorbed in the colon is approximately:

A. 30% B. 50%
C. 70% D. 90%

37. Total volume of water in stool is:

A. ~50 mL/day B. ~150 mL/day
C. ~250 mL/day D. ~500 mL/day

38. False about the physiology of colon is:

A. Aldosterone decreases colonic potassium secretion and this effect is blocked by spironolactone
B. Potassium chloride and bicarbonate are actively secreted into the lumen

C. Some forms of colitis impairs colonic absorption or produce secretion of chloride, such as collagenous and microscopic colitis and congenital chloridorrhea

D. In colon, sodium and chloride are actively absorbed via Na^+/H^+, Na^+/K^+, and Cl^-/HCO_3^- exchange

39. True statement is/are:

A. Colonic bacteria are rich in urease, which is important for urea recycling

B. When the liver cannot reuse the urea nitrogen absorbed by the colon, ammonia crosses the blood-brain barrier and produces "false" neurotransmitters, which results in hepatic coma

C. Antibiotics and lactulose decrease the amount of ammonia absorbed by lowering the concentration of bacteria and reducing the pH, respectively

D. All of the above

40. False about bile salts and colon is:

A. When the colonic absorptive capacity is exceeded, colonic bacteria conjugate bile acids

B. Choleretic diarrhea is seen early after right hemicolectomy as a transient phenomenon and more permanently after extensive ileal resection

C. The colon absorbs bile acids that escape absorption by the terminal ileum

D. Bile acids are passively transported across the colonic epithelium by non-ionic diffusion

41. Large bowel contents have a concentration of bacterial cells/gram:

A. 10^4 to 10^5 bacterial cells/gram

B. 10^7 to 10^8 bacterial cells/gram

C. 10^9 to 10^{10} bacterial cells/gram

D. 10^{11} to 10^{12} bacterial cells/gram

42. Bacterial cells contribute around:

A. 30% of fecal mass B. 50% of fecal mass

C. 70% of fecal mass D. 90% of fecal mass

43. False about dietary fiber and colon is:

A. The main source of energy for intestinal bacteria is dietary fiber, composed of complex carbohydrates

B. Dietary recommendations (i.e., "adding fiber") generally refer to bulking agents, such as lignin and psyllium, which are nonabsorbable and nonfermentable by colonic bacteria

C. Antibiotics disrupt cohabitation of bacterial flora, and decreased bacteria leads to less butyrate, which, in turn, negatively affects colonocyte function leading to diarrhea

D. Bulking agents decrease intracolonic pressures and decrease colonic transit time

44. False about SCFAs and colon is:

A. Butyrate may also play an important role in maintaining cellular health by arresting the proliferation of neoplastic colonocytes while paradoxically being trophic for normal colonocytes

B. Besides butyrate; acetate and propionate, are produced in the colon, with acetate being the most common of all 3

C. The production of acetate is reduced by nonabsorbable, nonfermentable dietary fiber, such as psyllium, which in turn has a beneficial effect on cholesterol levels

D. < 50% of the SCFAs produced are absorbed

45. In flatus, the gases produced by bacterial fermentation compose approximately:

A. 30% B. 50%

C. 70% D. 90%

46. False about probiotics and prebiotics is:

A. Probiotics can be defined as dietary supplements that contain live cultures of bacteria and/or yeast that are beneficial to colonic and host function

B. Probiotics may have widespread health benefits, including stimulation of immune function, anti-inflammatory effects, and suppression of enteropathogenic colonization

C. Prebiotics are digestible oligosaccharides that help the host by stimulating the growth of certain species of beneficial intestinal bacteria

D. Prebiotics are nutrients that support the growth of probiotic bacteria

47. False about colonic motility is:

A. Parasympathetic innervation is excitatory, and it reaches the colon via the vagus nerve and the rectum via the sacral nerves (S2–S4) through the pelvic plexus

B. Sympathetic fibers originate from lumber ventral roots (L2–L5), postganglionic hypogastric nerves, and the splanchnic nerves (T5–T12), which reach the colon and rectum through perivascular plexuses

C. High-amplitude propagated contractions (HAPCs) allow mixing, which promotes optimal absorption and are bursts of short-duration contractions
D. The interstitial cells of Cajal are the primary pacemaker cells governing the function of the enteric nervous system and are important for colonic motility

48. False about the physiology of defecation is:

A. Colonic transit is longer in men than in men and longer in postmenopausal than in premenopausal women
B. Supplementation with nonstarch polysaccharides shortens colonic transit time in individuals with idiopathic constipation
C. Normal defecation requires adequate colonic transit time, stool consistency and fecal continence
D. All of the above are true

PREOPERATIVE EVALUATION

49. True about preoperative bowel preparation is:

A. Mechanical bowel preparation combined with preoperative oral antibiotics is typically recommended for elective colorectal resections
B. Preoperative mechanical bowel preparation alone, without oral antibiotics, is generally not recommended for patients undergoing elective colorectal surgery
C. Preoperative oral antibiotics alone, without mechanical preparation, are generally not recommended for patients undergoing elective colorectal surgery
D. Preoperative enemas alone, without mechanical bowel preparation and oral antibiotics, are generally recommended for patients undergoing elective colorectal surgery

50. True about bowel stomas is:

A. Transverse loop colostomies should seldom be used, as they are large, very prone to prolapse, and can be difficult to maintain pouch adherence, frequently being located in an area around the patient's belt line or mid-upper abdomen
B. Loop ileostomies are often chosen for temporary diversion due to their lack of odor, ease of care and ease of closing
C. Loop descending or sigmoid colostomies can easily be closed
D. All of the above

51. Boundaries of "ostomy triangle" are all except:

A. Umbilicus
B. Pubic tubercle
C. Xiphisternum
D. Anterior superior iliac spine

52. False about colostomy is:

A. In obese individuals, the thickest part of the abdominal wall is often in the upper abdomen and hence colostomies should be created in upper abdomen
B. In constructing an end colostomy, typically it does not need to protrude > 0.5 to 1 cm above the level of the abdominal skin
C. Typically, create an aperture that will admit 2 fingers is adequate
D. Ascending colostomies tend to have a higher amount of liquid effluent, while descending and left-sided colostomies are usually preferable

53. True about ileostomies is:

A. Ileostomies are generally favored by colorectal surgeons for fecal diversion as they are easier to construct, especially in obese individuals
B. Ileostomy will empty continuously and has a high rate of associated chemical dermatitis due to the more alkaline pH associated with small bowel effluent as opposed to the stool of the colon
C. Ileostomy effluent usually has no odor, in contrast to colostomy effluent, which usually has odor associated with colonic flora
D. All of the above

54. Prior to hospital discharge, one should ensure that the 24-hour stoma output is:

A. < 5000 mL
B. < 1000 mL
C. < 1500 mL
D. < 2000 mL

ENHANCED RECOVERY PROTOCOLS

55. Which of the following is NOT a principle of Enhanced Recovery After Surgery (ERAS) protocols in colorectal surgery?

A. Multimodal analgesia
B. Hypothermia
C. Minimizing perioperative starvation
D. Early postoperative ambulation

56. Risk of developing a SSI postoperatively in Colorectal surgery patients is upto:

A. 5%
B. 10%
C. 20%
D. 40%

57. False about ERAS protocol is:

A. These protocols, also called fast-track or enhanced recovery after surgery protocols, have been shown to reduce complications, length of stay and cost of care without increasing readmission rates

B. Ostomy creation is an independent risk factor for increased postoperative length of stay and structured education has been shown to mitigate this risk

C. There is strong evidence to support the recommendation of a clear liquid diet up until 4 hours before the induction of anesthesia

D. Minimizing opioids is associated with earlier return of bowel function and shorter length of stay

58. The most common reason for readmission after an ileostomy creation is:

A. Skin irritation
B. Prolapse
C. Ischemic stricture
D. Dehydration

DIVERTICULAR DISEASE

59. False about Diverticular disease is:

A. The rectum is generally affected

B. The vast majority of diverticula in the colon are "false" diverticula (pulsion, pseudodiverticula), containing only the mucosa and muscularis mucosa

C. Diverticula are classically formed on the mesenteric side of the colonic wall in regions where vasa recta traverse through the muscular layer to provide blood to the mucosa

D. Diverticula are saccular outpouchings of the bowel wall

60. False about Diverticular disease is:

A. Intake of nuts, seeds and popcorn does not appear to increase the risk

B. Colonic diverticula are noted in approximately 40% of individuals between the ages of 50 and 60 years and in over 60% of individuals over the age of 80 years

C. > 25% of patients with diverticulosis will develop diverticulitis

D. Western dietary patterns high in red meat, fat, and refined grains are associated with an increased risk of the disease, whereas increased fiber intake, with abundant fruit, vegetables and whole grains, reduces the risk of diverticulitis

61. Adherence to a low-risk lifestyle could prevent the incident diverticulitis by:

A. 30%
B. 50%
C. 70%
D. 90%

62. Low-risk lifestyle changes for diverticular disease are all except:

A. 2 hours of vigorous activity per week

B. < 4 servings of red meat per week

C. History of smoking

D. Atleast 23 g of fiber per day

63. False about clinical evaluation of diverticular disease is:

A. Diverticular disease can manifest as diverticulitis, but it is also the most common reason for severe lower GI bleeding

B. Rectal bleeding is a common in the presentation of acute diverticulitis

C. Fever, change in bowel habits, anorexia and urinary urgency (in cases where the bladder is secondarily inflamed) are frequent

D. Signs and symptoms will generally result from the pericolonic inflammation

64. True about imaging of diverticular disease is:

A. Signs of diverticulitis on CT include the presence of diverticula, colonic wall thickening, pericolic fat stranding and abscess formation

B. Contrast studies, ultrasound and magnetic resonance imaging (MRI) have also been used, but currently, computed tomography (CT) has become the most useful examination to confirm the diagnosis, exclude other diagnoses and classify the severity of the disease

C. CT studies have the capacity to localize abscesses and fistulas and define the extent of the disease

D. CT scan has the ability to distinguish between grade 3 and grade 4

65. A patient has with diverticular disease with confined pericolic abscess on CT. As per Modified Hinchey classification system it is:

A. Stage Ia
B. Stage Ib
C. Stage II
D. Stage III

66. A patient has with diverticular disease with generalized purulent peritonitis. As per Modified Hinchey classification system it is:

A. Stage Ib
B. Stage II
C. Stage III
D. Stage IV

67. A patient has with diverticular disease has phlegmon on CT scan. As per Modified Hinchey classification system it is:

A. Stage Ia
B. Stage Ib
C. Stage II
D. Stage III

68. False about the management of complicated diverticulitis is:

A. In case of diverticulitis patients with fistulas; Cystoscopy will usually disclose inflammation at the site of the fistula
B. Fistulas to the small bowel will characteristically require resection and primary anastomosis
C. Patients with abscesses amenable to percutaneous drainage and responsive to treatment still require urgent surgery
D. In the case of the bladder, with small fistula openings, drainage of the bladder with a Foley catheter for 7 to 10 days will usually allow for healing

69. The most common type of fistula in diverticular disease is a:

A. Colovaginal fistula
B. Colovesical fistula
C. Colocutaneous fistula
D. Coloureteral fistula

70. False about diverticular disease and obstruction is:

A. Patients with recurrent and chronic diverticulitis can develop fibrosis of the colonic wall, leading to stricture formation
B. It is not important, prior to resection, to perform a colonoscopy
C. Patients with a complete obstruction unresponsive to therapy will require emergency surgery
D. Patients with a partial obstruction can usually be initially treated with a nasogastric tube for decompression, antibiotics, fluids and bowel rest

71. True about perforation in diverticular disease is:

A. Up to 50% of patients will never be reversed after Hartmann procedure
B. The mainstay of treatment in these cases has traditionally been the Hartmann procedure
C. Hinchey grades 3 and 4 are considered a surgical emergency
D. All of the above

72. False about the management of uncomplicated diverticulitis is:

A. The mainstay of treatment is based on pain medications, short-term alteration of diet and antibiotics
B. Upon recovery, it is recommended that patients undergo a colonoscopy after 4 to 8 weeks to exclude malignancy
C. Following the initial episode of acute, uncomplicated diverticulitis, 50% to 65% of individuals will have another episode
D. The aim of elective surgery is to remove the affected segment of the colon (usually the sigmoid colon) and to perform a primary anastomosis of the healthy remaining bowel

73. False about right-sided diverticulitis is:

A. It typically affects younger patients and may be challenging to diagnose as signs and symptoms are very similar to those of acute appendicitis
B. Patients who have recurrent episodes or complicated disease and patients with an uncertain diagnosis should be considered for resection with a right hemicolectomy
C. Differential diagnoses to be considered include Meckel's diverticulitis, cholecystitis, ischemic colitis, mesenteric adenitis, pyelonephritis and pelvic inflammatory disease
D. It is common in western countries but rare in the Asian countries

74. False about immunocompromised patients with diverticulitis is:

A. Immunocompromised patients who require emergency surgery and resection should probably not undergo primary anastomosis at the initial surgery because of their impaired immune system and healing
B. The prevalence of diverticulitis in these patients is more compared to the general population
C. Immunocompromised patients include transplant patients; patients with diabetes mellitus, renal failure, or cirrhosis; and patients being treated with systemic steroids and/or chemotherapy
D. Because of this risk, there should be a lower threshold for resection after a single attack of diverticulitis

75. Cecal diverticula are different from sigmoid diverticula in that:

A. Sigmoid diverticula are true diverticula while cecal diverticula are false diverticula

B. Cecal diverticulitis is usually distinguishable from cancer
C. Cecal diverticula are considered congenital in origin
D. Asymptomatic cecal diverticula found on barium enema or colonoscopy should be treated operatively because of the high incidence of complications

76. Which of the following is the most common cause of massive colonic bleeding?

A. CRC
B. Ulcerative colitis
C. Diverticulosis
D. Ischemic colitis

77. Which of the following is the least appropriate operative strategy for a patient presenting with sigmoid diverticulitis and localized peritonitis?

A. Total colectomy
B. Sigmoid colectomy with primary anastomosis and diverting ileostomy
C. Sigmoid colectomy with end colostomy and rectal stump
D. Drainage and ileostomy without resection

78. A 55-year-old man presents with left lower quadrant (LLQ) abdominal pain of 2-day duration, associated with constipation. On physical examination, he has tenderness localized to the LLQ with fullness in that area leukocyte count is 22,000 and temperature is 101.5°F. Which would be the best diagnostic study to evaluate this man?

A. Plain abdominal roentgenogram
B. Diagnostic laparoscopy
C. Computed tomography (CT) of the abdomen/pelvis with orally and intravenous (IV) contrast
D. Barium enema

79. Enteric fistulas may be a complication of diverticulitis. Which of the following statements is true?

A. Colocutaneous fistulas frequently occur spontaneously
B. Suspected colovesical fistulas are best confirmed with barium enema
C. Pneumaturia and faecaluria may also be present
D. Surgical correction of enteric fistulas is best accomplished in stages

80. Complications of diverticulitis include:

A. Carcinoma of the colon
B. Extraintestinal manifestations such as arthritis, iritis and skin rashes
C. Fistulisation to adjacent organs such as the bladder, with colovesical fistula
D. Arteriovenous fistulae of the intestine

81. A patient's CT scan reveals diverticulitis confined to the sigmoid colon. There is no associated pericolic abscess. What is best course of treatment?

A. Urgent surgical resection
B. Steroids
C. Bowel rest, nasogastric suction, IV fluids and broad spectrum antibiotics
D. Diverting colostomy

82. A 55-year-old woman presents with pain in the LLQ of the abdomen and fever of 102°F. On examination, she is found to be dehydrated and has tenderness in the LLQ. A CT scan shows a mass in the LLQ involving the sigmoid colon. There is a minimal amount of free fluid and no free air. What should the initial treatment of this patient include?

A. IV fluids, cefoxitin and nasogastric drainage
B. Immediate laparotomy
C. IV fluids, blood transfusion and laparotomy
D. IV fluids, penicillin and steroids

LARGE BOWEL OBSTRUCTION

83. False about Large bowel obstruction is:

A. The most common etiology of mechanical obstruction in the United States is colorectal cancer (CRC)
B. Large bowel obstruction, defined as bowel obstruction distal to the ligament of Treitz
C. Any portion of the colon that is not fixed to the retroperitoneum and that has an elongated mesentery has the potential for volvulus
D. Colonic volvulus is more common in Russia, Eastern Europe, Africa, the Middle East and India

84. The most common site of volvulus is the:

A. Sigmoid colon
B. Caecum
C. Transverse colon
D. Ascending colon

85. True about Large bowel obstruction is:

A. Closed-loop obstruction is commonly encountered in cases such as volvulus and strangulated hernias

B. Mechanical obstruction will generally present with increased peristalsis and low-grade colicky pain, but late, long-lasting obstruction may have decreased bowel sounds

C. Acute obstructions tend to present more dramatically with rapid onset of pain, distension, and abdominal tenderness, whereas patients with progressive obstruction may present with increasing constipation, pencil-thin stools and intermittent abdominal pain

D. All of the above

86. False about large bowel obstruction is:

A. The colonic gas originates both from swallowed air (around two thirds) and bacterial fermentation

B. Although most malignant obstructions occur in the proximal parts of the colon, the necrosis and perforation usually occur in the sigmoid colon

C. In incarcerated hernias and volvulus, pressure on the mesentery can compromise the blood supply initially obstructing venous return, and with increasing edema and inflammation, eventually occluding the arterial blood supply

D. Plain films of the abdomen can help in localizing the obstruction, demonstrating the degree of distension as well as the status of the ileocecal valve

87. False about diagnosis of large bowel obstruction is:

A. Digital rectal examination should be performed to inspect for neoplasms and for the presence of fecal impaction

B. Water-soluble and IV contrast-enhanced CT scans provide significant information revealing the location and etiology of the obstruction such as diverticulitis, IBD and extraluminal causes

C. CT can also provide clues regarding tissue ischemia and impending perforation

D. Plain films of the abdomen can help in localizing the obstruction, but does not demonstrate the degree of distension as well as the status of the ileocecal valve

88. Identify the typical sign in the given image:

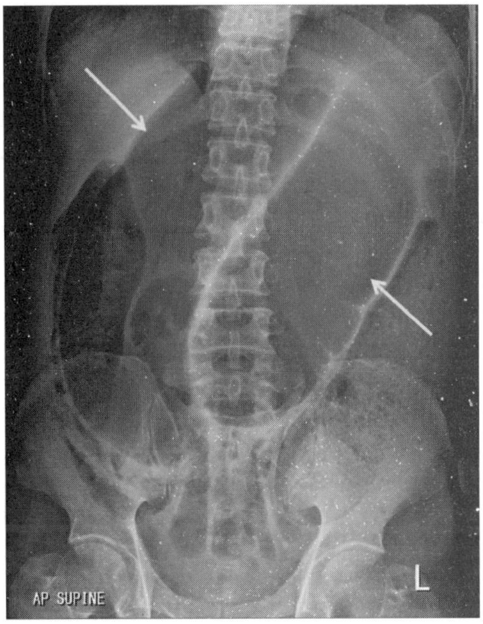

A. Coffee bean sign

B. Bent inner tube appearance

C. Kidney bean sign

D. All of the above

89. A 60-year-old otherwise healthy woman presents to the emergency department for acute onset of lower abdominal pain with associated nausea and emesis. Her previous surgical history includes a total hysterectomy. On examination, she is distended and peritonitic. Her vitals show tachycardia and hypotension, and lab results show bicarb of 14 and lactic acid of 4.8. The emergency department has the following CT plate to interpret. What is the diagnosis?

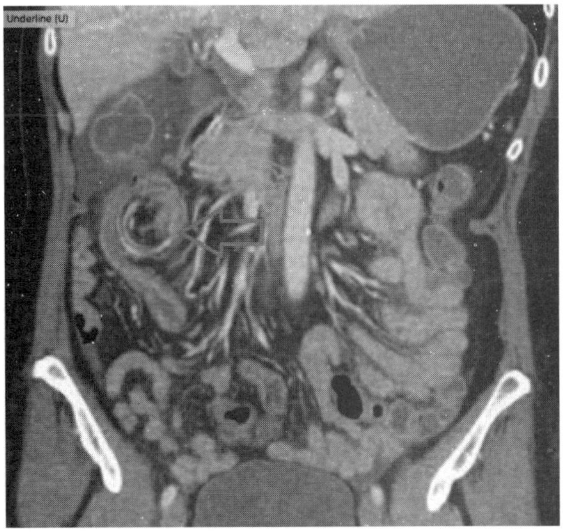

A. Caecal volvulus
B. Sigmoid volvulus
C. Pseudo obstruction
D. Sigmoid cancer

90. What is the optimal therapy for the patient in Q.89?

A. Subtotal colectomy with end ileostomy
B. Right hemicolectomy and primary anastomosis with or without diverting ileostomy
C. Intraoperative decompression followed by subtotal colectomy
D. Laparotomy, detorsion and cecostomy tube

91. True about the treatment of sigmoid volvulus is:

A. In patients with sigmoid volvulus, endoscopic decompression is often successful using either a rigid or flexible sigmoidoscope with placement of a rectal tube proximal to the point of torsion
B. If decompression is unsuccessful, patients require surgery with resection, colostomy and a Hartmann procedure
C. If decompression is successful, elective sigmoid resection with primary anastomosis should be performed due to the high rate of recurrence
D. All of the above

92. False about the treatment of large bowel obstruction is:

A. Hernias causing mechanical large bowel obstruction usually require surgery
B. Foreign bodies can usually be removed via surgery
C. Patients with obstruction as a result of active IBD will commonly respond initially to steroids
D. Paracolic abscesses can be drained percutaneously

93. Which statement is false regarding sigmoid volvulus?

A. Sigmoid volvulus is commonly seen in patients who are elderly, debilitated, chronically constipated, or on psychotropic medications
B. Mortality rates are lower when emergent decompression is performed before sigmoid resection
C. Nonoperative reduction of sigmoid volvulus is successful in 70%–80% of cases
D. If the gangrenous bowel is seen during decompression, a rectal tube should be placed to prevent recurrence

94. Which of the following is not a type of cecal volvulus?

A. An axial volvulus from clockwise twisting where the torsed cecum remains in the right lower quadrant
B. Upward folding of the cecum
C. Downward folding of the cecum
D. A torsion of the cecum and a portion of the terminal ileum resulting in a displacement of the cecum out of the right lower quadrant

95. A 65-year-old woman with a history of chronic constipation is transferred from a nursing home because of abdominal pain and marked abdominal distention. On examination, her abdomen is found to be distended and tender in the LLQ. What is the most likely diagnosis?

A. Appendicitis
B. Carcinoma of the colon
C. Volvulus of the sigmoid colon
D. Volvulus of the cecum

96. An elderly nursing home patient is brought to the hospital with recent onset of colicky abdominal pain, distension and obstipation on examination, the abdomen is markedly distended and tympanitic. There is no marked tenderness. Plain abdominal X-ray shows a markedly distended loop located mainly in the right upper quadrant. The likely diagnosis is:

A. Gallstone ileus
B. Sigmoid volvulus
C. Mesenteric vascular occlusion
D. Small-bowel obstruction

97. The standard initial therapy for acute sigmoid volvulus is:

A. Colonoscopy
B. Laparotomy to reduce the volvulus and replace the sigmoid colon to its normal position
C. IV neostigmine
D. Rigid sigmoidoscopy

COLONIC PSEUDO-OBSTRUCTION

98. False about colonic pseudo-obstruction is:

A. Dysregulation of the colonic autonomic innervation is hypothesized to play an important part
B. It is most commonly encountered among elderly and comorbid patients, classically following an acute illness on a background of neurologic, cardiac, or respiratory diseases
C. Systemic toxicity and peritoneal signs are common
D. It is characterized by acute colonic dilatation in the absence of a mechanical obstruction

99. Conditions associated with pseudo-obstruction include all except:

A. Hypertension
B. Diabetes mellitus
C. Solid organ transplants
D. Cytomegalovirus

100. Drugs associated with pseudo-obstruction include all except:

A. Anticholinergics
B. Oral hypoglycemic agents
C. Anti-Parkinson drugs
D. Opiates

101. False about the diagnosis of pseudo-obstruction is:

A. The presenting symptoms of the condition commonly include abdominal distension, pain, nausea and vomiting
B. A water-soluble contrast enema can't reliably distinguish between a mechanical obstruction and pseudo-obstruction
C. Plain abdominal radiographs typically demonstrate a distended colon, with the largest diameter usually encountered in the cecum and right colon, which can reach 10 to 12 cm in diameter
D. Lack of intestinal contractility is often associated with decreased or absent bowel sounds, but high-pitched, tinkling bowel sounds may also be encountered

102. Signs that may be indicative of colon ischemia, perforation, or impending perforation are all except:

A. Cecal dilation > 10 cm
B. Fever
C. Abdominal tenderness
D. Leukocytosis

103. False about the management of colonic pseudo-obstruction is:

A. Osmotic and stimulant laxatives should be tried as first line of management
B. Nonoperative, supportive care is initiated for patients with a cecal diameter that is < 12 cm without evidence of ischemia or perforation
C. In cases that do not improve with supportive care or with a cecal diameter of > 12 cm, but without systemic toxicity and abdominal tenderness, colonic decompression is indicated
D. Ambulation, prone positioning and knee-chest position to encourage passage of flatus can assist

104. False about the management of colonic pseudo-obstruction is:

A. Success rates for neostigmine treatment range from 60% to 94%, with recurrences observed in up to 31% of patients, with some patients requiring multiple drug administration
B. Neostigmine is the keystone of pharmacologic decompression therapy
C. Neostigmine is given as a 2 to 2.5 mg IV bolus injected over 3 to 5 minutes and results in significant parasympathetic stimulation causing strong colonic peristalsis that usually leads to subsequent flatus and bowel movements
D. Colonoscopic decompression should not be considered in patients with contraindications to neostigmine

INFLAMMATORY BOWEL DISEASE

105. False about IBD is:

A. The prevalence of IBD in Western countries is approximately 0.5% of the general population
B. Over 10% of patients with IBD have a family history of IBD
C. In Crohn's disease, smoking tends to suppress symptoms, whereas in UC, smoking tends to exacerbate symptoms
D. Antibiotic use in early life has also been thought to predispose to IBD, as has NSAID use

106. False about the clinical presentation of IBD is:

A. Diarrhea can be a presenting symptom in both diseases; however, this is typically more prevalent and severe in UC, where the diarrhea is characteristically blood
B. Roughly 25% of patients with UC will have associated perianal disease
C. Typical UC symptoms also include tenesmus and urgency as well as associated anemia
D. In Crohn's disease, symptoms of abdominal pain may predominate

107. False about extraintestinal manifestations of IBD is:

A. Arthritis is by far the most common extra-intestinal manifestation
B. Sclerosing cholangitis is estimated to affect approximately 50% of patients with IBD

C. Ankylosing spondylitis patients are HLA-B27 positive and may present in advanced cases with decreased cervical flexion, which has important anesthetic implications for intubation

D. It is estimated that up to half of IBD patients will have 1 or more extraintestinal manifestations

108. Which of the following scoring systems is used for endoscopic assessment of UC?

A. Barcelona Clinic Scoring System
B. Paris Clinic Scoring System
C. Tokyo Clinic Scoring System
D. Mayo Clinic Scoring System

109. As per Mayo Clinic Scoring System, a lesion that bleeds on touch is:

A. Grade 1 B. Grade 2
C. Grade 3 D. Grade 4

110. As per Mayo Clinic Scoring System, a lesion with significant bleeding and friability is:

A. Grade 1 B. Grade 2
C. Grade 3 D. Grade 4

111. False about endoscopic diagnosis of Crohn's disease is:

A. Crohn's disease ulcers are worse on the anti-mesenteric side of the bowel
B. Crohn's disease is more characterized by deeper punched-out appearing ulcerations
C. Crohn's disease can also affect the small bowel or upper GI tract
D. Regarding the distribution of Crohn's disease, the most common site of involvement in nearly half of patients is ileocolic, followed by colonic involvement

112. False about histologic evaluation of IBD is:

A. As a rule, inflammation in UC is restricted to the surface epithelium
B. In patients with UC, term "focal active enteritis" is used
C. In contrast, in patients with Crohn's disease, there is often transmural inflammation
D. In UC, colonic mucosal biopsies will typically show significant inflammation with the presence of multiple polymorphonuclear leukocytes within the lamina propria

113. Number of patients with IBD undetermined class are up to:

A. 5% - 10% B. 10% - 15%
C. 20% - 25% D. 35% - 50%

114. False about Aminosalicylates used in IBD is:

A. This medication is most effective for severe disease
B. Mesalamine (Pentasa) begins to dissolve in the stomach and releases drug throughout the GI tract, whereas Asacol begins to be released in the terminal ileum by means of a pH-dependent mechanism and coats the entire colon
C. The same medication in small-volume enema form (Rowasa enemas) can be administered also at bedtime
D. Suppository formulations are administered at bedtime

115. True about steroid use in IBD is:

A. Steroids are usually started at a high dose and then tapered quickly
B. In the outpatient setting, pulse therapy is usually given in the form of prednisone at doses starting at 40 to 60 mg/day, tapering by 5 to 10 mg at 2-week intervals until 10 mg/day is reached and then tapering by 5 mg every 2 weeks, at which time the drug is discontinued
C. In the hospital setting, 100 mg of hydrocortisone can be given intravenously every 6 to 8 hours depending on disease severity
D. All of the above

116. False about Immunomodulators used in IBD is:

A. When methotrexate is given, patients require folic acid supplementation
B. Thiopurine intramuscular dosing is particularly convenient in patients who have problems with significant diarrhea or absorption issues (e.g., short bowel syndrome)
C. Long-term thiopurine use is also associated with a higher risk of developing non-Hodgkin lymphoma than the general population
D. Thiopurines are a "steroid-sparing" class of medication that are usually begun once patients are placed on steroids and perhaps have been unsuccessful in weaning off steroids after 1 or 2 attempts at pulse therapy

117. False about biologics used in the treatment of inflammatory bowel disease is:

A. The first agent was Adalimumab, which was approved by the FDA
B. Anti-TNF-α antibody has been associated with a low risk of hepatosplenic T-cell lymphomas, particularly in young men who have been taking anti-TNF antibody therapy

in combination with other immunosuppressive therapy such as a thiopurine

C. Before starting these drugs, the patient should have either a tuberculin skin test or undergo testing with QuantiFERON gold assay as well as obtain a hepatitis profile

D. The side effects of these drugs include reactivation of infections including tuberculosis, histoplasmosis, actinomycosis and hepatitis

118. Classification used for assessment of symptom severity of UC is:

A. Harvey Bradshaw classification

B. Truelove and Witts classification

C. Mayo Clinic classification

D. Barcelona classification

119. Classification used for assessment of symptom severity of Crohn's disease is:

A. Harvey Bradshaw index

B. Truelove and Witts classification

C. Mayo Clinic scale

D. Barcelona classification

120. Harvey-Bradshaw Index of 15 is:

A. Remission

B. Mild disease

C. Moderate disease

D. Severe disease

121. For severe disease the Harvey-Bradshaw Index is:

A. >16 B. >15

C. >20 D. >24

122. For severe disease Crohn's disease activity index (CDAI) is:

A. CDAI >150 B. CDAI >250

C. CDAI >350 D. CDAI >450

123. Fulminant colitis is defined as all except:

A. Hypoalbuminemia < 3.5 g/dL^3

B. Leukocytosis > 12,000/dL^3

C. Temperature > 38°C

D. Tachycardia > 100/min

124. As a component of Fulminant colitis, the diameter of the transverse colon on a plain abdominal radiograph is:

A. > 5 cm B. > 8 cm

C. > 10 cm D. > 12 cm

125. True about Ulcerative Colitis is:

A. Patients with longstanding UC (>8 years) have a high risk of developing dysplasia or cancer, as do those who have sclerosing cholangitis

B. The finding of colonic dysplasia in patients with longstanding UC is an indication for surgery that has undergone significant change over the last 20 years

C. Overall, it is felt that approximately one fifth of the world's cancers arise in the setting of chronic inflammation

D. All of the above

126. The simplest and easiest pouch and the one with the least complications is the:

A. H Pouch B. W Pouch

C. S Pouch D. J Pouch

127. The length the limbs of the J pouch should be:

A. 5 cm B. 10 cm

C. 15 cm D. 25 cm

128. Common early complications of IPAA includes:

A. Ileal pouch–anal anastomotic sinuses

B. Ileal pouch–anal anastomotic fistulae

C. Pelvic sepsis

D. All of the above

129. A 22-year-old man in whom Crohn's disease has recently been diagnosed has just recovered from his first Crohn's flare-up. Currently, he has no perianal involvement. What medical therapy is not used as a first-line agent to maintain remission?

A. 6-Mercaptopurine B. Metronidazole

C. Mesalamine D. Prednisone

130. A 39-year-old man with a history of mild, long-standing ulcerative colitis controlled with sulfasalazine recently underwent routine colonoscopy that showed a lesion in the sigmoid colon. Pathologic evaluation reveals high-grade dysplasia. Which of the following is the best management option?

A. Sigmoid colectomy, provided that the rectum is minimally involved

B. Proctocolectomy with ileal pouch–anal anastomosis (IPAA)

C. Total abdominal colectomy with ileorectal anastomosis (IRA)

D. Total proctocolectomy with Brooke ileostomy

131. A 21-year-old woman is noted to have persistent bloody diarrhea, abdominal cramps and fever. Stool studies are negative for infectious diarrhea. Colonoscopy reveals friable mucosa in a continuous manner from the rectum to the sigmoid colon. No granulomas are found on biopsy. Which of the following statements is true regarding the most likely diagnosis in this patient?

A. Pseudopolyps and cobble stoning are common colonoscopic findings
B. Surgery is curative for this diagnosis
C. Rectal sparing is commonly seen on colonoscopy
D. Perianal fistulas are commonly found on rectal examination

132. A 28-year-old patient with severe ulcerative colitis undergoes a total proctocolectomy with IPAA. Four days after the operation, she develops fever, anal pain and tenesmus. Which of the following is the most likely diagnosis?

A. Small bowel obstruction
B. Pelvic sepsis
C. Ileoanal anastomotic stricture
D. Pouch–vaginal fistula

133. An 18-year-old man with a 2-year history of ulcerative colitis is admitted for an acute exacerbation of his disease. He is febrile and tachycardic with a heart rate of 135 beats/min. His blood pressure is stable. Laboratories show a leukocytosis of 12.3 × 10^3/L, and plain radiographs show moderate colonic distention to 7 cm in the transverse colon. What is the next step in the treatment of toxic megacolon in this patient?

A. Nasoenteric decompression, broad-spectrum antibiotics and intravenous steroids
B. Colonoscopic decompression
C. Emergency total abdominal colectomy with ileostomy
D. Diverting colostomy

134. Which of the following statements is correct?

A. Backwash ileitis is associated with ulcerative colitis
B. Diversion colitis is associated with ulcerative colitis and Crohn's colitis
C. Microscopic colitis is associated with Campylobacter infection
D. Metronidazole is used to treat acute ileitis caused by Yersinia infection

135. A 25-year-old male develops diarrhea and colicky abdominal pain. Ulcerative colitis is diagnosed on colonoscopy. Which of the following findings is consistent with the diagnosis?

A. The rectum is not involved
B. The disease is confluent, there are no skip areas in the colon and the rectum is involved
C. The full thickness of the bowel wall is involved
D. Microscopic examination of the mucosa reveals normal cells without evidence of dysplasia

136. A 35-year-old man has known ulcerative colitis. Which of the following is an indication for total proctocolectomy?

A. Occasional bouts of colic and diarrhea
B. Sclerosing cholangitis
C. Toxic megacolon
D. Arthritis

137. Ten years after diagnosis of total proctocolitis this patient undergoes colonscopy and biopsy reveals high-grade dysplasia in 2–10 specimens. What should the physician recommend?

A. Repeat colonoscopy in 1 year
B. Increase steroid dosage
C. Early repeat colonoscopy and biopsy area again
D. Total proctocolectomy

138. A 43-year-old woman undergoes investigation for colitis. In her history, it is noted that 20 years earlier she underwent a surgical procedure on the large intestine. The diagnosis is more likely to be Crohn's disease rather than ulcerative colitis because the previous operation was which of the following?

A. Performed in a young patient
B. Confined to the colon
C. Followed by improvement after bypass of the diseased segment
D. Followed by improvement because steroids were prescribed

139. A 43-year-old woman undergoes investigation for colitis. In her history, it is noted that 20 years earlier she underwent a surgical procedure on the large intestine. Is the diagnosis more likely to be ulcerative colitis rather than Crohn's disease because at the previous operation?

A. All layers of the bowel wall were involved
B. There was evidence of fistula formation
C. The serosa appeared normal on inspection, but the colon mucosa was extensively involved
D. Skip lesions were noted

140. A 54-year-old man with diarrhea is found to have ulcerative colitis. Colectomy should be advised in patients with ulcerative colitis who have symptoms that persist for more than which of the following?

A. 1 month
B. 6 months
C. 1–5 years
D. 10–20 years

141. A 48-year-old woman develops colon cancer. She is known to have a long history of ulcerative colitis. In ulcerative colitis, which of the following is a characteristic of colon cancer?

A. Occurs more frequently than in the rest of the population
B. Is more likely to occur when the ulcerative disease is confined to the left colon
C. Occurs equally in the right and left side
D. Has a synchronous carcinoma in 4–5% of cases

142. A 40-year-old man with a long history of bloody diarrhea presents with increased abdominal pain, vomiting and fever. On examination, he is found to be dehydrated and shows tachycardia and hypotension. The abdomen is markedly tender with guarding and rigidity. What is the most likely cause?

A. Toxic megacolon in ulcerative colitis
B. Small-bowel perforation from regional enteritis
C. Perforated carcinoma of the sigmoid colon
D. Volvulus of the sigmoid colon

143. Recurrence rate following surgery for Crohn's disease is higher in:

A. Patients who have already had 2 or more operations for fistulizing disease
B. It has been reported that Crohn patients who smoke are at higher risk of early disease recurrence
C. Patients < 30 years old
D. All of the above

INFECTIOUS COLITIS

144. False about C difficile infection is:

A. C difficile is an anaerobic, spore-forming, gram-negative bacillus
B. C difficile is the most common cause of healthcare-associated diarrhea and is considered to be a major source of health care-associated morbidity occurring in 2% of all hospital discharges for all diseases
C. Toxicogenic C difficile pathogens can produce A and B toxins, both of which have been associated with colitis
D. Binding of toxin A or B to colonocyte glycoprotein receptors leads to colonocyte death and release of inflammatory mediators

145. Risk factors for C difficile infection are:

A. Immunodeficiency
B. Chemotherapy treatment
C. Recent exposure to antibiotics
D. All of the above

146. False about C difficile infection is:

A. Patients with CDI can be categorized into asymptomatic colonization, nonsevere disease, severe disease and fulminant disease
B. Symptoms of CDI commonly begin 4 to 9 days after initiation of antibiotics but can commence 10 weeks or more after antibiotic treatment
C. Patients with IBD have increased rates of CDI, along with worse outcomes [HIV] and higher rates of colectomy
D. The most important risk factor for the development of a clinical infection is immunodeficiency

147. Patients with an increased risk for death from CDI include:

A. Acute renal failure
B. Hyperalbuminemia
C. Ribotype 027
D. Advanced age

148. Variables used in ATLAS Criteria includes all except:

A. Age
B. Leucocyte count
C. Serum BUN
D. Serum Albumin

149. False about diagnosis of CDI is:

A. Imaging is very useful for diagnosis as it is very specific
B. Classically raised, yellowish-white small (2–10 mm) plaques (pseudomembranes) can be observed in approximately half of patients with CDI
C. Flexible sigmoidoscopy may be helpful as a diagnostic modality for CDI
D. Laboratory testing is based on detection of C difficile toxins, C difficile antigen, or the bacteria itself

150. False about the treatment of CDI is:

A. Initial treatment includes stopping or minimizing previous antibiotics, parenteral fluids and correction of electrolytes
B. The use of antiperistaltic agents for the treatment of CDI should be promoted
C. Treatment options for recurrent episodes generally include changing antibiotics (from metronidazole to vancomycin or fidaxomicin from vancomycin)
D. Current guidelines recommend Fecal microbiota transplant (FMT) for patients with multiple recurrences of CDI, in whom antibiotic treatment has failed

151. True about Fecal microbiota transplant (FMT) is:

A. Reimplantation of normal gut bacteria, particularly bacteria resistant to C difficile from healthy donors can help restore normal gut biodiversity and correct the imbalance
B. Different routes of administration have been described in the literature including nasogastric, oral (frozen fecal microbial capsules), rectal enema and colonic per colonoscopy
C. The efficacy of FMT ranges from 77% to 100%, with multiple FMTs needed to achieve a good clinical response
D. All of the above

152. Monoclonal antibody against C difficile toxins B is:

A. Actoxumab
B. Bezlotoxumab
C. Rituximab
D. Abciximab

153. Monoclonal antibody against C difficile toxins A is:

A. Actoxumab
B. Bezlotoxumab
C. Eutaximab
D. Abciximab

154. A 73-year-old man undergoes an exploratory laparotomy and small bowel resection for small bowel obstruction. During his postoperative course, the patient develops diarrhea, abdominal tenderness and distention. He is diagnosed with a postoperative ileus. A stool specimen is sent that is positive for C difficile toxin. He is developing a significant leukocytosis, fever and elevated creatinine. What is the recommended treatment?

A. IV metronidazole and vancomycin via a rectal tube
B. IV vancomycin
C. Piperacillin-tazobactam
D. Metronidazole oral

OTHER COLONIC INFECTIONS

155. False about Campylobacter jejuni infection is:

A. Exposure to improperly prepared chicken or beef
B. Spiral, microaerophilic gram-positive rod
C. May mimic appendicitis or Crohn's disease
D. Commonly involves the sigmoid and descending colon

156. False about Shigella infection is:

A. Common cause for dysentery in developing countries
B. Often affects cecum and terminal ileum
C. Fever, abdominal pain, watery diarrhea that can progress to bloody diarrhea
D. Gram-negative, facultative anaerobe

ISCHEMIC COLITIS

157. False about Ischemic colitis is:

A. Ischemic colitis is considered a disease of large blood vessels and typically presents more dramatically, requiring vascular intervention
B. Patients undergoing aortic reconstructive surgery or abdominal surgery in which the IMA is ligated are also especially predisposed to colonic ischemia
C. The presence of a large arc of Riolan commonly indicates an obstruction of one of the major mesenteric arteries
D. Patients with low-flow states, as a result of heart failure or sepsis, are especially prone to develop ischemic colitis

158. Griffiths point is at:

A. Splenic flexure
B. Hepatic flexure
C. Rectosigmoid junction
D. Ileocolic junction

159. Sudeck's point is at:

A. Splenic flexure
B. Hepatic flexure
C. Rectosigmoid junction
D. Ileocolic junction

160. Ischemic colitis is significantly more common in all except:

A. Men
B. Patients with multiple comorbidities
C. Elderly patients
D. Women

161. False about the presentation and diagnosis of ischemic colitis is:

A. About 80% of the patients present with isolated right-sided ischemic colitis
B. Bleeding associated with ischemic colitis is usually minor and seldom requires blood transfusions
C. Presenting symptoms usually include sudden abdominal pain and cramping, tenesmus, and bloody diarrhea or hematochezia
D. The majority of patients with partial-thickness ischemia of a localized section of colon present with relatively nonspecific signs and symptoms

162. The most common affected region in ischemic colitis is:

A. Right colon
B. Left colon
C. Transverse colon
D. All are affected equally

163. What is the sign shown in the following radiograph?

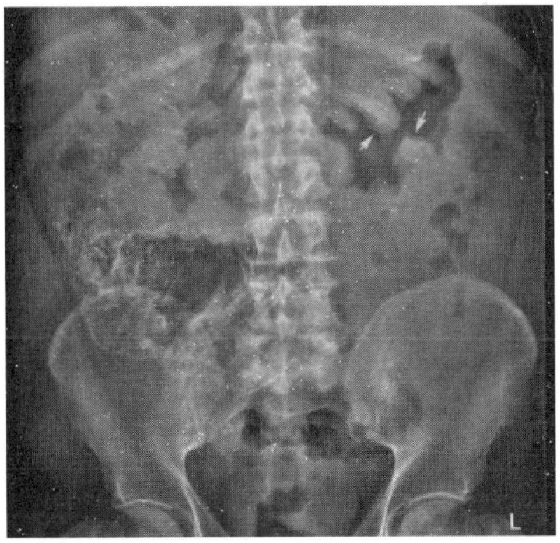

A. Pneumatosis coli
B. Thumbprinting
C. Portal and mesenteric venous gas
D. Gas under diaphragm

164. With regard to ischemic colitis, which of the following statements is true?

A. The most common symptoms are lower abdominal pain and bright red rectal bleeding
B. Occlusion of the major mesenteric vessels is the cause of ischemia in most cases
C. The splenic flexure and hepatic flexure are the most vulnerable areas of the colon
D. Nonoperative management is not justified because of the significant rates of perforation and peritonitis

165. What is true of colonic ischemia?

A. It occurs in a younger age group (40–60 years of age)
B. Patients with isolated right-sided ischemic colitis have a higher chance of requiring surgery and have a poorer prognosis
C. It usually causes severe abdominal pain
D. It results in the patient's appearing seriously ill

166. 3 days after undergoing an operation for an abdominal aortic aneurysm, a patient has moderate fever, abdominal pain and rectal bleeding. What is the most helpful investigation?

A. Angiography
B. Upper GI endoscopy
C. Abdominal ultrasound
D. Flexible endoscopy

167. Findings suggestive of ischemic colitis, although relatively nonspecific, includes:

A. Thumb printing
B. Pericolonic fat stranding
C. Segmental bowel thickening
D. All of the above

168. The gold standard for the diagnosis of ischemic colitis is:

A. CT scan
B. Flexible endoscopy
C. MRI
D. Angiography

169. False about the diagnosis of ischemic colitis is:

A. Early colonoscopy should be performed (within 48 hours), except in cases of acute peritonitis or in cases of suspected severe transmural ischemia
B. The "single-stripe sign", a single linear ulcer running along the longitudinal axis of the colon is rare but considered specific for ischemic colitis
C. Diagnostic endoscopy usually can distinguish between partial-thickness and full-thickness ischemia
D. All of the above are true

170. No. of patients that respond to non-operative conservative line of management in Ischemic Colitis is:

A. 20% B. 40%
C. 60% D. 80%

171. False about the treatment of Ischemic Colitis is:

A. The mainstay of treatment includes bowel rest, IV fluids and broad-spectrum antibiotics
B. Colonic ischemia can result in failure of the intestinal epithelial barrier with bacterial translocation leading to overt sepsis
C. Glucocorticoids should be always given unless treating a pre-existing disorder such as lupus or rheumatoid arthritis
D. Most episodes of ischemic colitis are mild and self-limiting

172. Conditions associated with ischemic colitis are:

A. Abdominal aortic aneurysm repair
B. Hypertension
C. Diabetes mellitus
D. All of the above

173. Drugs associated with ischemic colitis are:

A. Oral contraceptives
B. Sumatriptan
C. Opioids
D. All of the above

NEOPLASIA

174. True about colorectal cancer genetics is:

A. Mutator phenotype associated with Lynch syndrome, accounts for 5% of CRC
B. It is currently thought that Vogelstein's pathway accounts for approximately 60% of patients with CRC
C. The second major pathway accounting for approximately 35% of patients is the CpG island methylator phenotype cancer
D. All of the above

175. The most common initiating mutation in this CpG island methylator phenotype pathway involves a mutation of the:

A. CIMP gene B. BRAF gene
C. KRAS gene D. NRAS gene

176. The microsatellite instability (MSI) pathway is thought to be involved in up to:

A. 55% of early-stage CRCs
B. 35% of early-stage CRCs
C. 25% of early-stage CRCs
D. 15% of early-stage CRCs

177. True about Consensus Molecular Subtypes (CMS) is:

A. CMS1 cancers show a mesenchymal phenotype, prominent transforming growth factor-β activation, stromal invasion and angiogenesis
B. CMS2 cancers show an epithelial phenotype and exhibit marked WNT and MYC signaling activation
C. CMS3 cancers are hypermutated, microsatellite unstable and exhibit strong immune activation
D. CMS4 cancers are characterized by an epithelial phenotype and metabolic dysregulation

COLORECTAL POLYPS

178. True about polyps is:

A. Polyps can be characterized according to their endoscopic appearance into pedunculated or sessile
B. Polyps are usually asymptomatic, but may bleed or cause obstructive symptoms when large and some are precursors for cancer
C. Neoplastic polyps that have the potential to develop into CRC should be removed in order to reduce cancer risk
D. All of the above

179. False about Hyperplastic polyps is:

A. Consists of elongated colonic crypts with a papillary configuration of epithelial cells with atypia
B. < 5 mm
C. Small sessile lesions
D. All of the above are true

180. True about Inflammatory polyps is:

A. They do not have any intrinsic neoplastic potential but may be large, mimicking a neoplasm
B. Their significance is that they are found in diseased colons otherwise at risk for cancer and must be differentiated from neoplastic lesions
C. They are usually formed in an area of regeneration after full-thickness epithelial ulceration in which the new mucosa forms in an irregular polypoid configuration
D. All of the above

181. **Hamartomas are commonly related to a genetic syndrome such as:**
   A. Peutz-Jeghers syndrome (PJS)
   B. Juvenile polyposis syndrome
   C. PTEN hamartoma syndrome
   D. All of the above

182. **False about Serrated polyps is:**
   A. Patients with sessile serrated polyps and traditional serrated adenomas are recognized as having an increased risk of CRC
   B. These polyps should not be removed
   C. The development of CRC in these patients usually follows the serrated neoplasia pathway in contrast to the classic adenoma–carcinoma pathway seen in adenomatous polyps
   D. Sessile serrated polyps and traditional serrated adenomas are combinations of adenomatous and hyperplastic polyps

183. **True about Neoplastic Polyps is:**
   A. Tubular adenomas are characterized by branched tubular glands on histology
   B. Villous adenomas have long finger like projections of the surface epithelium
   C. Tubulovillous adenomas have elements of both types
   D. All of the above

184. **The most common type of neoplastic polyps is:**
   A. Tubulovillous adenoma
   B. Villous adenoma
   C. Tubular adenoma
   D. All of the above

185. **Patients with an advanced adenoma defined as:**
   A. Villous histology
   B. Size at least 1 cm
   C. High-grade dysplasia
   D. All of the above

186. **Incidence of carcinoma in a tubular adenoma < 1 cm is:**
   A. 5% B. 25%
   C. 50% D. 65%

187. **Incidence of carcinoma in a villous adenoma > 2 cm is:**
   A. 5% B. 25%
   C. 50% D. 65%

188. **As per Haggitt's classification level 2 is:**
   A. Carcinoma invading to the level of the neck
   B. Carcinoma invading into the submucosa, limited to the head of the polyp
   C. Carcinoma limited to the mucosa, carcinoma in situ
   D. Carcinoma invading any part of the stalk

189. **Carcinoma invading into the submucosa of the colon wall, below the level of the stalk, but above the muscularis propria is:**
   A. Haggitt's level 1 B. Haggitt's level 2
   C. Haggitt's level 3 D. Haggitt's level 4

190. **A 32-year-old male had sessile poly on his colonoscopy. On examination it invades into the upper third of the submucosa. What is the Haggitt's level?**
   A. Haggitt's level 1 B. Haggitt's level 2
   C. Haggitt's level 3 D. Haggitt's level 4

191. **A 32-year-old male had sessile poly on his colonoscopy. On examination it invades into the upper third of the submucosa. What is the Kikuchi's level?**
   A. Sm1 B. Sm2
   C. Sm3 D. Sm4

192. **As per American Gastroenterological Association, recommendations for repeat colonoscopy following endoscopic removal of a sessile serrated polyp < 10 mm is:**
   A. 6 months B. 3 years
   C. 10 years D. 5 years

193. **As per American Gastroenterological Association, recommendations for repeat colonoscopy following endoscopic removal of 9 mm hyperplastic polyp in rectum is:**
   A. 6 months B. 3 years
   C. 10 years D. 5 years

194. **As per American Gastroenterological Association, recommendations for repeat colonoscopy following endoscopic removal of a sessile serrated polyp >10 mm is:**
   A. 6 months B. 3 years
   C. 10 years D. 5 years

195. **A 52-year-old male had poly on his colonoscopy. He underwent piecemeal removal of polyp. As per American Gastroenterological Association, recommendations for repeat colonoscopy is:**

A. 6 months B. 3 years
C. 10 years D. 5 years

196. Which of the following neoplastic polyps is most likely to require surgical excision after a complete colonoscopic resection?

A. A 3 cm pedunculated carcinoma–containing adenomatous polyp with low-grade differentiation, no lymphovascular invasion, and no mucosal penetration that is resected piecemeal in 5 sessions
B. A 2 cm pedunculated carcinoma–containing adenomatous polyp with low-grade differentiation, positive lymphovascular invasion, and no mucosal penetration resected completely in one session
C. A 3 cm pedunculated hyperplastic polyp with no evidence of neoplasia
D. A 3 cm adenomatous noncancerous polyp with a 3 mm resection margin

197. A 30-year-old male is diagnosed with Peutz Jeghers syndrome. What findings is consistent with the diagnosis?

A. Adenomas
B. Hamartomas
C. Adenomatous polyps
D. Villoglandular polyps

198. A 64-year-old man has a benign lesion of the colon. He is informed that the lesion does not predispose to colon cancer. What is the lesion he has?

A. Ulcerative colitis
B. Villous adenoma
C. Hyperplastic polyp
D. Adenoma in familial polyposis

199. A 25-year-old man complains of rectal bleeding, weight loss and abdominal pain. He gives a history of similar complaints in his siblings as well as his mother. Findings on physical examination are unremarkable except for guaiac positive stool. What is the most likely diagnosis?

A. Peutz–Jeghers syndrome
B. Familial polyposis of the colon
C. Ulcerative colitis
D. Carcinoma of the stomach

200. FAP is a syndrome caused by germline mutation in the APC tumor suppressor gene which is responsible for regulation of β-catenin and located on:

A. Chromosome 9p21 B. Chromosome 5q21
C. Chromosome 9q21 D. Chromosome 5p21

201. In classic FAP, germline mutations in the APC gene are found in:

A. 10% to 20% B. 30% to 40%
C. 50% to 70% D. 80% to 90%

202. Number of patients with FAP who have a de novo mutation and thus have no family history is approximately:

A. 5% B. 15%
C. 25% D. 40%

203. In the absence of treatment in FAP patients, the lifetime risk for CRC is nearly:

A. 60% B. 80%
C. 90% D. 100%

204. If left untreated, patients with FAP develop CRC at an average age of around:

A. 33 years B. 39 years
C. 26 years D. 45 years

205. True about FAP is:

A. Patients with FAP may be asymptomatic or may present with bleeding, diarrhea, abdominal pain, or mucous discharge per rectum
B. Severe FAP is characterized by thousands of colorectal adenomas
C. FAP is characterized by early development of a wide range of colorectal adenomatous polyps after the second decade of life and many extracolonic manifestations
D. All of the above

206. In FAP patients, non-neoplastic gastric fundic gland polyps are a common finding in about:

A. 10% B. 30%
C. 50% D. 70%

207. Gastric adenomas present in patients with FAP are seen most commonly at:

A. Antrum B. Cardia
C. Fundus D. Body

208. In FAP patients, gastric adenomas are present in about:

A. 10% B. 30%
C. 50% D. 70%

209. In FAP patients, duodenal adenomas are present in about:

A. 1% to 5% B. 5% to 10%
C. 30% to 70% D. 80% to 90%

210. In FAP patients, the lifetime risk for duodenal cancer is:

A. 1% to 2% B. 4% to 10%
C. 10% to 20% D. 25% to 50%

211. The 2nd most common cause of death in FAP patients is:

A. Colorectal cancer
B. Duodenal cancer
C. Desmoid tumor
D. Adrenal adenomas

212. Classification used for duodenal polyps in familial adenomatous polyposis is:

A. Kikuchi classification
B. Haggitt's classification
C. Spigelman classification
D. Gardner's classification

213. False about Desmoid tumors in FAP is:

A. Desmoid tumors, together with duodenal polyposis and/or cancer, are the major causes of morbidity and mortality after proctocolectomy, leading to death in approximately 10% of patients
B. These tumors are associated with male gender and with a family history of desmoids
C. About half of FAP-associated desmoid tumors arise intraabdominally in the bowel mesentery and 40% develop in the abdominal wall
D. Desmoid tumors are histologically benign but locally invasive monoclonal proliferations of fibroblasts

214. Percentage of patients with FAP that will have desmoid tumor is:

A. 5% to 10% B. 10% to 15%
C. 20% to 30% D. 30% to 45%

215. The incidence of thyroid cancer in patients with FAP is:

A. 2% B. 5%
C. 10% D. 20%

216. In FAP patients, CHRPE is seen in:

A. 5% to 10% B. 10% to 25%
C. 30% to 45% D. 60% to 85%

217. Gardner syndrome includes all except:

A. Medulloblastoma
B. Epidermal inclusion cysts
C. Osteomas
D. Desmoid tumors

218. In FAP, genetic testing reveals an APC germline mutation in approximately:

A. 20% of cases B. 40% of cases
C. 60% of cases D. 80% of cases

219. Indications for genetic counselling referral and testing for FAP includes:

A. A family history of FAP
B. Extracolonic manifestation of FAP
C. Personal history of > 10 adenomas
D. All of the above

220. For individuals suspected of AFAP, gene testing is recommended if:

A. 5 or more cumulative colorectal adenomas are found
B. 10 or more cumulative colorectal adenomas are found
C. 20 or more cumulative colorectal adenomas are found
D. 50 or more cumulative colorectal adenomas are found

221. Colorectal screening in individuals of FAP affected families begins at age:

A. 8 B. 12
C. 20 D. 40

222. Screening of FAP includes:

A. Colorectal screening in individuals of affected families begins at age 12 and can be initiated with flexible proctosigmoidoscopy
B. Annual thyroid screening by ultrasound should be recommended to FAP patients
C. Patients at risk for AFAP should receive endoscopic screening with colonoscopy at ages 12, 15, 18 and 21 years, and then every 2 years
D. All of the above

223. In FAP, upper GI tract screening begins at:

A. 10 to 15 years of age
B. 15 to 20 years of age
C. 20 to 25 years of age
D. 30 to 40 years of age

224. The surgical options in the treatment of FAP are:

A. Proctocolectomy and IPAA
B. Subtotal colectomy and IRA
C. Proctocolectomy with end ileostomy
D. All of the above

225. Which of the following is AR in inheritance?

A. Attenuated FAP
B. MUTYH-associated polyposis
C. Classical FAP
D. Severe FAP

226. CRC risk in attenuated FAP is:

A. 40% B. 60%
C. 80% D. 100%

227. CRC risk in juvenile polyposis syndrome is:

A. 40% B. 60%
C. 80% D. 100%

228. CRC risk in Peutz-Jeghers polyposis is:

A. 40% B. 60%
C. 80% D. 100%

229. CRC risk in MAP is:

A. 40% B. 60%
C. 80% D. 100%

230. APC gene is associated with all except:

A. Classical FAP
B. MUTYH-associated polyposis
C. Attenuated FAP
D. Severe FAP

231. A patient was Stage III on Spiegelman's classification. What is the recommendation for his treatment and surveillance?

A. Repeat endoscopy in 2–3 years
B. Repeat endoscopy in 6–12 months and surgical evaluation
C. Repeat endoscopy in 10 years
D. Repeat endoscopy in 5 years

232. Timing of surgery in patients with familial polyposis with presence of symptoms is:

A. As soon as possible
B. 21–25 years of age
C. Delay surgery (after evaluating CRC risk)
D. Avoid as long as the patient remains in a strict surveillance program

233. FAP patients who should undergo IPAA are all except:

A. >20 synchronous adenomas
B. Large (>30 mm) adenomas
C. >100 synchronous adenomas
D. Adenoma with high-grade dysplasia

234. IRA should not be performed in patients with following except:

A. Rectum containing > 10 rectal adenomas
B. Adenomas with severe dysplasia
C. Adenomas >3 cm diameter
D. Presence of colon cancer

235. False about MUTYH-Associated Polyposis is:

A. CRC risk is increased 28 fold for individuals with biallelic MUTYH mutations, while the risk for monoallelic carriers appears to be only moderately increased
B. The syndrome is primarily characterized by multiple colorectal adenomas and an increased risk for CRC at a younger age (40–50 years of age)
C. Although most polyps in MAP are adenomas, patients can present with serrated polyps or a mixture of adenomas and serrated polyps
D. The diagnosis of MAP should be considered in patients presenting with colorectal polyposis (>100 lifetime adenomas)

236. MUTYH gene is located on:

A. Chromosome 1 B. Chromosome 5
C. Chromosome 9 D. Chromosome 10

237. False about MUTYH-Associated Polyposis is:

A. Approximately 20% of patients with MAP will have duodenal polyposis
B. Osteomas, desmoids and CHRPE are also associated with MAP
C. Indications for MUTYH gene testing: patients with 10 to 100 polyps, siblings of patients with biallelic MUTYH gene mutation, patients with early-onset CRC (< 44–55 years), or children of monoallelic or biallelic MUTYH gene mutation carriers
D. Rectal cancer is uncommon in MAP

238. True about Peutz-Jeghers syndrome is:

A. PJS is an autosomal-dominant hereditary cancer syndrome that carries a 39% lifetime risk of CRC characterized by benign hamartomatous, primarily GI, polyps, mucocutaneous pigmentation and a high predisposition to many intestinal and extraintestinal cancers

B. Nearly 90% of PJS patients will develop hamartomatous polyps

C. Polyps differ histologically from juvenile polyps in that they arise due to an overgrowth of the muscularis mucosa rather than the lamina propria

D. All of the above

239. Peutz-Jeghers Syndrome (PJS) patients have a risk of following cancers except:

A. Gastric cancer
B. Skin cancer
C. Colorectal cancer
D. Pancreatic cancer

240. PJS is caused by a mutation of the STK11/LKB1 gene located on chromosome:

A. 9p
B. 9q
C. 19p
D. 19q

241. World Health Organization criteria for PJS has all except:

A. Characteristic, prominent, mucocutaneous pigmentation with a family history of PJS

B. Any number of Peutz-Jeghers polyps and characteristic prominent, mucocutaneous pigmentation

C. Any number of PJ polyps with a family history of PJS

D. 5 or more histologically confirmed Peutz-Jeghers polyps

242. False about PJS patient's special surveillance is:

A. Pancreatic cancer screening involves endoscopic ultrasound or magnetic resonance cholangiopancreatography along with serum CA19-9 every 1 to 2 years starting at age 25 to 30 years

B. Women should have breast physical examinations every 6 months and yearly mammogram and breast MRI starting at age 45 years

C. Males should undergo annual testicular physical examination starting at age 10 years, and females should undergo an annual pelvic examination and Papanicolaou stain starting at age 18 to 20 years

D. Screening begins at 8 to 10 years of age with an evaluation of the small bowel

243. False about Juvenile polyposis syndrome is:

A. There is an increased cancer risk in afflicted individuals, with a malignant potential of at least 50% in patients with multiple juvenile polyps

B. JPS is clinically diagnosed when there are 5 or more juvenile polyps in the colorectum, multiple juvenile polyps throughout the GI tract, any number or juvenile polyps with a family history, or juvenile polyposis

C. SMAD4 (chromosome 18q) and BMPR1A (chromosome 10q), have been linked to JPS

D. Juvenile polyposis syndrome is an inherited autosomal-dominant pattern and is characterized by the development of hamartomatous intestinal polyps

244. Of all CRCs, HNPCC accounts for:

A. 1% to 2%
B. 3% to 5%
C. 5% to 10%
D. 10% to 25%

245. False about Lynch syndrome is:

A. It is an autosomal dominantly inherited syndrome characterized by a mutation in one of the DNA mismatch repair (MMR) genes

B. Mutations in MLH1 and MSH2 account for up to 20% of patients with Lynch syndrome

C. MSI is found in most (>90%) colon malignancies in patients with Lynch syndrome

D. Somatic mutations in the BRAF gene are noted in 15% of sporadic CRCs but not in Lynch syndrome tumors

246. Amsterdam II criteria includes all except:

A. One affected patient is a first-degree relative of the other two

B. 3 or more successive generations are affected

C. Familial adenomatous polyposis is excluded

D. Pathologic diagnosis of cancer is verified

247. False about Lynch syndrome is:

A. The estimated lifetime risk for CRC is 70% for men and 40% for women

B. Lynch syndrome–associated CRCs show a predilection for the right colon as compared to sporadic CRC

C. Compared with patients with AFAP or MAP, patients with Lynch syndrome develop few colorectal adenomas by the age of 50 years

D. Adenoma may progress to carcinoma within 5 to 10 years, compared with from 10 to 20 years in the general population

248. The most common extracolonic cancer in HNPCC is:

A. Endometrial adenocarcinoma

B. Ovarian CA
C. Glioblastoma
D. Sebaceous gland adenomas

249. Muir-Torre variant of Lynch syndrome includes all except:

A. Skin cancer
B. Sebaceous adenomas
C. Endometrial adenocarcinoma
D. Keratoacanthomas

250. Bethesda criteria for testing colorectal tumors for microsatellite instability (MSI) includes all except:

A. Colorectal cancer diagnosed in at least 3 first- or second-degree relatives with HNPCC-related tumors, regardless of age
B. Colorectal cancer with the MSI histology diagnosed in a patient before age 60 years
C. Colorectal cancer diagnosed in at least 1 first-degree relative with an HNPCC-related tumor in which one cancer was diagnosed < 50 years
D. Colorectal cancer diagnosed in a patient < 50 years

251. False about the screening in HNPCC is:

A. Screening for CRC by colonoscopy is recommended in persons at risk or those affected with Lynch syndrome every 1 to 2 years, beginning at 30 to 35 years of age or 2 to 5 years before the youngest age of diagnosis of CRC in the family if diagnosed before age 25 years
B. For the endometrial cancer, the screening should be offered to women at risk for or affected with Lynch syndrome by pelvic examination and endometrial sampling annually starting at age 30 to 35 years
C. Screening of ovarian cancer should be offered beginning at the same age as endometrial cancer
D. Screening for gastric cancer should be considered in persons with Lynch syndrome by esophagogastroduodenoscopy with gastric biopsy of the antrum at 30 to 35 years

252. With regard to the APC syndromes, which of the following statements is true?

A. Annual colonoscopic screening of family members should begin at the age of 25
B. Twenty-five percent of the offspring of an afflicted individual will have the disease
C. The risk for the development of colon cancer is approximately 50%
D. Periampullary tumors are an important cause of death

253. Which of the following is true about HNPCC (Lynch syndrome)?

A. It is inherited as an autosomal recessive trait
B. Most cancers in patients with HNPCC involve the right colon
C. The average age at diagnosis is 62 years
D. A segmental colectomy is frequently curative for these patients

254. Which statement is correct concerning intestinal polyposis syndromes?

A. Hamartomas are found in patients with both juvenile polyps and Peutz-Jeghers syndrome (PJS)
B. Familial polyposis syndrome often includes extraintestinal manifestations
C. Turcot syndrome often includes small bowel polyps
D. PJS, Gardner syndrome and Turcot syndrome are inherited in an autosomal recessive pattern

STAGING

255. Staging systems for CRC include all except:

A. Dukes classification
B. Modified Astler-Coller classification
C. Spiegelman's classification
D. AJCC staging system

SURGICAL TREATMENT OF COLORECTAL CANCER

256. Anatomic vascular landmarks when performing a colorectal resection includes all except:

A. The left colic artery originates about 5 cm distally to the origin of the IMA
B. The middle colic vessels originate from the superior mesenteric vessels at the level of the inferior margin of the pancreas
C. The inferior mesenteric vein can be easily identified at the level of the ligament of Treitz
D. The ileocolic pedicle originates from the superior mesenteric vessels just caudal to the second portion of the duodenum

257. Free margins recommended for colon cancer surgery is:

A. 2 cms
B. 5 cms
C. 8 cms
D. 10 cms

258. For rectal cancer, distal free margin recommended is:

A. 2 cms
B. 5 cms
C. 8 cms
D. 10 cms

259. True about surgical management of left-sided tumors is:

A. The inferior mesenteric vein is divided at the level of the ligament of Treitz
B. Left hemicolectomy includes the high ligation of the IMA at its origin
C. The IMA can also be ligated 2 to 3 cm more distally without compromising the oncologic outcome but lowering the risk of injuring the mesenteric and hypogastric nervous plexus
D. All of the above

260. Which of the following is the appropriate operation for a sigmoid cancer that has not metastasized?

A. Segmental resection of the sigmoid with 5 cm margins and high ligation of the sigmoid branch of the IMA
B. Resection of the entire sigmoid from the distal descending colon to the rectosigmoid junction, sparing the main left colic artery
C. Resection of the sigmoid and the descending colon, with high ligation of the IMA at its origin
D. Resection of the entire colon proximal to the lesion with IRA

261. A pedunculated 1.5 cm tubular adenoma is removed endoscopically from the sigmoid colon and found to contain well-differentiated adenocarcinoma extending to but not beyond the muscularis mucosae. The margin of resection is free of tumor. Select the best therapeutic option:

A. Observation only
B. Endoscopic fulguration of the polypectomy site
C. Operative colostomy and excision of the polypectomy site
D. Sigmoid colectomy

262. A 32-year-old woman presents to the emergency department with abdominal pain that has gradually increased over the past week. The patient has a history of FAP and underwent a total proctocolectomy with IPAA at age 20. She has 5 to 6 soft to loose bowel movements per day, which is normal for her. A CT scan reveals a 10 cm soft tissue mass in the middle abdomen, displacing the loop of small bowel to either side. Upon review of a CT scan from several years prior, the mass was present but has grown from 7 cm. What is the next step in initial management?

A. External beam radiation
B. Surgical debulking
C. Chemotherapy
D. Daily tamoxifen

263. A 64-year-old train conductor is diagnosed as having carcinoma confined to the descending colon. Before operation, what should be told?

A. He will most likely require a colostomy
B. He should have the cancer excised by cautery
C. He should undergo left hemicolectomy
D. Radiotherapy is the treatment of choice

264. An 83-year-old man is diagnosed on colonoscopy to have cancer of the colon. He refuses surgical intervention and after a 3 month follow up period is admitted to the emergency department with large-bowel obstruction. Carcinoma of the colon is most likely to obstruct if found in the:

A. Cecum
B. Ascending colon
C. Descending colon
D. Rectum

265. A 70-year-old man presents with pallor and breathlessness on exertion. He does not complain of abdominal pain. He has microcytic, hypochromic anemia. What is the most probable cause?

A. Carcinoma of the right colon
B. Peptic ulcer disease
C. Crohn's disease
D. Diverticulosis of the colon

OBSTRUCTING COLON CANCERS

266. False about management of left-sided colonic obstructions due to malignancies is:

A. In sigmoid and left colon obstructions, patients are commonly referred for urgent surgery
B. Endoscopic stenting as a bridge for surgery has also emerged as an attractive technique to relieve obstructions and permit elective surgery under more favorable conditions
C. Stenting has not been shown to permit higher rates of primary anastomosis, decreased wound infections, and a higher rate of completion of surgery laparoscopically
D. Stenting is contraindicated in suspected ischemic or perforated bowel

267. Clinical success of stenting in left-sided colonic obstructions due to malignancies is around:

A. 10% to 20%
B. 30% to 40%
C. 50% to 60%
D. 70% to 80%

RECTAL CANCER

268. False about the preoperative assessment of rectal cancer is:

A. Staging of the rectal cancer can be performed either with endorectal ultrasound or with MRI
B. Endorectal ultrasound is a much less expensive test, can be performed without sedation, and provides an accurate assessment of the T stage of a rectal cancer
C. With endorectal ultrasound the accuracy of lymph node detection is much more than the accuracy of detecting T stage
D. In order to obtain a meaningful study for rectal cancer staging, the MRI has to be performed according to a specific rectal cancer protocol in which the MRI is accessed in the same axis as the rectum

269. Among rectal cancer patients undergoing neoadjuvant chemoradiation, approximate patients that will achieve a "complete response" is:

A. 5%
B. 10%
C. 20%
D. 40%

270. Criteria for performing a local excision for a rectal cancer is:

A. Lesions that are mobile (not fixed)
B. Small lesions (< 2 cm in diameter)
C. Well-differentiated cancers within reach of the index finger
D. All of the above

271. False about local excision for a rectal cancer is:

A. T1 lesions are ideal, and patients with T2 or T3 lesions are not suitable, as the recurrence rate following local excision in this group of patients has been unacceptable
B. If a traditional local excision is performed, cautery is used to score a 1 cm margin around the lesion
C. Local excision is safe when performed for lesions that are located anterior to the rectum due to the presence of the mesorectum
D. If lesions are located in the anterior rectum in women, there is risk of iatrogenic rectovaginal fistula or, in the case of men, injury to the prostate

272. Following instrument shown is used for:

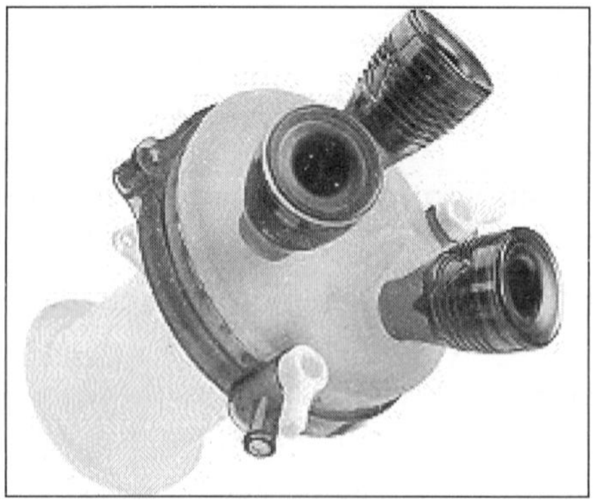

A. Transanal minimally invasive surgery (TAMIS)
B. Moh's procedure
C. Heald's procedure
D. Heller's procedure

273. False about Low Anterior Resection is:

A. After vascular division similar to left colectomies, the peritoneal reflection of the rectum is divided at the level of the sacral promontory and the rectum with its proximal mesorectum is gently pulled anteriorly entering the avascular "cotton candy" plane between the fascia of the mesorectum and the presacral fascia
B. Recent evidence demonstrates that the laparoscopic approach has similar results with regard to the quality of resection, clear circumferential margins and recurrence rate when compared to the open approach
C. For cancers located in the distal two thirds of the rectum, the dissection must be continued more distally, dissecting the rectum away from the prostate along the fascia of Denonvilliers
D. The diverting stoma is usually maintained for at least 12 weeks after surgery and is closed only after the perfect healing of the anastomosis has been confirmed with a gastrografin enema or with endoscopy

274. True about sphincter-sparing surgery procedures for low rectal cancers is:

A. In young and fit patients with good preoperative sphincter function, if the sphincters are not infiltrated with cancer and do not need to be sacrificed for oncologic reasons
B. With a standard mucosectomy, the distal mucosa is peeled off from the internal sphincter
C. Ideally, 1 to 2 cm of mucosa above the dentate line should be saved because this portion of

distal mucosa has a critical importance in rectal sensibility and consequently for postoperative functional outcomes

D. All of the above

275. APR carries intrinsic risk of higher recurrence rates of upto:

A. 25% B. 33%
C. 50% D. 66%

276. The retroileal transmesenteric route provides the colon with an additional length of:

A. 1 to 2 cm B. 5 to 8 cm
C. 4 to 5 cm D. 8 to 10 cm

277. The incidence of anastomotic leaks after coloanal anastomoses is up to:

A. 2% B. 10%
C. 20% D. 30%

278. Risk factors associated with postoperative dehiscence are all except:

A. Obesity
B. ASA score III to V
C. Female gender
D. Low extraperitoneal anastomoses

279. True about the treatment of colocolonic anastomosis is:

A. If the leak involves < one third of the anastomosis and the abdominal contamination is minimal, a diverting stoma may be sufficient
B. An ileocolic anastomosis in right-sided resections can be managed ideally by redo of the anastomosis, but if the patient is unstable, the anastomosis has to be dismantled and an end ileostomy constructed
C. Abdominal exploration allows peritoneal lavage and reposition of new drains if needed
D. All of the above

280. In colorectal surgeries, major bleeding with hemodynamic instability requiring active resuscitation, need of blood transfusion, and active treatment, can occur in up to:

A. 1% B. 4%
C. 10% D. 18%

281. After circular anastomoses, clinically significant strictures are those that present with obstructive symptoms and occur in:

A. 0.5% to 1% B. 1% to 2%
C. 4% to 10% D. 15% to 30%

282. Risk factors for strictures are all except:

A. Chemotherapy
B. Use of a small-diameter stapler
C. Ischemia
D. Anastomotic leaks

283. Amongst patients undergoing a low anterior resection, low anterior resection syndrome is seen in upto:

A. 20% B. 40%
C. 60% D. 80%

284. Low anterior resection syndrome includes:

A. Multiple fragmented bowel movements
B. Constipation and diarrhea
C. Incontinence
D. All of the above

285. False about low anterior resection syndrome is:

A. Most of the symptoms improve 10 years or more after the resection
B. It may be due to an injury of the internal sphincter, loss of sensitivity in the anorectal mucosa, loss or impairment of the rectoanal-inhibitory reflex, reduction of the capacity of the rectal reservoir, and/or loss of compliance of the transposed colon
C. Preventive technical mechanisms are currently used to improve LARS symptoms that aim to increase the capacity of the neorectum: anastomosis with a 5 to 6 cm colonic J-pouch or with a transverse coloplasty or side-to-end colorectal anastomosis
D. In a minority of highly symptomatic patients with low quality of life, after failure of conservative treatment, the construction of a stoma can be necessary as a definitive treatment

286. 5-year survival rate for patients with stage I colorectal cancer is approximately:

A. 45% B. 60%
C. 75% D. 90%

287. Patients with distant nonresectable metastases in colorectal cancer have a 5-year survival rate of about:

A. 2% B. 5%
C. 10% D. 15%

288. In patients with colorectal cancer and resectable liver metastases amenable to curative liver

resection with free margins and favorable clinical risk factors may have a 5-year survival rate up to:

A. 45%　　B. 60%
C. 75%　　D. 90%

289. **The majority of recurrences after resection of the primary colorectal tumor occur within the first:**

A. 1 year　　B. 2 years
C. 5 years　　D. 10 years

290. **In stage II colon cancer patients, the potential risk factors that can be considered as relative indications for chemotherapy are all except:**

A. Vascular and perineural invasion
B. Inadequate number of examined number lymph nodes (<16)
C. Poorly differentiated cancer (G3–4)
D. Obstruction or perforation

291. **False about postoperative treatment in colorectal cancer is:**

A. MSI is another relevant characteristic for oncologic postsurgical treatment in stage II disease
B. Adjuvant 5-FU treatment seems to have a detrimental effect on survival in stage III but not stage II colon cancer patients
C. MSI-H condition (deficient expression of MMR genes) is more frequent in stage II disease (22%) than in stages III (12%) and IV (3%) and does appear to have a favorable prognostic significance in stage II
D. All of the above are true

292. **True about postoperative management of stage III disease is:**

A. Low-risk patients were defined as pT3pN1 and high-risk patients, pT4 (any N) or N2
B. Adjuvant chemotherapy is indicated in stage III patients
C. With regard to the FOLFOX regimen, 6 months seems superior to 3 months, regardless of the risk group
D. All of the above

293. **True about the postoperative management of metastatic colorectal disease is:**

A. In older or unfit patients, unable to tolerate doublets, capecitabine with bevacizumab is an appropriate treatment
B. Anti-EGFR antibodies (panitumumab, cetuximab) can be used in pan-Ras wild-type and BRAF wild-type neoplasia
C. In left-sided primary tumors, the addition of cetuximab or panitumumab to FOLFOX/FOLFIRI could be the first line of treatment
D. All of the above

294. **The standard treatment in BRAF-mutated metastatic colorectal disease is the administration of:**

A. FOLFOX and bevacizumab
B. FOLFOXIRI and bevacizumab
C. FOLFOX and panitumumab
D. FOLFOXIRI and panitumumab

295. **A screening colonoscopy identifies a broad sessile villous appearing lesion of the rectum beginning 4 cm above the anal verge and extending 5 cm proximally. Biopsies show a villous adenoma with dysplasia. Endorectal ultrasound (EUS) shows that the muscularis propria is not involved. No suspicious lymph nodes are seen. Which of the following approaches is the most appropriate for the management of this patient?**

A. Repeated biopsies
B. Fulguration
C. Transanal excision
D. Abdominoperineal resection (APR)

296. **At the time of surgery for left colon obstruction, you find a thickened segment of colon with a narrow lumen and proximal bowel impacted with stool. There are no liver masses palpated. Which of the following is not an appropriate operative strategy for this patient?**

A. Strictureplasty
B. Left hemicolectomy and primary anastomosis following intraoperative colonic irrigation
C. Initial decompressive colostomy, bowel washout, and resection within 7 to 10 days
D. Primary left colectomy, colostomy, and either a Hartmann's pouch or mucous fistula

297. **Which of the following is true regarding EUS imaging?**

A. Sedation is required
B. The bowel must be prepared as for colonoscopy or colectomy
C. Scanning is best performed with a 3.0-MHz crystal
D. Image-guided needle biopsy of extraluminal nodules is safe

298. **Which of the following is the most important prognostic determinant of survival after treatment of CRC?**

A. Lymph node involvement
B. Transmural extension
C. Tumor size
D. Histologic differentiation

299. A patient presents with a recently diagnosed 3 cm rectal cancer with its lower edge 4 cm from the anorectal ring. EUS shows a tumor extending through the muscularis propria with three adjacent lymph nodes measuring 1 cm each. CT scan does not show any evidence of distant spread to the liver or lungs. Which of the following is the most appropriate treatment for this patient?

A. APR with colostomy
B. LAR with total mesocolon excision and anastomosis
C. Chemotherapy and radiation followed by resection
D. Preoperative external beam radiation therapy

300. A 62-year-old woman complains to her doctor of bright red blood per rectum, mixed with stool. On rectal examination, she is found to have a palpable mass at the tip of the finger. Proctoscopy shows the presence of a posterior 4 cm ulcerated mass that occupies 35% of the circumference beginning at 4 cm from the anorectal ring. A biopsy shows rectal adenocarcinoma, and a complete staging shows a T3 lesion and several enlarged lymph nodes, but no distant metastasis. Her carcinoembryonic antigen (CEA) level is normal. Select the most appropriate treatment for this patient:

A. Local excision
B. TEM excision
C. APR
D. Preoperative chemotherapy and radiation followed by resection

301. In which of the following settings should a low anterior resection (LAR) be performed?

A. A 56-year-old male with a circumferential villous adenoma beginning at the dentate line and extending 8 cm proximally
B. Palliation of obstructing rectal cancer just above the dentate line with minimal liver metastases in a 60-year-old female
C. An 80-year-old male with a large rectal cancer that produces anal pain and tenesmus and involves the anal sphincter
D. A 75-year-old male with urinary incontinence and a rectal cancer 5 cm above the dentate line

302. A 54-year-old man is referred by his physician for the evaluation of rectal bleeding. He admits to a recent history of constipation and rectal fullness. Colonoscopy showed a 3 cm mass starting 2 cm above the dentate line. Biopsies are consistent with a neuroendocrine cancer that contains a large amount of amine precursor (5-hydroxytryptophan). Which statement is correct regarding this tumor?

A. This tumor occurs at equal frequency in the colon and rectum
B. The incidence of invasive malignancy and metastases correlates with the location of the tumor
C. This tumor in the rectum frequently causes flushing, diarrhea and heat intolerance
D. Local excision for a rectal cancer should be done for small lesions (<2 cms)

303. Which of the following findings warrants APR?

A. A fixed circumferential adenocarcinoma just above the dentate line
B. An ulcerating adenocarcinoma whose lower edge is 7 cm from the dentate line, with infiltration and expansion of the second hypoechoic layer seen on ultrasound imaging
C. A 2 cm mobile adenocarcinoma arising in a villous adenoma 3 cm from the dentate line, with an intact second hypoechoic band seen on ultrasound imaging
D. A circumferential adenocarcinoma 12 cm from the anal verge

304. A 68-year-old dentist undergoes anterior resection (sigmoid resection) for cancer at the rectosigmoid junction. The tests performed before her surgery were colonscopy and biopsy. There were no other lesions detected with sigmoidoscopy or in the pathology specimen. Following operation, she requires which of the following within 2–3 months?

A. Bone scan
B. Colonoscopy
C. Repeat rectal examination and sigmoidoscopy
D. CT scan of the abdomen

305. A 64-year-old man undergoes CEA surveillance for cancer, because his brother and father both had colon cancer. What information should he be provided?

A. CEA is highly sensitive for diagnosis
B. Increases in CEA after resection may indicate tumor recurrence

C. If CEA is elevated preoperatively, it implies unresectable disease
D. CEA is highly specific for the presence of colon cancer

PELVIC FLOOR DISORDERS AND CONSTIPATION

306. The failure of the puborectalis and the external anal sphincter to relax during defecation is called:

A. Procidentia
B. Anismus
C. Rectocele
D. Polysmus

307. Normal resting pressure values of anus are:

A. 40 to 80 mm Hg
B. 40 to 80 cm of H_2O
C. 20 to 40 mm Hg
D. 20 to 40 cm of H_2O

308. The balloon expulsion test evaluates the ability of the patient to expel a balloon inflated with:

A. 50 to 60 cc of air
B. 50 to 60 cc of water
C. 50 to 60 cc of gas
D. All of the above

309. Normal pudendal nerve terminal motor latency times are:

A. 1.0 ± 0.2 milliseconds
B. 2.0 ± 0.2 milliseconds
C. 1.0 ± 0.1 milliseconds
D. 2.0 ± 0.1 milliseconds

310. In colonic transit time test, in the healthy population, percentage of the marker that should be expelled by day 5 is:

A. 20%
B. 60%
C. 40%
D. 80%

311. False about rectal prolapse is:

A. The rectal prolapse is a circumferential, full-thickness intussusception of the rectal wall
B. Men older than 50 years are 6 times more likely than women to develop rectal prolapse
C. Rectal prolapse is an uncommon condition that occurs in about 0.5% of the general population
D. Young patients (males and females) with prolapse often suffer from psychiatric diseases, such as autism or developmental delay, and take constipating medications

312. Anatomic defects are commonly found in patients with total rectal prolapse are:

A. Diastasis of the levator ani muscle
B. An abnormally deep cul-de-sac
C. A redundant sigmoid colon
D. All of the above

313. Risk factors of rectal procidentia include all except:

A. Age > 40 years
B. Male gender
C. Chronic diarrhea
D. Vaginal delivery

314. False about the symptoms of rectal prolapse are:

A. Symptoms include discomfort due to the prolapsed tissue, incontinence with drainage of mucous or blood and constipation
B. Up to 5% of patients with incontinence have also pudendal neuropathy with a prolonged pudendal nerve terminal motor latency
C. The other 25% to 50% of the patients and in particular those with intrarectal prolapse, report constipation or obstructed defecation
D. The majority (50%–75%) of patients with evident rectal prolapse complain of fecal incontinence

315. False about the diagnosis of rectal prolapse is:

A. Colonoscopy should be always performed to exclude the presence of CRC or other colonic pathology
B. Fluoroscopic or MRI defecography is an additional test to confirm the diagnosis of rectal prolapse and provides more information regarding coexisting disorders, such as rectocele cystocele, vaginal vault prolapse, enterocele and sigmoidocele
C. At rest, typical findings include a patulous anus with a lax sphincter
D. Endoanal ultrasound usually shows a thickening of the external anal sphincter

316. Modified Ripstein operation is also called as:

A. STARR procedure
B. Posterior mesh rectopexy
C. Ventral mesh rectopexy
D. Perineal proctectomy

317. The Altemeier procedure is also called as:

A. STARR procedure
B. Anterior mesh rectopexy
C. Ventral mesh rectopexy
D. Perineal proctectomy

318. The rectal prolapse procedure shown in the following image is:

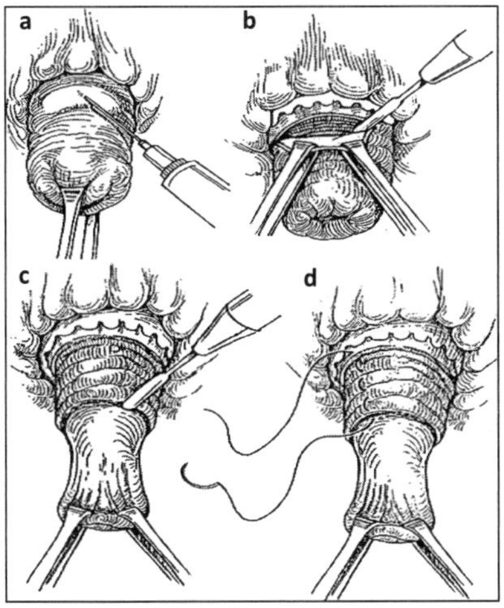

A. Delorme procedure
B. Altemeier procedure
C. STARR procedure
D. Posterior mesh rectopexy

319. The rectal prolapse procedure shown in the following image is:

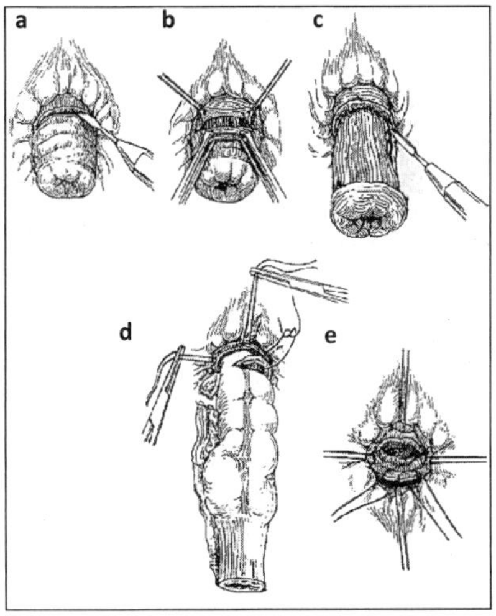

A. Delorme procedure
B. Altemeier procedure
C. STARR procedure
D. Posterior mesh rectopexy

320. False about Solitary rectal ulcer syndrome (SRUS) is:

A. 20% of patients have a single ulcer, while 40% of patients have multiple ulcers
B. SRUS is a disorder of young adults (30–40 years), with a slight male predominance
C. The cause is multifactorial and includes internal rectal prolapse and abnormal/paradoxical contraction of the puborectalis muscle
D. Symptoms reported by patients with SRUS include rectal bleeding, prolonged excessive straining, incomplete defecation/tenesmus, mucous discharge, perineal and abdominal pain and constipation

321. In Solitary rectal ulcer syndrome (SRUS), physical examination and anoscopy demonstrates:

A. 1 to 1.5-cm ulcer of the posterior rectal wall 3 to 10 cm from the anal verge
B. 2 to 2.5-cm ulcer of the posterior rectal wall 3 to 10 cm from the anal verge
C. 1 to 1.5-cm ulcer of the anterior rectal wall 3 to 10 cm from the anal verge
D. 2 to 2.5-cm ulcer of the anterior rectal wall 3 to 10 cm from the anal verge

322. False about the management of Solitary rectal ulcer syndrome (SRUS) is:

A. Histologic examination of biopsies shows characteristic findings: fibromuscular obliteration of the lamina propria, hypertrophied muscularis mucosae with muscular fibers between the crypts and glandular crypt abnormalities
B. Surgery is indicated only for highly symptomatic patients absolutely unresponsive to medical treatment
C. For patients with severe symptoms, medical treatment is usually effective
D. Surgical options include local excision of the ulcer, treatment of the rectal prolapse, or a defunctioning stoma for patients who have failed other options

323. The most common risk factors for rectocele are:

A. History of pregnancy and vaginal childbirth
B. History of hysterectomy
C. Advanced age
D. All of the above

324. False about the diagnosis of rectocele is:

A. The goal of surgery is to remove the redundant tissue of the rectocele and to strengthen the rectovaginal septum
B. Asymptomatic rectoceles do not need treatment, while patients with a symptomatic rectocele are initially managed with a bowel regimen and fiber products in order to improve defecation
C. The balloon expulsion tests can identify the inability to expel an inflated balloon from the rectum after 1 minute of sitting on a commode
D. Dynamic MRI and MRI defecography are limited by the fact that they are performed with the patient in the supine position

325. False about constipation is:

A. Constipation is a frequent condition that can affect more than 50% of population over 65

B. Hyperthyroidism and medication-induced constipation are common causes

C. Patients should be counselled to increase fluid intake up to 1.5 to 2 L/day and to increase the fiber content in diet

D. Several medical conditions can contribute to constipation, including metabolic, endocrine, neurologic and psychiatric disorders

326. According to Rome IV criteria, functional constipation is diagnosed if:

A. There are at least 2 of the following symptoms, during at least 25% of defecations, for at least 3 months - straining, lumpy, or hard stools; a sensation of incomplete evacuation

B. Loose stools rarely present without the use of laxatives

C. There are insufficient criteria for irritable bowel syndrome

D. All of the above

ANSWERS

1. **Ans: C. Internal anal sphincter is formed by the posterior part of the cloacal sphincter**

   Ref: Chapter No.52, Page No.1321

2. **Ans: A. Distal duodenum**

   Ref: Chapter No.52, Page No.1321

3. **Ans: B. Proximal one third of the transverse colon**

   Ref: Chapter No.52, Page No.1321

4. **Ans: B. Celiac artery**

   Ref: Chapter No.52, Page No.1321

5. **Ans: A. Superior mesenteric artery (SMA)**

   Ref: Chapter No.52, Page No.1321

6. **Ans: C. Inferior mesenteric artery (IMA)**

   Ref: Chapter No.52, Page No.1321

7. **Ans: B. Internal pudendal artery**

   Ref: Chapter No.52, Page No.1321

8. **Ans: C. 7.5 cm**

   Ref: Chapter No.52, Page No.1321

9. **Ans: B. The cecum has a thick wall compared to the rest of the colon and considering its large diameter**

   Ref: Chapter No.52, Page No.1321

10. **Ans: B. Caecum**

    Ref: Chapter No.52, Page No.1321

11. **Ans: C. 8 to 10 cm**

    Ref: Chapter No.52, Page No.1322

12. **Ans: A. Pelvic position**

    Ref: Chapter No.52, Page No.1322

13. **Ans: B. Retrocecal position**

    Ref: Chapter No.52, Page No.1322

14. **Ans: D. All of the above**

    Ref: Chapter No.52, Page No.1322

15. **Ans: B. 15 cm**

    Ref: Chapter No.52, Page No.1323

16. **Ans: C. 45 cm**

    Ref: Chapter No.52, Page No.1323

17. **Ans: B. Avascular plane of Toldt**

    Avascular plane of **Reeve:**

    - The avascular space, named as the space of Reeve, has been demonstrated to be an important anatomical landmark and should be identified at surgery.
    - Utilization of this space aids the ***recognition of structures close to the thyroid*** and can reduce morbidities of surgery which are associated with thyroid surgery.

    Avascular plane of **Brodel:**

    - The avascular plane of Brodel is the section of renal parenchyma ***between 2/3 anterior and 1/3 posterior kidney*** on the cross-section that is relatively avascular.
    - The reason for its relative avascularity is that it represents the plane where the ***anterior and posterior segmental*** renal artery ***branches meet.***
    - It is ***located just posterior to the lateral convex border of the kidney*** and permits a relatively safe access route to the pelvicalyceal system for nephrostomy ***insertion.***

    Avascular plane of **Heald:**

    - Dissection is along the avascular alveolar plane between the ***presacral and mesorectal fascia,*** described the ***'Holy Plane' of rectal surgery.***

    Ref: Chapter No.52, Page No.1323

    https://journals.sagepub.com/doi/pdf/10.1177/014107688808100904

    https://pubmed.ncbi.nlm.nih.gov/29160086/

18. **Ans: A. The greater omentum has 2 parts, the superior gastrocolic ligament composed of 4 serous layers, and the inferior portion, which is composed of 8 serous layers draping over the anterior abdominal cavity like an apron**

    Ref: Chapter No.52, Page No.1323

19. **Ans: C. Gastrocolic ligament to the body of stomach**

    Ref: Chapter No.52, Page No.1323

20. **Ans: C. The sigmoid is thinner and more mobile compared to the descending colon varying in length from 15 to 50 cm**

    Ref: Chapter No.52, Page No.1325

21. **Ans: B. Lower border of the L1 vertebra**

    Ref: Chapter No.52, Page No.1325

22. **Ans: B. 20%**

    Ref: Chapter No.52, Page No.1325

23. **Ans: B. L2–3 vertebrae (It is approximately 3 cm above the aortic bifurcation)**

    Ref: Chapter No.52, Page No.1325

24. **Ans: C. The Moskowitz artery**

    - The ***arc of Riolan,*** is also known as the ***mesenteric meandering artery (of Moskowitz)*** or ***central anastomotic mesenteric artery.***
    - It is an arterioarterial anastomosis between the ***superior and inferior mesenteric arteries.***

    Ref: Chapter No.52, Page No.1325

25. **Ans: A. Marginal artery of Drummond**

    - The marginal artery of Drummond, also known as the marginal artery of the colon, is a ***continuous arterial*** *circle* or *arcade along the inner border of the colon* formed by the anastomoses of the terminal branches of the ***superior mesenteric artery (SMA) and inferior mesenteric artery (IMA).***

- The marginal artery of **D**rummond runs **D**istally and the arc of **R**iolan p**R**oximally to the root of the mesentery.

Ref: Chapter No.52, Page No.1326

26. **Ans: B. The middle third of the rectum is totally extraperitoneal, extending from 1 to 5 cm above the dentate line**

Ref: Chapter No.52, Page No.1327

27. **Ans: B. 5 cm**

Ref: Chapter No.52, Page No.1327

28. **Ans: C. Waldeyer fascia (aka Rectosacral fascia)**

Ref: Chapter No.52, Page No.1328

29. **Ans: A. Presacral fascia**

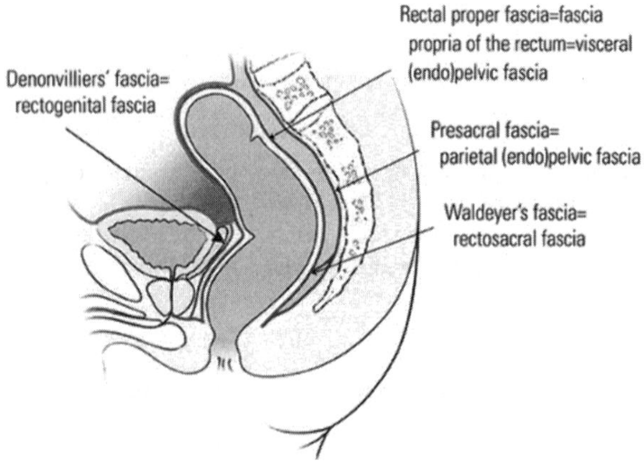

The relationship between fascia around the rectum:

- The **rectal proper fascia**, the fascia covering the mesorectum, is also called ***visceral endopelvic fascia***
- The **presacral fascia**, the fascia covering the sacrum, is also called the ***parietal endopelvic fascia***
- **Denonvilliers' fascia**, a dense membrane between the rectum and the seminal vesicles, is also called the ***rectogenital fascia***
- **Waldeyer's fascia** is a dense connective tissue layer between the posterior part of the rectal proper fascia and the presacral fascia at the ***S3 and S4 levels***

Ref: Chapter No.52, Page No.1328

30. **Ans: D. The inferior rectal arteries are branches of the external pudendal arteries**

Ref: Chapter No.52, Page No.1328

31. **Ans: D. All of the above**

Ref: Chapter No.52, Page No.1329

32. **Ans: B. The sympathetic innervation of the rectum is derived from sympathetic nerves exiting at the level of L4–5, forming the superior hypogastric plexus**

Ref: Chapter No.52, Page No.1329

33. **Ans: C. The ascending colon and descending colon are usually fixed to the retroperitoneum**

Ref: Chapter No.52, Page No.1321-1325

34. **Ans: D. Butyrate is a short-chain fatty acid and a bacterial fermentation product that is the main fuel for colonic epithelial cells**

Ref: Chapter No.52, Page No.1332

35. **Ans: C. Colon has the ability to absorb up to 2 L of fluid per day**

Ref: Chapter No.52, Page No.1330

36. **Ans: D. 90%**

Ref: Chapter No.52, Page No.1330

37. **Ans: B. ~150 mL/day**

Ref: Chapter No.52, Page No.1330

38. **Ans: A. Aldosterone decreases colonic potassium secretion and this effect is blocked by spironolactone**

Ref: Chapter No.52, Page No.1330-1331

39. **Ans: D. All of the above**

Ref: Chapter No.52, Page No.1330

40. **Ans: A. When the colonic absorptive capacity is exceeded, colonic bacteria conjugate bile acids**

Ref: Chapter No.52, Page No.1331

41. **Ans: D. 10^{11} to 10^{12} bacterial cells/gram**

Ref: Chapter No.52, Page No.1332

42. **Ans: B. 50% of fecal mass**

Ref: Chapter No.52, Page No.1332

43. **Ans: D. Bulking agents decrease intracolonic pressures and decrease colonic transit time**

Ref: Chapter No.52, Page No.1332

44. **Ans: D. < 50% of the SCFAs produced are absorbed**

Ref: Chapter No.52, Page No.1332

45. **Ans: B. 50%**

Ref: Chapter No.52, Page No.1332

46. **Ans: C. Prebiotics are digestible oligosaccharides that help the host by stimulating the growth of certain species of beneficial intestinal bacteria**

Ref: Chapter No.52, Page No.1333

47. **Ans: C. High-amplitude propagated contractions (HAPCs) allow mixing, which promotes optimal absorption and are bursts of short-duration contractions**

Ref: Chapter No.52, Page No.1333

48. **Ans: A. Colonic transit is longer in men than in men and longer in postmenopausal than in premenopausal women**

Ref: Chapter No.52, Page No.1333

49. **Ans: D. Preoperative enemas alone, without mechanical bowel preparation and oral antibiotics, are generally recommended for patients undergoing elective colorectal surgery**

The American Society of Colon and Rectal Surgeons Clinical Practice Guidelines for The Use of Bowel Preparation in Elective Colon and Rectal Surgery – 2019

1. *MBP combined with preoperative oral antibiotics is typically recommended for elective colorectal resections.*

   Grade of Recommendation: Strong recommendation based on moderate-quality evidence, 1B.

2. Preoperative ***MBP alone***, without oral antibiotics, is generally ***not recommended*** for patients undergoing elective colorectal surgery.

   Grade of Recommendation: Strong recommendation based on high-quality evidence, 1A.

3. Preoperative ***oral antibiotics alone***, without mechanical preparation, are generally ***not recommended*** for patients undergoing elective colorectal surgery.

   Grade of Recommendation: Weak recommendation based on low-quality evidence, 2C.

4. Preoperative ***enemas alone, without MBP and oral antibiotics***, are generally ***not recommended*** for patients undergoing elective colorectal surgery.

   Grade of Recommendation: Weak recommendation based on moderate-quality evidence, 2B.

Ref: Chapter No.52, Page No.1333-1334

https://fascrs.org/healthcare-providers/education/clinical-practice-guidelines

50. Ans: D. All of the above

Ref: Chapter No.52, Page No.1334

51. Ans: C. Xiphisternum

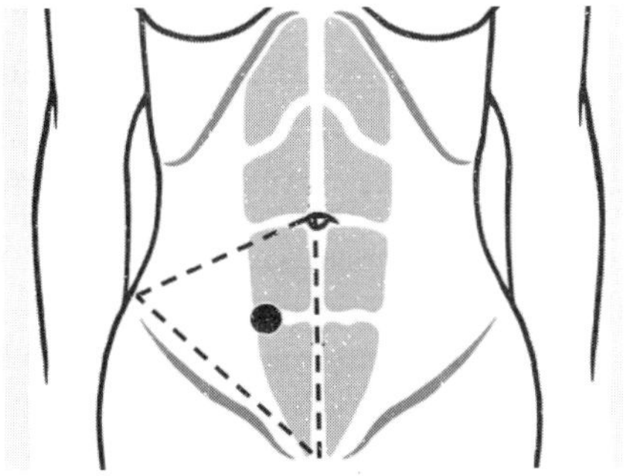

- In routine situations, marking begins with identifying the "ostomy triangle" bounded by the ***anterior superior iliac spine, the pubic tubercle, and the umbilicus.***
- The stoma, **ileostomy** traditionally on the ***right*** and colostomy on the ***left***, is placed in the center of this triangle, ***through the rectus muscle slightly below the umbilicus***.
- The site should be ***5 cm away*** from skin folds, prior scars or bony prominences, and the patient's belt line. This will allow for proper fitting of the stoma appliance.
- However, in difficult situations, such as a **large patient**, with a thick abdominal wall (particularly if there is a large abdominal pannus) marking ***superior to the umbilicus*** will facilitate both stoma creation (there is less fat above the umbilicus allowing for easier stoma construction) and stoma care (it is very difficult for obese patients to see stomas below their umbilicus).
- Individuals with disabilities, such as a spinal cord injury, should be marked in the position they spend most time, as this will facilitate appliance fitting and care.
- In making the stoma aperture in the abdominal wall, the ***rectus muscle is split*** and the ***rectus sheath is divided sharply.***

Stoma siting procedure as per **American Society of Colon and Rectal Surgeons (ASCRS)**

1. Gather items needed for the procedure: Marking pen, surgical marker, transparent film dressing, flat skin barrier (according to surgeon's preference and facility policy).
2. Explain stoma marking procedure to patient, and encourage patient participation and input.
3. Carefully examine patient's abdominal surface. Begin with patient fully clothed in sitting position with feet on floor. Observe the presence of belts, braces and any other ostomy appliances.
4. Examine patient's exposed abdomen in various positions (standing, lying, sitting and bending forward) to observe for creases, valleys, scars, folds, skin turgor and contour.
5. Draw an imaginary line where the surgical incision is going to be. Choose a point approximately ***2 inches*** from the surgical incision where 2 – 3 inches of flat adhesive barrier can be placed.
6. With patient lying on back identify the rectus muscle. (This can be done having the patient do a modified sit up (raise the head up off the bed). Placement within the rectus muscle can help to prevent peristomal hernia formation and/or prolapse.
7. Choose an area that is visible to the patient, and if possible, below the belt line to conceal the pouch.
8. If the abdomen is large, choose the apex of the mound or if the patient is extremely obese, place in the upper abdominal quadrants.
9. It may be desirable to mark sites on the right and left sides of the abdomen to prepare for a change in the surgical outcome (you may want to number your first choice as 1 #).
10. Clean the desired site with alcohol and allow to dry. Then proceed with marking the selected site with a surgical marker/pen. You may cover with transparent film dressing if desired to preserve the mark.
11. Once marked have the patient assume sitting, bending and lying position to assess and confirm best choice. It is important to have the patient confirm they can see the site.

Ref: Chapter No.52, Page No.1334

https://fascrs.org/ascrs/media/files/downloads/publications/stoma_sting_procedure.pdf

52. Ans: A. In obese individuals, the thickest part of the abdominal wall is often in the upper abdomen and hence colostomies should be created in upper abdomen

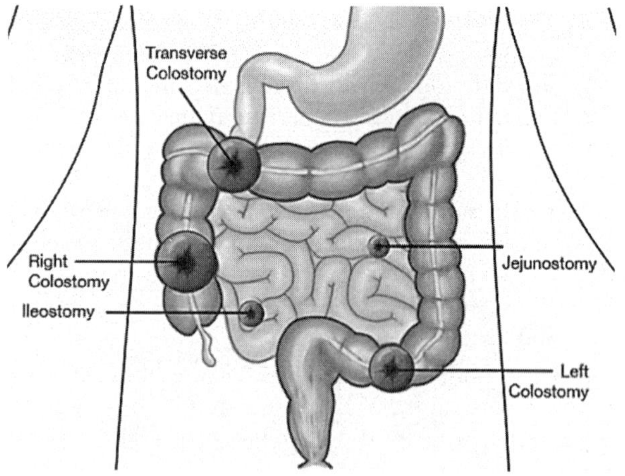

Ref: Chapter No.52, Page No.1335

53. **Ans: D. All of the above**

Ref: Chapter No.52, Page No.1335-1336

54. **Ans: B. < 1000 mL**

Ref: Chapter No.52, Page No.1335

55. **Ans: B. Hypothermia**

Ref: Chapter No.52, Page No.1336
https://link.springer.com/article/10.1007/s00268-018-4844-y

56. **Ans: C. 20%**

Ref: Chapter No.52, Page No.1336

57. **Ans: C. There is strong evidence to support the recommendation of a clear liquid diet up until 4 hours before the induction of anesthesia**

Ref: Chapter No.52, Page No.1336

58. **Ans: D. Dehydration**

Ref: Chapter No.52, Page No.1336

59. **Ans: A. The rectum is generally affected**

Ref: Chapter No.52, Page No.1337

60. **Ans: C. > 25% of patients with diverticulosis will develop diverticulitis**

Ref: Chapter No.52, Page No.1337

61. **Ans: B. 50%**

Ref: Chapter No.52, Page No.1337

62. **Ans: C. History of smoking**

Ref: Chapter No.52, Page No.1337

63. **Ans: B. Rectal bleeding is a common in the presentation of acute diverticulitis**

Ref: Chapter No.52, Page No.1338

64. **Ans: D. CT scan has the ability to distinguish between grade 3 and grade 4**

Ref: Chapter No.52, Page No.1338

65. **Ans: B. Stage Ib**

Ref: Chapter No.52, Page No.1338

66. **Ans: C. Stage III**

Ref: Chapter No.52, Page No.1338

67. **Ans: A. Stage Ia**

Ref: Chapter No.52, Page No.1338

68. **Ans: C. Patients with abscesses amenable to percutaneous drainage and responsive to treatment still require urgent surgery**

Ref: Chapter No.52, Page No.1338-1339

69. **Ans: B. Colovesical fistula**

Ref: Chapter No.52, Page No.1338

70. **Ans: B. It is not important, prior to resection, to perform a colonoscopy**

Ref: Chapter No.52, Page No.1339

71. **Ans: D. All of the above**

Ref: Chapter No.52, Page No.1339

72. **Ans: C. Following the initial episode of acute, uncomplicated diverticulitis, 50% to 65% of individuals will have another episode**

Ref: Chapter No.52, Page No.1339

73. **Ans: D. It is common in western countries but rare in the Asian countries**

Ref: Chapter No.52, Page No.1340

74. **Ans: B. The prevalence of diverticulitis in these patients is more compared to the general population**

Ref: Chapter No.52, Page No.1340

75. **Ans: C. Cecal diverticula are considered congenital in origin**

- Isolated cecal diverticula are usually ***true or congenital***. However, acquired diverticulosis may affect all parts of the colon (pan-diverticulosis).
- Cecal diverticulitis is ***relatively uncommon***, and ***80%*** of cases are initially diagnosed as *acute appendicitis or, occasionally, perforated cancer*.

Ref: Chapter No.52, Page No.1339
https://www.sciencedirect.com/science/article/pii/S2049080115000084

76. **Ans: C. Diverticulosis**

Ref: Chapter No.52, Page No.1337

77. **Ans: A. Total colectomy**

Ref: Chapter No.52, Page No.1339

78. **Ans: C. Computed tomography (CT) of the abdomen/pelvis with orally and intravenous (IV) contrast**

Ref: Chapter No.52, Page No.1338

79. **Ans: C. Pneumaturia and faecaluria may also be present**

Ref: Chapter No.52, Page No.1338

80. **Ans: C. Fistulisation to adjacent organs such as the bladder with colovesical fistula**

Ref: Chapter No.52, Page No.1338-1339

81. **Ans: C. Bowel rest, nasogastric suction, IV fluids, and broad spectrum antibiotics**

Ref: Chapter No.52, Page No.1339

82. **Ans: A. IV fluids, cefoxitin and nasogastric drainage**

Ref: Chapter No.52, Page No.1339

83. **Ans: B. Large bowel obstruction, defined as bowel obstruction distal to the ligament of Treitz**

Ref: Chapter No.52, Page No.1340

84. **Ans: A. Sigmoid colon**

Ref: Chapter No.52, Page No.1340

85. **Ans: D. All of the above**

Ref: Chapter No.52, Page No.1340

86. **Ans: B. Although most malignant obstructions occur in the proximal parts of the colon, the necrosis and perforation usually occur in the sigmoid colon**

Ref: Chapter No.52, Page No.1340

87. **Ans: D. Plain films of the abdomen can help in localizing the obstruction, but does not demonstrate the degree of distension as well as the status of the ileocecal valve**

Ref: Chapter No.52, Page No.1341

88. **Ans: D. All of the above**

Ref: Chapter No.52, Page No.1341

89. **Ans: A. Caecal volvulus (Whirl's sign seen in Caecal volvulus)**

Ref: Chapter No.52, Page No.1341

90. **Ans: B. Right hemicolectomy and primary anastomosis with or without diverting ileostomy**

Ref: Chapter No.52, Page No.1341-1342

91. **Ans: D. All of the above**

Ref: Chapter No.52, Page No.1342

92. **Ans: B. Foreign bodies can usually be removed via surgery**

Ref: Chapter No.52, Page No.1342

93. **Ans: D. If the gangrenous bowel is seen during decompression, a rectal tube should be placed to prevent recurrence**

Ref: Chapter No.52, Page No.1342

94. **Ans: C. Downward folding of the cecum**

In general, there are 3 different types of cecal volvulus:

- **Type 1:** This cecal volvulus forms by a ***clockwise axial twisting or torsion*** *of the* ***cecum*** along the long axis. The location of the cecal volvulus is in the ***right lower quadrant***.
- **Type 2:** This cecal volvulus develops from a ***twisting or torsion of a portion*** *of the* ***cecum and a portion of the terminal ileum***. The location of the cecum gets displaced to an ectopic location (typically ***left upper quadrant***) and is relocated in an inverted orientation. Traditionally, but not for all cases, a type 2 cecal volvulus will encounter a ***counter clockwise twist***.
- **Type 3:** This cecal volvulus (also known as ***cecal bascule***) is the ***upward folding of the cecum***. There is ***no axial twisting*** like with type 1 and type 2.

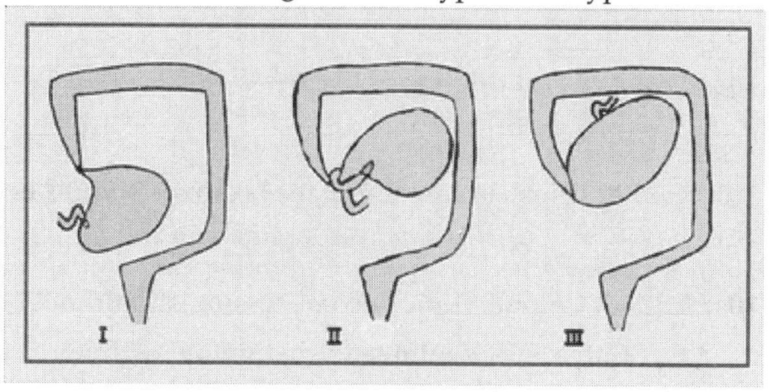

Type 1 and type 2, which involve axial torsion, account for approximately ***80%*** of all cecal volvuli.

Cecal bascules account for the remaining ***20%*** of cecal volvuli.

Ref: Chapter No.52, Page No.1342

https://www.ncbi.nlm.nih.gov/books/NBK470305/

https://link.springer.com/article/10.1007/s10140-007-0647-4/figures/1

95. **Ans: C. Volvulus of the sigmoid colon**

Ref: Chapter No.52, Page No.1342

96. **Ans: B. Sigmoid volvulus**

Ref: Chapter No.52, Page No.1342

97. **Ans: D. Rigid sigmoidoscopy**

- Bedside decompression with a flatus tube should only be carried out by experienced physicians, and ***under no circumstance against resistance***, as there is a risk of inadvertent iatrogenic perforation.
- The safest method to decompress the sigmoid colon is ***under direct vision with rigid or flexible sigmoidoscopy.***
- A successful decompression will immediately ***result in the evacuation of liquid and gas per rectum with subsequent resolution of the abdominal distension***, resulting in a soft abdomen.
- This resolution can be ***documented on a repeat abdominal radiograph.***
- It is important to ***assess the patient for sustained resolution*** once the flatus tube has been removed and the patient is started on oral intake, to avoid the volvulus recur before the patient is even discharged.

https://www.ncbi.nlm.nih.gov/books/NBK441925/#:~:text=Sigmoid%20volvulus%20is%20the%20most,a%20history%20of%20chronic%20constipation.

Ref: Chapter No.52, Page No.1342

98. **Ans: C. Systemic toxicity and peritoneal signs are common**

Ref: Chapter No.52, Page No.1342-1343

99. **Ans: A. Hypertension**

Ref: Chapter No.52, Page No.1343

100. Ans: B. Oral hypoglycemic agents

Ref: Chapter No.52, Page No.1343

101. Ans: B. A water-soluble contrast enema can't reliably distinguish between a mechanical obstruction and pseudo-obstruction

Ref: Chapter No.52, Page No.1343

102. Ans: A. Cecal dilation > 10 cm

Ref: Chapter No.52, Page No.1343

103. Ans: A. Osmotic and stimulant laxatives should be tried as first line of management

Ref: Chapter No.52, Page No.1343-1344

104. Ans: D. Colonoscopic decompression should not be considered in patients with contraindications to neostigmine

- **Catchpole Regimen:** Neostigmine regimen used in colonic pseudo-obstruction. The combined use of a sympathetic blocker followed by a cholinesterase inhibitor (neostigmine) to treat motility disorders was ***first documented by Catchpole*** in 1969.

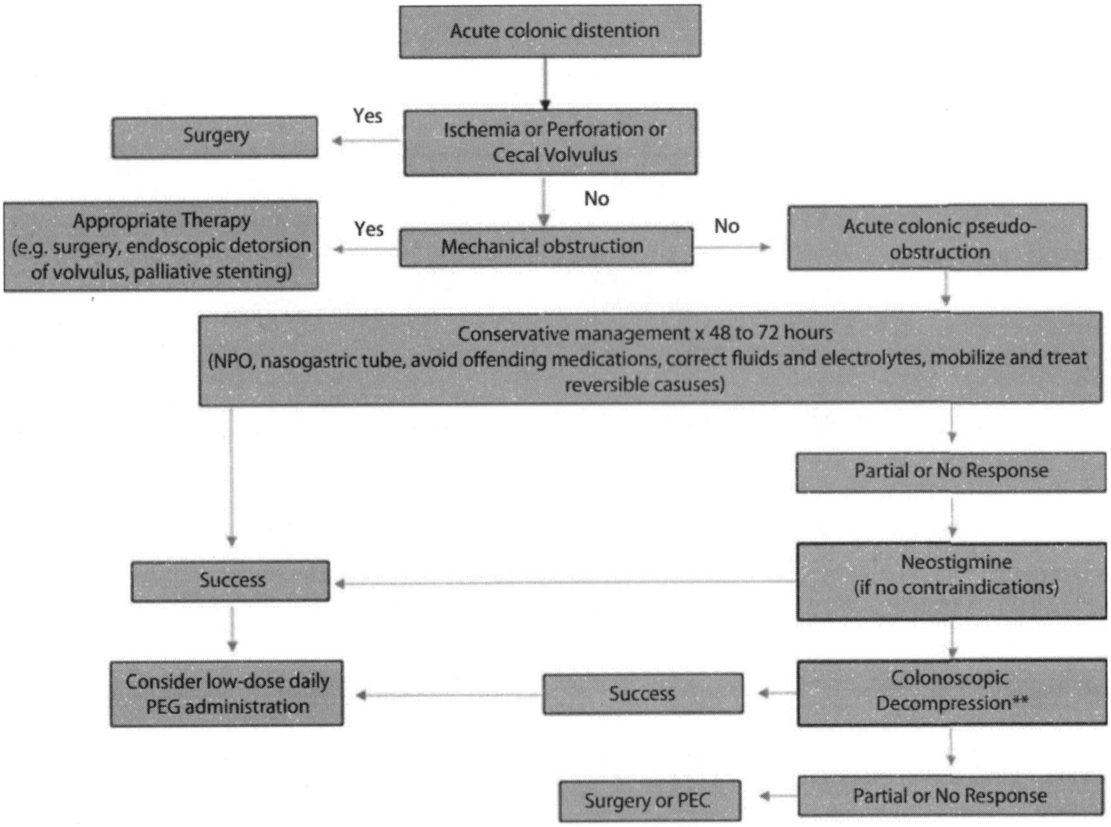

Ref: 1. Chapter No.52, Page No.1344
2. https://www.asge.org/docs/default-source/guidelines/american-society-for-gastrointestinal-endoscopy-guideline-on-the-role-of-endoscopy-in-the-management-of-acute-colonic-pseudo-obstruction-and-colonic-volvulus-2020-february-gie.pdf?sfvrsn=294db752_2
3. https://journals.co.za/doi/pdf/10.10520/AJA20785135_31858

105. Ans: C. In Crohn's disease smoking tends to suppress symptoms, whereas in UC, smoking tends to exacerbate symptoms

Ref: Chapter No.52, Page No.1344

106. Ans: B. Roughly 25% of patients with UC will have associated perianal disease

Ref: Chapter No.52, Page No.1344-1345

107. Ans: B. Sclerosing cholangitis is estimated to affect approximately 50% of patients with IBD

Ref: Chapter No.52, Page No.1346

108. Ans: D. Mayo Clinic Scoring System

Ref: Chapter No.52, Page No.1346

109. Ans: C. Grade 3

Ref: Chapter No.52, Page No.1346

110. Ans: D. Grade 4

Ref: Chapter No.52, Page No.1346

111. Ans: A. Crohn's disease ulcers are worse on the anti-mesenteric side of the bowel

Ref: Chapter No.52, Page No.1346

112. Ans: B. In patients with UC, term "focal active enteritis" is used

Ref: Chapter No.52, Page No.1346

113. Ans: B. 10% - 15%

Ref: Chapter No.52, Page No.1346

114. Ans: A. This medication is most effective for severe disease

Ref: Chapter No.52, Page No.1348

115. Ans: D. All of the above

Ref: Chapter No.52, Page No.1348-1349

116. Ans: B. Thiopurine intramuscular dosing is particularly convenient in patients who have problems with significant diarrhea or absorption issues (e.g., short bowel syndrome)

Ref: Chapter No.52, Page No.1349

117. Ans: A. The first agent was Adalimumab, which was approved by the FDA

Ref: Chapter No.52, Page No.1349

118. Ans: B. Truelove and Witts classification

FORMULA

- Diagnosis is mild when all six criteria are satisfied.
- Diagnosis is severe when criteria for frequency of bowel movement and ≥ 1 features of systemic upset (bolded) are satisfied.
- Diagnosis is moderate when variables fall between these criteria.

Severity of ulcerative colitis

Variable	**Mild**	**Moderate**	**Severe**
Bowel movements per day	<4	4-5	≥ 6
Blood in stool	None or no more than small amounts of blood	Between mild and severe	Visible blood
Pyrexia*	No	No	Yes
Pulse > 90 bpm	No	No	Yes
Anemia**	No	No	Yes
Erythrocyte sedimentation rate, mm/hr	≤ 30		> 30

* Defined as temperature ≥ 100.04 °F (37.8 °C).

** Defined as hemoglobin ≤ 10.5 g/dL (105 g/L).

Ref: Chapter No.52, Page No.1349
https://www.mdcalc.com/calc/10235/truelove-witts-severity-index-ulcerative-colitis#evidence

119. Ans: A. Harvey Bradshaw index [And Crohn's disease activity index (CDAI)]

Ref: Chapter No.52, Page No.1349

120. Ans: C. Moderate disease

Ref: Chapter No.52, Page No.1349

https://www.mdcalc.com/calc/10069/harvey-bradshaw-index-hbi-crohns-disease#evidence

121. Ans: A. >16

Harvey-Bradshaw Index (HBI) for Crohn's Disease

- Simpler than the CDAI, which requires symptoms ***over the past 7 days***.
- Shown to have 93% correlation with the CDAI in the original study (Harvey 1980).
- Since the ***CDAI requires a 7-day patient symptom diary***, the Harvey-Bradshaw Index was proposed as a modification of this scheme that only used clinical data.

Harvey-Bradshaw Index	Severity
<5	Remission
5-7	Mild disease
8-16	Moderate disease
>16	Severe disease

Ref: Chapter No.52, Page No.1349

https://www.mdcalc.com/calc/10069/harvey-bradshaw-index-hbi-crohns-disease#evidence

122. Ans: D. CDAI >450

Crohn's disease activity index (CDAI)

Score interpretation:

- **CDAI <150** is a marker of ***remission*** of Crohn's disease
- **CDAI >450** is a marker of ***severe*** Crohn's disease

Ref: Chapter No.52, Page No.1349

123. Ans: A. Hypoalbuminemia < 3.5 g/dL[3]

Ref: Chapter No.52, Page No.1349-1350

124. Ans: A. > 5 cm

Ref: Chapter No.52, Page No.1350

125. Ans: D. All of the above

Ref: Chapter No.52, Page No.1350

126. Ans: D. J Pouch

Ref: Chapter No.52, Page No.1352

127. Ans: C. 15 cm

Ref: Chapter No.52, Page No.1352

128. Ans: D. All of the above

Ref: Chapter No.52, Page No.1353-1354

129. Ans: D. Prednisone

Ref: Chapter No.52, Page No.1348

130. Ans: B. Proctocolectomy with ileal pouch–anal anastomosis (IPAA)

Ref: Chapter No.52, Page No.1352

131. Ans: B. Surgery is curative for this diagnosis

Ref: Chapter No.52, Page No.1352

132. Ans: B. Pelvic sepsis

Ref: Chapter No.52, Page No.1353

133. Ans: A. Nasoenteric decompression, broad-spectrum antibiotics and intravenous steroids

Ref: Chapter No.52, Page No.1352

134. Ans: A. Backwash ileitis is associated with ulcerative colitis

Ref: Chapter No.52, Page No.1352

135. Ans: B. The disease is confluent, there are no skip areas in the colon and the rectum is involved

Ref: Chapter No.52, Page No.1346

136. Ans: C. Toxic megacolon

Ref: Chapter No.52, Page No.1349-1350

137. Ans: D. Total proctocolectomy

Ref: Chapter No.52, Page No.1350

138. Ans: C. Followed by improvement after bypass of the diseased segment

- Crohn's disease differs from ulcerative colitis in that clinical improvement usually occurs when a diseased segment is excluded from the fecal stream

Ref: Chapter No.52, Page No.1352

139. Ans: C. The serosa appeared normal on inspection, but the colon mucosa was extensively involved

- In ulcerative colitis, the distal rectum and colon are primarily involved in continuity to the proximal extent of the lesion

Ref: Chapter No.52, Page No.1352

140. Ans: D. 10–20 years

Ref: Chapter No.52, Page No.1350

141. Ans: A. Occurs more frequently than in the rest of the population

Ref: Chapter No.52, Page No.1350

142. Ans: A. Toxic megacolon in ulcerative colitis

Ref: Chapter No.52, Page No.1344-1346

143. Ans: D. All of the above

Ref: Chapter No.52, Page No.1352

144. Ans: A. C difficile is an anaerobic, spore-forming, gram-negative bacillus

Ref: Chapter No.52, Page No.1355-1356

145. Ans: D. All of the above

Ref: Chapter No.52, Page No.1356

146. Ans: D. The most important risk factor for the development of a clinical infection is Immunodeficiency

Ref: Chapter No.52, Page No.1356

147. Ans: B. Hyperalbuminemia

Ref: Chapter No.52, Page No.1356

148. Ans: C. Serum BUN

ATLAS Criteria

Age

Treatment with systemic antibiotics during C diff infection therapy (≥1 day duration)

Leukocyte count

Serum Albumin

Serum Creatinine

ATLAS Score	Cure rate	Mortality
0	95.7%	0.0%
1	93.3%	0.0%
2	92.7%	0.0%
3	89.5%	3.6%
4	81.1%	4.2%
5	76.1%	8.7%
6	85.7%	10.9%
7	50.0%	14.3%
8	55.6%	56.0%
9	33.0%	
10	< 33.0%	> 56.0%

Ref: Chapter No.52, Page No.1356

149. Ans: A. Imaging is very useful for diagnosis as it is very specific

Ref: Chapter No.52, Page No.1356

150. Ans: B. The use of antiperistaltic agents for the treatment of CDI should be promoted

Ref: Chapter No.52, Page No.1356

151. Ans: D. All of the above

Ref: Chapter No.52, Page No.1356

152. Ans: B. Bezlotoxumab

Ref: Chapter No.52, Page No.1356

153. Ans: A. Actoxumab

Ref: Chapter No.52, Page No.1356

154. Ans: A. IV metronidazole and vancomycin via a rectal tube

Ref: Chapter No.52, Page No.1357

155. Ans: D. Commonly involves the sigmoid and descending colon

Ref: Chapter No.52, Page No.1358

156. Ans: B. Often affects cecum and terminal ileum

Ref: Chapter No.52, Page No.1358

157. Ans: A. Ischemic colitis is considered a disease of large blood vessels and typically presents more dramatically, requiring vascular intervention

Ref: Chapter No.52, Page No.1358

158. Ans: A. Splenic flexure

Ref: Chapter No.52, Page No.1358

159. Ans: C. Rectosigmoid junction

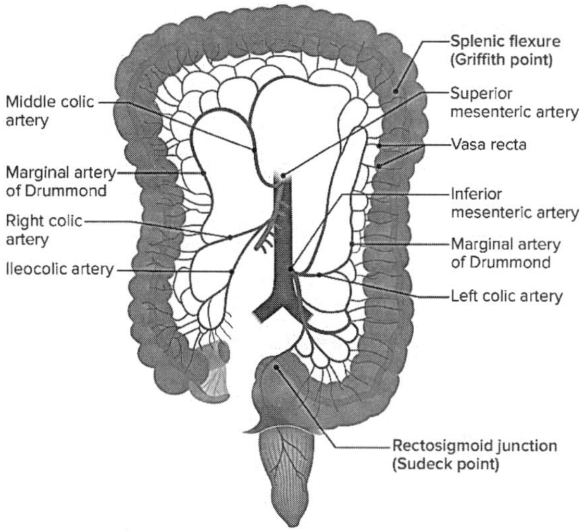

Ref: Chapter No.52, Page No.1359

160. Ans: A. Men

Ref: Chapter No.52, Page No.1359

161. Ans: A. About a 80% of the patients present with isolated right-sided ischemic colitis

Ref: Chapter No.52, Page No.1359

162. Ans: B. Left colon

Ref: Chapter No.52, Page No.1359

163. Ans: B. Thumbprinting

- **Thumbprinting** is a radiographic sign of large bowel wall thickening, usually caused by edema, related to an ***infective or inflammatory process (colitis)***

Ref: Chapter No.52, Page No.1359

164. Ans: A. The most common symptoms are lower abdominal pain and bright red rectal bleeding

Ref: Chapter No.52, Page No.1359

165. Ans: B. Patients with isolated right-sided ischemic colitis have a higher chance of requiring surgery and have a poorer prognosis

Ref: Chapter No.52, Page No.1359

166. Ans: D. Flexible endoscopy

Ref: Chapter No.52, Page No.1360

167. Ans: D. All of the above

Ref: Chapter No.52, Page No.1359

168. Ans: B. Flexible endoscopy

Ref: Chapter No.52, Page No.1360

169. Ans: C. Diagnostic endoscopy usually can distinguish between partial-thickness and full-thickness ischemia

Ref: Chapter No.52, Page No.1360

170. Ans: D. 80%

Ref: Chapter No.52, Page No.1360

171. Ans: C. Glucocorticoids should be always given unless treating a pre-existing disorder such as lupus or rheumatoid arthritis

Ref: Chapter No.52, Page No.1360

172. Ans: D. All of the above

Ref: Chapter No.52, Page No.1361

173. Ans: D. All of the above

Ref: Chapter No.52, Page No.1361

174. Ans: D. All of the above

Ref: Chapter No.52, Page No.1361-1362

175. Ans: B. BRAF gene

Ref: Chapter No.52, Page No.1364

176. Ans: D. 15% of early-stage CRCs

Ref: Chapter No.52, Page No.1364

177. Ans: B. CMS2 cancers show an epithelial phenotype and exhibit marked WNT and MYC signaling activation

Ref: Chapter No.52, Page No.1364

178. Ans: D. All of the above

Ref: Chapter No.52, Page No.1365

179. Ans: A. Consists of elongated colonic crypts with a papillary configuration of epithelial cells with atypia

Ref: Chapter No.52, Page No.1365

180. Ans: D. All of the above

Ref: Chapter No.52, Page No.1366

181. Ans: D. All of the above

Ref: Chapter No.52, Page No.1367

182. Ans: B. These polyps should not be removed

Ref: Chapter No.52, Page No.1367

183. Ans: D. All of the above

Ref: Chapter No.52, Page No.1367

184. Ans: C. Tubular adenoma

Ref: Chapter No.52, Page No.1367

185. Ans: D. All of the above

Ref: Chapter No.52, Page No.1367

186. Ans: A. 5%

Ref: Chapter No.52, Page No.1367

187. Ans: C. 50%

Ref: Chapter No.52, Page No.1367

188. Ans: B. Carcinoma invading into the submucosa, limited to the head of the polyp

Ref: Chapter No.52, Page No.1367

189. Ans: D. Haggitt's level 4

Ref: Chapter No.52, Page No.1368

190. Ans: D. Haggitt's level 4

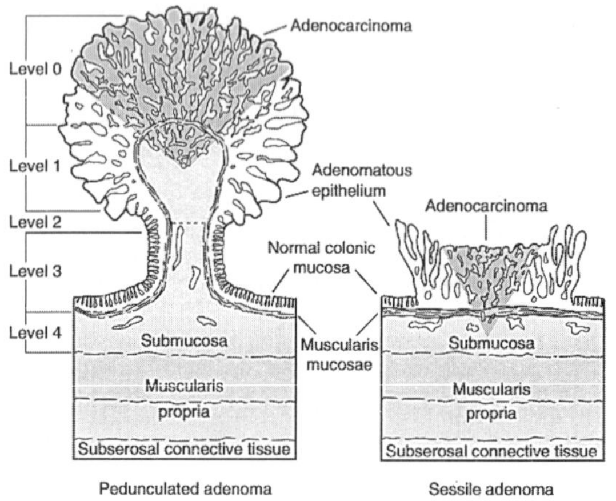

Ref: Chapter No.52, Page No.1368

191. Ans: A. Sm1

Ref: Chapter No.52, Page No.1368

192. Ans: D. 5 years

Ref: Chapter No.52, Page No.1369

193. Ans: C. 10 years

Ref: Chapter No.52, Page No.1369

194. Ans: B. 3 years

Ref: Chapter No.52, Page No.1369

195. Ans: A. 6 months

Ref: Chapter No.52, Page No.1369

196. Ans: B. A 2 cm pedunculated carcinoma–containing adenomatous polyp with low-grade differentiation, positive lymphovascular invasion, and no mucosal penetration resected completely in one session

Ref: Chapter No.52, Page No.1367

197. Ans: B. Hamartomas

Ref: Chapter No.52, Page No.1366

198. Ans: C. Hyperplastic polyp

Ref: Chapter No.52, Page No.1365

199. Ans: B. Familial polyposis of the colon

Ref: Chapter No.52, Page No.1368-1369

200. Ans: B. Chromosome 5q21

Ref: Chapter No.52, Page No.1368

201. Ans: D. 80% to 90%

Ref: Chapter No.52, Page No.1368

202. Ans: C. 25%

Ref: Chapter No.52, Page No.1368

203. Ans: D. 100%

Ref: Chapter No.52, Page No.1368

204. Ans: B. 39 years

Ref: Chapter No.52, Page No.1368

205. Ans: D. All of the above

Ref: Chapter No.52, Page No.1368-1369

206. Ans: C. 50%

Ref: Chapter No.52, Page No.1369

207. Ans: A. Antrum

Ref: Chapter No.52, Page No.1369

208. Ans: A. 10%

Ref: Chapter No.52, Page No.1369

209. Ans: C. 30% to 70% (there is a predilection for the *ampullary and periampullary regions*)

Ref: Chapter No.52, Page No.1369

210. Ans: B. 4% to 10%

Ref: Chapter No.52, Page No.1369

211. Ans: B. Duodenal cancer

Ref: Chapter No.52, Page No.1369

212. Ans: C. Spigelman classification

Ref: Chapter No.52, Page No.1369

213. Ans: B. These tumors are associated with male gender and with a family history of desmoids

Ref: Chapter No.52, Page No.1369-1370

214. Ans: B. 10% to 15%

Ref: Chapter No.52, Page No.1369

215. Ans: A. 2%

Ref: Chapter No.52, Page No.1370

216. Ans: D. 60% to 85%

Ref: Chapter No.52, Page No.1370

217. Ans: A. Medulloblastoma

Ref: Chapter No.52, Page No.1370

218. Ans: D. 80% of cases

Ref: Chapter No.52, Page No.1370

219. Ans: D. All of the above

Ref: Chapter No.52, Page No.1369

220. Ans: C. 20 or more cumulative colorectal adenomas are found

Ref: Chapter No.52, Page No.1370

221. Ans: B. 12

Ref: Chapter No.52, Page No.1370

222. Ans: D. All of the above

Ref: Chapter No.52, Page No.1370

223. Ans: C. 20 to 25 years of age

Ref: Chapter No.52, Page No.1370

224. Ans: D. All of the above

Ref: Chapter No.52, Page No.1370-1371

225. Ans: B. MUTYH-associated polyposis

Ref: Chapter No.52, Page No.1369

226. Ans: C. 80%

Ref: Chapter No.52, Page No.1369

227. Ans: A. 40%

Ref: Chapter No.52, Page No.1369

228. Ans: A. 40%

Ref: Chapter No.52, Page No.1369

229. Ans: C. 80%

Ref: Chapter No.52, Page No.1369

230. Ans: B. MUTYH-associated polyposis

Ref: Chapter No.52, Page No.1369

231. Ans: B. Repeat endoscopy in 6–12 months and surgical evaluation

Ref: Chapter No.52, Page No.1370

232. Ans: A. As soon as possible

Ref: Chapter No.52, Page No.1370

233. Ans: C. >100 synchronous adenomas

Ref: Chapter No.52, Page No.1371

234. Ans: A. Rectum containing > 10 rectal adenomas

Ref: Chapter No.52, Page No.1371

235. Ans: D. The diagnosis of MAP should be considered in patients presenting with colorectal polyposis (>100 lifetime adenomas)

Ref: Chapter No.52, Page No.1371

236. Ans: A. Chromosome 1

Ref: Chapter No.52, Page No.1371

237. Ans: B. Osteomas, desmoids and CHRPE are also associated with MAP

Ref: Chapter No.52, Page No.1372

238. Ans: D. All of the above

Ref: Chapter No.52, Page No.1372

239. Ans: B. Skin cancer

Ref: Chapter No.52, Page No.1372

240. Ans: C. 19p

Ref: Chapter No.52, Page No.1372

241. Ans: D. 5 or more histologically confirmed Peutz-Jeghers polyps

Ref: Chapter No.52, Page No.1372

242. Ans: B. Women should have breast physical examinations every 6 months and yearly mammogram and breast MRI starting at age 45 years

Ref: Chapter No.52, Page No.1372

243. Ans: A. There is an increased cancer risk in afflicted individuals, with a malignant potential of at least 50% in patients with multiple juvenile polyps

Ref: Chapter No.52, Page No.1372

244. Ans: B. 3% to 5%

Ref: Chapter No.52, Page No.1372

245. Ans: B. Mutations in MLH1 and MSH2 account for up to 20% of patients with Lynch syndrome

Ref: Chapter No.52, Page No.1372-1373

246. Ans: B. 3 or more successive generations are affected

Ref: Chapter No.52, Page No.1373

247. Ans: D. Adenoma may progress to carcinoma within 5 to 10 years, compared with from 10 to 20 years in the general population

Ref: Chapter No.52, Page No.1373

248. Ans: A. Endometrial adenocarcinoma

Ref: Chapter No.52, Page No.1373

249. Ans: C. Endometrial adenocarcinoma

Ref: Chapter No.52, Page No.1373

250. Ans: A. Colorectal cancer diagnosed in at least 3 first- or second-degree relatives with HNPCC-related tumors, regardless of age

Ref: Chapter No.52, Page No.1373

251. Ans: A. Screening for CRC by colonoscopy is recommended in persons at risk or those affected with Lynch syndrome every 1 to 2 years, beginning at 30 to 35 years of age or 2 to 5 years before the youngest age of diagnosis of CRC in the family if diagnosed before age 25 years

- CRC - *20 to 25 years*
- Endometrial cancer, ovarian cancer, urinary tract malignancies - ***30 to 35 years***

Ref: Chapter No.52, Page No.1373

252. Ans: D. Periampullary tumors are an important cause of death

Ref: Chapter No.52, Page No.1370

253. Ans: B. Most cancers in patients with HNPCC involve the right colon

Ref: Chapter No.52, Page No.1373

254. Ans: A. Hamartomas are found in patients with both juvenile polyps and Peutz-Jeghers syndrome (PJS)

Ref: Chapter No.52, Page No.1372

255. Ans: C. Spiegelman's classification

Ref: Chapter No.52, Page No.1374

256. Ans: A. The left colic artery originates about 5 cm distally to the origin of the IMA

Ref: Chapter No.52, Page No.1374

257. Ans: B. 5 cms

Ref: Chapter No.52, Page No.1375

258. Ans: A. 2 cms

- **In *ultra distal sphincter-sparing surgery* resections, a cancer-free margin of *1 cm* or, in selected cases, a free margin at frozen section examination can be accepted**

Ref: Chapter No.52, Page No.1375

259. Ans: D. All of the above

Ref: Chapter No.52, Page No.1377

260. Ans: B. Resection of the entire sigmoid from the distal descending colon to the rectosigmoid junction, sparing the main left colic artery

Ref: Chapter No.52, Page No.1377

261. Ans: A. Observation only

- This lesion is classified as ***carcinoma in situ*** or ***intramucosal adenocarcinoma*** and is treated adequately by endoscopic polypectomy

Ref: Chapter No.52, Page No.1368

262. Ans: D. Daily tamoxifen

Ref: Chapter No.52, Page No.1370

263. Ans: C. He should undergo left hemicolectomy

Ref: Chapter No.52, Page No.1377

264. Ans: C. Descending colon

Ref: Chapter No.52, Page No.1378

265. Ans: A. Carcinoma of the right colon

Ref: Chapter No.52, Page No.1374

266. Ans: C. Stenting has not been shown to permit higher rates of primary anastomosis, decreased wound infections, and a higher rate of completion of surgery laparoscopically

Ref: Chapter No.52, Page No.1378

267. Ans: D. 70% to 80%

Ref: Chapter No.52, Page No.1378

268. Ans: C. With endorectal ultrasound the accuracy of lymph node detection is much more than the accuracy of detecting T stage

Ref: Chapter No.52, Page No.1379

269. Ans: C. 20%

Ref: Chapter No.52, Page No.1380

270. Ans: D. All of the above

Ref: Chapter No.52, Page No.1380

271. Ans: C. Local excision is safe when performed for lesions that are located anterior to the rectum due to the presence of the mesorectum

Ref: Chapter No.52, Page No.1380

272. Ans: A. Transanal minimally invasive surgery (TAMIS) - GelPOINT Path

- ***Transanal minimally invasive surgery (TAMIS)*** is a technique that was originally devised as a hybrid between ***Transanal Endoscopic Microsurgery (TEM)*** and ***single-site laparoscopy*** for resection of rectal lesions
- It is categorized by the use of a single-site port transanally in combination with ordinary laparoscopic instruments, a laparoscopic camera lens, and a standard laparoscopic CO_2 insufflator for the purpose of performing endoluminal rectal surgery
- In the US, there are currently 2 FDA approved devices for transanal access for the TAMIS procedure– the **GelPOINT Path** (Applied Medical, Rancho Santa Margarita, CA) and the **SILS™ Port** (Covidien, Mansfield, MA)
- Pneumorectum is achieved using a typical laparoscopic tower with CO_2 for insufflation. Initial pressure settings should be between ***8-18 mmHg*** and can be increased if there is difficulty maintaining distention of the rectum for visualization
- General anesthesia with ***muscle paralysis is recommended*** to avoid collapse of the rectal wall which can occur with diaphragmatic breathing

Ref: Chapter No.52, Page No.1380

https://www.sages.org/publications/guidelines/clinical-spotlight-review-transanal-minimally-invasive-surgery-tamis/

273. Ans: D. The diverting stoma is usually maintained for at least 12 weeks after surgery and is closed only after the perfect healing of the anastomosis has been confirmed with a gastrografin enema or with endoscopy

Ref: Chapter No.52, Page No.1381-1382

274. Ans: D. All of the above

Ref: Chapter No.52, Page No.1382-1384

275. Ans: B. 33%

Ref: Chapter No.52, Page No.1385

276. Ans: C. 4 to 5 cm

Ref: Chapter No.52, Page No.1386

277. Ans: C. 20%

Ref: Chapter No.52, Page No.1386

278. Ans: C. Female gender

Ref: Chapter No.52, Page No.1386

279. Ans: D. All of the above

Ref: Chapter No.52, Page No.1386-1387

280. Ans: B. 4%

Ref: Chapter No.52, Page No.1387

281. Ans: C. 4% to 10%

Ref: Chapter No.52, Page No.1387

282. Ans: A. Chemotherapy

Ref: Chapter No.52, Page No.1387

283. Ans: D. 80%

Ref: Chapter No.52, Page No.1388

284. Ans: D. All of the above

Ref: Chapter No.52, Page No.1388

285. Ans: A. Most of the symptoms improve 10 years or more after the resection

Ref: Chapter No.52, Page No.1388

286. Ans: D. 90%

Ref: Chapter No.52, Page No.1388

287. Ans: B. 5%

Ref: Chapter No.52, Page No.1388

288. Ans: B. 60%

Ref: Chapter No.52, Page No.1388-1389

289. Ans: B. 2 years

Ref: Chapter No.52, Page No.1389

290. Ans: B. Inadequate number of examined number lymph nodes (<16)

Ref: Chapter No.52, Page No.1389

291. Ans: B. Adjuvant 5-FU treatment seems to have a detrimental effect on survival in stage III but not stage II colon cancer patients

Ref: Chapter No.52, Page No.1389

292. Ans: D. All of the above

Ref: Chapter No.52, Page No.1389

293. Ans: D. All of the above

Ref: Chapter No.52, Page No.1389

294. Ans: B. FOLFOXIRI and bevacizumab

Ref: Chapter No.52, Page No.1389

295. Ans: C. Transanal excision

Ref: Chapter No.52, Page No.1380

296. Ans: A. Strictureplasty

Ref: Chapter No.52, Page No.1375-1377

297. Ans: D. Image-guided needle biopsy of extraluminal nodules is safe

Ref: Chapter No.52, Page No.1374

298. Ans: A. Lymph node involvement

Ref: Chapter No.52, Page No.1374

299. Ans: C. Chemotherapy and radiation followed by resection

Ref: Chapter No.52, Page No.1378-1389

300. Ans: D. Preoperative chemotherapy and radiation followed by resection

Ref: Chapter No.52, Page No.1378-1389

301. Ans: D. A 75-year-old male with urinary incontinence and a rectal cancer 5 cm above the dentate line

Ref: Chapter No.52, Page No.1388

302. Ans: D. Local excision for a rectal cancer should be done for small lesions (<2 cms)

Ref: Chapter No.52, Page No.1380

303. Ans: A. A fixed circumferential adenocarcinoma just above the dentate line

Ref: Chapter No.52, Page No.1385

304. Ans: B. Colonoscopy

Ref: Chapter No.52, Page No.1389

305. Ans: B. Increases in CEA after resection may indicate tumor recurrence

Ref: Chapter No.52, Page No.1389

306. Ans: B. Anismus

Ref: Chapter No.52, Page No.1390

307. Ans: A. 40 to 80 mm Hg

Ref: Chapter No.52, Page No.1390

308. Ans: D. All of the above

Ref: Chapter No.52, Page No.1390

309. Ans: B. 2.0 ± 0.2 milliseconds

Ref: Chapter No.52, Page No.1390

310. Ans: D. 80%

Ref: Chapter No.52, Page No.1390

311. Ans: B. Men older than 50 years are 6 times more likely than women to develop rectal prolapse

Ref: Chapter No.52, Page No.1390

312. Ans: D. All of the above

Ref: Chapter No.52, Page No.1390

313. Ans: B. Male gender

Ref: Chapter No.52, Page No.1390

314. Ans: B. Up to 5% of patients with incontinence have also pudendal neuropathy with a prolonged pudendal nerve terminal motor latency

Ref: Chapter No.52, Page No.1392

315. Ans: D. Endoanal ultrasound usually shows a thickening of the external anal sphincter

Ref: Chapter No.52, Page No.1392

316. Ans: B. Posterior mesh rectopexy

Ref: Chapter No.52, Page No.1395

317. Ans: D. Perineal proctectomy

Ref: Chapter No.52, Page No.1394

318. Ans: A. Delorme procedure

Ref: Chapter No.52, Page No.1395

319. Ans: B. Altemeier procedure

Ref: Chapter No.52, Page No.1395

320. Ans: B. SRUS is a disorder of young adults (30–40 years), with a slight male predominance

Ref: Chapter No.52, Page No.1396

321. Ans: C. 1 to 1.5 cm ulcer of the anterior rectal wall 3 to 10 cm from the anal verge

Ref: Chapter No.52, Page No.1396

322. Ans: C. For patients with severe symptoms, medical treatment is usually effective

Ref: Chapter No.52, Page No.1396

323. Ans: D. All of the above

Ref: Chapter No.52, Page No.1396

324. Ans: C. The balloon expulsion tests can identify the inability to expel an inflated balloon from the rectum after 1 minute of sitting on a commode

Ref: Chapter No.52, Page No.1397

325. Ans: B. Hyperthyroidism and medication-induced constipation are common causes

Ref: Chapter No.52, Page No.1397

326. Ans: D. All of the above

Ref: Chapter No.52, Page No.1397

53

Anus

ANATOMY

1. **Length of anal canal is approximately:**

A. 2 cms B. 4 cms
C. 6 cms D. 8 cms

2. **False about anatomy of anal canal is:**

A. The proximal anal canal is typically lined by columnar epithelium and the distal anus by squamous epithelium
B. The anus appears as an anteroposterior slit-like cutaneous opening
C. The junction between the ectoderm and the endoderm, located at the midpoint of the anal canal, appears as an undulating demarcation referred to as the dentate line
D. Between the dentate line and the anal verge, the mucosa is lined by a modified squamous epithelium, similar to the epithelium of the skin, with hair follicles and glands

3. **False about anatomy of anal canal is:**

A. The submucosa in the area of the distal anal canal is formed by a discontinuous layer of thickened tissue creating hemorrhoidal "cushions," typically found in the left lateral, right anterior, and right posterior positions
B. The anal gland duct traverses the submucosal plane and its branches terminate within the internal anal sphincter or extend into the intersphincteric plane
C. These cushions generally receive their blood supply from 2 hemorrhoidal arteries distributed along the circumference of the distal rectum and anus
D. The mucosa above the dentate line appears pleated with longitudinal folds, known as the columns of Morgagni

4. **Number of anal glands is:**

A. 2 - 4 B. 4 - 8
C. 6 - 12 D. 10 - 16

5. **True about anatomy of anal canal is:**

A. Below the dentate line, blood supply and drainage are provided by the middle hemorrhoidal system
B. The internal anal sphincter is composed of autonomically innervated smooth muscle and contributes between 50% to 85% of the resting tone of the anal canal
C. Venous and lymphatic drainage above the dentate line flows into the external iliac vessels
D. Anatomically, the internal anal sphincter is a thickened continuation of the longitudinal layer of the muscularis propria of the distal rectum

6. **False about the musculature of anal canal is:**

A. The internal anal sphincter is unique because it can be controlled both by the autonomic nervous system and by voluntary contraction
B. The external anal sphincter is a funnel shaped structure composed of the pelvic floor muscles enveloping the distal rectum and anus
C. In response to increases in intraabdominal pressure or rectal distention, the external anal sphincter and puborectalis reflexively and voluntarily contract to prevent fecal leakage
D. Rectal sling originates at the pubis, passes around the rectum posteriorly, and returns to the pubis

7. **The external anal sphincter can be subjected to muscular fatigue with maximal voluntary contraction sustained for only:**

A. 10 to 20 seconds B. 20 to 40 seconds
C. 30 to 60 seconds D. 60 to 120 seconds

8. **False about the nerve supply of anal canal is:**
   A. The external anal sphincter is innervated on each side by the inferior rectal branch of the pudendal nerve (S2 and S3) and by the perineal branch of S4
   B. If the S1 - S3 nerve roots remain intact only on one side, the patient can't maintain control of the anal sphincters
   C. The internal anal sphincter is supplied by sympathetic (L5) and parasympathetic (S2, S3, and S4) nerves
   D. The rectal branch of the pudendal nerve transmits anal sensation, and it is thought to play a role in maintenance of anal continence

9. **Golgi-Mazzoni bodies are responsible for:**
   A. Touch
   B. Friction
   C. Pressure
   D. Temperature sensation

10. **Genital corpuscules are responsible for:**
   A. Touch
   B. Friction
   C. Pressure
   D. Temperature sensation

11. **False about the physiology of anal canal is:**
   A. The hemorrhoidal cushions alone provide a complete airtight and watertight seal
   B. Continence requires rectal wall compliance to accommodate the fecal material, appropriate neurogenic control of the pelvic floor muscles, and properly functioning internal and external sphincter muscles
   C. With defecation, the angle straightens, allowing downward force to be applied along the axis of the rectum and anus
   D. Distention of the rectum results in reflexive relaxation of the internal anal sphincter

12. **When defecation is deemed appropriate, the external anal sphincter relaxes together with the puborectalis muscle, which allows?**
   A. Straightening of the rectoanal angle
   B. Evacuation of fecal material
   C. Opening of the anal canal
   D. All of the above

13. **False about the presenting complaints of anal canal disorders is:**
   A. Anal pain or pressure is frequently a presenting complaint
   B. Acute pain of relatively short duration may suggest a thrombosed hemorrhoid
   C. Pain occurring even without defecation, especially with bleeding, could indicate malignancy
   D. Sharp, razor knife pain that occurs with bowel movements will almost always indicate an Fistula-in-ano

14. **Following image denotes which position of examination?**

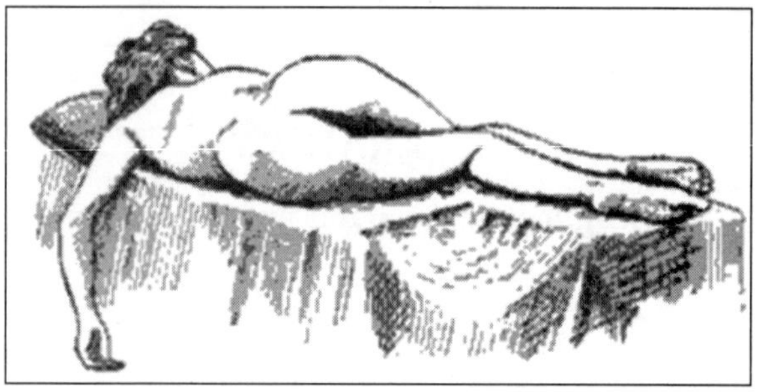

   A. Fowler's position
   B. Sim's position
   C. Lithotomy position
   D. Knee chest position

15. **Steps of per rectal examination involves all except:**
   A. In men, the prostate is palpated anteriorly; in women, the presence of a rectocele may be determined by gently flexing the examining finger anteriorly
   B. When asked to bear down, the patient is expected to reflexively contract their anal sphincter
   C. Gentle spreading of the buttocks will reveal the anal verge and anoderm
   D. Using the first phalanx of the examining finger, a sweep of the anal canal should be performed

16. **False about the imaging of anal canal disorders is:**
   A. Ultrasound can be a used to accurately estimate the degree of anal sphincter disruption and to outline the anatomy of a complex anal fistula
   B. Anorectal manometry provides a detailed physiologic assessment of anorectal function
   C. Computed tomography (CT) is more sensitive than Magnetic resonance imaging (MRI) for detecting pelvic lesions, and in defining the relationship to the pelvic muscular structures or pelvic sidewall
   D. MRI can be quite useful in detection and delineation of a complex fistula-in-ano

COMMON BENIGN DISORDERS OF THE ANUS

17. **Grade of hemorrhoids shown in the following image:**

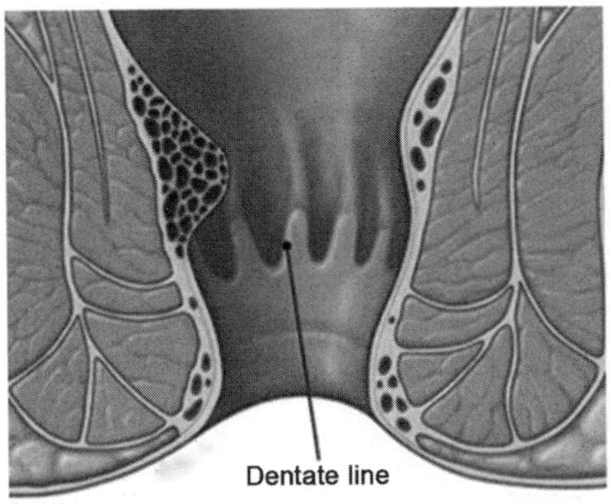

A. Grade 1
B. Grade 2
C. Grade 3
D. Grade 4

18. **A 38-year-old male came to OPD with complaints of bleeding per rectum. On examination hemorrhoids with bleeding and protrusion was present. Manual reduction was possible. Following is the image of the pathology. What is the grade of hemorrhoids?**

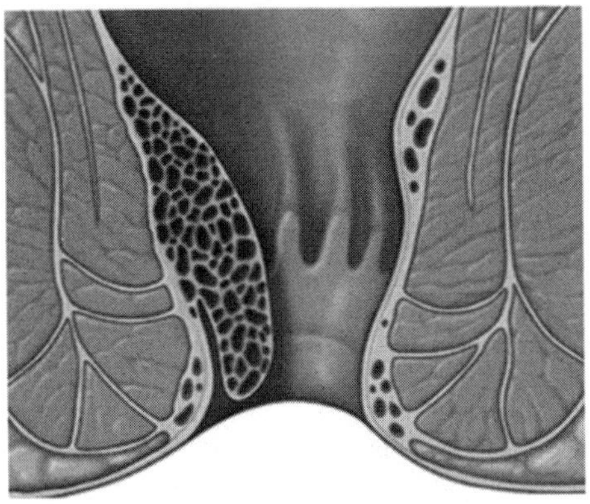

A. Grade 1
B. Grade 2
C. Grade 3
D. Grade 4

19. **False about internal hemorrhoids is:**

A. Painful bleeding associated with bowel movements with intermittent tissue protrusion is the most common complaint of patients with symptomatic internal hemorrhoids
B. The key etiologic factors contributing to the development of hemorrhoids include constipation and prolonged straining
C. A 6 to 8 weeks trial of medical management is usually indicated before considering more aggressive interventions
D. Anorectal examination should include visual inspection of the anus, digital rectal examination, and anoscopy to evaluate the extent of hemorrhoidal disease and search for other abnormalities

20. **False about rubber band ligation (RBL) in hemorrhoids is:**

A. Band ligation strangulates hemorrhoidal tissue, which results in ischemia and necrosis of the prolapsing mucosa, followed by scar fixation to the rectal wall
B. Hemorrhoidal rubber band ligation (RBL) is commonly the most effective option, and has been shown to be superior to sclerotherapy and infrared coagulation (IRC)
C. This procedure alleviates symptoms by decreasing the size of the hemorrhoidal cushion and increasing the fixation of the hemorrhoidal tissue to the rectal wall, thus minimizing hemorrhoidal prolapse
D. RBL is generally well-tolerated because the rubber band is placed distal to the dentate line

21. **False about sclerotherapy in hemorrhoids is:**

A. The most commonly used sclerosing agents are 5% phenol in almond or vegetable oil and sodium tetradecyl sulfate
B. Sclerotherapy is appropriately offered to anticoagulated patients or those receiving antiplatelet therapy, who are often not optimal candidates for RBL or surgical excision
C. Sclerotherapy is accomplished by injection of a sclerosing agent directly into the hemorrhoid, which results in fibrosis of the submucosa
D. Injection is performed into the submucosa at the base of a hemorrhoidal cushion, using approximately 10 ml of sclerosing agent

22. **False about external hemorrhoids is:**

A. Patients with thrombosed external hemorrhoids typically present with severe anal pain that may be relieved by sitting or defecation
B. Thrombectomy with evacuation of clot is often performed in the emergency department setting
C. External hemorrhoids are characterized by distended vascular tissue distal to the dentate line
D. Most patients will experience resolution of their symptoms within 72 hours after the onset of symptoms with conservative measures

23. **The most commonly used technique in surgical management of hemorrhoids is the:**

A. Stapled hemorrhoidopexy

B. Milligan-Morgan hemorrhoidectomy
C. Ferguson hemorrhoidectomy
D. Hill-Ferguson hemorrhoidectomy

24. **Open hemorrhoidectomy is also called as:**

A. Stapled hemorrhoidopexy
B. Milligan-Morgan hemorrhoidectomy
C. Ferguson hemorrhoidectomy
D. Hill-Ferguson hemorrhoidectomy

25. **True about closed hemorrhoidectomy steps is:**

A. The internal sphincter fibers should be identified and preserved
B. The hemorrhoid is excised with a diamond-shaped excision extending onto the anoderm, using a scalpel, scissors, or energy device
C. Complete hemostasis should be achieved with suture closure of the defect
D. All of the above

26. **Post operative care after hemorrhoidectomy is:**

A. Postoperative care should be aimed at maintaining regular bowel function with liberal use of milk of magnesia or polyethylene glycol laxatives to prevent constipation and impaction as needed
B. Pain is managed with sitz baths and judicious use of opioids
C. A feared complication of hemorrhoidectomy is pelvic sepsis
D. All of the above

27. **The most common complication after hemorrhoidectomy is:**

A. Hemorrhage
B. Pelvic sepsis
C. Acute urinary retention
D. Recurrence

28. **False about the surgical management of hemorrhoids is:**

A. Stapled hemorrhoidopexy utilizes a specially designed stapling device to create a mucosa-to-mucosa anastomosis, while removing redundant mucosa proximal to the dentate line
B. Like excisional hemorrhoidectomy, this technique can address external hemorrhoids
C. In Doppler-guided hemorrhoid artery ligation (HAL) there is no need for tissue excision, but mucosal pexy is required for patients with symptomatic hemorrhoidal prolapse
D. HAL was found to be cost-effective compared with RBL in terms of incremental cost per quality-adjusted life-year

29. **False about the anal fissure is:**

A. The most common symptom is sharp anal pain with defecation, often described by patients as the feeling of "passing pieces of glass or razor blades"
B. The majority of acute anal fissures need surgical management
C. An anal fissure is an elliptical or oval shaped tear in the anal canal starting at the anal verge and extending proximally for a varying length towards the dentate line
D. Symptoms are commonly cyclical in nature

30. **To be considered chronic, anal fissures should be present for:**

A. >2-4 weeks B. >6-8 weeks
C. >8-12 weeks D. >12-16 weeks

31. **Features of a chronic fissure include:**

A. Hypertrophied anal papilla
B. Skin tag or sentinel pile
C. The presence of exposed internal sphincter fibers at the base
D. All of the above

32. **The most common location of an anal fissure is the:**

A. Anterior midline B. Posterior midline
C. Left lateral D. Right lateral

33. **Anterior midline location of fissure is more common in:**

A. Women B. Men
C. Equal in both D. None

34. **The differential diagnosis of atypical fissures includes all except:**

A. Anal cancer B. Syphilis
C. Crohn's disease D. Chronic idiopathic

35. **True about the management of fissures is:**

A. Topical application of nitrates and calcium channel blockers are often used as an adjunct in nonoperative management
B. The majority of acute anal fissures resolve with medical management alone
C. The initial step in management should be to increase fluid and fiber ingestion as well as sitz baths and may include mineral oil or stool softeners to help with lubrication
D. All of the above

36. **False about Botulinum toxin use in fissure in ano is:**

A. Healing rates of 65% were reported when BT injection was combined with concurrent topical application of diltiazem
B. Injection can be done safely in the office or may be performed as an outpatient procedure with sedation
C. BT is associated with a modest increase in healing rates as second line therapy following unsuccessful treatment with topical agents
D. A typical dose of 20 to 100 IU of BT will produce relaxation lasting approximately 12 months

37. **The most common side effects of BT injection are:**

A. Urinary residual volume
B. Temporary incontinence to flatus
C. Heart block
D. Skin irritation

38. **False about Lateral internal sphincterotomy (LIS) is:**

A. The distal segment of the internal anal sphincter muscle is divided sharply for the length corresponding to that of the anal fissure
B. LIS has shown to be inferior to topical nitrates, calcium channel blockers, or BT
C. It induces sustained partial relaxation of the internal anal sphincter and reduces anal sphincter tone, enabling healing of the anal fissure
D. Reported rates of fecal incontinence after LIS rates range from 8% to 30% but is usually limited to minor episodes of incontinence to flatus

39. **False about perianal abscess is:**

A. Abscesses commonly expand by caudal extension to the anoderm (perianal abscess)
B. Is also referred to as a cryptoglandular abscess
C. Approximately 50% of perirectal abscesses occur due to other etiologies, such as Crohn disease, trauma, HIV, STDs, radiation therapy, or foreign body
D. Obstruction of the anal gland ducts leads to stasis, bacterial overgrowth, and ultimately abscesses that develop in the intersphincteric space

40. **True about perianal abscess is:**

A. Thorough digital rectal examination or anoscopic examination is often deferred in the acute setting owing to pain
B. If the diagnosis is in question, imaging with a pelvic CT or examination under anesthesia should be considered
C. Anal abscess typically present with the indolent onset of a constant, throbbing anal pain associated with localized swelling, erythema and fluctuance
D. All of the above

41. **True about the treatment of perianal abscess is:**

A. The drainage should be performed starting at the most fluctuant aspect of the abscess
B. Perianal abscess should be treated promptly by incision and drainage
C. The size of the incision should be generous and tailored to the size of the abscess
D. All of the above

42. **False about the treatment of perianal abscess is:**

A. If the abscess cavity is larger than 5 cm, one may consider placing counter incisions and bridge them with penrose drains
B. A well-drained abscess cavity typically needs require wet-to-dry dressing changes to achieve debridement
C. A well-drained perirectal abscess does not typically require treatment with antibiotics, as they have not been shown to improve healing times or reduce the recurrence rate
D. An alternative to a wide incision and drainage is inserting a drainage catheter that can be left in place for several weeks until the abscess resolves and then removed in the outpatient setting

43. **A perianal abscess wound is typically expected to completely heal within:**

A. 6 weeks B. 8 weeks
C. 10 weeks D. 12 weeks

44. **In perianal abscess, development of a chronic Fistula-in-ano occurs in up to:**

A. 10% B. 20%
C. 30% D. 50%

45. **Perianal abscess may recur in up to:**

A. 10% B. 20%
C. 30% D. 50%

46. **False about fistula-in-ano is:**

A. Fistula-in-ano results from persistent communication between the anal canal (internal opening) and perianal skin (external opening) following spontaneous or surgical drainage of a perianal abscess

B. Patients often report a cyclical pattern of pain and swelling, followed by drainage associated with relief of the symptoms
C. Multiple external openings, or a so-called "watering can perineum," should trigger suspicion of perianal Crohn's disease
D. If the course of the fistulous track remains unclear, a pelvic CT can be useful in identifying the location of the primary and secondary openings and delineate the anatomy of the fistula tracks

47. **Classification of Fistula-in-ano is based on:**
A. Goodsall classification
B. Park's classification
C. Morgan's classification
D. Ferguson's classification

48. **Rule that can be used as guide to predict the course of the fistula track and location of the internal opening is:**
A. Goodsall rule B. Park's rule
C. Morgan rule D. Ferguson rule

49. **Goodsall rule says all except:**
A. Fistulas with an external opening anterior to the anus typically track in a radial fashion directly into the anal canal
B. Exception is for those located at a distance >5 cm from the anal verge
C. Fistulas with an external opening posterior to the anus often track in a curvilinear fashion to a posterior midline internal opening
D. All of the above are true

50. **As per Park's classification most common type of Fistula-in-ano is:**
A. Type 1 B. Type 2
C. Type 3 D. Type 4

51. **As per Park's classification incidence of type 2 fistula is:**
A. 45% B. 30%
C. 15% D. 10%

52. **As per Park's classification incidence of type 4 fistula is:**
A. 5% B. 10%
C. 30% D. 45%

53. **False about the management of Fistula-in-ano is:**
A. Cutting seton has not been proven to shorten the tract over time
B. Simple short fistulas may be treated by lay-open fistulotomy
C. The preferred treatment of anal fistulas would ideally result in obliteration of the internal opening and all associated tracts without the need to divide any of the sphincter
D. In fistulas involving larger amounts of sphincter muscle, the initial treatment is often focused on controlling the fistula with a draining seton using a silastic vessel loop or a rubber band

54. **The recurrence rate for treatment of simple anal fistulas with fistulotomy is around:**
A. 2% B. 5%
C. 10% D. 20%

55. **True about rectovaginal fistula is:**
A. Rectovaginal fistula is an abnormal epithelial-lined communication between the rectum and vagina
B. Breakdown of the repair of a 3rd or 4th degree tear or infection can result in fistula development
C. The spectrum of presentation is from occasional passage of flatus to continuous drainage of stool through the vagina, causing marked irritation and embarrassing symptoms
D. All of the above

56. **The most common infectious cause of a high colovaginal fistula is:**
A. Malignancies
B. Crohn's diseases
C. Diverticular disease
D. Bartholin gland infections

57. **Definitive surgical repair of a low rectovaginal fistula is typically recommended after:**
A. 1 to 2 months B. 3 to 6 months
C. 6 to 8 months D. 12 to 18 months

58. **False about the treatment of rectovaginal fistula is:**
A. A draining seton, antibiotics, or fecal diversion may be necessary depending on the size, location, and etiology of the fistula
B. Both A and C
C. The most popular method of surgical repair is an endoanal sliding advancement flap
D. None

59. In endoanal sliding advancement flap, which is advanced to cover the anorectal side of the fistula contains:

A. Mucosa
B. Mucosa and submucosa
C. Mucosa, submucosa and circular muscle fibers
D. Mucosa, submucosa, circular and longitudinal muscle fibers

60. Martius flap is:

A. Gracilis interposition
B. Labial fat pad interposition
C. Episioproctotomy with sphincter interposition
D. Bioprosthetic fistula plugs

61. False about Pilonidal Sinus is:

A. Pilonidal disease is a common anorectal problem affecting young people, typically in their middle to late 20s
B. The foreign body reaction produced by trapped hair may lead to a hair-filled abscess cavity
C. Pilonidal disease is caused by shed hair drawn into the natal cleft by motion from the buttocks
D. Women are at higher risk because they tend to be more hirsute

62. Among the following associations with pilonidal disease, most common is:

A. Obesity
B. Sedentary occupation
C. Local irritation
D. Trauma

63. False about Pilonidal Sinus is:

A. The location of the abscess is distinctly different from a perirectal abscess, which is typically found near the anus
B. Majority of patients will initially present with an acute abscess caudal to the natal cleft
C. The presence of sinus openings along the midline of the natal cleft 4 to 8 cm from the anus is the hallmark finding in pilonidal disease
D. All of the above are true

64. False about treatment of Pilonidal Sinus is:

A. Complex or recurrent pilonidal disease my require transposition of healthy, well-vascularized tissue to close the defect
B. Trimming, shaving, waxing, or laser depilation has not been shown to be effective in preventing recurrence
C. Antibiotics may be an important adjunct in surgical treatment of pilonidal disease as bacterial colonization was found to range from 50% to 70%
D. The surrounding skin of the buttock, lower back and perianal region should meticulously depilated at the time of operation and maintained hair free

65. Which reconstructive technique is shown in the image, used in pilonidal sinus?

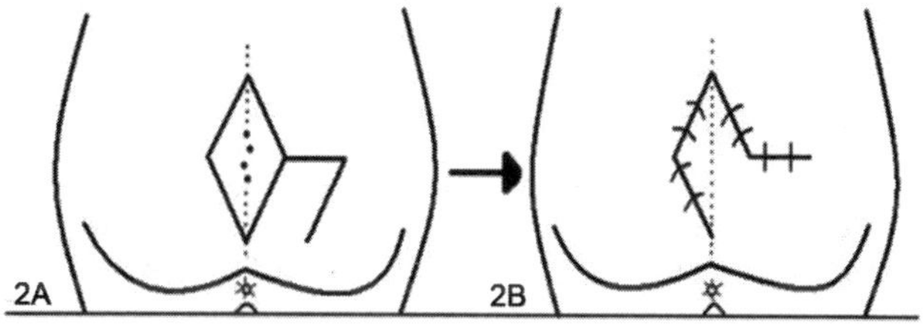

A. Z-plasty
B. Limberg flap
C. V-to-Y advancement flap
D. Karydakis flap

66. Which reconstructive technique is shown in the image, used in pilonidal sinus?

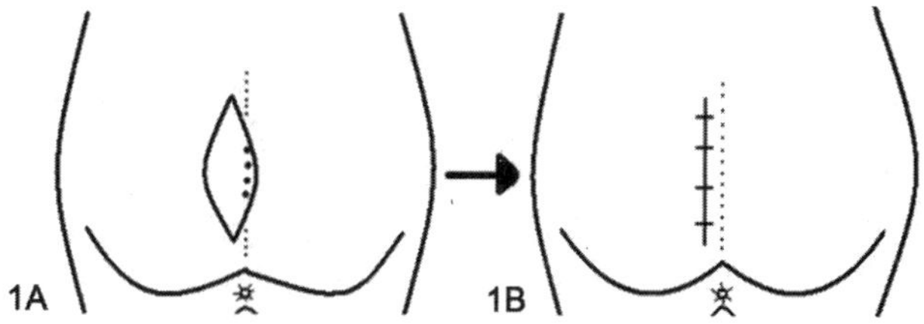

A. Z-plasty
B. Limberg flap
C. V-to-Y advancement flap
D. Karydakis flap

67. False about Sexually Transmitted Diseases is:

A. Human papillomavirus (HPV) is the most common STD
B. Both men who have sex with men (MSM) and heterosexual couples who engage in anal receptive intercourse are at increased risk
C. Serotypes 16 and 18 are found in benign warts
D. Complaints may include anal pain, tenesmus, urgency, purulent drainage and bleeding

68. False about HPV infection is:

A. Buschke-Lowenstein disease is a benign variant of HPV infection
B. The use of condoms lowers the risk of sexual transmission

C. The clearance rate following surgical removal ranges from 60% to 90%, with recurrence rates of 20% to 30%
D. Anal condyloma can be treated by topical agents such as imiquimod, podophyllin, and 5-fluorouracil (5-FU) or surgical methods such as tangential excision, cryotherapy, and fulguration

69. **Treatment of Herpes simplex virus proctitis is with:**
A. Acyclovir for 1 to 2 days
B. Acyclovir for 5 to 7 days
C. Acyclovir for 7 to 10 days
D. Acyclovir for 10 to 14 days

70. **Treatment of both Gonorrhea and Chlamydia is:**
A. Ceftriaxone 500 mg in a single I.M. dose + Azithromycin 500 mg orally in a single dose
B. Ceftriaxone 250 mg in a single I.M. dose + Azithromycin 1 g orally in a single dose
C. Doxycycline 100 mg orally twice daily for 14 days
D. Doxycycline 100 mg orally twice daily for 21 days

71. **Perianal condylomata lata is seen in:**
A. Primary syphilis
B. Secondary syphilis
C. Gonorrhoea
D. Herpes simplex virus

72. **Following anal intercourse, anorectal syphilis appears within _____ of exposure.**
A. 1 to 2 weeks B. 2 to 10 weeks
C. 10 to 16 weeks D. 18 to 24 weeks

73. **Debilitating ulcerating gummas are seen in:**
A. Primary syphilis B. Secondary syphilis
C. Tertiary syphilis D. HIV

74. **False about HIV and anorectal disease is:**
A. Clinical characteristics include a broad-based appearance, localization to the posterior midline and more proximally in the anal canal erosion into the submucosa and sphincters with decreased anal sphincter tone
B. Treatment is with anti-retroviral drugs
C. Idiopathic anal ulcers in HIV can be diagnosed after ruling out STDs and cancer
D. HIV infection is a common contributing factor to STDs and may result in certain HIV-specific anorectal disorders

75. **False about Anorectal Kaposi sarcoma is:**
A. Diagnosis is confirmed with serology
B. Anorectal Kaposi sarcoma presents with characteristic small, round, purple lesions and can be easily mistaken for hemorrhoids or other benign lesions
C. Intralesional chemotherapy and radiation are associated with lesion regression, improved cosmesis and palliation
D. Treatment with highly active antiretroviral therapy can induce rapid regression of the disease

76. **False about Hidradenitis Suppurativa is:**
A. The disease is thought to result from occlusion of the apocrine glands or the hair follicular duct
B. The distribution of disease, characteristic subcutaneous "pitlike" scarring, distorting contractures, and induration of the skin should be considered pathognomonic for advanced HS
C. Perineal disease is more commonly seen in women
D. Treatment is based on the stage of disease at presentation and ranges from medical therapy (antibiotics, antiandrogens and immuno-suppression) to more invasive procedures where total excision of all effected apocrine sweat gland areas may be required

77. **False about Perianal Crohn's disease is:**
A. The anti TNF-α antibody, infliximab, has been shown to be effective in preventing the progression of Crohn fistulizing disease
B. The diagnosis of Crohn's disease should be considered in those patients who have complex fistulas, especially located bilaterally, large "elephant ear" type skin tags
C. The mainstay of management in these patients is medications
D. Colonoscopy with ileal intubation will usually be sufficient to make the diagnosis

78. **In patients with Crohn's disease, anorectal disease is seen in:**
A. 20% B. 40%
C. 60% D. 80%

79. **False about treatment Perianal Crohn's disease is:**
A. Anal strictures are typically located at the top of anorectal ring and may be dilated if symptomatic

B. Fistulotomy may result in a nonhealing rectal wound and cause incontinence in these patients who often suffer with frequent, loose stools
C. Asymptomatic tags are common and should usually excised
D. In a long-standing perianal Crohn's disease, malignancy may develop and requires a high index of suspicion in patients with long-standing disease and unusual appearing fistulas, strictures, or ulcerations

80. **False about Fourth-Degree Hemorrhoids is:**
A. Patients with strangulated or acutely thrombosed internal hemorrhoids may present with severely painful and irreducible hemorrhoids
B. The goal of this treatment is to allow resolution of the acute crisis so that a less invasive treatment modality such as hemorrhoid banding can be performed at a later time once swelling has subsided
C. Patients who fail a limited trial of nonoperative management or those with strangulation and necrosis, require prompt operation and manual reduction of the strangulated hemorrhoids should be attempted once in this setting
D. Unless the tissue is necrotic, mucosa and anoderm should be preserved as much as possible to prevent postoperative anal stricture

81. **False about Fournier gangrene (FG) is:**
A. It is a fulminant form of necrotizing fasciitis of the perineal, genital, or perianal regions
B. FG has been associated with diabetes, chronic alcohol abuse, and immunosuppression, although it can occur in healthy patients without significant comorbidities
C. Bacterial infection results in microthrombosis of the small subcutaneous vessels leading to the development of gangrene of the overlying skin
D. The patient is likely to demonstrate signs of severe systemic illness, usually in proportion to the local extent of the disease

82. **False about the treatment of Fournier gangrene (FG) is:**
A. Treatment of FG requires an aggressive multimodal approach, including hemodynamic stabilization and broad-spectrum antibiotics
B. Urogenital infections tend to extend posteriorly along Bucks and Dartos fascia up to the Colles fascia, but are limited from the anal margin by the attachment of the Colles fascia to the perineal body
C. Split thickness skin grafts appear to be the treatment of choice in covering perineal and scrotal skin defects
D. FG is a surgical not a emergency

83. **False about Horseshoe Abscess is:**
A. Horseshoe ischiorectal abscess can result from the lateral spread of infection originating in the deep postanal space
B. Deep postanal space abscesses are almost always associated with an anterior midline fistula-in-ano
C. Drainage of the deep postanal space can be achieved by a midline incision between the coccyx and the anus
D. A fistula tract should be identified, and the lower half of the internal sphincter may be divided (Hanley procedure) or a seton placed through the fistula track

84. **The most common cause of fecal incontinence is:**
A. Neurological causes
B. Prior anal surgery
C. Colorectal cancer
D. Obstetric injury

85. **True about treatment of fecal incontinence is:**
A. Anal sphincter repair can be beneficial in patients with anal sphincter disruption secondary to traumatic childbirth or prior anal surgery
B. Colorectal cancer must be ruled out in those individuals with a recent change in bowel habits, particularly when blood per rectum is present
C. Medical therapy may include antidiarrheal agents, such as loperamide, which can slow down transit time and decrease the frequency of loose stools
D. All of the above

86. **False about constipation is:**
A. Constipation may occur because of a primary motor disorder involving the colon, rectum or anus, a defecation disorder, or as an adverse effect of medications
B. Polyethylene glycol solutions are typically safe and effective when these measures are inadequate
C. Prokinetics and secretagogues should be used in most patients

D. The Malone antegrade colonic enema procedure with construction of a small stoma from the appendix can allow for colonic irrigations and cleansing

87. A 65-year-old woman presents to your office reporting 1 year of fecal incontinence. She states that she experiences the loss of loose stools twice per week. She typically passes five loose or watery stools daily. She has a history of four vaginal deliveries including at least one episiotomy. She had a normal screening colonoscopy 1 year ago. The most appropriate initial treatment for these symptoms is:

A. Colostomy
B. Bulk-forming agents
C. Sacral nerve stimulation
D. Artificial bowel sphincter

NEOPLASMS

88. False about anal intraepithelial neoplasia (AIN) is:

A. It is characterized by metaplastic changes in the anal canal that are thought to be the precursor lesions to invasive anal carcinoma
B. Current treatments for AIN include ablative and topical therapies
C. Ablative therapies include surgical excision, IRC and thermal ablation
D. Currently available quadrivalent HPV vaccines have the potential to reduce anal cancer incidence if administered before initiation of sexual activity

89. Most cases of anal dysplasia are caused by the HPV, particularly the:

A. HPV-6 subtype
B. HPV-11 subtype
C. HPV-16 subtype
D. HPV-18 subtype

90. Squamous cell carcinoma (SCC) of the anal canal is most commonly associated with:

A. HIV infection
B. HPV infection
C. Genetic causes
D. Radiation

91. False about Squamous cell carcinoma (SCC) is:

A. Hematogenous spread of anal canal cancer occurs in fewer than 10% of cases
B. Liver metastases are more common than lung or bone metastases and usually occur in the setting of a tumor arising at the anorectal junction
C. Lymphatic spread occurs in 10% to 15% of patients, in the distribution of the perirectal and/or inguinal nodal basin
D. Men are more likely than women to suffer from anal cancer

92. True about imaging of Squamous cell carcinoma (SCC) of anal canal is:

A. MRI is considered the modality of choice for assessment of locoregional disease
B. CT is primarily used to evaluate for distant metastatic disease
C. PET/CT can help in differentiating residual viable anal cancer from post treatment necrosis and fibrosis
D. All of the above

93. False about the treatment of Squamous cell carcinoma (SCC) of anal canal is:

A. Combined modality therapy (CMT) with mitomycin C, 5-FU and radiotherapy (45–50.4 Gy) achieves a complete response in 64% to 86% of patients
B. After completion of CMT, it is recommended that a biopsy should be delayed for at least 3 months
C. A salvage abdominoperineal resection is required in up to 30% of cases
D. Distant metastasis is more common than locoregional relapse in anal cancer

94. Predictors of poor outcome following salvage surgery in anal canal cancer is/are all except:

A. Tumor size > 5 cm
B. Associated comorbidities
C. Adjacent organ involvement
D. Female gender

95. A 47-year-old man presents with a 2.5 cm anal mass arising just proximal to the dentate line, involving > 1/2 of the circumference of the anal canal, and fixed to the internal sphincter muscle. Biopsies show squamous cell carcinoma. Metastatic evaluation is negative. What treatment would you recommend for this patient?

A. Low anterior resection with coloanal anastomosis
B. High-resolution anoscopy
C. 5-Flourouricil, mitomycin C and radiation therapy
D. APR with colostomy

96. Large perineal wounds can be covered with tissue flaps like:

A. Pedicled omental flap
B. Gracilis flap
C. Gluteus maximus flap
D. All of the above

97. **Among all anal cancers, anal margin cancers account for about:**

A. 5% B. 10%
C. 15% D. 25%

98. **Fasle about Perianal Paget's disease is:**

A. Perianal Paget's disease is thought to correspond to an intraepithelial adenocarcinoma arising from dermal apocrine sweat glands
B. Patients with this condition tend to present with nonspecific symptoms such as pruritus, discharge, or bleeding
C. The recurrence rate can be as high as 70% to 90% at 5 years
D. Wide local excision is recommended for most patients

99. **No. of patients with anal margin Paget's disease harbouring a synchronous colorectal neoplasm is approximately:**

A. 10% B. 30%
C. 50% D. 75%

100. **False about Basal cell carcinoma (BCC) of the perianal region is:**

A. Women are predominantly affected (60%–80%)
B. About 30% of patients have a past history of BCC at other sites
C. This cancer originates from the stratum basale of the epidermis and pilosebaceous follicle units
D. Radiation, immunodeficiency, trauma, burns or chronic irritation, or infection may also play role in development of perianal BCC

101. **False about Basal cell carcinoma (BCC) of the perianal region is:**

A. Tumors < 2 cm are excised with at least a 1 cm margin
B. Perianal BCC has been shown to have an association with HPV infection
C. Large lesions with extension into the anal canal can be treated with radiation therapy and/or abdominoperineal resection
D. Larger lesions, without extension into the anal canal, are excised primarily but typically require coverage with skin grafts or flaps

102. **False about Malignant melanoma of the anal margin is:**

A. The anus is the 3rd most common site after skin and the eye
B. Amelanotic lesions occur in 30% of cases
C. Overall prognosis is very good
D. Wide local excision is usually recommended when feasible; patients with large lesions and/or extensive sphincter involvement generally require more aggressive surgery for local control

103. **False about Adenocarcinoma of anal canal is:**

A. Anal canal adenocarcinoma usually originates from the anal glands but may develop in longstanding fistula-in-ano
B. Staging workup includes pelvic MRI and CT scanning
C. Because of the mucosal location of the anal glands, anal adenomas are apparent early
D. Treatment is typically neoadjuvant chemoradiation followed by abdominoperineal resection for lesions larger than 2 cm

104. **Risk factors for anal canal adenocarcinoma include all except:**

A. Infection with HPV and HIV
B. Alcohol
C. Smoking
D. History of anoreceptive intercourse

105. **Characteristic MRI findings of anal canal adenocarcinoma is/are:**

A. Enhancing solid components
B. Fistula between the mass and the anus
C. Markedly hyperintense fluid on T2-weighted images
D. All of the above

ANSWERS

1. **Ans: B. 4 cms**

   Ref: Chapter No.53, Page No.1401

2. **Ans: D. Between the dentate line and the anal verge, the mucosa is lined by a modified squamous epithelium, similar to the epithelium of the skin, with hair follicles and glands**

   Ref: Chapter No.53, Page No.1401

3. **Ans: C. These cushions generally receive their blood supply from 2 hemorrhoidal arteries distributed along the circumference of the distal rectum and anus**

   Ref: Chapter No.53, Page No.1401

4. **Ans: C. 6 - 12**

   Ref: Chapter No.53, Page No.1401

5. **Ans: B. The internal anal sphincter is composed of autonomically innervated smooth muscle and contributes between 50% to 85% of the resting tone of the anal canal**

   Ref: Chapter No.53, Page No.1401

6. **Ans: A. The internal anal sphincter is unique because it can be controlled both by the autonomic nervous system and by voluntary contraction**

   Ref: Chapter No.53, Page No.1401-1403

7. **Ans: C. 30 to 60 seconds**

   Ref: Chapter No.53, Page No.1403

8. **Ans: B. If the S1 - S3 nerve roots remain intact only on one side, the patient can't maintain control of the anal sphincters**

   Ref: Chapter No.53, Page No.1403

9. **Ans: C. Pressure**

   Ref: Chapter No.53, Page No.1403

10. **Ans: B. Friction**

    Ref: Chapter No.53, Page No.1403

11. **Ans: A. The hemorrhoidal cushions alone provide a complete airtight and watertight seal**

    Ref: Chapter No.53, Page No.1403

12. **Ans: D. All of the above**

    Ref: Chapter No.53, Page No.1403

13. **Ans: D. Sharp, razor knife pain that occurs with bowel movements will almost always indicate an fistula in ano**

    Ref: Chapter No.53, Page No.1403

14. **Ans: B. Sim's position**

    Ref: Chapter No.53, Page No.1403

15. **Ans: B. When asked to bear down, the patient is expected to reflexively contract their anal sphincter**

    Ref: Chapter No.53, Page No.1403-1404

16. **Ans: C. Computed tomography (CT) is more sensitive than Magnetic resonance imaging (MRI) for detecting pelvic lesions, and in defining the relationship to the pelvic muscular structures or pelvic sidewall**

    Ref: Chapter No.53, Page No.1404

17. **Ans: A. Grade 1**

    Ref: Chapter No.53, Page No.1404

18. **Ans: C. Grade 3**

    Ref: Chapter No.53, Page No.1404

19. **Ans: A. Painful bleeding associated with bowel movements with intermittent tissue protrusion is the most common complaint of patients with symptomatic internal hemorrhoids**

    Ref: Chapter No.53, Page No.1404

20. **Ans: D. RBL is generally well-tolerated because the rubber band is placed distal to the dentate line**

    Ref: Chapter No.53, Page No.1404-1405

21. **Ans: D. Injection is performed into the submucosa at the base of a hemorrhoidal cushion, using approximately 10 ml of sclerosing agent**

    Ref: Chapter No.53, Page No.1405

22. **Ans: A. Patients with thrombosed external hemorrhoids typically present with severe anal pain that may be relieved by sitting or defecation**

    Ref: Chapter No.53, Page No.1405

23. **Ans: C. Ferguson hemorrhoidectomy**

    Ref: Chapter No.53, Page No.1406

24. **Ans: B. Milligan-Morgan hemorrhoidectomy**

    Ref: Chapter No.53, Page No.1406

25. **Ans: D. All of the above**

    Ref: Chapter No.53, Page No.1406

26. **Ans: D. All of the above**

    Ref: Chapter No.53, Page No.1406

27. **Ans: A. Hemorrhage**

    Ref: Chapter No.53, Page No.1406

28. **Ans: D. HAL was found to be cost-effective compared with RBL in terms of incremental cost per quality-adjusted life-year**

    Ref: Chapter No.53, Page No.1407

29. **Ans: B. The majority of acute anal fissures need surgical management**

    Ref: Chapter No.53, Page No.1407

30. **Ans: B. >6-8 weeks**

    Ref: Chapter No.53, Page No.1407

31. **Ans: D. All of the above**

    Ref: Chapter No.53, Page No.1407

32. Ans: B. Posterior midline

Ref: Chapter No.53, Page No.1407

33. Ans: A. Women

Ref: Chapter No.53, Page No.1407

34. Ans: D. Chronic idiopathic

Ref: Chapter No.53, Page No.1407

35. Ans: D. All of the above

Ref: Chapter No.53, Page No.1407-1408

36. Ans: D. A typical dose of 20 to 100 IU of BT will produce relaxation lasting approximately 12 months

Ref: Chapter No.53, Page No.1408

37. Ans: B. Temporary incontinence to flatus

Ref: Chapter No.53, Page No.1408

38. Ans: B. LIS has shown to be inferior to topical nitrates, calcium channel blockers, or BT

Ref: Chapter No.53, Page No.1408

39. Ans: C. Approximately 50% of perirectal abscesses occur due to other etiologies, such as Crohn disease, trauma, HIV, STDs, radiation therapy, or foreign body

Ref: Chapter No.53, Page No.1408

40. Ans: D. All of the above

Ref: Chapter No.53, Page No.1408

41. Ans: D. All of the above

Ref: Chapter No.53, Page No.1408

42. Ans: B. A well-drained abscess cavity typically needs require wet-to-dry dressing changes to achieve debridement

Ref: Chapter No.53, Page No.1408

43. Ans: A. 6 weeks

Ref: Chapter No.53, Page No.1408

44. Ans: D. 50%

Ref: Chapter No.53, Page No.1408

45. Ans: A. 10%

Ref: Chapter No.53, Page No.1408

46. Ans: D. If the course of the fistulous track remains unclear, a pelvic CT can be useful in identifying the location of the primary and secondary openings and delineate the anatomy of the fistula tracks

Ref: Chapter No.53, Page No.1408-1409

47. Ans: B. Park's classification

Ref: Chapter No.53, Page No.1409

48. Ans: A. Goodsall rule

Ref: Chapter No.53, Page No.1409

49. Ans: B. Exception is for those located at a distance >5 cm from the anal verge

Ref: Chapter No.53, Page No.1409

50. Ans: A. Type 1

Ref: Chapter No.53, Page No.1410

51. Ans: B. 30%

Ref: Chapter No.53, Page No.1410

52. Ans: A. 5%

Ref: Chapter No.53, Page No.1410

53. Ans: A. Cutting seton has not been proven to shorten the tract over time

Ref: Chapter No.53, Page No.1410

54. Ans: B. 5%

Ref: Chapter No.53, Page No.1410

55. Ans: D. All of the above

Ref: Chapter No.53, Page No.1410

56. Ans: C. Diverticular disease

Ref: Chapter No.53, Page No.1410

57. Ans: B. 3 to 6 months

Ref: Chapter No.53, Page No.1410

58. Ans: D. None

Ref: Chapter No.53, Page No.1410

59. Ans: C. Mucosa, submucosa and circular muscle fibers

Ref: Chapter No.53, Page No.1410-1411

60. Ans: B. Labial fat pad interposition

Ref: Chapter No.53, Page No.1411

61. Ans: D. Women are at higher risk because they tend to be more hirsute

Ref: Chapter No.53, Page No.1411

62. Ans: B. Sedentary occupation

Ref: Chapter No.53, Page No.1411

63. Ans: B. Majority of patients will initially present with an acute abscess caudal to the natal cleft

Ref: Chapter No.53, Page No.1411

64. Ans: B. Trimming, shaving, waxing, or laser depilation has not been shown to be effective in preventing recurrence

Ref: Chapter No.53, Page No.1411

65. Ans: B. Limberg flap

Ref: Chapter No.53, Page No.1411

66. Ans: D. Karydakis flap

Ref: Chapter No.53, Page No.1411

67. Ans: C. Serotypes 16 and 18 are found in benign warts

Ref: Chapter No.53, Page No.1411-1412

68. Ans: A. Buschke-Lowenstein disease is a benign variant of HPV infection

Ref: Chapter No.53, Page No.1412

69. **Ans: C. Acyclovir for 7 to 10 days**

Ref: Chapter No.53, Page No.1413

70. **Ans: B. Ceftriaxone 250 mg in a single I.M. dose + Azithromycin 1 g orally in a single dose**

Ref: Chapter No.53, Page No.1413-1415

71. **Ans: B. Secondary syphilis**

Ref: Chapter No.53, Page No.1414

72. **Ans: B. 2 to 10 weeks**

Ref: Chapter No.53, Page No.1415

73. **Ans: C. Tertiary syphilis**

Ref: Chapter No.53, Page No.1415

74. **Ans: B. Treatment is with anti-retroviral drugs**

Ref: Chapter No.53, Page No.1415

75. **Ans: A. Diagnosis is confirmed with serology**

Ref: Chapter No.53, Page No.1415

76. **Ans: C. Perineal disease is more commonly seen in women**

Ref: Chapter No.53, Page No.1415

77. **Ans: C. The mainstay of management in these patients is medications**

Ref: Chapter No.53, Page No.1415-1416

78. **Ans: D. 80%**

Ref: Chapter No.53, Page No.1415

79. **Ans: C. Asymptomatic tags are common and should usually excised**

Ref: Chapter No.53, Page No.1416

80. **Ans: C. Patients who fail a limited trial of nonoperative management or those with strangulation and necrosis, require prompt operation and manual reduction of the strangulated hemorrhoids should be attempted once in this setting**

Ref: Chapter No.53, Page No.1416

81. **Ans: D. The patient is likely to demonstrate signs of severe systemic illness, usually in proportion to the local extent of the disease**

Ref: Chapter No.53, Page No.1416

82. **Ans: D. FG is a surgical not an emergency**

Ref: Chapter No.53, Page No.1416-1417

83. **Ans: B. Deep postanal space abscesses are almost always associated with an anterior midline fistula-in-ano**

Ref: Chapter No.53, Page No.1417

84. **Ans: D. Obstetric injury**

Ref: Chapter No.53, Page No.1417

85. **Ans: D. All of the above**

Ref: Chapter No.53, Page No.1418

86. **Ans: C. Prokinetics and secretagogues should be used in most patients**

Ref: Chapter No.53, Page No.1418

87. **Ans: B. Bulk-forming agents**

Ref: Chapter No.53, Page No.1418

88. **Ans: A. It is characterized by metaplastic changes in the anal canal that are thought to be the precursor lesions to invasive anal carcinoma**

Ref: Chapter No.53, Page No.1419

89. **Ans: C. HPV-16 subtype**

Ref: Chapter No.53, Page No.1419

90. **Ans: B. HPV infection**

Ref: Chapter No.53, Page No.1420

91. **Ans: D. Men are more likely than women to suffer from anal cancer**

Ref: Chapter No.53, Page No.1420

92. **Ans: D. All of the above**

Ref: Chapter No.53, Page No.1421

93. **Ans: D. Distant metastasis is more common than locoregional relapse in anal cancer**

Ref: Chapter No.53, Page No.1421

94. **Ans: D. Female gender**

Ref: Chapter No.53, Page No.1421

95. **Ans: C. 5-Flourouricil, mitomycin C and radiation therapy**

Ref: Chapter No.53, Page No.1421

96. **Ans: D. All of the above**

Ref: Chapter No.53, Page No.1421

97. **Ans: D. 25%**

Ref: Chapter No.53, Page No.1421

98. **Ans: C. The recurrence rate can be as high as 70% to 90% at 5 years**

Ref: Chapter No.53, Page No.1421-1422

99. **Ans: C. 50%**

Ref: Chapter No.53, Page No.1421

100. **Ans: A. Women are predominantly affected (60%–80%)**

Ref: Chapter No.53, Page No.1422

101. **Ans: B. Perianal BCC has been shown to have an association with HPV infection**

Ref: Chapter No.53, Page No.1422

102. **Ans: C. Overall prognosis is very good**

Ref: Chapter No.53, Page No.1422

103. **Ans: C. Because of the mucosal location of the anal glands, anal adenomas are apparent early**

Ref: Chapter No.53, Page No.1422-1423

104. **Ans: B. Alcohol**

Ref: Chapter No.53, Page No.1422

105. **Ans: D. All of the above**

Ref: Chapter No.53, Page No.1422-1423

54

The Liver

HISTORICAL PERSPECTIVE

1. **The first physician to describe the essential anatomy of the blood vessels of the liver accurately was:**
   A. Hippocrates B. Francis Glisson
   C. Lortat-Jacob D. Couinaud

2. **Credit for the first anatomic liver resection is usually given to:**
   A. Hippocrates B. Francis Glisson
   C. Lortat-Jacob D. Couinaud

3. **Partial hepatectomy on normal livers is consistently performed with mortality rates of:**
   A. 1% - 2% B. 2% - 5%
   C. 5% - 10% D. 10% - 20%

ANATOMY AND PHYSIOLOGY

4. **False about the Gross Anatomy of liver is:**
   A. The liver is a solid gastrointestinal organ whose mass (1.2–1.6 kg) largely occupies the right upper quadrant of the abdomen
   B. The posterior surface straddles the inferior vena cava (IVC)
   C. Hepatic arterial blood and portal venous blood enter the liver at the hilum and branch throughout the liver as a single portal pedicle unit, which also includes a bile duct
   D. The umbilical fissure is on the inferior surface of the right liver and contains the right portal pedicle

5. **The liver is invested in peritoneum except for:**
   A. The gallbladder fossa
   B. Porta hepatis
   C. Posterior aspect of the liver on either side of the IVC in 2 wedge-shaped areas
   D. All of the above

6. **The ligamentum teres is:**
   A. Obliterated left umbilical vein
   B. Obliterated umbilical artery
   C. Obliterated sinus venosus
   D. Obliterated vitelline vein

7. **Ligamentum venosum is:**
   A. Obliterated left umbilical vein
   B. Obliterated umbilical artery
   C. Obliterated sinus venosus
   D. Obliterated vitelline vein

8. **False about development and embryology of liver is:**
   A. During embryogenesis, signals are transmitted from the cardiac mesenchyme and septum transversum
   B. Hematopoietic cells, Kupffer cells and connective tissue form from the endoderm of the septum transversum
   C. Hepatic cells develop cords and intermingle with the vitelline and umbilical veins to form hepatic sinusoids
   D. The molecules regulating embryogenesis are fibroblast growth factor, bone morphogenetic protein, Wnt, tissue growth factor beta

9. **During embryonic development, the liver primordium begins to form in the:**
   A. 2nd week B. 3rd week
   C. 5th week D. 8th week

10. **True among the following is:**
    A. The vitelline veins carry blood from the yolk sac to the sinus venosus and ultimately form a network of veins around the foregut (future duodenum) that drain into the developing hepatic sinusoid
    B. The sinus venosus, which empties into the fetal

heart, becomes the hepatocardiac channel and then the hepatic veins and retrohepatic IVC

C. The right umbilical vein ultimately disappears, and the left umbilical vein later drains directly into the hepatocardiac channel

D. All of the above

11. Umbilical veins begin to drain into hepatic sinusoids at:

A. 2nd week
B. 3rd week
C. 5th week
D. 8th week

12. Oval cells are:

A. Hepatic progenitor cells
B. Kupffer cells
C. Myofibroblastic mesenchymal cells
D. Vascular endothelial cells

13. Hepatic stellate cells:

A. Kupffer cells
B. Myofibroblastic mesenchymal cells
C. Vascular endothelial cells
D. Hepatic progenitor cells

14. False about functional anatomy of liver is:

A. The line of the main scissura is also known as Cantlie line

B. The main scissura contains the middle hepatic vein, which runs in an anteroposterior direction from the gallbladder fossa to the left side of the vena cava

C. The right liver has a visible fissure along its inferior surface called the umbilical fissure

D. The right liver is divided into anterior (segments V and VIII) and posterior (segments VI and VII) sectors by the right scissura, which contains the right hepatic vein

15. Portal triad is composed of all except:

A. Bile duct
B. Portal vein
C. Hepatic vein
D. Hepatic artery

16. False about functional anatomy of liver is:

A. The umbilical fissure is a scissura and contains a hepatic vein

B. The left liver is split into anterior (segments III and IV) and posterior (segment II, the only sector composed of a single segment) sectors by the left scissura

C. The left scissura runs posterior to the ligamentum teres and contains the left hepatic vein

D. All of the above are true

17. False among the following is:

A. The right portal triad has a short extrahepatic course of approximately 1 - 1.5 cm before entering the substance of the liver

B. The left portal triad has a long extrahepatic course of up to 3 to 4 cm and runs transversely along the base of segment IV in a peritoneal sheath

C. The continuation of the left portal triad runs posteriorly and cephalad in the umbilical fissure and gives branches to segments II and III

D. The caudate lobe (segment I) is the dorsal portion of the liver

18. False about caudate lobe is:

A. It embraces the IVC on its ventral surface and lies posterior to the left portal triad inferiorly and the left and middle hepatic veins superiorly

B. The main bulk of the caudate lobe is to the left of the IVC

C. The right portion of the caudate lobe lies in the lesser omental bursa and is covered anteriorly by the gastrohepatic ligament (lesser omentum) that separates it from segments II and III anteriorly

D. The vascular inflow and biliary drainage to the caudate lobe come from both the right and left pedicles

19. False about caudate lobe is:

A. Anomalous development of the liver is very commonly encountered

B. The right side of the caudate, the caudate process, largely derives its portal venous supply from the right portal vein

C. The left portion of the caudate derives its portal venous inflow from the left main portal vein

D. The posterior edge of the left side of the caudate terminates as a fibrous component that attaches to the crura of the diaphragm and also runs posteriorly, wrapping behind the IVC and attaching to segment VII of the right liver called caval ligament

20. Riedel lobe is:

A. Tongue of tissue extending superiorly off the right liver

B. Tongue of tissue extending inferiorly off the left liver

C. Tongue of tissue extending superiorly off the left liver

D. Tongue of tissue extending inferiorly off the right liver

21. Hepatic blood inflow provided by the portal vein is:

A. 25% B. 50%
C. 75% D. 90%

22. Liver's oxygen requirement provided by portal vein is:

A. 10% - 20% B. 20% - 50%
C. 50% - 70% D. 70% - 90%

23. Diameter of portal vein is:

A. 0.5 cm B. 0.8 cm
C. 1 cm D. 1.5 cm

24. False about the course of portal vein is:

A. Portal vein runs behind the 1st portion of the duodenum
B. In the hepatoduodenal ligament
C. Along the right border of the lesser omentum
D. Anterior to the CBD and proper hepatic artery

25. False about portal vein is:

A. There is usually a small caudate process branch off the main right portal vein or at the right portal vein bifurcation that comes off posteriorly to supply this portion of liver
B. The portal vein is the only vein with both tributaries and branches
C. The left branch of the portal vein runs transversely along the base of segment IV and into the umbilical fissure
D. The right portal vein has a long extrahepatic course

26. The most significant portosystemic collateral locations are all except:

A. The inferior hemorrhoidal plexus receives portal flow from inferior mesenteric vein tributaries and can form large hemorrhoids
B. The submucosal veins of the proximal stomach and distal esophagus receive portal flow from the short gastric veins and the left gastric vein
C. The umbilical and abdominal wall veins recanalize from flow through the umbilical vein in the ligamentum teres
D. All of the above are true

27. The standard configuration, where main portal vein divides into the left and right branches and the right portal vein then divides into right anterior and right posterior portal vein, is found in up to:

A. 30% B. 50%
C. 70% D. 90%

28. The most common variant configuration of portal veins is:

A. Right posterior portal vein originating as the first branch of portal vein
B. Portal vein trifurcation
C. A pulmonary vein may enter the portal vein
D. Congenital absence of the left branch of the portal vein

29. The hepatic artery provides approximately:

A. 25% of the hepatic blood flow and 50% to 60% of its oxygenation
B. 50% of the hepatic blood flow and 50% to 60% of its oxygenation
C. 25% of the hepatic blood flow and 30% to 50% of its oxygenation
D. 50% of the hepatic blood flow and 30% to 50% of its oxygenation

30. The common description of the arterial supply to the liver and biliary tree is present in approximately:

A. 30% B. 50%
C. 60% D. 80%

31. False about the hepatic artery is:

A. The left hepatic artery heads vertically toward the umbilical fissure to supply segments II, III and IV
B. The left hepatic artery usually also gives off a middle hepatic artery branch that heads toward the right side of the umbilical fissure and supplies segment IV
C. Hepatic vessels replaced to the superior mesenteric artery run behind the head of the pancreas
D. An accessory cystic artery can originate from the proper hepatic artery or gastroduodenal artery, where it runs posterior to the bile duct

32. Calot triangle has following boundaries except:

A. Cystic duct
B. Common bile duct
C. Common hepatic duct
D. Liver edge

33. Replaced or accessory right hepatic arteries come off the superior mesenteric artery and are present approximately:

A. 5% to 10%
B. 10% to 20%
C. 20% to 30%
D. 30% to 50%

34. A replaced or accessory left hepatic artery is present approximately:

A. 1% to 2%
B. 4% to 10%
C. 10% to 15%
D. 15% to 25%

35. A replaced or accessory left hepatic artery originates from the:

A. Superior mesenteric artery
B. Descending aorta
C. Right gastroepiploic artery
D. Left gastric artery

36. False about hepatic veins is:

A. The left hepatic vein runs in the left scissura between segments II and III and drains segments II and III
B. The right hepatic vein runs in the right scissura between the anterior and posterior sectors of the right liver and drains most of the right liver
C. The left and middle hepatic veins usually join extrahepatically and enter the left side of the IVC as a single vessel
D. A number of small posterior venous branches from the right posterior sector and caudate lobe drain directly into the IVC

37. Biliary drainage is through the left system only in up to:

A. 5%
B. 10%
C. 15%
D. 25%

38. Biliary drainage is through the right system only in up to:

A. 5%
B. 10%
C. 15%
D. 25%

39. The length of common bile duct is:

A. 5 to 7 cm
B. 7 to 10 cm
C. 10 to 15 cm
D. 15 to 20 cm

40. The diameter of common bile duct is:

A. 5 mm
B. 6 mm
C. 7 mm
D. 8 mm

41. Sphincter of Oddi is made up of all except:

A. The pancreatic sphincter, present to variable degrees, which surrounds the intraduodenal pancreatic duct
B. The sphincter choledochus, which is a circular muscle that regulates bile flow and the filling of the gallbladder
C. The sphincter ampullae, made up of circular muscle, which prevents duodenal reflux
D. All of the above are true

42. The most common variation of the hepatic duct confluence is:

A. Trifurcation at the confluence
B. Either of the right sectoral ducts drains into the common hepatic duct
C. Either of the right sectoral ducts drains into the left hepatic duct
D. Absence of right hepatic duct and drainage of right posterior sectoral duct into the cystic duct

43. Length of gallbladder is approximately:

A. 3 cms
B. 5 cms
C. 7 cms
D. 10 cms

44. The line in the image denotes:

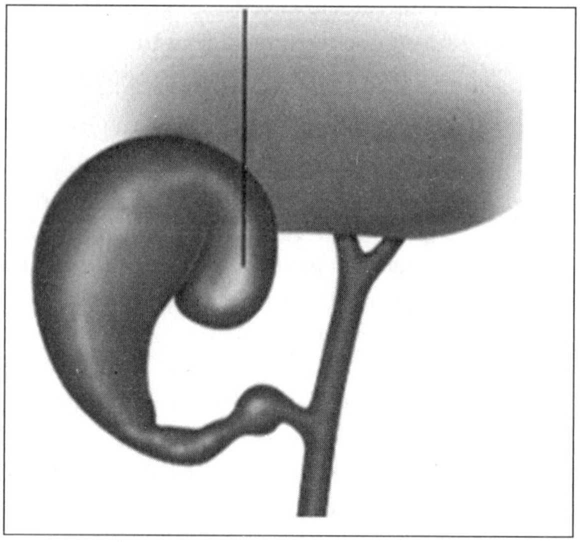

A. Hartmann pouch
B. Fold of Heister
C. Phrygian cap
D. None of the above

45. False about the gallbladder is:

A. The gallbladder can also have a long mesentery, which can predispose it to torsion
B. The cystic duct can also run a spiral course anteriorly or posteriorly and enter the left side of the common hepatic duct
C. Anomalies of the position of the gallbladder are more common
D. The venous drainage of the gallbladder empties into the veins that drain the bile duct and drains directly into the portal vein

46. **The supraduodenal and infrahilar bile ducts are predominantly supplied by 2 axial vessels that run at:**
   A. 2- and 8-O'clock positions
   B. 3- and 9-O'clock positions
   C. 4- and 10-O'clock positions
   D. 6- and 12-O'clock positions

47. **False about the innervation of the liver and biliary tract is:**
   A. Sympathetic fibers originating from T7 through T10
   B. Parasympathetic fibers from only right vagal nerve
   C. Acute distention of the liver, and thus the liver capsule, can result in right upper quadrant pain, which may be referred to the right shoulder
   D. The gallbladder and extrahepatic bile ducts receive innervation from sympathetic and parasympathetic fibers

48. **A hepatic lobule is made up of:**
   A. A central terminal hepatic venule surrounded by 4 to 6 terminal portal triads that form a polygonal unit
   B. A central terminal hepatic artery surrounded by 4 to 6 terminal portal triads that form a polygonal unit
   C. A central terminal hepatic venule surrounded by 10 to 12 terminal portal triads that form a polygonal unit
   D. A central terminal hepatic artery surrounded by 10 to 12 terminal portal triads that form a polygonal unit

49. **False about the functional unit anatomy of the liver is:**
   A. Hepatic lobule is made up of a central terminal hepatic venule surrounded by 4 to 6 terminal portal triads that form a polygonal unit
   B. Unit is lined on its periphery between each terminal portal triad by terminal portal triad branches
   C. Blood flows from the hepatic venule through the sinusoids into the terminal portal triad
   D. Bile is formed within the hepatocytes and empties into terminal canaliculi, which form on the lateral walls of the intercellular hepatocyte

50. **True about zones of hepatic lobular unit is:**
   A. Zone 1 - perivenular zone
   B. Zone 2 - intermediate zone
   C. Zone 3 - periportal zone
   D. Phenomenon of centrilobular necrosis from hypotension is because zone 1 is the most susceptible to decreases in oxygen delivery

51. **The hepatic sinusoids are 7 to 15 μm wide and can increase in size by up to:**
   A. 2 fold B. 5 fold
   C. 10 fold D. 20 fold

52. **Of the total hepatic cell mass, the sinusoidal endothelial cells account for:**
   A. 5% to 10% B. 15% to 20%
   C. 25% to 30% D. 35% to 40%

53. **False about hepatic stellate cells is:**
   A. Also called as ito cells
   B. These cells high in calcium content
   C. These cells are found in the space of Disse
   D. The major functions of these stellate cells include vitamin A storage and the synthesis of extracellular collagen and other extracellular matrix proteins

54. **Of the hepatic cellular mass, hepatocytes are complex multifunctional cells that make up:**
   A. 50% B. 60%
   C. 70% D. 80%

55. **False about the hepatocytes is:**
   A. Hepatocytes are arranged in single-cell-layer plates lined on either side by blood-filled sinusoids
   B. The monoclonal antibody HepPar1 (hepatocyte paraffin 1) identifies a unique antigen on hepatocyte mitochondria and is widely used to identify hepatocytes
   C. There are 100 mitochondria/hepatocytes occupying approximately 50% of the cell volume
   D. The bile canaliculi form a ring around the hepatocyte that drains into small bile ducts known as canals of Hering

56. **False about the hepatic lobule of liver is:**
   A. Sinusoids in the periportal zone are narrower and more tortuous, facilitating increased uptake of substrate by the hepatocytes in this area
   B. Sinusoids in zone 3 (perivenous) have larger fenestrations, allowing uptake of larger molecules

C. Glucose uptake and release, bile formation, and synthesis of albumin and fibrinogen take place in the perivenous zone
D. Glucose catabolism, xenobiotic metabolism, and synthesis of α1-antitrypsin and α-fetoprotein (AFP) occur in the perivenous zone

57. The location of the urea cycle enzymes in hepatic lobule is in:

A. Zone 1 B. Zone 2
C. Zone 3 D. Zone 4

58. Of the total cardiac output, hepatic blood flow represents about:

A. 15% B. 25%
C. 40% D. 50%

59. The most profound effect on hepatic blood flow is by:

A. Vitamins B. Proteins
C. Fats D. Carbohydrates

60. Portal pressure is generally:

A. 6 to 10 cm of H_2O B. 6 to 10 mm Hg
C. 2 to 4 cm of H_2O D. 2 to 4 mm Hg

61. The osmolality of bile is approximately:

A. 100 mOsmol/kg B. 200 mOsmol/kg
C. 300 mOsmol/kg D. 400 mOsmol/kg

62. False about bile formation is:

A. Bile is initially secreted by hepatocytes into the canaliculi through specialized microvilli containing lateral membranes of the hepatocytes that form the canaliculi
B. Bile acids are transported from the sinusoidal blood into the hepatocyte by ATP-requiring active transport
C. The major organic solutes in bile are bile acids, bile pigments, cholesterol and phospholipids
D. It is well recognized that bile flow has a non linear association with bile acid secretion

63. Daily secretion of bile is approximately:

A. 300 mL B. 500 mL
C. 1000 mL D. 1500 mL

64. True about biliary system is:

A. The gallbladder acts as the reservoir of the biliary tree, its function is to store bile in the fasting state
B. The gallbladder reabsorbs water, concentrating stored bile, and secretes mucin
C. Contraction of the gallbladder is mediated hormonally, largely through cholecystokinin, in response to a meal, with the simultaneous relaxation of the sphincter of Oddi and release of bile into the duodenum
D. All of the above

65. False about enterohepatic circulation is:

A. The primary bile salts cholic acid and chenodeoxycholic acid are produced in the liver from cholesterol and subsequently conjugated with glycine or taurine in the hepatocyte
B. Once secreted in the gut, the primary bile acids are modified by intestinal bacteria to form the secondary bile acids deoxycholic acid and lithocholic acid
C. Bile acids are reabsorbed actively into the jejunum and ileum
D. The bile acids re-enters the portal venous system, and up to 90% of the bile acids are extracted by hepatocytes

66. False about bilirubin metabolism is:

A. An early phase of heme breakdown, accounting for 20% of bilirubin, is from hemoproteins and occurs within 30 days of labelling with radioactive heme
B. A late phase of heme breakdown, accounting for 80% of bilirubin, is from senescent red blood cells and occurs approximately 110 days after administration of radioactive labeled heme
C. Bilirubin has long been known to be a toxic compound and is the agent responsible for neonatal encephalopathy and cochlear damage secondary to severe unconjugated hyperbilirubinemia
D. Free bilirubin can uncouple oxidative phosphorylation, inhibit ATPases, decrease glucose metabolism, and inhibit a broad spectrum of protein kinase activities

67. The glycogen content per kilogram of liver tissue is up to:

A. 25 g B. 45 g
C. 65 g D. 85 g

68. After fasting, hepatic glycogen is depleted and the liver shifts from glycogenolysis to gluconeogenesis after:

A. 12 hours B. 24 hours
C. 48 hours D. 72 hours

69. Fatty liver associated with alcohol intake has a number of causes; it is related to all except:

A. Decreased lipolysis
B. Relative starvation in the chronic alcoholic
C. Augmented esterification of hepatic fatty acids
D. Reduced oxygenation

70. False about protein metabolism is:

A. Excess amino acids not used in peripheral tissues are generally handled by the liver, in which they are oxidized for energy providing 10% of the liver's energy needs
B. Branched chain amino acids cannot be catabolized in the liver and are mostly dealt with by muscle
C. The liver is also responsible for the so-called acute-phase response, a synthetic response by protein to trauma or infection
D. Albumin is made exclusively in the liver and is the predominant serum binding protein

71. Warfarin acts in the liver by blocking activation of all of the following factors except:

A. X B. IX
C. II D. VIII

72. The shortest half-life of the coagulation factors is:

A. IV B. V
C. VIII D. VII

73. False about xenobiotics is:

A. Phase I reactions, through oxidation, reduction, and hydrolysis, increase the polarity and, thus, water solubility of compounds
B. Phase I reactions occur in the cytochrome P450 system
C. Phase II reactions generally act to create a less toxic or less active byproduct
D. Phase I reactions always detoxify chemicals

74. After partial hepatectomy, maximal hepatocyte DNA synthesis occurs in:

A. 14 - 24 hours B. 24 - 36 hours
C. 36 - 48 hours D. 48 - 72 hours

75. Liver specific enzyme is:

A. AST B. ALP
C. ALT D. GGT

76. False about liver function test is:

A. Alkaline phosphatase (ALP) is expressed in liver, bile ducts, bone, intestine, placenta, kidney and leukocytes
B. Elevations of ALT levels in hepatobiliary diseases are generally secondary to cholestasis or biliary obstruction
C. 5′-Nucleotidase is also found in a wide variety of organs in addition to the liver, but increased levels are fairly specific to hepatic disease
D. Gamma glutamyl transpeptidase (GGT) is also induced by alcohol intake and is elevated in biliary obstruction

77. Gamma glutamyl transpeptidase (GGT) is an enzyme in many organs in addition to the liver, such as all except:

A. Seminal vesicles B. Spleen
C. Pancreas D. Adrenals

78. False about albumin is:

A. Albumin is synthesized exclusively in the liver and can be used as a general measure of hepatic synthetic function
B. Because of the remarkable protein synthetic capacity of the liver, hypoalbuminemia is a marker of severe liver disease
C. Albumin level it is most helpful in acute liver disease
D. Albumin levels lacks sensitivity, and large decreases in hepatic function are required to be reflected in albumin levels

79. Autoimmune antibodies are used to diagnose primary biliary cirrhosis is:

A. Antimitochondrial antibodies
B. Antineutrophil antibodies
C. α1-Antitrypsin antibodies
D. None of the above

80. Autoimmune antibodies are used to diagnose primary sclerosing cholangitis is:

A. Antimitochondrial antibodies
B. Antineutrophil antibodies
C. α1-Antitrypsin antibodies
D. None of the above

81. False about the hepatic specific diagnostic tests is all except:

A. Technetium-99m (Tc 99m) galactosyl human serum albumin scintigraphy and Tc 99m mebrofenin hepatobiliary scintigraphy potentially identify patients at risk for postresectional liver failure who might benefit from liver-augmenting techniques
B. The aminopyrine breath test is based on cytochrome P450 clearance of radiolabeled aminopyrine

C. The galactose elimination test is based on the liver's role in phosphorylating galactose and converting it to fructose
D. The lidocaine clearance test yields similar information to the aminopyrine test because it is based on its clearance by the hepatic cytochrome P450 test

82. All of the following variables are seen in Child-Pugh classification except:
A. Bilirubin (mg/dL)
B. Creatinine (mg/dL)
C. Albumin (g/dL)
D. Ascites

83. Patients with a score of 8 point is:
A. Child-Pugh class A
B. Child-Pugh class B
C. Child-Pugh class C
D. Child-Pugh class D

PORTAL HYPERTENSION

84. Portal hypertension is defined by a portal pressure gradient:
A. > 5 cm of H_2O B. > 5 mm Hg
C. > 8 mm Hg D. > 8 cm of H_2O

85. Portal pressure gradient typically required to begin stimulating the development of portosystemic collateralization is:
A. 8–10 mm Hg B. 8–10 cm of H_2O
C. 10–12 mm Hg D. 10–12 cm of H_2O

86. False about the pathophysiology of portal hypertension is:
A. Increased hepatic vascular resistance caused by active vasoconstriction by norepinephrine and endothelin
B. Increased passive resistance secondary to fibrosis and regenerative nodules
C. Decreased portal venous inflow secondary to a hyperdynamic systemic circulation and splanchnic hyperemia
D. Splanchnic hormones, decreased sensitivity of the splanchnic vasculature to catecholamines, and increased production of nitrous oxide and prostacyclin may be involved

87. The most common cause of prehepatic portal hypertension is:
A. EHPVO
B. Portal vein thrombosis
C. Isolated splenic vein thrombosis
D. Budd-Chiari syndrome

88. In children, portal vein thrombosis as a cause of portal hypertension accounts for approximately:
A. 10% B. 20%
C. 30% D. 50%

89. In patients of cirrhosis, mortality due to variceal hemorrhage is:
A. 20% B. 33%
C. 50% D. 66%

90. The most common cause of intrahepatic presinusoidal hypertension is:
A. Alcoholic cirrhosis
B. Non-alcoholic cirrhosis
C. Schistosomiasis
D. Budd-Chiari syndrome

91. Posthepatic or postsinusoidal causes of portal hypertension is/are:
A. Constrictive pericarditis
B. Budd-Chiari syndrome
C. Heart failure
D. All of the above

92. False about variceal hemorrhage is:
A. Bleeding from esophagogastric varices is the single most life-threatening complication of portal hypertension
B. Approximately 20% of these deaths are caused by uncontrolled bleeding
C. The risk for death from bleeding is mainly related to the underlying hepatic functional reserve
D. Once bleeding is controlled, the greatest risk for rebleeding from varices is within the first few days after the onset of hemorrhage; the risk declines rapidly between that point and 6 weeks

93. False about the treatment of variceal bleeding is:
A. For acutely bleeding patients with portal hypertension, nonoperative treatments are generally used as a first-line approach
B. Endoscopic treatment (e.g., sclerosis or ligation) has become the mainstay of nonoperative treatment of acute hemorrhage
C. Pharmacotherapy can also be initiated, and trials have suggested that it may not be as effective as endoscopic treatment

D. TIPS has replaced operative shunts for managing acute variceal bleeding when pharmacotherapy and endoscopic treatment fail to control bleeding

94. Acute variceal bleeding episodes are successfully controlled by endoscopic measures in:

A. 20% to 30%
B. 50% to 60%
C. 70% to 80%
D. 80% to 90%

95. False about the endoscopic management of variceal bleeding is:

A. Sclerotherapy and band ligation of varices are the two main options available for control of acute variceal bleeding
B. Sclerotherapy is better than band ligation in the initial control of bleeding and is associated with fewer complications
C. Patients should be started on vasoactive drugs early, and endoscopy with band ligation is performed after initial resuscitation
D. Early endoscopy, preferably within 12 hours of admission, with an attempt at control of bleeding is recommended

96. False about the pharmacological management of variceal bleeding is:

A. Medical therapy should be initiated at the onset of variceal bleeding
B. Randomized trials have also shown that somatostatin and its longer-acting analogue octreotide are as efficacious as endoscopic treatment for control of acute variceal bleeding
C. In patients with variceal bleeding, antibiotic prophylaxis should not be initiated
D. Because of the adverse systemic effects of vasopressin, nitroglycerin should be simultaneously infused and then titrated to achieve blood pressure control

97. True about the variceal tamponade as a management of variceal bleeding is:

A. The major advantages of variceal tamponade using the Sengstaken Blakemore tube are immediate cessation of bleeding in more than 85% of patients
B. There are significant disadvantages of balloon tamponade, including frequent recurrent hemorrhage in up to 50% of patients after balloon deflation
C. Balloon tamponade is as effective as pharmacotherapy and endoscopic therapy in controlling acute variceal bleeding
D. All of the above

98. False about TIPS in management of variceal bleeding is:

A. TIPS has become the preferred treatment for acute variceal bleeding when pharmacotherapy and endoscopic treatment fail
B. With TIPS, a functional portacaval end-to-side shunt is established
C. TIPS is associated with risk of encephalopathy
D. TIPS is able to control bleeding in almost all patients

99. The most common situations requiring urgent or emergency surgery are all except:

A. Failure of long-term endoscopic therapy
B. After TIPS placement
C. Failure of acute endoscopic treatment
D. Hemorrhage from gastric varices or portal hypertensive gastropathy

100. The major disadvantage of emergency surgery is that operative mortality rates exceed:

A. 10%
B. 25%
C. 50%
D. 70%

101. After a patient has bled from varices, the likelihood of a repeated episode exceeds:

A. 40%
B. 50%
C. 60%
D. 70%

102. False about the prophylaxis of recurrent variceal bleeding is:

A. The combination of a beta blocker and long-acting nitrate has been shown to be less effective than variceal ligation
B. Combination therapy should be recommended as the first line of treatment for secondary prophylaxis of variceal bleeding
C. The combination of variceal ligation and pharmacotherapy with nonselective beta blockade is more effective than variceal ligation alone
D. Rebleeding and mortality rates also appear to be lower after variceal ligation

103. False about the interventional therapy as prophylaxis of recurrent variceal bleeding is:

A. TIPS is being increasingly used for definitive treatment of patients who bleed from portal hypertension
B. A major limitation of TIPS, however, is a high incidence (up to 50%) of shunt stenosis or shunt thrombosis within the first year

C. Shunt stenosis, which is usually secondary to neointimal hyperplasia and is less common than thrombosis

D. TIPS stenosis and occlusion have become less frequent with the use of PTFE-covered stents

104. TIPS dysfunction developed in ____ of patients.

A. 20%
B. 30%
C. 50%
D. 70%

105. False about TIPS is:

A. Encephalopathy was significantly more common in TIPS patients as compared to endoscopic therapy

B. TIPS is not effective for the treatment of medically intractable ascites

C. Group of patients in whom TIPS may be advantageous includes those with advanced hepatic functional decompensation

D. TIPS appears to be the ideal therapy when only short-term portal decompression is required

106. The most effective means of preventing recurrent hemorrhage in patients with portal hypertension is:

A. Endoscopy band ligation
B. Pharmacotherapy
C. Portosystemic shunts
D. Sclerotherapy

107. Eck fistula is:

A. Side-to-side portacaval shunt
B. End-to-side portacaval shunt
C. Portacaval interposition shunt
D. Conventional splenorenal shunt

108. The most common causes of death in medically treated is:

A. Renal failure
B. Accelerated hepatic failure
C. Irretractable ascites
D. Rebleeding

109. The most common causes of death in shunted patients is:

A. Renal failure
B. Accelerated hepatic failure
C. Irretractable ascites
D. Rebleeding

110. True about surgical therapy is:

A. Side-to-side shunts accelerate hepatic failure and lead to frequent post shunt encephalopathy

B. Side-to-side portosystemic shunts are the most effective shunt procedures for relieving ascites as well as for preventing recurrent variceal bleeding

C. A conventional splenorenal shunt that is of sufficient caliber to remain patent gradually dilates and eventually causes complete portal decompression and portal flow diversion

D. All of the above

111. False about distal splenorenal shunt is:

A. The distal splenorenal shunt consists of anastomosis of the distal end of the splenic vein to the left renal vein and interruption of all collateral vessels

B. The distal splenorenal shunt tends to aggravate relieve ascites

C. A splenic vein diameter < 7 mm is a relative contraindication to the procedure

D. A contraindication to a distal splenorenal shunt is prior splenectomy

112. False about partial portosystemic shunts is:

A. When the prosthetic graft is 10 mm or less in diameter, hepatic portal perfusion is preserved in most patients, at least during the early postoperative interval

B. In early experience with small-diameter prosthetic shunt is that <15% of shunts have thrombosed

C. Partial (8 mm in diameter) and nonselective (16 mm in diameter) interposition portacaval shunts have shown a lower frequency of encephalopathy after the partial shunt

D. The small-diameter interposition shunt was discovered to have a higher overall failure rate than TIPS

113. True about hepatic transplantation and portal hypertension is:

A. Transplantation in patients who have bled secondary to portal hypertension is the only therapy that addresses the underlying liver disease in addition to providing reliable portal decompression

B. Patients with variceal bleeding who are transplantation candidates include non-alcoholic cirrhotic patients

C. There is accumulating evidence that variceal bleeders with well compensated hepatic functional reserve are initially better served by nontransplantation strategies

D. All of the above

INFECTIOUS DISEASES

114. **False about pyogenic abscess is:**
   A. Pyogenic liver abscess is now mostly seen in patients in their 50s or 60s
   B. There is no significant gender, ethnic, or geographic differences in disease frequency
   C. The male-to-female ratio is approximately 10:1
   D. Comorbid conditions associated with pyogenic abscess are cirrhosis, diabetes, chronic renal failure, and a history of malignant disease

115. **The most common identifiable cause of hepatic abscess is:**
   A. Cryptogenic infections
   B. Caroli disease
   C. Biliary ascariasis
   D. Malignant obstruction

116. **The most common cause of pyogenic hepatic abscess in Asia is:**
   A. Malignant obstruction
   B. Intrahepatic stones
   C. Caroli disease
   D. Biliary tract surgery

117. **True about pyogenic abscess is:**
   A. Hepatic abscess has also been associated with colorectal malignant disease
   B. Prior biliary-enteric anastomosis has also been associated with hepatic abscess formation
   C. The incidence of gastrointestinal cancers was increased fourfold among patients with pyogenic liver abscess
   D. All of the above

118. **False about pyogenic abscess is:**
   A. Most hepatic abscesses involve the right hemiliver, accounting for about 75% of cases
   B. The left liver is involved in approximately 20% of the cases
   C. The caudate lobe is rarely involved ~5%
   D. Bilobar involvement with multiple abscesses is common

119. **True about pyogenic liver abscess is/are:**
   A. Anaerobic organisms are involved approximately 40% to 60% of the time
   B. Approximately 50% of hepatic abscesses are solitary
   C. Many hepatic abscesses are polymicrobial in nature and account for approximately 40% of cases
   D. All of the above

120. **The most common organisms cultured in pyogenic liver abscess is:**
   A. Streptococci
   B. Escherichia coli
   C. Staphylococcus aureus
   D. Enterococcus spp

121. **In pyogenic abscess, blood cultures are positive in approximately:**
   A. 20% to 30%
   B. 30% to 50%
   C. 50% to 60%
   D. 70% to 80%

122. **False about the clinical features of pyogenic hepatic abscess is:**
   A. The classic description of the presenting symptoms of hepatic abscess is fever, jaundice and right upper quadrant pain, tenderness to palpation
   B. The typical presentation is present in 50% of cases
   C. Fever, chills and abdominal pain are the most common presenting symptoms
   D. Involvement of the diaphragm may result in symptoms of cough or dyspnea

123. **False about the clinical features of pyogenic hepatic abscess is:**
   A. Jaundice is also found in approximately 50% of cases and is often secondary to underlying biliary disease
   B. On physical examination, fever and right upper quadrant tenderness are the most common findings
   C. Tenderness is present in 40% to 70% of patients
   D. Chest findings are often found in approximately 25% of patients

124. **False about endogenous endophthalmitis is:**
   A. It is a rare complication specific to Klebsiella hepatic abscesses
   B. This serious complication is more common in alcoholics
   C. It occurs in approximately 3% of cases
   D. The best chance to preserve visual function is with early diagnosis and treatment

125. **In pyogenic abscess, chest radiographs are abnormal approximately:**
   A. 10%
   B. 20%
   C. 50%
   D. 70%

126. In pyogenic abscess, the lab findings are:

A. The ALP level is mildly elevated in 80% of patients
B. Total bilirubin concentration is elevated in 20% to 50% of the time
C. Transaminases are mildly elevated in approximately 60% of patients
D. All of the above

127. False about the imaging in pyogenic liver abscess is:

A. Chest radiographs findings generally reflect subdiaphragmatic disease, such as an elevated right hemidiaphragm, right pleural effusion, or atelectasis
B. Ultrasound usually demonstrates a round or oval area that is more echogenic than the surrounding liver
C. Magnetic resonance imaging (MRI) can be helpful in distinguishing the cause of many hepatic masses and evaluating the biliary tree for pathologic changes
D. The abscess wall usually has an intense enhancement on contrast-enhanced CT

128. The sensitivity of ultrasound in diagnosing hepatic abscess is:

A. 50% to 65% B. 60% to 75%
C. 80% to 95% D. 95% to 100%

129. The sensitivity of CT in diagnosing hepatic abscess is:

A. 50% to 65% B. 60% to 75%
C. 80% to 95% D. 95% to 100%

130. False about the treatment of pyogenic abscess is:

A. Once the diagnosis of pyogenic hepatic abscess is suspected, broad-spectrum IV antibiotics should be started immediately to control ongoing bacteremia and its associated complications
B. Combinations such as ampicillin, an aminoglycoside, and metronidazole or a 3rd generation cephalosporin with metronidazole are appropriate
C. Surgery has become the treatment of choice for most patients
D. Relative contraindications to percutaneous catheter drainage include the presence of ascites, coagulopathy and proximity to vital structures

131. Success rates of percutaneous catheter drainage range from:

A. 50% to 60% B. 65% to 90%
C. 40% to 70% D. 20% to 50%

132. Success rate of percutaneous aspiration without the placement of an indwelling drain is:

A. 20% to 30% B. 30% to 50%
C. 60% to 90% D. 80% to 95%

133. Liver resection is occasionally required for hepatic abscess it may be required for all except:

A. Hepatolithiasis
B. Cholangitis
C. Infected hepatic malignant neoplasm
D. Intrahepatic biliary stricture

134. False about amoebic abscesses is:

A. Entamoeba dispar is the nonpathogenic form
B. E histolytica infections have estimated that as many as 55% of those in endemic regions are infected, although less than 50% are symptomatic
C. A female preponderance of more than 10:1 has been reported in almost all studies
D. Heavy alcohol consumption is commonly reported and may render the liver more susceptible to amoebic infection

135. False about the pathogenesis of amoebic abscesses is:

A. Humans are the principal host, and the main source of infection is human contact with a cyst-passing carrier
B. Amoebic liver abscesses are formed by progressing, localized hepatic necrosis producing a cavity containing acellular proteinaceous debris surrounded by a rim of invasive amoebic trophozoites
C. Children who lack antiamebic IgM have innate resistance to invasive amoebic infection
D. E histolytica trophozoites can lyse tissues through a complex set of events, including cell adherence, cell activation, and subsequent release of enzymes, resulting in necrosis

136. Most common symptom of amoebic liver abscess is:

A. Fever B. Abdominal pain
C. Jaundice D. Hepatomegaly

137. False about the clinical features of amoebic liver abscess is:

A. The duration of symptoms has been found to be typically less than 10 days

B. Approximately 25% of patients have diarrhea despite an obligatory colonic infection
C. Rupture into the peritoneum with peritonitis occurs frequently; it is more often with right-sided abscesses
D. Synchronous hepatic abscess is found in one third of patients with active amoebic colitis

138. False about the clinical features and diagnosis of amoebic liver abscess is:

A. Acute presentations are typically more dramatic, with high fevers, chills and significant abdominal tenderness
B. In the acute presentation, 80% of patients have multiple lesions, whereas with the chronic presentation, more than 50% of patients have a single right-sided lesion
C. The most useful laboratory evaluation is the measurement of circulating antiamebic antibodies, which are present in 90% to 95% of patients
D. An enzyme immunoassay has a reported sensitivity of 99% and specificity higher than 90% in patients with hepatic abscess

139. The most common LFT abnormality in amoebic liver abscess is an:

A. Elevated bilirubin
B. Elevated AST/ALT
C. Elevated PT-INR
D. Elevated ALP

140. False about imaging studies of amoebic abscess is:

A. Abdominal ultrasound has a reported accuracy of approximately 90% when it is combined with a typical history and clinical presentation
B. Plain chest radiographs are abnormal in approximately 80% of cases
C. Abdominal CT scanning is probably more sensitive than ultrasound and is helpful in differentiating amoebic from pyogenic abscess, with rim enhancement noted in the pyogenic abscess
D. Tc 99m liver scans, can be helpful in differentiating pyogenic from amoebic abscesses because the amoebic abscesses typically do not contain leukocytes and therefore do not light up on these scans

141. False about the treatment of amoebic abscess is:

A. The mainstay of treatment for amoebic abscesses is metronidazole (750 mg orally, three times daily for 10 days)
B. Clinical improvement is usually seen within 7 days after metronidazole
C. Emetine hydrochloride is effective against invasive amebiasis, particularly in the liver and has serious cardiac side effects
D. After treatment of the liver abscess, it is recommended that luminal agents such as iodoquinol, paromomycin, and diloxanide furoate be administered to treat the carrier state

142. False about risk of rupture in amoebic abscess is seen in:

A. Abscesses >5 cm in diameter has increased risk
B. Right liver lesion has increased risk
C. The size of the abscess appears to be the most important risk factor for rupture
D. Most peritoneal ruptures tend to be contained by the diaphragm, abdominal wall, or omentum, but rupture can fistulize into a hollow viscus

143. False about the rupture of amoebic abscess is:

A. Rupture into the pleural space usually results in a large and rapidly accumulated effusion that collapses the involved lung
B. Treatment of rupture into pleural space consists of thoracentesis
C. Right-sided abscess may rupture into the pericardium and can be manifested as an asymptomatic pericardial effusion or even tamponade
D. Rupture can occur into the bronchi and is usually self-limited with postural drainage and bronchodilators

144. False about the outcomes of amoebic abscess is:

A. The mortality for all patients with amoebic liver abscess is approximately 5%
B. When an abscess ruptures, mortality ranges from 6% to as high as 50%
C. Mortality appears to be affected by the addition of aspiration to metronidazole therapy or by chronicity of symptoms
D. The average time to radiologic resolution is 3 - 9 months and in some patients, it can take years

145. Factors independently associated with poor outcome of amoebic abscess are:

A. Encephalopathy
B. Elevated serum bilirubin level (>3.5 mg/dL)
C. Abscess volume > 1000 mL
D. Hypoalbuminemia (<2.0 g/dL)

146. False about hydatid disease is:

A. Humans contract the disease from dogs but there is no human-to-human transmission

B. In the human duodenum, the parasitic embryo releases an oncosphere containing hooklets that penetrate the mucosa, allowing access to the bloodstream

C. Echinococcus granulosus is the most common

D. The adult tapeworm is attached to the villi of the duodenum

147. False about hydatid disease is:

A. Pericyst or fibrous capsule derived from host tissues develops around the hydatid cyst

B. 3 weeks after infection, a visible hydatid cyst develops, which then slowly grows in a spherical manner

C. Calcification of a hydatid cyst, imply that the cyst is dead

D. Brood capsules are small, intracystic cellular masses in which future worm heads develop into scoleces

148. False about presentation of hydatid disease is:

A. Hydatid cysts are diagnosed in equal numbers of men and women at an average age of about 45 years

B. Rupture of the cyst into the biliary tree or bronchial tree or free rupture into the peritoneal, pleural, or pericardial cavities can occur

C. Approximately 75% of hydatid cysts are located in the left liver and are solitary

D. The most common presenting symptoms are abdominal pain, dyspepsia and vomiting

149. The most frequent sign in hydatid cyst is:

A. Hepatomegaly
B. Jaundice
C. Fever
D. Anemia

150. True about the imaging of hydatid cyst is:

A. Calcifications in the wall of the cyst are highly suggestive of hydatid disease and can be helpful in the diagnosis

B. A rosette appearance is seen when daughter cysts are present

C. In patients with suspected biliary involvement, ERCP or percutaneous transhepatic cholangiography may be necessary

D. All of the above

151. False about the treatment of hydatid cyst is:

A. The cyst is then unroofed, which can then be followed by a number of possibilities, including excision (or pericystectomy), marsupialization procedures, leaving the cyst open, drainage of the cyst, omentoplasty, and partial hepatectomy to encompass the cyst

B. In older patients with small, asymptomatic, densely calcified cysts, conservative management is appropriate

C. Recurrence rates after surgical treatment range from 1% to 20%

D. Treatment of echinococcosis with albendazole or mebendazole is effective at shrinking cysts in many patients with E. granulosus infection, and cyst disappearance occurs in well above 50% of patients

152. False about recurrent pyogenic cholangitis is:

A. RPC is a syndrome of repeated attacks of cholangitis secondary to biliary stones and strictures that involve the extrahepatic and intrahepatic ducts

B. The disease strikes at an early age (20–40 years) in patients from lower socioeconomic classes among Asians

C. Also called as Oriental cholangiohepatitis or hepatolithiasis

D. Men are predominantly affected

153. False about recurrent pyogenic cholangitis is:

A. The cause of RPC is unknown but is related to recurrent infection of biliary radicals with gut bacteria

B. An association between RPC and Clonorchis sinensis and Ascaris lumbricoides infection has been noted and a true causal relationship has been proven

C. An increased incidence of cholangiocarcinoma has been noted, but a causal relationship is difficult to prove

D. Strictures can be found anywhere in the biliary tree but usually involve the intrahepatic main hepatic ducts, most often the left hepatic duct

154. In recurrent pyogenic cholangitis gallbladder is involved only in approximately:

A. 5%
B. 20%
C. 40%
D. 75%

155. False about the presentation of recurrent pyogenic cholangitis is:

A. Presents with multiple bouts of fever, right upper quadrant abdominal pain and jaundice

B. Biliary obstruction is usually complete and therefore, marked jaundice and pruritus are common

C. A combination of ultrasound, CT and direct cholangiography is often necessary to evaluate these patients
D. Magnetic resonance cholangiopancreatography can combine cross-sectional imaging and cholangiography in one non-invasive test

156. False about the treatment of recurrent pyogenic cholangitis is:

A. Percutaneous transhepatic cholangioscopic lithotomy is generally used for poor-risk surgical patients and those who have failed to respond to surgical treatment
B. In an acute presentation, most patients improve with conservative management, allowing time for radiologic studies and planning of a definitive operation, which is the treatment of choice
C. The goal of operative approaches is to clear the biliary tree of stones and to bypass, resect, or enlarge strictures
D. Nonoperative approaches, such as percutaneous transhepatic cholangioscopic lithotomy, have been developed, and are now the treatment of choice

157. True about the surgical management of recurrent pyogenic cholangitis is:

A. In complicated cases, providing permanent access to the biliary tree for interventional radiologic procedures by extending the end of the Roux-en-Y hepaticojejunostomy to the skin or subcutaneous space has been a successful approach
B. Partial hepatectomy is advocated for patients with intrahepatic strictures, hepatic atrophy, liver abscess, or suspicion of cholangiocarcinoma
C. Partial hepatectomy is advocated for patients with intrahepatic strictures, hepatic atrophy, liver abscess, or suspicion of cholangiocarcinoma
D. All of the above

158. Long-term survival of recurrent pyogenic cholangitis is mostly related to the presence of cholangiocarcinoma, which is found in approximately:

A. 2% B. 5%
C. 10% D. 20%

NEOPLASMS

159. False about liver cell adenoma is:

A. Liver cell adenoma (LCA) is a benign proliferation of hepatocytes in the context of a normal liver
B. It is predominantly found in young women (aged 20–40 years) and is often associated with steroid hormone use, such as long-term oral contraceptive pill use
C. The female-to-male ratio is approximately 1:11
D. Male anabolic hormone use can also predispose to development of LCA

160. False about liver cell adenoma is:

A. LCAs are usually singular, but multiple lesions have been reported in 12% to 30% of cases
B. Cases with multiple adenomas are not associated with OCP use and do not have as dramatic a female preponderance
C. Bile ductules are not observed histologically, and the normal architecture of the liver is absent in these lesions
D. Histologically, bile ductules are observed and the normal architecture of the liver is present

161. Liver adenomatosis is defined by the presence of:

A. > 1 LCAs B. > 10 LCAs
C. > 50 LCAs D. > 100 LCAs

162. Highest risk of malignant transformation is observed in LCA with:

A. HNF1A mutation
B. β-catenin activation
C. Inflammatory adenoma
D. Sonic hedgehog activation

163. LCA with β-catenin mutations can be further classified, increased risk of hepatocellular carcinoma (HCC) degeneration is with:

A. Exon-3 mutation B. Exon-7 mutation
C. Exon-8 mutation D. Exon-11 mutation

164. False about the presentation of LCA is:

A. Because of intratumoral hemorrhage, the necrosis and fat component of LCA tends to be heterogeneous on CT
B. Patients with LCA present with symptoms approximately 50% to 75% of the time
C. Tumor markers are abnormal
D. Upper abdominal pain is common and may be related to hemorrhage into the tumor or local compressive symptoms

165. **True about liver cell adenoma is:**
   A. Hepatic adenomas with β-catenin activation should be considered for early surgical intervention
   B. The two major risks of LCA are rupture, with potentially life-threatening intraperitoneal hemorrhage and malignant transformation
   C. All instances of spontaneous rupture occurring in lesions 5 cm and larger
   D. All of the above

166. **Risk of rupture in LCAs has been estimated to be:**
   A. 10% - 20%
   B. 20% - 30%
   C. 30% - 50%
   D. 60% - 70%

167. **False about the treatment of LCA is:**
   A. Patients with asymptomatic LCAs taking OCPs can be watched for regression after stopping of the OCPs, although progression and rupture have been observed in this setting
   B. Behavior of LCAs during pregnancy has been unpredictable and resection before a planned pregnancy is usually recommended
   C. Margin status is important in resections and resection with a margin of 2 cm should be performed
   D. The risk of malignancy is low in lesions < 5 cm

168. **The most common benign tumor if liver is:**
   A. Adenoma
   B. Focal nodular hyperplasia
   C. Hemangioma
   D. Lipoma

169. **The 2nd most common benign tumor if liver is:**
   A. Adenoma
   B. Focal nodular hyperplasia
   C. Hemangioma
   D. Lipoma

170. **False about focal nodular hyperplasia is:**
   A. On microscopic examination, FNH contains cords of benign-appearing hepatocytes divided by multiple fibrous septa originating from a central scar
   B. FNH is characterized by a central fibrous scar with radiating septa, although no central scar is seen in approximately 15% of cases
   C. Typical hepatic vascularity is seen and typical biliary epithelium is found scattered throughout the lesion
   D. The central scar often contains a large artery that branches out into multiple smaller arteries in a spoke wheel pattern

171. **The most common theory is that FNH is related to a:**
   A. OCPs
   B. Female
   C. Developmental vascular malformation
   D. Alcohol

172. **False about imaging and diagnosis of FNH is:**
   A. Serum AFP levels are abnormal
   B. FNH typically shows strong hypervascularity in the arterial phase of CT or MRI with central nonenhancing scar
   C. Physical examination is usually unrevealing and mild abnormalities of liver function may be found
   D. On occasion, histologic confirmation is necessary and resection is recommended for definitive diagnosis

173. **False about treatment of FNH is:**
   A. Asymptomatic patients with typical radiologic features do not require treatment
   B. Rupture, bleeding and infarction are exceedingly rare, and malignant degeneration of FNH has never been reported
   C. Careful observation of symptomatic FNH with serial imaging is not reasonable because symptoms never resolve in a most of the cases
   D. Because FNH is a benign diagnosis, resection must be performed, with minimal morbidity and mortality

174. **False about hemangioma is:**
   A. It occurs in women more than in men (3:1 ratio) and at a mean age of approximately 45 years
   B. They are usually solitary and > 5 cm in diameter, and they occur with incidence more common in left hemiliver
   C. Cavernous hemangiomas have been associated with FNH and are also theorized to be congenital vascular malformations
   D. The enlargement of hemangiomas is by ectasia rather than by neoplasia

175. **Giant hemangiomas are:**
   A. > 2 cm
   B. > 5 cm
   C. > 10 cm
   D. > 15 cm

176. **False about liver hemangioma is:**
   A. Symptoms ascribed to a liver hemangioma mandate a search for other disease because an

alternative cause of symptoms will be found in approximately 50% of cases

B. Involution or thrombosis of hemangiomas can result in dense fibrotic masses that may be difficult to differentiate from malignant tumor

C. Hemangiomas are usually asymptomatic and found incidentally on imaging studies

D. Spontaneous rupture of liver hemangiomas is common

177. Kasabach-Merritt syndrome is:

A. Syndrome of thrombocytosis and consumptive coagulopathy

B. Syndrome of thrombocytopenia and consumptive coagulopathy

C. Syndrome of leukopenia and consumptive coagulopathy

D. Syndrome of leukocytosis and consumptive coagulopathy

178. False about the diagnosis and imaging of hemangioma is:

A. The preferred approach to resection is enucleation with arterial inflow control

B. CT and MRI are usually sufficient if a typical peripheral nodular enhancement pattern is seen

C. Biopsy is recommended

D. Isotope-labeled red blood cell scans are an accurate test but are rarely necessary if high-quality CT and MRI are available

179. Indications for resection of hemangioma is/are:

A. Development of the Kasabach-Merritt syndrome

B. Rupture

C. Significant change in size

D. All of the above

180. False about liver hemangioma in children is:

A. Large hemangiomas in children can result in congestive heart failure secondary to arteriovenous shunting

B. Usually solitary and can involve other organs

C. Symptomatic childhood hemangiomas may be treated with therapeutic embolization and medical therapy should be initiated for congestive heart failure

D. Resection may be necessary for symptomatic lesions or rupture

181. False about benign liver tumors is:

A. Macroregenerative nodules, previously known as adenomatous hyperplasia, are single or multiple, well-circumscribed, bile stained, bulging surface nodules that occur primarily in cirrhotics and have malignant potential

B. Nodular regenerative hyperplasia has malignant potential and is associated with cirrhosis

C. Fatty tumors of the liver include primary lipomas, myelolipomas, angiolipomas and angiomyolipomas

D. Inflammatory pseudotumors of the liver are localized masses of inflammatory cells that can mimic a neoplasm

182. False about hepatocellular carcinoma is:

A. HCC is the most common primary malignant neoplasm of the liver

B. HCV is the most common cause of HCC in united states, accounting for more than half of all cases in the United States

C. Risk of HCC is further increased in obese patients and in those with non-alcoholic fatty liver disease and non-alcoholic steatohepatitis

D. HCC is 2 to 8 times more common in women than in men in low and high incidence areas

183. The most common cause of HCC worldwide is:

A. Alcoholic cirrhosis

B. Hepatitis B

C. Hepatitis C

D. Vinyl chloride

184. False about Hepatitis B and HCC is:

A. Cirrhosis is a prerequisite for the development of HBV-related HCC

B. The HBV has no known oncogenes, but insertional mutagenesis into hepatocytes may be a contributing factor to the development of HCC

C. Estimated relative risks of 5 to 100 for the development of HCC in HBV-infected individuals

D. Chronic HBV infection accounts for up to 50% of the world's cases of HCC and most of the cases of childhood HCC

185. False about Hepatitis C and HCC is:

A. HCV is an DNA virus that integrates into the host genome

B. HBV and HCV infections are both independent risk factors for the development of HCC but probably act synergistically when an individual is infected with both viruses

C. Factors associated with a more rapid progression include male gender, chronic alcohol use and older age at the time of infection

D. The rate of HCC among HCV-infected persons ranges from 1% to 3% over 30 years, and in individuals with HCV related cirrhosis, HCC develops at an annual rate of 1%–4%

186. **False about cirrhosis and HCC is:**

A. HBV infection and hemochromatosis are associated with higher risk of HCC

B. Alcohol and primary biliary cirrhosis are associated with a lower risk of HCC

C. Cirrhosis is required for the development of HCC, and hepatocarcinogenesis is an inevitable result of cirrhosis

D. Cirrhotic livers with higher DNA replication rates are associated with the development of HCC

187. **False about risk factors of HCC is:**

A. With chronic exposure, aflatoxin acts as a carcinogen and increases the risk of HCC

B. Cigarette smoking has been linked to the development of HCC, but the evidence is not consistent

C. Wilson disease, have also been implicated as risk factors for HCC

D. Alcohol causes cirrhosis but and has been shown to be directly carcinogenic in hepatocytes

188. **Thorotrast has been associated with:**

A. Angiosarcoma B. Cholangiosarcoma
C. HCC D. All of the above

189. **False about the clinical presentation of HCC is:**

A. Patients presenting with HCC are men 50 to 60 years of age who complain of right upper quadrant abdominal pain and weight loss and have a palpable mass

B. In countries endemic for HBV, presentation at a younger age is common and probably related to childhood infection

C. Small, incidentally noted tumors have become a more common presentation because of the knowledge of specific risk factors and screening programs

D. HCC can commonly be manifested as a rupture, with the sudden onset of abdominal pain followed by hypovolemic shock secondary to intraperitoneal bleeding

190. **HCCs manifest with paraneoplastic syndrome, all except:**

A. Hyperglycemia B. Hypercalcemia
C. Hypoglycemia D. Erythrocytosis

191. **False about the imaging of HCC is:**

A. Ultrasound plays a significant role in screening and early detection of HCC

B. Contrast enhanced CT and MRI protocols aimed at diagnosing HCC take advantage of the hypervascularity of these tumors, and arterial phase images are critical to assess the extent of disease adequately

C. Typical imaging criteria for HCC include rapid venous enhancement followed by washout in the delayed phase

D. Detection of bland or tumor thrombus in the portal or hepatic venous system is also important

192. **False about AFP and HCC is:**

A. AFP levels are particularly useful in monitoring treated patients for recurrence after normalization of levels

B. AFP measurements have low sensitivity and specificity

C. AFP is specific to HCC

D. Specificity and positive predictive values of AFP improve with higher cut-off levels (e.g., 400 ng/mL) but at the cost of sensitivity

193. **False about the evaluation of HCC is:**

A. Percutaneous fine-needle aspiration of HCC does run a small risk of tumor cell spillage (estimated to be ~1%) and rupture or bleeding

B. HCC largely metastasizes to the lung, bone and peritoneum

C. Preoperative chest CT is not mandatory

D. Liver resection is considered the treatment of choice for HCC and the risk of post-operative liver failure and death must be considered

194. **The risk of post operative liver failure and death is related to:**

A. Portal hypertension

B. Functional liver reserve

C. The degree of cirrhosis

D. All of the above

195. **True about the HCC treatment and Child-Pugh class is:**

A. Child-Pugh class A patients can usually tolerate some extent of liver resection

B. Child-Pugh class B patients to be candidates for operation, but they are generally borderline and therapy must be individualized

C. Child Pugh class C patients are not candidates for resectional therapy
D. All of the above

196. Staging laparoscopy has been used as a staging tool in HCC and doing it avoids nontherapeutic laparotomy in:

A. 10% B. 20%
C. 40% D. 50%

197. False about Cancer of the Liver Italian Program score is:

A. Score ranges from 0 to 6
B. A score of 4 to 6 is generally considered advanced disease
C. It is the most well-validated staging system
D. Presence of portal vein thrombosis gives 2 points

198. Which of the following is not a variable used in Cancer of the Liver Italian Program score?

A. AFP level
B. Tumor histology
C. Child-Pugh class
D. Portal vein thrombosis

199. The Okuda staging system considers all except:

A. Tumor involving > 50% of the liver
B. Presence of ascites
C. Bilirubin level > 3 mg/dL
D. Albumin level < 2 g/dL

200. Chinese University Prognostic Index includes all except:

A. Ascites
B. TNM stage
C. Levels of AST/ALT
D. Symptoms

201. False about the pathology of HCC is:

A. The pushing type of HCC is usually not resectable
B. The hanging type of HCC is connected to the liver by a small vascular stalk and is easily resected without sacrifice of a significant amount of adjacent nonneoplastic liver tissue
C. Infiltrative type of HCC, tends to invade vascular structures, even at a small size
D. The pushing type of HCC is well demarcated and often contains a fibrous capsule and characterized by growth that displaces vascular structures rather than invading them

202. False about the treatment of HCC is:

A. Preoperative portal vein embolization is an effective strategy to increase the volume and function of the FLR
B. Multifocal tumors and major vascular invasion are generally associated with a poor outcome
C. When possible, complete excision of HCC by partial hepatectomy or by total hepatectomy and liver transplantation is the treatment of choice
D. Only 40% to 50% of patients are considered to have resectable disease

203. The most commonly cited negative prognostic factors are all except:

A. Vascular invasion
B. Tumor size
C. Margin < 2 cm
D. Cirrhosis

204. True about transplantation in treatment of HCC is:

A. Patients with advanced cirrhosis (Child class B and C) and early-stage HCC should be considered for transplantation
B. Orthotopic liver transplantation is the ideal treatment for HCC because it addresses the liver dysfunction and cirrhosis and the HCC
C. Refinements in patient selection - namely, patients with single tumors smaller than 5 cm or no more than three tumors 3 cm in size have resulted in improved outcomes
D. All of the above

205. With a single application of Percutaneous ethanol injection (PEI), tumors up to what size can be ablated?

A. 1 cm B. 2 cm
C. 5 cm D. 7 cm

206. False about ablation of HCC is:

A. Percutaneous ethanol injection (PEI) is a useful technique for ablating small tumors
B. The tumor is killed by a combination of cellular dehydration, coagulative necrosis and vascular thrombosis
C. Percutaneous injection of acetic acid is a technique similar to PEI but has weak necrotizing abilities, making it less useful in septated tumors
D. Long-term survival after PEI for tumors smaller than 5 cm has been reported to range from 24% to 40%

207. False about cryotherapy as an ablative technique used in HCC is:

A. Cryotherapy is usually performed at laparotomy or laparoscopically, and it can't be performed with percutaneous techniques
B. Advantage is that the ice ball formed is easily monitored with ultrasound
C. Disadvantages include a heat sink effect, limiting the usefulness of freezing near major blood vessels
D. Reported 2-year survival rates for cryoablation of HCC range from 30% to 60%

208. False about radiofrequency ablation (RFA) as an ablative technique used in HCC is:

A. The procedure can easily be performed percutaneously with low complication rates
B. Temperatures higher than 80°C is reached and immediate cell death is seen
C. RFA is also limited by the protective effect of blood vessels and does not ablate well in these areas
D. RFA probes reportedly are able to ablate tumors as large as 7 cm

209. True about transarterial embolization in HCC is:

A. Metaanalysis has confirmed an overall survival advantage from the embolization strategies
B. Percutaneous transarterial embolization can induce ischemic necrosis in HCC, resulting in response rates as high as 50%
C. Intraarterial injections of iodine-131 with Ethiodol or yttrium-90 in glass microspheres have also been used to deliver localized radiation to HCCs
D. All of the above

210. True about systemic therapies in HCC is:

A. Sorafenib is best tolerated in patients with Child-Pugh class A cirrhosis
B. Systemic chemotherapy with a variety of agents has been ineffective and has had a minimal role in the treatment of HCC
C. Liver transplantation is applicable only if the tumor is 5 cm or smaller or there are two or three tumors, the largest of which is 3 cm or smaller
D. All of the above

211. False about Fibrolamellar HCC is:

A. The tumor generally occurs in younger patients without a history of cirrhosis
B. The tumor is usually well demarcated and encapsulated and may have a central fibrotic area
C. Fibrolamellar HCC does produces AFP
D. On histologic evaluation, fibrolamellar HCC is composed of large polygonal tumor cells embedded in a fibrous stroma, forming lamellar structures

212. Fibrolamellar HCC produces:

A. AFP
B. Neurotensin
C. Chromogranin A
D. HCG

213. False about the management of fibrolamellar HCC is:

A. Recurrence after resection is uncommon
B. Fibrolamellar HCC has a better prognosis than HCC
C. The gain of kinase activity may have a role in the pathogenesis of fibrolamellar HCC
D. Resection of lymph node metastases and recurrent disease has been advocated because of a lack of alternative therapy and the possibility of long-term survival

214. False about the childhood HCC is:

A. Childhood HCC is a distinct entity that represents almost 50% of pediatric liver tumors
B. There is a high incidence of multifocality, vascular invasion and extrahepatic metastases
C. Complete resection is the only potentially curative treatment
D. It has a relatively poor long-term survival rates of 10% to 20%

215. False about the variants of HCC is:

A. HCC can be manifested as a mixed hepatocellular cholangiocellular tumor, with cellular differentiation of both types are present
B. Mixed tumors tend to have a prognosis that is worse than for standard HCC
C. Some HCCs show evidence of sarcomatoid differentiation and are referred to as a sarcomatoid variant or carcinosarcoma and tend to produce AFP
D. The clear cell variant may have a better prognosis than standard HCC

216. False about Intrahepatic Cholangiocarcinoma is:

A. Most of these tumors (40% to 60%) involve the biliary confluence (Klatskin tumor)
B. Jaundice occurs commonly
C. Intrahepatic Cholangiocarcinoma is the 2nd most common primary hepatic neoplasm

D. The most common symptoms are right upper abdominal pain and weight loss

217. The most common risk factors for the development of cholangiocarcinoma (all types) were:

A. Choledochal cyst disease
B. Hepatolithiasis
C. Primary sclerosing cholangitis
D. All of the above

218. False about the diagnosis and imaging of IHC is:

A. IHC is a diagnosis of exclusion, and a search for a primary tumor with upper and lower gastrointestinal endoscopy and cross-sectional imaging of the chest, abdomen, and pelvis should be carried out
B. On CT and MRI, IHC is seen as a focal hepatic mass that may be associated with peripheral biliary dilation
C. Unlike HCC there is persistent enhancement on arterial phases due to the fibrotic nature of cholangiocarcinoma
D. Unlike in HCC, the AFP levels are normal, although CEA or CA 19-9 levels can be elevated in some cases

219. True about the treatment of HCC is:

A. Complete resection is the treatment of choice for IHC
B. Due to large tumor size and invasion into the surrounding structures, major hepatectomies with or without resection of surrounding organs may be required for achieving a margin negative resection
C. Factors associated with a poor outcome include multifocality, lymph node metastases, vascular invasion and positive margins
D. All of the above

220. False about hepatoblastoma is:

A. The median age at presentation is 18 months, and almost all cases occur before the age of 3 years
B. Hepatoblastoma is the most common primary hepatic tumor of childhood
C. Serum AFP levels are elevated in 40% to 50% of patients and is not a useful marker for therapeutic response
D. Hepatoblastoma has been associated with the familial polyposis syndrome

221. True about liver sarcomas is:

A. Angiosarcoma is probably the best-described primary hepatic sarcoma because of its well-known association with vinyl chloride or Thorotrast exposure
B. Any liver sarcoma must always be considered metastatic lesions until proven otherwise
C. Angiosarcoma typically is manifested as multiple hepatic masses and can appear in childhood
D. All of the above

222. True about metastatic liver tumors is:

A. Metastatic adenocarcinoma to the liver of unknown primary is often a primary IHC, and this diagnosis must always be kept in mind
B. The liver is a common site of metastases from gastrointestinal tumor
C. The most common malignant tumors of the liver are metastatic lesions
D. All of the above

223. False about the colorectal metastases to liver is:

A. Up to 60% of these patients will develop metastases during the course of their disease
B. Liver metastases can present synchronously or metachronously
C. Mild elevations in LFT results is common in metastatic colorectal cancer to the liver and is effective as a screening tool
D. A rising CEA level on serial examinations and a new solid mass on imaging studies are diagnostic of metastatic disease

224. Of the colorectal hepatic metastatic patients, the no of patients who are candidates for a potentially curative liver resection is:

A. 2% to 5%
B. 5% to 10%
C. 20% to 30%
D. 30% to 50%

225. False about the work up of colorectal metastasis of liver is:

A. Chest CT is performed and has high yield
B. Colonoscopy should be performed if it has been longer than 1 year since the last examination to rule out local recurrence or metachronous colorectal lesions
C. Routine use of PET does not significantly affect outcomes among patients with potentially resectable colorectal cancer liver metastasis
D. Complete abdominal and pelvic cross-sectional imaging must also be performed to rule out extrahepatic disease

226. Based on PET CT findings, the number of patients who have a change in management in colorectal metastasis to liver is:

A. 5% B. 25%
C. 10% D. 30%

227. Staging laparoscopy in colorectal metastasis to liver avoids nontherapeutic laparotomy in:

A. 5% B. 10%
C. 20% D. 33%

228. Preoperative factors that are most influential on outcome of hepatic resection in cases of colorectal cancer metastasis to liver are all except:

A. CEA level > 200 ng/mL
B. > 3 tumors
C. Lymph node positive primary
D. Size > 5 cm

229. True about the hepatic arterial infusion (HAI) chemotherapy use in colorectal cancer metastasis to liver is:

A. There is clearly a higher response rate for liver tumors with HAI therapy compared with systemic therapy
B. Regional infusion of chemotherapeutic agents such as fluorodeoxyuridine has hepatic extraction rates of 90%, providing high local concentrations with minimal systemic toxicity
C. The rationale for adjuvant hepatic artery chemotherapy is based on the fact that liver metastases derive most of their blood supply from the hepatic artery
D. All of the above

230. Combinations of chemotherapy and complete resection of hepatic metastases are associated with long-term survival in up to:

A. 10% to 20% B. 30% to 40%
C. 50% to 60% D. 70% to 80%

231. False about Neuroendocrine Metastases to liver is:

A. Insulinomas and carcinoid tumors metastasize to the liver commonly
B. ^{68}Ga-DOTA PET/CT provides higher resolution than octreotide scan, thus allowing better localization and greater sensitivity (82%–100%) and specificity (67%–100%) for neuroendocrine metastases
C. Long-acting somatostatin analogues are useful for alleviating hormonal symptoms and may have a cytostatic role as well
D. If preoperative staging suggests that at least 90% of tumor can be removed without prohibitive operative risk, surgical cytoreduction is reasonable

232. Best prognosis for liver resection in metastatic liver lesions is with:

A. Sarcoma
B. Melanoma
C. Genitourinary tumors
D. Breast tumor

233. False about the simple cysts of liver is:

A. They are generally spherical or ovoid and can be as large as 20 cm
B. Simple cysts are a relatively common finding in adults and are mostly asymptomatic incidental radiologic findings
C. In 90% of cases, the cysts are singular
D. Simple cysts are generally regarded as congenital malformations

234. False about the management of simple cysts of liver is:

A. Ultrasound is a helpful test of choice to confirm a single, thin-walled simple cyst
B. Surgical therapy is achieved by fenestration or unroofing of the portion of the cyst that is extrahepatic
C. The most common complication is intracystic bleeding and complications are very common
D. Hydatid disease, cystadenoma, and metastatic neuroendocrine tumor are the most important differential diagnoses to consider

235. False about Cystadenoma of the liver is:

A. The fluid contained in these cysts is usually serous
B. Cystadenoma of the liver is a rare neoplasm that generally is manifested as a large cystic mass, usually 10 to 20 cm
C. The epithelium often forms polypoid or papillary projections
D. Cystadenoma of the liver mainly affects women older than 40 years

236. False about management of Cystadenoma of the liver is:

A. Ultrasound usually demonstrates a cystic structure with varying wall thickness, nodularity, septations and fluid-filled locules

B. Cystadenomas tend to grow slowly but never progress to cystadenocarcinomas
C. Although many cystadenomas are asymptomatic, symptoms can include abdominal pain, anorexia, nausea and abdominal distention
D. All of the above are true

237. In patients with polycystic liver disease, prevalence of liver cysts in those older than 60 years, it is:

A. 20% B. 40%
C. 60% D. 80%

238. False about polycystic liver disease is:

A. In those younger than 20 years, the prevalence of liver cysts is 0%
B. When liver cysts are present in patients with adult polycystic kidney disease, they are always multiple in number
C. Due to the large number of liver cysts, hepatic parenchyma and function is not preserved
D. Liver transplantation is used only with progressive disease after fenestration or resection with liver or renal dysfunction

239. Most blood loss during a liver resection comes from the:

A. Portal vein B. Hepatic veins
C. Hepatic artery D. Phrenic arteries

240. Most complications and deaths after hepatic resection were seen in:

A. Cirrhotics with HCC
B. Extensive resections
C. Complex biliary tumors
D. All of the above

241. Bile leaks are a problem in cases requiring complex biliary reconstruction but can also occur in approximately:

A. 5% to 10% B. 10% to 20%
C. 25% to 30% D. 30% to 50%

242. Left hemihepatectomy, involves all of the following segments except:

A. I B. II
C. III D. IV

243. Right trisectionectomy, involves:

A. Segments VI–VIII
B. Segments V–VIII
C. Segments IV–VIII
D. Segments III–VIII

244. Left trisectionectomy, involves which segments:

A. III, IV, V, VI, VIII B. II, III, IV, V, VIII
C. IV, V, VI, VII, VIII D. III, IV, V, VI, VII

245. In normal noncirrhotic livers, resections are tolerated up to;

A. 75% B. 60%
C. 70% D. 80%

246. The risk of hepatic dysfunction is minimal if the reduction of functional liver parenchyma is:

A. Less than 60% B. Less than 50%
C. Less than 40% D. Less than 30%

HEMOBILIA

247. The most common causes of hemobilia is:

A. Tumors B. Iatrogenic trauma
C. Gallstones D. Vascular disorders

248. False about hemobilia is:

A. Hemobilia is defined as bleeding into the biliary tree from an abnormal communication between a blood vessel and bile duct
B. Hemobilia secondary to accidental trauma is more common with penetrating than with blunt abdominal trauma
C. Percutaneous liver biopsy results in hemobilia in < 1% of cases
D. The gallbladder can be a source of bleeding from trauma, gallstones, or acalculous cholecystitis

249. False about clinical presentation of hemobilia is:

A. Arterial hemobilia is the most common source
B. Portal venous bleeding into the biliary tree is common and often dramatic
C. Blood clots in the biliary tree can masquerade as stones if hemobilia goes unrecognized
D. An interesting aspect of hemobilia is the tendency for delayed presentations, up to weeks after the inciting causal event

250. The classic triad of symptoms and signs of hemobilia is all except:

A. Upper gastrointestinal hemorrhage
B. Anemia
C. Jaundice
D. Upper abdominal pain

251. False about diagnostic workup of hemobilia is;

A. Once hemobilia is suspected, the first evaluation should be upper gastrointestinal endoscopy

B. Upper endoscopy is diagnostic of hemobilia in only approximately 90% of cases
C. Arterial angiography is now recognized as the test of choice when significant hemobilia is suspected
D. Cholangiography demonstrates blood clots in the biliary tree that may appear as stringy defects or smaller spherical defects that may be difficult to distinguish from stones

252. False about management of hemobilia is:
A. The second line of therapy for major hemobilia was transarterial embolization, and success rates of 50% to 60%
B. Surgery is indicated when conservative therapy and transarterial embolization have failed
C. Hemorrhage from the gallbladder or hemorrhagic cholecystitis mandates cholecystectomy
D. The management of hemobilia after percutaneous transhepatic biliary drainage usually consists of removal of the catheter or replacement with larger catheters but may require transarterial embolization

VIRAL HEPATITIS AND THE SURGEON

253. False about viral hepatitis is:
A. It is the most common cause of liver disease worldwide
B. HAV and HEV are both responsible for forms of epidemic hepatitis and are transmitted through the fecal-oral route
C. HCV has a DNA genome
D. HDV requires the presence of HBV coinfection for replication and infectivity and can alter the clinical course of HBV infection

254. False about the diagnosis of viral hepatitis is:
A. HBsAg is a secretory protein that is a marker of HBV replication and infectivity
B. HBsAg is the hallmark of the diagnosis of HBV infection and appears in the serum 1 to 10 weeks after infection
C. Anti-HBc antibodies are detectable early after infection and persist after recovery and in chronic infections
D. Anti-HBs antibodies are also induced by the HBV vaccine

255. Chronic HBV infection is the persistence of HBsAg in the serum beyond:
A. 18 months
B. 6 months
C. 3 months
D. 12 months

256. The most accurate way of assessing HBV activity is:
A. Quantification of HBeAg
B. Quantification of HBsAg
C. Quantification of HBV DNA
D. Quantification of Anti-HBc

257. False about HBV infection is:
A. There is a particularly high incidence in male homosexuals and heterosexuals with multiple sexual partners
B. Horizontal transmission among children is common and is probably related to minor breaks in the skin and mucous membranes
C. HBV is the most commonly transmitted virus among healthcare personnel and transmission is usually patient to patient or patient to worker
D. Needle-stick risk has been related to HBsAg positivity

258. False about Hepatitis C is:
A. Health care workers have higher carrier rates than the general public
B. No identifiable risk factors are found in 10% to 20% of HCV cases
C. Transmission among healthcare workers is usually related to needle-stick incidents and the risk of transmission is higher than that of HBV and HIV
D. Currently, less than 2% of acute infections are caused by transfusions, and the risk of transfusion associated transmission is estimated to be about 1 in 10,000

259. False about the clinical presentation of hepatitis B infection is:
A. Stable form of HBV DNA is responsible for its persistence in infected hepatocytes
B. Clinical symptoms usually disappear within 12 months
C. Approximately 70% of patients with acute HBV infection have subclinical or anicteric hepatitis
D. The constitutional symptoms last about 10 days and are followed by jaundice in 30% of patients

260. False about chronic HBV infection is:
A. Risk of chronic HBV infection is related to immunocompetence and age
B. 10% of children and 50% of infants will develop chronic disease
C. Progression to cirrhosis is marked by hepatic synthetic dysfunction and often cytopenias, related to hypersplenism

D. The effect of age on HBV persistence is most likely due to difference in immune maturity between adults and young children

261. Extrahepatic manifestations of HBV infection, caused by circulating immune complexes, occur in approximately:

A. 5% to 10%
B. 10% to 20%
C. 20% to 30%
D. 30% to 50%

262. False about HCV infection is:

A. In general, 80% of cases occur 5 to 12 weeks after infection
B. HCV infection are at risk for development of cirrhosis and HCC
C. Jaundice occurs in more than 50% of patients, but fulminant hepatic failure caused by HCV is extremely uncommon
D. Extrahepatic manifestations, such as autoimmune disorders and lymphoma, can occur with HCV infection and are likely related to circulating immune complexes

263. Chronic HCV infection develops in approximately:

A. 25%
B. 33%
C. 50%
D. 66%

264. False about Hepatitis E infection is:

A. Cholestatic type of hepatitis is seen in more than 90% of patients
B. Pregnant women tend to have a more severe clinical course; mortality rates range from 5% to 25%
C. The incubation period of HEV infection ranges from 2 to 9 weeks
D. The most common form of illness is acute icteric hepatitis

265. In HEV infection, jaundice is present in more than:

A. 60%
B. 70%
C. 80%
D. 90%

266. False about prevention of viral hepatitis is:

A. CDC recommends a 4-dose HBV vaccination for all children, with the first dose being administered preferably within 72 hours after birth followed by 3 subsequent booster doses
B. Effective prevention of HBV infection prevents HDV infection
C. HEV infection prophylaxis has focused on sanitary measures, particularly strategies aimed at drinking water
D. The only effective preventive strategy for HCV infection relies on public health principles aimed at the major risk factors for transmission

267. True about the treatment of viral hepatitis is:

A. Treatment of HAV or HEV infection is supportive in nature and is generally aimed at correcting dehydration and providing adequate calorie intake
B. Interferon-alfa and the nucleoside analogue lamivudine used to be the only two approved therapies for the treatment of HBV
C. Treatment of chronic HCV infection is by the introduction of direct-acting antivirals (e.g., ledipasvir, sofosbuvir) that target specific non-structural proteins of HCV
D. All of the above

ANSWERS

1. **Ans: B. Francis Glisson**

Ref: Chapter No.54, Page No.1425

2. **Ans: C. Lortat-Jacob**

Ref: Chapter No.54, Page No.1425

3. **Ans: A. 1% - 2%**

Ref: Chapter No.54, Page No.1426

4. **Ans: D. The umbilical fissure is on the inferior surface of the right liver and contains the right portal pedicle**

Ref: Chapter No.54, Page No.1426

5. **Ans: D. All of the above**

Ref: Chapter No.54, Page No.1426.

6. **Ans: A. Obliterated left umbilical vein**

Ref: Chapter No.54, Page No.1426

7. **Ans: C. Obliterated sinus venosus**

Ref: Chapter No.54, Page No.1426

8. **Ans: B. Hematopoietic cells, Kupffer cells and connective tissue form from the endoderm of the septum transversum**

Ref: Chapter No.54, Page No.1427

9. **Ans: B. 3rd week**

Ref: Chapter No.54, Page No.1427

10. **Ans: D. All of the above**

Ref: Chapter No.54, Page No.1427

11. **Ans: C. 5th week**

Ref: Chapter No.54, Page No.1427

12. **Ans: A. Hepatic progenitor cells**

Ref: Chapter No.54, Page No.1427

13. **Ans: B. Myofibroblastic mesenchymal cells**

Ref: Chapter No.54, Page No.1427

14. **Ans: C. The right liver has a visible fissure along its inferior surface called the umbilical fissure**

Ref: Chapter No.54, Page No.1427

15. **Ans: C. Hepatic vein**

Ref: Chapter No.54, Page No.1427

16. **Ans: A. The umbilical fissure is a scissura and contains a hepatic vein**

Ref: Chapter No.54, Page No.1427

17. **Ans: C. The continuation of the left portal triad runs posteriorly and cephalad in the umbilical fissure and gives branches to segments II and III**

Ref: Chapter No.54, Page No.1427-1428

18. **Ans: C. The right portion of the caudate lobe lies in the lesser omental bursa and is covered anteriorly by the gastrohepatic ligament (lesser omentum) that separates it from segments II and III anteriorly**

Ref: Chapter No.54, Page No.1428

19. **Ans: A. Anomalous development of the liver is very commonly encountered**

Ref: Chapter No.54, Page No.1428

20. **Ans: D. Tongue of tissue extending inferiorly off the right liver**

Ref: Chapter No.54, Page No.1428

21. **Ans: C. 75%**

Ref: Chapter No.54, Page No.1428

2. **Ans: C. 50% - 70%**

Ref: Chapter No.54, Page No.1428

23. **Ans: C. 1 cm**

Ref: Chapter No.54, Page No.1429

24. **Ans: D. Anterior to the CBD and proper hepatic artery**

Ref: Chapter No.54, Page No.1429

25. **Ans: D. The right portal vein has a long extrahepatic course**

Ref: Chapter No.54, Page No.1429

26. **Ans: A. The inferior hemorrhoidal plexus receives portal flow from inferior mesenteric vein tributaries and can form large hemorrhoids**

Ref: Chapter No.54, Page No.1429

27. **Ans: C. 70%**

Ref: Chapter No.54, Page No.1429

28. **Ans: B. Portal vein trifurcation**

Ref: Chapter No.54, Page No.1429-1430

29. **Ans: C. 25% of the hepatic blood flow and 30% to 50% of its oxygenation**

Ref: Chapter No.54, Page No.1430

30. **Ans: C. 60%**

Ref: Chapter No.54, Page No.1430

31. **Ans: D. An accessory cystic artery can originate from the proper hepatic artery or gastroduodenal artery, where it runs posterior to the bile duct**

Ref: Chapter No.54, Page No.1430-1432

32. **Ans: B. Common bile duct**

Ref: Chapter No.54, Page No.1430

33. **Ans: B. 10% to 20%**

Ref: Chapter No.54, Page No.1431

34. **Ans: C. 4% to 10%**

Ref: Chapter No.54, Page No.1432

35. **Ans: D. Left gastric artery**

Ref: Chapter No.54, Page No.1432

36. **Ans: C. The left and middle hepatic veins usually join extrahepatically and enter the left side of the IVC as a single vessel**

Ref: Chapter No.54, Page No.1432

37. **Ans: C. 15%**

Ref: Chapter No.54, Page No.1434

38. **Ans: A. 5%**

Ref: Chapter No.54, Page No.1434

39. **Ans: C. 10 to 15 cm**

Ref: Chapter No.54, Page No.1434

40. **Ans: B. 6 mm**

Ref: Chapter No.54, Page No.1434

41. **Ans: C. The sphincter ampullae, made up of circular muscle, which prevents duodenal reflux**

Ref: Chapter No.54, Page No.1434

42. **Ans: B. Either of the right sectoral ducts drains into the common hepatic duct**

Ref: Chapter No.54, Page No.1435

43. **Ans: D. 10 cms**

Ref: Chapter No.54, Page No.1434

44. **Ans: C. Phrygian cap**

Ref: Chapter No.54, Page No.1434

45. **Ans: D. The venous drainage of the gallbladder empties into the veins that drain the bile duct and drains directly into the portal vein**

Ref: Chapter No.54, Page No.1434-1435

46. **Ans: B. 3- and 9-O'clock positions**

Ref: Chapter No.54, Page No.1434

47. **Ans: B. Parasympathetic fibers from only right vagal nerve**

Ref: Chapter No.54, Page No.1435

48. **Ans: A. A central terminal hepatic venule surrounded by 4 to 6 terminal portal triads that form a polygonal unit**

Ref: Chapter No.54, Page No.1436

49. **Ans: C. Blood flows from the hepatic venule through the sinusoids into the terminal portal triad**

Ref: Chapter No.54, Page No.1436

50. **Ans: B. Zone 2 - intermediate zone**

Ref: Chapter No.54, Page No.1436

51. **Ans: C. 10 fold**

Ref: Chapter No.54, Page No.1436

52. **Ans: B. 15% to 20%**

Ref: Chapter No.54, Page No.1436

53. **Ans: B. These cells high in calcium content**

Ref: Chapter No.54, Page No.1436

54. **Ans: B. 60%**

Ref: Chapter No.54, Page No.1437

55. **Ans: C. There are 100 mitochondria/hepatocytes occupying approximately 50% of the cell volume**

Ref: Chapter No.54, Page No.1437

56. **Ans: C. Glucose uptake and release, bile formation, and synthesis of albumin and fibrinogen take place in the perivenous zone**

Ref: Chapter No.54, Page No.1438

57. **Ans: C. Zone 3**

Ref: Chapter No.54, Page No.1438

58. **Ans: B. 25%**

Ref: Chapter No.54, Page No.1439

59. **Ans: D. Carbohydrates**

Ref: Chapter No.54, Page No.1439

60. **Ans: B. 6 to 10 mm Hg**

Ref: Chapter No.54, Page No.1439

61. **Ans: C. 300 mOsmol/kg**

Ref: Chapter No.54, Page No.1439

62. **Ans: D. It is well recognized that bile flow has a non linear association with bile acid secretion**

Ref: Chapter No.54, Page No.1439

63. **Ans: D. 1500 mL**

Ref: Chapter No.54, Page No.1439

64. **Ans: D. All of the above**

Ref: Chapter No.54, Page No.1439

65. **Ans: C. Bile acids are reabsorbed actively into the jejunum and ileum**

Ref: Chapter No.54, Page No.1440

66. **Ans: A. An early phase of heme breakdown, accounting for 20% of bilirubin, is from hemoproteins and occurs within 30 days of labelling with radioactive heme**

Ref: Chapter No.54, Page No.1440

67. **Ans: C. 65 g**

Ref: Chapter No.54, Page No.1440

68. **Ans: C. 48 hours**

Ref: Chapter No.54, Page No.1440

69. **Ans: A. Decreased lipolysis**

Ref: Chapter No.54, Page No.1441

70. **Ans: A. Excess amino acids not used in peripheral tissues are generally handled by the liver, in which they are oxidized for energy providing 10% of the liver's energy needs**

Ref: Chapter No.54, Page No.1441

71. **Ans: D. VIII**

Ref: Chapter No.54, Page No.1442

72. **Ans: D. VII**

Ref: Chapter No.54, Page No.1442

73. **Ans: D. Phase I reactions always detoxify chemicals**

Ref: Chapter No.54, Page No.1442

74. **Ans: B. 24 - 36 hours**

Ref: Chapter No.54, Page No.1442

75. **Ans: C. ALT**

Ref: Chapter No.54, Page No.1442

76. **Ans: B. Elevations of ALT levels in hepatobiliary diseases are generally secondary to cholestasis or biliary obstruction**

Ref: Chapter No.54, Page No.1442-1443

77. **Ans: D. Adrenals**

Ref: Chapter No.54, Page No.1443

78. **Ans: C. Albumin level it is most helpful in acute liver disease**

Ref: Chapter No.54, Page No.1443

79. **Ans: A. Antimitochondrial antibodies**

Ref: Chapter No.54, Page No.1443

80. **Ans: B. Antineutrophil antibodies**

Ref: Chapter No.54, Page No.1443

81. **Ans: C. The galactose elimination test is based on the liver's role in phosphorylating galactose and converting it to fructose**

Ref: Chapter No.54, Page No.1443

82. **Ans: B. Creatinine (mg/dL)**

Ref: Chapter No.54, Page No.1443

83. **Ans: B. Child-Pugh class B**

Ref: Chapter No.54, Page No.1444

84. **Ans: B. > 5 mm Hg**

Ref: Chapter No.54, Page No.1444

85. **Ans: A. 8–10 mm Hg**

Ref: Chapter No.54, Page No.1444

86. **Ans: C. Decreased portal venous inflow secondary to a hyperdynamic systemic circulation and splanchnic hyperemia**

Ref: Chapter No.54, Page No.1444

87. **Ans: B. Portal vein thrombosis**

Ref: Chapter No.54, Page No.1444

88. **Ans: D. 50%**

Ref: Chapter No.54, Page No.1444

89. **Ans: B. 33%**

Ref: Chapter No.54, Page No.1445

90. **Ans: C. Schistosomiasis**

Ref: Chapter No.54, Page No.1445

91. **Ans: D. All of the above**

Ref: Chapter No.54, Page No.1445

92. **Ans: B. Approximately 20% of these deaths are caused by uncontrolled bleeding**

Ref: Chapter No.54, Page No.1445

93. **Ans: C. Pharmacotherapy can also be initiated and trials have suggested that it may not be as effective as endoscopic treatment**

Ref: Chapter No.54, Page No.1445

94. **Ans: D. 80% to 90%**

Ref: Chapter No.54, Page No.1445

95. **Ans: B. Sclerotherapy is better than band ligation in the initial control of bleeding and is associated with fewer complications**

Ref: Chapter No.54, Page No.1445

96. **Ans: C. In patients with variceal bleeding, antibiotic prophylaxis should not be initiated**

Ref: Chapter No.54, Page No.1445

97. **Ans: D. All of the above**

Ref: Chapter No.54, Page No.1445-1446

98. **Ans: B. With TIPS, a functional portacaval end-to-side shunt is established**

Ref: Chapter No.54, Page No.1446

99. **Ans: B. After TIPS placement**

Ref: Chapter No.54, Page No.1446

100. **Ans: B. 25%**

Ref: Chapter No.54, Page No.1446

101. **Ans: D. 70%**

Ref: Chapter No.54, Page No.1446

102. **Ans: A. The combination of a beta blocker and long-acting nitrate has been shown to be less effective than variceal ligation**

Ref: Chapter No.54, Page No.1446-1447

103. **Ans: C. Shunt stenosis, which is usually secondary to neointimal hyperplasia and is less common than thrombosis**

Ref: Chapter No.54, Page No.1447

104. Ans: C. 50%

Ref: Chapter No.54, Page No.1447

105. Ans: B. TIPS is not effective for the treatment of medically intractable ascites

Ref: Chapter No.54, Page No.1447-1448

106. Ans: C. Portosystemic shunts

Ref: Chapter No.54, Page No.1448

107. Ans: B. End-to-side portacaval shunt

Ref: Chapter No.54, Page No.1448

108. Ans: D. Rebleeding

Ref: Chapter No.54, Page No.1448

109. Ans: B. Accelerated hepatic failure

Ref: Chapter No.54, Page No.1448

110. Ans: D. All of the above

Ref: Chapter No.54, Page No.1448-1449

111. Ans: B. The distal splenorenal shunt tends to aggravate relieve ascites

Ref: Chapter No.54, Page No.1449

112. Ans: D. The small-diameter interposition shunt was discovered to have a higher overall failure rate than TIPS

Ref: Chapter No.54, Page No.1450

113. Ans: D. All of the above

Ref: Chapter No.54, Page No.1450-1451

114. Ans: C. The male-to-female ratio is approximately 10:1

Ref: Chapter No.54, Page No.1451-1452

115. Ans: A. Cryptogenic infections

Ref: Chapter No.54, Page No.1453

116. Ans: B. Intrahepatic stones

Ref: Chapter No.54, Page No.1453

117. Ans: D. All of the above

Ref: Chapter No.54, Page No.1453

118. Ans: D. Bilobar involvement with multiple abscesses is common

Ref: Chapter No.54, Page No.1453-1454

119. Ans: D. All of the above

Ref: Chapter No.54, Page No.1454

120. Ans: B. Escherichia coli

Ref: Chapter No.54, Page No.1454

121. Ans: B. 30% to 50%

Ref: Chapter No.54, Page No.1454

122. Ans: B. The typical presentation is present in 50% of cases

Ref: Chapter No.54, Page No.1454

123. Ans: A. Jaundice is also found in approximately 50% of cases and is often secondary to underlying biliary disease

Ref: Chapter No.54, Page No.1454

124. Ans: B. This serious complication is more common in alcoholics

Ref: Chapter No.54, Page No.1454

125. Ans: C. 50%

Ref: Chapter No.54, Page No.1454

126. Ans: D. All of the above

Ref: Chapter No.54, Page No.1454

127. Ans: B. Ultrasound usually demonstrates a round or oval area that is more echogenic than the surrounding liver

Ref: Chapter No.54, Page No.1455

128. Ans: C. 80% to 95%

Ref: Chapter No.54, Page No.1455

129. Ans: D. 95% to 100%

Ref: Chapter No.54, Page No.1455

130. Ans: C. Surgery has become the treatment of choice for most patients

Ref: Chapter No.54, Page No.1455-1456

131. Ans: B. 65% to 90%

Ref: Chapter No.54, Page No.1456

132. Ans: C. 60% to 90%

Ref: Chapter No.54, Page No.1456

133. Ans: B. Cholangitis

Ref: Chapter No.54, Page No.1457

134. Ans: C. A female preponderance of more than 10:1 has been reported in almost all studies

Ref: Chapter No.54, Page No.1457

135. Ans: C. Children who lack antiamebic IgM have innate resistance to invasive amoebic infection

Ref: Chapter No.54, Page No.1457

136. Ans: B. Abdominal pain

Ref: Chapter No.54, Page No.1458

137. Ans: C. Rupture into the peritoneum with peritonitis occurs frequently; it is more often with right-sided abscesses

Ref: Chapter No.54, Page No.1457-1458

138. Ans: B. In the acute presentation, 80% of patients have multiple lesions, whereas with the chronic presentation, more than 50% of patients have a single right-sided lesion

Ref: Chapter No.54, Page No.1458

139. Ans: C. Elevated PT-INR

Ref: Chapter No.54, Page No.1458

140. Ans: B. Plain chest radiographs are abnormal in approximately 80% of cases

Ref: Chapter No.54, Page No.1458-1459

141. Ans: B. Clinical improvement is usually seen within 7 days after metronidazole

Ref: Chapter No.54, Page No.1459

142. Ans: B. Right liver lesion has increased risk

Ref: Chapter No.54, Page No.1459

143. Ans: C. Right-sided abscess may rupture into the pericardium and can be manifested as an asymptomatic pericardial effusion or even tamponade

Ref: Chapter No.54, Page No.1459

144. Ans: C. Mortality appears to be affected by the addition of aspiration to metronidazole therapy or by chronicity of symptoms

Ref: Chapter No.54, Page No.1459

145. Ans: C. Abscess volume > 1000 mL

Ref: Chapter No.54, Page No.1459

146. Ans: D. The adult tapeworm is attached to the villi of the duodenum

Ref: Chapter No.54, Page No.1460

147. Ans: C. Calcification of a hydatid cyst, imply that the cyst is dead

Ref: Chapter No.54, Page No.1460

148. Ans: C. Approximately 75% of hydatid cysts are located in the left liver and are solitary

Ref: Chapter No.54, Page No.1460

149. Ans: A. Hepatomegaly

Ref: Chapter No.54, Page No.1460

150. Ans: D. All of the above

Ref: Chapter No.54, Page No.1460-1461

151. Ans: D. Treatment of echinococcosis with albendazole or mebendazole is effective at shrinking cysts in many patients with E. granulosus infection, and cyst disappearance occurs in well above 50% of patients

Ref: Chapter No.54, Page No.1461

152. Ans: D. Men are predominantly affected

Ref: Chapter No.54, Page No.1461

153. Ans: B. An association between RPC and Clonorchis sinensis and Ascaris lumbricoides infection has been noted and a true causal relationship has been proven

Ref: Chapter No.54, Page No.1461

154. Ans: B. 20%

Ref: Chapter No.54, Page No.1461

155. Ans: B. Biliary obstruction is usually complete, and therefore, marked jaundice and pruritus are common

Ref: Chapter No.54, Page No.1461-1462

156. Ans: D. Nonoperative approaches, such as percutaneous transhepatic cholangioscopic lithotomy, have been developed, and are now the treatment of choice

Ref: Chapter No.54, Page No.1462

157. Ans: D. All of the above

Ref: Chapter No.54, Page No.1462

158. Ans: C. 10%

Ref: Chapter No.54, Page No.1462

159. Ans: C. The female-to-male ratio is approximately 1:11

Ref: Chapter No.54, Page No.1463

160. Ans: D. Histologically, bile ductules are observed and the normal architecture of the liver is present

Ref: Chapter No.54, Page No.1463

161. Ans: B. > 10 LCAs

Ref: Chapter No.54, Page No.1463

162. Ans: B. β-catenin activation

Ref: Chapter No.54, Page No.1463

163. Ans: A. Exon-3 mutation

Ref: Chapter No.54, Page No.1463

164. Ans: C. Tumor markers are abnormal

Ref: Chapter No.54, Page No.1463

165. Ans: D. All of the above

Ref: Chapter No.54, Page No.1463

166. Ans: C. 30% - 50%

Ref: Chapter No.54, Page No.1463

167. Ans: C. Margin status is important in resections, and resection with a margin of 2 cm should be performed

Ref: Chapter No.54, Page No.1463

168. Ans: C. Hemangioma

Ref: Chapter No.54, Page No.1463

169. Ans: B. Focal nodular hyperplasia

Ref: Chapter No.54, Page No.1463

170. Ans: C. Typical hepatic vascularity is seen, and typical biliary epithelium is found scattered throughout the lesion

Ref: Chapter No.54, Page No.1463

171. Ans: C. Developmental vascular malformation

Ref: Chapter No.54, Page No.1463

172. Ans: A. Serum AFP levels are abnormal

Ref: Chapter No.54, Page No.1463

173. Ans: C. Careful observation of symptomatic FNH with serial imaging is not reasonable because symptoms never resolve in a most of the cases

Ref: Chapter No.54, Page No.1464

174. Ans: B. They are usually solitary and > 5 cm in diameter, and they occur with incidence more common in left hemiliver

Ref: Chapter No.54, Page No.1464

175. Ans: B. > 5 cm

Ref: Chapter No.54, Page No.1464

176. Ans: D. Spontaneous rupture of liver hemangiomas is common

Ref: Chapter No.54, Page No.1464

177. Ans: B. Syndrome of thrombocytopenia and consumptive coagulopathy

Ref: Chapter No.54, Page No.1464

178. Ans: C. Biopsy is recommended

Ref: Chapter No.54, Page No.1464

179. Ans: D. All of the above

Ref: Chapter No.54, Page No.1464

180. Ans: B. Usually solitary and can involve other organs

Ref: Chapter No.54, Page No.1464

181. Ans: B. Nodular regenerative hyperplasia has malignant potential and is associated with cirrhosis

Ref: Chapter No.54, Page No.1464-1465

182. Ans: D. HCC is 2 to 8 times more common in women than in men in low and high incidence areas

Ref: Chapter No.54, Page No.1465

183. Ans: B. Hepatitis B

Ref: Chapter No.54, Page No.1465

184. Ans: A. Cirrhosis is a prerequisite for the development of HBV-related HCC

Ref: Chapter No.54, Page No.1465

185. Ans: A. HCV is an DNA virus that integrates into the host genome

Ref: Chapter No.54, Page No.1466

186. Ans: C. Cirrhosis is required for the development of HCC and hepatocarcinogenesis is an inevitable result of cirrhosis

Ref: Chapter No.54, Page No.1466

187. Ans: D. Alcohol causes cirrhosis but and has been shown to be directly carcinogenic in hepatocytes

Ref: Chapter No.54, Page No.1466

188. Ans: D. All of the above

Ref: Chapter No.54, Page No.1466

189. Ans: D. HCC can commonly be manifested as a rupture, with the sudden onset of abdominal pain followed by hypovolemic shock secondary to intraperitoneal bleeding

Ref: Chapter No.54, Page No.1466

190. Ans: A. Hyperglycemia

Ref: Chapter No.54, Page No.1466

191. Ans: C. Typical imaging criteria for HCC include rapid venous enhancement followed by washout in the delayed phase

Ref: Chapter No.54, Page No.1466

192. Ans: C. AFP is specific to HCC

Ref: Chapter No.54, Page No.1466-1477

193. Ans: C. Preoperative chest CT is not mandatory

Ref: Chapter No.54, Page No.1467

194. Ans: D. All of the above

Ref: Chapter No.54, Page No.1467

195. Ans: D. All of the above

Ref: Chapter No.54, Page No.1467

196. Ans: B. 20%

Ref: Chapter No.54, Page No.1467

197. Ans: D. Presence of portal vein thrombosis gives 2 points

Ref: Chapter No.54, Page No.1468

198. Ans: B. Tumor histology

Ref: Chapter No.54, Page No.1468

199. Ans: D. Albumin level < 2 g/dL

Ref: Chapter No.54, Page No.1468

200. Ans: C. Levels of AST/ALT

Ref: Chapter No.54, Page No.1468

201. Ans: A. The pushing type of HCC is usually not resectable

Ref: Chapter No.54, Page No.1468

202. Ans: D. Only 40% to 50% of patients are considered to have resectable disease

Ref: Chapter No.54, Page No.1468-1469

203. Ans: C. Margin < 2 cm

Ref: Chapter No.54, Page No.1469

204. Ans: D. All of the above

Ref: Chapter No.54, Page No.1469

205. Ans: B. 2 cm

Ref: Chapter No.54, Page No.1469

206. Ans: C. Percutaneous injection of acetic acid is a technique similar to PEI but has weak necrotizing abilities, making it less useful in septated tumors

Ref: Chapter No.54, Page No.1469

207. Ans: A. Cryotherapy is usually performed at laparotomy or laparoscopically, and it can't be performed with percutaneous techniques

Ref: Chapter No.54, Page No.1469

208. Ans: B. Temperatures higher than 80°C. is reached and immediate cell death is seen

Ref: Chapter No.54, Page No.1469

209. Ans: D. All of the above

Ref: Chapter No.54, Page No.1469

210. Ans: D. All of the above

Ref: Chapter No.54, Page No.1470

211. Ans: C. Fibrolamellar HCC does produces AFP

Ref: Chapter No.54, Page No.1470

212. Ans: B. Neurotensin

Ref: Chapter No.54, Page No.1470

213. Ans: A. Recurrence after resection is uncommon

Ref: Chapter No.54, Page No.1470

214. Ans: A. Childhood HCC is a distinct entity that represents almost 50% of pediatric liver tumors

Ref: Chapter No.54, Page No.1471

215. Ans: C. Some HCCs show evidence of sarcomatoid differentiation and are referred to as a sarcomatoid variant or carcinosarcoma and tend to produce AFP

Ref: Chapter No.54, Page No.1471

216. Ans: B. Jaundice occurs commonly

Ref: Chapter No.54, Page No.1471

217. Ans: D. All of the above

Ref: Chapter No.54, Page No.1471

218. Ans: C. Unlike HCC there is persistent enhancement on arterial phases due to the fibrotic nature of cholangiocarcinoma

Ref: Chapter No.54, Page No.1471

219. Ans: D. All of the above

Ref: Chapter No.54, Page No.1472

220. Ans: C. Serum AFP levels are elevated in 40% to 50% of patients and is not a useful marker for therapeutic response

Ref: Chapter No.54, Page No.1472

221. Ans: D. All of the above

Ref: Chapter No.54, Page No.1472

222. Ans: D. All of the above

Ref: Chapter No.54, Page No.1472

223. Ans: C. Mild elevations in LFT results is common in metastatic colorectal cancer to the liver and is effective as a screening tool

Ref: Chapter No.54, Page No.1472-1473

224. Ans: B. 5% to 10%

Ref: Chapter No.54, Page No.1473

225. Ans: A. Chest CT is performed and has high yield

Ref: Chapter No.54, Page No.1473

226. Ans: B. 25%

Ref: Chapter No.54, Page No.1473

227. Ans: B. 10%

Ref: Chapter No.54, Page No.1473

228. Ans: B. > 3 tumors

Ref: Chapter No.54, Page No.1474

229. Ans: D. All of the above

Ref: Chapter No.54, Page No.1476

230. Ans: C. 50% to 60%

Ref: Chapter No.54, Page No.1476

231. Ans: A. Insulinomas and carcinoid tumors metastasize to the liver commonly

Ref: Chapter No.54, Page No.1476-1477

232. Ans: C. Genitourinary tumors

Ref: Chapter No.54, Page No.1477

233. Ans: C. In 90% of cases, the cysts are singular

Ref: Chapter No.54, Page No.1477

234. Ans: C. The most common complication is intracystic bleeding and complications are very common

Ref: Chapter No.54, Page No.1477

235. Ans: A. The fluid contained in these cysts is usually serous

Ref: Chapter No.54, Page No.1477-1478

236. Ans: B. Cystadenomas tend to grow slowly but never progress to cystadenocarcinomas

Ref: Chapter No.54, Page No.1478

237. Ans: D. 80%

Ref: Chapter No.54, Page No.1478

238. Ans: C. Due to the large number of liver cysts, hepatic parenchyma and function is not preserved

Ref: Chapter No.54, Page No.1478

239. Ans: B. Hepatic veins

Ref: Chapter No.54, Page No.1478

240. Ans: D. All of the above

Ref: Chapter No.54, Page No.1478

241. Ans: B. 10% to 20%

Ref: Chapter No.54, Page No.1478

242. Ans: A. I

Ref: Chapter No.54, Page No.1479

243. Ans: C. Segments IV–VIII

Ref: Chapter No.54, Page No.1479

244. Ans: B. II, III, IV, V, VIII

Ref: Chapter No.54, Page No.1479

245. Ans: D. 80%

Ref: Chapter No.54, Page No.1479

246. Ans: B. Less than 50%

Ref: Chapter No.54, Page No.1479

247. Ans: B. Iatrogenic trauma

Ref: Chapter No.54, Page No.1481

248. Ans: B. Hemobilia secondary to accidental trauma is more common with penetrating than with blunt abdominal trauma

Ref: Chapter No.54, Page No.1480-1481

249. Ans: B. Portal venous bleeding into the biliary tree is common and often dramatic

Ref: Chapter No.54, Page No.1481

250. Ans: B. Anemia

Ref: Chapter No.54, Page No.1481

251. Ans: B. Upper endoscopy is diagnostic of hemobilia in only approximately 90% of cases

Ref: Chapter No.54, Page No.1481

252. Ans: A. The second line of therapy for major hemobilia was transarterial embolization and success rates of 50% to 60%

Ref: Chapter No.54, Page No.1481

253. Ans: C. HCV has a DNA genome

Ref: Chapter No.54, Page No.1482-1483

254. Ans: A. HBsAg is a secretory protein that is a marker of HBV replication and infectivity

Ref: Chapter No.54, Page No.1483

255. Ans: B. 6 months

Ref: Chapter No.54, Page No.1483

256. Ans: C. Quantification of HBV DNA

Ref: Chapter No.54, Page No.1483

257. Ans: D. Needle-stick risk has been related to HBsAg positivity

Ref: Chapter No.54, Page No.1484

258. Ans: B. No identifiable risk factors are found in 10% to 20% of HCV cases

Ref: Chapter No.54, Page No.1484

259. Ans: B. Clinical symptoms usually disappear within 12 months

Ref: Chapter No.54, Page No.1484

260. Ans: B. 10% of children and 50% of infants will develop chronic disease

Ref: Chapter No.54, Page No.1484-1485

261. Ans: B. 10% to 20%

Ref: Chapter No.54, Page No.1485

262. Ans: C. Jaundice occurs in more than 50% of patients, but fulminant hepatic failure caused by HCV is extremely uncommon

Ref: Chapter No.54, Page No.1485

263. Ans: D. 66%

Ref: Chapter No.54, Page No.1485

264. Ans: A. Cholestatic type of hepatitis is seen in more than 90% of patients

Ref: Chapter No.54, Page No.1485

265. Ans: D. 90%

Ref: Chapter No.54, Page No.1485

266. Ans: A. CDC recommends a 4-dose HBV vaccination for all children, with the first dose being administered preferably within 72 hours after birth followed by 3 subsequent booster doses

Ref: Chapter No.54, Page No.1485

267. Ans: D. All of the above

Ref: Chapter No.54, Page No.1486

55

Biliary System

ANATOMY AND PHYSIOLOGY

1. **Anatomic variations in biliary anatomy occur in up to:**

   A. 10% B. 15%
   C. 20% D. 30%

2. **False about the anatomy of biliary system is:**

   A. The left hepatic duct retains a shorter transverse extrahepatic portion and travels under the edge of segment IV before diving before joining the bifurcation
   B. Bile ducts, either intrahepatic or extrahepatic, lie superior to the corresponding portal vein, which in turn are lateral and inferior to the arterial supply
   C. The left duct drains segments I, II, III, and IV, with the most distal branch draining segment IVA
   D. The drainage of the right duct system includes segments V, VI, VII and VIII

3. **False about the anatomy of biliary system is:**

   A. The cystic duct can range from 1 to 5 cm in length and drains at an acute angle into the CBD
   B. It is 7 to 10 cm in length, holds 30 to 60 mL of bile as a reservoir, and is divided into neck, infundibulum with Hartmann pouch, body and fundus
   C. The valves of Heister, which are folds of mucosa oriented in spiral pattern within the fundus of gallbladder, function to retain bile in the gallbladder until contraction in response to enteric stimulation
   D. The gallbladder is a partially intraperitoneal structure that lies attached to the under surface of the liver on segments IVB and V

4. **False about the anatomy of biliary system is:**

   A. The insertion of cystic duct marks the separation of the CBD (below) from the common hepatic duct (above)
   B. The CBD is divided into three portions: supraduodenal, retroduodenal, and the pancreatic portion, which is the most inferior portion, encompassed by head of pancreas
   C. The CBD ends in the 3rd portion of duodenum at the ampulla of Vater
   D. There are generally no vascular structures overlying bile ducts at confluence of hepatic ducts at the hilar plate, allowing exposure of the bifurcation by incision at the base of segment IV and lifting the liver off these structures and the technique, called lowering hilar plate, is used to expose the proximal extrahepatic biliary tree

5. **False about the vascular anatomy of biliary system is:**

   A. The blood supply to the entire biliary tree is solely arterial as contrasted with the hepatic parenchyma
   B. The blood supply of the common hepatic duct and CBD comes from the left hepatic and cystic artery
   C. The cystic artery normally arises from the right hepatic artery
   D. The cystic artery can pass posterior or anterior to the CBD to supply the gallbladder

6. **Borders of triangle of calot are all except:**

   A. Cystic artery
   B. Edge of the liver
   C. Cystic duct
   D. Common hepatic duct

7. **An accessory or replaced right hepatic artery occur in:**
   A. 10% B. 15%
   C. 20% D. 30%

8. **Lymph node associated with cystic artery is:**
   A. Couinaud's node B. Calot's node
   C. Glisson's node D. Hartmann's node

9. **Content of triangle of calot is:**
   A. Cystic artery B. Right hepatic duct
   C. Cystic duct D. Common bile duct

10. **The blood supply to the CBD comes from all except:**
   A. Posterosuperior pancreaticoduodenal artery
   B. Gastroduodenal artery
   C. Anterosuperior pancreaticoduodenal artery
   D. Retroduodenal artery

11. **During palpation of the hepatoduodenal ligament, a pulsation is felt dorsal and slightly to the right of the common bile duct (CBD). Which of the following does this pulsation most likely represent?**
   A. A normal common hepatic artery
   B. A normal right hepatic artery
   C. A replaced right hepatic artery
   D. A gastroduodenal artery

12. **Which of the following anatomic features may contribute to stricture formation after injury to the CBD?**
   A. The blood supply to the supraduodenal bile duct has a longitudinal pattern
   B. The blood supply to the supraduodenal bile duct has a lateral pattern
   C. The blood supply to the supraduodenal bile duct has a segmental end-artery arrangement
   D. The blood supply to the CBD is derived primarily from the common hepatic artery

13. **False statement is:**
   A. The smallest functional unit of liver is the hepatic lobule
   B. Hepatic lobule is created by 4 to 6 portal triads and identified by its central terminal hepatic venules
   C. The liver makes only a small amount of the total bile salt pool used on a daily basis because most bile salts are recycled after use in the intestinal lumen, known as the enterohepatic circulation
   D. Bile salts combine to form spherical pockets, known as micelles and the salts themselves provide osmotic activity

14. **If a patient has complete bile duct obstruction, which of the following does not occur?**
   A. Triglyceride absorption
   B. Vitamin K absorption
   C. Cholesterol synthesis
   D. Bilirubin conjugation

15. **Conjugated bile acids are primarily absorbed in the intestine by which of the following mechanisms?**
   A. Active transport in the colon
   B. Passive transport in the colon
   C. Active transport in the ileum
   D. Passive transport in the ileum

16. **Cholic acid is converted by bacteria to which of the following secondary bile acids?**
   A. Deoxycholic acid
   B. Chenodeoxycholic acid
   C. Lithocholic acid
   D. Ursodeoxycholic acid

17. **False statement among the following is:**
   A. After passage into the intestinal tract and reabsorption by the terminal ileum, bile acids are transported back to the liver for recycling bound to albumin
   B. The passage of reabsorbed bile salts bound to albumin through the space of Disse allows uptake into the hepatocyte in an efficient process that involves sodium cotransport and sodium-independent pathways
   C. > 25% of bile salts are lost each day in the stool
   D. The transport of bile salts across the canalicular membrane remains the rate-limiting step in bile salt excretion

18. **False statement among the following is:**
   A. Bile pigment gives the color of bile and, when converted to urobilinogen by bacterial enzymes, gives stool its characteristic color
   B. Bile pigments such as bilirubin are breakdown products of hemoglobin and myoglobin
   C. The major lipid components of bile are phospholipids and cholesterol
   D. After a cholecystectomy when the speed of the enterohepatic circulation of bile decreases

19. Biliary synthesis per day is:

A. 0.1–0.2 g/d
B. 0.2–0.6 g/d
C. 0.8–1.2 g/d
D. 1.5–2.0 g/d

20. False statement among the following is:

A. The passage of fat, protein, and acid into the duodenum induces CCK secretion from duodenal epithelial cells
B. CCK causes gallbladder contraction, with intraluminal pressures up to 300 mm Hg
C. Coordinated with gallbladder contraction, the relaxation of this sphincter allows evacuation of up to 70% of the gallbladder contents within 2 hours of CCK secretion
D. Vagal activity also induces gallbladder emptying and is a more powerful stimulus to gallbladder contraction than CCK

BILIARY TREE PATHOPHYSIOLOGY

21. In jaundice, to see yellowish discolouration on sclera, level of bilirubin must reach:

A. 2.0 mg/dL
B. 2.5 mg/dL
C. 3.5 mg/dL
D. 5.0 mg/dL

22. In jaundice, to see yellowish discolouration on skin, level of bilirubin must reach:

A. 2.0 mg/dL
B. 2.5 mg/dL
C. 3.5 mg/dL
D. 5.0 mg/dL

23. False about ultrasound in evaluation of biliary tract is:

A. Transabdominal ultrasound is a sensitive, inexpensive, reliable and reproducible test to evaluate most of the biliary tree
B. It is seen as the study of choice for the initial evaluation of jaundice or symptoms of biliary disease
C. Ultrasound has a high specificity and sensitivity for cholelithiasis or gallstones
D. Most gallstones don't move with positional changes in the patient

24. Following image shows a US image of a 24-year-old female with pain in RHC. What is the most probable diagnosis?

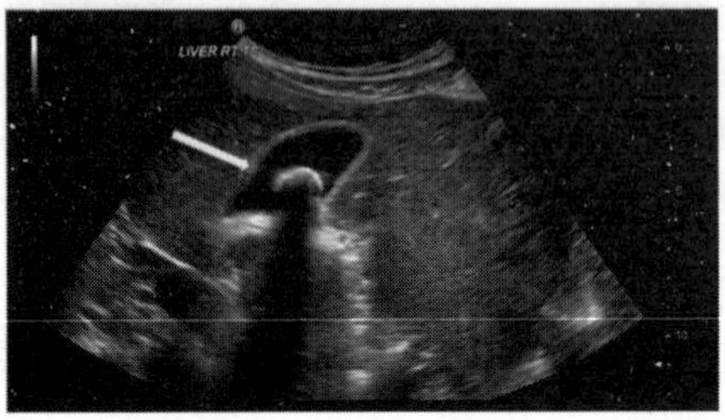

A. Cholecystitis
B. Cholelithiasis
C. Porcelain gallbladder
D. Gallbladder polyp

25. Following image shows a US image of a 34-year-old female with pain in RHC. She had tenderness and guarding in RHC on examination. What is the most probable diagnosis?

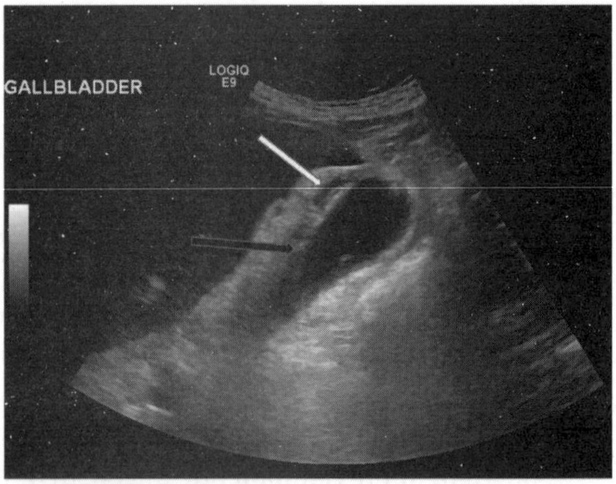

A. Cholecystitis
B. Cholelithiasis
C. Porcelain gallbladder
D. Gallbladder polyp

26. Following image shows a US image of a 54-year-old female with pain in RHC. What is the most probable diagnosis?

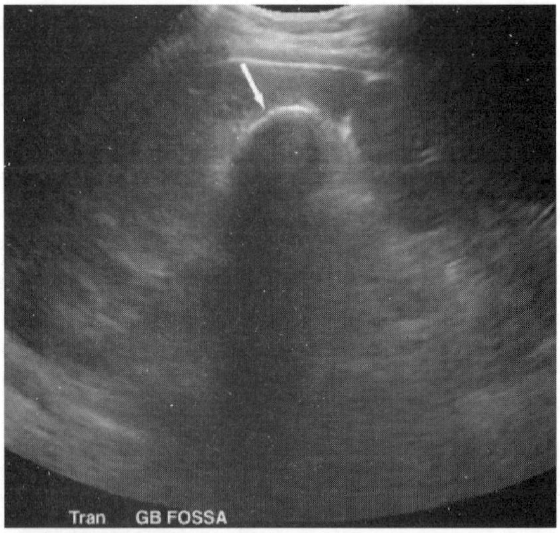

A. Cholecystitis
B. Cholelithiasis
C. Porcelain gallbladder
D. Gallbladder polyp

27. False about a hepatic iminodiacetic acid (HIDA) scan is:

A. As a nuclear medicine test, the test demonstrates physiologic flow and provides fine anatomic detail, but can't identify gallstones
B. Hepatic iminodiacetic acid (HIDA) scan, can be used to evaluate the physiologic secretion of bile
C. The scan will identify obstruction of the biliary tree and bile leaks, which may be useful in the postoperative setting
D. HIDA scans can be used to determine gallbladder function because the injection of CCK during a scan will document physiologic ejection of the gallbladder

28. HIDA demonstrates obstruction of the cystic duct, as seen in acute cholecystitis; if after injection of the dye there is failure to fill the gallbladder after:

A. 1 hour B. 2 hours
C. 4 hours D. 6 hours

29. False about biliary tract imaging among the following is:

A. CT provides superior anatomic information than USG and therefore is indicated when more anatomic delineation is required
B. Because most gallstones are radiographically hyperdense to bile, many will be distinguishable from bile
C. Ultrasound is operator dependent and provides no anatomic reconstruction of the biliary tree, CT can be used to identify the cause and site of biliary obstruction
D. When performed for the evaluation of hepatic or pancreatic parenchyma or possible neoplastic processes, CT is invaluable in preoperative planning, and the use of arterial phase, portal venous phase, and delayed phase imaging, known as a triple-phase CT, has essentially replaced diagnostic angiography of the liver

30. False about biliary tract imaging among the following is:

A. Magnetic resonance imaging (MRI) uses the water in bile to delineate the biliary tree and thus provides superior anatomic definition of the intrahepatic and extrahepatic biliary tree and pancreas
B. Endoscopic retrograde cholangiopancreatography (ERCP) is an invasive test using endoscopy and fluoroscopy to inject contrast material through the ampulla to image the biliary tree
C. Percutaneous transhepatic cholangiography (PTC) is a non-invasive procedure used to evaluate the biliary tree
D. PTC can decompress biliary obstruction and stent obstructions non-operatively and can provide anatomic information for biliary reconstruction

31. ERCP carries a complication rate of up to:

A. 5% B. 10%
C. 20% D. 25%

32. True about biliary tract imaging among the following is:

A. With the injection catheter inserted through the cystic duct during a cholecystectomy or through another point in the biliary tree, intraoperative cholangiography can help delineate anomalous biliary anatomy
B. Endoscopic ultrasound is valuable in the assessment of distal CBD and ampulla
C. Radial echoendoscopes are most useful for providing a tomographic evaluation, whereas linear echoendoscopes can guide interventions such as needle biopsies under real-time ultrasound guidance
D. All of the above

33. Indications for selective cholangiography are all except:

A. Pain at time of operation
B. Abnormal hepatic function panel
C. Elderly patient
D. Inability to perform postoperative endoscopic retrograde cholangiopancreatography

34. FDG PET scan's use in biliary tract disease is:

A. Demonstrating carcinomatosis
B. Differentiate benign and malignant lesions
C. Detect recurrence
D. Identify metastatic disease

BENIGN BILIARY DISEASE

35. The most common disease of gallbladder and biliary tree is:

A. Biliary Dyskinesia B. Cholelithiasis
C. Choledocholithiasis D. Choledochal cyst

36. Cholelithiasis is the most common disease of gallbladder and biliary tree, affecting:

A. 1% to 5% of the population
B. 5% to 10% of the population

C. 10% to 15% of the population
D. 20% to 25% of the population

37. Black pigment stones occur in:

A. High fatty diet
B. Hemolytic diseases
C. Disorder of biliary motility
D. All of the above

38. Gallstones associated to with biliary tract infections are:

A. Black stone
B. Brown stones
C. Yellow stones
D. Grey stones

39. Factors that explain most gallstone formation includes all except:

A. Concentration of bile in the gallbladder
B. Gallbladder hypermotility
C. Supersaturation of secreted bile
D. Crystal nucleation

40. False among the following about cholelithiasis is:

A. 50% to 60% of patients with asymptomatic stones will develop symptoms within 20 years
B. Gallstones often remain asymptomatic, only found incidentally on imaging
C. Stones that do not obstruct the cystic duct or pass through the entire biliary tree into the intestines without impaction do not cause symptoms
D. Biliary colic, caused by temporary blockage of the cystic duct, tends to occur after a meal in which the secretion of CCK leads to gallbladder contraction

41. Percentage of patients with asymptomatic gallstones that develop complications is:

A. 1%
B. 5%
C. 10%
D. 15%

42. Higher risk of gallbladder cancer among the following is all except:

A. Long common channel of bile and pancreatic ducts
B. Calcified gallbladder wall
C. Large (>2.5 cm) gallstones
D. All of the above

43. In gallstone disease, extracorporeal shock wave lithotripsy has a recurrence rate of approximately:

A. 10%
B. 15%
C. 20%
D. 25%

44. With medical treatment of gallstones (dissolution strategies), recurrence rates are up to:

A. 20%
B. 40%
C. 50%
D. 70%

45. False about chronic cholecystitis is:

A. Recurrent attacks of biliary colic, with permanent occlusion of the cystic duct, can cause inflammation and scarring of the neck of the gallbladder and cystic duct
B. The diagnosis of chronic cholecystitis relies on a history consistent with biliary tract disease
C. The presentation is that of symptomatic cholelithiasis, or biliary colic
D. Patients with sufficient symptoms from gallstones should undergo elective cholecystectomy

46. In chronic cholecystitis, biliary colic is associated with food intake in:

A. 10%
B. 30%
C. 50%
D. 70%

47. Which of the following is not a part of the process of cholesterol gallstone formation?

A. Supersaturation of bile with cholesterol
B. Bilirubin deconjugation
C. Crystal nucleation
D. Aggregation of cholesterol monomers

48. A 22-year-old female presents to your office with postprandial epigastric pain. Which of the following sonographic findings is not a feature of gallstone disease?

A. Hyperechoic intraluminal structure
B. Mobility of the intraluminal structure
C. Shadowing posterior to the structure
D. Acoustic enhancement posterior to the structure

49. False about acute calculous cholecystitis is:

A. In chronic cholecystitis or biliary colic, the blockage is temporary and repetitive, while in acute cholecystitis, the blockage does not resolve, leading to inflammation with edema and subserosal hemorrhage
B. Tokyo Guidelines is the most common grading system evaluating severity of cholecystitis
C. Acute cholecystitis becomes acute gangrenous cholecystitis and, when complicated by infection with a gas-forming organism, acute emphysematous cholecystitis
D. All of the above

50. False about the presentation of acute calculous cholecystitis is:

A. The inflammatory changes in the gallbladder wall are manifested as fever and right upper quadrant pain

B. Biliary colic in the absence of infection and inflammation is not associated with any reproducible physical examination finding or systemic symptom

C. AAST EGS categorizes acute cholecystitis into 3 grades

D. Mild elevations of alkaline phosphatase, bilirubin, and transaminase levels and leukocytosis support the diagnosis of acute cholecystitis

51. Ultrasonography is a sensitive, inexpensive and reliable tool for the diagnosis of acute cholecystitis, with a:

A. Sensitivity of 95% and specificity of 95%

B. Sensitivity of 95% and specificity of 85%

C. Sensitivity of 85% and specificity of 85%

D. Sensitivity of 85% and specificity of 95%

52. False about the treatment of acute cholecystitis is:

A. Patients are given nothing by mouth, and intravenous (IV) fluids and parenteral antibiotics are started

B. Cholecystectomy, whether open or laparoscopic, is the treatment of choice for acute cholecystitis

C. Early in the disease process (within the 1st week), cholecystectomy can be performed laparoscopically with equivalent or improved morbidity, mortality and length of stay as well as a similar conversion rate to open cholecystectomy

D. All of the above

53. After the initial episode of acute cholecystitis, an interval cholecystectomy is performed at approximately:

A. 2 weeks B. 4 weeks

C. 6 weeks D. 10 weeks

54. In cases of acute cholecystitis, Tokyo Guidelines are used to predict:

A. Prognosis

B. Used as a guideline to plan the management

C. Rate of conversion or bail-out procedure

D. All of the above

55. False about choledocholithiasis is:

A. CBD stones, or choledocholithiasis, are generally symptomatic, and are seen in up to 50% of patients undergoing biliary imaging

B. Primary common duct stones arise de novo in the bile duct, and secondary common duct stones pass from the gallbladder into the bile duct

C. Primary common duct stones are generally brown pigment stones, a combination of precipitated bile pigments and cholesterol

D. Brown pigment stones are associated with bacterial infections where free bilirubin is formed by hydrolyzing enzymes released by bacteria and then precipitates

56. After cholecystectomy, retained stones are secondary stones found in bile duct within:

A. 6 months B. 1 year

C. 2 years D. 5 years

57. Retained stones occur in:

A. 1% to 2% of patients

B. 5% to 7% of patients

C. 10% to 15% of patients

D. 20% to 25% of patients

58. Charcot triad has all except:

A. Hypotension

B. Right upper quadrant pain

C. Jaundice

D. Fever

59. Reynolds pentad has all except:

A. Hypotension

B. Mental status changes

C. Leucocytosis

D. Fever

60. False about the diagnosis of choledocholithiasis is:

A. Biliary type pain, jaundice, an abnormal liver function panel, and a dilated bile duct, usually > 8 mm, are all highly suggestive of choledocholithiasis

B. Even without symptoms of biliary colic, a dilated bile duct in the presence of gallstones suggests choledocholithiasis

C. Magnetic resonance cholangiopancreatography (MRCP), is sensitive (>80%) and specific (>90%) in identifying CBD stones

D. ERCP is also highly sensitive and specific for choledocholithiasis

61. **ERCP is the therapeutic procedure by clearing the duct in:**

A. >75% of patients during first procedure and in 90% with repeated ERCP
B. >50% of patients during first procedure and in 70% with repeated ERCP
C. >75% of patients during first procedure and in 100% with repeated ERCP
D. >50% of patients during first procedure and in 90% with repeated ERCP

62. **A sphincterotomy with a balloon sweep has complication rate of:**

A. < 1% to 3%
B. < 5% to 8%
C. < 10% to 12%
D. < 15% to 20%

63. **Indications for preoperative ERCP include:**

A. Cholangitis
B. Biliary pancreatitis
C. Patients with multiple comorbidities
D. All of the above

64. **True about the treatment for choledocholithiasis is:**

A. Treatment for choledocholithiasis is generally ERCP or CBD exploration, which can be performed via laparoscopic or open technique
B. Endoscopic sphincterotomy with stone extraction is effective for the treatment of choledocholithiasis
C. >50% of patients managed by ERCP without cholecystectomy will have recurrent symptoms of biliary tract disease
D. All of the above

65. **The most common causes of failure of ERCP are all except:**

A. Multiple stones
B. Large stones (> 2.5 cm)
C. Altered gastric or duodenal anatomy such as Roux-en-Y
D. Extrahepatic stones

66. **False about gallstone pancreatitis is:**

A. When a stone passes from the bile duct through the ampulla into the duodenum, this may cause secondary injury to the pancreas
B. Symptoms usually persist even after passage of stone
C. To prevent a future episode of gallstone pancreatitis, a cholecystectomy is warranted; this is generally recommended during the same hospitalization, just before discharge
D. In most cases of gallstone pancreatitis, the pancreatitis is not self-limited

67. **False about gallstone ileus is:**

A. Gallstone ileus is a mechanical intestinal obstruction secondary to a gallstone
B. The most common site for obstruction is in 4th part of duodenum
C. Usually happens in older patients and can be caused by inflammation or simply pressure necrosis
D. Pneumobilia, which may sometimes be identified only by CT scan, is a ubiquitous finding because the fistula that permitted a stone to pass into the duodenum allows air to enter the biliary tree

68. **False about the treatment of gallstone ileus is:**

A. The site of impaction is at risk of perforation, so signs of ischemia mandate resection
B. Approximately 50% of patients have multiple large stones, so the remainder of the small intestine should be inspected
C. A second operation for the cholecystectomy can be considered to avoid the possibility of future biliary complications
D. Palpation of the remaining small intestine should be performed to exclude a second stone that could cause recurrent obstruction

69. **False about acute acalculous cholecystitis is:**

A. Critically ill patients with acalculous cholecystitis may not have right upper quadrant pain and any fever with unknown origin in critically ill patients, especially with pericholecystic fluid and gallbladder wall thickening on imaging should raise suspicion for this disorder
B. HIDA scan is diagnostic for acalculous cholecystitis but can have false-positive result
C. < 10% of these patients improve with a cholecystostomy tube and interval cholecystectomy is always necessary
D. Treatment of acalculous cholecystitis is similar to that of calculous cholecystitis with cholecystectomy being therapeutic

70. **Risk factors for acute acalculous cholecystitis are except:**

A. Diabetes
B. Burns and trauma
C. Short term use of total parenteral nutrition
D. Immunosuppression

71. After CCK administration in a patient without stone, ejection fraction diagnostic of biliary dyskinesia is:

A. < 33% at 20 minutes B. < 33% at 30 minutes
C. < 66% at 20 minutes D. < 66% at 30 minutes

72. False about biliary dyskinesia is:

A. Biliary dyskinesia is a functional disorder of the biliary tree, generally defined by gallbladder dysmotility
B. Rome criteria helps in defining and diagnosing this functional disorder
C. It is usually a diagnosis of exclusion
D. < 65% of patients show improvement in symptoms after cholecystectomy

73. In patients with objective evidence of sphincter of Oddi dysfunction, division of the sphincter will improve or resolve the pain in:

A. 20% to 40% B. 40% to 60%
C. 60% to 80% D. 80% to 100%

74. False about sphincter of Oddi dysfunction is:

A. Similar to dyskinesia, sphincter of Oddi dysfunction is a functional disorder of the biliary tree
B. It is caused by a structurally or physiologically abnormal sphincter with higher tone and failing to relax, manifested by pain, and recurrent pancreatitis with a usually normal liver function panel
C. Risk factor includes acute pancreatitis
D. Therapy consists of endoscopic sphincterotomy or transduodenal sphincteroplasty with approximately equivalent results from the two approaches

75. The diagnosis of sphincter of Oddi dysfunction should be suspected in patients with biliary pain and a common duct diameter of:

A. > 8 mm B. > 10 mm
C. > 12 mm D. > 14 mm

76. Sphincter manometry has been used to make the diagnosis of sphincter of Oddi dysfunction and the sphincter pressure that predicts good response to therapy is:

A. > 20 mm Hg B. > 40 mm Hg
C. > 60 mm Hg D. > 80 mm Hg

77. False about primary sclerosing cholangitis (PSC) is:

A. It is an idiopathic disorder and considered an autoimmune process affecting the biliary tree
B. The course of PSC is characterized by progressive chronic cholestasis and advances at an unpredictable rate to biliary cirrhosis and eventually death from liver failure
C. Approximately 50% of patients have elevated perinuclear antineutrophil cytoplasmic antibodies and the severity of disease correlates to titer levels
D. Abnormal liver function tests in a patient observed for inflammatory bowel disease should suggest PSC

78. PSC is associated with autoimmune disorders, most common of them being:

A. Riedel thyroiditis
B. Ulcerative colitis
C. Crohn's disease
D. Rheumatoid arthritis

79. True about primary sclerosing cholangitis (PSC) is:

A. PSC is associated with cholangiocarcinoma and distinguishing the strictures of PSC fibrosis from those of cholangiocarcinoma can be challenging
B. Imaging with cholangiography demonstrates a multifocal diffuse dilation and stricturing of the intrahepatic and/or extrahepatic biliary trees called "beading" or "chain of lakes" and is characteristic of PSC
C. Liver biopsy tends to show an onion skin concentric periductal fibrosis
D. All of the above

80. False about the treatment of primary sclerosing cholangitis (PSC) is:

A. Ursodeoxycholic acid is commonly used as medical therapy for PSC and has demonstrated some improvement in liver function tests
B. In the symptomatic patient, endoscopic therapy, consisting of balloon dilation of the dominant strictures, has been shown to alleviate pruritus, to reduce likelihood of cholangitis and even to prolong survival
C. Surgical treatment options include biliary reconstruction in asymptomatic patients with focal extrahepatic disease in some cases
D. Orthotopic liver transplantation appears to be the only lifesaving option for patients with progressive hepatic dysfunction from PSC

81. After liver transplantation, percentage of PSC patients that develop recurrent biliary strictures, suggestive of recurrence of disease in the donor liver is:

A. 5% to 10%
B. 10% to 30%
C. 30% to 40%
D. 50% to 70%

82. False about biliary strictures is:

A. Any inflammatory of ischemic process along the length of the CBD may cause an extrahepatic stricture
B. Intrahepatic strictures are usually a result of cholangiohepatitis and/or ischemic events
C. The most common reason is iatrogenic and postcholecystectomy
D. Chronic pancreatitis can cause strictures in the intrapancreatic portion of CBD and are usually small (0.5– 1 cm) with gradually tapered narrowing

83. Incidence of biliary stricture reported in postcholecystectomy patient is:

A. 0.1% to 1%
B. 1% to 10%
C. 2.5% to 5%
D. 15% to 20%

84. True about the management of biliary strictures is:

A. Endoscopic and percutaneous therapy can provide long-term success in > 50% of patients
B. ERCP with sphincterotomy, balloon dilation and stent placement is generally regarded as primary treatment for benign bile duct strictures to make the diagnosis and potentially to treat the process
C. When endoscopic treatment fails, surgical management with anastomosis of the biliary tree to a Roux-en-Y jejunal limb has success rates of up to 90%
D. All of the above

85. Type of Mirizzi syndrome that has no Fistula is:

A. Type II
B. Type I
C. Type III
D. Type IV

86. Following image shows which type of choledochal cyst?

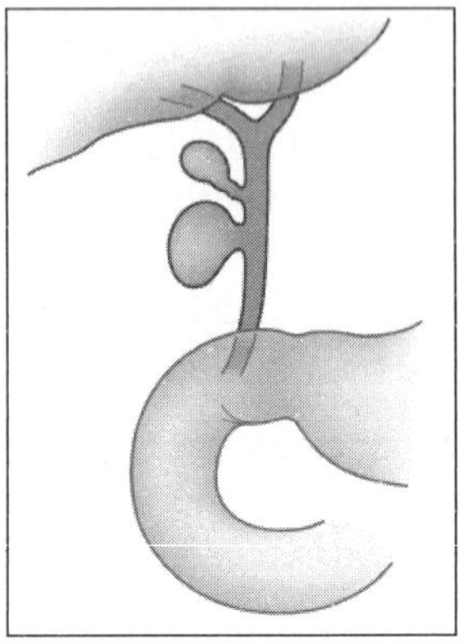

A. Type I
B. Type II
C. Type III
D. Type IV

87. Following image shows which type of choledochal cyst?

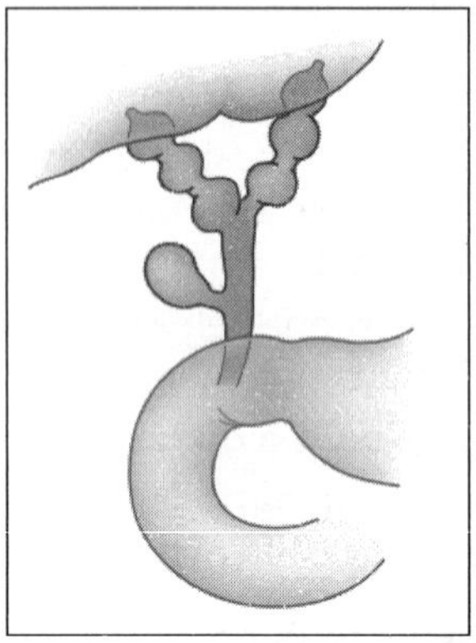

A. Type V
B. Type II
C. Type III
D. Type IV

88. Following image shows which type of choledochal cyst?

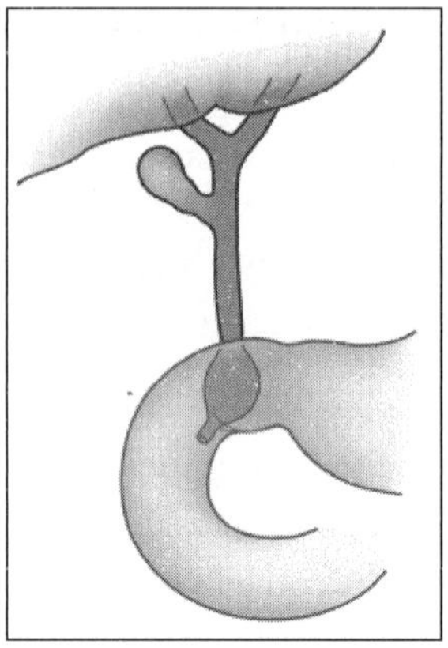

A. Type I
B. Type II
C. Type III
D. Type IV

89. Following image shows which type of choledochal cyst?

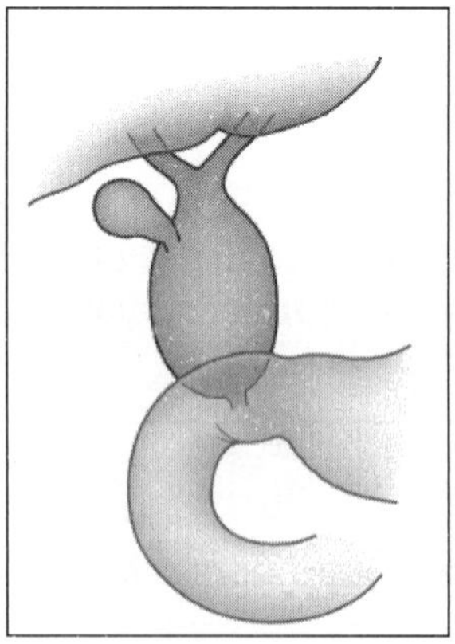

A. Type I
B. Type II
C. Type III
D. Type IV

90. False about choledochal cyst is:

A. It is a rare disorder, occurring in less than 1/100,000 patients
B. It occurs more frequently in female patients and in Asian populations
C. It is not a premalignant condition
D. Type V cysts, also known as Caroli disease, involve the intrahepatic ducts only

91. In patients with choledochal cysts, anomalous pancreatobiliary junction (APBJ) is seen in up to:

A. 30% B. 50%
C. 70% D. 90%

92. False about choledochal cyst is:

A. Types II and III almost never present with APBJ and are associated with minimal risk of malignancy
B. APBJ is seen in up to 90% of patients with choledochal cysts, but almost exclusively in types I and IV
C. Jaundice is the most consistent symptom, sometimes accompanied with right upper quadrant pain and rarely a palpable mass
D. The incidence of malignancy most commonly occurs in the 7th decade and almost exclusively occurring in types II and III

93. The risk of malignancy in choledochal cyst is around:

A. 1% and 3% B. 5% and 30%
C. 30% and 45% D. 55% and 70%

94. False about the treatment of choledochal cyst is:

A. Type I cysts are treated by complete surgical excision, cholecystectomy and Roux-en-Y hepaticojejunostomy
B. Type II cysts should be managed with ERCP
C. Because the pathogenesis of type III cysts is not clear and almost always does not involve APBJ, endoscopic drainage may suffice
D. Type IV cysts affecting only the extrahepatic bile ducts are managed similarly to type I cysts, with excision and hepaticojejunostomy

95. True about polypoid lesions of the gallbladder is:

A. Adenomyomatosis is seen as a sessile lesion, commonly in the fundus, with characteristic microcysts within the lesion and is frequently > 1 cm
B. Cholesterol polyps appear as pedunculated echogenic lesions of the gallbladder, are usually < 1 cm and are frequently multiple
C. Asymptomatic lesions < 10 mm with no other risk factors and no ultrasonographic features suggesting malignant disease can be observed with serial ultrasonography
D. All of the above

96. Of all polypoid disorders of gallbladder, true polyps (benign growths in the wall of the gallbladder) account for around:

A. 2% B. 5%
C. 10% D. 20%

97. True about benign biliary masses is:

A. The lesions occur in the periampullary duct, so a transduodenal approach can be used
B. Intraductal papillary neoplasms include mucin producing neoplasms, adenomas, papillomas and papillomatosis
C. Inflammatory lesions of the biliary tree, known as pseudotumors or benign fibrosing disease, may be mistaken for cholangiocarcinoma
D. All of the above

98. Which surgeon performed the world's first laparoscopic cholecystectomy?

A. Karl Langenbuch B. Phillippe Mouret
C. William B Saye D. Eric Mühe

99. In this transverse laparoscopic ultrasound scan of the hepatoduodenal ligament. What structure is labeled by the straight black arrow?

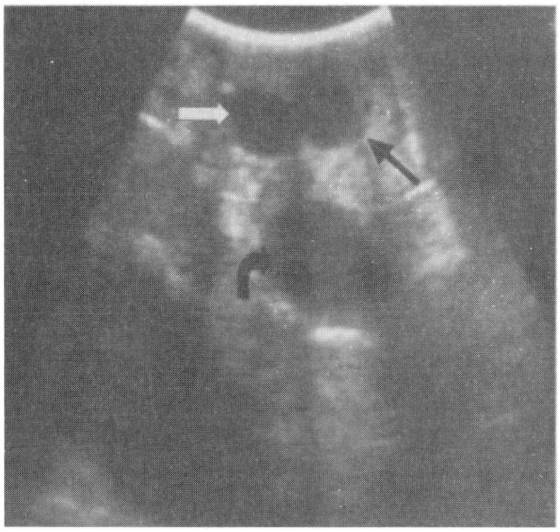

A. CBD
B. Cystic duct
C. Common hepatic artery
D. Right hepatic artery

100. True about laparoscopic cholecystectomy is:

A. Laparoscopic surgery results in smaller incisions, less pain, and shorter hospitalization when compared to traditional open cholecystectomy, which has significantly increased the number of these procedures done worldwide

B. Laparoscopic cholecystectomy has a 0.1% to 0.5% mortality and 2% to 3% morbidity

C. The standard way is the 4-port technique, usually 1 large port that will be used as extraction site, typically placed around umbilicus, and three, 5-mm or even smaller ports for dissection

D. All of the above

101. Contraindication to laparoscopic cholecystectomy is:

A. Old age

B. Coagulopathy

C. Inability to tolerate general anesthesia

D. End-stage liver disease with portal hypertension

102. 5 mm ports in laparoscopic cholecystectomy are all except:

A. Subxiphoid location

B. Right anterior axillary line

C. Palmer's point

D. Right midclavicular line

103. As per SAGES strategy that surgeons can employ to adopt a universal culture of safety for cholecystectomy to and minimize the risk of bile duct injury includes all except:

A. Use the Critical View of Safety (CVS) method of identification of the cystic duct and cystic artery

B. Consider an Intra-operative Momentary Pause during laparoscopic cholecystectomy prior to clipping, cutting or transecting any ductal structures

C. Understand the potential for aberrant anatomy in all cases

D. Make limited use of cholangiography or other methods to image the biliary tree intraoperatively

104. False about Open Cholecystectomy is:

A. Open cholecystectomy is generally performed after conversion from the laparoscopic approach, for patients who have a contraindication to the laparoscopic approach, or as a step during another operation, such as a pancreaticoduodenectomy

B. Open cholecystectomy can be performed through a midline or right subcostal incision

C. When it is performed for severe cholecystitis, the dissection of the gallbladder of the liver bed may be associated with substantial blood loss, but with removal of the infected gallbladder and packing of the area, the bleeding is usually well controlled

D. All of the above

105. Which of the following is/are bailout procedures for surgical management of cholecystitis?

A. Fundus first procedure (retrograde),

B. Subtotal cholecystectomy

C. Conversion to open

D. All of the above

106. False about Open CBD Exploration is:

A. Transduodenal sphincteroplasty must be the procedure of choice when impacted stones at the ampulla cannot be removed through choledochotomy or several stones are impacted in a nondilated tree

B. With dilated bile ducts, multiple distal impacted stones, a distal duct stricture with stones, intrahepatic stones, or primary bile duct stones drainage procedures provide more successful long-term outcomes

C. Open exploration carries a low morbidity (8%–15%) and mortality (1%–2%), with a low rate of retained stones (<5%)

D. The downside of choledochojejunostomy is a process known as sump syndrome

107. On the ampulla, the pancreatic duct usually enters at the:

A. 2 O'clock position

B. 5 O'clock position

C. 7 O'clock position

D. 11 O'clock position

108. False about the management of intrahepatic stones, is:

A. Percutaneous drainage catheters may be left in place and upsized to perform percutaneous stone extraction

B. With intrahepatic stones, the transhepatic approach to cholangiography is generally more successful

C. Liberal use of choledochoscopy at the time of a drainage procedure ensures removal of all current stones and this approach allows a stone clearance rate of < 50%

D. Long-term management of intrahepatic stones must be carefully tailored to the disease but frequently requires hepaticojejunostomy for optimal biliary drainage

109. False about Laparoscopic CBD Exploration is:

A. The 2 common laparoscopic approaches to explore the CBD for stone removal are the transcystic approach and choledochotomy

B. In the transcystic approach, using the Seldinger technique after balloon dilation, a flexible choledochoscope, or alternately a flexible ureteroscope, is passed into the cystic duct

C. Choledochotomy approach is technically easier

D. Both approaches are successful at stone removal, with most studies showing a 75% to 95% rate of stone clearance

110. Laparoscopic cholecystectomy is most strongly contraindicated in which of the following situations?

A. Pregnancy

B. Previous upper abdominal surgery

C. Known CBD stones

D. Recent myocardial infarction (MI) with severe coronary artery disease noted on cardiac catheterization, requiring full anticoagulation

111. Which of the following statements about "infundibular technique" is true?

A. The CBD can be mistaken for the cystic duct when obtaining this view

B. It requires dissection of the cystic plate over the bottom third of the gallbladder

C. It has been shown to prevent bile duct injuries

D. It facilitates identification of the anatomy in the hepatocystic triangle

112. A 65-year-old female presents with RUQ pain, nausea and vomiting. Her temperature is 38°C., heart rate (HR) is 115 beats/min, and blood pressure is (BP) 88/62 mmHg; she is saturating 92% on 2-L nasal cannula. Her abdominal examination is significant for a positive Murphy's sign. Laboratory values are significant for a white blood cell (WBC) count of 19,000/mm^3 and a normal total bilirubin. Ultrasound shows a gallbladder wall of 5 mm, pericholecystic fluid, gallstones and a CBD diameter of 4 mm. She is admitted to the surgical intensive care unit (SICU), IV fluids and vasopressors are started and antibiotics are administered. Which is the most appropriate surgical management?

A. Percutaneous cholecystectomy tube placement followed by cholecystectomy before hospital discharge

B. Emergent cholecystectomy

C. Percutaneous cholecystostomy tube placement followed by cholecystectomy in 3 months

D. Percutaneous cholecystostomy tube placement and cholecystectomy only if her symptoms recur

113. A 27-year-old female presents with RUQ pain, which started 12 hours ago. Her vitals are normal, and her examination is significant for RUQ tenderness without peritonitis. Laboratory values are significant for a WBC count of 12,000/mm^3 and normal total bilirubin. Ultrasound shows a gallbladder wall of 4 mm, pericholecystic fluid, gallstones and a CBD diameter of 3 mm. Which is the most appropriate surgical treatment?

A. IV fluids, antibiotics and interval elective cholecystectomy in 1 month after her symptoms resolve

B. ERCP with sphincterotomy for biliary decompression

C. Cholecystectomy within 72 hours of onset of symptoms

D. Percutaneous cholecystostomy tube placement

114. A 36-year-old male presents with RUQ pain, nausea and vomiting, which started 5 days ago. His vitals are significant for a HR of 106 beats/min and BP 126/75 mm Hg. His examination is significant for RUQ tenderness and positive Murphy's sign, but no peritonitis. Laboratory values are significant for a WBC count of 19,000/mm^3 and normal total bilirubin. Ultrasound shows a gallbladder wall of 5 mm, pericholecystic fluid, gallstones and a CBD diameter of 3 mm. Which is the most appropriate surgical treatment?

A. Percutaneous cholecystostomy tube placement

B. Immediate cholecystectomy

C. ERCP with sphincterotomy for biliary decompression

D. IV fluids, antibiotics and interval elective cholecystectomy in 3 months after his symptoms resolve

115. A 46-year-old male presents with 2 days of RUQ pain. His labs are significant for a WBC count of 15,000/mm^3. His ultrasound notes numerous gallstones with wall thickening

and pericholecystic fluid. On examination, his temperature is 99.5°F and he has a positive Murphy's sign. What is the best management for this individual?

A. Early laparoscopic cholecystectomy
B. Interval cholecystectomy after 6 weeks
C. IV antibiotics
D. Percutaneous cholecystostomy tube

116. With regard to acalculous cholecystitis, which of the following statements is true?

A. It most commonly affects elderly patients in an outpatient setting
B. The primary pathophysiologic feature involves gallbladder stasis
C. HIDA scan results are usually normal
D. Ultrasound imaging of the gallbladder is usually normal

117. The pertinent area of a plain X-ray film of the abdomen of a 78-year-old diabetic man with RUQ pain is shown in the image. Which of the following is the appropriate next step?

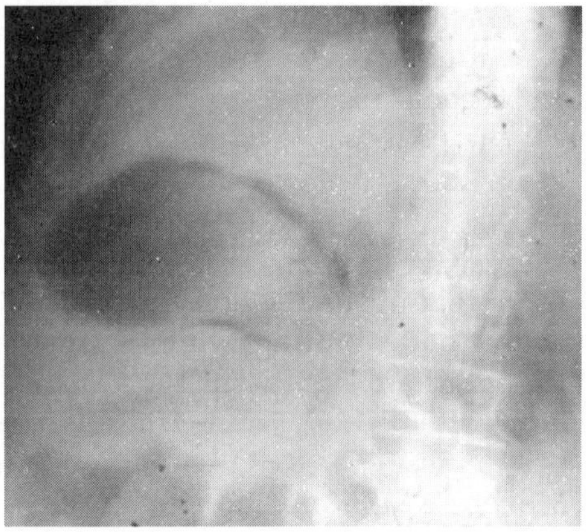

A. Ultrasound imaging of the gallbladder
B. CT scan
C. HIDA scan
D. Cholecystectomy

118. A 68-year-old male presented to the hospital with chronic cholecystitis. He was taken to the operating room for a laparoscopic cholecystectomy. Intraoperatively, the critical view of safety could not be obtained due to dense adhesions in the hepatocystic triangle. Which is the most reasonable next operative step?

A. Obtain the infundibular view and then proceed with cholecystectomy
B. Proceed with subtotal fenestrating cholecystectomy
C. Proceed with subtotal reconstituting cholecystectomy
D. Both C and D

119. When compared with standard three-or four-port laparoscopic cholecystectomy, single-incision laparoscopic surgery (SILS) is associated with which of the following?

A. Decreased rate of trocar site hernias
B. Increased bile duct injuries
C. Decreased pain
D. Increased operative time

120. Ultrasound of the gallbladder demonstrates a 5 mm hyperechoic focus along the gallbladder wall that does not move or produce shadowing and that has a "comet tail" echo pattern behind it. What is the most likely diagnosis?

A. Adenomatous polyp B. Cholesterol polyp
C. Gallstone D. Adenomyomatosis

121. With regard to adenomyomatosis of the gallbladder, which of the following statements is true?

A. It is a premalignant lesion
B. It results from chronic inflammation
C. It is frequently > 1 cm
D. It is rarely associated with cholelithiasis and cholecystitis

122. A 73-year-old female presents with acute onset of abdominal distention, pain, nausea and vomiting. She has no previous surgeries. She has no abdominal or inguinal hernias on examination. Abdominal X-ray shows dilated small bowel with air-fluid levels and Pneumobilia. The obstruction is most likely at which site?

A. Pylorus B. Duodenum
C. Jejunum D. Ileocecal valve

123. With regard to the management of a patient with gallstone ileus, which of the following statements is true?

A. Initial tube decompression and nonoperative management allow spontaneous stone passage in one-third of patients
B. Operative treatment attempts to displace the stone into the colon without enterotomy
C. Operative treatment involves enterotomy proximal to the site of obstruction
D. Cholecystectomy and fistula repair at the time of stone removal are contraindicated

124. With regard to balloon dilation of benign biliary strictures, which of the following statements is true?

A. Dilation can be performed via the transhepatic or endoscopic route
B. Repeated dilations are not often required
C. Perforation of the bile duct is the most frequent complication
D. Better success is obtained with anastomotic strictures than with primary duct strictures

125. Definitive treatment of a patient with sclerosing cholangitis and biliary cirrhosis involves which of the following?

A. Ursodeoxycholic acid
B. Endoscopic balloon dilation and stenting
C. Extrahepatic bile duct resection and transhepatic stenting
D. Hepatic transplantation

126. True about bile duct injury is:

A. Studies have suggested that misperception of the anatomy is a much more common factor in iatrogenic injury than surgical skill
B. More than 80% of bile duct injuries occur during cholecystectomy
C. The use of a 30-degree laparoscope provides adequate visualization of the critical view of safety during laparoscopic cholecystectomy
D. All of the above

127. Following image shows what type of bile duct injury?

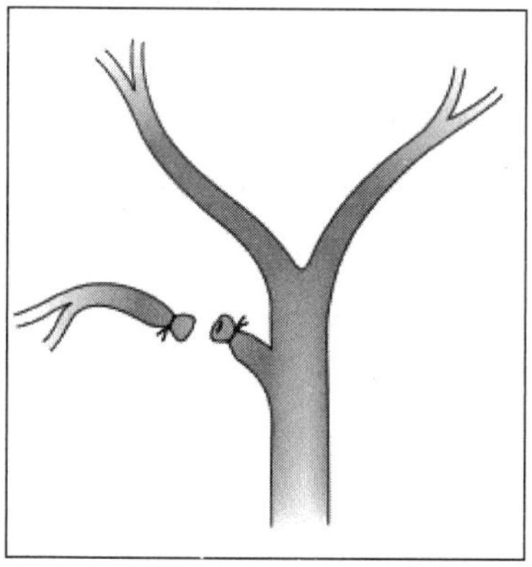

A. Strasberg's type A
B. Strasberg's type B
C. Strasberg's type C
D. Strasberg's type D

128. Following image shows what type of bile duct injury?

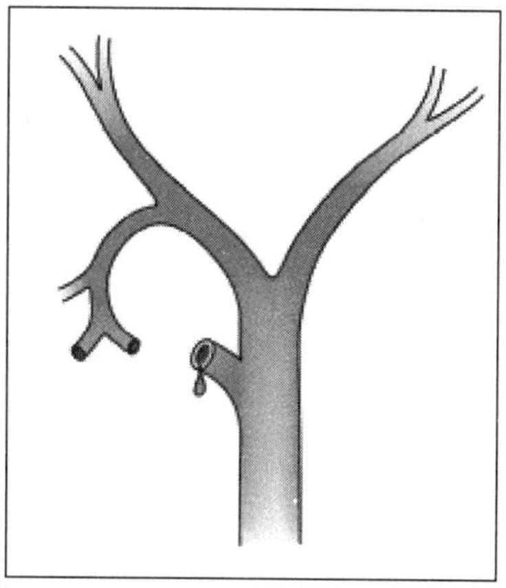

A. Strasberg's type A
B. Strasberg's type B
C. Strasberg's type C
D. Strasberg's type D

129. Following image shows what type of bile duct injury?

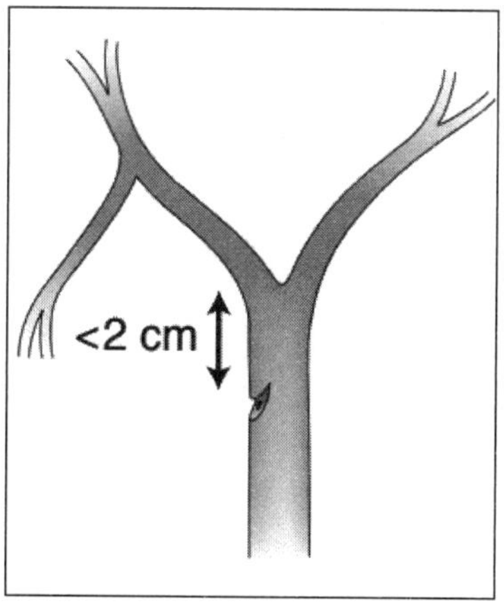

A. Bismuth's type 1
B. Bismuth's type 2
C. Bismuth's type 3
D. Bismuth's type 4

130. Following image shows what type of bile duct injury?

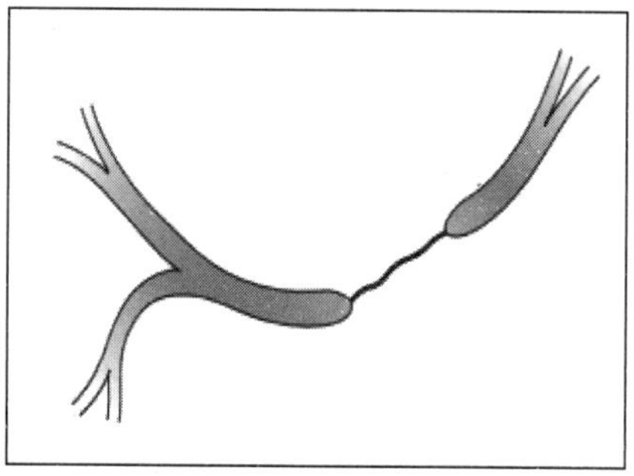

A. Bismuth's type 5
B. Bismuth's type 2
C. Bismuth's type 3
D. Bismuth's type 4

131. Following image shows what type of bile duct injury?

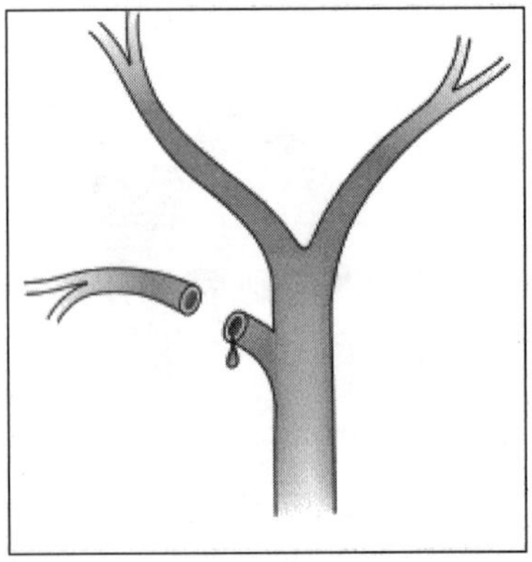

A. Strasberg's type A
B. Strasberg's type B
C. Strasberg's type C
D. Strasberg's type D

132. Following image shows what type of bile duct injury?

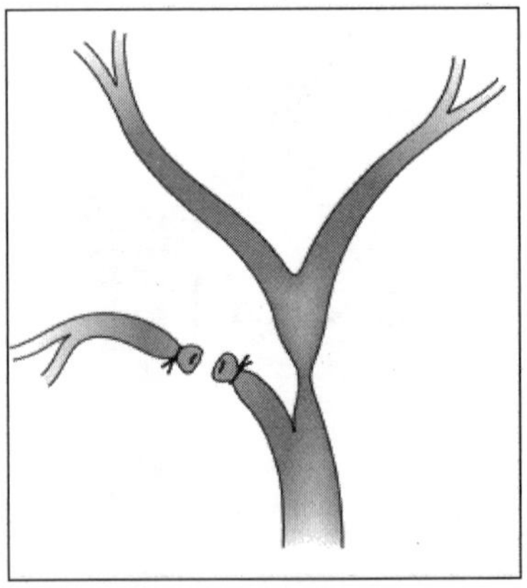

A. Bismuth's type 5
B. Bismuth's type 2
C. Bismuth's type 3
D. Bismuth's type 4

133. False about the management of bile duct injury recognized at the time of cholecystectomy is:

A. Defects > 1 cm defect between the ends of the bile duct, requiring reanastomosis to the gastrointestinal tract
B. Goals for the immediate treatment of bile duct injury include maintenance of ductal length, elimination of any bile leakage that would affect subsequent management and creation of a tension-free repair
C. Ducts smaller than 7 mm that by cholangiography drain only a single segment or subsegment of the liver and simple ligation may suffice for management
D. Defects < 1 cm and not near the hepatic duct bifurcation can be repaired by mobilization and end-to-end anastomosis of the bile duct

134. Goals of therapy in iatrogenic bile duct injury include:

A. Control of infection, limiting inflammation: Parenteral antibiotics and percutaneous drainage of periportal fluid collections
B. Clear and thorough delineation of entire biliary anatomy with ERCP or MRCP or PTC
C. Reestablishment of biliary-enteric continuity
D. All of the above

135. True about the presentation of bile duct injury identified after cholecystectomy is:

A. The diagnosis of iatrogenic bile duct injury should be suspected in any patient who presents with new or increasing symptoms after a laparoscopic cholecystectomy
B. Persistent or worsening postprandial pain, shoulder pain, malaise and/or fever must raise the suspicion of a bile duct injury
C. Without a site for external drainage, bile leakage can be manifested as a biloma, whether sterile or infected, or with biliary ascites
D. All of the above

136. In the setting of a bile duct injury, percentage of patients that will have concomitant unrecognized vascular injuries is:

A. 5% or more
B. 10% or more
C. 20% or more
D. 40% or more

137. What is the most common anatomic reason for a type B (Strasberg classification) bile duct injury during a laparoscopic cholecystectomy?

A. A short cystic duct
B. An aberrant right hepatic duct
C. A replaced right hepatic artery
D. A replaced left hepatic artery

138. Balloon dilation can treat bile duct strictures and this approach is successful in up to:

A. 10%
B. 30%
C. 50%
D. 70%

139. False about biliary leak is:

A. Fevers, chills, right upper quadrant pain, jaundice, leakage of bile from an incision or into a drain, or persistent anorexia or bloating are common signs and symptoms
B. Patients will generally present within 1 month of cholecystectomy as the bile collects and becomes clinically manifested

C. If the leak is from a cystic duct stump, sphincterotomy with stenting of the common duct will allow the leak to seal without need for surgical management
D. Persistence of a bile leak longer than 6 weeks should raise the suspicion of an unrecognized bile duct injury

140. False about lost gallstones during cholecystectomy is:

A. Pigmented stones, a high number of stones, less experienced surgeons performing the surgery, and severe cholecystitis are all risk factors
B. Most dropped stones settle into the Morison pouch or the retrohepatic space along the abdominal wall, which may develop into a chronic abscess in this location
C. Lost stones necessitate conversion to an open operation
D. Treatment includes extensive irrigation, significant attempt to retrieve lost stones, course of antibiotics, documentation of the perforation in the operative notes, and clear communication with the patient of the small possibility of delayed presentation from erosion or abscess

141. Accidental opening of the gallbladder with spillage of stones during cholecystectomy occurs in:

A. 10% to 20% B. 20% to 40%
C. 40% to 50% D. 50% to 70%

142. True about postcholecystectomy pain is:

A. Although unusual, pain similar to biliary colic may persist or recur after cholecystectomy
B. Recurrence of pain, if it is associated with other system findings of jaundice, fever, or chills within days to weeks after cholecystectomy suggests a secondary choledocholithiasis or a bile leak
C. Postoperative bile duct strictures, which usually are manifested with jaundice, are generally identified within the first year after cholecystectomy and may be manifested with pain or fever if only one lobar duct is obstructed
D. All of the above

143. False about acute cholangitis is:

A. With obstruction from a stone, bactibilia can be identified in up to 90% of patients
B. The most common pathogens include Klebsiella, E. coli, Enterobacter, Pseudomonas and Citrobacter spp
C. Hepatocellular injury from the infection and inflammation elevate serum transaminase and alkaline phosphatase levels
D. CT should be the first screening test and will commonly show dilation of the biliary tree

144. The classic Charcot triad of fever, jaundice and right upper quadrant pain in acute cholangitis can be seen in:

A. < 90% B. < 70%
C. < 50% D. < 30%

145. The least common finding in Charcot's triad is:

A. Right upper quadrant pain
B. Jaundice
C. Hypotension
D. Fever

146. False about the treatment of acute cholangitis is:

A. Adequate hydration and IV antibiotics should be started immediately
B. Endoscopic or percutaneous drainage achieves this goal with more morbidity than surgical intervention
C. If endoscopic and percutaneous means are unavailable or unsuccessful, surgical drainage consists of common duct exploration with placement of a T tube
D. Given the unstable nature of the patient, definitive surgical treatment of the cause is deferred until the patient is stabilized, the cholangitis is treated and the diagnosis is confirmed

147. False about recurrent pyogenic cholangitis is:

A. The chronicity of the infection and inflammation places these patients at risk for the development of cholangiocarcinoma
B. Recurrent pyogenic cholangitis is caused by cholangiohepatitis or intrahepatic stones
C. Recurrent pyogenic cholangitis tends to occur in the 5th to 6th decade of life, affecting men more than women
D. The clinical presentation is that of cholangitis with fever, right upper quadrant pain and jaundice

148. False about recurrent pyogenic cholangitis is:

A. Diagnosis is usually made by a combination of CT or MRCP with ERCP
B. In the setting of an acute attack surgical therapy is always needed

C. Given the risk of cholangiocarcinoma, disease affecting predominantly 1 lobe should be resected in patients with adequate hepatic reserve

D. The goals of surgical therapy are threefold: (1) remove all stones; (2) bypass, enlarge, or resect the strictures; and (3) provide adequate biliary drainage

MALIGNANT BILIARY DISEASE

149. True about Gallbladder cancer is:

A. Gallbladder cancer is an aggressive malignant disease and carries an extremely poor prognosis

B. Gallbladder cancer generally occurs in the sixth and seventh decades of life and is 2 to 3 times more common in women than in men

C. The highest incidence in women from India and Pakistan

D. All of the above

150. False about the causes of Gallbladder cancer is:

A. The presence of gallstones is considered to be the primary risk factor, and larger stones (>3 cm) carry an increased risk of cancer development

B. > 80% of patients with gallbladder cancer have cholelithiasis, and gallbladder cancer is approximately 7 times more common in patients with gallstones than in those without stones

C. The type of stone correlates with incidence of gallbladder cancer; highest with brown stones

D. Extensive calcification of the wall of the gallbladder, termed porcelain gallbladder, carries a risk of cancer development

151. In patients with porcelain gallbladder, malignant disease occurs in:

A. < 5% B. < 10%
C. < 20% D. < 40%

152. False about the Gallbladder cancer is:

A. Gallbladder cancer spreads via lymphatics, hematogenously, and notoriously into the peritoneal cavity or along biopsy or surgical wound tracts

B. Most tumors have an infiltrative pattern and spread in a subserosal plane and can invade the entire gallbladder wall and even into the porta hepatis

C. A small subset of gallbladder cancers are of the papillary subtype and carry a poor prognosis

D. Nodular types tend to grow as a more circumscribed mass and can invade the liver

153. True about the presentation of CA Gallbladder is:

A. Weight loss, jaundice, or an abdominal mass is associated with later stages of disease

B. 90% of gallbladder cancers originate in the fundus or body of the gallbladder, most do not produce symptoms until the disease is advanced

C. Symptoms of acute cholecystitis, with obstruction of the neck of the gallbladder, may portend a better prognosis because patients with these symptoms may present with earlier stages of disease

D. All of the above

154. Most gallbladder carcinomas have systemic disease at the time of presentation, with distant metastases in:

A. 10% B. 20%
C. 40% D. 70%

155. T staging of a gallbladder mass with the tumor invading the perimuscular connective tissue on the hepatic side with no extension into the liver is:

A. T2a B. T2b
C. T3 D. T4

156. T staging of a gallbladder mass invading hepatic artery is:

A. T2a B. T2b
C. T3 D. T4

157. T staging of a gallbladder mass invading colon and no invasion of any other surrounding organs is:

A. T2a B. T2b
C. T3 D. T4

158. T staging of a gallbladder tumor that perforates the serosa (visceral peritoneum) is:

A. T2a B. T2b
C. T3 D. T4

159. T staging of a gallbladder tumor that directly invades the liver is:

A. T2a B. T2b
C. T3 D. T4

160. T staging of a gallbladder tumor invading the muscular layer is:

A. T1b
B. T2a
C. T2b
D. T3

161. **A gallbladder tumor invading the portal vein, no lymph nodal involvement and distant mets has stage as:**

A. IIIA
B. IIIB
C. IVA
D. IVB

162. **True about the diagnosis of gallbladder cancer is:**

A. Ultrasonographic findings of gallbladder cancer include an irregularly shaped lesion in the subhepatic space, heterogeneous mass in the gallbladder lumen and asymmetrically thickened gallbladder wall
B. PET can also be a valuable adjunct in searching for metastatic disease or when CT or MRI provides limited information about the primary tumor
C. Cross-sectional imaging with CT or MRI is an important part of the preoperative assessment of gallbladder cancer and can provide critical information on the local extent of disease and whether distant metastases are present
D. All of the above

163. **The most consistent predictors of malignancy in gallbladder polyps are all except:**

A. Female sex
B. Age > 50 years
C. Size > 1 cm
D. Single polyp

164. **Cholecystectomy is generally recommended for polyps measuring:**

A. >5 mm
B. >1 cm
C. >2 cm
D. >4 cm

165. **True about the management of gallbladder cancer after cholecystectomy is:**

A. With T1a lesions, in which the carcinoma penetrates the lamina propria but does not invade the muscle layer, cholecystectomy suffices for therapy
B. Extended cholecystectomy is generally recommended for all patients who are medically fit with T1b or greater level of invasion
C. In patients with T2 lesions, in which the cancer extends past the muscularis but not beyond the serosa, a similar approach with radical cholecystectomy is indicated
D. All of the above

166. **False about the management of patients suspected of having gallbladder cancer preoperatively is:**

A. In the setting of metastatic disease, nonoperative strategies should be used to palliate symptoms
B. Radical resection in the setting of T3 and T4 lesions includes at least segments IVB and V but more often requires a central hepatectomy, including all of segments IV, V and VIII
C. Direct extension of tumor into adjacent structures such as the hepatic flexure is a contraindication to resection
D. Debulking without the possibility of complete resection has no role in the management of gallbladder cancer

167. **High-risk lesions in CA gallbladder is:**

A. Positive lymph nodes
B. T4 tumors
C. R1 resection
D. All of the above

168. **The likelihood of nodal disease in CA gallbladder T1a lesions is:**

A. < 1%
B. < 3%
C. < 8%
D. < 15%

169. **Ultrasound imaging demonstrates a 15 mm polypoid lesion in the gallbladder of an asymptomatic 60 years old patient. Which of the following best describes the recommended treatment?**

A. Observation with repeated ultrasound studies in 6 months
B. Cholecystectomy
C. Cholecystectomy if the patient is female
D. Cholecystectomy only if symptoms develop

170. **A 63 years old female undergoes a laparoscopic cholecystectomy for symptomatic cholelithiasis. The pathology report states that there is a focus of carcinoma which invades, but does not penetrate through, the lamina propria. What is the most appropriate management?**

A. Laparoscopic resection of the gallbladder fossa
B. Open extended cholecystectomy including segment 4b and 5 liver resection as well as removal of porta hepatis lymph nodes
C. Cholecystectomy is sufficient
D. Radiation and chemotherapy

171. **False about Cholangiocarcinoma is:**

A. The incidence of cholangiocarcinoma is rising worldwide and is now the second most common primary cancer of the liver behind hepatocellular carcinoma

B. More than two thirds of all cholangiocarcinomas involve the distal biliary tree known as a Klatskin tumor
C. Congenital lesions, such as choledochal cysts, predispose to the development of cholangiocarcinoma from exposure of the biliary epithelium to toxic pancreatic secretions
D. The incidence of cholangiocarcinoma is estimated between 10% and 20% if the cyst is not resected by age 20 years old

172. In the West, the most common risk factor for cholangiocarcinoma is:

A. Primary sclerosing cholangitis
B. Cigarette smoking
C. Thorotrast
D. Clonorchis sinensis

173. False about the presentation of cholangiocarcinoma is:

A. Painless jaundice is a common symptom, but patients with unilobar obstruction of a bile duct may present with unilateral lobar atrophy and subsequent contralateral lobar hypertrophy
B. Cholangiocarcinoma causing obstruction at or below the hepatic bifurcation tends to be manifested at later stages than intrahepatic cholangiocarcinoma
C. Cholangiocarcinoma tends to extend in a submucosal route, with associated perineural invasion, but constant pain on presentation suggests more advanced disease
D. With obstruction of the biliary tree, the common manifestations of direct hyperbilirubinemia, such as pruritus, dark urine and steatorrhea, can be seen

174. False about the diagnosis of cholangiocarcinoma is:

A. Tumor markers, including carcinoembryonic antigen and carbohydrate antigen 19-9, are reliable for diagnosis of cholangiocarcinoma
B. Cross-sectional imaging by triphasic CT allows not only assessment of metastatic disease but also evaluation of resectability
C. Tissue diagnosis before resection in operative patients is unnecessary
D. Establishment of a tissue diagnosis is important only when the patient is not a surgical candidate

175. False about the management of cholangiocarcinoma is:

A. More than 80% of patients undergoing exploration have historically had findings precluding resection, such as peritoneal metastases, hepatic metastases, or locally advanced lesions
B. An extensive neoadjuvant therapy protocol followed by transplantation has shown promising results in tightly controlled trials where hilar cholangiocarcinoma occurs in the setting of underlying liver disease
C. Surgical management of proximal cholangiocarcinoma involves resection of regional nodal tissue and en bloc resection of the CBD with hepatic parenchyma as necessary to achieve negative margins
D. Distal cholangiocarcinoma is managed by pancreaticoduodenectomy

176. As per Bismuth-Corlette classification of tumor involvement following image is:

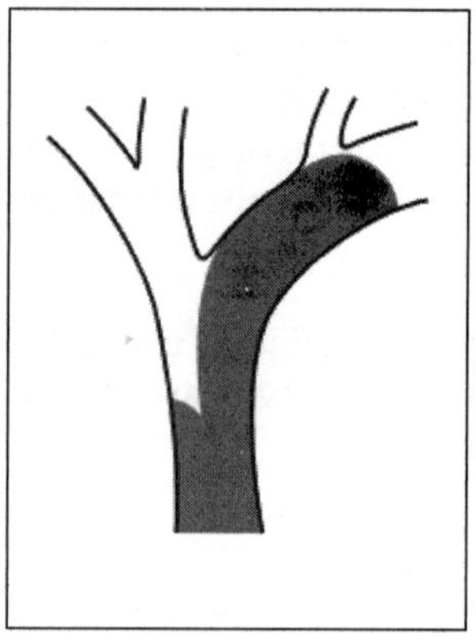

A. Type I
B. Type II
C. Type IIIa
D. Type IIIb

177. As per Bismuth-Corlette classification of tumor involvement following image is:

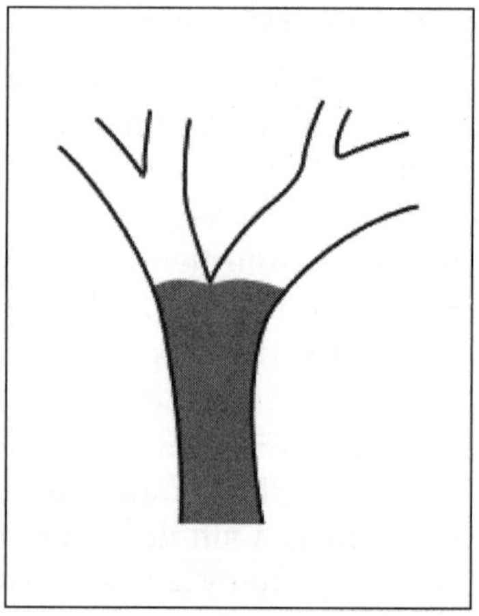

A. Type I
B. Type II
C. Type IIIa
D. Type IIIb

178. As per Bismuth-Corlette classification of tumor involvement following image is:

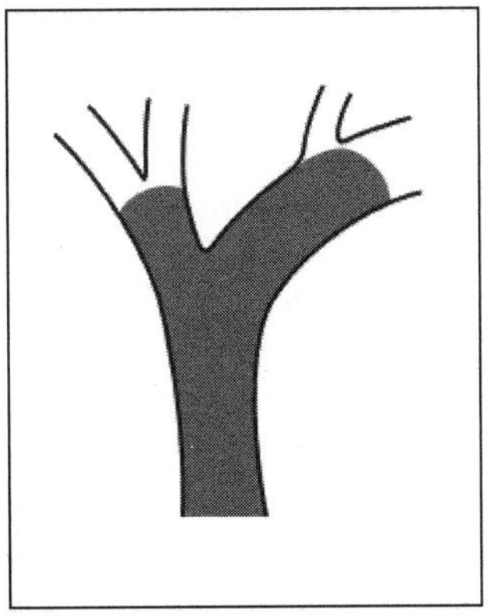

A. Type IV
B. Type II
C. Type IIIa
D. Type IIIb

179. True about the management of proximal cholangiocarcinoma is:

A. Types I and II lesions are treated with common duct resection, cholecystectomy, and a 5- to 10-mm margin of resection
B. Negative margin status is the most important variable associated with outcome
C. Types III and IV lesions may involve complex resection and reconstruction of the portal vein, hepatic artery, or both
D. All of the above

180. A Solitary intrahepatic bile duct tumor with intrahepatic vascular invasion has T stage as:

A. T1
B. T2
C. T3
D. T4

181. Any lymph nodal involvement in intrahepatic bile duct cancer is:

A. Stage I
B. Stage II
C. Stage IIIA
D. Stage IIIB

182. A perihilar bile duct tumor invading unilateral branches of the hepatic artery has T stage as:

A. T2a
B. T2b
C. T3
D. T4

183. A distal bile duct tumor involving the common hepatic artery has T staging as:

A. T1
B. T2
C. T3
D. T4

184. A distal bile duct tumor invading the bile duct wall with a depth of 11 mm has T staging as:

A. T1
B. T2
C. T3
D. T4

185. False statement among the following about cholangiocarcinoma is:

A. Surgical palliation has not been shown to prolong survival or but reduce complication rates
B. The goals of palliation should include relief of jaundice, alleviation of pain, and relief of duodenal obstruction, if necessary
C. Placement of a self-expandable metallic stent provides a durable solution
D. For distal cholangiocarcinomas, ERCP is the preferred route of nonoperative biliary drainage, whereas PTC is more useful for proximal lesions

ANSWERS

1. **Ans: D. 30%**

Ref: Chapter No.55, Page No.1489

2. **Ans: A. The left hepatic duct retains a shorter transverse extrahepatic portion and travels under the edge of segment IV before diving before joining the bifurcation**

Ref: Chapter No.55, Page No.1489

3. **Ans: C. The valves of Heister, which are folds of mucosa oriented in spiral pattern within the fundus of gallbladder, function to retain bile in the gallbladder until contraction in response to enteric stimulation**

Ref: Chapter No.55, Page No.1489

4. **Ans: C. The CBD ends in the 3rd portion of duodenum at the ampulla of Vater**

Ref: Chapter No.55, Page No.1489

5. **Ans: B. The blood supply of the common hepatic duct and CBD comes from the left hepatic and cystic artery**

Ref: Chapter No.55, Page No.1489-1490

6. **Ans: A. Cystic artery**

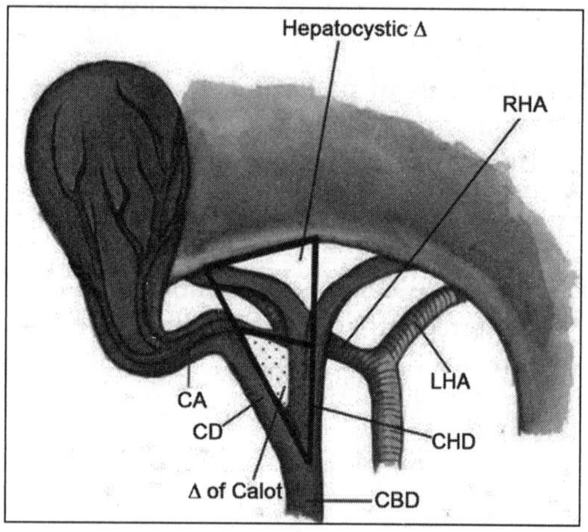

Ref: Chapter No.55, Page No.1490

7. **Ans: C. 20%**

Ref: Chapter No.55, Page No.1490

8. **Ans: B. Calot's node**

Ref: Chapter No.55, Page No.1490

9. **Ans: A. Cystic artery**

Ref: Chapter No.55, Page No.1490

10. **Ans: C. Anterosuperior pancreaticoduodenal artery**

Ref: Chapter No.55, Page No.1491

11. **Ans: C. A replaced right hepatic artery**

Ref: Chapter No.55, Page No.1490

12. **Ans: A. The blood supply to the supraduodenal bile duct has a longitudinal pattern**

The portion of the bile duct supplied by the ***longitudinal vessels*** receives most of its arterial blood supply from below, thus ***rendering the proximal portion of the duct subject to ischemia*** after injury or transection.

Ref: 1. Chari RS, Shah SA. Biliary system. In: Townsend CM, Beauchamp RD, Evers BM, et al., eds. Sabiston Textbook of Surgery: The Biological Basis of Modern Surgical Practice. 18th ed. Philadelphia: WB Saunders; 2008.

2. Mullholland MW, Lillemoe KD, Doherty GM, et al., eds. Greenfield's Surgery: Scientific Principles and Practice, Hepatobiliary and Portal Venous System Section. 4th ed. Philadelphia: Lippincott Williams & Wilkins; 2006.

3. Blumgart LH. Surgery of the Liver, Biliary Tract and Pancreas. 4th ed. Edinburgh: Churchill-Livingstone; 2006.

13. **Ans: D. Bile salts combine to form spherical pockets, known as micelles and the salts themselves provide osmotic activity**

The ***cations*** that are secreted into the biliary tree along with the ***bile salt anion*** provide the *osmotic load to draw water into the duct* and to increase flow to keep bile electrochemically neutral.

Ref: Chapter No.55, Page No.1491-1492

14. **Ans: B. Vitamin K absorption**

Ref: Chapter No.55, Page No.1492

15. **Ans: C. Active transport in the ileum**

Conjugated forms are absorbed by an ***active transport mechanism*** in the terminal ileum.

Ref: Chapter No.55, Page No.1492

16. **Ans: A. Deoxycholic acid**

The secondary bile acids ***deoxycholic acid*** and ***lithocholic acid*** are formed in the intestine as the result of bacterial enzyme activity.

Ref: Chapter No.55, Page No.1492

17. **Ans: C. > 25% of bile salts are lost each day in the stool**

Ref: Chapter No.55, Page No.1492

18. **Ans: D. After a cholecystectomy when the speed of the enterohepatic circulation of bile decreases**

Ref: Chapter No.55, Page No.1492

19. **Ans: B. 0.2–0.6 g/d**

Ref: Chapter No.55, Page No.1492

20. **Ans: D. Vagal activity also induces gallbladder emptying and is a more powerful stimulus to gallbladder contraction than CCK**

Ref: Chapter No.55, Page No.1493

21. **Ans: B. 2.5 mg/dL**

Ref: Chapter No.55, Page No.1493

22. **Ans: D. 5.0 mg/dL**

Ref: Chapter No.55, Page No.1493

23. **Ans: D. Most gallstones don't move with positional changes in the patient**

Ref: Chapter No.55, Page No.1493

24. **Ans: B. Cholelithiasis**

Sagittal ultrasound image of the gallbladder which demonstrates the typical appearance of a ***gallstone that is hyperechoic with posterior acoustic shadowing*** (arrow).

Ref: Chapter No.55, Page No.1493

25. **Ans: A. Cholecystitis**

Sagittal ultrasound image of the gallbladder which contains hyperechoic gallstones. There is ***gallbladder wall thickening (black arrow)*** and ***pericholecystic fluid (white arrow)*** consistent with ***acute calculous cholecystitis.***

Ref: Chapter No.55, Page No.1494

26. **Ans: C. Porcelain gallbladder**

Ultrasound image of porcelain gallbladder. The ***curvilinear sharp echogenic focus*** (arrow) combined with ***substantial posterior shadowing*** helps confirm this diagnosis.

Ref: Chapter No.55, Page No.1494

27. **Ans: A. As a nuclear medicine test, the test demonstrates physiologic flow and provides fine anatomic detail, but can't identify gallstones**

Ref: Chapter No.55, Page No.1494

28. **Ans: B. 2 hours**

Ref: Chapter No.55, Page No.1494

29. **Ans: B. Because most gallstones are radiographically hyperdense to bile, many will be distinguishable from bile**

Ref: Chapter No.55, Page No.1494-1495

30. **Ans: C. Percutaneous transhepatic cholangiography (PTC) is a non-invasive procedure used to evaluate the biliary tree**

Ref: Chapter No.55, Page No.1495

31. **Ans: B. 10%**

Ref: Chapter No.55, Page No.1495

32. **Ans: D. All of the above**

Ref: Chapter No.55, Page No.1496

33. **Ans: C. Elderly patient**

Ref: Chapter No.55, Page No.1496

34. **Ans: A. Demonstrating carcinomatosis**

Ref: Chapter No.55, Page No.1496

35. **Ans: B. Cholelithiasis**

Ref: Chapter No.55, Page No.1497

36. **Ans: C. 10% to 15% of the population**

Ref: Chapter No.55, Page No.1497

37. **Ans: B. Hemolytic diseases**

Ref: Chapter No.55, Page No.1497

38. **Ans: B. Brown stones**

Ref: Chapter No.55, Page No.1497

39. **Ans: B. Gallbladder hypermotility**

Ref: Chapter No.55, Page No.1497

40. **Ans: A. 50% to 60% of patients with asymptomatic stones will develop symptoms within 20 years**

Ref: Chapter No.55, Page No.1497

41. **Ans: A. 1%**

Ref: Chapter No.55, Page No.1497

42. **Ans: D. All of the above**

Ref: Chapter No.55, Page No.1498

43. **Ans: C. 20%**

Ref: Chapter No.55, Page No.1498

44. **Ans: C. 50%**

Ref: Chapter No.55, Page No.1498

45. **Ans: A. Recurrent attacks of biliary colic, with permanent occlusion of the cystic duct, can cause inflammation and scarring of the neck of the gallbladder and cystic duct**

Ref: Chapter No.55, Page No.1498

46. **Ans: C. 50%**

Ref: Chapter No.55, Page No.1498

47. **Ans: B. Bilirubin deconjugation**

Ref: Chapter No.55, Page No.1497

48. **Ans: D. Acoustic enhancement posterior to the structure**

The 3 ***sonographic criteria*** for gallstones are:

(1) The presence of a hyperechoic intraluminal focus
(2) ***Shadowing posterior*** to that focus
(3) Movement of the focus with changes in position of the patient

Ref: Chapter No.55, Page No.1493-1494

49. **Ans: D. All of the above**

Ref: Chapter No.55, Page No.1499

50. **Ans: C. AAST EGS categorizes acute cholecystitis into 3 grades**

Ref: Chapter No.55, Page No.1499

51. **Ans: D. Sensitivity of 85% and specificity of 95%**

Ref: Chapter No.55, Page No.1499

52. **Ans: D. All of the above**

Ref: Chapter No.55, Page No.1500

53. **Ans: C. 6 weeks**

Ref: Chapter No.55, Page No.1500

54. **Ans: D. All of the above**

Ref: Chapter No.55, Page No.1500

55. **Ans: A. CBD stones, or choledocholithiasis, are generally symptomatic, and are seen in up to 50% of patients undergoing biliary imaging**

Ref: Chapter No.55, Page No.1500

56. **Ans: C. 2 years**

Ref: Chapter No.55, Page No.1500

57. **Ans: A. 1% to 2% of patients**

Ref: Chapter No.55, Page No.1500

58. **Ans: A. Hypotension**

Ref: Chapter No.55, Page No.1500

59. **Ans: C. Leucocytosis**

Ref: Chapter No.55, Page No.1500

60. **Ans: C. Magnetic resonance cholangiopancreatography (MRCP), is sensitive (>80%) and specific (>90%) in identifying CBD stones**

Ref: Chapter No.55, Page No.1501

61. **Ans: A. >75% of patients during first procedure and in 90% with repeated ERCP**

Ref: Chapter No.55, Page No.1501

62. **Ans: B. < 5% to 8%**

Ref: Chapter No.55, Page No.1501

63. **Ans: D. All of the above**

Ref: Chapter No.55, Page No.1501

64. **Ans: D. All of the above**

Ref: Chapter No.55, Page No.1502

65. **Ans: D. Extrahepatic stones**

Ref: Chapter No.55, Page No.1502

66. **Ans: D. In most cases of gallstone pancreatitis, the pancreatitis is not self-limited**

Ref: Chapter No.55, Page No.1502

67. **Ans: B. The most common site for obstruction is in 4th part of duodenum**

Ref: Chapter No.55, Page No.1502

68. **Ans: B. Approximately 50% of patients have multiple large stones, so the remainder of the small intestine should be inspected**

Ref: Chapter No.55, Page No.1502

69. **Ans: C. < 10% of these patients improve with a cholecystostomy tube and interval cholecystectomy is always necessary**

Ref: Chapter No.55, Page No.1502-1503

70. **Ans: C. Short term use of total parenteral nutrition**

Ref: Chapter No.55, Page No.1503

71. **Ans: A. < 33% at 20 minutes**

Ref: Chapter No.55, Page No.1503

72. **Ans: D. < 65% of patients show improvement in symptoms after cholecystectomy**

Ref: Chapter No.55, Page No.1503

73. **Ans: C. 60% to 80%**

Ref: Chapter No.55, Page No.1503

74. **Ans: C. Risk factor includes acute pancreatitis**

Ref: Chapter No.55, Page No.1503

75. **Ans: C. > 12 mm**

Ref: Chapter No.55, Page No.1503

76. **Ans: B. > 40 mm Hg**

Ref: Chapter No.55, Page No.1503

77. **Ans: C. Approximately 50% of patients have elevated perinuclear antineutrophil cytoplasmic antibodies, and the severity of disease correlates to titer levels**

Ref: Chapter No.55, Page No.1503

78. **Ans: B. Ulcerative colitis**

Ref: Chapter No.55, Page No.1503

79. **Ans: D. All of the above**

Ref: Chapter No.55, Page No.1503-1504

80. **Ans: C. Surgical treatment options include biliary reconstruction in asymptomatic patients with focal extrahepatic disease in some cases (it is done *in symptomatic patients*)**

Ref: Chapter No.55, Page No.1504

81. **Ans: B. 10% to 30%**

Ref: Chapter No.55, Page No.1504

82. **Ans: D. Chronic pancreatitis can cause strictures in the intrapancreatic portion of CBD and are usually small (0.5–1 cm) with gradually tapered narrowing**

Ref: Chapter No.55, Page No.1504

83. **Ans: A. 0.1% to 1%**

Ref: Chapter No.55, Page No.1504

84. **Ans: D. All of the above**

Ref: Chapter No.55, Page No.1504

85. **Ans: B. Type I**

Obstruction of the bile duct from an inflammatory process is the *hallmark* of this syndrome.

	Type I	Type II	Type III	Type IV	Type V
Description	Impacted stone at cystic duct or gallbladder neck	Stone erodes	Fistula eroding 1/3 to 2/3 of CBD circumference	Fistula completely involves/obliterates CBD wall	Cholecystoenteric fistula + any type ± gallstone ileus
Cholecystobiliary fistula presence	No	Yes	Yes	Yes	Yes and no
Management	Partial or total cholecystectomy; CBD exploration not typically required	Cholecystectomy plus fistula closure (suture, T-tube or choledochoplasty)	Choledochoplasty or bilioenteric anastomosis depending on fistula	Bilioenteric anastomosis (typically choledocho-jejunostomy)	Cholecystectomy with excision of fistula

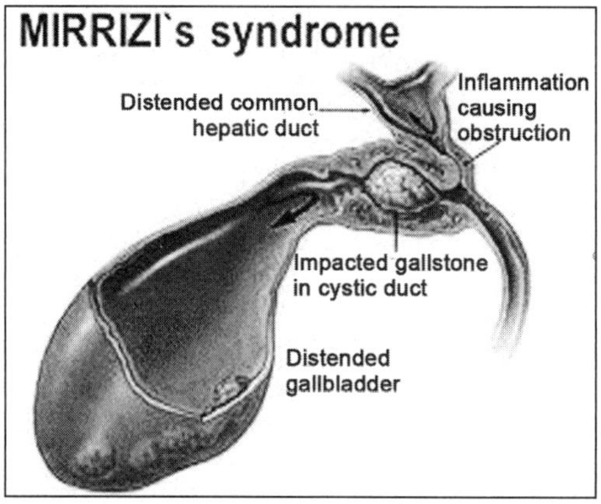

Ref: https://www.ncbi.nlm.nih.gov/books/NBK482491/#:~:text=Mirizzi%20syndrome%20is%20a%20rare,similar%20to%20symptoms%20of%20cholecystitis

86. Ans: B. Type II

Ref: Chapter No.55, Page No.1505

87. Ans: A. Type V

Ref: Chapter No.55, Page No.1505

88. Ans: C. Type III

Ref: Chapter No.55, Page No.1505

89. Ans: A. Type I

Ref: Chapter No.55, Page No.1505

90. Ans: C. It is not a premalignant condition

Ref: Chapter No.55, Page No.1504-1505

91. Ans: D. 90%

Ref: Chapter No.55, Page No.1505

92. Ans: D. The incidence of malignancy most commonly occurs in the 7th decade and almost exclusively occurring in types II and III

Ref: Chapter No.55, Page No.1505

93. Ans: B. 5% and 30%

Ref: Chapter No.55, Page No.1505

94. Ans: B. Type II cysts should be managed with ERCP

Ref: Chapter No.55, Page No.1505

95. Ans: D. All of the above

Ref: Chapter No.55, Page No.1506

96. Ans: B. 5%

Ref: Chapter No.55, Page No.1506

97. Ans: D. All of the above

Ref: Chapter No.55, Page No.1506

98. Ans: D. Eric Mühe

Ref: Chapter No.55, Page No.1506

99. Ans: C. Common hepatic artery

In the transverse plane, the structures of the hepatoduodenal ligament have a **"Mickey Mouse"** configuration.

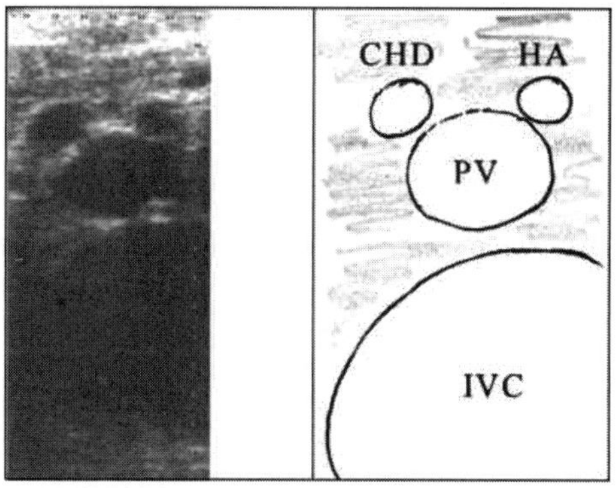

Ref: https://radiopaedia.org/articles/hepatoduodenal-ligament

100. Ans: D. All of the above

Ref: Chapter No.55, Page No.1506

101. Ans: A. Old age

Ref: Chapter No.55, Page No.1506

102. Ans: C. Palmer's point

Ref: Chapter No.55, Page No.1506

103. Ans: D. Make limited use of cholangiography or other methods to image the biliary tree intraoperatively

SAGES SAFE CHOLECYSTECTOMY PROGRAM

The following are ***6 suggested strategies*** surgeons can employ to adopt a universal culture of safety for cholecystectomy to and minimize the risk of bile duct injury.

1. Use the **Critical View of Safety (CVS)** method of identification of the cystic duct and cystic artery during laparoscopic cholecystectomy. **3 criteria** are required to achieve the CVS:
   - The ***hepatocystic triangle*** is cleared of fat and fibrous tissue. The hepatocystic triangle is defined as the triangle formed by the cystic duct, the common hepatic duct, and inferior edge of the liver. The common bile duct and common hepatic duct do not have to be exposed.
   - ***The lower one third of the gallbladder is separated from the liver to expose the cystic plate.*** The cystic plate is also known as liver bed of the gallbladder and lies in the gallbladder fossa.
   - ***Two and only two structures should be seen entering the gallbladder.***
   - Confirming the CVS – the CVS can be confirmed using a ***Doublet View***.
2. Understand the potential for ***aberrant anatomy in all cases***.
3. Make ***liberal use of cholangiography*** or other methods to image the biliary tree intraoperatively.
4. Consider an ***Intra-operative Momentary Pause*** during laparoscopic cholecystectomy ***prior to clipping, cutting or transecting any ductal structures***.
5. Recognize when the dissection is approaching a zone of significant risk and halt the dissection before entering the zone. Finish the operation by a safe method other than cholecystectomy if conditions around the gallbladder are too dangerous.
   - Consider ***laparoscopic subtotal cholecystectomy or cholecystostomy tube placement***, and/or ***conversion to an open procedure*** based on the judgment of the attending surgeon.
6. Get ***help from another surgeon*** when the dissection or conditions are difficult.

Ref: https://www.sages.org/safe-cholecystectomy-program

104. Ans: D. All of the above

Ref: Chapter No.55, Page No.1508

105. Ans: D. All of the above

Ref: Chapter No.55, Page No.1506

106. Ans: D. The downside of choledochojejunostomy is a process known as sump syndrome

Ref: Chapter No.55, Page No.1508-1509

107. Ans: B. 5 O'clock position

Ref: Chapter No.55, Page No.1509

108. Ans: C. Liberal use of choledochoscopy at the time of a drainage procedure ensures removal of all current stones and this approach allows a stone clearance rate of < 50%

Ref: Chapter No.55, Page No.1510

109. Ans: C. Choledochotomy approach is technically easier

Ref: Chapter No.55, Page No.1510

110. Ans: D. Recent myocardial infarction (MI) with severe coronary artery disease noted on cardiac catheterization, requiring full anticoagulation

Ref: Chapter No.55, Page No.1506

111. Ans: A. The CBD can be mistaken for the cystic duct when obtaining this view

The **infundibular technique** involves ***encircling the cystic duct and tracing it up to the characteristic funnel-shaped junction with the gallbladder.***

Ref: Strasberg SM, Hertl M, Soper NJ. An analysis of the problem of biliary injury during laparoscopic cholecystectomy. J Am Coll Surg. 1995;180: 101–125

112. Ans: C. Percutaneous cholecystostomy tube placement followed by cholecystectomy in 3 months

The patient presents with ***grade III (severe) cholecystitis*** as evidence by organ dysfunction (hypotension). The recommended initial treatment is percutaneous cholecystostomy tube placement.

Ref: Chapter No.55, Page No.1503
https://pubmed.ncbi.nlm.nih.gov/29045062/

113. Ans: C. Cholecystectomy within 72 hours of onset of symptoms

The patient in presents with ***grade I (mild) cholecystitis***, and cholecystectomy is recommended within 72 h since the onset of symptoms.

Ref: Chapter No.55, Page No.1500
https://pubmed.ncbi.nlm.nih.gov/29045062/

114. Ans: B. Immediate cholecystectomy

The patient presents with ***grade II (moderate) cholecystitis***; the recommended treatment is immediate cholecystectomy or biliary drainage if the patient is at a high surgical risk.

Ref: Chapter No.55, Page No.1500
https://pubmed.ncbi.nlm.nih.gov/29045062/

115. Ans: A. Early laparoscopic cholecystectomy

Ref: Chapter No.55, Page No.1500

116. Ans: B. The primary pathophysiologic feature involves gallbladder stasis

Ref: Chapter No.55, Page No.1502

117. Ans: D. Cholecystectomy

It is a case of **Emphysematous cholecystitis.**

Ref: Chapter No.55, Page No.1500

118. Ans: D. Both C and D

Ref: Chapter No.55, Page No.1508

119. Ans: D. Increased operative time

Ref: Chapter No.55, Page No.1506

120. Ans: B. Cholesterol polyp

Ref: Chapter No.55, Page No.1506

121. Ans: C. It is frequently > 1 cm

Ref: Chapter No.55, Page No.1506

122. Ans: D. Ileocecal valve

Ref: Chapter No.55, Page No.1502

123. Ans: C. Operative treatment involves enterotomy proximal to the site of obstruction

Ref: Chapter No.55, Page No.1502

124. Ans: A. Dilation can be performed via the transhepatic or endoscopic route

Ref: Chapter No.55, Page No.1504

125. Ans: D. Hepatic transplantation

Ref: Chapter No.55, Page No.1504

126. Ans: D. All of the above

Ref: Chapter No.55, Page No.1511

127. Ans: B. Strasberg's type B (Injury to a sectoral duct, causing obstruction of portion of the biliary system)

Ref: Chapter No.55, Page No.1511

128. Ans: A. Strasberg's type A (Injury to small ducts in continuity with the biliary system with a leak in the duct of Luschka or the cystic duct)

Ref: Chapter No.55, Page No.1511

129. Ans: B. Bismuth's type 2 (Bismuth type 4: destruction of the biliary confluence)

Ref: Chapter No.55, Page No.1511

130. Ans: D. Bismuth's type 4 (Bismuth type 4: destruction of the biliary confluence)

Ref: Chapter No.55, Page No.1511

131. Ans: C. Strasberg's type C (Injury to a sectoral duct with bile leak; leak from a duct not continuous with the biliary system)

Ref: Chapter No.55, Page No.1511

132. Ans: A. Bismuth's type 5

Ref: Chapter No.55, Page No.1511

133. Ans: C. Ducts smaller than 7 mm that by cholangiography drain only a single segment or subsegment of the liver and simple ligation may suffice for management

Ref: Chapter No.55, Page No.1511-1512

134. Ans: D. All of the above

Ref: Chapter No.55, Page No.1512

135. Ans: D. All of the above

Ref: Chapter No.55, Page No.1512

136. Ans: C. 20% or more

Ref: Chapter No.55, Page No.1512

137. Ans: B. An aberrant right hepatic duct

Ref: Chapter No.55, Page No.1511

138. Ans: D. 70%

Ref: Chapter No.55, Page No.1513

139. Ans: B. Patients will generally present within 1 month of cholecystectomy as the bile collects and becomes clinically manifested

Ref: Chapter No.55, Page No.1514

140. Ans: C. Lost stones necessitate conversion to an open operation

Ref: Chapter No.55, Page No.1514

141. Ans: B. 20% to 40%

Ref: Chapter No.55, Page No.1514

142. Ans: D. All of the above

Ref: Chapter No.55, Page No.1514

143. Ans: D. CT should be the first screening test and will commonly show dilation of the biliary tree

Ref: Chapter No.55, Page No.1515

144. Ans: C. < 50%

Ref: Chapter No.55, Page No.1515

145. Ans: B. Jaundice

Ref: Chapter No.55, Page No.1515

146. Ans: B. Endoscopic or percutaneous drainage achieves this goal with more morbidity than surgical intervention

Ref: Chapter No.55, Page No.1515

147. Ans: C. Recurrent pyogenic cholangitis tends to occur in the 5th to 6th decade of life, affecting men more than women

Ref: Chapter No.55, Page No.1515

148. Ans: B. In the setting of an acute attack surgical therapy is always needed

Ref: Chapter No.55, Page No.1515-1516

149. Ans: D. All of the above

Ref: Chapter No.55, Page No.1516

150. Ans: C. The type of stone correlates with incidence of gallbladder cancer; highest with brown stones

Ref: Chapter No.55, Page No.1516

151. Ans: B. < 10%

Ref: Chapter No.55, Page No.1516

152. Ans: C. A small subset of gallbladder cancers are of the papillary subtype and carry a poor prognosis

Ref: Chapter No.55, Page No.1516

153. Ans: D. All of the above

Ref: Chapter No.55, Page No.1516

154. Ans: C. 40%

Ref: Chapter No.55, Page No.1516

155. Ans: B. T2b

Ref: Chapter No.55, Page No.1517

156. Ans: D. T4

Ref: Chapter No.55, Page No.1517

157. Ans: C. T3

Ref: Chapter No.55, Page No.1517

158. Ans: C. T3

Ref: Chapter No.55, Page No.1517

159. Ans: C. T3

Ref: Chapter No.55, Page No.1517

160. Ans: A. T1b

Ref: Chapter No.55, Page No.1517

161. Ans: C. IVA

Ref: Chapter No.55, Page No.1517

162. Ans: D. All of the above

Ref: Chapter No.55, Page No.1517

163. Ans: A. Female sex

Ref: Chapter No.55, Page No.1518

164. Ans: B. >1 cm

Ref: Chapter No.55, Page No.1518

165. Ans: D. All of the above

Ref: Chapter No.55, Page No.1519

166. Ans: C. Direct extension of tumor into adjacent structures such as the hepatic flexure is a contraindication to resection

Ref: Chapter No.55, Page No.1519

167. Ans: D. All of the above

Ref: Chapter No.55, Page No.1519

168. Ans: B. < 3%

Ref: Chapter No.55, Page No.1518

169. Ans: B. Cholecystectomy

Ref: Chapter No.55, Page No.1518

170. Ans: C. Cholecystectomy is sufficient

Ref: Chapter No.55, Page No.1519

171. Ans: B. More than two thirds of all cholangiocarcinomas involve the distal biliary tree known as a Klatskin tumor

Ref: Chapter No.55, Page No.1519

172. Ans: A. Primary sclerosing cholangitis

Ref: Chapter No.55, Page No.1520

173. Ans: B. Cholangiocarcinoma causing obstruction at or below the hepatic bifurcation tends to be manifested at later stages than intrahepatic cholangiocarcinoma

Ref: Chapter No.55, Page No.1520

174. Ans: A. Tumor markers, including carcinoembryonic antigen and carbohydrate antigen 19-9, are reliable for diagnosis of cholangiocarcinoma

Ref: Chapter No.55, Page No.1520

175. Ans: A. More than 80% of patients undergoing exploration have historically had findings precluding resection, such as peritoneal metastases, hepatic metastases, or locally advanced lesions

Ref: Chapter No.55, Page No.1520-1524

176. Ans: D. Type IIIb

Ref: Chapter No.55, Page No.1524

177. Ans: B. Type II

Ref: Chapter No.55, Page No.1524

178. Ans: A. Type IV

Ref: Chapter No.55, Page No.1524

179. Ans: D. All of the above

Ref: Chapter No.55, Page No.1522

180. Ans: B. T2

Ref: Chapter No.55, Page No.1521

181. Ans: D. Stage IIIB

Ref: Chapter No.55, Page No.1521

182. Ans: C. T3

Ref: Chapter No.55, Page No.1522

183. Ans: D. T4

Ref: Chapter No.55, Page No.1523

184. Ans: B. T2

Ref: Chapter No.55, Page No.1523

185. Ans: A. Surgical palliation has not been shown to prolong survival or but reduce complication rates

Ref: Chapter No.55, Page No.1524

56

Exocrine Pancreas

ANATOMY

1. **Weight of pancreas is:**
   A. 25 – 50 g
   B. 50 – 75 g
   C. 75 – 125 g
   D. 125 – 200 g

2. **False about pancreas is:**
   A. The head lies to the right of midline within the C loop of the duodenum, immediately posterior to the inferior vena cava at the confluence of the renal vein
   B. The body and tail of the pancreas then extend across the midline, anterior to Gerota fascia and slightly cephalad, terminating within the splenic hilum
   C. It lies in the retroperitoneum just anterior to the first lumbar vertebra
   D. The uncinate process extends from the head of the pancreas behind the superior mesenteric vein (SMV) and terminates adjacent to the superior mesenteric artery (SMA)

3. **False about arterial blood supply of pancreas is:**
   A. The neck, body and tail receive arterial supply from the splenic arterial system
   B. The head and uncinate process are supplied by the pancreaticoduodenal arteries
   C. The superior pancreatic artery then runs along the inferior border of the pancreas, terminating at its tail
   D. Terminal branches of superior and inferior pancreaticoduodenal arteries join each other to form the arcade, which supplies the head and uncinate process of the pancreas and the duodenum

4. **False about venous drainage of pancreas is:**
   A. The body and tail are drained through the splenic venous system
   B. The anterior and posterior inferior pancreaticoduodenal veins enter the SMV along the superior border of the uncinate process
   C. The posterior superior pancreaticoduodenal vein enters the SMV laterally at the superior border of the neck of the pancreas
   D. Head of the pancreas draining into the anterior and posterior pancreaticoduodenal veins

EMBRYOLOGY

5. **The exocrine pancreas begins development during the ________ week of gestation.**
   A. 2nd
   B. 3rd
   C. 4th
   D. 5th

6. **False about embryology is:**
   A. The dorsal develops into the superior head, neck, body and tail of the mature pancreas
   B. Between the fourth and eighth weeks of gestation, the ventral bud rotates posteriorly in a clockwise fashion to fuse with the dorsal bud
   C. Dorsal and ventral buds appear from the mesoderm
   D. The ventral bud will become the inferior part of the head and uncinate process of the gland

7. **The major exocrine drainage pathway of the pancreas is:**
   A. Duct of Vater
   B. Duct of Wirsung
   C. Duct of Santorini
   D. None of the above

8. **Incidence in general population affected by pancreas divisum is:**
   A. 5%
   B. 10%
   C. 20%
   D. 25%

9. **Expression of Arx favors:**
   A. δ cell differentiation
   B. α/PP cell differentiation
   C. β cell differentiation
   D. All of the above

10. **Expression of Pax-4 favors:**
    A. β vs δ cell differentiation
    B. α/PP cell differentiation
    C. None
    D. All of the above

11. **Critical role in exocrine differentiation is:**
    A. Hedgehog B. PTF1
    C. Neurogenin 3 D. PDX1

12. **False about annular pancreas is:**
    A. Associated with other congenital defects, including Down syndrome, malrotation, intestinal atresia and cardiac malformations
    B. Annular pancreas results from aberrant migration of the ventral pancreas bud, which leads to circumferential or near-circumferential pancreas tissue surrounding the second portion of the duodenum
    C. If symptoms of obstruction occur, surgical bypass through duodenojejunostomy is performed instead of dividing the pancreatic tissue
    D. All of the above are true

13. **Treatment of asymptomatic adenocarcinoma arising in ectopic pancreas tissue is:**
    A. Chemotherapy
    B. Trimodality treatment
    C. Resection is not necessary
    D. Whipple's procedure

14. **Treatment of choice of annular pancreas is:**
    A. Duodenoduodenostomy
    B. Duodenojejunostomy
    C. Hepaticojejunostomy
    D. Pancreatojejunostomy

15. **Most common site of ectopic pancreas is:**
    A. Stomach
    B. Duodenum
    C. Meckel's diverticulum
    D. Jejunum

PHYSIOLOGY

16. **Acinar cells are responsible for ___ of exocrine pancreas.**
    A. 4% B. 85%
    C. 2% D. 10%

17. **Percentage of exocrine pancreas is composed of the epithelial duct system and blood vessels:**
    A. 4% B. 85%
    C. 2% D. 10%

18. **Pancreatic secretory tryps in inhibitor is encoded by:**
    A. SPINK1 gene B. PRSS1 gene
    C. SPINK2 gene D. PRSS2 gene

19. **The optimal pH for the function of chymotrypsin and trypsin is:**
    A. 7.0 to 8.0 B. 6.0 to 8.0
    C. 8.5 to 10.0 D. 8.0 to 9.0

20. **The optimal pH for the function of amylase is:**
    A. 8.0 B. 7.0
    C. 6.0 D. 9.0

21. **The optimal pH for the function of lipase is:**
    A. 7.0 to 7.5 B. 7.0 to 9.0
    C. 6.0 to 7.0 D. 7.0

22. **Cephalic phase in pancreatic secretion is responsible for _______ of daily secretion.**
    A. 10% B. 20% to 25%
    C. 40% to 60% D. 65% to 70%

23. **The most important phase of pancreatic secretion is the:**
    A. Intestinal phase B. Cephalic phase
    C. Gastric phase D. All of the above

24. **Intestinal phase in pancreatic secretion is responsible for ________ of daily secretion.**
    A. 10% B. 20% to 25%
    C. 40% to 60% D. 65% to 70%

25. **Intestinal phase in pancreatic secretion is mediated by:**
    A. Vagovagal reflex B. Acetylcholine
    C. Secretin and CCK D. All of the above

26. **Gastric phase in pancreatic secretion is mediated by:**

A. Vagovagal reflex
B. Acetylcholine
C. Secretin and CCK
D. All of the above

27. Gastric phase in pancreatic secretion is responsible for _______ of daily secretion.

A. 10%
B. 20% to 25%
C. 40% to 60%
D. 65% to 70%

28. Effect exerted by CCK is all except:

A. CCK induces the relaxation of the sphincter of Oddi
B. CCK potentiates the effects of secretin but not vice versa
C. CCK travels through the bloodstream and induces the release of pancreatic enzymes by acinar cells
D. CCK induces local duodenal vagovagal reflexes that cause the release of acetylcholine, vasoactive intestinal peptide and gastrin-releasing peptide, which promotes the release of pancreatic enzymes

29. CCK is released by:

A. B cells
B. D cells
C. I cells
D. A cells

ACUTE PANCREATITIS

30. False about acute pancreatitis is:

A. 10% to 20% of patients have a rapidly progressive inflammatory response associated with prolonged length of hospital stay and significant morbidity and mortality
B. The highest mortality rates in this group of patients are those who present with multiple organ dysfunction syndrome
C. Most patients develop a severe course
D. Patients with mild pancreatitis have a mortality rate of less than 1%, but in severe pancreatitis, this increases up to 10% to 50%

31. Mortality after late phase is often caused by:

A. Vascular complications
B. Cardiac complications
C. Renal complications
D. Septic complications

32. False about pathophysiology of acute pancreatitis is:

A. It is the cytosolic cathepsin B that then induces apoptosis or necrosis, leading to acinar cell death
B. The inflammatory cascade is self-limited in approximately 80% to 90% of patients
C. Immunolocalization studies have shown that after 15 minutes of pancreatic injury, both zymogen granules and lysosomes colocalize inside the acinar cells
D. The mortality seen in the early phase of pancreatitis is the result of this multiorgan failure

33. Most common cause of acute pancreatitis is:

A. Gallstones
B. Alcohol
C. Blunt abdominal trauma
D. Autoimmune

34. In pediatric patients most common cause of acute pancreatitis is:

A. Gallstones
B. Alcohol
C. Blunt abdominal trauma
D. Autoimmune

35. The overall incidence of acute pancreatitis in patients with symptomatic gallstone disease is:

A. 1%
B. 5%
C. 15%
D. 25%

36. False about biliary pancreatitis is:

A. It is seen more frequently in men between 50 and 70 years of age
B. Obstructive theory: pancreatic injury is the result of excessive pressure inside the pancreatic duct
C. The overall incidence of AP in patients with symptomatic gallstone disease is 3% to 8%
D. Common channel theory: proposes that stones become impacted in the ampulla of Vater and form a common channel that allows bile salt reflux into the pancreas

37. 2nd most common cause of acute pancreatitis is:

A. Gallstones
B. Alcohol
C. Blunt abdominal trauma
D. Autoimmune

38. False about alcohol induced acute pancreatitis is:

A. Compared with non-smokers, the relative risk of alcohol-induced pancreatitis in smokers is 4.9

B. It accounts for 35% of cases and is more prevalent in young men - 30–45 years of age
C. Heavy ethanol abuse (>100 g/day for at least 5 years), smoking and genetic predisposition are risk factors
D. Only 50% to 60% of patients who drink alcohol develop acute pancreatitis

39. Alcohol's deleterious effects in the pancreas and its mechanism of injury is all except:

A. Impaired pancreatic cell repair due to dysregulation in developmental factors PDX1, PTF1a and Notch
B. Trigger proinflammatory pathways via upregulation of nuclear factor κB (NF-κB), TNF-α and IL-1
C. Increased autophagy possibly due to dysregulation of cathepsin L and B
D. A shift in cell death caused by apoptosis to necrosis by increase in caspase 3/8 activity

40. Most common complication after ERCP is:

A. Duodenal perforation
B. Acute pancreatitis
C. Bile duct injury
D. Cholangitis

41. Incidence of acute pancreatitis after ERCP is:

A. 2% B. 5%
C. 10% D. 12%

42. False about acute pancreatitis after ERCP is:

A. The incidence of this complication after ERCP could be as high as 15% in high-risk patients
B. AP occurs more frequently in patients who have undergone therapeutic procedures compared with diagnostic procedures
C. To prevent ERCP-induced pancreatitis, use indomethacin
D. The clinical course is moderate to severe in 20% to 25% of patients

43. Post ERCP pancreatitis is more common in all except:

A. Young individuals
B. Female patients
C. Elderly male
D. Patients with prior history of ERCP induced pancreatitis

44. The common agents causing acute pancreatitis is/are:

A. Metronidazole B. Valproic acid
C. Sulfonamides D. All of the above

45. Triglyceride levels that can acute pancreatitis are:

A. >100 mg/dL B. >200 mg/dL
C. >500 mg/dL D. >1000 mg/dL

46. False about acute pancreatitis and hypertriglyceridemia/hypercalcemia is:

A. Hypercalcemia is postulated to induce pancreatic injury through the activation of trypsinogen to trypsin and intraductal precipitation of calcium
B. Hypertriglyceridemia secondary to hypothyroidism, diabetes mellitus, and alcohol induces acute pancreatitis
C. A triglyceride level higher than 2000 mg/dL confirms the diagnosis
D. It is more common in patients with type I, II or V hyperlipidemia

47. False about clinical manifestation of acute pancreatitis is:

A. 50% of patients have nausea or vomiting that typically relieves the pain
B. Significant abdominal distention associated with generalized rebound and abdominal rigidity is present in severe pancreatitis
C. The cardinal symptom of AP is epigastric or periumbilical pain that radiates to the back
D. Dehydration, poor skin turgor, tachycardia, hypotension and dry mucous membranes are commonly seen in patients with acute pancreatitis

48. The serum half-life of amylase is:

A. 3 hours B. 6 hours
C. 10 hours D. 18 hours

49. Levels of amylase normalise after:

A. 1–2 days B. 3–5 days
C. 5–8 days D. 8–14 days

50. Levels of lipase normalise after:

A. 1–2 days B. 3–5 days
C. 5–8 days D. 8–14 days

51. The diagnosis of AP includes:

A. Abdominal pain consistent with AP (acute onset of a persistent, severe, epigastric pain often radiating to the back
B. Characteristics findings of pancreatitis by imaging

C. 3X or higher elevation of serum amylase or lipase levels above the upper laboratory limit of normal
D. All of the above

52. In the diagnosis of acute biliary pancreatitis the elevation of alanine aminotransferase levels in the serum in the context of AP confirmed by high pancreatic enzyme levels has a positive predictive value of:

A. 75% B. 80%
C. 90% D. 95%

53. False about imaging in acute pancreatitis is:

A. In the setting of gallstone pancreatitis, endoscopic ultrasound (EUS) may play an important role in the evaluation of persistent choledocholithiasis
B. Contrast-enhanced computed tomography (CT) is currently the best modality for evaluation of the pancreas
C. MRI is also useful to evaluate the extent of necrosis, inflammation and presence of free fluid
D. In patients in whom persistent choledocholithiasis is confirmed by EUS, ERCP is needed for confirmation

54. Indications for CT in acute pancreatitis includes all except:

A. Failure to respond to conservative treatment
B. Diagnostic uncertainty
C. Clinical deterioration
D. Every patient at admission

55. Which of the following is not seen in Ranson's prognostic criteria for gallstone pancreatitis?

A. Base deficit >5 mEq/L
B. Aspartate aminotransferase level >250 IU/L
C. PaO_2 <60 mm Hg
D. Blood glucose level >220 mg/dL

56. Which of the following is not seen in Ranson's prognostic criteria for gallstone pancreatitis?

A. Age >55 years
B. White blood cell count >18,000 cells/mm^3
C. Hematocrit: decrease >10%
D. Serum calcium level

57. Which of the following is not seen in Ranson's prognostic criteria for non-gallstone pancreatitis?

A. Lactate dehydrogenase level >350 IU/L
B. Base deficit >4 mEq/L
C. Blood urea nitrogen level: increase >2 mg/dL
D. Blood glucose level >200 mg/dL

58. Severe pancreatitis has a Ranson score of:

A. ≥2 B. ≥3
C. ≥4 D. ≥5

59. False among the following is:

A. The Ranson score has a low positive predictive value (50%) and high negative predictive value (90%)
B. APACHE II has a positive predictive value of 43% and a negative predictive value of 89%
C. CRP level are measured within 48 hours after the onset of symptoms and not at admission
D. Mild pancreatitis can have organ failure lasting less than 48 hours

60. False about severe pancreatitis is:

A. An APACHE II score of ≥8 defines severe pancreatitis
B. Ranson score ≥3 defines severe pancreatitis
C. A CRP level of 150 mg/mL or higher defines severe pancreatitis
D. Severe pancreatitis is characterized by organ failure lasting beyond 24 hours

61. Computed Tomography Severity Index (CTSI) of a pancreatic lesion with Single fluid collection and 30%–50% pancreatic necrosis is:

A. 5 B. 6
C. 7 D. 8

62. Computed Tomography Severity Index (CTSI) of a pancreatic lesion with presence of gas and 70% pancreatic necrosis is:

A. 7 B. 8
C. 9 D. 10

63. Computed Tomography Severity Index (CTSI) of a pancreatic lesion with peripancreatic fat inflammatory changes and 25% pancreatic necrosis is:

A. 3 B. 4
C. 5 D. 7

64. CTSI of 5 has mortality rate of:

A. 3% B. 6%
C. 17% D. 35%

65. Not a criteria of systemic inflammatory response syndrome (SIRS) is:

A. Temperature >38.3°C
B. Respiratory rate of >20 breaths/min
C. Heart rate: >100 beats/min
D. WBC count of <4,000 cells/mL

66. C-reactive protein (CRP) is an inflammatory marker that peaks:

A. 12 - 24 hours B. 24 - 48 hours
C. 48 - 72 hours D. 72 - 96 hours

67. Organ Failure, as defined by Atlanta criteria for acute pancreatitis is all except:

A. Shock (systolic blood pressure <90 mm Hg)
B. Gastrointestinal bleeding (>500 mL/24 hours)
C. Pulmonary insufficiency (PaO_2 <60 mm Hg)
D. Renal failure (creatinine level >2 mg/dL before fluid resuscitation)

68. Not a criteria of systemic complication as defined by Atlanta criteria for acute pancreatitis is:

A. Fibrinogen <1 g/liter
B. Calcium level ≤7.5 mg/dL
C. Fibrin split products >80 μg/dL
D. Platelet count ≤50,000

69. False about treatment of acute pancreatitis is:

A. 5% DNS may be the best fluid for initial resuscitation
B. Patients should receive supplementary oxygen to maintain arterial saturation above 95%
C. Narcotics are usually preferred, especially morphine
D. Patients with AP require continuous pulse oximetry

70. False among the following about ERCP is:

A. ERCP is only indicated for patients who develop cholangitis and those with persistent bile duct obstruction demonstrated by other imaging modalities
B. Routine use of ERCP is not indicated for patients with mild pancreatitis because the bile duct obstruction is usually transient and resolves within 48 hours after the onset of symptoms
C. ERCP with sphincterotomy is a safe alternative to prevent recurrent biliary pancreatitis
D. All of the above are true

71. In the absence of definitive treatment, percentage of patients with acute biliary pancreatitis will have recurrent disease is:

A. 5% B. 10%
C. 30% D. 50%

72. The presence of acute peripancreatic fluids collection during an episode of acute pancreatitis has been described in:

A. 10% to 15% of patients
B. 20% to 30% of patients
C. 30% to 55% of patients
D. 60% to 75% of patients

73. False about peripancreatic fluid collections is:

A. Acute decompensation or failure to improve after 10 to 14 days may suggest infection and consideration should be given to CT-guided fluid sampling
B. In contrast to pseudocysts and cystic neoplasia of the pancreas, fluid collections are not surrounded or encased by epithelium or fibrotic capsule
C. Drainage (percutaneous or endoscopic) and IV administration of antibiotics should be instituted if infection is present
D. Acute peripancreatic fluids collections are simple in nature and after 6 weeks are referred to as a pseudocyst

74. Antibiotics known to penetrate pancreatic necrosis include:

A. Metronidazole B. Carbapenems
C. Macrolides D. Quinolones

75. False about Pancreatic Necrosis and Infected Necrosis is:

A. Infected necrotic collection should be suspected in patients with prolonged fever, elevated white blood cell count, or progressive clinical deterioration
B. Infection of acute necrotic collection is associated with bacterial translocation usually involving enteric flora
C. Contrast-enhanced CT is the most reliable technique to diagnose acute necrotic collection
D. Acute necrotic collection typically seen as areas of low attenuation (>40–50 HU) after the IV injection of contrast material

76. No. of patients with acute pancreatitis who develop acute necrotic collection is:

A. 10% B. 20%
C. 30% D. 50%

77. The main complication of acute necrotic collection is:

A. Colonic perforation B. Bleeding
C. Infection D. Pancreatic fistula

78. Indications for intervening in sterile necrotizing pancreatitis includes all except:

A. Failure to improve clinically with conservative management
B. Intermittent pain
C. Symptomatic biliary obstruction
D. Enteric obstruction

79. False about pathophysiology of pancreatic necrosis infection is:

A. Transient episodes of bacteremia are associated with pancreatic necrosis infection
B. The acute inflammatory injury that occurs during the first 48 to 72 hours causes mucosal ischemia and reperfusion injury
C. Local contamination after interventional procedures such as endoscopic retrograde cholangiopancreatography is not responsible for necrosis infection
D. Mucosal ischemia also produces an increase in the permeability of intestinal cells, which is initiated 72 hours after the acute episode but typically peaks one week later

80. The overall mortality rate after open necrosectomy is:

A. 10% to 15% B. 15% to 20%
C. 25% to 30% D. 40% to 50%

81. In patients who have peripancreatic fluid collections after acute pancreatitis, pancreatic pseudocysts occur in:

A. 1% - 5% B. 5% - 15%
C. 20% - 30% D. 30% - 50%

82. False about pancreatic pseudocyst is:

A. The fibrotic reaction typically requires at least 4 to 8 weeks to develop
B. Up to 10% of patients with pancreatic pseudocysts will develop symptoms
C. The capsule of a pseudocyst is composed of collagen and granulation tissue, and it is not lined by epithelium
D. Characteristic features of pancreatic pseudocysts include high amylase levels associated with the absence of mucin and low carcinoembryonic antigen (CEA) levels

83. Spontaneous regression after pseudocyst formation after acute pancreatitis is:

A. 10% B. 30%
C. 50% D. 70%

84. Spontaneous regression after pseudocyst formation after acute pancreatitis is not seen in:

A. No evidence of pancreatic duct obstruction
B. Located in the tail
C. Pseudocysts smaller than 4 cm in diameter
D. Communication with the main pancreatic duct

85. False about the treatment of pseudocyst after acute pancreatitis is:

A. Pancreatic pseudocysts located in the tail of the pancreas that are in close contact with the duodenum are treated with a cystoduodenostomy
B. After initial resolution, pseudocyst formation may recur in up to 12% of cases during long-term follow-up
C. Pancreatic pseudocysts closely attached to the stomach should be treated with a cystogastrostomy
D. Surgical cyst enterostomy is successful in achieving immediate cyst drainage in more than 90% of cases

86. Complications of pancreatic pseudocysts includes:

A. Rupture into the abdominal cavity
B. Pancreatic-pleural fistula
C. Bile duct and duodenal obstruction
D. All of the above

87. False about pancreatic ascites is:

A. Suspected in patients who have an episode of AP, who develop significant abdominal distention and have free intraabdominal fluid
B. Treatment consists of abdominal drainage combined with endoscopic placement of a pancreatic stent across the disruption
C. Failure of abdominal drainage therapy requires surgical treatment; it consists of distal resection and closure of the proximal stump
D. Diagnostic paracentesis typically demonstrates normal amylase and lipase levels

88. False about pancreatic-pleural fistula is:

A. Symptoms that suggest this condition include dyspnea, abdominal pain, cough, and chest pain

B. It is more common after alcoholic pancreatitis and in 70% of patients is associated with pancreatic pseudocysts
C. Amylase levels above 10,000 IU in the pleural fluid confirm the diagnosis
D. Initial treatment requires chest drainage, parenteral nutritional support, and administration of octreotide and up to 60% of patients respond to this therapy

89. Pseudoaneurysm formation as a vascular complication after acute pancreatitis is seen in:

A. SMA
B. Splenic artery
C. Gastroduodenal artery
D. Cystic artery

90. Most common vessel to have vascular thrombosis after acute pancreatitis is:

A. Splenic artery
B. Splenic vein
C. Renal vein
D. Right gastric artery

CHRONIC PANCREATITIS

91. False statement among the following is:

A. 30% to 70% of heavy drinkers develop chronic pancreatitis
B. The histologic hallmark of chronic pancreatitis is the persistent inflammation and irreversible fibrosis associated with atrophy of the pancreatic parenchyma
C. Prolonged alcohol abuse is the most important risk factor associated with chronic pancreatitis
D. In up to 20% of patients, a clear cause cannot be documented and cases are considered to be idiopathic

92. The most common cause of chronic pancreatitis is:

A. Gallstones
B. Alcohol
C. Autoimmune
D. Viral infection

93. True about alcohol's effect on pancreas is:

A. Increases glycoprotein 2 secretion in pancreatic juice
B. Increases the total protein concentration in the pancreatic juice
C. Promotes the synthesis and secretion of lithostathine by acinar cells
D. All of the above

94. True about alcohol's effect on pancreas is:

A. It has also been shown that alcohol and some of its metabolites (e.g., acetaldehyde) cause activation of PSCs
B. Acetaldehyde, another alcohol metabolite, causes direct acinar injury
C. Chronic alcohol consumption is associated with enhanced NF-κB activity, decreased perfusion in the microcirculation of the pancreas, and increased intracellular calcium levels
D. All of the above

95. False about smoking and chronic pancreatitis is:

A. Smoking increases the risk of alcohol-induced chronic pancreatitis
B. The risk of pancreatic calcifications and diabetes mellitus is not increased in patients who smoke compared with non-smokers
C. Active smokers develop chronic pancreatitis at a younger age compared with non-smokers
D. All of the above are true

96. PRSS1 is located on:

A. Chromosome 3
B. Chromosome 5
C. Chromosome 7
D. Chromosome 11

97. False about gene mutations and chronic pancreatitis is:

A. PRSS1 mutations have been documented in hereditary pancreatitis but are uncommon in other forms of chronic pancreatitis
B. Mutations in the cationic trypsinogen gene, also known as protease serine 1 (PRSS1) gene, are common in hereditary chronic pancreatitis
C. SPINK1 mutations are present in 10% to 20% of healthy patients
D. Mutation in human chymotrypsin C gene has been found to be associated with development of chronic pancreatitis

98. SPINK1 mutations are more prevalent in all except:

A. Hereditary pancreatitis
B. Alcoholic pancreatitis
C. Idiopathic pancreatitis
D. Tropical pancreatitis

99. Most common type of autoimmune pancreatitis is:

A. Type 1
B. Type 2
C. Type 3
D. Type 4

100. False about autoimmune pancreatitis is:

A. Type 2, a pancreatic specific disorder, not associated with immunoglobulin G4

B. In type 2, the pancreas is infiltrated by neutrophils, lymphocytes and plasma cells that destroy and obliterate the epithelium in the pancreatic duct
C. Type 1, which is the pancreatic manifestation of an immunoglobulin G4-related disease
D. Autoimmune pancreatitis is more common in women than in men

101. Type 1 autoimmune pancreatitis is characterized by all except:

A. Dense, periductal lymphoplasmacytic infiltrates
B. Obliterative endarteritis
C. Storiform fibrosis
D. Obliterative venulitis

102. Cassava ingestion is associated with:

A. Alcoholic pancreatitis
B. Idiopathic pancreatitis
C. Tropical pancreatitis
D. Autoimmune pancreatitis

103. Tropical pancreatitis is associated with:

A. Cassava ingestion B. SPINK1 mutation
C. PRSS1 mutation D. Both A and B

104. SPINK1 mutations is present with tropical pancreatitis in ______ of patients.

A. 5% to 10% B. 25% to 40%
C. 45% to 50% D. 50% to 70%

105. False about clinical manifestation of chronic pancreatitis is:

A. In severe cases, diseases associated with fat-soluble vitamin deficiency, such as bleeding, osteopenia and osteoporosis, can develop
B. At least 50% of the gland needs to be dysfunctional before steatorrhea, diarrhea and other symptoms of malabsorption develop
C. Exocrine insufficiency occurs in 80% to 90% of patients with long-standing chronic pancreatitis
D. Pain is the primary manifestation of chronic pancreatitis

106. No. of patients with chronic pancreatitis who will have clinical manifestations of diabetes mellitus is:

A. 10% - 20% B. 30% - 50%
C. 40% - 80% D. 80% - 90%

107. No. of patients in chronic pancreatitis have Jaundice or cholangitis is:

A. 5% to 10% B. 10% - 20%
C. 30% - 50% D. 40% - 80%

108. The most common CT findings in chronic pancreatitis is:

A. Pancreatic calcifications
B. Dilated pancreatic duct
C. Parenchymal atrophy
D. Pseudocyst

109. False about imaging and diagnosis of chronic pancreatitis is:

A. MRCP with secretin injection is particularly useful to evaluate intraductal strictures and pancreatic duct disruption
B. CT has a sensitivity of 55% to 85% and a specificity of 70% to 80% for the diagnosis of chronic pancreatitis
C. ERCP should be considered a therapeutic modality in patients who develop pancreatic duct complications amenable to endoscopic therapy
D. Histologic evidence of inflammation, atrophy and fibrosis is the gold standard for the diagnosis of chronic pancreatitis

110. The most accurate technique to diagnose chronic pancreatitis in patients with minimal change disease or in the early stages is:

A. CT scan B. MRI
C. EUS D. USG

111. As per Rosemont's consensus consistent diagnosis of chronic pancreatitis is done by all except:

A. 1 major A criterion + major B criterion
B. 1 major A criterion + $\geq$2 or more minor criteria
C. 2 major A criteria
D. All of the above can be used

112. Minor Criteria as per Rosemont's consensus and parenchymal features is all except:

A. Hyperechoic, nonshadowing foci $\geq$3 mm in length and width
B. Lobularity including three or more non-contiguous lobules in the head
C. Pancreatic cysts $\geq$2 mm in short axis
D. At least three strands

113. The diagnosis of steatorrhea is established when the stool fat content exceeds:

A. 3 g/day B. 5 g/day
C. 7 g/day D. 9 g/day

114. The diagnosis of severe pancreatic exocrine insufficiency is established when fecal elastase 1 concentration below:

A. 400 μg/g B. 300 μg/g
C. 200 μg/g D. 100 μg/g

115. The diagnosis of pancreatic exocrine insufficiency is established when fecal elastase 1 concentration below:

A. 400 μg/g B. 300 μg/g
C. 200 μg/g D. 100 μg/g

116. False among the following is:

A. Moderate to severe pain that does not respond to non-steroidal anti-inflammatory drugs should be treated with tramadol
B. Nonsteroidal anti-inflammatory drugs are the first line of treatment
C. For patients with unrelenting pain, celiac neurolysis has been attempted with sustained success in those with chronic pancreatitis
D. All of the above are true

117. False about endoscopic treatment in chronic pancreatitis is:

A. Extracorporeal shock wave lithotripsy followed by therapeutic ERCP may be required for the treatment of large impacted stones
B. ERCP is the primary modality for treating symptomatic pancreatic duct obstruction with dilation and polyethylene stent placement
C. Biliary obstruction caused by chronic pancreatitis occurs in 10% of patients and is best treated with endoscopic treatment
D. Endoscopic stone extraction should be considered for patients with pain and pancreatic duct dilation secondary to stones

118. Dilated pancreatic duct is defined as diameter >7 mm:

A. >5 mm B. >7 mm
C. >9 mm D. >11 mm

119. Pancreatic duct dilation secondary to duct stones when accompanied by intractable pain, the condition is best treated with:

A. Frey's procedure B. Puestow procedure
C. Whipple's procedure D. Berger's procedure

120. The modified Puestow procedure provides palliation of pain in ______ of cases.

A. 20% B. 40%
C. 60% D. 80%

121. In focal inflammatory mass in pancreas without significant dilation of the pancreatic duct, once malignant disease is ruled out with percutaneous or EUS biopsy, treatment is by:

A. Pancreaticoduodenectomy
B. Duodenum-preserving pancreatic head resection
C. Lateral pancreaticojejunostomy
D. Longitudinal pancreaticojejunostomy

122. Duodenum-preserving pancreatic head resection is also known as:

A. Frey's procedure
B. Puestow procedure
C. Whipple's procedure
D. Berger's procedure

123. Diffuse glandular involvement without dilation of the pancreatic duct is treated by:

A. Lateral pancreaticojejunostomy
B. Longitudinal pancreaticojejunostomy
C. Total pancreatectomy
D. Duodenum-preserving pancreatic head resection

124. False about the management of biliary strictures is:

A. Significant biliary obstruction occurs in 20% of patients
B. IV fluid and antibiotic therapy and temporary bile duct decompression with plastic stents is indicated for patients who present with cholangitis
C. Pancreaticoduodenectomy is indicated for patients in whom malignant disease cannot be excluded before surgery
D. Chronic scarring and fibrosis of the head of the pancreas result in external compression of the intrapancreatic portion of the common bile duct

125. Incidence of pseudocyst of pancreas after chronic pancreatitis is:

A. 5% to 10% B. 15% to 30%
C. 30% to 40% D. 50% to 70%

126. Spontaneous pancreatic pseudocyst regression after chronic pancreatitis is seen in:

A. 5% B. 10%
C. 30% D. 70%

CYSTIC NEOPLASMS OF THE PANCREAS

127. Serous cystic neoplasms (SCNs) have a predilection for:

A. Head of the pancreas
B. Tail of the pancreas
C. Body of the pancreas
D. Neck of the pancreas

128. False about Serous cystic neoplasms (SCNs) is:

A. On gross inspection, SCNs are small, poorly circumscribed masses
B. Central calcification, with radiating septa giving the sunburst appearance, is a radiographic sign on CT in 10% to 20% of patients
C. Patients commonly present with vague abdominal pain and less frequently with weight loss and obstructive jaundice
D. More common in females

129. False about management of Serous cystic neoplasms (SCNs) is:

A. In select patients with large (>4 cm) or rapidly growing lesions, resection of an SCN is appropriate
B. Patients with a tumor smaller than 4 cm are more likely to be symptomatic
C. Serous cystic tumors are generally considered benign, pancreatectomy is suggested when the diagnosis of malignant disease is uncertain or in symptomatic serous cystadenomas
D. Microscopic examination reveals multiloculated, glycogen-rich small cysts

130. False about mucinous cystic neoplasms (MCNs) is:

A. MCNs contain mucin-producing epithelium and are identified histologically by the presence of mucin-rich cells and ovarian-like stroma surrounding the cyst
B. Frequently seen in elderly men
C. These tumors span the histologic spectrum from benign to invasive carcinomas
D. Staining for estrogen and progesterone is positive in most cases

131. False about management of mucinous cystic neoplasms (MCNs) is:

A. Fluid analyses provide accurate diagnosis in up to 40% of cases
B. Pancreatic resection is the standard treatment for MCNs
C. FNA with cyst fluid analysis of MCNs demonstrates mucin-rich aspirate, high CEA levels (>192 ng/mL) and low amylase
D. The radiologic characteristic of an MCN on a CT scan is the presence of a solitary cyst, which may have fine septations and be surrounded by a rim of calcification

132. All of the following are suggestive of malignancy on cross-sectional imaging except:

A. Presence of eggshell calcification
B. Larger tumor size
C. Mural nodule
D. All of the above

133. No of patients with mucinous cystic neoplasms (MCNs) with history of pancreatitis is:

A. 5%
B. 10%
C. 20%
D. 40%

134. False about Intraductal Papillary Mucinous Neoplasm (IPMNs) is:

A. Neoplasia that affects only the small side branches is termed side branch or branch duct IPMN (BD-IPMN)
B. Involvement of the main pancreatic duct is termed main duct IPMN
C. IPMNs of the pancreas are mucinous epithelial neoplasms, which arise from the main pancreatic ducts or branch ducts or both
D. All of the above are true

135. Worrisome features of IPMN is all except:

A. Lymphadenopathy
B. Main duct 5–9 mm
C. Pancreatitis
D. Enhancing mural nodule >5 mm

136. High risk features of IPMN is all except:

A. Jaundice
B. Main duct >1 cm
C. BD-IPMN >3 cm
D. Enhancing mural nodule >5 mm

137. False about Branched Duct-IPMN is:

A. All cysts with worrisome features on CT or MRI should undergo EUS
B. Asymptomatic patients with cysts larger than 3 cm should be strongly considered for surgical resection
C. All cysts with high-risk features should be resected

D. Cysts smaller than 3 cm generally have a low risk for malignancy and therefor are most appropriate for surveillance

138. The risk of invasive malignant disease in the setting of BD-IPMN is approximately:

A. 2% to 3%
B. 10% to 15%
C. 30% to 50%
D. 50% to 70%

139. The risk of invasive malignant disease in the setting of MD-IPMN is approximately:

A. 2% to 3%
B. 10% to 15%
C. 30% to 50%
D. 50% to 70%

140. False about Main Duct-IPMN is:

A. Current guidelines suggest that main duct dilation of more than 5 mm is consistent with a diagnosis of MD-IPMN
B. Elevation of the CEA level is predictive of invasive malignant disease
C. Surgical resection is the cornerstone of treatment
D. Thick mucinous secretions can be seen oozing from a patulous papilla on endoscopic evaluation

141. False about the treatment of IPMN is:

A. For MD-IPMN in the absence of diffuse polyps or enhancing nodules in the main duct, total pancreatectomy is preferred
B. In BD-IPMN, resection should target the lesion of concern
C. Following resection, surveillance of the remnant pancreas is advocated due to risk of recurrence of IPMN or invasive malignancy
D. Survival outcomes are significantly better in patients with IPMNs than in patients with pancreatic duct adenocarcinoma

ADENOCARCINOMA OF THE EXOCRINE PANCREAS

142. False about pancreatic cancer is:

A. Overall, less than 8% of individuals will survive 5 years beyond their diagnosis
B. The risk of pancreatic cancer increases with age beyond the sixth decade; the mean age at diagnosis is 72 years
C. Men are affected slightly more commonly than women, with a 1.3 :1 incidence
D. 10 years are required for the acquisition of metastatic ability in pancreatic cancer

143. Pancreatic ductal adenocarcinoma risk in CDKN2A mutation is:

A. 40-fold
B. 30-fold
C. 20-fold
D. 10-fold

144. Pancreatic ductal adenocarcinoma risk in BRCA2 mutation is:

A. 20-fold
B. 10-fold
C. 8-fold
D. 4-fold

145. Pancreatic ductal adenocarcinoma risk in STK11 mutation is:

A. 100-fold
B. 50-fold
C. 40-fold
D. 30-fold

146. Increase in the risk for development of pancreatic cancer in individuals with hereditary pancreatitis is:

A. 100-fold
B. 50-fold
C. 40-fold
D. 30-fold

147. 30-fold increase in risk of Pancreatic ductal adenocarcinoma is:

A. PRSS1
B. MLH1
C. CFTR
D. APC

148. Pancreatic ductal adenocarcinoma risk in MLH1 mutation is:

A. 20-fold
B. 10-fold
C. 8-fold
D. 4-fold

149. False about smoking and Pancreatic ductal adenocarcinoma is:

A. The risk of pancreatic cancer persists many years beyond smoking cessation
B. The most notable risk factor is related to smoking
C. There seems to be a non-linear association, with pancreatic cancer incidence
D. On average, smokers face a 3x increase in risk for development of pancreatic cancer compared with non-smokers

150. False about risk factors of pancreatic ductal adenocarcinoma is:

A. The association with pancreatic cancer is strong if the new diagnosis of diabetes is made in those who are elderly and those who do not have family history of diabetes
B. Increased risk of pancreatic cancer is present in patients with inheritable inflammatory disease of the pancreas, namely, hereditary pancreatitis and cystic fibrosis

C. Patients with new onset diabetes have higher incidence of pancreatic cancer
D. The diagnosis of diabetes may precede the diagnosis of pancreatic cancer by up to 5 years

151. Family members of familial pancreatic cancer kindreds are at an _______ increased risk for development of pancreatic cancer.

A. 40-fold B. 30-fold
C. 18-fold D. 10-fold

152. True about PanIN in the following is:

A. The development of papillary architecture defines PanIN-1B, but it is otherwise identical to PanIN-1A
B. PanIN-2 denotes the progression from simple papillary growth to evidence of nuclear atypia not seen in PanIN-1B
C. PanIN-1A is histologically characterized by the presence of columnar, mucin-producing ductal epithelium that maintains basally located homogeneous nuclei without atypia
D. All of the above

153. False about pancreatic adenocarcinoma is:

A. Approximately 90% of PDACs demonstrate loss of p16 function
B. Mutation of the KRAS2 oncogene is one of the earliest genetic abnormalities identified in the progression of PanIN to PDAC
C. Loss of SMAD4, which normally functions as a downstream mediator related to TGF-β, leads to increased inhibition of cell growth and proliferation
D. The KRAS2 oncogene is activated in more than 95% of pancreatic cancers and is thought to be the initiating event in tumorigenesis

154. The defining presenting symptom of patients with PDACs in the periampullary region is:

A. Hematemesis B. Pain
C. Jaundice D. Weight loss

155. False about periampullary PDAC among the following is:

A. Periumbilical lymphadenopathy may be palpable also known as Sister Mary Joseph node
B. A palpable distended gallbladder can be identified in approximately two third of patients with periampullary PDAC
C. Perirectal tumor involvement may be palpable through digital rectal examination, referred to as Blumer shelf
D. New onset diabetes in an elderly patient with weight loss may be an early presenting symptom of pancreatic cancer

156. False about the diagnosis of PDAC is:

A. 10% to 15% of individuals do not have elevation of the CA 19-9 level, a finding that has been associated with blood Lewis antigen negative status and is caused by a lack of the fucosyltransferase gene
B. Normalization of CA 19-9 after neoadjuvant therapy has been suggested as an important prognostic factor
C. CA 19-9 is most sensitive for pancreatic adenocarcinoma
D. MRI has become the imaging modality of choice for the evaluation of suspected pancreatic cancer

157. False about diagnosis of pancreatic cancer is:

A. ERCP is frequently used in the assessment of the jaundiced patient because of its ability to perform a biopsy and to palliate jaundice
B. CT is the imaging study of choice for the evaluation of lesions arising in the pancreas
C. Pancreatic adenocarcinoma is typically seen as a hypoattenuating lesion during the portal venous phase of the imaging
D. Brush cytology has a sensitivity and specificity that are far superior to those of FNAC, with a diagnostic accuracy of 92% to 95%

158. FDG PET alters clinical planning in more than:

A. 5% of cases B. 10% of cases
C. 20% of cases D. 40% of cases

159. As per NCCN, borderline resectable as tumors are tumors that exhibit all except:

A. Common hepatic artery (abutment or encasement) without extension to the celiac axis or hepatic artery bifurcation
B. Hepatic artery involvement: common hepatic artery (abutment or encasement) without extension to the celiac axis or hepatic artery bifurcation
C. Solid tumor contact with SMV or portal vein of more than 180 degrees
D. Portal vein involvement

160. In pancreatic adenocarcinoma diagnostic laparoscopy identifies additional unresectable disease in up to:

A. 10% of cases B. 30% of cases
C. 50% of cases D. 70% of cases

161. False about surgical technique in pancreatic cancer is:

A. The duodenum is divided at least 2 cm distal to the pylorus
B. Resections that compromise less than 70% of the venous diameter can be closed primarily
C. The right gastroepiploic vein is ligated at its confluence with the SMV, allowing the SMV to be dissected from the inferior border and posterior neck of the pancreas
D. Before division of the GDA, the vessel is temporarily occluded, and blood flow through the distal common hepatic artery is ensured using a Doppler device

162. A feeding jejunostomy can be considered in selected patients with significant preoperative malnutrition with albumin levels of:

A. <2.0 g/dl B. <2.5 g/dl
C. <3.0 g/dl D. <3.5 g/dl

163. The pancreaticojejunostomy is created in:

A. 1 layer, posterior, with a duct to mucosa anastomosis
B. 2 layers, anterior and posterior, with a duct to mucosa anastomosis
C. 2 layers, anterior and posterior, with a mucosa-to-mucosa anastomosis
D. 1 layer, posterior, with a mucosa-to-mucosa anastomosis

164. DIPLOMA trial compared:

A. Open vs robotic approach of surgery
B. Laparoscopic vs robotic approach of surgery
C. Open vs endoscopic approach of surgery
D. Open only

165. Most common complication after pancreaticoduodenectomy is:

A. Pancreas fistula
B. Intra-abdominal abscess
C. Wound infection
D. Delayed gastric emptying

166. Anastomotic leaks from the hepaticojejunostomy and duodenojejunostomy occur after Whipple's procedure is:

A. <5% B. <10%
C. <20% D. <25%

167. According to International Study Group on Pancreatic Fistula Classification of Pancreatic Fistulas after pancreatic surgery, sepsis is seen in:

A. Grade A B. Grade B
C. Grade C D. Grade D

168. According to International Study Group on Pancreatic Fistula Classification of Pancreatic Fistulas after pancreatic surgery, signs of infections are not seen in:

A. Grade A B. Grade B
C. Grade C D. Grade D

169. Achilles heel of the Whipple procedure is:

A. Hepaticojejunostomy
B. Pancreaticojejunostomy
C. Choledochojejunostomy
D. Gastrojejunostomy

170. No. of patients found to have lymph node involvement at the time of the Whipple procedure is:

A. 25% to 30% B. 45% to 60%
C. 75% to 80% D. 60% to 70%

171. False about the treatment of pancreatic cancer is:

A. Irreversible electroporation preserves collagen rich structures such as blood vessels and ducts, while killing tumor cells
B. Antecolic duodenojejunostomy may improve gastric emptying compared with the retrocolic technique
C. Open pancreaticoduodenectomy remains the standard of care
D. Use of a surgical drain should not be considered standard of care

172. Which study showed adjuvant combination of gemcitabine and capecitabine is superior to gemcitabine alone?

A. ESPAC-3 B. ESPAC-4
C. ESPAC-1 D. GITSG

173. Which study showed adjuvant gemcitabine improves disease-free survival compared with observation?

A. CONKO-001 B. RTOG 97-04
C. ESPAC-1 D. GITSG

174. PRODIGE 24 trial, true is:

A. The median disease-free survival was nearly 9 months longer in the mFOLFIRINOX arm compared to the gemcitabine arm
B. Patients with surgical resected pancreatic cancer were randomized to receive either modified regimen of 5-FU, leucovorin,

irinotecan, and oxaliplatin (mFOLFIRINOX) or gemcitabine for 6 months

C. Median overall survival was 54 months for the mFOLFIRINOX arm and 35 months for gemcitabine arm

D. All of the above

175. No. of patients with pancreatic cancer present with locally advanced or metastatic disease is:

A. 20% B. 40%
C. 60% D. 80%

176. False about Biliary Obstruction after pancreatic cancer is:

A. ERCP with metal stent placement provides excellent palliation of jaundice, and at high-volume university centers, successful biliary drainage is possible in more than 50% of cases

B. For patients who are found at laparotomy to have unresectable disease or those for whom nonsurgical measures have failed, a surgical biliary-enteric bypass may be performed by Roux-en-Y hepaticojejunostomy

C. Palliation of biliary obstruction is commonly required for patients who are not candidates for surgical resection

D. In patients for whom endoscopic palliation is impossible, percutaneous biliary drainage with subsequent internalization may be required

177. No. of patients with locally advanced pancreatic cancer that will develop gastric outlet obstruction is:

A. 20% B. 40%
C. 60% D. 80%

178. False about pain relief in pancreatic cancer is:

A. Celiac nerve block procedure involves injecting a combination of 3 mL of 0.25% bupivacaine and 10 mL of absolute alcohol into each celiac plexus

B. CT-guided percutaneous neurolysis may also be performed

C. Palliation of pain is paramount for optimizing the quality of life for patients and should be a primary goal for physicians

D. Neurolysis can be achieved through EUS guidance with pain relief expected in 50% of patients

PANCREATIC TRAUMA

179. As per American Association for the Surgery of Trauma pancreatic injury grading, distal transection or pancreatic parenchymal injury with ductal injury is:

A. GRADE II B. GRADE III
C. GRADE IV D. GRADE V

180. As per American Association for the Surgery of Trauma pancreatic injury grading, pancreatic parenchymal injury involving the ampulla is:

A. GRADE II B. GRADE III
C. GRADE IV D. GRADE V

181. False about pancreatic trauma is:

A. The most reliable test to demonstrate pancreatic duct integrity is ERCP

B. Undiagnosed pancreatic injuries are associated with significant complications such as intra-abdominal abscess, fistula and fluid collections in 60% of patients

C. Up to 50% of deaths occur within the 24 to 48 hours after trauma and most are related to hypovolemic shock

D. Isolated pancreatic amylase measurement is not recommended because up to 40% of patients with transected pancreatic duct have normal serum amylase levels

ANSWERS

1. **Ans: C. 75 – 125 g**

Ref: Chapter No.56, Page No. 1528

2. **Ans: A. The head lies to the right of midline within the C loop of the duodenum, immediately posterior to the inferior vena cava at the confluence of the renal vein**

Ref: Chapter No.56, Page No. 1528

3. **Ans: C. The superior pancreatic artery then runs along the inferior border of the pancreas, terminating at its tail**

Ref: Chapter No.56, Page No. 1528

4. **Ans: B. The anterior and posterior inferior pancreatico-duodenal veins enter the SMV along the superior border of the uncinate process**

Ref: Chapter No.56, Page No. 1528-1529

5. **Ans: C. 4th**

Ref: Chapter No.56, Page No. 1529

6. **Ans: C. Dorsal and ventral buds appear from the mesoderm**

Ref: Chapter No.56, Page No. 1529

7. **Ans: B. Duct of Wirsung**

Ref: Chapter No.56, Page No. 1530

8. **Ans: B. 10%**

Ref: Chapter No.56, Page No. 1531

9. **Ans: B. α/PP cell differentiation**

Ref: Chapter No.56, Page No. 1531

10. **Ans: A. β vs δ cell differentiation**

Ref: Chapter No.56, Page No. 1531

11. **Ans: D. PDX1**

Ref: Chapter No.56, Page No. 1531

12. **Ans: D. All of the above are true**

Ref: Chapter No.56, Page No. 1531

13. **Ans: C. Resection is not necessary**

Ref: Chapter No.56, Page No. 1531

14. **Ans: B. Duodenojejunostomy**

Ref: Chapter No.56, Page No. 1531

15. **Ans: A. Stomach**

Ref: Chapter No.56, Page No. 1531

16. **Ans: B. 85%**

Ref: Chapter No.56, Page No. 1531

17. **Ans: A. 4%**

Ref: Chapter No.56, Page No. 1531

18. **Ans: A. SPINK1 gene**

Ref: Chapter No.56, Page No. 1532

19. **Ans: D. 8.0 to 9.0**

Ref: Chapter No.56, Page No. 1533

20. **Ans: B. 7.0**

Ref: Chapter No.56, Page No. 1533

21. **Ans: B. 7.0 to 9.0**

Ref: Chapter No.56, Page No. 1533

22. **Ans: B. 20% to 25%**

Ref: Chapter No.56, Page No. 1533

23. **Ans: A. Intestinal phase**

Ref: Chapter No.56, Page No. 1533

24. **Ans: D. 65% to 70%**

Ref: Chapter No.56, Page No. 1533

25. **Ans: C. Secretin and CCK**

Ref: Chapter No.56, Page No. 1533

26. **Ans: A. Vagovagal reflex**

Ref: Chapter No.56, Page No. 1533

27. **Ans: A. 10%**

Ref: Chapter No.56, Page No. 1533

28. **Ans: B. CCK potentiates the effects of secretin but not vice versa**

Ref: Chapter No.56, Page No. 1533

29. **Ans: C. I cells**

Ref: Chapter No.56, Page No. 1533

30. **Ans: C. Most patients develop a severe course**

Ref: Chapter No.56, Page No. 1533

31. **Ans: D. Septic complications**

Ref: Chapter No.56, Page No. 1533

32. **Ans: D. The mortality seen in the early phase of pancreatitis is the result of this multiorgan failure**

Ref: Chapter No.56, Page No. 1534

33. **Ans: A. Gallstones**

Ref: Chapter No.56, Page No. 1534

34. **Ans: C. Blunt abdominal trauma**

Ref: Chapter No.56, Page No. 1534

35. **Ans: B. 5%**

Ref: Chapter No.56, Page No. 1534

36. **Ans: A. It is seen more frequently in men between 50 and 70 years of age**

Ref: Chapter No.56, Page No. 1534

37. **Ans: B. Alcohol**

Ref: Chapter No.56, Page No. 1534

38. **Ans: D. Only 50% to 60% of patients who drink alcohol develop acute pancreatitis**

Ref: Chapter No.56, Page No. 1534

39. **Ans: D. A shift in cell death caused by apoptosis to necrosis by increase in caspase 3/8 activity**

Ref: Chapter No.56, Page No. 1534

40. **Ans: B. Acute pancreatitis**

Ref: Chapter No.56, Page No. 1535

41. **Ans: B. 5%**

Ref: Chapter No.56, Page No. 1535

42. **Ans: D. The clinical course is moderate to severe in 20% to 25% of patients**

Ref: Chapter No.56, Page No. 1535

43. **Ans: C. Elderly male**

Ref: Chapter No.56, Page No. 1535

44. **Ans: D. All of the above**

Ref: Chapter No.56, Page No. 1535

45. **Ans: D. >1000 mg/dL**

Ref: Chapter No.56, Page No. 1535

46. **Ans: B. Hypertriglyceridemia secondary to hypothyroidism, diabetes mellitus and alcohol induces acute pancreatitis**

Ref: Chapter No.56, Page No. 1535

47. **Ans: A. 50% of patients have nausea or vomiting that typically relieves the pain**

Ref: Chapter No.56, Page No. 1535

48. **Ans: C. 10 hours**

Ref: Chapter No.56, Page No. 1535

49. **Ans: B. 3–5 days**

Ref: Chapter No.56, Page No. 1535

50. **Ans: D. 8–14 days**

Ref: Chapter No.56, Page No. 1535

51. **Ans: D. All of the above**

Ref: Chapter No.56, Page No. 1535

52. **Ans: D. 95%**

Ref: Chapter No.56, Page No. 1535

53. **Ans: D. In patients in whom persistent choledocholithiasis is confirmed by EUS, ERCP is needed for confirmation**

Ref: Chapter No.56, Page No. 1536

54. **Ans: D. Every patient at admission**

Ref: Chapter No.56, Page No. 1536

55. **Ans: C. PaO_2 <60 mm Hg**

Ref: Chapter No.56, Page No. 1536

56. **Ans: A. Age >55 years**

Ref: Chapter No.56, Page No. 1536

57. **Ans: C. Blood urea nitrogen level: increase >2 mg/dL**

Ref: Chapter No.56, Page No. 1536

58. **Ans: B. ≥ 3**

Ref: Chapter No.56, Page No. 1536

59. **Ans: D. Mild pancreatitis can have organ failure lasting less than 48 hours**

Ref: Chapter No.56, Page No. 1536-1537

60. **Ans: D. Severe pancreatitis is characterized by organ failure lasting beyond 24 hours**

Ref: Chapter No.56, Page No. 1536-1537

61. **Ans: C. 7**

Ref: Chapter No.56, Page No. 1537

62. **Ans: D. 10**

Ref: Chapter No.56, Page No. 1537

63. **Ans: B. 4**

Ref: Chapter No.56, Page No. 1537

64. **Ans: B. 6%**

Ref: Chapter No.56, Page No. 1537

65. **Ans: C. Heart rate: >100 beats/min**

Ref: Chapter No.56, Page No. 1537

66. **Ans: C. 48 - 72 hours**

Ref: Chapter No.56, Page No. 1537

67. **Ans: D. Renal failure (creatinine level >2 mg/dL before fluid resuscitation)**

Ref: Chapter No.56, Page No. 1537

68. **Ans: D. Platelet count $\leq$50,000**

Ref: Chapter No.56, Page No. 1537

69. **Ans: A. 5% DNS may be the best fluid for initial resuscitation**

Ref: Chapter No.56, Page No. 1537

70. **Ans: D. All of the above are true**

Ref: Chapter No.56, Page No. 1538

71. **Ans: C. 30%**

Ref: Chapter No.56, Page No.1538

72. **Ans: C. 30% to 55% of patients**

Ref: Chapter No.56, Page No.1538

73. **Ans: D. Acute peripancreatic fluids collections are simple in nature and after 6 weeks are referred to as a pseudocyst**

Ref: Chapter No.56, Page No.1538

74. **Ans: C. Macrolides**

Ref: Chapter No.56, Page No.1538

75. **Ans: D. Acute necrotic collection typically seen as areas of low attenuation (>40–50 HU) after the IV injection of contrast material**

Ref: Chapter No.56, Page No.1538

76. **Ans: B. 20%**

Ref: Chapter No.56, Page No.1538

77. **Ans: C. Infection**

Ref: Chapter No.56, Page No.1538

78. **Ans: B. Intermittent pain**

Ref: Chapter No.56, Page No.1539

79. **Ans: C. Local contamination after interventional procedures such as endoscopic retrograde cholangiopancreatography is not responsible for necrosis infection**

Ref: Chapter No.56, Page No.1539

80. **Ans: C. 25% to 30%**

Ref: Chapter No.56, Page No.1540

81. **Ans: B. 5% - 15%**

Ref: Chapter No.56, Page No.1540

82. **Ans: B. Up to 10% of patients with pancreatic pseudocysts will develop symptoms**

Ref: Chapter No.56, Page No.1540

83. **Ans: D. 70%**

Ref: Chapter No.56, Page No.1540

84. **Ans: D. Communication with the main pancreatic duct**

Ref: Chapter No.56, Page No.1540

85. **Ans: A. Pancreatic pseudocysts located in the tail of the pancreas that are in close contact with the duodenum are treated with a cystoduodenostomy**

Ref: Chapter No.56, Page No.1540

86. **Ans: D. All of the above**

Ref: Chapter No.56, Page No.1540

87. **Ans: D. Diagnostic paracentesis typically demonstrates normal amylase and lipase levels**

Ref: Chapter No.56, Page No.1540-1541

88. **Ans: C. Amylase levels above 10,000 IU in the pleural fluid confirm the diagnosis**

Ref: Chapter No.56, Page No.1541

89. **Ans: B. Splenic artery**

Ref: Chapter No.56, Page No.1541

90. **Ans: B. Splenic vein**

Ref: Chapter No.56, Page No.1541

91. **Ans: A. 30% to 70% of heavy drinkers develop chronic pancreatitis**

Ref: Chapter No.56, Page No.1541-1542

92. **Ans: B. Alcohol**

Ref: Chapter No.56, Page No.1542

93. **Ans: D. All of the above**

Ref: Chapter No.56, Page No.1542

94. **Ans: D. All of the above**

Ref: Chapter No.56, Page No.1542

95. **Ans: B. The risk of pancreatic calcifications and diabetes mellitus is not increased in patients who smoke compared with non-smokers**

Ref: Chapter No.56, Page No.1542

96. **Ans: C. Chromosome 7**

Ref: Chapter No.56, Page No.1542

97. **Ans: C. SPINK1 mutations are present in 10% to 20% of healthy patients**

Ref: Chapter No.56, Page No.1542

98. **Ans: D. Tropical pancreatitis**

Ref: Chapter No.56, Page No.1542

99. **Ans: A. Type 1**

Ref: Chapter No.56, Page No.1542

100. **Ans: D. Autoimmune pancreatitis is more common in women than in men**

Ref: Chapter No.56, Page No.1542

101. **Ans: B. Obliterative endarteritis**

Ref: Chapter No.56, Page No.1542

102. **Ans: C. Tropical pancreatitis**

Ref: Chapter No.56, Page No.1543

103. **Ans: D. Both A and B**

Ref: Chapter No.56, Page No.1543

104. **Ans: C. 45% to 50%**

Ref: Chapter No.56, Page No.1543

105. **Ans: B. At least 50% of the gland needs to be dysfunctional before steatorrhea, diarrhea and other symptoms of malabsorption develop**

Ref: Chapter No.56, Page No.1543

106. **Ans: C. 40% - 80%**

Ref: Chapter No.56, Page No.1543

107. **Ans: A. 5% to 10%**

Ref: Chapter No.56, Page No.1543

108. Ans: B. Dilated pancreatic duct

Ref: Chapter No.56, Page No.1543

109. Ans: B. CT has a sensitivity of 55% to 85% and a specificity of 70% to 80% for the diagnosis of chronic pancreatitis

Ref: Chapter No.56, Page No.1543-1544

110. Ans: C. EUS

Ref: Chapter No.56, Page No.1544

111. Ans: B. 1 major A criterion + ≥2 or more minor criteria

Ref: Chapter No.56, Page No.1544

112. Ans: B. Lobularity including three or more non-contiguous lobules in the head

Ref: Chapter No.56, Page No.1544

113. Ans: C. 7 g/day

Ref: Chapter No.56, Page No.1544

114. Ans: D. 100 µg/g

Ref: Chapter No.56, Page No.1544

115. Ans: C. 200 µg/g

Ref: Chapter No.56, Page No.1544

116. Ans: C. For patients with unrelenting pain, celiac neurolysis has been attempted with sustained success in those with chronic pancreatitis

Ref: Chapter No.56, Page No.1544

117. Ans: C. Biliary obstruction caused by chronic pancreatitis occurs in 10% of patients and is best treated with endoscopic treatment

Ref: Chapter No.56, Page No.1545

118. Ans: B. >7 mm

Ref: Chapter No.56, Page No.1545

119. Ans: B. Puestow procedure

Ref: Chapter No.56, Page No.1545

120. Ans: D. 80%

Ref: Chapter No.56, Page No.1545

121. Ans: B. Duodenum-preserving pancreatic head resection

Ref: Chapter No.56, Page No.1546

122. Ans: D. Berger's procedure

Ref: Chapter No.56, Page No.1546

123. Ans: C. Total pancreatectomy

Ref: Chapter No.56, Page No.1546

124. Ans: A. Significant biliary obstruction occurs in 20% of patients

Ref: Chapter No.56, Page No.1546

125. Ans: C. 30% to 40%

Ref: Chapter No.56, Page No.1546

126. Ans: B. 10%

Ref: Chapter No.56, Page No.1546

127. Ans: A. Head of the pancreas

Ref: Chapter No.56, Page No.1547

128. Ans: A. On gross inspection, SCNs are small, poorly circumscribed masses

Ref: Chapter No.56, Page No.1547

129. Ans: B. Patients with a tumor smaller than 4 cm are more likely to be symptomatic

Ref: Chapter No.56, Page No.1547

130. Ans: B. Frequently seen in elderly men

Ref: Chapter No.56, Page No.1547

131. Ans: A. Fluid analyses provide accurate diagnosis in up to 40% of cases

Ref: Chapter No.56, Page No.1547-1548

132. Ans: D. All of the above

Ref: Chapter No.56, Page No.1547

133. Ans: C. 20%

Ref: Chapter No.56, Page No.1547

134. Ans: D. All of the above are true

Ref: Chapter No.56, Page No.1548

135. Ans: D. Enhancing mural nodule >5 mm

Ref: Chapter No.56, Page No.1549

136. Ans: C. BD-IPMN >3 cm

Ref: Chapter No.56, Page No.1549

137. Ans: D. Cysts smaller than 3 cm generally have a low risk for malignancy and therefor are most appropriate for surveillance

Ref: Chapter No.56, Page No.1549

138. Ans: B. 10% to 15%

Ref: Chapter No.56, Page No.1549

139. Ans: C. 30% to 50%

Ref: Chapter No.56, Page No.1549

140. Ans: B. Elevation of the CEA level is predictive of invasive malignant disease

Ref: Chapter No.56, Page No.1550-1551

141. Ans: A. For MD-IPMN in the absence of diffuse polyps or enhancing nodules in the main duct, total pancreatectomy is preferred

Ref: Chapter No.56, Page No.1551

142. Ans: D. 10 years are required for the acquisition of metastatic ability in pancreatic cancer

Ref: Chapter No.56, Page No.1551

143. Ans: A. 40-fold

Ref: Chapter No.56, Page No.1552

144. Ans: B. 10-fold

Ref: Chapter No.56, Page No.1552

145. Ans: A. 100-fold

Ref: Chapter No.56, Page No.1552

146. Ans: B. 50-fold

Ref: Chapter No.56, Page No.1552

147. Ans: C. CFTR

Ref: Chapter No.56, Page No.1552

148. Ans: C. 8-fold

Ref: Chapter No.56, Page No.1552

149. Ans: C. There seems to be a non-linear association, with pancreatic cancer incidence

Ref: Chapter No.56, Page No.1552

150. Ans: D. The diagnosis of diabetes may precede the diagnosis of pancreatic cancer by up to 5 years

Ref: Chapter No.56, Page No.1552

151. Ans: C. 18-fold

Ref: Chapter No.56, Page No.1553

152. Ans: D. All of the above

Ref: Chapter No.56, Page No.1553

153. Ans: C. Loss of SMAD4, which normally functions as a downstream mediator related to TGF-β, leads to increased inhibition of cell growth and proliferation

Ref: Chapter No.56, Page No.1553

154. Ans: C. Jaundice

Ref: Chapter No.56, Page No.1553

155. Ans: B. A palpable distended gallbladder can be identified in approximately two third of patients with periampullary PDAC

Ref: Chapter No.56, Page No.1554

156. Ans: D. MRI has become the imaging modality of choice for the evaluation of suspected pancreatic cancer

Ref: Chapter No.56, Page No.1554

157. Ans: D. Brush cytology has a sensitivity and specificity that are far superior to those of FNAC, with a diagnostic accuracy of 92% to 95%

Ref: Chapter No.56, Page No.1554-1555

158. Ans: B. 10% of cases

Ref: Chapter No.56, Page No.1555

159. Ans: D. Portal vein involvement

Ref: Chapter No.56, Page No.1555

160. Ans: B. 30% of cases

Ref: Chapter No.56, Page No.1555

161. Ans: B. Resections that compromise less than 70% of the venous diameter can be closed primarily

Ref: Chapter No.56, Page No.1556

162. Ans: D. <3.5 g/dl

Ref: Chapter No.56, Page No.1556

163. Ans: B. 2 layers, anterior and posterior, with a duct to mucosa anastomosis

Ref: Chapter No.56, Page No.1556

164. Ans: A. Open vs robotic approach of surgery

Ref: Chapter No.56, Page No.1557

165. Ans: D. Delayed gastric emptying

Ref: Chapter No.56, Page No.1558

166. Ans: A. <5%

Ref: Chapter No.56, Page No.1558

167. Ans: C. Grade C

Ref: Chapter No.56, Page No.1559

168. Ans: A. Grade A

Ref: Chapter No.56, Page No.1559

169. Ans: B. Pancreaticojejunostomy

Ref: Chapter No.56, Page No.1559

170. Ans: C. 75% to 80%

Ref: Chapter No.56, Page No.1559

171. Ans: D. Use of a surgical drain should not be considered standard of care

Ref: Chapter No.56, Page No.1560

172. Ans: B. ESPAC-4

Ref: Chapter No.56, Page No.1561

173. Ans: A. CONKO-001

Ref: Chapter No.56, Page No.1561

174. Ans: D. All of the above

Ref: Chapter No.56, Page No.1561

175. Ans: D. 80%

Ref: Chapter No.56, Page No.1562

176. Ans: A. ERCP with metal stent placement provides excellent palliation of jaundice, and at high-volume university centers, successful biliary drainage is possible in more than 50% of cases

Ref: Chapter No.56, Page No.1562

177. Ans: A. 20%

Ref: Chapter No.56, Page No.1562

178. Ans: D. Neurolysis can be achieved through EUS guidance with pain relief expected in 50% of patients

Ref: Chapter No.56, Page No.1563

179. Ans: B. GRADE III

Ref: Chapter No.56, Page No.1563

180. Ans: C. GRADE IV

Ref: Chapter No.56, Page No.1563

181. Ans: C. Up to 50% of deaths occur within the 24 to 48 hours after trauma, and most are related to hypovolemic shock

Ref: Chapter No.56, Page No.1563

57

The Spleen

SPLENIC ANATOMY

1. **Weight of spleen is:**
   A. 100 g B. 150 g
   C. 250 g D. 300 g

2. **The spleen develops from mesenchymal cells in the:**
   A. Ventral mesogastrium at 5 weeks
   B. Dorsal mesogastrium at 5 weeks
   C. Ventral mesogastrium at 7 weeks
   D. Dorsal mesogastrium at 7 weeks

3. **Spleen in the left lower thorax is normally protected by ribs:**
   A. 9, 10 and 11 B. 8, 9 and 10
   C. 8 and 9 D. 6, 7 and 8

4. **False about splenic anatomy is:**
   A. The gastrosplenic ligament carries the short gastric vessels in its superior aspect and the left gastroepiploic in its inferior aspect
   B. The tail of the pancreas abuts the splenic hilum in 70% of individuals
   C. The splenorenal ligament houses the splenic artery and vein as well as the tail of the pancreas
   D. In patients with portal hypertension, the splenophrenic and splenocolic ligaments are relatively vascular

5. **False about the vascular anatomy of spleen is:**
   A. The magistral type, which branches into terminal and polar arteries near the hilum of the spleen
   B. The splenic artery is a tortuous vessel that gives off multiple branches (16–18 branches) to the pancreas as it travels along its posterior aspect
   C. The magistral type of splenic arterial anatomy occurs in 70% of individuals compared with the distributed type (30%)
   D. The splenic artery branches to approximately 5 to 6 polar arteries and 6 short gastric arteries

6. **Patients without portal hypertension will have following structures avascular relatively:**
   A. Splenophrenic ligament
   B. Gastrocolic ligament
   C. Gastrosplenic ligament
   D. Splenorenal ligament

7. **Splenorenal ligament contains which of these structures?**
   A. Splenic artery B. Splenic vein
   C. Tail of pancreas D. All of the above

8. **True about splenic vein include all except:**
   A. Splenic vein leaves hilum and travels anteriorly to pancreas
   B. Sinusoids merge into venules and drain veins that finally form splenic vein
   C. Joins with pancreatic branches and often the inferior mesenteric vein
   D. Forms portal vein with superior mesenteric vein

9. **Which of the following make up white pulp of spleen?**
   A. Arterioles B. Lymphatic sheaths
   C. Capillaries D. Venules

SPLENIC FUNCTION

10. **Under normal conditions, spleen has no hematopoietic function after:**
    A. 4th months B. 5th months
    C. 6th months D. 7th months

11. Patients with splenomegaly are able to sequestrate large volume of platelets up to:

A. 50% B. 60%
C. 70% D. 80%

12. True among the following is:

A. In the open system, the blood flows through the arterioles and then trickles through a sieve-like parenchyma made up of reticuloendothelial cells into the splenic sinuses before draining into the venous system
B. In the closed system, blood flows directly from arteries to veins
C. Abnormal erythrocytes that result from hemoglobinopathies such as sickle cell anemia, hereditary spherocytosis, thalassemia, or pyruvate kinase deficiency (PKD) are also trapped and destroyed by the spleen
D. All of the above

13. Howell-Jolly bodies are:

A. Nuclear remnant
B. Spur cells
C. Iron granules
D. Denatured hemoglobin

14. Pappenheimer bodies are:

A. Target cells
B. Spur cells
C. Iron granules
D. Denatured hemoglobin

15. Heinz bodies are:

A. Target cells
B. Spur cells
C. Iron granules
D. Denatured hemoglobin

16. Life of RBCs is:

A. 60 days B. 75 days
C. 90 days D. 120 days

17. Asplenic patients usually have all except:

A. Reduced functional antibody levels
B. Subnormal Ig M levels
C. Increased tuftsin levels
D. All of the above

18. Which of the following biological substances are removed by spleen in normal individuals?

A. Heinz bodies
B. Spherocytes
C. Howell-Jolly bodies
D. Pappenheimer bodies

SPLENECTOMY

19. The most common hematologic indication for splenectomy is:

A. Hereditary spherocytosis
B. ITP
C. Sickle cell anemia
D. Thalassemia

20. False about ITP among the following is:

A. Intracerebral hemorrhage is a common and sometimes fatal presentation
B. ITP is characterized by a low platelet count below 100 × 10^9/L despite normal bone marrow
C. The typical presentation of ITP is characterized by purpura, epistaxis and gingival bleeding
D. Immunoglobulin G autoantibodies directed towards the platelet membranes are believed to be responsible for platelet destruction within the reticuloendothelial system

21. Chronic ITP is duration of:

A. >3 months B. >6 months
C. >12 months D. >24 months

22. False about ITP among the following is:

A. Bacterial infection, specifically Helicobacter pylori, has also been linked to infection-related thrombocytopenia that improves with eradication
B. Drug-induced thrombocytopenia is thought to occur rarely, in approximately 20 to 40 cases/million users of common medications, such as trimethoprim-sulfonamide and quinine
C. ITP is predominantly a disease of young men
D. The diagnosis of primary ITP involves the exclusion of other relatively common causes of thrombocytopenia

23. False about the management of ITP is:

A. Splenectomy is the treatment of choice for patients with incomplete response to glucocorticoid treatment and for pregnant women in the 2nd trimester of pregnancy who have also failed to respond to steroid treatment or intravenous immune globulin therapy
B. Patients with slightly lower platelet counts, between 30,000 and 50,000/mm^3, may be observed but with more routine follow-up

C. It is not necessary to proceed to splenectomy for patients who have platelet counts higher than 30,000/mm^3, who have had ITP for longer than 3 months
D. Asymptomatic patients with platelet counts higher than 50,000/mm^3 may be observed without further intervention

24. In symptomatic patients, initial medical treatment of patients is started when platelet counts are below:

A. 100,000/mm^3 B. 50,000/mm^3
C. 30,000/mm^3 D. 10,000/mm^3

25. In asymptomatic patients, initial medical treatment of patients is started when platelet counts are below:

A. 100,000/mm^3 B. 50,000/mm^3
C. 30,000/mm^3 D. 10,000/mm^3

26. Among the patients treated with steroids, how many patients will experience a complete response?

A. 12.5% B. 25%
C. 50% D. 75%

27. With significant mucous membrane bleeding, hospitalization may be required for patients with ITP whose platelets counts remain below:

A. 50,000/mm^3 B. 20,000/mm^3
C. 10,000/mm^3 D. 5,000/mm^3

28. Intravenous immune globulin is important for the treatment of acute bleeding; the usual dose is:

A. 1 g/kg body weight/day × 2 days
B. 2 g/kg body weight/day × 2 days
C. 1 g/kg body weight/day × 3 days
D. 2 g/kg body weight/day × 3 days

29. Intravenous immune globulin increases platelet count within:

A. 2 days B. 3 days
C. 2 weeks D. 3 weeks

30. Drug-induced thrombocytopenia is seen in all except:

A. Cimetidine B. Vancomycin
C. Cephalosporin D. Sulfonamides

31. Viral infections causing thrombocytopenia is all except:

A. HCV B. EBV
C. HIV D. HBV

32. Cause of thrombocytopenia is pregnancy is:

A. Preeclampsia
B. Gestational thrombocytopenia
C. HELLP syndrome
D. All of the above

33. Medical options for refractory ITP includes:

A. Rituximab (375 mg/m^2/week intravenously for 4 weeks)
B. Oral dexamethasone (40 mg/day for 4 days)
C. Thrombopoietin receptor antagonists (eltrombopag, romiplostim)
D. All of the above

34. The treatment of choice for ITP is splenectomy in:

A. Thrombocytopenia refractory to glucocorticoid treatment
B. Patients who require toxic doses of steroid to achieve remission
C. Severe thrombocytopenia with counts below 30,000/mm^3 for 4 weeks
D. Patients who have incomplete response to glucocorticoid treatment

35. Post splenectomy in ITP, false statement is:

A. Long-term failure rate of laparoscopic splenectomy at approximately 8%
B. Most patients will exhibit improved platelet counts within 21 days postoperatively
C. Evaluation for a missed accessory spleen must be undertaken in patients who experience a relapse
D. Durable platelet responses are associated with patients who have platelet counts of 150,000/mm^3 by postoperative day 3 or more than 500,000/mm^3 by postoperative day 10

36. No. of symptomatic patients of HIV infection who will develop ITP:

A. 5% to 10% B. 10% to 20%
C. 20% to 40% D. 0% to 70%

37. The most common Hereditary anemia is:

A. Hereditary xerocytosis
B. Hereditary pyropoikilocytosis
C. Hereditary elliptocytosis
D. Hereditary spherocytosis

38. False about Hereditary spherocytosis is:

A. The most common resulting clinical features are moderate hemolytic anemia, occasionally with jaundice, folate deficiency and splenomegaly

B. Hereditary spherocytosis is usually transmitted as an autosomal dominant disease
C. Splenectomy should be delayed until the age of five years to preserve immunologic function of the spleen and to reduce the risk of OPSI
D. The preoperative workup should include ultrasound evaluation; if gallstones are present, cholecystectomy is not performed

39. Hereditary spherocytosis is thought to be most commonly caused by mutation of genes affecting the production of the RBC cytoskeleton proteins such as:

A. Band 4.1
B. Spectrin
C. Band 3
D. Ankryin

40. Splenectomy is indicated in cases of severe hereditary anemia, except:

A. Hereditary xerocytosis
B. Hereditary pyropoikilocytosis
C. Hereditary elliptocytosis
D. Hereditary spherocytosis

41. True about ITP are all except:

A. Low platelet counts
B. Autoantibodies causing disordered platelet destruction
C. Megakaryocytes are present
D. Abnormal bone marrow

42. Pyruvate kinase deficiency (PKD), false statement is:

A. PKD causes chronic hemolysis compared to G6PD deficiency, which is more episodic
B. PKD is an autosomal recessive disease caused by a mutation to the pyruvate kinase L/R (PKLR gene)
C. PKD is the most common enzymopathy
D. There is a role for splenectomy in PKD

43. Sickle cell disease is a point mutation in the beta globin gene resulting a single amino acid substitution of:

A. Valine for glutamic acid in the 7th position of the alpha chain of hemoglobin A
B. Glutamic acid for valine in the 7th position of the β chain of hemoglobin A
C. Glutamic acid for valine in the 6th position of the alpha chain of hemoglobin A
D. Valine for glutamic acid in the 6th position of the β chain of hemoglobin A

44. False about sickle cell anemia is:

A. Hypersplenism related to sickle cell disease is characterized by anemia, leukopenia and thrombocytopenia requiring transfusions
B. Splenectomy is usually indicated after the 2nd attack to prevent subsequent attacks
C. Symptomatic massive splenomegaly that interferes with daily activities may also be improved by splenectomy
D. Acute splenic sequestration crises are life-threatening disorders in children with sickle cell disease or sickle-Beta thalassemia

45. False about splenic abscess is:

A. These patients present with fever, abdominal pain and a tender enlarged spleen
B. Most patients with splenic abscesses will have a leukocytosis as well as thrombocytosis and Howell-Jolly bodies, indicating a functional asplenia
C. Salmonella and Enterobacter spp. are common pathogens
D. These patients are always managed conservatively

46. False about Hodgkin's lymphoma is:

A. Hodgkin's lymphoma usually affects young adults in their 20s and 30s with a second peak in adults over the age of 50
B. Hodgkin's lymphoma is a not fluorodeoxy-glucose-avid lymphoma
C. It is a group of malignant conditions that are characterized by the presence of Reed-Sternberg cells on histology
D. Splenectomy for Hodgkin's lymphoma is currently rarely indicated, however it may be performed for symptomatic splenomegaly

47. False about non-Hodgkin's lymphoma is:

A. Staging relies mostly on integrated PET/CT
B. Ideally, biopsy is obtained after initiation of steroid therapy
C. Non-Hodgkin's lymphoma is a group of malignant neoplasms derived from progenerates of B cell, T cell, mature B cells and mature T cells
D. Splenomegaly or hypersplenism is a common occurrence during the course of non-Hodgkin's lymphoma

48. Splenectomy is indicated for non-Hodgkin's lymphoma patients with:

A. Anemia associated with hypersplenism

B. Massive splenomegaly
C. Thrombocytopenia associated with hypersplenism
D. All of the above

49. False about hairy cell leukaemia is:

A. It is characterized by splenomegaly, pancytopenia, and neoplastic mononuclear cells in the peripheral blood and normal bone marrow
B. Treatment for cytopenias or splenomegaly typically begins with first line therapy with purine analogue chemotherapy
C. The male-to-female ratio is approximately 4:5
D. Patients with diffusely involved bone marrow without massive splenomegaly are less responsive to splenectomy

50. Most of second malignant neoplasms after hairy cell leukaemia are solid tumors, such as all except:

A. Skin cancers
B. Prostate cancer
C. Brain cancer
D. Lung cancer

51. False about Chronic lymphocytic leukemia (CLL) is:

A. Medical treatment is reserved for fit patients with symptomatic disease and advanced Rai stages
B. Chronic lymphocytic leukemia (CLL) is the most common leukemia in the western world
C. High-risk CLL involves lymphocytosis and lymphadenopathy in any site
D. The Rai system helps clinicians determine when therapy should be started

52. False about Chronic myelogenous leukemia (CML) is:

A. Peripheral blood smear analysis shows leukocytosis of white blood cell count up to 100,000/µL with white blood cell count from myeloblasts to mature neutrophils
B. Symptomatic splenomegaly and hypersplenism in CML can't be effectively treated with splenectomy
C. The gold standard for the diagnosis of CML is a chromosomal marker, the Philadelphia chromosome, is caused by the fusion of fragments of chromosomes Abelson gene (ABL1) 9q34 and breakpoint cluster region gene (BCR) on chromosome 22q11.2
D. The BCR-ABL gene product is the target for therapy with tyrosine kinase inhibitors (imatinib, dasatinib and nilotinib)

53. The most common tumor involving the spleen is:

A. Hemangiomas
B. Angiosarcomas
C. Lymphoma
D. Lymphangiomas

54. False among the following is:

A. Patients with angiosarcomas may present with splenomegaly, hemolytic anemia, ascites, pleural effusions, or even spontaneous splenic rupture
B. Secondary metastatic splenic neoplasms are very common
C. Splenic hamartomas are rare and are usually composed of malformed disorganized red pulp elements
D. Metastases are often asymptomatic but may be associated with splenomegaly and even splenic rupture

55. False about splenic parasitic cysts is:

A. Treatment of choice is medical management
B. Rupture of the cyst and expulsion of contents into the abdomen may precipitate anaphylactic shock
C. As with hydatid cysts of the liver, the cysts may be sterilized by injection of a 3% sodium chloride solution, alcohol, or 0.5% silver nitrate
D. Parasitic cysts occur in areas of endemic hydatid disease

56. Most common cyst of spleen is:

A. Traumatic cyst
B. Epidermoid cyst
C. Hydatid cyst
D. Lymphatic cyst

57. False about true splenic cysts is:

A. Total or partial splenectomy may provide appropriate treatment
B. True splenic cysts are often symptomatic
C. Rarely, splenic cysts are manifested with acute symptoms related to rupture, hemorrhage, or infection
D. Diagnosis is best made by CT, and operative intervention is indicated for those with symptomatic or large cysts

58. Amount of the spleen that appears to be sufficient to protect against pneumococcal pneumonia is:

A. 25%
B. 50%
C. 70%
D. 90%

59. False about nonparasitic pseudocysts is:

A. Pseudocysts of the spleen are not lined with epithelium

B. Radiologic imaging usually reveals a smooth, unilocular, thick-walled lesion, sometimes with focal calcifications
C. Nonparasitic pseudocysts represent the remaining 70% to 80% of nonparasitic splenic cysts
D. Asymptomatic, small (<4 cm) pseudocysts require treatment

60. False about splenic abscess is:

A. Approximately 70% of splenic abscesses result from hematogenous spread of the infective organism from another location
B. Splenomegaly is typically present
C. The mortality rate for splenic abscess ranges from 15% to 20% in previously healthy patients with single unilocular lesions up to 80% for multiple abscesses in immunocompromised patients
D. CT is the preferred method for diagnosis; however, the diagnosis can also be made with ultrasound

61. False about management of splenic abscess is:

A. In one third of adult patients, the abscess is multilocular
B. Multilocular lesions, are usually treated with splenectomy, drainage of the left upper quadrant and antibiotics
C. In two third of children, the abscess is unilocular
D. Unilocular abscesses are often amenable to percutaneous drainage, along with antibiotics, with high success rates for unilocular lesions

62. False about wandering spleen is:

A. In multiparous women, hormonal changes and abdominal laxity lead to an acquired defect in splenic attachments
B. A non-contrasted spleen or whorled appearance of the vascular pedicle provides additional evidence for the condition and may be helpful in choosing splenopexy or splenectomy
C. USG of the abdomen provides confirmation of the diagnosis, with the spleen located outside its usual position
D. Failure to form these attachments is thought to arise from lack of fusion of the dorsal mesogastrium to the posterior abdominal wall during embryogenesis

63. False about Elective Laparoscopic Splenectomy is:

A. Laparoscopic splenectomy is now the preferred method for resecting the spleen
B. Laparoscopic splenectomy has been reported for most splenic diseases and is the preferred method for most situations, barring trauma or cases of massive splenomegaly
C. Laparoscopic splenectomy can be completed in approximately 90% of patients
D. CT scan is reliable in detecting accessory splenic tissue and surgical exploration at the time of surgery is essential to avoid disease recurrence in ITP

64. Vaccinations after splenectomy is for:

A. S pneumoniae
B. H1N1 virus
C. N meningitidis
D. Haemophilus influenzae

65. In elective splenectomy, vaccination is done at least ______ before splenectomy.

A. 7 days
B. 10 days
C. 14 days
D. 21 days

66. False about operative technique of laparoscopic splenectomy is:

A. The tail of the pancreas, which is within 1 cm of the splenic hilum in 75% of patients and touches the hilum in 30%, should be well visualized as the stapler is applied to avoid injury
B. The gastrosplenic ligament is opened, and the tail of the pancreas is confirmed to be free of splenic tissue
C. Laparoscopic splenectomy is considered the gold standard for normal size spleen
D. A 3 cm cuff of peritoneum is left along the lateral aspect of the spleen, which can then be grasped to facilitate lateral retraction

67. Predictors of technical difficulties and post-operative complications with a minimally invasive approach are all except:

A. Surgeons experience
B. Etiology of disease
C. Splenic size >19 cm
D. Older patients

68. False about post operative complications after splenectomy is:

A. Gastric perforation at the lesser curvature of the stomach
B. Pancreatic leak is typically managed with percutaneous drainage with or without ERCP & sphincterotomy to reduce resistance forward flow of pancreatic secretions

C. Complications in the immediate postoperative period are usually related to postoperative bleeding due to slipped ligature from the hilar vessels
D. Thromboembolism is one of the most serious complications after splenectomy

69. False about abdominal venous thrombosis is:

A. Abdominal venous thrombosis referred as post splenectomy thrombosis of the splenic, mesenteric, and portal veins (PST-SMPv) has an incidence of 20% to 30%
B. Presentation is usually with nonspecific postoperative gastrointestinal symptoms of abdominal pain and ascites
C. Splenic size and myeloproliferative disorder are the main risk factors
D. Management is usually medical with systemic anticoagulation

70. Risk factors of overwhelming post splenectomy infection (OPSI) is all except:

A. Thalassemia major
B. Older age
C. Idiopathic thrombocytopenia
D. Sick cell anemia

71. False about OPSI is:

A. The risk is greatest in patients with thalassemia major and sickle cell disease
B. OPSI is the most common fatal late complication of splenectomy
C. OPSI is typically caused by polysaccharide encapsulated organisms, such as S pneumoniae, N meningitidis and H influenzae with S pneumoniae
D. Most infections occurred more than 10 years after splenectomy

72. In OPSI, the mortality rate is:

A. 5% - 10%   B. 20% - 30%
C. 40% - 50%   D. 50% - 70%

73. Survivors of OPSI often have a long and complicated hospital course with multiple sequelae, such as all except:

A. Blindness from meningitis
B. Peripheral gangrene requiring amputation
C. Mastoid osteomyelitis
D. Cardiac valvular destruction

74. False about post splenectomy vaccination is:

A. These vaccines should be ideally given 10 to 12 weeks prior to elective splenectomy and at least 14 days prior to surgery
B. The CDC recommended that all splenectomy patients, including those with hereditary spherocytosis, be revaccinated and re-educated between 2 and 6 years after splenectomy
C. All asplenic or hyposplenic patients should receive seasonal influenza vaccination, measles, mumps and rubella, varicella and tetanus diphtheria pertussis
D. If the patient did not receive these vaccines before surgery such as in emergency surgery, vaccine should be given 10 days after splenectomy or upon discharge whichever comes first

75. Currently in an adult, the standard of care for asplenic and hyposplenism patients includes immunization with all except:

A. Even with vaccination, oral antibiotic prophylaxis with penicillin V or amoxicillin should be considered for children under 2 years of age or high-risk postsplenectomy patients
B. Immunologically naive: PCV13 followed by PPSV23 8 weeks later; repeat PPSV23 every 5 years
C. MPSV4, meningococcal 4-valent polysaccharide; repeat MenACWY every 5 years
D. Hib 2 doses

76. The second choice of prophylaxis of OPSI would be a:

A. Amoxycillin plus clavulanate
B. Oral penicillin
C. Macrolide
D. Carbapenems

ANSWERS

1. **Ans: C. 250 g**

Ref: Chapter No.57, Page No.1566

2. **Ans: B. Dorsal mesogastrium at 5 weeks**

Ref: Chapter No.57, Page No.1566

3. **Ans: A. 9, 10 and 11**

Ref: Chapter No.57, Page No.1566

4. **Ans: B. The tail of the pancreas abuts the splenic hilum in 70% of individuals**

Ref: Chapter No.57, Page No.1566

5. **Ans: C. The magistral type of splenic arterial anatomy occurs in 70% of individuals compared with the distributed type (30%)**

Ref: Chapter No.57, Page No.1566

6. **Ans: A. Splenophrenic ligament**

Ref: Chapter No.57, Page No.1566

7. **Ans: D. All of the above**

Ref: Chapter No.57, Page No.1566

8. **Ans: A. Splenic vein leaves hilum and travels anteriorly to pancreas**

Ref: Chapter No.57, Page No.1566-1567

9. **Ans: B. Lymphatic sheaths**

Ref: Chapter No.57, Page No.1566-1567

10. **Ans: B. 5th month**

Ref: Chapter No.57, Page No.1567

11. **Ans: D. 80%**

Ref: Chapter No.57, Page No.1567

12. **Ans: D. All of the above**

Ref: Chapter No.57, Page No.1567-1568

13. **Ans: A. Nuclear remnant**

Ref: Chapter No.57, Page No.1567

14. **Ans: C. Iron granules**

Ref: Chapter No.57, Page No.1567

15. **Ans: D. Denatured hemoglobin**

Ref: Chapter No.57, Page No.1567

16. **Ans: D. 120 days**

Ref: Chapter No.57, Page No.1568

17. **Ans: C. Increased tuftsin levels**

Ref: Chapter No.57, Page No.1569

18. **Ans: B. Spherocytes**

Ref: Chapter No.57, Page No.1569

19. **Ans: B. ITP**

Ref: Chapter No.57, Page No.1569

20. **Ans: A. Intracerebral hemorrhage is a common and sometimes fatal presentation**

Ref: Chapter No.57, Page No.1570

21. **Ans: C. >12 months**

Ref: Chapter No.57, Page No.1570

22. **Ans: C. ITP is predominantly a disease of young men**

Ref: Chapter No.57, Page No.1570

23. **Ans: C. It is not necessary to proceed to splenectomy for patients who have platelet counts higher than 30,000/mm^3, who have had ITP for longer than 3 months**

Ref: Chapter No.57, Page No.1570-1571

24. **Ans: B. 50,000/mm^3**

Ref: Chapter No.57, Page No.1570

25. **Ans: C. 30,000/mm^3**

Ref: Chapter No.57, Page No.1570

26. **Ans: B. 25%**

Ref: Chapter No.57, Page No.1570

27. **Ans: B. 20,000/mm^3**

Ref: Chapter No.57, Page No.1570

28. **Ans: A. 1 g/kg body weight/day × 2 days**

Ref: Chapter No.57, Page No.1570

29. **Ans: B. 3 days**

Ref: Chapter No.57, Page No.1570

30. **Ans: C. Cephalosporin**

Ref: Chapter No.57, Page No.1571

31. **Ans: D. HBV**

Ref: Chapter No.57, Page No.1571

32. **Ans: D. All of the above**

Ref: Chapter No.57, Page No.1571

33. **Ans: D. All of the above**

Ref: Chapter No.57, Page No.1571

34. **Ans: C. Severe thrombocytopenia with counts below 30,000/ mm3 for 4 weeks**

Ref: Chapter No.57, Page No.1571

35. **Ans: B. Most patients will exhibit improved platelet counts within 21 days postoperatively**

Ref: Chapter No.57, Page No.1571

36. **Ans: B. 10% to 20%**

Ref: Chapter No.57, Page No.1571

37. **Ans: D. Hereditary spherocytosis**

Ref: Chapter No.57, Page No.1571

38. **Ans: D. The preoperative workup should include ultrasound evaluation; if gallstones are present, cholecystectomy is not performed**

Ref: Chapter No.57, Page No.1572

39. **Ans: A. Band 4.1**

Ref: Chapter No.57, Page No.1572

40. **Ans: A. Hereditary xerocytosis**

Ref: Chapter No.57, Page No.1572

41. **Ans: D. Abnormal bone marrow**

Ref: Chapter No.57, Page No.1570

42. **Ans: C. PKD is the most common enzymopathy**

Ref: Chapter No.57, Page No.1572

43. **Ans: D. Valine for glutamic acid in the 6th position of the β chain of hemoglobin A**

Ref: Chapter No.57, Page No.1572

44. **Ans: B. Splenectomy is usually indicated after the 2nd attack to prevent subsequent attacks**

Ref: Chapter No.57, Page No.1572

45. **Ans: D. These patients are always managed conservatively**

Ref: Chapter No.57, Page No.1573

46. **Ans: B. Hodgkin's lymphoma is a not fluorodeoxyglucose-avid lymphoma**

Ref: Chapter No.57, Page No.1573

47. **Ans: B. Ideally, biopsy is obtained after initiation of steroid therapy**

Ref: Chapter No.57, Page No.1573

48. **Ans: D. All of the above**

Ref: Chapter No.57, Page No.1573

49. **Ans: A. It is characterized by splenomegaly, pancytopenia, and neoplastic mononuclear cells in the peripheral blood and normal bone marrow**

Ref: Chapter No.57, Page No.1573

50. **Ans: C. Brain cancer**

Ref: Chapter No.57, Page No.1573

51. **Ans: C. High-risk CLL involves lymphocytosis and lymphadenopathy in any site**

Ref: Chapter No.57, Page No.1573

52. **Ans: B. Symptomatic splenomegaly and hypersplenism in CML can't be effectively treated with splenectomy**

Ref: Chapter No.57, Page No.1574

53. **Ans: C. Lymphoma**

Ref: Chapter No.57, Page No.1574

54. **Ans: B. Secondary metastatic splenic neoplasms are very common**

Ref: Chapter No.57, Page No.1574

55. **Ans: A. Treatment of choice is medical management**

Ref: Chapter No.57, Page No.1574

56. **Ans: C. Hydatid cyst**

Ref: Chapter No.57, Page No.1574

57. **Ans: B. True splenic cysts are often symptomatic**

Ref: Chapter No.57, Page No.1574

58. **Ans: A. 25%**

Ref: Chapter No.57, Page No.1574

59. **Ans: D. Asymptomatic, small (<4 cm) pseudocysts require treatment**

Ref: Chapter No.57, Page No.1574-1575

60. **Ans: B. Splenomegaly is typically present**

Ref: Chapter No.57, Page No.1575

61. **Ans: C. In two third of children, the abscess is unilocular**

Ref: Chapter No.57, Page No.1575

62. **Ans: C. USG of the abdomen provides confirmation of the diagnosis, with the spleen located outside its usual position**

Ref: Chapter No.57, Page No.1575

63. **Ans: D. CT scan is reliable in detecting accessory splenic tissue and surgical exploration at the time of surgery is essential to avoid disease recurrence in ITP**

Ref: Chapter No.57, Page No.1575

64. **Ans: B. H1N1 virus**

Ref: Chapter No.57, Page No.1575-1576

65. **Ans: C. 14 days**

Ref: Chapter No.57, Page No.1576

66. **Ans: D. A 3-cm cuff of peritoneum is left along the lateral aspect of the spleen, which can then be grasped to facilitate lateral retraction**

Ref: Chapter No.57, Page No.1577

67. **Ans: B. Etiology of disease**

Ref: Chapter No.57, Page No.1577-1578

68. **Ans: A. Gastric perforation at the lesser curvature of the stomach**

Ref: Chapter No.57, Page No.1578

69. **Ans: A. Abdominal venous thrombosis referred as post splenectomy thrombosis of the splenic, mesenteric, and portal veins (PST-SMPv) has an incidence of 20% to 30%**

Ref: Chapter No.57, Page No.1578

70. **Ans: B. Older age**

Ref: Chapter No.57, Page No.1579

71. **Ans: D. Most infections occurred more than 10 years after splenectomy**

Ref: Chapter No.57, Page No.1579

72. **Ans: C. 40% - 50%**

Ref: Chapter No.57, Page No.1579

73. **Ans: A. Blindness from meningitis**

Ref: Chapter No.57, Page No.1579

74. **Ans: D. If the patient did not receive these vaccines before surgery such as in emergency surgery, vaccine should be given 10 days after splenectomy or upon discharge whichever comes first**

Ref: Chapter No.57, Page No.1579

75. **Ans: D. Hib 2 doses**

Ref: Chapter No.57, Page No.1580

76. **Ans: C. Macrolide**

Ref: Chapter No.57, Page No.1580

58

Lung, Chest Wall and Mediastinum

1. **All are true about chest wall anatomy except:**
   A. The primary muscles include the diaphragm and intercostal muscles
   B. Intercostal spaces contain the intercostal bundles that travel along the lower edge of each rib
   C. Tertiary system of muscles provides ventilatory assistance through fixation of the upper extremities
   D. The 7th to 10th ribs coalesce into the costal arch

2. **All of the following comprise secondary respiratory muscle group except:**
   A. Sternocleidomastoid
   B. Pectoralis major
   C. Serratus posterior
   D. Levatores costarum

3. **Which is incorrect about anatomic relation of chest structures?**
   A. The angle of Louis is a superficial anatomic landmark for the level of the carina
   B. The trachea in adults is approximately 12 cm long with 18 to 22 cartilaginous rings
   C. The cricoid is the only complete cartilaginous ring in the trachea
   D. The azygos vein arches over the proximal right pulmonary artery as it travels from anterior to posterior

4. **All of the following arteries supply trachea except:**
   A. Inferior thyroid artery
   B. Ascending pharyngeal artery
   C. Supreme intercostals artery
   D. Internal thoracic artery

5. **All are true about lung embryology except:**
   A. The true alveolar stage occurs from approximately 7 months to term
   B. Alveolar proliferation continues till age of 10 years
   C. There are 23 generations of bronchi between the trachea and terminal alveoli
   D. There are 10 bronchopulmonary segments on each side

6. **Number of bronchopulmonary segments in left lung:**
   A. 7 B. 8
   C. 9 D. 10

7. **Which of the following is false statement?**
   A. Flow of lymph from the left lower lobe may drain to the right mediastinal lymph node
   B. The pulmonary parenchyma has vagal nerve supply
   C. Thoracic duct enters into the chest through the aortic hiatus in an anterolateral position
   D. Thoracic duct crosses over to the left at the level of T5

PREOPERATIVE EVALUATION

8. **Recommended smoking abstinence before operative procedure is:**
   A. 2 weeks B. 4 weeks
   C. 8 weeks D. 12 weeks

9. **Which is false regarding pulmonary function assessment?**
   A. FEV1 is the most commonly used as an indicator of postoperative pulmonary reserve
   B. Predicted postoperative FEV 30% or less increases post-operative morbidity
   C. DLCO levels less than 40% are associated with increased perioperative risk
   D. In restrictive disease, the FEV1/FVC ratio is low

10. **58 years old patient with COPD had complain of breathlessness. Evaluation reveals a 4 cm right lower lobe adenocarcinoma. After negative EBUS of mediastinum, he referred for right lower lobectomy. Preoperative evaluation of lung function reveals FEV1 of 45% and a DLCO of 35%. What is the next most appropriate step in management?**
    A. No further testing as he is not a surgical candidate
    B. Cardiopulmonary exercise stress testing
    C. A 6-minute walk test
    D. Surgical resection

11. **Following parameters are measured during cardiopulmonary exercise testing except:**
    A. ECG
    B. Heart rate
    C. FEV1
    D. Minute ventilation

12. **Maximal oxygen consumption (VO_2 max) less than____ considered as high risk for perioperative morbidity.**
    A. 5 mL/Kg/min
    B. 10 mL/Kg/min
    C. 15 mL/Kg/min
    D. 20 mL/Kg/min

13. **Which is incorrect about thoracotomy approach?**
    A. In posterolateral thoracotomy, chest is typically entered through the fifth interspace
    B. A vertical axillary incision approach provides excellent hilar visualization
    C. A median sternotomy can spread the sternum approximately 8 to 10 cm
    D. Both internal mammary arteries are preserved during clamshell incision

CONGENITAL LESIONS

14. **What is the most common cause of pulmonary hypoplasia?**
    A. Oligohydramnios
    B. Bochdalek hernia
    C. Scimitar syndrome
    D. Prune-belly syndrome

15. **Which is incorrect about congenital lesions of lung?**
    A. Unilateral agenesis of lung occurs more frequently on the left
    B. Hyaline membrane disease is frequent in infants of diabetic mothers
    C. Bronchogenic cysts have communication with trachea or bronchus
    D. Lobar emphysema is the most commonly resected congenital cystic lesion

16. **All are true about bronchogenic cysts except:**
    A. Bronchogenic cysts become completely separated from the trachea
    B. Frequently found as an asymptomatic mass on routine CXRs
    C. They are located in the superior mediastinum
    D. Excision is recommended in all symptomatic cysts

17. **Most common location of bronchogenic cysts:**
    A. Superior mediastinum
    B. Anterior mediastinum
    C. Mid mediastinum
    D. Lung parenchyma

18. **Which is incorrect concerning lobar emphysema?**
    A. It affects the upper lobes predominately
    B. It rarely occurs after 6 months of age
    C. Lobar emphysema is the most commonly resected congenital cystic lesion
    D. Treatment of choice is wedge resection

19. **"Stocker classification" is used for:**
    A. Bronchogenic cysts
    B. Congenital cystic adenomatoid malformations
    C. Bronchopulmonary sequestration
    D. Pulmonary arteriovenous malformations

20. **Which is most common type of congenital cystic adenomatoid malformations?**
    A. Type I
    B. Type II
    C. Type III
    D. Type IV

21. **Pleuropulmonary blastoma is strongly associated with which type of congenital cystic adenomatoid malformations?**
    A. Type I
    B. Type II
    C. Type III
    D. Type IV

22. **Which is false regarding bronchopulmonary sequestration?**
    A. It is an area of embryonic lung tissue, separate from the tracheobronchial tree
    B. Blood supply is from an anomalous systemic artery from the aorta
    C. Intralobar sequestration are more common and occurs within the lower lobes predominately
    D. Extralobar sequestration is more common in female patients

23. Which is the most common congenital pulmonary lesion?

A. Bronchogenic cysts
B. Tracheoesophageal fistula
C. Bronchial atresia
D. Tracheal stenosis

24. Which is incorrect about congenital tracheobronchial lesions?

A. The lung tissue distal to the bronchial atresia becomes emphysematous
B. The left upper lobe is the most frequently involved of all lobes within the lung in bronchial atresia
C. Complete circular tracheal rings causing stenosis are commonly associated with a pulmonary artery sling
D. Collapse of greater than 50% of the tracheal lumen during expiration is consistent with tracheomalacia

25. Idiopathic hyperlucent lung seen in:

A. Congenital cystic adenomatoid malformations
B. Swyer James syndrome
C. Osler-Weber-Rendu syndrome
D. Scimitar syndrome

26. Which is incorrect about congenital pulmonary vascular lesions?

A. Macleod syndrome may cause an auto pneumonectomy and idiopathic hyperlucent lung
B. Scimitar syndrome is associated with hypoplastic left lung
C. Hereditary hemorrhagic telangiectasia is associated with Osler-Weber-Rendu syndrome
D. Large arteriovenous malformations tend to be subpleural in location

27. All are true about pulmonary vascular sling except:

A. Aberrant left pulmonary artery arises from the right pulmonary artery
B. It courses between the trachea and the esophagus
C. Many patients are asymptomatic
D. Complete circular tracheal rings are commonly associated

28. Which is false about vascular ring anomalies of aorta?

A. The most common vascular ring is a double aortic arch
B. The left arch is the dominant arch
C. Barium swallow is investigation of choice
D. Bronchoscopy or esophagoscopy are routine before intervention

LUNG CANCER

29. Which cancer is the leading cause of death in women?

A. Stomach B. Lung
C. Breast D. Pancreas

30. Which cancer is the leading cause of death in men?

A. Stomach B. Lung
C. Prostate D. Colorectal

31. 5-year survival of locally advanced lung cancer is:

A. 5% B. 10%
C. 20% D. 30%

32. Which cancer is associated with radon exposure?

A. Nasopharyngeal cancer
B. Lung cancer
C. Bladder cancer
D. Leukemia

33. Which is the most common histologic type of lung cancer?

A. Squamous cell cancer B. Adenocarcinoma
C. Small cell cancer D. Large call carcinoma

34. Which is incorrect concerning adenocarcinoma of the lung?

A. Majority of adenocarcinomas are peripherally located
B. Adenocarcinoma more frequently metastasize to the central nervous system
C. Pure lepidic type growth is adenocarcinoma in situ
D. Adenocarcinoma may be more readily detected on sputum cytology

35. Which of the following histopathologic type of adenocarcinoma of the lung has lowest recurrence rate?

A. Acinar B. Papillary
C. Lepidic D. Solid

36. What is false about squamous cell carcinomas of the lung?

A. Keratinization and intercellular bridges are characteristics of SCC

B. Two thirds of these tumors are peripherally located
C. SCC are prone to undergo central necrosis and cavitation
D. SCC may be more readily detected on sputum cytology

37. All are true concerning neuroendocrine carcinomas of the lung except:

A. These tumors are centrally located
B. They are aggressive and have early distant metastasis
C. More frequent metastases to the bone and CNS
D. Radiation therapy is standard treatment

38. Adenocarcinoma of the lung frequently metastasize to:

A. Bone B. Brain
C. Adrenal D. Liver

39. Which is wrong statement about the National Lung Screening Trial (NSLT)?

A. Patients with 30 pack-years or more of cigarette smoking, either current smokers or had recently quit, were included
B. Patients aged 55 to 74 years were eligible for screening
C. Patients required annual screening with a CXR or low-dose CT scan for 7 years
D. A 20% reduction in mortality rate in high risk population screened with low-dose helical CT scan

40. Which is false regarding screening recommendations of the lung cancer?

A. NCCN recommends low-dose helical CT as screening modality
B. For individuals aged 55 to 74 years with a 30 or more pack-year history of smoking tobacco who currently smoke or former smoker
C. For individuals aged 50 years or older with a 10 or more pack-year history of smoking tobacco who are either current or former smokers
D. Individuals having risk for lung cancer is greater than 1.3%

41. Neurologic paraneoplastic syndromes are frequently associated with which type of lung cancer?

A. Squamous cell cancer
B. Adenocarcinoma
C. Small cell cancer
D. Large call carcinoma

42. Which is incorrect about management of lung cancer?

A. Solitary pulmonary nodule which is radiologically stable on CT scan over a minimum of 2 years are very likely to be benign
B. Paraneoplastic syndromes are due to distant metastasis from small cell carcinoma of the lung
C. Bronchoscopy is recommended before any planned pulmonary resection
D. Malignant pleural effusion is a contraindication to resection

43. Wedge pulmonary resection is recommended in which of the following condition?

A. Undiagnosed solitary pulmonary nodule
B. Stage IA3 SCC with positive pleural fluid cytology
C. Stage IB NSCLC
D. Pancoast tumor

44. At the time of diagnosis, mediastinal lymph node metastases are present in ______% of patients with lung cancer.

A. 15 - 20% B. 25 - 30%
C. 40 - 50% D. 50 - 60%

45. MRI brain in case of lung cancer is recommended in following conditions except:

A. Any patient with Stage III lung cancer
B. Lepidic adenocarcinoma
C. Small cell carcinoma
D. Pancoast tumor

46. All are true about nodal staging of lung cancer except:

A. CT has a sensitivity of 57% to 79% for mediastinal lymph node assessment in NSCLC
B. PET-CT for mediastinal lymph node metastases being more accurate in larger (T2) tumors and in smaller (<1 cm) lymph nodes
C. Cervical mediastinoscopy is commonly performed for biopsy of bilateral paratracheal and subcarinal lymph nodes
D. A left anterior mediastinotomy is used to gain access to the aortopulmonary window or anterior mediastinum lymph nodes

47. A 45 years old patient presents with clinically staged IIIA (T2a N2 M0) left upper lobe NSCLC. Which is appropriate management?

A. EBUS should be performed for pathologic diagnosis

B. Mediastinal lymph nodes sampling at the time of resection
C. Refer for definitive chemotherapy
D. Mediastenoscopy has better diagnostic accuracy than EBUS

48. Patient presents NSCLC with > 1cm anterior mediastinal lymph nodes (N2). Which is appropriate investigation for pathologic diagnosis?

A. Mediastenocopy
B. Mediastenotomy
C. EBUS
D. Esophageal ultrasound

49. Patient presents NSCLC with > 1cm hilar lymph nodes (N1). Which is appropriate investigation for pathologic diagnosis?

A. Mediastenocopy
B. Mediastenotomy
C. EBUS
D. Esophageal ultrasound

50. Subcarinal lymph nodes has lymph node station of:

A. Level 5 B. Level 6
C. Level 7 D. Level 8

51. Patients with lung cancer have metastatic adrenal involvement in _____% of cases at presentation.

A. 7% B. 14%
C. 21% D. 28%

52. What is the T stage for a patient with a 6 cm peripheral lung adenocarcinoma?

A. T1c B. T2a
C. T2b D. T3

53. Which of the following is not included in T2 stage?

A. Tumor >3 cm but ≤5 cm
B. Involvement of main bronchus and carina
C. Visceral pleura invasion
D. Obstructive pneumonitis involving whole lung

54. 4 cm tumor with invasion of lobar bronchus on bronchoscopy is staged as:

A. T1b B. T2a
C. T2b D. T3

55. All of the following constitute stage T3 of the lung cancer except:

A. Primary tumor associated with separate tumor nodule(s) in the same lobe
B. Superior sulcus tumors
C. Parietal pericardium invasion
D. Recurrent laryngeal nerve involvement

56. All of the following constitute stage T3 of the lung cancer except:

A. Tumor >5 cm but ≤7 cm in greatest dimension
B. Chest wall invasion
C. Carina invasion
D. Phrenic nerve

57. All of the following constitute stage T4 of the lung cancer except:

A. Involvement of carina
B. Separate tumor nodule(s) in a different ipsilateral lobe than that of the primary tumor
C. Diaphragmatic invasion
D. Parietal pericardial invasion

58. All of the following constitute stage T4 of the lung cancer except:

A. Tumor >7 cm in greatest dimension
B. Mediastinal invasion
C. Involvement of main bronchus
D. Recurrent laryngeal nerve involvement

59. Which of the following are N3 lymph nodes in case of lung cancer staging?

A. Contralateral mediastinal
B. Subcarinal
C. Contralateral hilar
D. Ipsilateral scalene

60. A 5 cm NSCLC with ipsilateral hilar lymph nodes and malignant pleural effusion is staged as:

A. T1c N2 M1b B. T2a N1 M1a
C. T2b N1 M1a D. T2a N2 M1b

61. Which of the following does not constitute M1a metastatic stage?

A. Separate tumor nodule(s) in a different ipsilateral lobe than that of the primary tumor
B. Malignant pericardial effusion
C. Pleural nodules
D. Malignant pleural effusion

62. A 3 cm pure lepidic adenocarcinoma of the lung has T stage:

A. T1a(mi) B. Tis
C. T1b D. T1c

63. **Patient presents with 5 cm NSCLC with parietal pleural invasion, contralateral mediastinal lymph nodes and evidence of pleural nodules is staged as:**

A. Stage IIIA B. Stage IIIB
C. Stage IIIC D. Stage IVA

64. **A 4 cm NSCLC in right upper lobe with anterior chest wall invasion and ipsilateral mediastinal lymph node involvement is staged as:**

A. Stage IIB B. Stage IIIA
C. Stage IIIB D. Stage IVA

65. **A right sided 3 cm NSCLC with involvement of main stem bronchus associated with separate tumor nodule in the same lobe and involvement of ipsilateral hilar lymph nodes is staged as:**

A. Stage IIB B. Stage IIIA
C. Stage IIIB D. Stage IVA

66. **N1 nodal stations for lung cancer involves nodal levels:**

A. 5 – 9 B. 7 – 14
C. 10 – 14 D. 12 – 14

67. **Wrongly matched nodal stations of lung cancer:**

A. Level 1 – Supraclavicular
B. Level 3p – Retrotracheal
C. Level 5 – Subaortic
D. Level 9 – Hilar

68. **Wrongly matched nodal stations of lung cancer:**

A. Level 7 – Subcarinal
B. Level 9 – Pulmonary ligament
C. Level 11 – Hilar
D. Level 12 – Lobar

69. **In case of lung cancer, hilar lymph nodes have nodal station:**

A. Level 9 B. Level 10
C. Level 11 D. Level 12

70. **A 60-year-old male presents with biopsy-proven lung adenocarcinoma, but no mediastinal disease is found on PET/CT. Which of the following characteristics does not require mediastinal lymph node sampling prior to definitive treatment?**

A. Centrally located T1 tumor
B. Peripherally located T2 tumor
C. CT-positive mediastinal lymph nodes that have no PET avidity
D. None of the above

71. **Segmentectomy may be offered in following patient:**

A. Pure lepidic adenocarcinoma
B. Peripheral Stage I tumor with a low activity on PET/CT
C. Undiagnosed solitary pulmonary nodule
D. Centrally located NSCLC < 3 cm

72. **A healthy 45-year-old male, with normal pulmonary function, presents with left arm pain. CT scan shows a 3 cm irregular mass at the apex of the right lung involving the first and second ribs anteriorly. Transthoracic needle biopsy demonstrates primary lung adenocarcinoma. PET scan and mediastinoscopy demonstrate no metastatic disease. What is the best initial treatment for this patient?**

A. Right upper lobectomy with en bloc chest wall resection
B. Induction chemotherapy and radiation
C. Definitive chemotherapy and radiation
D. Right en bloc chest wall resection, mediastinal lymph node dissection, and adjuvant chest wall radiation

73. **Which is false regarding management of NSCLC?**

A. Anatomical resection with lobectomy and mediastinal lymph node dissection is standard for stage I and II NSCLC
B. Stereotactic body radiation therapy has equal efficacy as surgical resection in stage I NSCLC
C. All patients staged IB and IIB should be considered for adjuvant chemotherapy after resection
D. Induction chemoradiotherapy followed by resection may be advocated in stage IIIA NSCLC

74. **Which of the following targeted therapy is used for NSCLC?**

A. Erlotinib B. Osimertinib
C. Vandetanib D. Pazopanib

75. **Which is most commonly mutated gene is squamous cell carcinoma of the lung?**

A. CDKN2A B. p53
C. EGFR D. KRAS

76. **Immunotherapy is most effective in lung tumors with following characteristics except:**

A. High levels PD-L1 expression
B. NSCLC associated with smoking

C. NSCLC with EGFR mutations
D. Defective DNA repair mechanisms

77. Most frequently associated driver mutations in NSCLC:

A. BRAF B. EGFR
C. MET D. ALK

78. 70 years old male presented with symptoms of dyspnea at rest. Evaluation reveals right upper lobe NSCLC with multiple bilateral mediastinal lymph nodal involvement and right sided pleural effusion. Pleural fluid cytometry shows presence of malignant cells. What is the initial best step of management?

A. Definitive chemotherapy and radiotherapy
B. Placement of tunneled indwelling pleural catheter
C. Pleurodesis
D. Right pneumonectomy followed by chemotherapy

TRACHEA

79. Which is false about tracheal anatomy?

A. The trachea extends from C6 to T4 level
B. The location of the carina is at the level of the angle of Louis
C. The tracheal wall consists of up to 20 incomplete rings of elastic cartilage
D. 50% reduction of the inner diameter increases the airflow resistance sixteen fold

80. A patient who had prolonged endotracheal intubation presented with worsening dyspnea and stridor. Bronchoscopy shows 70% obliteration of tracheal lumen. What is standard treatment for this patient?

A. Tracheal dilatation
B. Internal stent placement
C. Laser resection
D. Resection of stenotic part and end-to-end anastomosis

81. Which is the most common malignancy of trachea?

A. Squamous cell cancer
B. Adenoid cystic carcinoma
C. Pleomorphic adenoma
D. Mucoepidermoid carcinoma

82. Following primary cancers may show hematogenous spread to trachea except:

A. Breast B. Liver
C. Colon D. Melanoma

83. Which is incorrect regarding squamous cell carcinoma of trachea?

A. SCCs often present with hemoptysis
B. Up to 10% can be multifocal
C. The peak incidence is in the sixth to seventh decade primarily in smokers
D. Perineural invasion and extension along vascular structures is very common

84. All are true regarding adenoid cystic carcinoma of trachea except:

A. Well-differentiated, slow-growing neoplasms
B. ACCs typically form polypoid lesions in the trachea
C. Perineural invasion and extension along vascular structures is very common
D. ACCs rarely show recurrence or metastasis

85. Which is false about adenoid cystic carcinoma of trachea?

A. Often present with hemoptysis
B. It affects men and women equally
C. Usually affects nonsmokers
D. The peak incidence occurs in the fourth and fifth decade of life

86. Maximum length of trachea that can be resected during primary anastomosis is ______ cm.

A. 4 cm B. 5 cm
C. 6 cm D. 7 cm

87. Which of the following statement is incorrect regarding management of primary tracheal tumor?

A. Bronchoscopy is mandatory to obtain a tissue diagnosis
B. Complete surgical resection is the treatment of choice for malignant tracheal tumors
C. Postoperative radiotherapy improves survival for patients with completely resected tumors
D. Involvement of the trachea because of local extension from bronchogenic carcinoma may contraindicate resection

88. Most common location of tracheobronchial injury in blunt trauma:

A. Just below cricoid cartilage
B. Cervical tracheal rings
C. Within 2 cm of carina
D. Right main bronchus

89. 35 years old patient of presents with blunt trauma to neck. Which is false regarding management?

A. Early airway assessment followed by definitive airway protection is the key step
B. Chest roentgenogram and chest CT scan are the first step in diagnosis
C. Bronchoscopy is the most important procedure to exactly locate and assess tracheobronchial injuries
D. Immediate exploration of neck wounds should be avoided in blunt neck injuries

90. Which thoracotomy approach gives excellent exposure for carina and proximal left mainstem bronchus?

A. Axillary incision
B. Left thoracotomy
C. Right thoracotomy
D. Left posterolateral thoracotomy

91. Following are the contraindications for tracheal repair except:

A. Permanent tracheostomy for patients with amyotrophic lateral sclerosis
B. Use of high-dose steroids
C. Recent tracheostomy
D. Patients with poor pulmonary reserve

PULMONARY INFECTIONS

92. Surgery is indicated for lung abscess in following conditions except:

A. Persistent cavity $\geq$4 cm
B. Failure to clear sepsis after 8 weeks of medical therapy
C. Hemoptysis
D. To exclude malignancy

93. Which of the following is false statement about pulmonary diseases?

A. Bronchiectasis is abnormal and permanent dilation of the bronchi
B. Lobectomy is the most frequently performed surgery in bronchiectasis
C. Broncholithiasis often cause massive hemoptysis
D. Resection is indicated if pneumonic consolidation persists over 6 to 8 weeks

94. Which is incorrect about broncholithiasis?

A. Sudden bleeding caused by erosion of a small bronchial artery by a spicule in the calcified node
B. Bleeding usually stops with sedation and antitussive therapy
C. Bronchoscopy is possible during a bleeding episode to localize the site of the bleeding
D. Chest CXR is usually diagnostic

95. Surgical intervention needed in case of MDR-TB with following conditions except:

A. Presence of extensive drug resistance requiring therapy more than nine months
B. Massive hemoptysis
C. Persistently positive sputum cultures beyond four to six months of antituberculous therapy
D. Persistent bronchopleural fistula

96. Which is most common opportunistic infection in immunocompromised patient?

A. Candida
B. Pneumocystis
C. Aspergillus
D. Actinomyces

97. All are true about aspergillosis except:

A. Aspergillosis characterized by coarse fragmented septa and hyphae
B. Aspergilloma is the most common form of aspergillosis
C. Patients with aspergilloma fungus balls are at high risk for fatal hemorrhage
D. CXR may demonstrate a crescent radiopacity next to a rounded mass

98. Which is false about pulmonary opportunistic infections?

A. Histoplasma usually causes mediastinal lymph node enlargement
B. In endemic areas, coccidioidomycosis is a frequent cause of lung nodules
C. Any patient diagnosed with pulmonary cryptococcosis should undergo lumbar puncture
D. Operative therapy is recommended for all diagnosed echinococcal pulmonary cysts

MASSIVE HEMOPTYASIS

99. Criteria for massive hemoptysis:

A. $\geq$ 600 ml of blood loss in 24 hours
B. Bleeding >100 mL/Hr
C. Bleeding > 250 mL over 3-4 hours
D. Both A and B

100. Which is most common cause of massive hemoptysis?

A. Bronchiectasis
B. Bronchogenic carcinoma
C. Lung infections
D. Trauma

101. Which is preferred initial investigation of choice in case of massive hemoptysis?

A. Rigid bronchoscopy
B. Flexible bronchoscopy
C. Pulmonary arteriography
D. HRCT chest

EMPHYSEMA AND DIFFUSE LUNG DISEASE

102. All are true concerning emphysematous lung disease except:

A. Emphysema is defined as dilation and destruction of the terminal air spaces
B. Emphysema predominantly involve lower lobes
C. On pulmonary angiography, bullae are vacant and do not contain vessels
D. Simple removal of the symptomatic bullae alone is required with preservation of lung parenchyma

103. What is causative agent for Farmer lung?

A. Nocardia B. Aspergillus
C. Actinomyces D. Mucormycosis

104. Which is the causative agent for Silo filler's disease?

A. NO_2 gas B. Kerosene
C. H_2S gas D. CCl_4 gas

PULMONARY METASTASIS AND MISCELLANEOUS TUMORS

105. Which of the following factor does not affect decision of pulmonary metastasectomy?

A. Extrapulmonary metastases
B. Control of primary tumor
C. Pulmonary reserve
D. Tumor histology

106. Which is false regarding neuroendocrine tumors of lung?

A. Carcinoid tumors rise from Kulchitsky cells in bronchial epithelium
B. Atypical carcinoids are more common in lobar bronchi
C. Carcinoid syndrome is common manifestation
D. Anatomic resection with lobectomy is standard

107. Most common benign tumor of the lung:

A. Hamartoma B. Papilloma
C. Fibroma D. Hemangioma

108. Popcorn appearance on chest radiograph is characteristically seen in:

A. Hemangioma
B. Lymphangiomyomatosis
C. Hamartoma
D. Plasma cell granuloma

109. Following are the features of papilloma of bronchus except:

A. Squamous epithelial origin
B. Occur in childhood
C. Probably viral etiology
D. Resection is curative

110. Tumorlets seen in lung specimen are:

A. Hamartomas
B. Epithelial proliferative lesions
C. Micrometastases
D. Infectious microcysts

CONGENITAL DEFORMITIES OF CHEST WALL

111. Most common congenital chest wall defect:

A. Pectus excavatum
B. Pectus carinatum
C. Pouter pigeon breast
D. Cleft sternum

112. Which is incorrect regarding pectus excavatum deformity?

A. Occurs in 1 of 400 children
B. Male : female ratio is 4:1
C. It may be asymmetric with left sided predominance
D. Pectus excavatum repair is recommended in 15-16 years of age

113. Haller index is used in cases of:

A. Pectus excavatum B. Pectus carinatum
C. Poland syndrome D. Cleft sternum

114. Surgical indications for pectus excavatum:

A. Significant body image issues
B. Haller index on CT scan of greater than 3

C. Caliper measurement depth of greater than 2.5 cm
D. All of the above

115. Ravitch procedure is used for:

A. Pectus excavatum
B. Pectus carinatum
C. Pouter pigeon breast
D. Cleft sternum

116. All are true about Nuss technique except:

A. Minimally invasive operation for the correction of pectus excavatum
B. A convex stainless steel bar is placed under the sternum
C. Single lateral thoracic incision is required
D. The bar is removed after 3 years

117. Which is false regarding pectus carinatum deformity?

A. Keel chest is the most frequent variety pyramidal chest
B. Corrective bracing is successful in more than 80% of patients
C. The timing for repair of should be when patients have finished their teenage growth spurt
D. Robicsek procedure is used for repair

118. Robicsek procedure is used for which chest wall deformity repair?

A. Pectus excavatum
B. Pectus carinatum
C. Pouter pigeon breast
D. Cleft sternum

CHEST WALL TUMORS

119. Which is incorrect statement concerning chest wall tumors?

A. 60% of primary chest wall tumors are malignant
B. They are more likely malignant in the extremes of age
C. Tissue biopsy is usually mandatory to confirm the diagnosis
D. Recommended negative margin for resection is 2 cm

120. 45 years old male presented with 4 cm chest wall mass. Evaluation reveals diagnosis of solitary plasmacytoma. What is the appropriate management?

A. En block resection of chest wall
B. Chemotherapy followed by resection
C. Radiotherapy alone
D. Combined chemoradiation therapy

121. Which is most common malignant bone tumor of chest wall?

A. Osteosarcoma
B. Chondrosarcoma
C. Ewing sarcoma
D. Hemangiosarcoma

122. Tietze syndrome is associated with:

A. Enchondroma of ribs
B. Adenomyosis of breast
C. Costochondritis
D. Superficial thrombophlebitis

THORACIC OUTLET SYNDROME

123. Which of the following test is not used in the diagnosis of thoracic outlet syndrome?

A. Allen test
B. Write's test
C. Roos test
D. Halsted test

124. Identify the structures related to A, B and C in the following figure:

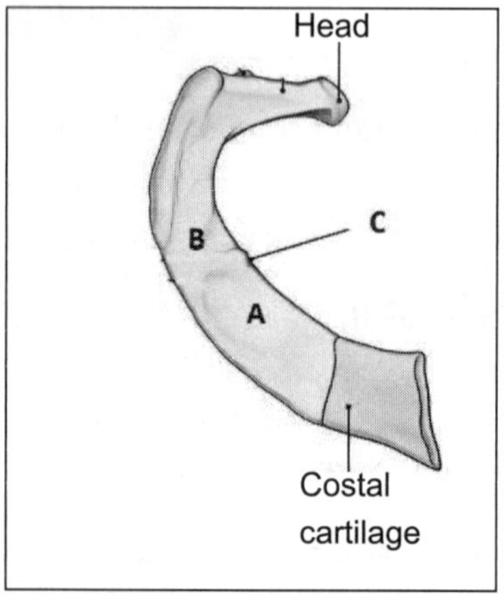

A. A – Subclavian artery, B – Subclavian vein, C – Lower trunk of brachial plexus
B. A – Subclavian artery, B – Subclavian vein, C – Scalene medius
C. A – Subclavian vein, B – Subclavian artery, C – Scalene anterior
D. A – Subclavian vein, B – Subclavian artery, C – Lower trunk of brachial plexus

125. Which is incorrect regarding thoracic outlet syndrome?

A. Middle-aged women are most commonly affected
B. Neurogenic manifestations are reported in more than 90% of cases

C. Paget-Schroetter syndrome is caused by venous compression at thoracic outlet
D. Surgery is the primary treatment

PLEURA

126. Which of the following is the cause of transudative pleural effusion?

A. Pancreatitis
B. Mesothelioma
C. Uremia
D. Pulmonary embolism

127. Minimum amount of pleural fluid detected by chest radiography:

A. 150 ml B. 200 ml
C. 250 ml D. 300 ml

128. Minimum amount of pleural fluid detected on clinical examination:

A. 300 ml B. 400 ml
C. 250 ml D. 600 ml

129. Open drainage or Eloesser flap is recommended for following conditions except:

A. Chronic empyema with residual pleural space
B. Bronchopleural fistula
C. Esophageal perforation
D. Post-lobectomy empyema

130. Following are causes of chylothorax except:

A. Iatrogenic
B. Neoplasms
C. Collagen vascular disease
D. Infectious

131. Which is false about management of chylothorax?

A. Analysis of pleural fluid with chylomicrons confirms the diagnosis
B. Conservative measures such as medium-chain triglyceride diet or TPN and octreotide are initially indicated
C. If conservative measures fail, operative intervention may be considered after 14 days
D. Placement of olive oil or ice cream by nasogastric tube at the time of the operation may identify area of thoracic duct disruption

132. A 22 years old tall, thin male presents with spontaneous pneumothorax on right side. Patient had history of similar episode 6 months back and had chest tube placed. What is the appropriate treatment for this patient?

A. Needle aspiration and discharge
B. Chest tube insertion
C. Lobectomy
D. Apical wedge resection and pleurodesis

133. Which of the following is incorrect about malignant pleural mesothelioma?

A. It is strongly associated with asbestos exposure
B. Long latency period of 15–40 years exists between primary exposure and disease development
C. The diagnosis is made with pleural biopsy
D. Extrapleural pneumonectomy is the procedure of choice

MEDIASTINUM

134. Which is most common anterior mediastinal neoplasm in adults?

A. Lymphoma B. Thymoma
C. Germ cell tumors D. Teratoma

135. Which is most common primary tumors of mediastinum?

A. Lymphoma B. Thymoma
C. Neurogenic tumors D. Teratoma

136. All of the following mediastinal tumors are found in the anterior mediastinum except

A. Lymphoma B. Seminoma
C. Ganglioneuroma D. Thyroid tumors

137. Which is most common neurogenic tumor of mediastinum?

A. Neurofibroma B. Schwannoma
C. Ganglioneuroma D. Paraganglioma

138. Which is most common neurogenic tumor of children?

A. Neurofibroma B. Paraganglioma
C. Ganglioneuroma D. Neuroblastoma

139. All are associated with thymomas except:

A. Myasthenia gravis
B. Red cell aplasia
C. Hypergammaglobulinemia
D. Smooth muscle degeneration

140. What is diagnostic modality of choice in mediastinal masses?

A. Chest radiograph B. CT scan
C. MRI D. EUS

141. A chest X-ray of a 30 years old male, for complaints of dyspnea and cough, shows a 5 cm mediastinal mass in the anterior mediastinum and confirmed by CT. AFP levels are raised. What is the probable diagnosis?

A. Lymphoma
B. Teratoma
C. Seminoma
D. Nonseminomatous germ cell tumor

142. A 30 years old patient presents with upper extremity swelling, fatigue, weight loss and dyspnea. CXR shows multiple superior mediastinal masses and confirmed on CT. LDH and ALP levels are raised. What is probable diagnosis?

A. Thymoma B. Germ cell tumor
C. Lymphoma D. Pancoast tumor

143. Which is incorrect about primary mediastinal cysts?

A. They account for approximately 20% of mediastinal masses
B. Majority are asymptomatic
C. Bronchogenic cysts are most common
D. Pericardial cyst occur in the cardiophrenic angle mostly on the left side

PRIMARY MEDIASTINAL NEOPLASMS

144. Which is false regarding thymoma?

A. Peak incidence is in the third to fifth decades
B. The most common syndrome associated is myasthenia gravis
C. Type A being the most indolent subtype
D. Primary surgical resection alone is sufficient

145. Masaoka-Koga staging system is used for:

A. Neuroblastoma B. Thymoma
C. Lymphoma D. Germ cell tumors

146. Which is most common extragonadal primary site of germ cell tumors?

A. Superior mediastinum
B. Middle mediastinum
C. Posterior mediastinum
D. Retroperitoneum

147. Which is most common primary germ cell tumor of mediastinum?

A. Teratoma
B. Seminoma
C. Choriocarcinoma
D. Yolk sac tumor

148. AFP is raised in which type of germ cell tumors?

A. Teratoma B. Seminoma
C. Yolk sac tumor D. Choriocarcinoma

149. Hematologic malignancies are associated with which of the following tumors?

A. Thymoma
B. Neurogenic tumors
C. Mediastinal nonseminomatous germ cell tumors
D. Testicular germ cell tumors

150. Which is incorrect concerning mediastinal primary nonseminomatous germ cell tumors?

A. They are more aggressive tumors and more frequently disseminated at the time of diagnosis
B. They are radiosensitive
C. Treatment of nonseminomatous tumors currently is with cisplatin and etoposide-based regimens
D. The pathology of the resected post chemotherapy specimen appears to be the most significant predictor of survival

151. All are true about neurogenic tumors of mediastinum except:

A. Most of neurogenic tumors are benign in children
B. Many of these tumors are asymptomatic
C. During resection of dumbbell tumors, the intraspinal component should be removed first
D. A separate transthoracic approach is needed for resection of the intrathoracic component

152. Which is false concerning neuroblastoma?

A. Neuroblastomas originate from the sympathetic nervous system
B. The most common location for a neuroblastoma is in the posterior mediastinum
C. Most of these tumors occur in children 4 years old or younger
D. These are highly invasive neoplasms that have frequently metastasized before diagnosis

153. All of the following are associated with Carney syndrome except:

A. Pulmonary chondroma
B. Atrial myxoma
C. Gastric leiomyosarcoma
D. Extra-adrenal paraganglioma

154. Which is false regarding paragangliomas?

A. They represents less than 2% of all pheochromocytomas
B. Most are found in the paravertebral sulcus
C. Extra-adrenal paragangliomas have elevated epinephrine levels
D. I-131 MIBG scintigraphy is used particularly when the tumors are hormonally active

155. Needle biopsy is non-diagnostic in which of the mediastinal tumors?

A. Germ cell tumors
B. Lymphoma
C. Neuroendocrine tumor
D. Leiomyosarcoma

156. Thymic neuroendocrine tumors are commonly associated with:

A. Hyperparathyroidism
B. Myasthenia gravis
C. Cushing's syndrome
D. Carcinoid syndrome

ANSWERS

1. **Ans: D. The 7th to 10th ribs coalesce into the costal arch**
   Ref: Chapter No. 58, Page No. 1585
2. **Ans: B. Pectoralis major**
   Ref: Chapter No. 58, Page No. 1585
3. **Ans: D. The azygos vein arches over the proximal right pulmonary artery as it travels from anterior to posterior**
   Ref: Chapter No. 58, Page No. 1586
4. **Ans: B. Ascending pharyngeal artery**
   Ref: Chapter No. 58, Page No. 1586
5. **Ans: D. There are 10 bronchopulmonary segments on each side**
   Ref: Chapter No. 58, Page No. 1586-87
6. **Ans: B. 8**
   Ref: Chapter No. 58, Page No. 1587
7. **Ans: B. The pulmonary parenchyma has vagal nerve supply**
   Ref: Chapter No. 58, Page No. 1587
8. **Ans: B. 4 weeks**
   Ref: Chapter No. 58, Page No. 1588
9. **Ans: D. In restrictive disease, the FEV1/FVC ratio is low**
   Ref: Chapter No. 58, Page No. 1588
10. **Ans: B. Cardiopulmonary exercise stress testing**
    Ref: Chapter No. 58, Page No. 1588
11. **Ans: C. FEV1**
    Ref: Chapter No. 58, Page No. 1588
12. **Ans: B. 10 mL/Kg/min**
    Ref: Chapter No. 58, Page No. 1588
13. **Ans: D. Both internal mammary arteries are preserved during clamshell incision**
    Ref: Chapter No. 58, Page No. 1589-90
14. **Ans: B. Bochdalek hernia**
    Ref: Chapter No. 58, Page No. 1590
15. **Ans: C. Bronchogenic cysts have communication with trachea or bronchus**
    Ref: Chapter No. 58, Page No. 1591
16. **Ans: C. They are located in the superior mediastinum**
    Ref: Chapter No. 58, Page No. 1591
17. **Ans: C. Mid mediastinum**
    Ref: Chapter No. 58, Page No. 1591
18. **Ans: D. Treatment of choice is wedge resection**
    Ref: Chapter No. 58, Page No. 1591
19. **Ans: B. Congenital cystic adenomatoid malformations**
    Ref: Chapter No. 58, Page No. 1591
20. **Ans: A. Type I**
    Ref: Chapter No. 58, Page No. 1591
21. **Ans: D. Type IV**
    Ref: Chapter No. 58, Page No. 1591
22. **Ans: D. Extralobar sequestration is more common in female patients**
    Ref: Chapter No. 58, Page No. 1591
23. **Ans: B. Tracheoesophageal fistula**
    Ref: Chapter No. 58, Page No. 1592
24. **Ans: D. Collapse of greater than 50% of the tracheal lumen during expiration is consistent with tracheomalacia**
    Ref: Chapter No. 58, Page No. 1592-93
25. **Ans: B. Swyer James syndrome**
    Ref: Chapter No. 58, Page No. 1593
26. **Ans: B. Scimitar syndrome is associated with hypoplastic left lung**
    Ref: Chapter No. 58, Page No. 1593
27. **Ans: C. Many patients are asymptomatic**
    Ref: Chapter No. 58, Page No. 1593
28. **Ans: B. The left arch is the dominant arch**
    Ref: Chapter No. 58, Page No. 1593
29. **Ans: B. Lung**
    Ref: Chapter No. 58, Page No. 1594
30. **Ans: B. Lung**
    Ref: Chapter No. 58, Page No. 1594
31. **Ans: A. 5%**
    Ref: Chapter No. 58, Page No. 1594
32. **Ans: B. Lung cancer**
    Ref: Chapter No. 58, Page No. 1594
33. **Ans: B. Adenocarcinoma**
    Ref: Chapter No. 58, Page No. 1595
34. **Ans: D. Adenocarcinoma may be more readily detected on sputum cytology**
    Ref: Chapter No. 58, Page No. 1595
35. **Ans: C. Lepidic**
    Ref: Chapter No. 58, Page No. 1595

36. **Ans: B. Two thirds of these tumors are peripherally located**

Ref: Chapter No. 58, Page No. 1595

37. **Ans: D. Radiation therapy is standard treatment**

Ref: Chapter No. 58, Page No. 1595

38. **Ans: B. Brain**

Ref: Chapter No. 58, Page No. 1595

39. **Ans: C. Patients required annual screening with a CXR or low-dose CT scan for 7 years**

Ref: Chapter No. 58, Page No. 1595

40. **Ans: C. For individuals aged 50 years or older with a 10 or more pack-year history of smoking tobacco who are either current or former smokers**

Ref: Chapter No. 58, Page No. 1596

41. **Ans: C. Small cell cancer**

Ref: Chapter No. 58, Page No. 1596

42. **Ans: B. Paraneoplastic syndromes are due to distant metastasis from small cell carcinoma of the lung**

Ref: Chapter No. 58, Page No. 1596

43. **Ans: A. Undiagnosed solitary pulmonary nodule**

Ref: Chapter No. 58, Page No. 1596

44. **Ans: B. 25 - 30%**

Ref: Chapter No. 58, Page No. 1597

45. **Ans: B. Lepidic adenocarcinoma**

Ref: Chapter No. 58, Page No. 1597

46. **Ans: B. PET-CT for mediastinal lymph node metastases being more accurate in larger (T2) tumors and in smaller (<1 cm) lymph nodes**

Ref: Chapter No. 58, Page No. 1598

47. **Ans: A. EBUS should be performed for pathologic diagnosis**

Ref: Chapter No. 58, Page No. 1598

48. **Ans: B. Mediastenotomy**

Ref: Chapter No. 58, Page No. 1598

49. **Ans: C. EBUS**

Ref: Chapter No. 58, Page No. 1598

50. **Ans: C. Level 7**

Ref: Chapter No. 58, Page No. 1598

51. **Ans: A. 7%**

Ref: Chapter No. 58, Page No. 1598

52. **Ans: D. T3**

Ref: Chapter No. 58, Page No. 1599

53. **Ans: B. Involvement of main bronchus and carina**

Ref: Chapter No. 58, Page No. 1599

54. **Ans: C. T2b**

Ref: Chapter No. 58, Page No. 1599

55. **Ans: D. Recurrent laryngeal nerve involvement**

Ref: Chapter No. 58, Page No. 1599

56. **Ans: C. Carina invasion**

Ref: Chapter No. 58, Page No. 1599

57. **Ans: D. Parietal pericardial invasion**

Ref: Chapter No. 58, Page No. 1599

58. **Ans: C. Involvement of main bronchus**

Ref: Chapter No. 58, Page No. 1599

59. **Ans: B. Subcarinal**

Ref: Chapter No. 58, Page No. 1599

60. **Ans: C. T2b N1 M1a**

Ref: Chapter No. 58, Page No. 1599

61. **Ans: A. Separate tumor nodule(s) in a different ipsilateral lobe than that of the primary tumor**

Ref: Chapter No. 58, Page No. 1599

62. **Ans: B. Tis**

Ref: Chapter No. 58, Page No. 1599

63. **Ans: D. Stage IVA**

Ref: Chapter No. 58, Page No. 1599-1600

64. **Ans: C. Stage IIIB**

Ref: Chapter No. 58, Page No. 1599-1600

65. **Ans: B. Stage IIIA**

Ref: Chapter No. 58, Page No. 1599-1600

66. **Ans: C. 10 – 14**

Ref: Chapter No. 58, Page No. 1602

67. **Ans: D. Level 9 – Hilar**

Ref: Chapter No. 58, Page No. 1602

68. **Ans: C. Level 11 – Hilar**

Ref: Chapter No. 58, Page No. 1602

69. **Ans: B. Level 10**

Ref: Chapter No. 58, Page No. 1602

70. **Ans: D. None of the above**

Ref: Chapter No. 58, Page No. 1604

71. **Ans: D. Centrally located NSCLC < 3 cm**

Ref: Chapter No. 58, Page No. 1604

72. **Ans: B. Induction chemotherapy and radiation**

Ref: Chapter No. 58, Page No. 1606

73. **Ans: B. Stereotactic body radiation therapy has equal efficacy as surgical resection in stage I NSCLC**

Ref: Chapter No. 58, Page No. 1602-04

74. **Ans: B. Osimertinib**

Ref: Chapter No. 58, Page No. 1606

75. **Ans: B. p53**

Ref: Chapter No. 58, Page No. 1607

76. **Ans: C. NSCLC with EGFR mutations**

Ref: Chapter No. 58, Page No. 1607

77. **Ans: B. EGFR**

Ref: Chapter No. 58, Page No. 1608

78. **Ans: B. Placement of tunneled indwelling pleural catheter**

Ref: Chapter No. 58, Page No. 1608

79. **Ans: C. The tracheal wall consists of up to 20 incomplete rings of elastic cartilage**

Ref: Chapter No. 58, Page No. 1608-09

80. **Ans: D. Resection of stenotic part and end-to-end anastomosis**

Ref: Chapter No. 58, Page No. 1609

81. **Ans: A. Squamous cell cancer**

Ref: Chapter No. 58, Page No. 1609

82. **Ans: B. Liver**

Ref: Chapter No. 58, Page No. 1609

83. **Ans: D. Perineural invasion and extension along vascular structures is very common**

Ref: Chapter No. 58, Page No. 1609

84. **Ans: D. ACCs rarely show recurrence or metastasis**

Ref: Chapter No. 58, Page No. 1609

85. **Ans: A. Often present with hemoptysis**

Ref: Chapter No. 58, Page No. 1610

86. **Ans: B. 5 cm**

Ref: Chapter No. 58, Page No. 1610

87. **Ans: C. Postoperative radiotherapy improves survival for patients with completely resected tumors**

Ref: Chapter No. 58, Page No. 1610

88. **Ans: C. Within 2 cm of carina**

Ref: Chapter No. 58, Page No. 1610

89. **Ans: D. Immediate exploration of neck wounds should be avoided in blunt neck injuries**

Ref: Chapter No. 58, Page No. 1610

90. **Ans: C. Right thoracotomy**

Ref: Chapter No. 58, Page No. 1610

91. **Ans: D. Patients with poor pulmonary reserve**

Ref: Chapter No. 58, Page No. 1611

92. **Ans: A. Persistent cavity ≥4 cm**

Ref: Chapter No. 58, Page No. 1614

93. **Ans: C. Broncholithiasis often cause massive hemoptysis**

Ref: Chapter No. 58, Page No. 1613-14

94. **Ans: D. Chest CXR is usually diagnostic**

Ref: Chapter No. 58, Page No. 1614

95. **Ans: A. Presence of extensive drug resistance requiring therapy more than nine months**

Ref: Chapter No. 58, Page No. 1614

96. **Ans: C. Aspergillus**

Ref: Chapter No. 58, Page No. 1614

97. **Ans: D. CXR may demonstrate a crescent radiopacity next to a rounded mass**

Ref: Chapter No. 58, Page No. 1615

98. **Ans: D. Operative therapy is recommended for all diagnosed echinococcal pulmonary cysts**

Ref: Chapter No. 58, Page No. 1615

99. **Ans: D. Both A and B**

Ref: Chapter No. 58, Page No. 1616

100. **Ans: C. Lung infections**

Ref: Chapter No. 58, Page No. 1616

101. **Ans: B. Flexible bronchoscopy**

Ref: Chapter No. 58, Page No. 1616

102. **Ans: B. Emphysema predominantly involve lower lobes**

Ref: Chapter No. 58, Page No. 1617

103. **Ans: C. Actinomyces**

Ref: Chapter No. 58, Page No. 1618

104. **Ans: A. NO_2 gas**

Ref: Chapter No. 58, Page No. 1618

105. **Ans: D. Tumor histology**

Ref: Chapter No. 58, Page No. 1618

106. **Ans: C. Carcinoid syndrome is common manifestation**

Ref: Chapter No. 58, Page No. 1619

107. **Ans: A. Hamartoma**

Ref: Chapter No. 58, Page No. 1619

108. **Ans: C. Hamartoma**

Ref: Chapter No. 58, Page No. 1619

109. **Ans: D. Resection is curative**

Ref: Chapter No. 58, Page No. 1619

110. **Ans: B. Epithelial proliferative lesions**

Ref: Chapter No. 58, Page No. 1620

111. **Ans: A. Pectus excavatum**

Ref: Chapter No. 58, Page No. 1620

112. **Ans: C. It may be asymmetric with left sided predominance**

Ref: Chapter No. 58, Page No. 1620

113. Ans: A. Pectus excavatum

Ref: Chapter No. 58, Page No. 1620

114. Ans: D. All of the above

Ref: Chapter No. 58, Page No. 1620

115. Ans: A. Pectus excavatum

Ref: Chapter No. 58, Page No. 1621

116. Ans: C. Single lateral thoracic incision is required

Ref: Chapter No. 58, Page No. 1621

117. Ans: D. Robicsek procedure is used for repair

Ref: Chapter No. 58, Page No. 1621

118. Ans: A. Pectus excavatum

Ref: Chapter No. 58, Page No. 1622

119. Ans: D. Recommended negative margin for resection is 2 cm

Ref: Chapter No. 58, Page No. 1623

120. Ans: C. Radiotherapy alone

Ref: Chapter No. 58, Page No. 1623

121. Ans: B. Chondrosarcoma

Ref: Chapter No. 58, Page No. 1623

122. Ans: C. Costochondritis

Ref: Chapter No. 58, Page No. 1626

123. Ans: A. Allen test

Ref: Chapter No. 58, Page No. 1627

124. Ans: C. A – Subclavian vein, B – Subclavian artery, C – Scalene anterior

Ref: Chapter No. 58, Page No. 1627

125. Ans: D. Surgery is the primary treatment

Ref: Chapter No. 58, Page No. 1627

126. Ans: D. Pulmonary embolism

Ref: Chapter No. 58, Page No. 1629

127. Ans: D. 300 ml

Ref: Chapter No. 58, Page No. 1629

128. Ans: C. 500 ml

Ref: Chapter No. 58, Page No. 1629

129. Ans: C. Esophageal perforation

Ref: Chapter No. 58, Page No. 1630

130. Ans: C. Collagen vascular disease

Ref: Chapter No. 58, Page No. 1631

131. Ans: C. If conservative measures fail, operative intervention may be considered after 14 days

Ref: Chapter No. 58, Page No. 1631

132. Ans: D. Apical wedge resection and pleurodesis

Ref: Chapter No. 58, Page No. 1631

133. Ans: D. Extrapleural pneumonectomy is the procedure of choice

Ref: Chapter No. 58, Page No. 1632

134. Ans: B. Thymoma

Ref: Chapter No. 58, Page No. 1633

135. Ans: C. Neurogenic tumors

Ref: Chapter No. 58, Page No. 1633

136. Ans: C. Ganglioneuroma

Ref: Chapter No. 58, Page No. 1633

137. Ans: B. Schwannoma

Ref: Chapter No. 58, Page No. 1633

138. Ans: C. Ganglioneuroma

Ref: Chapter No. 58, Page No. 1633

139. Ans: C. Hypergammaglobulinemia

Ref: Chapter No. 58, Page No. 1634

140. Ans: B. CT scan

Ref: Chapter No. 58, Page No. 1634

141. Ans: D. Nonseminomatous germ cell tumor

Ref: Chapter No. 58, Page No. 1634

142. Ans: C. Lymphoma

Ref: Chapter No. 58, Page No. 1634

143. Ans: D. Pericardial cyst occur in the cardiophrenic angle mostly on the left side

Ref: Chapter No. 58, Page No. 1634

144. Ans: D. Primary surgical resection alone is sufficient

Ref: Chapter No. 58, Page No. 1635

145. Ans: B. Thymoma

Ref: Chapter No. 58, Page No. 1635

146. Ans: A. Superior mediastinum

Ref: Chapter No. 58, Page No. 1635

147. Ans: A. Teratoma

Ref: Chapter No. 58, Page No. 1635

148. Ans: C. Yolk sac tumor

Ref: Chapter No. 58, Page No. 1637

149. Ans: C. Mediastinal nonseminomatous germ cell tumors

Ref: Chapter No. 58, Page No. 1637

150. Ans: B. They are radiosensitive

Ref: Chapter No. 58, Page No. 1637

151. Ans: A. Most of neurogenic tumors are benign in children

Ref: Chapter No. 58, Page No. 1637

152. Ans: B. The most common location for a neuroblastoma is in the posterior mediastinum

Ref: Chapter No. 58, Page No. 1637

153. Ans: B. Atrial myxoma

Ref: Chapter No. 58, Page No. 1638

154. Ans: C. Extra-adrenal paragangliomas have elevated epinephrine levels

Ref: Chapter No. 58, Page No. 1638

155. Ans: B. Lymphoma

Ref: Chapter No. 58, Page No. 1638

156. Ans: C. Cushing's syndrome

Ref: Chapter No. 58, Page No. 1638

59

Congenital Heart Disease

ANATOMY AND DIAGNOSIS

1. **According to Anderson nomenclature, congenitally corrected transposition is described as:**
   A. Atrial situs solitus with atrioventricular concordance and ventriculoarterial discordance
   B. Atrial situs solitus with atrioventricular discordance and ventriculoarterial discordance
   C. Atrial situs inversus with atrioventricular concordance and ventriculoarterial discordance
   D. Atrial situs inversus with atrioventricular discordance and ventriculoarterial discordance

2. **Modified Blalock – Taussig shunt includes:**
   A. Right subclavian artery to pulmonary artery anastomosis
   B. Left subclavian artery to main pulmonary trunk anastomosis
   C. Use of prosthetic interposition graft
   D. Left pulmonary artery to descending aorta shunt

3. **What is heterotaxy syndrome of heart?**
   A. Absent or deranged sinoatrial node
   B. Atrioventricular accessory pathway
   C. Absent or deranged atrioventricular node
   D. Bundle of hiss abnormality

4. **What is radiation dose of CT chest?**
   A. 1 – 3 mSv B. 3 – 5 mSv
   C. 5 – 7 mSv D. 9 – 11 mSv

5. **What is radiation dose of CT coronary angiography?**
   A. 3 – 5 mSv B. 5 – 7 mSv
   C. 7 – 9 mSv D. 9 – 11 mSv

6. **Which is false regarding normal physiology of heart?**
   A. The 'c' wave of atrial pressure corresponds to A-V valve closure
   B. Filling or end-diastolic pressures in both ventricles are between 2 and 10 mm Hg
   C. In normal hearts, there is a small, physiologically insignificant left-to-right shunt
   D. The physiologic shunt represents less than 5% of the cardiac output

7. **What is normal pulmonary artery systolic pressure?**
   A. 1 to 5 mm Hg B. 2 to 10 mm Hg
   C. 15 to 30 mm Hg D. 90 to 110 mm Hg

8. **Pulmonary vascular resistant is calculated using following parameters except:**
   A. Pulmonary artery pressure
   B. Right ventricular pressure
   C. Left atrial pressure
   D. Pulmonary blood flow

PATENT DUCTUS ARTERIOSUS

9. **All are associated with increased pulmonary blood flow except:**
   A. Patent Ductus arteriosus
   B. A-V canal defect
   C. Truncus arteriosus
   D. Tetralogy of Fallot

10. **Which is false regarding patent ductus arteriosus?**
   A. PDA is found in 1 in 2000 term neonates
   B. Ductal flow is from the pulmonary artery to the aorta during gestation
   C. It is completely closed in most infants by 2 to 3 weeks of age
   D. Endocarditis risk is very low for PDA

11. Which is incorrect statement about management of PDA?

A. A large unrestricted PDA can proceeds to irreversible Eisenmenger syndrome
B. Closure is recommended for all PDAs
C. The gold standard is surgery, usually through a left anterolateral thoracotomy
D. Medical treatment with indomethacin, 0.2 mg/kg for ≥1 kg on day 1, then 0.1 mg/kg daily for days 2–7 oral or IV over 1 hour can be given

12. Indomethacin treatment in neonates is associated with:

A. Pulmonary fibrosis
B. Hepatotoxicity
C. Necrotizing enterocolitis
D. Myocardial ischemia

13. Indomethacin in neonates has following side effects except:

A. Necrotizing enterocolitis
B. Renal toxicity
C. Intracranial hemorrhage
D. Pulmonary fibrosis

AORTOPULMONARY SEPTAL DEFECT

14. Which is incorrect about aortopulmonary septal defect?

A. A failure of complete separation of the embryologic common arterial trunk into the aorta and pulmonary artery
B. Type I is common arterial trunk
C. Type III is associated with a separate origin of the right pulmonary artery from the aorta
D. Surgical exposure of aortopulmonary septal defect includes a transverse incision in the ascending aorta

ATRIAL SEPTAL DEFECT (ASD)

15. Most common atrial septal defect is:

A. Ostium primum B. Ostium secundum
C. Sinus venosus D. Membranous

16. All are true regarding atrial septal defects except:

A. ASD is a congenital cardiac lesions occurring in 13 of every 10,000 live births
B. The most frequently encountered ASD is a result of incomplete closure of the septum primum
C. Pulmonary vascular disease is a typical finding in secundum ASDs
D. Most recommend ASD closure in patients before school age

17. Identify following defect noted by "A":

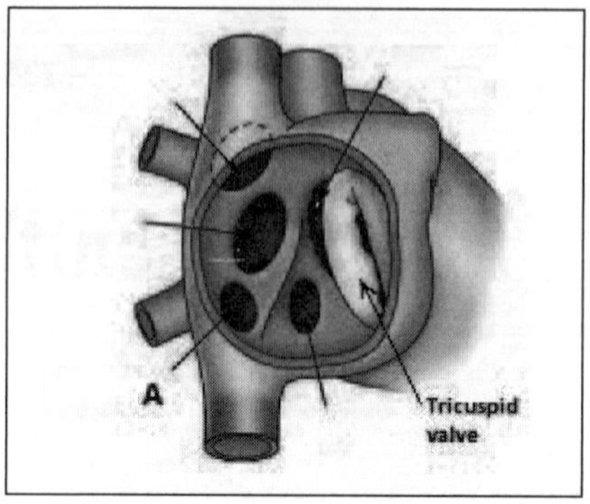

A. Ostium prium ASD
B. Ostium secundum ASD
C. Coronary sinus ASD
D. Sinus venosus ASD

18. Which atrial septal defect is associated with total anomalous pulmonary venous return?

A. Ostium prium ASD
B. Ostium secundum ASD
C. Coronary sinus ASD
D. Sinus venosus ASD

19. Scimitar syndrome is related to:

A. Atrioventricular canal defect
B. Total anomalous pulmonary venous return
C. Transposition of the great arteries
D. Pulmonary artery slings

20. Identify the marked structure:

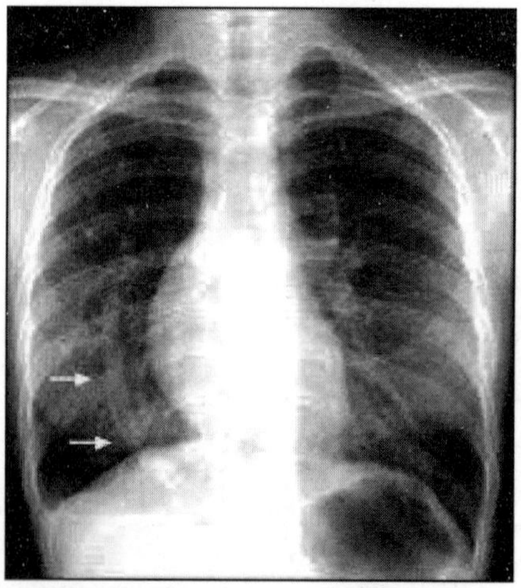

A. Pulmonary sequestration
B. Right aortic arch
C. Total anomalous pulmonary venous return
D. Duplication of IVC

21. Warden procedure for anomalous pulmonary venous return involves:

A. SVC translocation
B. SVC reconstruction with intervening graft
C. IVC translocation
D. IVC reconstruction with intervening graft

VENTRICULAR SEPTAL DEFECT (VSD)

22. Which is false regarding ventricular septal defect?

A. Outlet VSD exhibit a potential for spontaneous closure
B. Swiss cheese pattern is seen with muscular VSD
C. All subarterial VSDs should be closed surgically
D. It carries lifelong risk for endocarditis

23. Which type of VSD exhibit potential for spontaneous closure?

A. Perimembranous VSD
B. Subarterial VSD
C. Inlet VSD
D. Trabecular VSD

24. Indications for surgical closure of VSD includes following factors except:

A. Size of the VSD B. Location of VSD
C. Degree of shunting D. Associated lesions

ATRIOVENTRICULAR SEPTAL DEFECT

25. Which is incorrect about atrioventricular septal defect?

A. It occurs in approximately 1 in every 2100 live births
B. The A-V valve tissue is always abnormal
C. Complete AVSDs are frequently seen in patients with trisomy 18
D. The ASD in this defect is termed a primum ASD

26. Which chromosomal anomaly is most commonly associated with atrioventricular septal defect?

A. Trisomy 18 B. Trisomy 21
C. Turner syndrome D. Trisomy 13

27. Rastelli classification is used for

A. TAPVC
B. Transposition of great vessels
C. Complete A-V canal defect
D. Persistent truncus arteriosus

28. Which of the following is not associated with atrioventricular septal defect?

A. Abnormal A-V valve tissue
B. Displaced AV node and bundle of Hiss
C. Secundum VSD
D. Variable chordal support

29. Which is incorrect about atrioventricular septal defect?

A. Rastelli type A defect, with superior leaflet and chordal support committed to the right side of the ventricular septum
B. Surgical repair is recommended in infancy usually before 6 months of age
C. The ASD in this defect is termed a primum ASD which is distinctly separate from the ovale fossa
D. The critical component of the repair lies in the valve repair

PERSISTENT ARTERIAL TRUNK

30. Which is false about persistent truncus arteriosus?

A. It occurs in approximately 1 in 10,000 live births
B. It is associated with a restrictive perimembranous VSD
C. The condition is classified by the relationship of the origins of the pulmonary arteries
D. Type IV truncus arteriosus is a form of pulmonary atresia with VSD

31. Which chromosomal anomaly associated with persistent truncus arteriosus?

A. Chromosome 16 B. Chromosome 18
C. Chromosome 21 D. Chromosome 22

32. Which is not associated with persistent truncus arteriosus?

A. Interruption of the aortic arch
B. DiGeorge syndrome
C. Pulmonary vascular disease
D. Ductal-independence

33. Following are associated with DiGeorge syndrome except:

A. Transposition of great vessels
B. Thymic aplasia
C. Hypocalcemia
D. Abnormal T cell function

34. Interruption of the aortic arch is associated in _____% of newborns presenting with truncus arteriosus.

A. 5% B. 15%
C. 25% D. 35%

35. Classification system used for persistent truncus arteriosus:

A. Van Praagh classification
B. Rastelli classification
C. David – Miller classification
D. Anderson classification

36. Classification system used for persistent truncus arteriosus:

A. Rastelli classification
B. Collett and Edwards classification
C. David – Miller classification
D. Anderson classification

37. Contegra conduit used for the repair of truncus arteriosus is made up of:

A. Aortic valved homograft
B. Pulmonary valved homograft
C. Porcine jugular vein valved conduit
D. Bovine jugular vein valved conduit

TOTAL ANOMALOUS PULMONARY VENOUS RETURN

38. Which is false regarding total anomalous pulmonary venous return?

A. It occurs in 1 in every 10,000 live births
B. In most common variation of supracardiac TAPVR, the vertical vein courses anterior to the left pulmonary artery to join the left innominate vein
C. In intracardiac TAPVR, the pulmonary veins drain into the right atrium
D. Infracardiac TAPVR variation is almost always obstructed

39. In infracardiac TAPVR, anomalous pulmonary drains into which vein?

A. Supradiaphragmatic IVC
B. Retrohepatic IVC
C. Ductus venosus
D. Intrahepatic IVC

40. Cor Triatriatum is described as:

A. Pulmonary veins enter into coronary sinus
B. Pulmonary veins enter a chamber posterior to left atrium
C. Pulmonary veins enter a chamber posterior to right atrium
D. Pulmonary veins enter into a diverticulum of left atrium

41. Which is most common anomalous systemic venous drainage?

A. Absence of right SVC B. Persistent left SVC
C. Interrupted IVC D. Duplication of IVC

TETRALOGY OF FALLOT

42. What is the incidence of tetralogy of Fallot?

A. 1 in 500 B. 1 in 2500
C. 1 in 5000 D. 1 in 25000

43. What is anatomic hallmark of Tetralogy of Fallot?

A. Malalignment VSD
B. Aortic override
C. Right ventricular outflow tract obstruction
D. Right ventricular hypertrophy

44. Blalock-Taussig shunt includes:

A. Anastomosis of the right subclavian artery to the divided right pulmonary artery
B. Anastomosis of the left subclavian artery to the divided left pulmonary artery
C. Anastomosis of the left pulmonary artery to the descending aorta
D. Anastomosis of the right pulmonary artery to the ascending aorta

45. Tetralogy of Fallot does not include:

A. Perimembranous, pressure-nonrestrictive VSD
B. Right-to-left shunt
C. Ductal independence
D. Lifelong follow up

46. Palliative BT shunt for TOF is done in which of the following condition?

A. Asymptomatic < 4 kg
B. Asymptomatic > 3 months
C. Symptomatic < 4 kg
D. Symptomatic < 3 months

PULMONARY ATRESIA

47. Which is false about pulmonary atresia with intact ventricular septum?

A. It is ductal dependent condition
B. It may be associated with right ventricle dependent coronary circulation
C. Palliative BT shunt may be required to promote single ventricle pathway

D. Atrial septostomy (balloon) required to allow left-to-right shunting

48. Which is incorrect regarding pulmonary atresia with VSD?

A. It is associated atretic pulmonary valve
B. Lungs are variably perfused by collateral vessels originating from the descending aorta and brachiocephalic vessels
C. Collateral arteries have a propensity to develop severe stenoses
D. The goal of surgical therapy is biventricular repair

TRANSPOSITION OF GREAT ARTERIES (TGA)

49. What is incidence of TGA?

A. 2 in 100 B. 2 in 1000
C. 2 in 10000 D. 2 in 100000

50. TGA with VSD is not associated with which of the following condition?

A. Aortic arch hypoplasia
B. Coarctation of aorta
C. Subaortic stenosis
D. Pulmonary atresia

51. Which procedure involves atrial switch operation with creation of intraatrial baffles using a patch channel?

A. Senning procedure B. Mustard procedure
C. Lecompte procedure D. Starnes procedure

52. Which procedure involves infolding of the native atrial wall and interatrial septum to create atrial switch?

A. Senning procedure B. Mustard procedure
C. Lecompte procedure D. Starnes procedure

53. Which is incorrect regarding transposition of great vessels anomaly?

A. TGA with pulmonary atresia have ductal-dependent pulmonary blood flow
B. Echocardiography is the primary diagnostic modality for TGA
C. Atrial switch operation as the surgical treatment of choice for patients with TGA
D. Arterial switch operation is offered to all patients with TGA regardless of the coronary branching pattern

54. What is the procedure of choice for TGA anomaly?

A. Atrial switch procedure
B. Arterial switch operation
C. Double switch procedure
D. Ross procedure

55. Lecompte maneuver is performed during which procedure?

A. Atrial switch procedure
B. Arterial switch operation
C. Ross procedure
D. Interrupted aortic arch repair

56. What is preferred time of arterial switch operation in case of TGA with intact ventricular septum?

A. 1 – 2 weeks B. 2 – 4 weeks
C. 4 – 6 weeks D. 6 – 8 weeks

57. Rastelli procedure is performed for:

A. Atrioventricular septal defect
B. Total anomalous pulmonary venous return
C. Transposition of great vessels
D. Double outlet right ventricle

58. All of the following procedures are done for TGA except:

A. Arterial switch operation
B. Rastelli procedure
C. REV procedure
D. Norwood operation

DOUBLE OUTLET RIGHT VENTRICLE

59. What is Taussig-Bing anomaly?

A. Subaortic VSD
B. Subpulmonary VSD
C. Sinus venousus ASD
D. Coronary sinus ASD

60. What is the procedure of choice for Taussig-Bing anomaly?

A. Ross procedure
B. Starnes procedure
C. Arterial switch operation
D. Norwood procedure

ccTGA

61. Which of the following is not associated with congenitally corrected TGA?

A. VSD
B. Subpulmonic stenosis
C. ASD
D. Ebsteinoid left A-V valve

62. Which is false regarding congenitally corrected TGA with intact ventricular septum?

A. Usually asymptomatic
B. Associated with complete heart block
C. Require arterial switch operation
D. Retraining of left ventricle for 6 months before definitive surgery

63. Which procedure is performed for congenitally corrected TGA anomaly?

A. Arterial switch operation
B. Double switch procedure
C. Ross procedure
D. Fontan operation

LEFT VENTRICULAR OUTFLOW TRACT OBSTRUCTION

64. Which is false about aortic valve replacement in case of congenital severe aortic stenosis?

A. Heterograft aortic valve extended durability in children
B. Aortic homograft does not require anticoagulation
C. Pulmonary autograft aortic root replacement is known as Ross procedure
D. Ross procedure exhibit the potential for somatic growth

65. Ross procedure for left ventricular outlet obstruction involves:

A. Valve sparing aortic root replacement
B. Aortic root replacement with pulmonary autograft
C. Prosthetic heterograft for aortic root replacement
D. Intraventricular baffle creation to bypass left ventricular outlet obstruction

66. What is false about fibromuscular subaortic stenosis?

A. Asymmetrical protrusion of the interventricular septum into the outflow tract
B. Membrane is often concentric
C. Densely adherent to the septum and mitral valve
D. Treated with balloon dilation

67. Which is wrong regarding tunnel subaortic stenosis?

A. More severe form of LVOTO
B. Aortic annular hyperplasia
C. It may require aortic root–enlarging procedure known as Konno procedure
D. It may be presented as a part of Shone complex

AORTIC ARCH ANOMALIES

68. Following are characteristics of infantile coarctation of aorta except:

A. Large PDA
B. Preductal aortic coarctation
C. Predominantly left-to-right flow
D. Coarctation occurs distal to the aortic isthmus

69. Which is incorrect about coarctation of aorta?

A. It occurs in 3 of every 10,000 live births
B. Coarctation is classified relative to its association with the ligamentum arteriosus and aortic arch
C. Echocardiography is now the primary diagnostic modality
D. Balloon dilation is as effective as surgical repair

70. Following lesions are associated with Shone complex, except:

A. Mitral stenosis
B. Left ventricular hypoplasia
C. Subaortic stenosis
D. Atrial myxoma

71. Waldhausen method for coarctation of aorta repair involves:

A. End-to-end primary anastomosis of aorta
B. Subclavian flap aortoplasty
C. Prosthetic Patch augmentation
D. Extended resection with primary anastomosis

72. Which is false about interrupted aortic arch (IAA) anomaly?

A. IAA is classified based on the level of the interruption
B. Type A occurs proximal to the left subclavian artery
C. Frequent finding of an aberrant right subclavian artery from the descending aorta
D. Survival for patients with IAA is initially predicated on ductal patency

SINGLE VENTRICLE

73. Which is false regarding tricuspid atresia?

A. Tricuspid atresia occurs in 1 of every 10,000 live births
B. It may be presented with pulmonary overcirculation
C. Single left ventricle with normally related or transposed great vessels
D. Blalock shunt is constructed preferably to the morphologic left pulmonary artery

74. Pott's shunt is:

A. Left Subclavian artery-to-branch pulmonary artery
B. Side-to-side left pulmonary artery to descending aorta
C. Side-to-side right pulmonary artery to ascending aorta
D. Side-to-side right pulmonary artery to innominate artery with prosthetic graft

75. Waterson shunt is:

A. Left subclavian artery-to-branch pulmonary artery
B. Side-to-side left pulmonary artery to descending aorta
C. Side-to-side right pulmonary artery to ascending aorta
D. Side-to-side right pulmonary artery to innominate artery with prosthetic graft

76. Which of the following is not associated with hypoplastic left heart syndrome?

A. Absent ascending aorta
B. Pulmonary overcirculation
C. Ductal-dependence
D. Shone complex

77. Following maneuvers increases pulmonary vascular resistance except:

A. Hypoventilation
B. Low inspired oxygen concentration
C. Carbon dioxide supplementation
D. Hypothermia

78. Following procedures are performed for hypoplastic left heart syndrome except:

A. Norwood procedure B. Takeuchi procedure
C. Sano procedure D. Fontan procedure

79. Sano procedure for HLHS involves:

A. Blalock shunt
B. Right ventricle-pulmonary artery conduit
C. Pulmonary banding with ductal stent placement
D. Intracardiac baffle for cavopulmonary shunt

80. Which is false about hybrid procedure for HLHS?

A. Palliative procedure
B. Preferred in high risk patients
C. Blalock shunt
D. Stent placement for ductal patency

81. What is the procedure of choice for patients with single ventricle?

A. Norwood procedure
B. Sano procedure
C. Fontan procedure
D. Cardiac transplant

82. Fontan circulation depends on following factors except:

A. Right atrial pressure
B. AV valve function
C. Aortic valve function
D. Ventricular function

83. Which is incorrect about Fontan shunt?

A. It is procedure of choice for single ventricle syndrome
B. Active blood flow occurs through Fontan circuit
C. Fontan shunt involves total cavopulmonary connection
D. It predisposes to systemic congestive symptoms

84. Which palliative shunt is used as intervening stage during Fontan operation?

A. Blalock shunt B. Glenn shunt
C. Pott shunt D. Waterson shunt

85. Which is false regarding Glenn shunt?

A. It is used as intervening stage of palliation for single ventricle patients
B. It is bidirectional shunt
C. Involves superior cavopulmonary anastomosis
D. Patients are fully saturated post procedure

86. Identify the shunt procedure shown in the following figure:

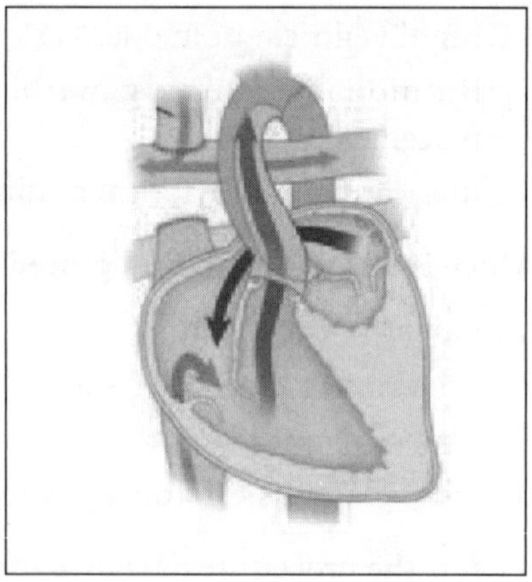

A. Modified Blalock-Taussig shunt
B. Sano shunt
C. Glenn shunt
D. Fontan shunt

87. Following are the complications of Fontan shunt except:

A. Chronic hepatic congestion
B. Protein losing enteropathy
C. Venous stasis syndrome
D. Cerebral encephalopathy

MISCELLANEOUS ANOMALIES

88. What is the location of Kommerell diverticulum?

A. At the base of left subclavian artery
B. At the base of anomalous left subclavian artery
C. At the base of right subclavian artery
D. At the base of anomalous right subclavian artery

89. Which is the most common form of complete ring anomaly?

A. Right aortic arch
B. Double aortic arch
C. Right arch with anomalous left subclavian artery
D. Right arch with mirror image branching

90. Which is false regarding aberrant right subclavian artery?

A. Most common form of partial aortic arch anomaly
B. It arises distal to the left subclavian artery with a left arch
C. It passes between the trachea and the esophagus
D. Posterior and leftward origin of the innominate artery from a left arch causes compression of the trachea

91. Which is incorrect statement about pulmonary artery sling?

A. It occurs when the left pulmonary artery arises from the right pulmonary artery
B. It passes anterior to the trachea
C. It causes tracheal compression or stenosis
D. Esophageal compression does not occur

92. All are true about management of vascular rings except:

A. Documentation of a ring is an indication for surgery in children
B. Older patients are often asymptomatic
C. Echocardiography is the first investigation
D. MRI provides complete anatomic detail

93. First choice of investigation for vascular rings:

A. Echocardiography
B. Barium swallow
C. CT angiography
D. MR angiography

94. All are true about anomalous left coronary artery rising from pulmonary artery (ALCAPA) except:

A. Suspected in patients having dilated cardiomyopathy with mitral regurgitation
B. PDA ligation or closure of a VSD can be fatal
C. The echocardiogram is usually diagnostic
D. Ligation of the ALCAPA can be safely done

95. Takeuchi procedure is performed for:

A. Single ventricle
B. ALCAPA
C. TAPVR
D. Double aortic arch

96. Takeuchi procedure involves:

A. Direct reimplantation of the coronary artery into the ascending aorta
B. Coronary artery tunnel creation
C. Use of intervening homograft
D. Arterial switch reconstruction

97. Following are complications associated with Takeuchi tunnel procedure except:

A. Tunnel stenosis
B. Aortic valve damage
C. Anastomotic leak
D. Left ventricular outlet obstruction

98. Coronary artery aneurysms are associated with:

A. Takayasu arteritis
B. Kawasaki disease
C. Polyarteritis nodosa
D. Wegener's granulomatosis

EBSTEIN ANOMALY

99. All are associated with Ebstein anomaly except:

A. ASD
B. VSD
C. Pulmonary atresia
D. ccTGA

100. Which is false regarding Ebstein anomaly?

A. Atrialization of the right ventricle
B. Variable pulmonary outflow obstruction
C. The anterior leaflet remains large and sail-like
D. In older patients, cyanosis and heart failure are contraindications to intervene

101. Starnes operation is performed for:

A. Mitral valve regurgitation
B. Ebstein's anomaly
C. Congenital aortic stenosis
D. Tricuspid atresia

102. Carpentier procedure is used for:

A. Left ventricular outlet obstruction
B. Right ventricular outlet obstruction
C. Ebstein's anomaly
D. Double-orifice mitral valve repair

103. All are types of subvalvular mitral stenosis except:

A. Parachute mitral valve
B. Double orifice mitral valve
C. Hammock valve
D. Absence of papillary muscle

ANSWERS

1. **Ans: B. Atrial situs solitus with atrioventricular discordance and ventriculoarterial discordance**

   Ref: Chapter No. 59, Page No. 1643

2. **Ans: C. Use of prosthetic interposition graft**

   Ref: Chapter No. 59, Page No. 1643

3. **Ans: A. Absent or deranged sinoatrial node**

   Ref: Chapter No. 59, Page No. 1644

4. **Ans: C. 5 – 7 mSv**

   Ref: Chapter No. 59, Page No. 1645

5. **Ans: D. 9 – 11 mSv**

   Ref: Chapter No. 59, Page No. 1645

6. **Ans: C. In normal hearts, there is a small, physiologically insignificant left-to-right shunt**

   Ref: Chapter No. 59, Page No. 1645

7. **Ans: C. 15 to 30 mm Hg**

   Ref: Chapter No. 59, Page No. 1645

8. **Ans: B. Right ventricular pressure**

   Ref: Chapter No. 59, Page No. 1646

9. **Ans: D. Tetralogy of Fallot**

   Ref: Chapter No. 59, Page No. 1647

10. **Ans: D. Endocarditis risk is very low for PDA**

    Ref: Chapter No. 59, Page No. 1647

11. **Ans: C. The gold standard is surgery, usually through a left anterolateral thoracotomy**

    Ref: Chapter No. 59, Page No. 1647

12. **Ans: C. Necrotizing enterocolitis**

    Ref: Chapter No. 59, Page No. 1647

13. **Ans: D. Pulmonary fibrosis**

    Ref: Chapter No. 59, Page No. 1647

14. **Ans: B. Type I is common arterial trunk**

    Ref: Chapter No. 59, Page No. 1648-49

15. **Ans: B. Ostium secundum**

    Ref: Chapter No. 59, Page No. 1648

16. **Ans: C. Pulmonary vascular disease is a typical finding in secundum ASDs**

    Ref: Chapter No. 59, Page No. 1649

17. **Ans: D. Sinus venosus ASD**

    Ref: Chapter No. 59, Page No. 1649

18. **Ans: D. Sinus venosus ASD**

    Ref: Chapter No. 59, Page No. 1650

19. **Ans: B. Total anomalous pulmonary venous return**

    Ref: Chapter No. 59, Page No. 1650

20. **Ans: C. Total anomalous pulmonary venous return**

    Ref: Chapter No. 59, Page No. 1650

21. **Ans: A. SVC translocation**

Ref: Chapter No. 59, Page No. 1650

22. **Ans: A. Outlet VSD exhibit a potential for spontaneous closure**

Ref: Chapter No. 59, Page No. 1650

23. **Ans: A. Perimembranous VSD**

Ref: Chapter No. 59, Page No. 1650

24. **Ans: B. Location of VSD**

Ref: Chapter No. 59, Page No. 1650

25. **Ans: C. Complete AVSDs are frequently seen in patients with trisomy 18**

Ref: Chapter No. 59, Page No. 1651

26. **Ans: B. Trisomy 21**

Ref: Chapter No. 59, Page No. 1651

27. **Ans: C. Complete A-V canal defect**

Ref: Chapter No. 59, Page No. 1651

28. **Ans: C. Secundum VSD**

Ref: Chapter No. 59, Page No. 1651

29. **Ans: A. Rastelli type A defect, with superior leaflet and chordal support committed to the right side of the ventricular septum**

Ref: Chapter No. 59, Page No. 1651

30. **Ans: B. It is associated with a restrictive perimembranous VSD**

Ref: Chapter No. 59, Page No. 1652

31. **Ans: D. Chromosome 22**

Ref: Chapter No. 59, Page No. 1653

32. **Ans: D. Ductal-independence**

Ref: Chapter No. 59, Page No. 1653

33. **Ans: A. Transposition of great vessels**

Ref: Chapter No. 59, Page No. 1653

34. **Ans: C. 25%**

Ref: Chapter No. 59, Page No. 1653

35. **Ans: A. Van Praagh classification**

Ref: Chapter No. 59, Page No. 1653

36. **Ans: B. Collett and Edwards classification**

Ref: Chapter No. 59, Page No. 1653

37. **Ans: D. Bovine jugular vein valved conduit**

Ref: Chapter No. 59, Page No. 1653

38. **Ans: C. In intracardiac TAPVR, the pulmonary veins drain into the right atrium**

Ref: Chapter No. 59, Page No. 1654

39. **Ans: C. Ductus venosus**

Ref: Chapter No. 59, Page No. 1654

40. **Ans: B. Pulmonary veins enter a chamber posterior to left atrium**

Ref: Chapter No. 59, Page No. 1654

41. **Ans: B. Persistent left SVC**

Ref: Chapter No. 59, Page No. 1655

42. **Ans: B. 1 in 2500**

Ref: Chapter No. 59, Page No. 1655

43. **Ans: A. Malalignment VSD**

Ref: Chapter No. 59, Page No. 1656

44. **Ans: B. Anastomosis of the left subclavian artery to the divided left pulmonary artery**

Ref: Chapter No. 59, Page No. 1656

45. **Ans: C. Ductal independence**

Ref: Chapter No. 59, Page No. 1656-57

46. **Ans: C. Symptomatic < 4 kg**

Ref: Chapter No. 59, Page No. 1659

47. **Ans: D. Atrial septostomy (balloon) required to allow left-to-right shunting**

Ref: Chapter No. 59, Page No. 1658-59

48. **Ans: A. It is associated atretic pulmonary valve**

Ref: Chapter No. 59, Page No. 1659

49. **Ans: C. 2 in 10000**

Ref: Chapter No. 59, Page No. 1659

50. **Ans: C. Subaortic stenosis**

Ref: Chapter No. 59, Page No. 1659

51. **Ans: B. Mustard procedure**

Ref: Chapter No. 59, Page No. 1660

52. **Ans. A. Senning procedure**

Ref: Chapter No. 59, Page No. 1660

53. **Ans: C. Atrial switch operation as the surgical treatment of choice for patients with TGA**

Ref: Chapter No. 59, Page No. 1660

54. **Ans: B. Arterial switch operation**

Ref: Chapter No. 59, Page No. 1660

55. **Ans: B. Arterial switch operation**

Ref: Chapter No. 59, Page No. 1660

56. **Ans: A. 1 – 2 weeks**

Ref: Chapter No. 59, Page No. 1661

57. **Ans: C. Transposition of great vessels**

Ref: Chapter No. 59, Page No. 1661

58. **Ans: D. Norwood operation**

Ref: Chapter No. 59, Page No. 1661

59. **Ans: B. Subpulmonary VSD**

Ref: Chapter No. 59, Page No. 1661

60. **Ans: C. Arterial switch operation**

Ref: Chapter No. 59, Page No. 1661

61. **Ans: C. ASD**

Ref: Chapter No. 59, Page No. 1662

62. **Ans: C. Require arterial switch operation**

Ref: Chapter No. 59, Page No. 1662-63

63. **Ans: B. Double switch procedure**

Ref: Chapter No. 59, Page No. 1663

64. **Ans: A. Heterograft aortic valve extended durability in children**

Ref: Chapter No. 59, Page No. 1664

65. **Ans: B. Aortic root replacement with pulmonary autograft**

Ref: Chapter No. 59, Page No. 1664

66. **Ans: D. Treated with balloon dilation**

Ref: Chapter No. 59, Page No. 1664

67. **Ans: B. Aortic annular hyperplasia**

Ref: Chapter No. 59, Page No. 1665

68. **Ans: C. Predominantly left-to-right flow**

Ref: Chapter No. 59, Page No. 1665

69. **Ans: D. Balloon dilation is as effective as surgical repair**

Ref: Chapter No. 59, Page No. 1665-66

70. **Ans: D. Atrial myxoma**

Ref: Chapter No. 59, Page No. 1665

71. **Ans: B. Subclavian flap aortoplasty**

Ref: Chapter No. 59, Page No. 1666

72. **Ans: B. Type A occurs proximal to the left subclavian artery**

Ref: Chapter No. 59, Page No. 1666

73. **Ans: D. Blalock shunt is constructed preferably to the morphologic left pulmonary artery**

Ref: Chapter No. 59, Page No. 1667

74. **Ans: B. Side-to-side left pulmonary artery to descending aorta**

Ref: Chapter No. 59, Page No. 1667

75. **Ans: C. Side-to-side right pulmonary artery to ascending aorta**

Ref: Chapter No. 59, Page No. 1667

76. **Ans: A. Absent ascending aorta**

Ref: Chapter No. 59, Page No. 1667

77. **Ans: D. Hypothermia**

Ref: Chapter No. 59, Page No. 1668

78. **Ans: B. Takeuchi procedure**

Ref: Chapter No. 59, Page No. 1669-70

79. **Ans: B. Right ventricle-pulmonary artery conduit**

Ref: Chapter No. 59, Page No. 1670

80. **Ans: C. Blalock shunt**

Ref: Chapter No. 59, Page No. 1670

81. **Ans: C. Fontan procedure**

Ref: Chapter No. 59, Page No. 1671

82. **Ans: A. Right atrial pressure**

Ref: Chapter No. 59, Page No. 1671

83. **Ans: B. Active blood flow occurs through Fontan circuit**

Ref: Chapter No. 59, Page No. 1671

84. **Ans: B. Glenn shunt**

Ref: Chapter No. 59, Page No. 1671

85. **Ans: D. Patients are fully saturated post procedure**

Ref: Chapter No. 59, Page No. 1671

86. **Ans: C. Glenn shunt**

Ref: Chapter No. 59, Page No. 1671

87. **Ans: D. Cerebral encephalopathy**

Ref: Chapter No. 59, Page No. 1671

88. **Ans: B. At the base of anomalous left subclavian artery**

Ref: Chapter No. 59, Page No. 1672

89. **Ans: B. Double aortic arch**

Ref: Chapter No. 59, Page No. 1672

90. **Ans: C. It passes between trachea and esophagus**

Ref: Chapter No. 59, Page No. 1672

91. **Ans: B. It passes anterior to the trachea**

Ref: Chapter No. 59, Page No. 1672

92. **Ans: C. Echocardiography is the first investigation**

Ref: Chapter No. 59, Page No. 1673

93. **Ans: B. Barium swallow**

Ref: Chapter No. 59, Page No. 1673

94. **Ans: D. Ligation of the ALCAPA can be safely done**

Ref: Chapter No. 59, Page No. 1674

95. **Ans: B. ALCAPA**

Ref: Chapter No. 59, Page No. 1674

96. **Ans: B. Coronary artery tunnel creation**

Ref: Chapter No. 59, Page No. 1674

97. **Ans: D. Left ventricular outlet obstruction**

Ref: Chapter No. 59, Page No. 1675

98. **Ans: B. Kawasaki disease**

Ref: Chapter No. 59, Page No. 1675

99. **Ans: B. VSD**

Ref: Chapter No. 59, Page No. 1675

100. **Ans: D. In older patients, cyanosis and heart failure are contraindications to intervene**

Ref: Chapter No. 59, Page No. 1675

101. **Ans: B. Ebstein's anomaly**

Ref: Chapter No. 59, Page No. 1675

102. **Ans: C. Ebstein's anomaly**

Ref: Chapter No. 59, Page No. 1675

103. **Ans: B. Double orifice mitral valve**

Ref: Chapter No. 59, Page No. 1675

60

Coronary Artery Disease

ANATOMY AND PHYSIOLOGY

1. **All are true regarding vascular anatomy of the heart except:**
   A. The left coronary artery (LCA) arises from the posteriorly located left coronary sinus
   B. The right coronary artery (RCA) arises from the anteriorly located right coronary sinus
   C. LAD supplies more than 50% of the LV mass
   D. The diagonal branches of the LAD supply the anterolateral wall of the right ventricle

2. **Following vessels constitute trifurcation of the left coronary artery except:**
   A. Left anterior descending
   B. Circumflex coronary
   C. Acute marginal artery
   D. Ramus intermedius

3. **Obtuse marginal artery is a branch of:**
   A. Left anterior descending
   B. Circumflex coronary artery
   C. Posterior descending artery
   D. Right coronary artery

4. **Following are branches of right coronary artery except:**
   A. Acute marginal artery
   B. Posterior descending artery
   C. Diagonal arteries
   D. Right posterolateral artery

5. **Which is incorrect regarding coronary anatomy?**
   A. The AV node artery arises from the LCA in approximately 90% of patients
   B. The sinoatrial node artery arises from the proximal RCA in 50% of patients
   C. The source of the PDA is often used clinically to define dominance of circulation in the heart
   D. All the epicardial conductance vessels and septal perforators play a crucial role in oxygen and nutrient exchange

6. **Major arterial supply to the AV node is by:**
   A. Left coronary artery
   B. Right coronary artery
   C. Left anterior descending artery
   D. Posterior descending artery

7. **Which is false about venous drainage of the heart?**
   A. The coronary sinus lies within the posterior AV groove
   B. The coronary sinus receives 50% of coronary venous blood
   C. The thebesian veins drain directly into the cardiac chambers
   D. The anterior right ventricular veins form the small cardiac vein

8. **Which is incorrect regarding myocardial perfusion?**
   A. During resting conditions, coronary blood flow autoregulated over a pressure range of 90–150 mm Hg
   B. Normal coronary blood flow averages 225 mL/min
   C. Normal coronary blood flow delivers 0.1 mL/g/min of oxygen to the myocardium
   D. Under normal conditions, more than 75% of the delivered oxygen is extracted in the coronary capillary bed

9. **Following are features of coronary blood flow except:**
   A. Coronary blood flow is 0.7–0.9 mL per gram of myocardium per minute

B. Coronary sinus blood is the most deoxygenated blood in the body
C. 80% blood flow occurs during diastole
D. Flow-limited oxygen supply

HISTORY OF CABG

10. Who developed cardiopulmonary bypass machine?

A. DeBakey B. Gibbon
C. Buckberg D. Sabiston

11. Who performed first successful coronary artery bypass grafting using GSV?

A. DeBakey B. Vineberg
C. Sones D. Sabiston

12. Who introduced beating-heart coronary artery bypass grafting?

A. Sones B. Buckberg
C. Subramanian D. Sondergaard

13. Who introduced blood cardioplegia solution for arrested myocardial protection?

A. Cooley B. Subramanian
C. Sondergaard D. Buckberg

ATHEROSCLEROTIC CAD

14. Which of the following are false regarding atherosclerotic CAD?

A. Intramyocardial arteries are the most susceptible
B. Statin treatment was associated with improved survival in all age groups
C. C-reactive protein is a biomarker of inflammation and CAD
D. Inflammatory response is involved in all stages of the disease

15. Which heart vessels are most susceptible to atherosclerotic changes?

A. Intramyocardial arteries
B. Epicardial conductance vessels
C. Left anterior descending artery
D. Main coronary arteries

16. Following are risk factors for atherosclerotic plaque rupture except:

A. Soft lipid core
B. Thin fibrous cap
C. Increased plaque neovascularity
D. Concentric lesion

17. Which is incorrect about coronary artery obstruction?

A. 75% atherosclerotic plaques of the coronary arteries are eccentric
B. Concentric lesion are more prone to plaque rupture
C. Coronary blood flow is significantly compromised when the cross-sectional area of the vessel has decreased by 75% or more
D. A 90% reduction in luminal diameter results in resting angina

18. VSD or ventricular wall rupture occurs after how many days following MI?

A. 12 to 24 hours B. 2 to 3 days
C. 5 to 7 days D. 7 to 10 days

19. Which is false about exercise stress test?

A. Bruce protocol is used for exercise stress test
B. Five 3-minute bouts of treadmill exercise with increasing METs
C. 12 metabolic equivalents of energy expenditure needed for complete test
D. Low sensitivity in multivessel disease

20. Which is incorrect statement concerning Bruce protocol?

A. Five 3-minute bouts of treadmill exercise with increasing METs
B. Comprises 7 stages
C. 12 metabolic equivalents of energy expenditure needed for complete test
D. It is used for pharmacologic stress test

21. Following are limitations of exercise tolerance test except:

A. Single vessel disease
B. Abnormal baseline ECG
C. Premenopausal women
D. Duration of exercise

22. Following are advantages of stress echocardiography except:

A. Higher sensitivity and specificity
B. Identification of structural cardiac abnormalities
C. Evaluation of perfusion with contrast agents
D. Quantitative image analysis

23. Following are advantages of stress SPECT perfusion imaging except:

A. Higher sensitivity and specificity
B. Evaluation of perfusion and function

C. Anatomic correlates of the coronary vessels
D. Quantitative image analysis

24. Which of the following agent is used for stress SPECT perfusion imaging?

A. Lutetium 177
B. Iodine 123
C. Thallium 201
D. Indium 111

25. Following are pharmacologic stress agents used during CAD detection except:

A. Dopamine
B. Dipyridamole
C. Adenosine
D. Regadenoson

26. Which of the following pharmacologic stress agent can be given as bolus injection?

A. Dobutamine
B. Dipyridamole
C. Adenosine
D. Regadenoson

27. All are true statement regarding coronary CT angiography except:

A. Planning of grafting sites for CABG
B. Detects vessel wall calcification and the course of coronary arteries
C. It has high negative predictive value for obstructive CAD
D. It cannot assess arterial remodeling and non calcified plaques

28. What is gold standard imaging for CAD?

A. Coronary CT angiography
B. Coronary catheterization
C. MR perfusion imaging
D. 99 Tc SPECT perfusion imaging

29. All are true regarding coronary catheterization except:

A. Coronary catheterization is the "gold standard" for diagnosis of CAD
B. Luminal diameter reduction of at least 70% is considered to be significant stenosis
C. There is marked variation in interobserver reliability
D. It helps to interpret functional significance of a given coronary stenosis

30. Left main disease is defined as left main stem coronary artery stenosis of at least:

A. 40%
B. 50%
C. 60%
D. 70%

31. Fractional Flow Reserve below_____ is considered significant ischemia-producing lesions.

A. 0.85
B. 0.75
C. 0.65
D. 0.50

32. Following criteria are used to describe physiologically significant lesions:

A. Fractional Flow Reserve <0.75
B. IVUS minimum luminal diameter of 2.8
C. IVUS minimum luminal area of 6 mm^2
D. Luminal diameter reduction of at least 50%

CORONARY ARTERY REVASCULARIZATION

33. What is the only class Ia indication for PCI?

A. Stable IHD
B. Acute STEMI
C. Acute NSTEMI
D. Prior episode of MI

34. Following are class I indications for CABG except:

A. Unprotected Left Main coronary
B. Three-Vessel Disease
C. Two-Vessel Disease with Proximal LAD Artery Disease
D. CAD with LVEF 35% to 50%

35. Which of the following statement is false about coronary revascularization?

A. CABG offers a survival advantage over medical therapy for patients with LCA or three-vessel CAD
B. PCI does not lower the long-term risk of MI
C. Relief of angina is more effective with CABG than with PCI
D. PCI improves survival in stable patients

36. All are true about coronary revascularization procedures except:

A. More survival benefits after CABG as compared to PCI
B. Incidence of MI was similar following CABG and PCI
C. Relief of angina was more effective with CABG than with PCI
D. Repeated coronary revascularization is required more often after PCI

37. SYNTAX Trial was done for:

A. CABG and DES implantation in patients with three-vessel or left main disease
B. Mitral valve repair vs replacement for acquired mitral valve disease
C. CABG and PCI in acute myocardial ischemia
D. Open repair vs TEVAR in aortic arch disease

38. SYNTAX score includes following variables of stenotic lesion except:

A. Location B. Severity
C. Extent D. Complexity

39. Which is false statement regarding SYNTAX Trial?

A. Low SYNTAX score indicates less complicated anatomic CAD
B. SYNTAX score is considered high if > 33 points
C. Similar benefits with CABG and DES in patients with low SYNTAX score
D. The occurrence of major adverse cardiac events correlated with the SYNTAX score following both CABG and PCI procedures

40. Which of the following trial does not compare benefits of CABG and PCI?

A. SYNTAX trial B. NOBLE trial
C. STICH trial D. EXCEL trial

41. Which Trial compared the effects of CABG and medical therapy in patients of ischemic LV dysfunction?

A. PRECOMBAT trial B. STICH trial
C. NOBLE trial D. EXCEL trial

42. Which of the following factor favors the choice of repeat CABG over PCI in a patient with previous CABG?

A. Limited areas of ischemia
B. Patent graft to the LAD artery
C. Multiple diseased bypass grafts
D. Comorbid conditions

43. What is the target door-to-balloon time in treating acute MI?

A. 30 minutes B. 45 minutes
C. 60 minutes D. 90 minutes

44. What is the target door-to-needle time in treating acute MI?

A. 30 minutes B. 45 minutes
C. 60 minutes D. 90 minutes

45. All are true statements about management of CAD except:

A. PCI and thrombolytics have equal survival benefits as an initial treatment for acute STEMI
B. Immediate CABG is an independent predictor of mortality in cases of acute MI
C. The longer the door-to-balloon time, the higher the mortality risk
D. Symptoms of acute coronary syndrome are more likely to be reduced with a revascularization procedure than with medical therapy

46. Which of the following is incorrect regarding cardiopulmonary bypass technique?

A. Venous reservoir collects blood by using rotator pump
B. Median sternotomy is most common approach
C. The priming solution consists of a balanced salt solution
D. Distal anastomosis is carried out before proximal anastomosis of graft

47. Which is false about cardioplegia solution?

A. It is potassium enriched solution
B. Oxygenated blood is mixed with cardioplegia solution in a 4:1 ratio
C. It is administered as pre-warmed solution
D. It may be administered retrograde through the coronary sinus

48. Ratio of oxygenated blood to the cardioplegia solution used in CPB is:

A. 2:1 B. 3:1
C. 4:1 D. 5:1

49. What is the oxygen consumption of a patient on CPB at normal temperatures?

A. 20 to 40 $mL/min/m^2$
B. 50 to 80 $mL/min/m^2$
C. 80 to 120 $mL/min/m^2$
D. 120 to 150 $mL/min/m^2$

50. The mean oxygen consumption of the body decreases by _____% for every 10°C decrease in body temperature.

A. 30% B. 40%
C. 50% D. 60%

51. Which is false regarding CPB procedure?

A. Cold cardioplegia solution injected into the coronary circulation to arrest and to protect the heart
B. Patient is systemically heparinized with 300 U/kg after cannulation
C. An activated clotting time should be maintained for more than 450 seconds throughout CPB
D. Centrifugal pump is preferred to reduce hemolysis and to maintain non-turbulent flow

52. Which type of conduit achieves best patency rates with CABG?

A. Great saphenous vein
B. Left internal mammary artery
C. Radial artery
D. Gastroepiploic artery

53. All are true concerning internal mammary artery (IMA) graft in CABG except:

A. The long-term patency rate of the Left IMA graft has been shown to be approximately 80% at 10 years
B. The best patency rates are achieved when the Left IMA is used as an in situ pedicled graft
C. Skeletonization of the bilateral IMA grafts may reduce the wound complication rate
D. No-touch technique is used for harvesting the IMA

54. Which conduit is more prone for the development of graft atherosclerosis?

A. Great saphenous vein
B. Left internal mammary artery
C. Radial artery
D. Right Gastroepiploic artery

55. Regarding patency of conduits used for CABG, correct is:

A. GSV > LIMA > Radial artery > right gastroepiploic artery
B. LIMA > GSV > Radial artery > right gastroepiploic artery
C. LIMA > GSV > right gastroepiploic artery > Radial artery
D. LIMA > Radial artery > GSV > right gastroepiploic artery

56. Which of the following vessel is not used for CABG?

A. Radial artery
B. Right gastroepiploic artery
C. Cephalic vein
D. Great saphenous vein

57. All are risk factors for deep sternal infection with bilateral IMA graft except:

A. Diabetes B. Severe PVD
C. Hypertension D. Morbid obesity

58. Heparin dosage used for heparinization during CPB:

A. 1 mg/Kg B. 3 mg/Kg
C. 10 mg/Kg D. 30 mg/Kg

59. Axillary artery cannulation is achieved with an 8 mm graft anastomosed ____ to axillary artery.

A. End to end B. Side to end
C. End to side D. Side to side

60. Which is false about CPB procedure?

A. Aortic cannula has angulated tip for laminar flow of blood
B. Dual-stage venous cannula is inserted into right atrium for venous drainage
C. The venous drainage is a passive siphon aided by gravity
D. The first stage of venous cannula has the fenestrated basket that usually rests at the entrance of IVC

61. All are true about cardioplegia solution use during CPB except:

A. Potassium cardioplegia solution is used to arrest the heart during systole
B. Homogeneous distribution of cardioplegia solution is achieved with retrograde administration
C. Sump drain functions to decompress the left ventricle while the heart is arrested
D. Additional doses are usually administered every 15 to 20 minutes

62. Which is incorrect statement regarding graft anastomoses during CABG?

A. End to side distal anastomosis is technically the most challenging step
B. The LIMA to left descending artery anastomosis is the first one to be performed
C. Construction of the proximal anastomoses done last
D. The patient is warmed back to physiologic temperature before constructing proximal anastomosis

63. All are true regarding intra-aortic balloon pump except:

A. The IABP is a special Silastic balloon with a capacity of 40 to 60 mL
B. It is positioned in the descending aorta just beyond the origin of the left subclavian artery
C. The balloon inflation is timed to occur at the dicrotic notch of the arterial line tracing
D. The use of IABP is absolutely contraindicated in patients with aortic aneurysm

64. Absolute contraindication for the use of IABP:

A. Aortic aneurysm
B. Aortic regurgitation
C. Pulmonary hypertension
D. Peripheral vascular disease

POST OPERATIVE CARE OF CABG

65. Which is false about the parameters to be achieved in post-operative period of CABG?

A. Maintaining perfusion pressure of 60–80 mm Hg
B. Mixed venous oxygenation should be kept at 60%
C. Maintaining hemoglobin level higher than 8 g/dL
D. Keeping blood glucose levels below 140 mg/dL

66. Which is false about the parameters to be achieved in post-operative period of CABG?

A. Maintaining core body temperature higher than 36.5°C
B. Maintaining hemoglobin level > 8 g/dL in older patients or those with severe cerebrovascular disease
C. Maintaining a sinus or perfusing rhythm at a rate of 70 to 100 beats/min
D. Keeping blood glucose levels below 180 mg/dL

67. What is the mortality rate following CABG?

A. 3% B. 6%
C. 9% D. 15%

68. Following are the causes of immediate post operative bleeding:

A. Hypothermia
B. Platelet dysfunction
C. Inadequate protamine reversal
D. Emergency procedure

69. Indication for mediastinal exploration following CABG procedure are all except:

A. Bleeding of more than 500 mL in the first hour
B. Persistent bleeding of more than 200 mL/hr for 4 hours
C. Pericardial tamponade
D. Evidence of hemothorax on radiograph

70. All are true about regarding development of neurological deficit following CABG except:

A. Age and hypertension are consistent risk factors
B. Type I deficit is a focal neurologic deficit
C. Type II deficit is manifested as nonspecific encephalopathy
D. Atherosclerosis of the aorta, diabetes are risk factors for type II deficit

71. Which conduit use for CABG procedure is associated with higher risk of mediastinitis?

A. Left internal mammary artery
B. Bilateral internal mammary artery
C. Great saphenous vein
D. Right gastroepiploic artery

72. What is the incidence of deep sternal wound infection following CABG?

A. 2% B. 5%
C. 8% D. 14%

ALTERNATIVE METHODS FOR MYOCARDIAL REVASCULARIZATION

73. Which is false regarding the method of hypothermic fibrillary arrest?

A. It avoids the use of the aortic cross-clamp
B. It is useful alternative in patients with an extensively calcified aorta
C. Once CPB is initiated; the patient is cooled to 32°C
D. It is contraindicated in patients with significant aortic valve incompetence

74. Patient having LVEF <40% is undergoing CABG, which of the following method is preferred?

A. CPB with cardioplegic arrest
B. CPB with hypothermic fibrillary arrest
C. On-Pump Beating-Heart Bypass
D. Off-Pump Coronary Artery Bypass Grafting

75. Advantage of Off-Pump Coronary Artery Bypass Grafting is:

A. Improved long-term patency
B. Lower incidence of major cardiac events
C. Lower risk of fluid shift complications
D. Decreased need of re-intervention

76. Fork-octopus for stabilizing the heart is used during:

A. CPB with cardioplegic arrest
B. CPB with hypothermic fibrillary arrest
C. On-Pump Beating-Heart Bypass
D. Off-Pump Coronary Artery Bypass Grafting

77. Following trials are based on Off-Pump Coronary Artery Bypass Grafting except:

A. ROOBY Trial
B. GOPCADE Trial
C. SMART Trial
D. NOBLE Trial

78. Which is false regarding minimally Invasive Direct Coronary Artery Bypass?

A. Anterolateral thoracotomy or subxiphoid approach
B. Robot assisted procedure
C. Performed on the beating heart
D. Limited revascularization territory

79. Following scores are used for cardiac surgery risk assessment:

A. STS score
B. EuroSCORE
C. RCR Index
D. All of the above

80. All are true regarding Transmyocardial Laser Revascularization therapy except:

A. Recommended for patients with an LVEF greater than 0.30 and refractory angina
B. It is always used as an adjunct therapy
C. It uses a high-energy laser beam to create myocardial transmural channels
D. It causes local cardiac denervation and anginal relief

81. What is hybrid procedure of coronary revascularization?

A. Use of LIMA and GSV for multivessel anastomosis
B. LIMA to LAD anastomosis at multiple level
C. Minimally invasive LIMA to LAD anastomosis in conjunction with PCI
D. LIMA to LAD anastomosis with prosthetic graft

82. Following factors increases the risk of reoperation of CABG except:

A. Absence of an IMA graft
B. Older age at the time of the index operation
C. NYHA class III angina
D. Prior incomplete revascularization

COMPLICATIONS OF CAD

83. False statement regarding left ventricular aneurysm:

A. Most common cause is transmural MI following acute LAD artery occlusion
B. Patients may develop an aneurysm as early as 48 hours after infarction
C. Two thirds of patients are symptomatic
D. The risk of thromboembolism is low, so long-term anticoagulation is not recommended

84. Most common cause of death following ventricular aneurysm:

A. Arrhythmias
B. Recurrent MI
C. Chronic heart failure
D. Ventricular rupture

85. Post-infarction VSD is manifested within ____ days.

A. 2 to 4
B. 5 to 7
C. 7 to 10
D. 10 to 14

86. Which is incorrect regarding post infarction VSD?

A. The defect is more common in men than in women (3:2)
B. VSD that occurs in the first 6 days after an infarct is considered acute
C. The VSD is usually located in the anterior or apical aspect of the ventricular septum
D. Patients should be treated early with closure of the defect and concomitant CABG

87. Post-infarct VSD is considered acute, when it occurs within period of:

A. 6 hours
B. 6 days
C. 6 weeks
D. 6 months

88. Which is incorrect concerning acute ischemic mitral regurgitation?

A. Acute ischemic MR may result from papillary muscle necrosis and rupture
B. It is caused by occlusion of the overlying epicardial arteries
C. Three to six times more often involvement of the posterior papillary muscle
D. Prompt surgical intervention involves mitral valve repair and concomitant CABG

ANSWERS

1. **Ans: D. The diagonal branches of the LAD supply the anterolateral wall of the right ventricle**

   Ref: Chapter No. 60, Page No. 1680

2. **Ans: C. Acute marginal artery**

   Ref: Chapter No. 60, Page No. 1680

3. **Ans: B. Circumflex coronary artery**

   Ref: Chapter No. 60, Page No. 1680

4. **Ans: C. Diagonal arteries**

   Ref: Chapter No. 60, Page No. 1680

5. **Ans: A. The AV node artery arises from the LCA in approximately 90% of patients**

   Ref: Chapter No. 60, Page No. 1680

6. **Ans: B. Right coronary artery**

   Ref: Chapter No. 60, Page No. 1680

7. **Ans: B. The coronary sinus receives 50% of coronary venous blood**

   Ref: Chapter No. 60, Page No. 1680

8. **Ans: A. During resting conditions, coronary blood flow autoregulated over a pressure range of 90–150 mm Hg**

   Ref: Chapter No. 60, Page No. 1680

9. **Ans: C. 80% blood flow occurs during diastole**

   Ref: Chapter No. 60, Page No. 1680

10. **Ans: B. Gibbon**

    Ref: Chapter No. 60, Page No. 1680

11. **Ans: A. DeBakey**

    Ref: Chapter No. 60, Page No. 1681

12. **Ans: C. Subramanian**

    Ref: Chapter No. 60, Page No. 1681

13. **Ans: D. Buckberg**

    Ref: Chapter No. 60, Page No. 1681

14. **Ans: A. Intramyocardial arteries are the most susceptible**

    Ref: Chapter No. 60, Page No. 1681-82

15. **Ans: B. Epicardial conductance vessels**

    Ref: Chapter No. 60, Page No. 1681

16. **Ans: D. Concentric lesion**

    Ref: Chapter No. 60, Page No. 1682

17. **Ans: B. Concentric lesion are more prone to plaque rupture**

    Ref: Chapter No. 60, Page No. 1682

18. **Ans: D. 7 to 10 days**

    Ref: Chapter No. 60, Page No. 1683

19. **Ans: D. Low sensitivity in multivessel disease**

    Ref: Chapter No. 60, Page No. 1684

20. **Ans: D. It is used for pharmacologic stress test**

    Ref: Chapter No. 60, Page No. 1684

21. **Ans: D. Duration of exercise**

    Ref: Chapter No. 60, Page No. 1684

22. **Ans: D. Quantitative image analysis**

    Ref: Chapter No. 60, Page No. 1684

23. **Ans: C. Anatomic correlates of the coronary vessels**

    Ref: Chapter No. 60, Page No. 1684

24. **Ans: C. Thallium 201**

    Ref: Chapter No. 60, Page No. 1684

25. **Ans: A. Dopamine**

    Ref: Chapter No. 60, Page No. 1684

26. **Ans: D. Regadenoson**

    Ref: Chapter No. 60, Page No. 1684

27. **Ans: D. It cannot assess arterial remodeling and non calcified plaques**

    Ref: Chapter No. 60, Page No. 1685

28. **Ans: B. Coronary catheterization**

    Ref: Chapter No. 60, Page No. 1685

29. **Ans: D. It helps to interpret functional significance of a given coronary stenosis**

    Ref: Chapter No. 60, Page No. 1685

30. **Ans: B. 50%**

    Ref: Chapter No. 60, Page No. 1685

31. **Ans: B. 0.75**

    Ref: Chapter No. 60, Page No. 1686

32. **Ans: D. Luminal diameter reduction of at least 50%**

    Ref: Chapter No. 60, Page No. 1686

33. **Ans: B. Acute STEMI**

    Ref: Chapter No. 60, Page No. 1686

34. **Ans: D. CAD with LVEF 35% to 50%**

    Ref: Chapter No. 60, Page No. 1687

35. **Ans: D. PCI improves survival in stable patients**

    Ref: Chapter No. 60, Page No. 1688

36. **Ans: A. More survival benefits after CABG as compared to PCI**

    Ref: Chapter No. 60, Page No. 1688

37. **Ans: A. CABG and DES implantation in patients with three-vessel or left main disease**

Ref: Chapter No. 60, Page No. 1688

38. **Ans: D. Complexity**

Ref: Chapter No. 60, Page No. 1688

39. **Ans: D. The occurrence of major adverse cardiac events correlated with the SYNTAX score following both CABG and PCI procedures**

Ref: Chapter No. 60, Page No. 1688

40. **Ans: C. STICH trial**

Ref: Chapter No. 60, Page No. 1689

41. **Ans: B. STICH trial**

Ref: Chapter No. 60, Page No. 1689

42. **Ans: C. Multiple diseased bypass grafts**

Ref: Chapter No. 60, Page No. 1690

43. **Ans: D. 90 minutes**

Ref: Chapter No. 60, Page No. 1690

44. **Ans: A. 30 minutes**

Ref: Chapter No. 60, Page No. 1690

45. **Ans: A. PCI and thrombolytics have equal survival benefits as an initial treatment for acute STEMI**

Ref: Chapter No. 60, Page No. 1690

46. **Ans: A. Venous reservoir collects blood by using rotator pump**

Ref: Chapter No. 60, Page No. 1692

47. **Ans: C. It is administered as pre-warmed solution**

Ref: Chapter No. 60, Page No. 1692

48. **Ans: C. 4:1**

Ref: Chapter No. 60, Page No. 1692

49. **Ans: C. 80 to 120 mL/min/m^2**

Ref: Chapter No. 60, Page No. 1693

50. **Ans: C. 50%**

Ref: Chapter No. 60, Page No. 1693

51. **Ans: B. Patient is systemically heparinized with 300 U/kg after cannulation**

Ref: Chapter No. 60, Page No. 1693

52. **Ans: B. Left internal mammary artery**

Ref: Chapter No. 60, Page No. 1693

53. **Ans: A. The long-term patency rate of the Left IMA graft has been shown to be approximately 80% at 10 years**

Ref: Chapter No. 60, Page No. 1693-94

54. **Ans: A. Great saphenous vein**

Ref: Chapter No. 60, Page No. 1694

55. **Ans: D. LIMA > Radial artery > GSV > right gastro-epiploic artery**

Ref: Chapter No. 60, Page No. 1695

56. **Ans: C. Cephalic vein**

Ref: Chapter No. 60, Page No. 1695

57. **Ans: C. Hypertension**

Ref: Chapter No. 60, Page No. 1695

58. **Ans: B. 3 mg/Kg**

Ref: Chapter No. 60, Page No. 1695

59. **Ans: C. End to side**

Ref: Chapter No. 60, Page No. 1695

60. **Ans: D. The first stage of venous cannula has the fenestrated basket that usually rests at the entrance of IVC**

Ref: Chapter No. 60, Page No. 1696

61. **Ans: A. Potassium cardioplegia solution is used to arrest the heart during systole**

Ref: Chapter No. 60, Page No. 1696

62. **Ans: B. The LIMA to left descending artery anastomosis is the first one to be performed**

Ref: Chapter No. 60, Page No. 1696-97

63. **Ans: D. The use of IABP is absolutely contraindicated in patients with aortic aneurysm**

Ref: Chapter No. 60, Page No. 1698

64. **Ans: B. Aortic regurgitation**

Ref: Chapter No. 60, Page No. 1698

65. **Ans: D. Keeping blood glucose levels below 140 mg/dL**

Ref: Chapter No. 60, Page No. 1699

66. **Ans: B. Maintaining hemoglobin level > 8 g/dL in older patients or those with severe cerebrovascular disease**

Ref: Chapter No. 60, Page No. 1699

67. **Ans: A. 3%**

Ref: Chapter No. 60, Page No. 1699

68. **Ans: D. Emergency procedure**

Ref: Chapter No. 60, Page No. 1700

69. **Ans: D. Evidence of hemothorax on radiograph**

Ref: Chapter No. 60, Page No. 1700

70. **Ans: D. Atherosclerosis of the aorta, diabetes are risk factors for type II deficit**

Ref: Chapter No. 60, Page No. 1700

71. **Ans: B. Bilateral internal mammary artery**

Ref: Chapter No. 60, Page No. 1700

72. **Ans: A. 2%**

Ref: Chapter No. 60, Page No. 1700

73. **Ans: C. Once CPB is initiated, the patient is cooled to 32°C**

Ref: Chapter No. 60, Page No. 1701

74. **Ans: C. On-Pump Beating-Heart Bypass**

Ref: Chapter No. 60, Page No. 1701

75. **Ans: C. Lower risk of fluid shift complications**

Ref: Chapter No. 60, Page No. 1702

76. **Ans: D. Off-Pump Coronary Artery Bypass Grafting**

Ref: Chapter No. 60, Page No. 1702

77. **Ans: D. NOBLE Trial**

Ref: Chapter No. 60, Page No. 1702

78. **Ans: B. Robot assisted procedure**

Ref: Chapter No. 60, Page No. 1702

79. **Ans: D. All of the above**

Ref: Chapter No. 60, Page No. 1703

80. **Ans: B. It is always used as an adjunct therapy**

Ref: Chapter No. 60, Page No. 1703

81. **Ans: C. Minimally invasive LIMA to LAD anastomosis in conjunction with PCI**

Ref: Chapter No. 60, Page No. 1703

82. **Ans: B. Older age at the time of the index operation**

Ref: Chapter No. 60, Page No. 1704

83. **Ans: C. Two thirds of patients are symptomatic**

Ref: Chapter No. 60, Page No. 1704

84. **Ans: A. Arrhythmias**

Ref: Chapter No. 60, Page No. 1704

85. **Ans: A. 2 to 4**

Ref: Chapter No. 60, Page No. 1705

86. **Ans: B. VSD that occurs in the first 6 days after an infarct is considered acute**

Ref: Chapter No. 60, Page No. 1705

87. **Ans: C. 6 weeks**

Ref: Chapter No. 60, Page No. 1705

88. **Ans: D. Prompt surgical intervention involves mitral valve repair and concomitant CABG**

Ref: Chapter No. 60, Page No. 1706

61

Valvular Heart Disease

HISTORY

1. **Who performed first successful closed digital mitral valve commissurotomy?**
   A. Elliot Cutler B. Henry Souttar
   C. Charles Bailey D. Theodore Tuffier

2. **Who performed first mechanical dilation of aortic valve using an instrument?**
   A. Henry Souttar B. Theodore Tuffier
   C. Russell Brock D. Charles Bailey

3. **Who performed first successful implantation of a prosthetic aortic valve?**
   A. Charles Bailey B. Charles Hufnagel
   C. Harken D. Albert Starr

4. **Who performed first successful in situ aortic valve replacement?**
   A. Charles Hufnagel B. Albert Starr
   C. Harken D. Gibbon

5. **Who performed first prosthetic replacement of the mitral valve?**
   A. Albert Starr B. Harken
   C. Gibbon D. Charles Hufnagel

6. **Who developed cardiopulmonary bypass machine?**
   A. Albert Starr B. Gibbon
   C. Bernard D. Henry Souttar

VALVE ANATOMY

7. **Wrongly matched of the following:**
   A. Fibrosa – fibrillar collagen
   B. Spongiosa – proteoglycans
   C. Atrialis – elastin
   D. Ventricularis – glycosaminoglycans

8. **Cusps are made up of following structures except:**
   A. Hinge B. Annulus
   C. Coapting surface D. Lannulae

9. **Nodes of Aranti are present at:**
   A. Mitral valve
   B. Aortic valve
   C. Chordae tendineae
   D. Pericardium

10. **False regarding anatomy of the mitral valve:**
    A. The mitral valve proper has two leaflets possessing approximately equal surface area
    B. Anterior leaflet originates from approximately the anterior two third of the valve annulus
    C. The posterior mitral leaflet is less wide
    D. The mitral valve is supported by an anterior and posterior papillary muscle

11. **Incorrect regarding anatomy of tricuspid valve:**
    A. Anterior leaflet is the largest
    B. Large anterior papillary muscle sends chordae to the anterior and posterior leaflets
    C. The anterior and posterior leaflets each have three scallops due to indentations
    D. There is no formal septal papillary muscle

12. **Septal RV wall provides chordae tendinae to:**
    A. Only to septal leaflet
    B. Anterior and posterior leaflets
    C. Anterior and septal leaflets
    D. Posterior and septal leaflets

13. **Which of the following is incorrect about anatomic relations of cardiac valves?**
    A. Posterior cusp of aortic valve is non coronary cusp

B. The atrioventricular node lies just beneath the commissure between the non-coronary and right coronary aortic leaflets
C. The atrioventricular node and bundle of His lie deep to the posteromedial commissure of the mitral valve
D. The atrioventricular node lies in the base of "Koch triangle"

14. What is the location of circumflex coronary artery?

A. Anterior interventricular groove
B. Right atrioventricular groove
C. Left atrioventricular groove
D. Posterior interventricular groove

15. Anatomic location of the AV node is:

A. Beahr's triangle B. Koch's triangle
C. Joll triangle D. Sherren triangle

16. All are the boundaries of "Koch triangle" except:

A. Septal leaflet of the tricuspid valve
B. The tendon of Todaro
C. Coronary sinus
D. Posterior cusp of aortic valve

ETIOLOGY AND PATHOLOGY

17. What is the most common cause of valvular heart disease?

A. Acquired degenerative disease
B. Rheumatic heart disease
C. Congenital anomaly
D. Ischemic disease

18. Most commonly involved cardiac valve in rheumatic heart disease:

A. Mitral valve B. Tricuspid valve
C. Aortic valve D. Pulmonary valve

19. Most common valvular lesion caused by rheumatic heart disease:

A. Mitral stenosis
B. Mitral regurgitation
C. Tricuspid regurgitation
D. Aortic stenosis

20. RHD is caused by which host cardiac protein molecular mimicry?

A. Type IV collagen B. Laminin
C. Fibronectin D. Perlecan

21. Which is false concerning rheumatic heart disease?

A. It is caused by Group A beta-hemolytic streptococcal infection acquired during the first decade of life
B. Molecular mimicry between streptococcal proteins and host cardiac protein laminin
C. "Fish mouth" funnel valve is characteristic lesion of acute RHD
D. Clinically apparent heart failure typically develops from these RHD lesions in the third or fourth decade

22. "Fish mouth" funnel valve is characteristic lesion of:

A. Mitral stenosis
B. Mitral regurgitation
C. Mixed mitral valve lesion
D. Annulus fibrosis lesion

23. Which valvular heart lesion most commonly requires surgical intervention?

A. Mitral regurgitation B. Aortic stenosis
C. Aortic regurgitation D. Pulmonary stenosis

24. What is the most common cause of aortic stenosis?

A. Congenital bicuspid valve
B. Rheumatic heart disease
C. Degenerative disease
D. Endocarditis

25. All are true regarding bicuspid aortic valve except:

A. It is present in 1% to 2% of the population
B. It is most common congenital valve lesion
C. It more commonly found in females
D. Degenerative disease of bicuspid aortic valves occur earlier than it does with tricuspid valves

26. "Wear and tear disease" or "senile disease" of aortic valve is associated with:

A. Bicuspid valve
B. Atherosclerosis
C. Rheumatic heart disease
D. Endocarditis

27. What is false regarding aortic valve stenotic lesion?

A. Aortic valvular stenosis is the most common form of valvular heart disease requiring surgical intervention
B. Aortic stenosis is almost always acquired

C. Prevalence of aortic stenosis increases with the age
D. Aortic stenosis occurs in 50% to 60% of patients born with bicuspid aortic valves

28. Carpentier classification is used for which valvular heart disease?

A. Aortic regurgitation
B. Mitral regurgitation
C. Mitral stenosis
D. Tricuspid regurgitation

29. Which is false concerning mitral regurgitation (MR)?

A. MR is the most frequent form of valve dysfunction overall
B. Degenerative changes to the mitral valve apparatus are the most common cause
C. Typically found in old patients
D. Posterior papillary muscle is more susceptible to coronary ischemia

30. According to Carpentier classification of mitral regurgitation, functional MR is classified as:

A. Type I lesion B. Type II lesion
C. Type IIIa lesion D. Type IIIb lesion

31. Most common myxomatous disease leading to mitral regurgitation:

A. Marfan disease
B. Ehlers-Danlos disease
C. Barlow disease
D. Scleroderma

32. According to Carpentier classification of mitral regurgitation, connective tissue disorder causing excessive leaflet motion are classified as:

A. Type I lesion B. Type II lesion
C. Type IIIa lesion D. Type IIIb lesion

33. False about Barlow disease is:

A. Redundant, "billowing" valve leaflets
B. Chordae rupture
C. Occurs in young women
D. Click-murmur syndrome

34. All are true about fibroelastic deficiency syndrome except:

A. Thinned leaflets
B. Chordal rupture
C. Prolapse or flail of the middle posterior leaflet cusp (P2)
D. Presents in younger patients

35. According to Carpentier classification of mitral regurgitation, wrongly matched of the following:

A. Type I lesion –Annular dilation
B. Type II lesion – Leaflet or subvalvular deformations resulting in excessive leaflet motion
C. Type IIIa lesion – Restricted closure
D. Type IIIb lesion – Ischemic or functional MR

36. Lesions causing restricted systolic motion of leaflets are classified according to Carpentier classification of mitral regurgitation as:

A. Type I lesion B. Type II lesion
C. Type IIIa lesion D. Type IIIb lesion

37. Following are causes of aortic root dilatation:

A. Cystic medial necrosis
B. Loeys Dietz syndrome
C. Congenital bicuspid valve
D. All of the above

38. Following are the causes of aortic valve regurgitation:

A. Connective tissue disorders
B. Congenital bicuspid valve
C. Endocarditis
D. All of the above

39. Libman-Sacks lesions are seen with:

A. Rheumatic valve disease
B. Systemic lupus erythematosus
C. Myxomatous degeneration
D. Syphilitic aortitis

40. Following are causes of functional tricuspid regurgitation except:

A. RV failure
B. Left sided ventricular dysfunction
C. Pulmonary hypertension
D. Carcinoid syndrome

41. What is most common cause of tricuspid stenosis?

A. Rheumatic heart disease
B. Carcinoid syndrome
C. Congenital anomaly
D. Degenerative disease

42. Carpentier Type IIIa lesion involves all of the following except:

A. Leaflet thickening
B. Leaflet calcification

C. Rupture of papillary muscle
D. Chordal thickening

43. Following conditions lead to Carpentier Type II lesion except:

A. Degenerative valve disease
B. Endocarditis
C. Chronic Rheumatic disease
D. Trauma

44. Carpentier Type IIIa lesion of MR is caused by:

A. Fibroelastic deficiency
B. Dilated cardiomyopathy
C. Carcinoid heart disease
D. Endocarditis

45. Ideal actin-myosin alignment occurs at a sarcomere length of:

A. 1.1 micrometers B. 2.2 micrometers
C. 3.3 micrometers D. 4.4 micrometers

MITRAL STENOSIS (MS)

46. Which is false statement regarding pathological changes of MS?

A. Normal sized mitral valve has 4–6 cm^2 cross-sectional area
B. Normal left atrial pressure is typically less than 10 to 15 mm Hg
C. Valve orifice of less than 2 cm^2 is classified as severe MS
D. Pulmonary edema develops at a left atrial pressure of 25 mm Hg

47. Severe MS is defined as the mitral valve cross-sectional area less than:

A. 2.5 cm^2 B. 2 cm^2
C. 1.5 cm^2 D. 1 cm^2

48. Which is incorrect statement regarding symptoms of MS?

A. MS patients may remain asymptomatic for many years
B. Thromboembolization will occur in 5% of patients with MS
C. Half of all thromboembolic events will involve the cerebral circulation
D. MS causes systemic congestive symptoms

49. MS murmur is characterized by all except:

A. High-pitched
B. Diastolic murmur with presystolic accentuation
C. High-pitched "opening snap"
D. Best heard at the apex with the patient in the left lateral decubitus position

50. Graham Steell diastolic murmur is seen with which cardiac valvular lesion?

A. Mitral stenosis
B. Mitral regurgitation
C. Aortic regurgitation
D. Pulmonary regurgitation

51. Following radiographic findings are consistent with MS except:

A. Straightening of the left cardiac border
B. Inverted 3 sign
C. Double shadow in the cardiac silhouette
D. Elevated left main stem bronchus

52. Patient presented with dyspnea and orthopnea. On chest auscultation diastolic murmur was heard at apex. ECG shows characteristic P mitrale wave. What is the probable diagnosis of this patient?

A. Mitral stenosis
B. Mitral regurgitation
C. Aortic regurgitation
D. Aortic stenosis

53. All are true about echocardiography in MS diagnosis except:

A. 3D echocardiography provides further definition of valve morphology and function
B. Orifice area can be measured by planimetry
C. Mitral valve area can also be determined based upon the pressure half-time, the time in which the transvalvular velocity decreases by half
D. Pressure half-time will be shortened with increasing severity of stenosis

54. $CHADS_2VASc$ score is used for:

A. Antihypertensive therapy
B. Anticoagulation therapy
C. Arrhythmia treatment
D. Surgical intervention for heart block

55. $CHADS_2$ score includes all of the following variables except:

A. Hypertension
B. Congestive heart failure
C. Age ≥ 75 years
D. Sex category

56. According to $CHADS_2$ score, 2 points are given for:

A. Age ≥ 75 years
B. Prior stroke or thromboembolism
C. Hypertension
D. Congestive heart failure

57. According to $CHADS_2$ VASc score, 2 points are given for:

A. Age ≥ 75 years
B. Hypertension
C. Sex category (female)
D. Congestive heart failure

58. Following variables are included in HAS-BLED score except:

A. Diabetes mellitus
B. Stroke
C. Labile INR
D. Abnormal renal/liver function

59. Following are correct components of HAS-BLED score except:

A. Elderly > 75 years
B. Drugs/alcohol use
C. Abnormal renal/liver function
D. Bleeding history or predisposition

60. Following are the indications for surgical intervention of MS except:

A. Asymptomatic severe MS
B. Moderate or severe MS undergoing cardiac surgery for other reasons
C. Severe MS with recurrent embolic events while on anticoagulation
D. MS with valve area < 1 cm^2

61. Wilkins echocardiographic criteria is used for which valvular heart lesion?

A. Mitral stenosis B. Mitral regurgitation
C. Aortic regurgitation D. Aortic stenosis

62. Wilkins echocardiographic criteria is used for which procedure?

A. Open surgical repair of mitral valve
B. Mitral valve replacement
C. Percutaneous balloon mitral commissurotomy
D. Mitraclip application

63. Percutaneous balloon mitral commissurotomy is indicated in following valve conditions except:

A. Presence of mobile leaflets
B. Noncalcified thin valve
C. Moderate MR
D. Absence of LA thrombus

64. All are true about Percutaneous balloon mitral commissurotomy (PBMC) except:

A. PBMC patient selection is based upon Wilkins echocardiographic criteria
B. Wilkins score ranges between 4 and 16
C. PBMC is likely to be successful with a score of 10 or less
D. Successful PBMC is defined as a post-dilation valve area of more than 1.5 cm^2 with MR less than 2/4, is achieved in over 80% of patients

65. Percutaneous balloon mitral commissurotomy (PBMC) is recommended in patients with Wilkins score of:

A. ≤ 8 B. ≥ 8
C. ≤ 10 D. ≥ 10

66. Wilkins criteria for mitral valve includes following variables except:

A. Valve mobility
B. Leaflet thickening
C. Valve calcification
D. Subvalvular apparatus thinning

MITRAL REGURGITATION (MR)

67. Following features are consistent with severe MR except:

A. Effective regurgitant orifice of at least 0.4 cm^2
B. Regurgitant volume of at least 60 mL
C. Regurgitant fraction of at least 30%
D. Holosystolic eccentric jet

68. Following features are consistent with severe MR except:

A. Vena contract larger than 7 mm
B. Central MR jet larger than 40% of LA area
C. Regurgitant fraction of at least 30%
D. Regurgitant volume of at least 40 mL

69. Which of the following is not a class I indication for MR surgery?

A. Asymptomatic patients with chronic severe primary MR
B. Asymptomatic primary MR with LV ejection fraction [LVEF] 30%–60%

C. Asymptomatic primary MR with LV end systolic diameter [LVESD] ≥40 mm
D. Symptomatic patients and an LVEF < 30%

70. Which of the following is a class I indication for MR repair?

A. Asymptomatic chronic primary severe MR without LV dysfunction who exhibit a progressive increase in LV size or decrease in EF
B. Asymptomatic patients with preserved LV function in whom a 95% chance of successful repair with <1% mortality is predicted
C. Asymptomatic MR patients with preserved LV function having new onset atrial fibrillation
D. Chronic moderate primary MR undergoing cardiac surgery for other indications

71. All are true regarding mitral valve repair surgery except:

A. Repair of the mitral valve is preferred over mitral valve replacement for patients with primary MR
B. Mitral repair has reoperations rates less than 10% at 10 years
C. Ring annuloplasty is now generally indicated with all mitral valve repairs
D. Better overall LV remodeling or survival for patients undergoing repair as compared to replacement

AORTIC STENOSIS (AS)

72. Following are class I indications of aortic valve replacement surgery for AS except:

A. Symptomatic severe, high-gradient AS
B. Asymptomatic severe AS and reduced LVEF (<50%)
C. Patient with severe AS, undergoing cardiac surgery for another indication
D. Asymptomatic severe AS with preserved LVEF (≥50%), but rapid disease progression

73. Which of the following is false statement regarding Aortic stenosis?

A. The normal aortic valve orifice measures 3 to 5 cm^2
B. Two-thirds of patients who progress to severe AS develop myocardial ischemia
C. Myocardial hypertrophy precipitates early ventricular diastolic dysfunction
D. The onset of symptoms occurs when the valve orifice area decreases to approximately 1.5 cm^2

74. What is the earliest symptom of Aortic stenosis?

A. Angina
B. Syncope
C. Dyspnea
D. Heart failure

75. Following are characteristics of Aortic stenosis except:

A. Crescendo-decrescendo ejection murmur
B. Murmur best heard along the left sternal border that radiates to carotid arteries
C. Pulsus parvus et tardus
D. Box shaped heart on chest radiograph

76. Boot shaped heart on chest radiograph is seen in:

A. Total anomalous pulmonary venous return
B. Aortic stenosis
C. Ebstein anomaly
D. Transposition of great vessels

77. Following are Doppler echocardiographic features of Severe Aortic stenosis except:

A. Doppler velocity >4 m/sec
B. Mean aortic valve gradient >40 mm Hg
C. Valve area < 1 cm^2
D. LV end systolic diameter >40 mm

78. All are true about survival following Aortic stenosis except:

A. Mean survival after the appearance of angina is about 10 years
B. Survival is less than 3 years after the onset of syncope
C. Only 1 to 2 years survival, once the heart failure symptoms develop
D. Sudden death may also occur in symptomatic patients at a rate of 2% per month

79. Which is incorrect regarding transcatheter aortic valve replacement (TAVR) for AS?

A. TAVR is indicated in symptomatic, severe AS and prohibitive surgical risk with a predicted post-TAVR survival >12 months
B. Reasonable alternative to surgical AVR for symptomatic, severe AS and high surgical risk
C. Preferred in elderly patients suitable for transfemoral access
D. TAVR is indicated for asymptomatic severe aortic stenosis with LVEF < 50%

80. All are true about Percutaneous balloon aortic valvuloplasty (PBAV) except:

A. As a bridge to surgical or trans-catheter aortic valve replacement

B. For patients with severe AS who are severely symptomatic
C. For patients requiring urgent noncardiac major surgery
D. Hemodynamically stable patients requiring cardiac surgery for other indications

AORTIC INSUFFICIENCY (AI)

81. Following are the causes of acute AI except:

A. Infective endocarditis
B. Myocardial infarction
C. Trauma
D. Aortic dissection

82. Which of the following are class I indications for aortic valve replacement surgery in patients with AI?

A. Symptomatic AI regardless of LVEF
B. Asymptomatic severe chronic AI and reduced LVEF (<50%)
C. Severe AR with or without symptoms while undergoing cardiac surgery for other indication
D. Severe AI and preserved LVEF (≥50%), but progressive severe LV dilation (LVEDD >65 mm)

83. Following are the characteristic findings of AI except:

A. Peripheral water-hammer pulses
B. Decrescendo diastolic murmur best heard with patient sitting up and leaning forward
C. The murmur is increased by maneuvers such as squatting or hand-grip
D. Mid-diastolic Graham Steell murmur

84. Wrongly matched clinical finding of AI:

A. Corrigan pulse - bounding carotid pulse
B. de Musset sign - head bobbing with each heartbeat
C. Quincke sign - pulsation of the uvula
D. Traube sign - "pistol shot" auscultated with compression of the femoral artery

85. Diastolic Austin-Flint murmur is seen in which valvular lesion?

A. Mitral stenosis
B. Aortic regurgitation
C. Tricuspid stenosis
D. Pulmonary regurgitation

86. Following are echocardiographic findings of AI except:

A. Regurgitant jet width ≥50% of the LV outflow tract
B. >0.6 cm vena contracta
C. Regurgitant fraction ≥50%
D. An effective regurgitant orifice area ≥0.3 cm^2

87. Use of intra-aortic balloon pump is absolutely contraindicated in:

A. Mitral regurgitation B. Aortic stenosis
C. Aortic regurgitation D. Aortic aneurysm

88. Which procedure involves aortic valve replacement with a pulmonary auto graft and heterograft substitution of the native pulmonic valve?

A. Rastelli procedure
B. Ross procedure
C. Norwood procedure
D. Carpentier procedure

RIGHT SIDED VALVE DISEASE

89. Which is most prevalent right sided valvular disease?

A. Primary TR B. Functional TR
C. Tricuspid stenosis D. Pulmonary stenosis

90. Following are causes of primary TR except:

A. Carcinoid disease
B. Injuries resulting from pacemaker implantation
C. Endocarditis
D. Ischemic disease

91. Carvallo sign, a holosystolic murmur that increases with inspiration is seen with:

A. Patent truncus arteriosus
B. Tricuspid regurgitation
C. Pulmonary stenosis
D. Ventricular septal defect

92. Tricuspid annular dilation is considered when annular diameter of greater than:

A. 30 mm B. 40 mm
C. 50 mm D. 60 mm

93. Which is incorrect about management of tricuspid valve lesions?

A. Concomitant tricuspid valve surgery in patients having severe TR, who are undergoing left-heart surgery
B. Tricuspid valve repair is generally preferred to replacement whenever possible

C. Valve replacement should be considered for functional TR due to leaflet tethering and RV remodeling
D. Asymptomatic patients with isolated TS are best treated with valve replacement

OPERATIVE APPROACHES

94. What is operative mortality following cardiac valvular surgery?

A. 3% B. 9%
C. 15% D. 21%

95. Following risk factors are considered in EuroSCORE except:

A. Age > 60 years
B. Male sex
C. Recent MI within 90 days
D. Unstable angina

96. Following risk scoring systems are used for cardiac surgeries:

A. STS score B. EuroSCORE
C. EACTS D. All of the above

97. Which valvular lesion is associated with highest surgical mortality risk?

A. Mitral regurgitation
B. Aortic regurgitation
C. Isolated tricuspid regurgitation
D. Pulmonary stenosis

98. Which approach gives greater exposure of mitral valve?

A. Left lateral atriotomy approach
B. Right atriotomy approach
C. Superior septal approach
D. Left ventricular approach

99. Commonly used approach for exposure of mitral valve:

A. Left lateral atriotomy approach
B. Right atriotomy approach
C. Superior septal approach
D. Left ventricular approach

100. Which approach gives greater exposure of mitral valve?

A. Left lateral atriotomy approach
B. Right atriotomy approach
C. Superior septal approach
D. Left ventricular approach

101. Which post-surgical complication has higher rate of occurrence following aortic valve surgery as compared to mitral valve surgery?

A. Reoperation for bleeding
B. Permanent stroke
C. Deep sternal infection
D. Longer postoperative hospital stay

102. Valve-sparing root replacement involving reimplantation of the native valve inside a Dacron graft is:

A. Starnes procedure B. Takeuchi procedure
C. David procedure D. Ross procedure

103. Which is wrong statement regarding prosthetic valves?

A. Lifelong anticoagulation required
B. Recommended aspirin dose of 325 mg daily
C. Prosthetic valve endocarditis (PVE), which is 50 times more likely to occur
D. Failure rates may be higher in younger patients

104. Recommended anticoagulation therapy following bioprosthetic valve replacement is:

A. 1 month B. 6 months
C. 12 months D. Lifelong

105. What is the most common cause of prosthetic valve endocarditis?

A. Strep. pyogenes
B. Strep. viridans
C. Staph. aureus
D. Staph. epidermidis

106. PARTNER Trial is related to:

A. Valve sparing aortic root replacement
B. Transcatheter aortic valve replacement
C. Percutaneous mitral valve repair
D. Percutaneous mitral valve commissurotomy

107. False regarding transcatheter aortic valve replacement surgery:

A. Provide long-term relief of AS
B. TAVR was non-inferior to SAVR for symptomatic patients with severe AS
C. Indicated for patients with a predicted post-procedural survival less than 12 months
D. Complications of paravalvular regurgitation, valve thrombosis remain higher after TAVR than SAVR

108. False statement about MitraClip system:

A. Percutaneous mitral valve therapy
B. Catheter-based clip delivery system through femoral artery
C. Edge-to-edge "Alfieri" leaflet repair
D. The reduction of severe MR is less effective than surgical therapy

109. Patient presented with dyspnea on exertion and pulmonary congestion. On chest auscultation high pitched holosystolic murmur was heard at apex radiating to axilla. Patient has undergone following procedure:

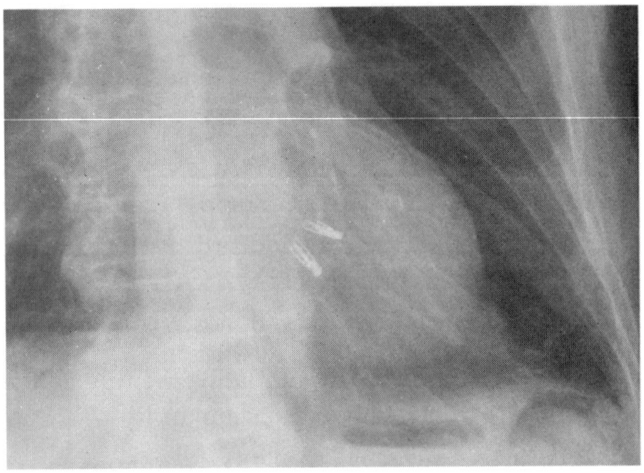

Identify the procedure.

A. Transcatheter aortic valve replacement
B. Percutaneous ventricular septal defect closure
C. MitraClip application
D. Open mitral valve repair surgery

110. Identify the following structure:

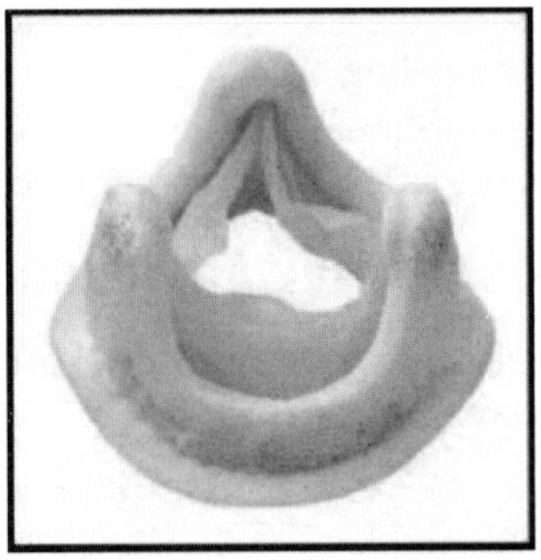

A. Starr-Edward valve B. St Jude's valve
C. Bjork-Shilley valve D. Porcine valve

111. Identify the structure "A" shown in the following image:

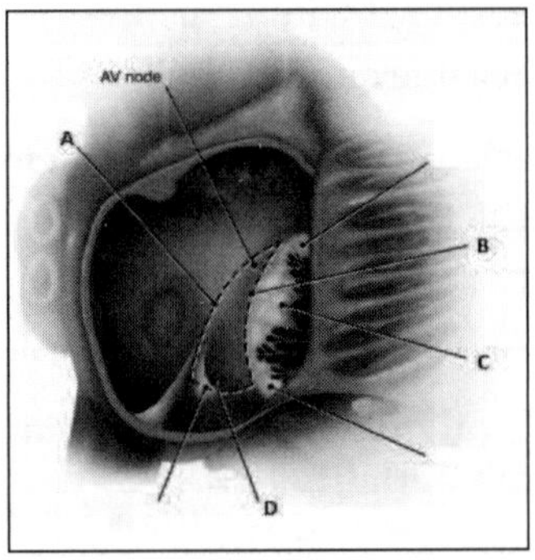

A. Septal leaflet of tricuspid valve
B. Bundle of His
C. Tendon of Todaro
D. Coronary sinus

ANSWERS

1. **Ans: B. Henry Souttar**
Ref: Chapter No. 61, Page No. 1711

2. **Ans: C. Russell Brock**
Ref: Chapter No. 61, Page No. 1712

3. **Ans: B. Charles Hufnagel**
Ref: Chapter No. 61, Page No. 1712

4. **Ans: C. Harken**
Ref: Chapter No. 61, Page No. 1712

5. **Ans: A. Albert Starr**
Ref: Chapter No. 61, Page No. 1712

6. **Ans: B. Gibbon**
Ref: Chapter No. 61, Page No. 1712

7. **Ans: D. Ventricularis – glycosaminoglycans**
Ref: Chapter No. 61, Page No. 1712

8. **Ans: B. Annulus**
Ref: Chapter No. 61, Page No. 1712

9. **Ans: B. Aortic valve**
Ref: Chapter No. 61, Page No. 1712

10. **Ans: B. Anterior leaflet originates from approximately the anterior two third of the valve annulus**
Ref: Chapter No. 61, Page No. 1712

11. **Ans: C. The anterior and posterior leaflets each have three scallops due to indentations**
Ref: Chapter No. 61, Page No. 1712

12. **Ans: C. Anterior and septal leaflets**
Ref: Chapter No. 61, Page No. 1713

13. **Ans: D. The atrioventricular node lies in the base of "Koch triangle"**
Ref: Chapter No. 61, Page No. 1713

14. **Ans: C. Left atrioventricular groove**
Ref: Chapter No. 61, Page No. 1713

15. **Ans: B. Koch's triangle**
Ref: Chapter No. 61, Page No. 1713

16. **Ans: D. Posterior cusp of aortic valve**
Ref: Chapter No. 61, Page No. 1713

17. **Ans: B. Rheumatic heart disease**
Ref: Chapter No. 61, Page No. 1714

18. **Ans: A. Mitral valve**
Ref: Chapter No. 61, Page No. 1714

19. **Ans: A. Mitral stenosis**
Ref: Chapter No. 61, Page No. 1714

20. **Ans: B. Laminin**
Ref: Chapter No. 61, Page No. 1714

21. **Ans: C. "Fish mouth" funnel valve is characteristic lesion of acute RHD**
Ref: Chapter No. 61, Page No. 1714

22. **Ans: C. Mixed mitral valve lesion**
Ref: Chapter No. 61, Page No. 1714

23. **Ans: B. Aortic stenosis**
Ref: Chapter No. 61, Page No. 1714

24. **Ans: C. Degenerative disease**
Ref: Chapter No. 61, Page No. 1714

25. **Ans: C. It more commonly found in females**
Ref: Chapter No. 61, Page No. 1716

26. **Ans: B. Atherosclerosis**
Ref: Chapter No. 61, Page No. 1716

27. **Ans. D. Aortic stenosis occurs in 50% to 60% of patients born with bicuspid aortic valves**
Ref: Chapter No. 61, Page No. 1716

28. **Ans: B. Mitral regurgitation**
Ref: Chapter No. 61, Page No. 1716

29. **Ans: C. Typically found in old patients**
Ref: Chapter No. 61, Page No. 1717

30. **Ans: D. Type IIIb lesion**
Ref: Chapter No. 61, Page No. 1717

31. **Ans: A. Marfan's disease**
Ref: Chapter No. 61, Page No. 1717

32. **Ans: B. Type II lesion**
Ref: Chapter No. 61, Page No. 1717

33. **Ans: B. Chordae rupture**
Ref: Chapter No. 61, Page No. 1717

34. **Ans: D. Presents in younger patients**
Ref: Chapter No. 61, Page No. 1717

35. **Ans: C. Type IIIa lesion – Restricted closure**
Ref: Chapter No. 61, Page No. 1717-1718

36. **Ans: C. Type IIIa lesion**
Ref: Chapter No. 61, Page No. 1718

37. **Ans: D. All of the above**
Ref: Chapter No. 61, Page No. 1718

38. **Ans: D. All of the above**

Ref: Chapter No. 61, Page No. 1718-1719

39. **Ans: B. Systemic lupus erythematosus**

Ref: Chapter No. 61, Page No. 1720

40. **Ans: D. Carcinoid syndrome**

Ref: Chapter No. 61, Page No. 1720

41. **Ans: A. Rheumatic heart disease**

Ref: Chapter No. 61, Page No. 1720

42. **Ans: C. Rupture of papillary muscle**

Ref: Chapter No. 61, Page No. 1721

43. **Ans: C. Chronic Rheumatic disease**

Ref: Chapter No. 61, Page No. 1721

44. **Ans: C. Carcinoid heart disease**

Ref: Chapter No. 61, Page No. 1721

45. **Ans: B. 2.2 micrometers**

Ref: Chapter No. 61, Page No. 1721

46. **Ans: C. Valve orifice of less than 2 cm^2 is classified as severe MS**

Ref: Chapter No. 61, Page No. 1722

47. **Ans: C. 1.5 cm^2**

Ref: Chapter No. 61, Page No. 1722

48. **Ans: B. Thromboembolization will occur in 5% of patients with MS**

Ref: Chapter No. 61, Page No. 1722

49. **Ans: A. High-pitched**

Ref: Chapter No. 61, Page No. 1722-1723

50. **Ans: A. Mitral stenosis**

Ref: Chapter No. 61, Page No. 1723

51. **Ans: B. Inverted 3 sign**

Ref: Chapter No. 61, Page No. 1723

52. **Ans: A. Mitral stenosis**

Ref: Chapter No. 61, Page No. 1723

53. **Ans: D. Pressure half-time will be shortened with increasing severity of stenosis**

Ref: Chapter No. 61, Page No. 1723

54. **Ans: B. Anticoagulation therapy**

Ref: Chapter No. 61, Page No. 1723

55. **Ans: D. Sex category**

Ref: Chapter No. 61, Page No. 1723

56. **Ans: B. Prior stroke or thromboembolism**

Ref: Chapter No. 61, Page No. 1723

57. **Ans: A. Age $\geq$ 75 years**

Ref: Chapter No. 61, Page No. 1723

58. **Ans: A. Diabetes mellitus**

Ref: Chapter No. 61, Page No. 1723

59. **Ans: A. Elderly > 75 years**

Ref: Chapter No. 61, Page No. 1723

60. **Ans: A. Asymptomatic severe MS**

Ref: Chapter No. 61, Page No. 1724

61. **Ans: A. Mitral stenosis**

Ref: Chapter No. 61, Page No. 1724

62. **Ans: C. Percutaneous mitral balloon commissurotomy**

Ref: Chapter No. 61, Page No. 1724

63. **Ans: C. Moderate MR**

Ref: Chapter No. 61, Page No. 1724

64. **Ans: C. PBMC is likely to be successful with a score of 10 or less**

Ref: Chapter No. 61, Page No. 1724

65. **Ans: A. $\leq$ 8**

Ref: Chapter No. 61, Page No. 1724

66. **Ans: D. Subvalvular apparatus thinning**

Ref: Chapter No. 61, Page No. 1724

67. **Ans: C. Regurgitant fraction of at least 30%**

Ref: Chapter No. 61, Page No. 1725

68. **Ans: D. Regurgitant volume of at least 40 mL**

Ref: Chapter No. 61, Page No. 1725

69. **Ans: D. Symptomatic patients and an LVEF < 30%**

Ref: Chapter No. 61, Page No. 1726

70. **Ans: D. Chronic moderate primary MR undergoing cardiac surgery for other indications**

Ref: Chapter No. 61, Page No. 1726

71. **Ans: D. Better overall LV remodeling or survival for patients undergoing repair as compared to replacement**

Ref: Chapter No. 61, Page No. 1727-1728

72. **Ans: D. Asymptomatic severe AS with preserved LVEF ($\geq$50%), but rapid disease progression**

Ref: Chapter No. 61, Page No. 1728

73. **Ans: D. The onset of symptoms occurs when the valve orifice area decreases to approximately 1.5 cm^2**

Ref: Chapter No. 61, Page No. 1729

74. **Ans: A. Angina**

Ref: Chapter No. 61, Page No. 1729

75. **Ans: D. Box shaped heart on chest radiograph**

Ref: Chapter No. 61, Page No. 1729

76. **Ans: B. Aortic stenosis**

Ref: Chapter No. 61, Page No. 1729

77. **Ans: D. LV end systolic diameter >40 mm**

Ref: Chapter No. 61, Page No. 1729

78. **Ans: A. Mean survival after the appearance of angina is about 10 years**

Ref: Chapter No. 61, Page No. 1730

79. **Ans: D. TAVR is indicated for asymptomatic severe aortic stenosis with LVEF < 50%**

Ref: Chapter No. 61, Page No. 1731

80. **Ans. D. Hemodynamically stable patients requiring cardiac surgery for other indications**

Ref: Chapter No. 61, Page No. 1731

81. **Ans: B. Myocardial infarction**

Ref: Chapter No. 61, Page No. 1730

82. **Ans: D. Severe AI and preserved LVEF (≥50%), but progressive severe LV dilation (LVEDD >65 mm)**

Ref: Chapter No. 61, Page No. 1728

83. **Ans. D. Mid-diastolic Graham Steell murmur**

Ref: Chapter No. 61, Page No. 1731

84. **Ans: C. Quincke sign - pulsation of the uvula**

Ref: Chapter No. 61, Page No. 1731

85. **Ans: B. Aortic regurgitation**

Ref: Chapter No. 61, Page No. 1731

86. **Ans: A. Regurgitant jet width ≥50% of the LV outflow tract**

Ref: Chapter No. 61, Page No. 1732

87. **Ans: C. Aortic regurgitation**

Ref: Chapter No. 61, Page No. 1732

88. **Ans: B. Ross procedure**

Ref: Chapter No. 61, Page No. 1732

89. **Ans: B. Functional TR**

Ref: Chapter No. 61, Page No. 1732

90. **Ans: D. Ischemic disease**

Ref: Chapter No. 61, Page No. 1732

91. **Ans: B. Tricuspid regurgitation**

Ref: Chapter No. 61, Page No. 1732

92. **Ans: B. 40 mm**

Ref: Chapter No. 61, Page No. 1732

93. **Ans: D. Asymptomatic patients with isolated TS are best treated with valve replacement**

Ref: Chapter No. 61, Page No. 1733-1734

94. **Ans: A. 3%**

Ref: Chapter No. 61, Page No. 1733

95. **Ans: B. Male sex**

Ref: Chapter No. 61, Page No. 1734

96. **Ans: D. All of the above**

Ref: Chapter No. 61, Page No. 1734

97. **Ans: C. Isolated tricuspid regurgitation**

Ref: Chapter No. 61, Page No. 1735

98. **Ans: C. Superior septal approach**

Ref: Chapter No. 61, Page No. 1735

99. **Ans: A. Left lateral atriotomy approach**

Ref: Chapter No. 61, Page No. 1735

100. **Ans: B. Right atriotomy approach**

Ref: Chapter No. 61, Page No. 1735

101. **Ans: C. Deep sternal infection**

Ref: Chapter No. 61, Page No. 1735

102. **Ans: C. David procedure**

Ref: Chapter No. 61, Page No. 1737

103. **Ans: B. Recommended aspirin dose of 325 mg daily**

Ref: Chapter No. 61, Page No. 1737-1739

104. **Ans: B. 6 months**

Ref: Chapter No. 61, Page No. 1739

105. **Ans. C. Staph. aureus**

Ref: Chapter No. 61, Page No. 1739

106. **Ans: B. Transcatheter Aortic Valve Replacement**

Ref: Chapter No. 61, Page No. 1740

107. **Ans: C. Indicated for patients with a predicted post-procedural survival less than 12 months**

Ref: Chapter No. 61, Page No. 1740

108. **Ans: B. Catheter-based clip delivery system through femoral artery**

Ref: Chapter No. 61, Page No. 1740

109. **Ans: C. MitraClip application**

Ref: Chapter No. 61, Page No. 1740

110. **Ans: D. Porcine valve**

Ref: Chapter No. 61, Page No. 1739

111. **Ans: C. Tendon of Todaro**

Ref: Chapter No. 61, Page No. 1739

62

The Aorta

1. **Which of the following is incorrect about aortic development?**
   A. Aorta and its major branches formation begins in the third week of gestation
   B. Two ventral pairs fuse to form the aortic sac and the dorsal pairs fuse to form the descending thoracoabdominal aorta
   C. Embryologic aortic arches develop in a cephalocaudal fashion, they regress in the opposite order
   D. The aortic arches completely disappear by 6 weeks

2. **What is wrong about development of aortic arches?**
   A. Normal left-sided aortic arch requires regression of segment 1
   B. Right-sided aortic arch will occur with regression of segment 5
   C. Regression of segment 2 results in a left-sided arch with an aberrant right subclavian artery
   D. Right-sided arch with an aberrant left subclavian artery will occur with regression of segment 3

3. **Society for vascular surgery (SVS) divides aorta in "zones" on the basis of:**
   A. Extent of disease
   B. Endograft placement
   C. Endoleak
   D. Severity of malperfusion

4. **Crawford classification is used for which of the following?**
   A. Aortic blunt injury
   B. Thoracic aortic aneurysm
   C. Abdominothoracic aorta dissection
   D. Abdominothoracic aortic aneurysm

5. **Extent IV according to Crawford classification involves which part of aorta?**
   A. Descending thoracic aorta and abdominal aorta to the level of the celiac artery
   B. Entire thoracic and abdominal aorta
   C. Entire abdominal aorta
   D. Thoracic and abdominal aorta from 6th ICS to renal arteries

6. **Extent II according to Crawford classification involves which part of aorta?**
   A. Descending thoracic aorta and abdominal aorta to the level of the celiac artery
   B. Entire thoracic and abdominal aorta
   C. Entire abdominal aorta
   D. Thoracic and abdominal aorta from 6th ICS to renal arteries

7. **Which of the following classification system is not used for aortic dissection?**
   A. DeBakey classification
   B. Stanford classification
   C. Penn classification
   D. Crawford classification

8. **Which of the following type involves only ascending aortic dissection?**
   A. Type I DeBakey
   B. Type II DeBakey
   C. Type III DeBakey
   D. Type B Stanford

9. **Type IIIa DeBakey involves which part of aortic dissection?**
   A. Entire ascending, arch and to some extent descending aorta
   B. Ascending aorta only
   C. Descending thoracic aorta only
   D. Descending aorta

10. Subacute aortic dissection occurs during:

A. < 24 hours
B. 2 – 7 days
C. 8 – 30 days
D. 30 – 60 days

11. Number of landing zones upto descending thoracic aorta:

A. 3
B. 4
C. 5
D. 6

12. Penn classification of AD is divided into sub-groups:

A. 2
B. 3
C. 4
D. 5

13. Which of the following is not used to characterize aortic aneurysm?

A. An increase in size of more than 25% above the normal arterial diameter
B. Aneurysms of the ascending aorta as 4.7 cm in men and 4.2 cm in women
C. Aneurysms of the descending aorta as 3.7 cm in men and 3.3 cm in women
D. Aneurysms of the infrarenal aorta as 3.0 cm in men and 2.7 cm in women

14. What is the cause of mycotic aneurysms?

A. Atherosclerosis
B. Bacterial infection
C. Fungal infection
D. Trauma

15. Risk factors for development of aneurysm are all except:

A. Age
B. Female gender
C. Concurrent aneurysm
D. Marfan's syndrome

16. Risk factors for development of aneurysm are all except:

A. Tobacco
B. Hypertension
C. Hyperlipidemia
D. Diabetes

17. Which of the following is a risk factor for development of aneurysm?

A. Female gender
B. Black race
C. Diabetes
D. Height

18. Ortner syndrome is caused by:

A. Compression superior vena cava
B. Impingement of left recurrent laryngeal nerve
C. Compression of the left main stem bronchus
D. Dysphagia due to compression of esophagus

19. Which of the following is wrong statement?

A. The incidence of abdominal aortic aneurysm range from 3% to 10%
B. Aneurysms may be asymptomatic
C. Ultrasound is a good screening tool in AAA management
D. Transesophageal echocardiogram (TEE) is useful in seeing ascending aorta proximal to innominate artery

20. All are risk factors for aneurismal rupture except:

A. Female gender
B. Higher mean blood pressure
C. Renal transplantation
D. Size of aneurysm

21. Which of the following is risk factor for aneurismal rupture?

A. Male
B. Female
C. Hypertension
D. Family history

22. Which of the following is false regarding diagnosis of aortic aneurysm?

A. CT angiography is best tool for anatomic information, calcification and analysis for operative planning
B. Magnetic resonance angiography provides rapid 3D imaging of the aorta but needs ECG-gating
C. Contrast-enhanced ultrasound is particularly useful in patients after endovascular aneurysm repair (EVAR)
D. Current guidelines recommend one-time screening of all men aged 65 years or more

23. Gadolinium is associated with which of the following complication?

A. Glomerulosclerosis
B. Glomerulonephritis
C. Nephrogenic systemic fibrosis
D. Acute tubular necrosis

24. Which of the following is incorrect concerning aneurismal management?

A. Size and symptoms are important in determining the management of aortic aneurysms
B. Medical therapy prevents aneurismal dilatation or even cause regression
C. ACE inhibitors, ARBs drugs has been shown to be choice in aneurismal patients
D. Statin therapy improves survival following repair and prevents enlargement

25. What is the expansion rate of AAA in current smokers?

A. 1.2 mm/year
B. 1 mm/year
C. 0.7 mm/year
D. 0.4 mm/year

26. Which is not the recommendation for screening of aortic aneurysm?

A. One-time screening of all men aged 65 years and older

B. All men aged 55 years and older with a family history of AAA

C. Recommended against routine screening in nonsmoking women

D. Recommend routine screening in women who smoke

27. What is the size criteria for surgical intervention of abdominal aortic aneurysm?

A. 45 mm B. 50 mm
C. 55 mm D. 60 mm

28. Which of the following is incorrect statement for surgical intervention?

A. Ascending aortic aneurysm with Marfan syndrome of size ≥ 50 mm

B. Ascending aortic aneurysm of size > 45 mm patients requiring aortic valve repair

C. Aortic arch aneurysm producing signs or symptoms of local compression having size >40 mm

D. Descending thoracic aorta aneurysm with size ≥ 55 mm for TEVAR

29. Screening is not recommended for aneurismal size of:

A. < 1.5 cm B. < 2.6 cm
C. < 3 cm D. < 3.4 cm

30. Which is the mainstay of treatment for ascending and arch of aorta aneurysms?

A. Medical therapy B. TEVAR
C. Open surgical repair D. Any of the above

31. All are important factors for TEVAR except:

A. Size of aneurismal sac

B. Neck size and angulation of the aneurysm

C. Length of the aneurysm

D. Calcification

32. Which is wrongly matched concerning endoleak?

A. Type I – seal zone leak

B. Type 2 - retrograde flow from lumbar and/or inferior mesenteric arteries

C. Type 3 - component separation

D. Type 4 - expanding aneurysm without demonstrable blood flow

33. Expanding aneurysm without demonstrable blood flow is classified as which type of endoleak?

A. Type I B. Type II
C. Type IV D. Type V

34. Which is most common type of early endoleak after EVAR?

A. Type IA B. Type IB
C. Type II D. Type III

35. IMPROVE trial was based on:

A. Aortic dissection repair

B. Abdominal aortic injury

C. EVAR for ruptured aneurysm

D. Endoleak after EVAR

36. Which of the following is incorrect about aortic dissection (AD)?

A. Acute AD is the most common clinical emergency involving the aorta

B. Men are more frequently diagnosed with an AD

C. Type A ADs occur more commonly

D. Acute use of cocaine predisposes to AD

37. Loeys-Dietz syndrome is associated which condition?

A. Aortic aneurysm B. Aortic dissection
C. IVC thrombosis D. SVC thrombosis

38. Marfan syndrome is caused by which gene defect?

A. Elastin B. Fibrillin-1
C. COL1A2 D. FKBP14

39. Illicit drug use of cocaine and methamphetamine associated with:

A. Type A aortic aneurysm

B. Type B aortic aneurysm

C. Type A aortic dissection

D. Type B aortic dissection

40. What is the sensitivity and specificity of CT for confirmation of aortic dissection?

A. 80% and 90% B. 90% and 95%
C. 95% and 100% D. 100% and 100%

41. Which of the following is least useful in aortic dissection diagnosis?

A. CT

B. MRI

C. Transthoracic echocardiogram

D. Transesophageal echocardiogram

42. "Triple rule out" conditions on CT imaging includes all except:

A. Aortic dissection
B. Pulmonary embolism
C. Carotid artery thrombosis
D. Coronary artery calcification

43. "Frozen elephant trunk technique" as hybrid approach is used for repair of:

A. Type A aortic aneurysm
B. Type B aortic aneurysm
C. Type A aortic dissection
D. Type B aortic dissection

44. Patient presented with acute aortic dissection just distal to subclavian artery origin. Patient has no comorbidities and is stable with normal lactate, RFT and LFT. What is the appropriate management of this patient?

A. Observation with serial TEE examination
B. Selective beta blocker therapy
C. EVAR procedure
D. Open aortic repair

45. Patient presented with acute onset chest pain. Radiographic examination shows descending aortic dissection with extramural hematoma. What is appropriate management of this patient?

A. Selective beta blocker therapy
B. TEVAR procedure
C. Open surgical repair
D. Transfemoral aortic balloon placement

46. Which of the following trial is not related to TEVAR and medical treatment comparison?

A. IMPROVE Trial
B. ADSORB Trial
C. INSTEAD Trial
D. INSTEAD-XL Trial

47. PETTICOAT technique was initially described as an adjunct to TEVAR for:

A. Uncomplicated Type A aortic dissection
B. Complicated Type A aortic dissection
C. Uncomplicated Type B dissection
D. Complicated Type B dissection

48. Which is incorrect concerning intramural aortic hematoma?

A. It is a subadventitial lesion usually involving the outer third of the media
B. A slight predominance seen in women compared to men
C. Type B IMH occurs more frequently than Type A IMH
D. Marfan's syndrome or other connective tissue disorders have risk in development of IMH

49. Which statement is false regarding IMH?

A. Sine qua non for diagnosis requires the localized or circumferential thickened aortic wall > 5 mm with no detectable blood flow on CT imaging
B. Type A IMH typically requires emergent TEVAR management
C. Uncomplicated Type B IMH is managed with initial medical therapy and surveillance
D. Complicated Type B IMH requires TEVAR or open surgical management

50. Which of the following is incorrect about penetrating aortic ulcer (PAU)?

A. PAU involves both the intima and media, arising from an ulceration of an atherosclerotic plaque
B. PAU occurs more frequently in the thoracic aorta in women and more frequently in the abdominal aorta in men
C. Pain is presenting symptom in patients with PAU
D. Early intervention of PAU recommended when the greatest diameter is larger than 20 mm or the neck is larger than 10 mm

51. What is the most common site of aortic injury?

A. Root of aorta
B. Arch of aorta
C. Isthmus of aorta
D. At diaphragmatic opening

52. Which is wrongly matched about aortic injury grades?

A. Grade I – Intimal tear
B. Grade II – Intramural hematoma
C. Grade III – Aortic dissection
D. Grade IV – Aortic rupture

53. What is gold standard investigation for blunt aortic injury?

A. CT angiography
B. Aortogram
C. Intravascular ultrasonography
D. MR angiography

54. What is preferred management for Grade II BTAI with hemodynamically stable patient?

A. Observation with serial radiographic imaging
B. Selective beta blocker therapy

C. TEVAR repair
D. Open surgical repair

55. Selective cerebral perfusion can be maintained by cannulation of which vessel during CPB?

A. Root of aorta
B. Axillary artery
C. Femoral artery
D. Apex of left ventricle

56. Advantages of axillary artery access over femoral artery during CPB are all except:

A. Rapid percutaneous access
B. Selective cerebral perfusion
C. Avoids atheroembolism
D. Prevents false lumen perfusion

57. "Samurai technique" of arterial access during CPB is:

A. Direct access through apex of left ventricle
B. Access via surgical cut-down of femoral artery
C. Direct cannulation through transection of the ascending aorta
D. Echo-guided cannulation of ascending aorta/arch

58. Period of circulatory arrest achieved with profound hypothermia (<14°C):

A. 10 – 20 mins B. 20 – 30 mins
C. 30 – 40 mins D. 40 – 50 mins

59. Which of the following is valve sparing aortic root replacement procedure?

A. Bentall procedure B. David procedure
C. Ross procedure D. Rastelli procedure

60. "Florida sleeve technique" is used for which procedure?

A. Graft – aortic root anastomosis
B. Aortic cannulation
C. Aortic valve replacement
D. Coronary reimplantation

61. Which is incorrect about open aortic repair?

A. TEVAR is not applicable to patients with Marfan disease
B. Open surgical procedures require cardio-pulmonary bypass
C. Acute changes in neurologic status, an immediate drainage of 30 to 40 ccs of CSF may salvage the spinal cord
D. Spinal cord perfusion pressure depends on mean aortic pressure and central venous pressure

62. Rate of CSF drain to preserve spinal perfusion pressure during aortic surgery:

A. 5 – 10 cc/hr B. 10 – 20 cc/hr
C. 20 – 30 cc/hr D. 30 – 40 cc/hr

63. Which is false about open infrarenal abdominal aneurysm repair?

A. Open repair can be performed through a transabdominal or retroperitoneal approach without entering the thorax
B. Omentum and transverse colon is retracted cephalad and the small intestines are retracted to the patient's right
C. If back bleeding is scant the IMA should be suture ligated
D. Graft anastomosis is done first proximally and then distally

64. Zone 3 for graft landing zone corresponds to which portion of aorta?

A. Proximal to the left common carotid artery
B. Proximal to the origin of the left SCA
C. Proximal descending thoracic aorta less than 2 cm from the left SCA
D. Greater than 2 cm from the left SCA and extends to the proximal portion of the descending aorta

65. Size of access vessel diameter required for TEVAR device delivery:

A. 5 mm B. 6 mm
C. 7 mm D. 8 mm

66. Indications for left subclavian revascularization are all except:

A. Absent left vertebral artery
B. Patent LIMA-LAD bypass
C. History of arm ischemia
D. Incomplete vertebrobasilar system

67. What is major complication of TEVAR procedure?

A. Endoleak
B. Disruption of access vessel
C. Infection
D. Graft dislodgement

ANSWERS

1. **Ans: D. The aortic arches completely disappear by 6 weeks**

   Ref: Chapter No. 62, Page No. 1744

2. **Ans: B. Right-sided aortic arch will occur with regression of segment 5**

   Ref: Chapter No. 62, Page No. 1744

3. **Ans: B. Endograft placement**

   Ref: Chapter No. 62, Page No. 1745

4. **Ans: D. Abdominothoracic aortic aneurysm**

   Ref: Chapter No. 62, Page No. 1745

5. **Ans: C. Entire abdominal aorta**

   Ref: Chapter No. 62, Page No. 1745

6. **Ans: B. Entire thoracic and abdominal aorta**

   Ref: Chapter No. 62, Page No. 1745

7. **Ans: D. Crawford classification**

   Ref: Chapter No. 62, Page No. 1745

8. **Ans: B. Type II DeBakey**

   Ref: Chapter No. 62, Page No. 1745

9. **Ans: C. Descending thoracic aorta only**

   Ref: Chapter No. 62, Page No. 1745

10. **Ans: C. 8 – 30 days**

    Ref: Chapter No. 62, Page No. 1746

11. **Ans: C. 5**

    Ref: Chapter No. 62, Page No. 1747

12. **Ans: C. 4**

    Ref: Chapter No. 62, Page No. 1747

13. **Ans: A. An increase in size of more than 25% above the normal arterial diameter**

    Ref: Chapter No. 62, Page No. 1747-1748

14. **Ans: B. Bacterial infection**

    Ref: Chapter No. 62, Page No. 1748

15. **Ans: B. Female gender**

    Ref: Chapter No. 62, Page No. 1748

16. **Ans: D. Diabetes**

    Ref: Chapter No. 62, Page No. 1748

17. **Ans: D. Height**

    Ref: Chapter No. 62, Page No. 1748

18. **Ans: B. Impingement of left recurrent laryngeal nerve**

    Ref: Chapter No. 62, Page No. 1748

19. **Ans: D. Transesophageal echocardiogram (TEE) is useful in seeing ascending aorta proximal to innominate artery**

    Ref: Chapter No. 62, Page No. 1749

20. **Ans: D. Size of aneurysm**

    Ref: Chapter No. 62, Page No. 1749

21. **Ans: B. Female**

    Ref: Chapter No. 62, Page No. 1749

22. **Ans: B. Magnetic resonance angiography provides rapid 3D imaging of the aorta but needs ECG-gating**

    Ref: Chapter No. 62, Page No. 1749

23. **Ans: C. Nephrogenic systemic fibrosis**

    Ref: Chapter No. 62, Page No. 1749

24. **Ans: C. ACE inhibitors, ARBs drugs has been shown to be choice in aneurismal patients**

    Ref: Chapter No. 62, Page No. 1749

25. **Ans: D. 0.4 mm/year**

    Ref: Chapter No. 62, Page No. 1749

26. **Ans: D. Recommend routine screening in women who smoke**

    Ref: Chapter No. 62, Page No. 1750

27. **Ans: C. 55 mm**

    Ref: Chapter No. 62, Page No. 1750

28. **Ans: C. Aortic arch aneurysm producing signs or symptoms of local compression having size >40 mm**

    Ref: Chapter No. 62, Page No. 1750

29. **Ans: B. < 2.6 cm**

    Ref: Chapter No. 62, Page No. 1750

30. **Ans: C. Open surgical repair**

    Ref: Chapter No. 62, Page No. 1751

31. **Ans: A. Size of aneurismal sac**

    Ref: Chapter No. 62, Page No. 1751

32. **Ans: D. Type 4 - expanding aneurysm without demonstrable blood flow**

    Ref: Chapter No. 62, Page No. 1751

33. **Ans: D. Type V**

    Ref: Chapter No. 62, Page No. 1751

34. **Ans: C. Type II**

    Ref: Chapter No. 62, Page No. 1751

35. **Ans: C. EVAR for ruptured aneurysm**

    Ref: Chapter No. 62, Page No. 1751

36. **Ans: D. Acute use of cocaine predisposes to AD**

    Ref: Chapter No. 62, Page No. 1752

37. **Ans: B. Aortic dissection**

Ref: Chapter No. 62, Page No. 1752

38. **Ans: B. Fibrillin-1**

Ref: Chapter No. 62, Page No. 1752

39. **Ans: D. Type B aortic dissection**

Ref: Chapter No. 62, Page No. 1752

40. **Ans: D. 100% and 100%**

Ref: Chapter No. 62, Page No. 1752

41. **Ans: C. Transthoracic echocardiogram**

Ref: Chapter No. 62, Page No. 1752

42. **Ans: C. Carotid artery thrombosis**

Ref: Chapter No. 62, Page No. 1752

43. **Ans: C. Type A aortic dissection**

Ref: Chapter No. 62, Page No. 1753

44. **Ans: B. Selective beta blocker therapy**

Ref: Chapter No. 62, Page No. 1753

45. **Ans: B. TEVAR procedure**

Ref: Chapter No. 62, Page No. 1753

46. **Ans: A. IMPROVE Trial**

Ref: Chapter No. 62, Page No. 1753

47. **Ans: D. Complicated Type B dissection**

Ref: Chapter No. 62, Page No. 1753

48. **Ans: A. It is a subadventitial lesion usually involving the outer third of the media**

Ref: Chapter No. 62, Page No. 1753

49. **Ans: B. Type A IMH typically requires emergent TEVAR management**

Ref: Chapter No. 62, Page No. 1754

50. **Ans: C. Pain is presenting symptom in patients with PAU**

Ref: Chapter No. 62, Page No. 1754

51. **Ans: C. Isthmus of aorta**

Ref: Chapter No. 62, Page No. 1754

52. **Ans: C. Grade III – Aortic dissection**

Ref: Chapter No. 62, Page No. 1755

53. **Ans: A. CT angiography**

Ref: Chapter No. 62, Page No. 1755

54. **Ans: C. TEVAR repair**

Ref: Chapter No. 62, Page No. 1755

55. **Ans: B. Axillary artery**

Ref: Chapter No. 62, Page No. 1756

56. **Ans: A. Rapid percutaneous access**

Ref: Chapter No. 62, Page No. 1756

57. **Ans: C. Direct cannulation through transection of the ascending aorta**

Ref: Chapter No. 62, Page No. 1756

58. **Ans: C. 30 – 40 mins**

Ref: Chapter No. 62, Page No. 1756

59. **Ans: B. David procedure**

Ref: Chapter No. 62, Page No. 1757

60. **Ans: D. Coronary reimplantation**

Ref: Chapter No. 62, Page No. 1757

61. **Ans: C. Acute changes in neurologic status, an immediate drainage of 30 to 40 ccs of CSF may salvage the spinal cord**

Ref: Chapter No. 62, Page No. 1758

62. **Ans: B. 10 – 20 cc/hr**

Ref: Chapter No. 62, Page No. 1758

63. **Ans: C. If back bleeding is scant the IMA should be suture ligated**

Ref: Chapter No. 62, Page No. 1759

64. **Ans: C. Proximal descending thoracic aorta less than 2 cm from the left SCA**

Ref: Chapter No. 62, Page No. 1759

65. **Ans: D. 8 mm**

Ref: Chapter No. 62, Page No. 1760

66. **Ans: A. Absent left vertebral artery**

Ref: Chapter No. 62, Page No. 1760

67. **Ans: B. Disruption of access vessel**

Ref: Chapter No. 62, Page No. 1760

63

Peripheral Arterial Disease

PRESENTATION AND PATHOPHYSIOLOGY

1. What is the major risk factor for development of PAD?

A. Aging B. Hypertension
C. Hyperlipidemia D. Diabetes

2. Chronic limb threatening ischemia includes all except:

A. Rest pain B. Ischemic ulcer
C. Claudication D. Gangrene

3. Patient presented with lower right limb rest pain. Pain aggravates on prolonged limb elevation. What is probable diagnosis?

A. Venous insufficiency
B. Arterial occlusion
C. Prolapsed vertebral disc
D. Chronic limb threatening ischemia

4. What is the strongest risk factor for development of PAD?

A. Age B. Diabetes
C. Hypertension D. Current smoking

5. Which of the following is incorrect?

A. Vasculogenic claudication typically resolves with a short period of rest
B. Neurogenic claudication is variable in onset and it requires a change in position for symptom resolution
C. Nerve root compression can take a long time for recovery, may arise from standing alone, often relieved by changes in spine position
D. Venous claudication occurs during or after exercise and relives by leg elevation

6. Diagnosis of PAD requires anckle-brachial index:

A. < 0.3 B. < 0.7
C. < 0.9 D. > 1.2

7. Factors responsible for falsely elevated ABI are all except:

A. Advanced age B. Diabetes
C. Hypertension D. Medial calcinosis

8. Toe-brachial index of ____ indicates hemodynamically significant PAD.

A. ≤ 0.3 B. ≤ 0.5
C. ≤ 0.7 D. ≤ 0.9

9. Patient presented with lower limb rest pain which relieved by dangling the foot off the bed. Patient has diminished pulse in lower limb. Which of the following parameter does not support the diagnosis of the above condition?

A. ABI less than 0.4
B. An ankle systolic pressure less than 50 mm Hg
C. A systolic toe pressure less than 30 mm Hg
D. Transcutaneous partial pressure of oxygen ($TcPO_2$) less than 60 mm Hg

10. Buerger's disease is also called as:

A. Giant cell arteritis
B. Polyarteritis nodosa
C. Thromboangiitis obliterans
D. Pseudoxanthoma elasticum

11. Which of the following is false statement?

A. The elastic arteries are the aorta and the pulmonary arteries
B. The muscular arteries are distributive in nature
C. Elastic arteries are thicker relative to their diameters than the muscular arteries
D. Capillary bed are generally less than 300 microns in diameter

12. What is characteristic feature of fatty streaks?

A. Fibrous cap
B. Foam cells

C. Necrotic debris
D. Platelets aggregation

13. What is the earliest hallmark of vessel injury?
A. Vascular spasm
B. Dysfunction of endothelium
C. Thrombus formation
D. Capillary leak

14. Which of the following is incorrect regarding atherosclerotic disease?
A. Atherosclerosis tends to develop at specific, anatomic locations within the arterial tree
B. Patients with claudication will be found to have single level disease
C. PAD associated with diabetes more frequently have involvement of the deep femoral (profunda) artery and the infrapopliteal arteries
D. Pedal vessels are often spared among patients with end-stage renal disease

MANAGEMENT

15. Which is incorrect regarding medical management of atherosclerotic disease?
A. Antithrombotic therapy is strongly recommended for all patients with PAD
B. The mainstay of medical therapy is clopidogrel monotherapy
C. High-intensity statin therapy have direct anti inflammatory effect and help in atherosclerotic plaque stability
D. The specific goal is to maintain a Hemoglobin A1c level of less than 7%

16. Which of the following risk factor causes more of proximal atherosclerotic disease?
A. Age
B. Diabetes
C. End stage renal disease
D. Smoking

17. General recommendation for exercise duration in PAD patient is:
A. 10 to 15 minutes of exercise, 4 times per week
B. 15 to 20 minutes of exercise, 4 times per week
C. 30 to 45 minutes of exercise, 3 times per week
D. 45 to 60 minutes of exercise, 3 times per week

18. Which of the following is false regarding diabetic foot ulcers?
A. About one in four patients with diabetes will develop a foot ulcer during their lifetime
B. 40% of diabetes-related amputations are preceded by a diabetic foot ulcer
C. 49%–66% of people with DFUs have detectable underlying PAD
D. Diabetic wound with PAD increases likelihood of revascularization procedure

19. PEDIS classification does not include which of the following?
A. Perfusion
B. Extent/size
C. Tissue loss
D. Ischemia

20. Fontaine classification is used for:
A. Vasculitis
B. Venous ulcer
C. Critical limb ischemia
D. Lymphedema

21. Critical limb ischemia is classified by:
A. Fontaine classification
B. Rutherford classification
C. WIfI classification
D. All of the above

22. Which of the following is incorrect regarding WIfI classification?
A. This classification is applicable to patients without diabetes
B. It is based on three major factors: wound, ischemia, and foot infection
C. WIfI is a limb staging system and limb must be staged at presentation
D. WIfI has been shown to have prognostic value in predicting amputation risk as well as likelihood of revascularization

23. Which is wrong about WIfI classification?
A. It includes in total 3 grades for each factor
B. Increase in wound class increases risk of amputation
C. Infected wound with PAD increases likelihood revascularization
D. Infection grade 3 requires amputation regardless of other factors

24. Grade 3 ischemic limb according to WIfI includes all except:
A. ABI < 0.4
B. Ankle pressure < 50 mm Hg
C. Toe pressure < 40 mm Hg
D. Transcutaneous oxygen concentration < 30 mm Hg

25. Critical limb threatening ischemia is defined by all except:

A. It includes limb ischemia caused by acute and chronic conditions

B. Ischemic rest pain with confirmatory hemodynamic measurements

C. Diabetic foot ulcer or any lower limb ulcer present for at least two weeks

D. Gangrene involving any part of the lower limb or foot

26. Critical limb threatened ischemia term is applied specifically in relation with:

A. Acute thrombosis

B. Atherosclerosis

C. Vasculitides

D. Venous disease

27. Best modality for anatomic delineation in case of lower limb CLTI:

A. Duplex

B. CT angiography

C. MR angiography

D. Catheter angiography

28. Which is wrong about management of CLTI?

A. Limb staging is done with the WIfI classification system

B. PLAN system estimates risk of intervention as well as short- and long-term mortality

C. GLASS classifies the limb disease burden from the bifurcation of aorta to the foot

D. TAP is selected by the operator and is a continuous route of inline flow from groin to foot

ENDOVASCULAR THERAPY VS SURGICAL THERAPY

29. BASIL Trial was done for:

A. Medical therapy vs open surgical bypass for PAD

B. Medical therapy vs endovascular therapy for PAD

C. Endovascular therapy vs open surgical bypass for PAD

D. Medical therapy vs Endovascular therapy vs open surgical bypass

30. Which is false regarding management of PAD?

A. Open bypass is still preferable in long segment, extensive aortoiliac and femoropopliteal lesions

B. Restenosis rates are lower after EVT

C. CLTI often have long segment and multilevel disease which has inferior patency rates after endovascular intervention

D. Endovascular therapy is strongly indicated for patients with medical comorbidities and short life expectancy

31. GLASS system is based on following variables except:

A. Extent of disease

B. Presence of total occlusion

C. Involvement of main vessels and branches

D. Presence of collaterals

32. Grade 3 according to GLASS includes all of the following except:

A. Total length SFA disease >2/3 (>20 cm) length

B. Non-flush chronic total occlusion 10-20 cm long

C. Short popliteal stenosis 2-5 cm

D. Popliteal disease extending into trifurcation

33. What is the most common complication of endovascular therapy?

A. Access site complications

B. Restenosis

C. Erosion

D. Rupture

34. Any chronic total occlusion of tibioperoneal trunk is classified by which grade of GLASS system?

A. Grade 1 B. Grade 2

C. Grade 3 D. Grade 4

35. Revascularization is not indicated for which grade of WIfI classification?

A. Grade 1 B. Grade 2

C. Grade 3 D. Grade 4

36. Which is the incorrect statement regarding open surgical management of PAD?

A. Nonoperative management is appropriate and initially preferable for claudication

B. The primary indication for performing infrainguinal bypass in selected claudicants is to prevent limb loss

C. Major amputation in patients with claudication occurring in only 5%

D. Majority with CLTI require intervention to decrease the risk of limb loss

37. All are true about surgical bypass for PAD except:

A. The anteroposterior foot view is extremely important

B. Conduit selection is the most critical factor for successful outcome
C. Duplex ultrasound is adequate to determine the quality of autologous veins
D. Autologous vein is most preferred conduit for infrainguinal bypass

38. Which is not used to replace infected aortic graft?

A. Expanded PTFE
B. Rifampicin bonded Dacron
C. Femoral vein
D. Cryopreserved artery

39. Which of the following is false about aortofemoral bypass surgery?

A. Outflow target either the common femoral arteries or the profunda femoris arteries bilaterally
B. Optimal inflow site is almost always just inferior to the renal arteries
C. Clamp applied side to side rather than from front to back
D. The needle is directed from inside the artery to out when performing arterial anastomoses

40. Which of the following is immediate complication seen after aortofemoral bypass?

A. Limb thrombosis
B. Aortoenteric fistula
C. Anastomotic pseudoaneurysm
D. Buttock and pelvic necrosis

41. Which is false about autologous venous conduit?

A. In situ vein graft avoids full length GSV harvesting
B. Nonreversed vein requires full vein harvesting, tunneling of the graft and valve lysis
C. Reversing the vein avoids the need for valve lysis
D. Reversed vein conduits are inferior to other techniques

SURVEILLANCE

42. All are true regarding surveillance of endovascular therapy except:

A. Duplex ultrasound surveillance (DUS) within the first month after EVT is recommended
B. Society for Vascular Surgery guideline suggests continued clinical follow up at 3 months and then subsequently at 6-month intervals
C. Peak systolic velocity greater than 500 cm/sec considered as stenotic area
D. Routine DUS is currently not recommended beyond 1 month in the absence of recurrent symptoms

43. Which is not true regarding open surgical bypass graft surveillance?

A. Open surgical therapy has no established guidelines for clinical and imaging surveillance
B. Early postoperative assessment within 4 weeks of open intervention is recommended
C. The purpose of vein graft surveillance is to prevent loss of primary patency
D. The most common cause of vein graft failure is an intrinsic vein graft stenosis due to intimal hyperplasia

44. All of the following are risk factors for graft thrombosis except:

A. Peak systolic velocity greater than 300 cm/s
B. Velocity ratio greater than 3.5 at the site of a stenosis
C. Globally low peak systolic graft flow velocity less than 45 cm/s
D. A drop in ABI greater than 0.3

45. Patency is maintained over a specified time interval without reintervention on the graft itself or its anastomoses is known as:

A. Primary patency
B. Assisted primary patency
C. Secondary patency
D. Failed patency

46. Successful reintervention on a patent but restenotic graft is termed as:

A. Primary patency
B. Assisted primary patency
C. Secondary patency
D. Failed patency

47. Successful re-canalization of occluded graft is termed as:

A. Primary patency
B. Assisted primary patency
C. Secondary patency
D. Failed patency

ANSWERS

1. **Ans: A. Aging**
Ref: Chapter No. 63, Page No. 1767

2. **Ans: C. Claudication**
Ref: Chapter No. 63, Page No. 1767

3. **Ans: D. Chronic limb threatening ischemia**
Ref: Chapter No. 63, Page No. 1767

4. **Ans: D. Current smoking**
Ref: Chapter No. 63, Page No. 1768

5. **Ans: B. Neurogenic claudication is variable in onset and it requires a change in position for symptom resolution**
Ref: Chapter No. 63, Page No. 1768

6. **Ans: C. < 0.9**
Ref: Chapter No. 63, Page No. 1769

7. **Ans: C. Hypertension**
Ref: Chapter No. 63, Page No. 1769

8. **Ans: C. $\leq$ 0.7**
Ref: Chapter No. 63, Page No. 1769

9. **Ans: D. Transcutaneous partial pressure of oxygen ($TcPO_2$) less than 60 mm Hg**
Ref: Chapter No. 63, Page No. 1769

10. **Ans: C. Thromboangiitis obliterans**
Ref: Chapter No. 63, Page No. 1769

11. **Ans: C. Elastic arteries are thicker relative to their diameters than the muscular arteries**
Ref: Chapter No. 63, Page No. 1769

12. **Ans: B. Foam cells**
Ref: Chapter No. 63, Page No. 1769

13. **Ans: B. Dysfunction of endothelium**
Ref: Chapter No. 63, Page No. 1769

14. **Ans: D. Pedal vessels are often spared among patients with end-stage renal disease**
Ref: Chapter No. 63, Page No. 1769-1770

15. **Ans: B. The mainstay of medical therapy is clopidogrel monotherapy**
Ref: Chapter No. 63, Page No. 1770

16. **Ans: D. Smoking**
Ref: Chapter No. 63, Page No. 1771

17. **Ans: D. 45 to 60 minutes of exercise, 3 times per week**
Ref: Chapter No. 63, Page No. 1771

18. **Ans: B. 40% of diabetes-related amputations are preceded by a diabetic foot ulcer**
Ref: Chapter No. 63, Page No. 1771-1772

19. **Ans: D. Ischemia**
Ref: Chapter No. 63, Page No. 1772

20. **Ans: C. Critical limb ischemia**
Ref: Chapter No. 63, Page No. 1772

21. **Ans: D. All of the above**
Ref: Chapter No. 63, Page No. 1772

22. **Ans: A. This classification is applicable to patients without diabetes**
Ref: Chapter No. 63, Page No. 1772

23. **Ans: A. It includes in total 3 grades for each factor**
Ref: Chapter No. 63, Page No. 1772

24. **Ans: C. Toe pressure < 40 mm Hg**
Ref: Chapter No. 63, Page No. 1773

25. **Ans: A. It includes limb ischemia caused by acute and chronic conditions**
Ref: Chapter No. 63, Page No. 1774

26. **Ans: B. Atherosclerosis**
Ref: Chapter No. 63, Page No. 1774

27. **Ans: D. Catheter angiography**
Ref: Chapter No. 63, Page No. 1774

28. **Ans: C. GLASS classifies the limb disease burden from the bifurcation of aorta to the foot**
Ref: Chapter No. 63, Page No. 1774

29. **Ans: C. Endovascular therapy vs open surgical bypass for PAD**
Ref: Chapter No. 63, Page No. 1775

30. **Ans: B. Restenosis rates are lower after EVT**
Ref: Chapter No. 63, Page No. 1776

31. **Ans: D. Presence of collaterals**
Ref: Chapter No. 63, Page No. 1777

32. **Ans: D. Popliteal disease extending into trifurcation**
Ref: Chapter No. 63, Page No. 1777

33. **Ans: A. Access site complications**
Ref: Chapter No. 63, Page No. 1778

34. **Ans. D. Grade 4**
Ref: Chapter No. 63, Page No. 1778

35. **Ans: A. Grade 1**

Ref: Chapter No. 63, Page No. 1782

36. **Ans: B. The primary indication for performing infrainguinal bypass in selected claudicants is to prevent limb loss**

Ref: Chapter No. 63, Page No. 1782

37. **Ans: A. The anteroposterior foot view is extremely important**

Ref: Chapter No. 63, Page No. 1782

38. **Ans: A. Expanded PTFE**

Ref: Chapter No. 63, Page No. 1784

39. **Ans: C. Clamp applied side to side rather than from front to back**

Ref: Chapter No. 63, Page No. 1784-1786

40. **Ans: D. Buttock and pelvic necrosis**

Ref: Chapter No. 63, Page No. 1786

41. **Ans: D. Reversed vein conduits are inferior to other techniques**

Ref: Chapter No. 63, Page No. 1787

42. **Ans: C. Peak systolic velocity greater than 500 cm/sec considered as stenotic area**

Ref: Chapter No. 63, Page No. 1788

43. **Ans: A. Open surgical therapy has no established guidelines for clinical and imaging surveillance**

Ref: Chapter No. 63, Page No. 1788

44. **Ans: D. A drop in ABI greater than 0.3**

Ref: Chapter No. 63, Page No. 1788

45. **Ans: A. Primary patency**

Ref: Chapter No. 63, Page No. 1788

46. **Ans: B. Assisted primary patency**

Ref: Chapter No. 63, Page No. 1788

47. **Ans: C. Secondary patency**

Ref: Chapter No. 63, Page No. 1788

64

Vascular Trauma

EVALUATION AND MANAGEMENT

1. **Which of the following statement is wrong about vascular trauma?**
   - A. High velocity (>2500 ft/sec) gun shot causes extensive tissue damage with creation of temporary cavity
   - B. Close-range shotgun wounds are defined as within 9 feet and are devastating
   - C. Partially transected arteries and veins cause much more extensive hemorrhage
   - D. An arteriovenous fistula typically occurs after penetrating trauma that causes injury to both an artery and a vein

2. **Which of the following is not a 'hard findings' requiring immediate intervention?**
   - A. Pulsatile bleeding
   - B. Palpable thrill or audible bruit
   - C. Moderate hemorrhage
   - D. Expanding hematoma

3. **Which of the following is not a 'soft findings' regarding vascular trauma?**
   - A. Moderate hemorrhage
   - B. Proximity fracture or dislocation
   - C. Wounds in proximity neck vessels with unexplained hemorrhagic shock
   - D. Evidence of extremity ischemia

4. **Which is most specific investigation in extremity vascular injury?**
   - A. Doppler color flow
   - B. CT angiography
   - C. Catheter arteriography
   - D. Arterial fluoroscopy

5. **Operative therapy required for all of the following except:**
   - A. Thrombosis
   - B. Arteriovenous fistula
   - C. Symptoms of chronic ischemia
   - D. Small pseudoaneurysm

6. **What is the mainstay treatment of active solid organ hemorrhage?**
   - A. Conservative management
   - B. Intra-arterial catheter directed embolization
   - C. Damage control surgery
   - D. Elective laparotomy

7. **What is gold standard for the distal extremity vascular injury repair?**
   - A. Clamp and ligation
   - B. Endovascular stent placement
   - C. Autologous vein graft
   - D. PTFE graft transposition

8. **Blood products can be used during massive hemorrhage protocol:**
   - A. Type O-positive packed cells and type O fresh-frozen plasma
   - B. Type O-positive packed cells and type AB fresh-frozen plasma
   - C. Type O-negative packed cells and type O fresh-frozen plasma
   - D. Type O-negative packed cells and type AB fresh-frozen plasma

9. **Intravenous heparin can be used in which of the following traumatic injury?**
   - A. Head injury
   - B. Torso injury
   - C. Pelvic injury
   - D. Isolated extremity trauma

10. **Chest injuries with life-threatening hemorrhage are best approached through which incision?**

A. Median sternotomy
B. Anterolateral thoracotomy
C. Posterolateral thoracotomy
D. Axillary

11. **Which of the following is wrong statement?**

A. Control at the site of injury is the first priority in the exposure of vascular injuries
B. More generous incisions are used to manage vascular injuries
C. A medial incision from the proximal to distal popliteal space is appropriate in popliteal vascular injury
D. Dividing the inguinal ligament, pectoralis major and removing the mid clavicle may be done in vascular trauma

12. **Which of the following arteries can be ligated in extremity?**

A. Brachial artery
B. Popliteal artery
C. Superficial Femoral artery
D. Posterior tibial artery

13. **All of the following arteries can be ligated except:**

A. Celiac artery
B. Superior mesenteric artery
C. Inferior mesenteric artery
D. Subclavian artery

14. **Which of the following vessel can be safely ligated in vascular trauma?**

A. Superficial femoral artery
B. Profunda femoris artery
C. Popliteal artery
D. Brachial artery

15. **Which is false regarding autologous vein graft for vascular trauma?**

A. Most preferred graft is autologous great saphenous vein
B. It is compliant with the normal pulsatile flow of an artery
C. It is thrombogenic
D. It has superior long-term patency compared to prosthetic graft

16. **Which vascular grafts have high risk of infection and thrombosis?**

A. Great saphenous vein
B. Cephalic vein
C. PTFE graft
D. Dacron graft

17. **Which is false regarding use of PTFE graft for vascular repair?**

A. It has shown improved patency and low infection rates
B. PTFE is inferior to vein for popliteal and more distal vessels
C. PTFE grafts of less than 3 mm should not be used
D. PTFE and vein grafts must be covered

18. **What is most common cause of preventable limb loss after revascularization?**

A. Thrombosis
B. Failure to do fasciotomy
C. Bleeding
D. Infection

19. **Which is false statement regarding compartment syndrome?**

A. Calf compartment syndrome is the most common indication for fasciotomy
B. The first clinical findings are pain and loss of light touch sensation
C. The loss of arterial pulses is a late finding
D. Fasciotomy is performed when compartment pressure exceeds 32 mm Hg

20. **It is safest to perform fasciotomy if compartment pressure exceeds:**

A. 20 mm Hg
B. 25 mm Hg
C. 30 mm Hg
D. 35 mm Hg

SPECIFIC INJURIES

21. **Which of the following is incorrect regarding head and neck vascular injury?**

A. Blunt trauma to the carotid and vertebral arteries, collectively known as blunt cerebrovascular injuries
B. Blunt cerebrovascular injuries are often occult and asymptomatic
C. Zone I of neck is cephalad from the angle of the mandible
D. In a stable patient with a vascular injury in zone 1 or zone 3, vascular imaging is mandatory

22. **Denver criteria is used for which of the following?**

A. SMA injury
B. Cervical fracture

C. Aortic injury
D. Blunt cerebrovascular injury

23. All are associated with blunt cerebrovascular injury except:

A. Basilar skull fracture
B. Cervical spine fracture
C. Blunt neck trauma from hanging
D. Undisplaced midface fractures

24. Carotid artery is more commonly injured at vertebral level:

A. C1 and C4 B. C2 and C4
C. C4 and C6 D. C2 and C6

25. Pseudoaneurysm formation after blunt vascular injury is classified as:

A. Grade I B. Grade II
C. Grade III D. Grade IV

26. Median sternotomy gives best exposure of following structures except:

A. Proximal innominate
B. Proximal right subclavian
C. Proximal right carotid
D. Proximal left carotid

27. Which approach is used for left subclavian artery proximal control and definitive repair?

A. Median sternotomy
B. Right anterior thoracotomy
C. Left anterior thoracotomy
D. Posterolateral thoracotomy

28. Which of the following is correct?

A. 3rd intercostal space anterolateral thoracotomy provides exposure for proximal control in supraclavicular injuries
B. Distal control of the carotid arteries is obtained by median sternotomy with cervical extension
C. Distal subclavian arterial control is obtained through a supraclavicular incision
D. All of the above

29. Which incision is not used in emergency thoracotomy?

A. Left anterolateral thoracotomy
B. Right anterolateral thoracotomy
C. Posterolateral thoracotomy
D. Sternotomy

30. Which of the following is incorrect about blunt thoracic aortic injury?

A. The aorta is typically injured at locations of root of the aorta and ligamentum arteriosum
B. Confirmatory diagnosis is by HRCT chest
C. SBP of less than 100 mm Hg and heart rate below 90 beats/min are maintained
D. Open repair with partial cardiopulmonary bypass have a competitively low rate of paraplegia

31. Which is false statement of the following?

A. Penetrating injuries to the abdominal aorta are best exposed and repaired with a left medial visceral rotation
B. The inferior vena cava is exposed with a right medial visceral rotation
C. Anterior or lateral surfaces of the vena cava can most often be repaired primarily
D. Hemodynamically stable patients, the vena cava can be ligated or shunted

32. Which of the following is false?

A. The common and external iliac arteries can be ligated
B. Injuries to the internal iliac artery can be routinely ligated
C. Simple injuries to the iliac veins should be repaired with primary venorrhaphy
D. Complex repairs of destructive injuries to the iliac veins should not be attempted

33. Fullen classification is used for:

A. Renal artery injury B. IVC injury
C. SMA injury D. IMA injury

34. Zone III injury to SMA is beyond:

A. Pancreaticoduodenal artery
B. Right colic artery
C. Middle colic artery
D. Ileocolic artery

35. Nephrectomy is necessary in all conditions except:

A. Combined renal artery and vein injury
B. Right renal vein ligation
C. Left renal vein ligation
D. AAST grade V injury

36. Which is most affected nerve in upper extremity arterial injury?

A. Ulnar nerve B. Radial nerve
C. Medial nerve D. Axillary nerve

37. Which is false statement about extremity vascular trauma?

A. The vein should be repaired first in combined arterial and venous injury
B. Fasciotomy in the case of prolonged ischemia must always be considered
C. The popliteal artery is at particularly high risk of injury after dislocation of the knee
D. Injuries at the level of the tibial vessels are best managed by ligation if one of the three calf vessels are patent

38. **Number of compartments present in thigh:**

A. 2 B. 3
C. 4 D. 5

39. **Risk of thrombosis after vascular repair is maximum in:**

A. 12 hours B. 24 hours
C. 48 hours D. 72 hours

40. **The most common cause of amputation after vascular injury:**

A. Thrombosis
B. Compartment syndrome
C. Nerve ischemia
D. Infection

ANSWERS

1. **Ans: B. Close-range shotgun wounds are defined as within 9 feet and are devastating**
Ref: Chapter No. 64, Page No. 1793

2. **Ans: C. Moderate hemorrhage**
Ref: Chapter No. 64, Page No. 1794

3. **Ans: D. Evidence of extremity ischemia**
Ref: Chapter No. 64, Page No. 1794

4. **Ans: C. Catheter arteriography**
Ref: Chapter No. 64, Page No. 1794

5. **Ans: D. Small pseudoaneurysm**
Ref: Chapter No. 64, Page No. 1794

6. **Ans: B. Intra-arterial catheter directed embolization**
Ref: Chapter No. 64, Page No. 1796

7. **Ans: C. Autologous vein graft**
Ref: Chapter No. 64, Page No. 1797

8. **Ans: D. Type O-negative packed cells and type AB fresh-frozen plasma**
Ref: Chapter No. 64, Page No. 1798

9. **Ans: D. Isolated extremity trauma**
Ref: Chapter No. 64, Page No. 1798

10. **Ans: B. Anterolateral thoracotomy**
Ref: Chapter No. 64, Page No. 1799

11. **Ans: A. Control at the site of injury is the first priority in the exposure of vascular injuries**
Ref: Chapter No. 64, Page No. 1799

12. **Ans: D. Posterior tibial artery**
Ref: Chapter No. 64, Page No. 1800

13. **Ans: B. Superior mesenteric artery**
Ref: Chapter No. 64, Page No. 1800

14. **Ans: B. Profunda femoris artery**
Ref: Chapter No. 64, Page No. 1800

15. **Ans: C. It is thrombogenic**
Ref: Chapter No. 64, Page No. 1800

16. **Ans: D. Dacron graft**
Ref: Chapter No. 64, Page No. 1800

17. **Ans: C. PTFE grafts of less than 3 mm should not be used**
Ref: Chapter No. 64, Page No. 1800

18. **Ans: B. Failure to do fasciotomy**
Ref: Chapter No. 64, Page No. 1800

19. **Ans: D. Fasciotomy is performed when compartment pressure exceeds 32 mm Hg**
Ref: Chapter No. 64, Page No. 1800-1801

20. **Ans: B. 25 mm Hg**
Ref: Chapter No. 64, Page No. 1801

21. **Ans: C. Zone I of neck is cephalad from the angle of the mandible**
Ref: Chapter No. 64, Page No. 1801

22. **Ans: D. Blunt cerebrovascular injury**
Ref: Chapter No. 64, Page No. 1801

23. **Ans: D. Undisplaced midface fractures**
Ref: Chapter No. 64, Page No. 1801

24. **Ans: D. C2 and C6**
Ref: Chapter No. 64, Page No. 1801

25. **Ans: C. Grade III**
Ref: Chapter No. 64, Page No. 1802

26. **Ans: D. Proximal left carotid**
Ref: Chapter No. 64, Page No. 1802

27. **Ans: D. Posterolateral thoracotomy**

Ref: Chapter No. 64, Page No. 1802

28. **Ans: D. All of the above**

Ref: Chapter No. 64, Page No. 1802

29. **Ans: C. Posterolateral thoracotomy**

Ref: Chapter No. 64, Page No. 1802

30. **Ans: C. SBP of less than 100 mm Hg and heart rate below 90 beats/min are maintained**

Ref: Chapter No. 64, Page No. 1802

31. **Ans: D. Hemodynamically stable patients, the vena cava can be ligated or shunted**

Ref: Chapter No. 64, Page No. 1804

32. **Ans: A. The common and external iliac arteries can be ligated**

Ref: Chapter No. 64, Page No. 1804

33. **Ans: C. SMA injury**

Ref: Chapter No. 64, Page No. 1804

34. **Ans: C. Middle colic artery**

Ref: Chapter No. 64, Page No. 1804

35. **Ans: C. Left renal vein ligation**

Ref: Chapter No. 64, Page No. 1805

36. **Ans: C. Medial nerve**

Ref: Chapter No. 64, Page No. 1805

37. **Ans: D. Injuries at the level of the tibial vessels are best managed by ligation if one of the three calf vessels are patent**

Ref: Chapter No. 64, Page No. 1805-1806

38. **Ans: B. 3**

Ref: Chapter No. 64, Page No. 1806

39. **Ans: C. 48 hours**

Ref: Chapter No. 64, Page No. 1807

40. **Ans: C. Nerve ischemia**

Ref: Chapter No. 64, Page No. 1807

65

Venous Disease

ANATOMY

1. **Which of the following statement is incorrect about superficial leg veins?**
   A. The dorsal venous arch is continuous with the great saphenous vein medially and the small saphenous vein laterally
   B. Saphenous sheath is present below the deep fascia of the leg
   C. Most commonly, the small saphenous vein terminates within a lateral branch of the thigh, bypassing the classic saphenopopliteal junction
   D. Vein of Giacomini, connects the small saphenous vein with the great saphenous vein

2. **Which is not the tributary of the great saphenous vein at saphenous opening?**
   A. External pudendal vein
   B. Superficial circumflex iliac vein
   C. Superficial epigastric vein
   D. Superficial inguinal vein

3. **What is correct regarding deep venous system of leg?**
   A. Medial and lateral plantar veins drain into the posterior tibial vein
   B. Dorsalis pedis veins on the dorsum of the foot form the paired anterior tibial veins
   C. Bilateral gastrocnemius veins empty into the popliteal vein distal to the point of entry of the small saphenous vein
   D. Popliteal vein enters a window in the adductor longus to continue as femoral vein

4. **Intergemellar vein drains into:**
   A. Posterior tibial vein
   B. Anterior tibial vein
   C. Popliteal vein
   D. Common femoral vein

5. **'May vein' is present at:**
   A. Perforator at soleus point
   B. Perforator at gastrocnemius point
   C. Peroneal perforator
   D. Lateral ankle perforator

6. **Dodd perforator are present at:**
   A. Distal 1/3rd of leg B. Below knee
   C. Above knee D. Mid thigh

7. **Perforators present in Gaiters area of leg:**
   A. Dodd B. Boyd
   C. Cockett D. Hunter

8. **Which of the following is wrong about perforators of leg?**
   A. Perforator valves prevent reflux from the deep to the superficial venous system
   B. Cockett perforators connect the posterior arch and posterior tibial veins
   C. Boyd perforators connect the great saphenous and popliteal vein
   D. Dodd perforators connect the great saphenous and superficial femoral vein

9. **Which is wrong statement?**
   A. Veins contain mainly elastin
   B. No valves are present in the superior vena cava and inferior vena cava
   C. Venous system functions as capacitance vessels
   D. Veins can withstand large volume shifts without significant changes in pressure

10. **Incorrect statement of the following:**
    A. In the upright position, the resting venous pressure of the foot reflects the hydrostatic pressure from the upright column of blood
    B. The normally functioning valves in the venous system prevent retrograde flow

C. During calf muscle contraction, the venous pressure of the foot and ankle increases dramatically
D. The pressures developing in the muscle compartments during exercise range from 150 to 200 mm Hg

VENOUS INSUFFICIENCY

11. All of the following are the primary venous insufficiency except:

A. Venous ectasias
B. Absence of venous valve
C. Klippel-Trénaunay syndrome
D. May-Thurner syndrome

12. All are risk factors for varicose veins expect:

A. Age
B. Prolonged standing
C. Male gender
D. Multiparity

13. Which among the following is false statement regarding risk factors for venous insufficiency?

A. Advancing age appears to be an important significant risk factor
B. Estrogen and progesterone have profound effects on venous functions
C. Development of varicose vein has autosomal recessive inheritance
D. Klippel-Trénaunay syndrome has venous and lymphatic abnormality

14. May-Thurner syndrome causes:

A. Arterial claudication
B. Venous claudication
C. Neurogenic leg pain
D. Testicular pain

15. Patient has dull aching pain in lower leg. Cramping pain develops during or after exercise but it subsides on rest or leg elevation. What is most probable cause?

A. Peripheral arterial disease
B. Prolapsed vertebral disc
C. Compartment syndrome
D. Deep venous thrombosis

16. Telangiectasia are present in which layer?

A. Intradermal
B. Subdermal
C. Subcutaneous tissue
D. Fascial layer

17. Which of the following is associated with leg telangiectasia?

A. Lupus erythematosus
B. Dermatomyositis
C. Xeroderma pigmentosum
D. All of the above

18. What is the cause of nutcracker syndrome?

A. Compression of left iliac vein by right iliac artery
B. Compression of left iliac vein by left iliac artery
C. Compression of left renal vein between aorta and SMA
D. Compression of SMV by duodenum

19. Which of the following is not feature of venous insufficiency?

A. Telangiectasias are less than 3 mm intradermal venules
B. Posterior calf varicose veins tend to originate from the small saphenous vein
C. Venous ulcers are painful and appear at the lateral malleolus
D. Corona phlebectatica or venous flare, usually located at the medial malleolus or the dorsum of the foot

20. What is the diagnostic modality to confirm pelvic congestion syndrome?

A. USG pelvis
B. CECT pelvis
C. TRUS
D. MR venography

21. Which of the following is advanced sign of venous insufficiency?

A. Atrophie blanche
B. Corona phlebectatica
C. Hyperpigmentation
D. Varicosity

22. "Champagne bottle leg" is characteristic of which of the following?

A. Lymphedema
B. Venous insufficiency
C. Peripheral arterial disease
D. Cellulitis

23. Lipodermatosclerosis is a feature of

A. Varicose veins
B. Advanced venous insufficiency
C. Venous ulcer
D. Lipedema

24. **Which is the best modality for venous insufficiency?**
    A. Brodie Trendelenburg test
    B. Duplex imaging
    C. Phlebography
    D. MRI venography

25. **Which frequency probe is used for venous imaging by USG?**
    A. 3 – 5 Hz B. 5 – 7.5 Hz
    C. 7.5 – 10 Hz D. 10 – 14 Hz

26. **Which is wrong statement regarding phlebography?**
    A. Phlebography is useful in the diagnosis and treatment of primary venous insufficiency
    B. Ascending phlebography is performed by injection of contrast material into a superficial pedal vein after a tourniquet is applied at the ankle
    C. Ascending phlebography differentiate primary from secondary venous insufficiency
    D. Descending phlebography is performed with retrograde injection of contrast material into the deep venous system at the groin or popliteal fossa

27. **Which of the following is incorrect statement about venous insufficiency diagnosis?**
    A. Perthes test is done for superficial veins insufficiency of lower leg
    B. Duplex examination needs to be done with standing because in supine position, venous valves remain open
    C. Significant perforator reflux is defined as a diameter of more than 3.5 mm and a reflux time of 500 milliseconds or longer
    D. MRI venography is an excellent test to evaluate for pelvic congestion syndrome

28. **CEAP classification is used for:**
    A. Chronic limb ischemia
    B. Venous disease
    C. Lymphedema
    D. Vasculitis

29. **CEAP classification stratifies venous disease based on all except:**
    A. Congenital
    B. Etiology
    C. Anatomy
    D. Pathology

TREATMENT

30. **Compression pressure used for patients with combined chronic venous disease and peripheral arterial disease is:**
    A. 10 – 20 mm Hg B. 20 – 30 mm Hg
    C. 30 – 40 mm Hg D. 40 – 50 mm Hg

31. **Class II compression stocking (USA standard) delivers pressure of:**
    A. 20 – 30 mm Hg B. 30 – 40 mm Hg
    C. 40 – 50 mm Hg D. 50 – 60 mm Hg

32. **Which of the following is not included in C1 grade of CEAP classification?**
    A. Telangiectasia B. Reticular veins
    C. Varicose veins D. Malleolar flare

33. **Varicose veins are included in which clinical grade of CEAP classification?**
    A. C1 B. C2
    C. C3 D. C4

34. **Lipodermatosclerosis is included in which clinical class of CEAP classification?**
    A. C2 B. C3
    C. C4 D. C5

35. **Venous ulcers are included in which clinical class of CEAP classification?**
    A. C3 B. C4
    C. C5 D. C6

36. **Unna boot is used for treating which condition?**
    A. Diabetic foot
    B. Venous ulcers
    C. Congenital talipes equinovarus foot
    D. Below knee amputation

37. **Unna boot uses triple layer compression dressing impregnated with:**
    A. Zinc oxide
    B. Copper sulphate
    C. Hydrogen peroxide
    D. Silver

38. **Eschar Trial was done for:**
    A. Arterial disease B. Venous disease
    C. Burns D. Diabetic foot ulcer

39. **Which of the following is contraindication for sclerotherapy?**
    A. Pregnancy
    B. Acute DVT

C. Acute thrombophlebitis
D. All of the above

40. Sclerosants used for sclerotherapy:

A. Hypertonic saline
B. Sodium tetradecyl sulfate
C. Polidocanol
D. All of the above

41. Which is wrong statement regarding sclerotherapy?

A. Injection should begin proximally and proceed distally
B. The amount injected at one site needs to be limited to less than 1 mL
C. Patients are able to perform regular activities immediately post-therapy
D. Abstain from direct sun exposure and airline travel for 2 weeks

42. What is the maximum volume of sclerosant can be used at a one setting?

A. 4 ml
B. 6 ml
C. 8 ml
D. 10 ml

43. What is maximum volume of hypertonic saline used for sclerotherapy?

A. 4 ml
B. 6 ml
C. 8 ml
D. 10 ml

44. Most success has been achieved with which newer technique for telangiectasia?

A. High-intensity pulsed light
B. Holmium laser
C. Nd:YAG laser treatment
D. KTP laser

45. What is incorrect about laser treatment of telangiectasia?

A. Neodymium: yttrium-aluminium-garnet laser uses wavelength of 1064 nm
B. Laser treatment does tend to be more painful
C. Laser treatment can be used in conjunction with injection sclerotherapy
D. Laser treatment can used to treat the larger branches of veins

46. Which of the following is correct statement concerning telangiectasia?

A. Sclerosants cause periphlebitis reaction, which acts to obliterate the vein segment
B. Preprocedural preparation of the patient is recommended
C. Laser therapy cannot be used in conjunction with injection sclerotherapy
D. Patients are advised not to ambulate during the first 24 hours

47. Who introduced saphenous vein invagination and stripping?

A. Mayo
B. Keller
C. Kistner
D. Babcock

48. Who introduced use of external stripper to remove the saphenous vein?

A. Mayo
B. Keller
C. Kistner
D. Babcock

49. Which of the following is incorrect regarding saphenous vein stripping technique?

A. Great saphenous vein stripped from groin to ankle under spinal anesthesia
B. Small saphenous vein stripping requires placing the patient in the prone position
C. Stripping of the small saphenous should be done only to the level of the midcalf
D. The incidence of neovascularization after high ligation and stripping of the great saphenous vein exceeds 30%

50. Great saphenous vein is stripped in which direction?

A. Knee to groin
B. Groin to knee
C. Ankle to groin
D. Groin to ankle

51. What is not true about endovenous ablation?

A. Minimal invasive procedure
B. Outpatient procedure with local anesthesia
C. No need of withholding anti coagulants
D. Risk of neovascularization

52. Which of the following is incorrect statement about EVLA therapy?

A. Patients who are receiving anticoagulation should remain on their standard regimen
B. All antiplatelet medications can be continued throughout the procedural course
C. An acute occlusive DVT is an absolute contraindication
D. Procedure requires spinal anesthesia

53. What type of anesthesia is used for EVLA therapy?

A. General anesthesia
B. Spinal anesthesia
C. Tumescent anesthesia
D. Bier's block

54. Contents of tumescent anesthesia are all except:

A. Bupivacaine

B. Sodium bicarbonate
C. Epinephrine
D. Normal saline

55. Which of the following is wrong about EVLA?
A. Radiofrequency ablation uses heat energy which is delivered at a temperature of 120°C
B. The radiofrequency directly injures the vein wall endothelium, resulting in collagen contraction and thrombosis of the treated vein
C. EVLA uses wavelength 1470 nm which delivers energy to the blood itself
D. 20 mm halo of tumescent anesthesia is required along the entire course of vein

56. Which of the following is incorrect about endovenous heat induced thrombosis (EHIT)?
A. Protective flush prevents postprocedural development of EHIT
B. EHIT becomes sonographically echogenic after 48 hours
C. EHIT appears to have a low propensity to propagate or to embolize
D. Complete resolution of EHIT usually seen within 7 to 10 days

57. Smallest size of the needle that can be used for USG guided sclerotherapy:
A. 18 G B. 22 G
C. 24 G D. 25 G

58. Which among the following is false regarding treatment of varicosities?
A. Mechanical chemical ablation involves concomitant injection of a liquid sclerosant
B. Ambulatory phlebectomy involves 1 cm incisions to retrieve vein and resect
C. Powered phlebectomy (TriVex) is used to treat extensive secondary branch varicosities
D. TriVex involves the use of resector that transects the veins and then removes through a high-suction tubing system

59. First successful major vein reconstruction was done by:
A. Mayo B. Linton
C. Kistner D. Palma

60. Venous reconstruction option includes:
A. Palma's venous bypass
B. Direct valvuloplasty of Kistner
C. Venous segment transfer of Kistner
D. All of the above

61. Which of the following procedure is not performed for deep venous insufficiency?
A. Linton procedure
B. Foam sclerotherapy
C. Endoscopic subfascial perforator ligation
D. Kistner procedure

DEEP VEIN THROMBOSIS

62. What is most common site of initiation of venous thrombosis?
A. Iliac veins B. Femoral vein
C. Popliteal vein D. Soleal sinuses

63. Which of the following does not cause hyper-coagulable state?
A. Factor V Leiden deficiency
B. Prothrombin gene mutation
C. Antithrombin III deficiency
D. Homocysteinemia

64. Which of the following is wrong about DVT?
A. Stasis has been shown to be a causative factor for DVT
B. Protein C or Protein S deficiency requires lifelong anticoagulation
C. Venous thrombosis occurs in veins that are distant from the site of operation
D. The recurrence rate of DVT with anticoagulation has been noted to be 6% to 7%

65. What is the incidence of post thrombotic syndrome after DVT?
A. 10% B. 10 – 20%
C. 20 – 50% D. > 50%

66. What are the risk factor for post thrombotic syndrome?
A. Persistent leg symptoms after acute DVT
B. Extensive DVT involving the iliofemoral system
C. Recurrent ipsilateral DVT
D. All of the above

67. Which of the following is incorrect statement regarding DVT diagnosis?
A. Homan sign refers to pain in the calf on dorsiflexion of the foot
B. Massively swollen leg with pitting edema and blanching called as phlegmasia alba dolens
C. Phlegmasia cerulea dolens occurs due to compromised venous outflow

D. Compression therapy remains the mainstay of treatment for post thrombotic syndrome

68. Which of the following is incorrect about diagnosis of DVT?

A. Impedance plethysmography shows prolongation of the outflow wave in a case of venous thrombosis
B. Negative D-dimer test has a high negative predictive value in suspected DVT case
C. Test of choice for the diagnosis of DVT is duplex ultrasound
D. Venous thrombosis is suspected on duplex if any segment of the venous system fails to demonstrate decreased flow on compression

69. All are true regarding DVT prophylaxis except:

A. Major surgery or prolonged immobility of >3 days require prophylactic anticoagulation therapy
B. The practice of having a patient out of bed into a chair is one of the most thrombogenic positions
C. Dose of 5000 units unfractionated heparin subcutaneously every 12 hours is most effective
D. LMWH is considered the optimal method of prophylaxis for moderate- and high-risk patients

70. All are true about LMWH except:

A. LMWH inhibits factor Xa and IIa activity in ratio 1:1 to 4:1
B. LMWH has a short plasma half-life
C. No laboratory monitoring is necessary
D. LMWH in head-injured and trauma patients have also proved the safety of LMWH with no increase in any major bleeding

71. What is recurrence rate of untreated lower limb DVT?

A. 10% B. 20%
C. 30% D. 40%

72. Dose of heparin used to treat DVT is:

A. 18 units/kg IV bolus followed by 80 units/kg/hr
B. 80 units/kg IV bolus followed by 18 units/kg/hr
C. 8 units/kg IV bolus followed by 18 units/kg/hr
D. 80 units/kg IV bolus followed by 8 units/kg/hr

73. Which INR goal needs to be achieved to prevent DVT recurrence?

A. 1 to 1.5 B. 1.5 to 2
C. 2 to 3 D. 3 to 4

74. Recommended period of anticoagulation therapy for DVT:

A. 1 month B. 3 months
C. 6 months D. 12 months

75. What is false regarding thrombolysis therapy?

A. Preservation of valve function and lesser chance for development of PTS
B. ATTRACT trial recommends catheter directed thrombolysis for proximal iliofemoral involvement
C. In patients with phlegmasia, thrombolysis is advocated for relief of significant venous obstruction
D. Long-term anticoagulation is not required

76. Which of the following statement is wrong concerning upper extremity DVT?

A. Pulmonary embolism occurs in up to one third of all patients with an upper extremity DVT
B. Paget-Schroetter syndrome develop effort thrombosis of the extremity caused by compression of the superior vena cava
C. Classic presentation involves a young athlete who uses the upper extremity in a repetitive motion
D. Diagnosis of idiopathic upper extremity DVT warrants evaluation for an undetected malignant neoplasm

77. Paget-Schroetter syndrome is due to the thrombosis of which vein?

A. Subclavian B. Superior vena cava
C. Common Iliac D. Femoral

78. What is the primary cause of upper extremity DVT?

A. Paget-Schroetter syndrome
B. Malignancy
C. Thrombophilia
D. Stewart Treves syndrome

79. Following are the causes of secondary upper extremity DVT except:

A. Cervical rib
B. Indwelling central venous catheter
C. Pacemaker
D. Thrombophilia

80. What is gold standard investigation for pulmonary thromboembolism?

A. CT angiography
B. Pulmonary angiography

C. MR angiography
D. Transesophageal echocardiography

81. All are indications for vena cava filter placement except:

A. Contraindication to systemic anticoagulation
B. Pulmonary hypertension due to chronic embolism
C. Propagating iliofemoral venous thrombus
D. Previous episode of DVT

82. All are indications for retrievable IVC filter placement except:

A. High-risk trauma patient
B. During venous thrombolytic therapy
C. Extensive iliocaval thrombosis
D. Recurrent thromboembolism

83. Which is wrong statement regarding superficial thrombophlebitis?

A. The condition is self-limiting
B. Duplex ultrasonography is recommended to confirm diagnosis
C. The initial treatment of noncomplicated thrombophlebitis involves conservative therapy
D. Superficial thrombophlebitis involving a ≥2 cm great saphenous vein segment is a mid-treatment dose of LMWH for 6 weeks

84. Patient presented with superficial thrombophlebitis of great saphenous vein extending upto saphenofemoral junction. What is appropriate management?

A. Local heparin application
B. NSAID and compression therapy
C. LMWH subcutaneously for 6 weeks
D. Great saphenous vein excision

85. What is Mondor's disease?

A. Migratory thrombophlebitis secondary to Ca breast
B. Superficial thrombophlebitis of breast veins
C. Lymphangitis of breast
D. Deep venous thrombosis of breast

86. Migratory thrombophlebitis is characteristically seen with which cancer?

A. Breast
B. Colon
C. Tail of pancreas
D. Stomach

ANSWERS

1. **Ans: B. Saphenous sheath is present below the deep fascia of the leg**

   Ref: Chapter No. 65, Page No. 1812

2. **Ans: D. Superficial inguinal vein**

   Ref: Chapter No. 65, Page No. 1812

3. **Ans: D. Popliteal vein enters a window in the adductor longus to continue as femoral vein**

   Ref: Chapter No. 65, Page No. 1813

4. **Ans: C. Popliteal vein**

   Ref: Chapter No. 65, Page No. 1813

5. **Ans: B. Perforator at gastrocnemius point**

   Ref: Chapter No. 65, Page No. 1814

6. **Ans: C. Above knee**

   Ref: Chapter No. 65, Page No. 1814

7. **Ans: C. Cockett**

   Ref: Chapter No. 65, Page No. 1814

8. **Ans: C. Boyd perforators connect the great saphenous and popliteal vein**

   Ref: Chapter No. 65, Page No. 1814

9. **Ans: A. Veins contain mainly elastin**

   Ref: Chapter No. 65, Page No. 1814

10. **Ans: C. During calf muscle contraction, the venous pressure of the foot and ankle increases dramatically**

    Ref: Chapter No. 65, Page No. 1815

11. **Ans: D. May-Thurner syndrome**

    Ref: Chapter No. 65, Page No. 1815

12. **Ans: C. Male gender**

    Ref: Chapter No. 65, Page No. 1815

13. **Ans: C. Development of varicose vein has autosomal recessive inheritance**

    Ref: Chapter No. 65, Page No. 1815

14. **Ans: B. Venous claudication**

    Ref: Chapter No. 65, Page No. 1816

15. **Ans: D. Deep venous thrombosis**

    Ref: Chapter No. 65, Page No. 1816

16. **Ans: A. Intradermal**

    Ref: Chapter No. 65, Page No. 1816

17. **Ans: D. All of the above**

    Ref: Chapter No. 65, Page No. 1816

18. **Ans: C. Compression of left renal vein between aorta and SMA**

    Ref: Chapter No. 65, Page No. 1816

19. **Ans: C. Venous ulcers are painful and appear at the lateral malleolus**

    Ref: Chapter No. 65, Page No. 1816-1817

20. **Ans: D. MR venography**

    Ref: Chapter No. 65, Page No. 1816

21. **Ans: C. Hyperpigmentation**

    Ref: Chapter No. 65, Page No. 1816

22. **Ans: B. Venous insufficiency**

    Ref: Chapter No. 65, Page No. 1817

23. **Ans: B. Advanced venous insufficiency**

    Ref: Chapter No. 65, Page No. 1817

24. **Ans: B. Duplex imaging**

    Ref: Chapter No. 65, Page No. 1817

25. **Ans: C. 7.5 – 10 Hz**

    Ref: Chapter No. 65, Page No. 1817

26. **Ans: A. Phlebography is useful in the diagnosis and treatment of primary venous insufficiency**

    Ref: Chapter No. 65, Page No. 1818

27. **Ans: A. Perthes test is done for superficial veins insufficiency of lower leg**

    Ref: Chapter No. 65, Page No. 1817-18

28. **Ans: B. Venous disease**

    Ref: Chapter No. 65, Page No. 1818

29. **Ans: A. Congenital**

    Ref: Chapter No. 65, Page No. 1818

30. **Ans: C. 30 – 40 mm Hg**

    Ref: Chapter No. 65, Page No. 1818

31. **Ans: A. 20 – 30 mm Hg**

    Ref: Chapter No. 65, Page No. 1818

32. **Ans: C. Varicose veins**

    Ref: Chapter No. 65, Page No. 1819

33. **Ans: B. C2**

    Ref: Chapter No. 65, Page No. 1819

34. **Ans: C. C4**

    Ref: Chapter No. 65, Page No. 1819

35. **Ans: D. C6**

    Ref: Chapter No. 65, Page No. 1819

36. **Ans: B. Venous ulcers**

Ref: Chapter No. 65, Page No. 1820

37. **Ans: A. Zinc oxide**

Ref: Chapter No. 65, Page No. 1820

38. **Ans: B. Venous disease**

Ref: Chapter No. 65, Page No. 1820

39. **Ans: D. All of the above**

Ref: Chapter No. 65, Page No. 1821

40. **Ans: D. All of the above**

Ref: Chapter No. 65, Page No. 1821

41. **Ans: B. The amount injected at one site needs to be limited to less than 1 mL**

Ref: Chapter No. 65, Page No. 1821

42. **Ans: A. 4 ml**

Ref: Chapter No. 65, Page No. 1821

43. **Ans: D. 10 ml**

Ref: Chapter No. 65, Page No. 1821

44. **Ans: C. Nd:YAG laser treatment**

Ref: Chapter No. 65, Page No. 1821

45. **Ans: D. Laser treatment can used to treat the larger branches of veins**

Ref: Chapter No. 65, Page No. 1821

46. **Ans: A. Sclerosants cause periphlebitis reaction, which acts to obliterate the vein segment**

Ref: Chapter No. 65, Page No. 1821

47. **Ans: B. Keller**

Ref: Chapter No. 65, Page No. 1821

48. **Ans: A. Mayo**

Ref: Chapter No. 65, Page No. 1821

49. **Ans: A. Great saphenous vein stripped from groin to ankle under spinal anesthesia**

Ref: Chapter No. 65, Page No. 1822

50. **Ans: B. Groin to knee**

Ref: Chapter No. 65, Page No. 1822

51. **Ans: D. Risk of neovascularization**

Ref: Chapter No. 65, Page No. 1822

52. **Ans: D. Procedure requires spinal anesthesia**

Ref: Chapter No. 65, Page No. 1822

53. **Ans: C. Tumescent anesthesia**

Ref: Chapter No. 65, Page No. 1822

54. **Ans: A. Bupivacaine**

Ref: Chapter No. 65, Page No. 1823

55. **Ans: D. 20 mm halo of tumescent anesthesia is required along the entire course of vein**

Ref: Chapter No. 65, Page No. 1823

56. **Ans: B. EHIT becomes sonographically echogenic after 48 hours**

Ref: Chapter No. 65, Page No. 1824

57. **Ans: D. 25 G**

Ref: Chapter No. 65, Page No. 1824

58. **Ans: B. Ambulatory phlebectomy involves 1-cm incisions to retrieve vein and resect**

Ref: Chapter No. 65, Page No. 1824

59. **Ans: D. Palma**

Ref: Chapter No. 65, Page No. 1826

60. **Ans: D. All of the above**

Ref: Chapter No. 65, Page No. 1826

61. **Ans: B. Foam sclerotherapy**

Ref: Chapter No. 65, Page No. 1826

62. **Ans: D. Soleal sinuses**

Ref: Chapter No. 65, Page No. 1827

63. **Ans: A. Factor V Leiden deficiency**

Ref: Chapter No. 65, Page No. 1827

64. **Ans: A. Stasis has been shown to be a causative factor for DVT**

Ref: Chapter No. 65, Page No. 1827

65. **Ans: C. 20 – 50%**

Ref: Chapter No. 65, Page No. 1828

66. **Ans: D. All of the above**

Ref: Chapter No. 65, Page No. 1828

67. **Ans: C. Phlegmasia cerulea dolens occurs due to compromised venous outflow**

Ref: Chapter No. 65, Page No. 1828

68. **Ans: D. Venous thrombosis is suspected on duplex if any segment of the venous system fails to demonstrate decreased flow on compression**

Ref: Chapter No. 65, Page No. 1828

69. **Ans: C. Dose of 5000 units unfractionated heparin subcutaneously every 12 hours is most effective**

Ref: Chapter No. 65, Page No. 1829

70. **Ans: B. LMWH has a short plasma half-life**

Ref: Chapter No. 65, Page No. 1829

71. **Ans: C. 30%**

Ref: Chapter No. 65, Page No. 1829

72. **Ans: B. 80 units/kg IV bolus followed by 18 units/kg/hr**

Ref: Chapter No. 65, Page No. 1829

73. **Ans: C. 2 to 3**

Ref: Chapter No. 65, Page No. 1829

74. **Ans: B. 3 months**

Ref: Chapter No. 65, Page No. 1829

75. **Ans: D. Long-term anticoagulation is not required**

Ref: Chapter No. 65, Page No. 1830

76. **Ans: B. Paget-Schroetter syndrome develop effort thrombosis of the extremity caused by compression of the superior vena cava**

Ref: Chapter No. 65, Page No. 1830

77. **Ans: A. Subclavian**

Ref: Chapter No. 65, Page No. 1830

78. **Ans: A. Paget-Schroetter syndrome**

Ref: Chapter No. 65, Page No. 1830

79. **Ans: A. Cervical rib**

Ref: Chapter No. 65, Page No. 1830

80. **Ans: B. Pulmonary angiography**

Ref: Chapter No. 65, Page No. 1830

81. **Ans: D. Previous episode of DVT**

Ref: Chapter No. 65, Page No. 1831

82. **Ans: D. Recurrent thromboembolism**

Ref: Chapter No. 65, Page No. 1831

83. **Ans: D. Superficial thrombophlebitis involving a ≥2 cm great saphenous vein segment is a mid-treatment dose of LMWH for 6 weeks**

Ref: Chapter No. 65, Page No. 1831

84. **Ans: C. LMWH subcutaneously for 6 weeks**

Ref: Chapter No. 65, Page No. 1831

85. **Ans: B. Superficial thrombophlebitis of breast veins**

Ref: Chapter No. 65, Page No. 1831

86. **Ans: C. Tail of pancreas**

Ref: Chapter No. 65, Page No. 1831

66

Lymphatics

1. **Which of the following is wrong about lymphatic development?**
   A. Jugular lymph sacs develop in sixth week of gestation
   B. Cisterna chyli develop in eighth week
   C. Thoracic duct develop during the 12th week
   D. Lymphangiogenesis is regulated by the VEGF C and D

2. **Lymphangiogenesis is regulated by all except:**
   A. VEGF A B. VEGF C
   C. VEGFR 3 D. Neuropilin 2

3. **Hereditary lymphedema-distichiasis syndrome is associated with which gene mutation?**
   A. FOXC2 B. SOX18
   C. RAMP1 D. VEGFR 3

4. **Hypotrichosis-lymphedema-telangiectasia is associated with which mutation?**
   A. FOXC2 B. SOX18
   C. RAMP1 D. VEGFR3

5. **All are correct statements regarding function of lymphatics except:**
   A. Terminal lymphatic capillaries absorb lymph
   B. Collecting vessels serve primarily as conduits for lymph transport
   C. Lymph nodes represent the first line of the immune system
   D. Terminal lymphatics have does not allow entry of large macromolecules, cells and microbes

6. **Lymphatics are present in which of the following:**
   A. Epidermis B. Dermis
   C. Cornea D. Cartilage

7. **Lymphatics are absent in:**
   A. CNS B. Muscle
   C. Tendon D. All of the above

8. **Forward flow of lymph is mainly maintained by:**
   A. Muscle activity
   B. Thoracic negative pressure
   C. Intrinsic contractility
   D. Transmitted arterial pulsations

9. **Non pitting edema is first seen in which stage of lymphedema?**
   A. Stage I B. Stage II
   C. Stage III D. Stage IV

10. **Which statement is false regarding lymphedema?**
    A. The vessels are incompetent and tortuous in lymphatic hyperplasia
    B. In the latent phase, there is clinical evidence of reducible edema on elevation
    C. In the second stage, tissue edema is nonpitting and skin fibrosis is more apparent
    D. Edema is irreversible at third stage of lymphedema

11. **Tree trunk appearance of lower limb is seen in which condition?**
    A. Venous disorder B. Arterial disease
    C. Lipedema D. Lymphedema

12. **"Tree trunk" pattern and "buffalo hump" is seen in which stage of lymphedema?**
    A. Latent stage B. Stage I
    C. Stage II D. Stage III

13. All are signs of advanced lymphatic disease except:

A. Stemmer sign
B. Lichenification
C. Peau de orange
D. Hyperkeratosis

14. Positive 'Stemmer sign' is seen in which stage of lymphedema?

A. Latent stage
B. Stage I
C. Stage II
D. Stage III

15. Which of the following is false regarding lipedema?

A. It is bilateral and non-pitting
B. No skin changes and the enlargement is not affected by elevation
C. Typically found in obese women
D. Edema is greatest at feet

16. What is the most common cause of unilateral leg edema?

A. Lymphedema
B. Venous disease
C. Arterial disease
D. Infection

17. Which is the most common primary lymphedema?

A. Congenital lymphedema
B. Lymphedema precox
C. Milroy disease
D. Lymphedema tarda

18. Primary lymphedema with onset before 1 year of age is called:

A. Congenital lymphedema
B. Milroy disease
C. Lymphedema tarda
D. Lymphedema precox

19. Familial primary lymphedema with onset before 1 year of age is called:

A. Congenital lymphedema
B. Milroy disease
C. Meige disease
D. Lymphedema precox

20. Wrongly matched of the following:

A. Familial lymphedema between age 1 to 35 years – Lymphedema precox
B. Primary lymphedema between age 1 to 35 years – Meige disease
C. Primary lymphedema beyond age of 35 years – Lymphedema tarda
D. None of the above

21. What is the most common worldwide cause of secondary lymphedema?

A. Surgery
B. Filariasis
C. Tumor
D. Trauma

22. What is the diagnostic test of choice for suspicion of lymphedema?

A. Direct contrast Lymphangiography
B. Lymphoscintigraphy
C. Plethysmography
D. CT lymphangiography

23. Which statement regarding lymphoscintigraphy is false?

A. It can differentiate between primary and secondary lymphedemas
B. It is simple, safe and reproducible
C. 5 mCi of radioiodinated human albumin or technetium-99m–labeled sulfur colloid is injected at 1st web space of foot
D. The amount of radioactivity is measured at the inguinal nodes 30 and 60 minutes after injection

24. What value of radioactivity on lymphoscintigraphy is diagnostic of lymphedema?

A. More than 2% of total dose at 60 minutes
B. Less than 1.6% of total dose at 60 minutes
C. More than 0.6% of total dose at 30 minutes
D. Less than 0.3% of total dose at 30 minutes

25. Which condition shows inguinal node radioactivity more than 2% on lymphoscintigraphy?

A. Filariasis
B. Lymphadenectomy
C. Venous disease
D. Arterial disease

26. Which of the following is wrong regarding lymphedema evaluation?

A. It is prerequisite to rule out neoplastic involvement of lymphatic for diagnosing primary lymphedema
B. Lymphoscintigraphy differentiate lymphedema from other causes of limb swelling
C. The degree of edema involving the lower extremity affects the rate of clearance of the isotope
D. Direct contrast lymphangiography provides anatomical details of lymphatics

27. Contrast agent used in MR lymphangiography:

A. Gadoterate meglumine

B. Gadopentate dimeglumine
C. Gadobenate dimeglumine
D. Gadoxetate disodium

28. **Pressure delivered by ideal compression garment for treatment of lymphedema is:**

A. 10 – 15 mm Hg B. 18 – 24 mm Hg
C. 25 – 30 mm Hg D. 30 – 60 mm Hg

29. **Incorrect statement about decongestive physical therapy:**

A. The technique is initiated on the normal contralateral side of the body
B. The affected extremity is massaged in a segmental fashion initiated with distal zone
C. Therapy is appropriate for patients with all stages of lymphedema
D. Lifelong maintenance is imperative to maintain reduction

30. **Which of the following is not an indication for surgical intervention of lymphedema?**

A. Stage II or stage III lymphedema
B. Severe functional impairment
C. Single episode of lymphangitis
D. Failed medical therapy

31. **A 40 years old patient undergone inguinal lymphadenectomy following which he has developed lymphedema of left leg. What will be appropriate procedure of choice for this patient?**

A. Benzopyrones drug therapy
B. Compression bandages
C. Lymphatic reconstruction
D. Homan procedure

32. **Which is false about Kontoleon procedure for lymphedema?**

A. A choice of procedure for patients with recalcitrant stage II and early stage III lymphedema
B. Flaps about 1 to 2 cm thick are elevated anteriorly and posteriorly
C. The sural nerve is preserved
D. The excision is usually performed in one stage with graft coverage

33. **Staged subcutaneous excision below skin flaps involved in which lymphedema procedure?**

A. Homan B. Charles
C. Thompson D. Sistrunk

34. **Single stage circumferential excision upto deep fascia with skin grafting is done in which lymphedema procedure?**

A. Homan B. Charles
C. Thompson D. Sistrunk

35. **What is most common cause of chylothorax?**

A. Malignancy B. Iatrogenic
C. Tuberculosis D. Filariasis

36. **Patient has lung cancer with pleural effusion. Pleural tap shows chylomicrons and triglycerides level 150 mg/dl. He has persistent drainage despite chemotherapy. What will be next appropriate management?**

A. TPN with octreotide therapy
B. VATS for thoracic duct repair
C. Lymphangiographic embolization of thoracic duct
D. Pleurodesis

37. **What is the most common cause of chyloperitoneum in children?**

A. Iatrogenic
B. Congenital lymphatic abnormality
C. Malignancy
D. Filariasis

38. **What is the most common cause of chyloperitoneum in adults?**

A. Iatrogenic
B. Congenital lymphatic abnormality
C. Malignancy
D. Filariasis

39. **Which of the following is false regarding cystic hygroma?**

A. They are capillary lymphangiomas
B. Commonly occur in the neck or the axilla
C. Majority are present at birth
D. Treatment of choice is surgical excision

40. **What is the latent period for development of Stewart Treves syndrome in lymphedema?**

A. 2 years B. 5 years
C. 10 years D. 20 years

ANSWERS

1. **Ans: C. Thoracic duct develop during the 12th week**
Ref: Chapter No. 66, Page No. 1834
2. **Ans: A. VEGF A**
Ref: Chapter No. 66, Page No. 1834
3. **Ans: A. FOXC2**
Ref: Chapter No. 66, Page No. 1834
4. **Ans: B. SOX18**
Ref: Chapter No. 66, Page No. 1834
5. **Ans: D. Terminal lymphatics have does not allow entry of large macromolecules, cells and microbes**
Ref: Chapter No. 66, Page No. 1834
6. **Ans: B. Dermis**
Ref: Chapter No. 66, Page No. 1835
7. **Ans: D. All of the above**
Ref: Chapter No. 66, Page No. 1835
8. **Ans: C. Intrinsic contractility**
Ref: Chapter No. 66, Page No. 1835
9. **Ans: B. Stage II**
Ref: Chapter No. 66, Page No. 1836
10. **Ans: B. In the latent phase, there is clinical evidence of reducible edema on elevation**
Ref: Chapter No. 66, Page No. 1836
11. **Ans: D. Lymphedema**
Ref: Chapter No. 66, Page No. 1836
12. **Ans: C. Stage II**
Ref: Chapter No. 66, Page No. 1836
13. **Ans: A. Stemmer sign**
Ref: Chapter No. 66, Page No. 1836
14. **Ans: C. Stage II**
Ref: Chapter No. 66, Page No. 1836
15. **Ans: D. Edema is greatest at feet**
Ref: Chapter No. 66, Page No. 1836
16. **Ans: B. Venous disease**
Ref: Chapter No. 66, Page No. 1836
17. **Ans: B. Lymphedema precox**
Ref: Chapter No. 66, Page No. 1836
18. **Ans: A. Congenital lymphedema**
Ref: Chapter No. 66, Page No. 1836
19. **Ans: B. Milroy disease**
Ref: Chapter No. 66, Page No. 1836
20. **Ans: D. None of the above**
Ref: Chapter No. 66, Page No. 1836
21. **Ans: B. Filariasis**
Ref: Chapter No. 66, Page No. 1836
22. **Ans: B. Lymphoscintigraphy**
Ref: Chapter No. 66, Page No. 1837
23. **Ans: A. It can differentiate between primary and secondary lymphedemas**
Ref: Chapter No. 66, Page No. 1837
24. **Ans: D. Less than 0.3% of total dose at 30 minutes**
Ref: Chapter No. 66, Page No. 1837
25. **Ans: C. Venous disease**
Ref: Chapter No. 66, Page No. 1837
26. **Ans: C. The degree of edema involving the lower extremity affects the rate of clearance of the isotope**
Ref: Chapter No. 66, Page No. 1837
27. **Ans: C. Gadobenate dimeglumine**
Ref: Chapter No. 66, Page No. 1837
28. **Ans: D. 30 – 60 mm Hg**
Ref: Chapter No. 66, Page No. 1838
29. **Ans: B. The affected extremity is massaged in a segmental fashion initiated with distal zone**
Ref: Chapter No. 66, Page No. 1838
30. **Ans: C. Single episode of lymphangitis**
Ref: Chapter No. 66, Page No. 1839
31. **Ans: C. Lymphatic reconstruction**
Ref: Chapter No. 66, Page No. 1839
32. **Ans: D. The excision is usually performed in one stage with graft coverage**
Ref: Chapter No. 66, Page No. 1839
33. **Ans: A. Homan**
Ref: Chapter No. 66, Page No. 1839
34. **Ans: B. Charles**
Ref: Chapter No. 66, Page No. 1839
35. **Ans: B. Iatrogenic**
Ref: Chapter No. 66, Page No. 1839
36. **Ans: D. Pleurodesis**
Ref: Chapter No. 66, Page No. 1840
37. **Ans: B. Congenital lymphatic abnormality**
Ref: Chapter No. 66, Page No. 1840
38. **Ans: C. Malignancy**
Ref: Chapter No. 66, Page No. 1840
39. **Ans: A. They are capillary lymphangiomas**
Ref: Chapter No. 66, Page No. 1841
40. **Ans: C. 10 years**
Ref: Chapter No. 66, Page No. 1841

67

Pediatric Surgery

PHYSIOLOGY AND NUTRITION

1. **Ambient temperature maintained in OT at:**
   A. 18°C B. 23°C
   C. 28°C D. 30°C

2. **Use of Indomethacin in premature infants is:**
   A. Closure of ductus venous
   B. Closure of ductus arteriosus
   C. Prevention of pulmonary hypertension
   D. Relaxation of vascular smooth muscles

3. **About fetal respiratory function false is:**
   A. Tidal volume of 6 to 10 mL/kg
   B. Infants are obligate nasal breathers
   C. Neonatal lung has higher type II pneumocytes
   D. Lecithin - sphingomyelin ratio is used to determine fetal lung maturity

4. **Ideal replacement solution for gastric losses in pediatric patient:**
   A. 5% Dextrose in 0.9% NS with 10 mEq/L potassium
   B. 5% Dextrose in 0.9% NS with 20 mEq/L potassium
   C. 5% Dextrose in 0.45% NS with 10 mEq/L potassium
   D. 5% Dextrose in 0.45% NS with 20 mEq/L potassium

5. **Hypovolemia due to acute blood loss corrected with following except:**
   A. Packed red cells B. Plasma
   C. Normal saline D. 5% Albumin

6. **Ideal enteral calorie requirement of infant:**
   A. 100 calories/kg/day
   B. 120 calories/kg/day
   C. 150 calories/kg/day
   D. 180 calories/kg/day

7. **In infants with unconjugated hyperbilirubinemia caution required with administration of:**
   A. Glucose B. Protein
   C. Fat D. Amino acids

8. **Infants tolerate starvation upto:**
   A. 2-3 days B. 5-7 days
   C. 10-14 days D. 21 days

9. **Ideal treatment of TPN-associated cholestasis:**
   A. Reducing TPN volume
   B. Restoring enteral nutrition
   C. Use of omega-3 fatty acids
   D. Use of medium chain triglycerides

HEAD AND NECK LESIONS

10. **Common location of epidermoid cysts:**
    A. Face B. Scalp
    C. Back D. Chest

11. **Which of the following is incorrect about epidermoid cyst?**
    A. Slow growing benign lesion
    B. Common location is lateral corner of eyebrow
    C. They are often osteolytic
    D. It is always symptomatic

12. **Which of the following is false about Cat-scratch disease?**
    A. It is self-limited infectious disease
    B. It is caused by gram negative Bartonella henselae

C. It is characterized by painless regional lymphadenopathy
D. History of exposure to cats is not always present

13. Incorrect about cystic hygroma:

A. Multiloculated cysts due to lymphatic malformation
B. Most involve jugular lymph sacs in posterior neck region
C. Diagnosed with prenatal USG or MRI
D. Aggressive and radical resection required

14. Most common location of Thyroglossal cyst:

A. At base of tongue
B. Above hyoid bone
C. Just below hyoid bone
D. Thyroid gland

15. Which of the following is incorrect about thyroglossal duct remnant?

A. It originates at the base of the tongue at the foramen caecum
B. Thyroid diverticulum develops as a lateral ectodermal thickening at the foramen caecum
C. Thyroglossal duct remnant exists with the central portion of the hyoid bone
D. Failure of normal caudal migration of the thyroid gland results in a lingual thyroid

16. Gold standard treatment for Thyroglossal duct cysts:

A. Swensen procedure
B. Duhamel procedure
C. Sistrunk procedure
D. Dunhill procedure

17. Which of the following is not removed in Sistrunk procedure?

A. Thyroglossal cyst
B. Patent thyroglossal tract
C. Hyoid bone
D. Thyroid gland

18. False regarding branchial clefts remnants:

A. Branchial cleft remnants present as lateral neck masses
B. The second branchial cleft anomalies are the most common type
C. External ostium of these remnants is located along the anterior border of the sternocleidomastoid muscle
D. Third branchial cleft remnants have associated sinuses or fistulas in the suprasternal notch

19. Which of the following is incorrect about branchial clefts remnants?

A. Structures of the head and neck are derived from six pairs of branchial arches
B. First branchial anomalies are typically located in the upper neck near the mandible
C. Second branchial anomalies located at posterior border of sternocleidomastoid
D. Third branchial cleft remnants usually are located in the suprasternal notch or clavicular region

20. Second branchial cleft fistula ends in:

A. External auditory canal
B. Tonsillar fossa or other nasopharyngeal spaces
C. Suprasternal notch
D. Anterior border of sternocleidomastoid

PULMONARY

21. Indications for neonatal extracorporeal membrane oxygenation (ECMO) include:

A. Meconium aspiration
B. Respiratory distress syndrome
C. Congenital diaphragmatic hernia
D. All of the above

22. Most common indication of ECMO with highest survival:

A. Meconium aspiration
B. Congenital diaphragmatic hernia
C. Respiratory distress syndrome
D. Primary pulmonary HTN

23. Criteria for application of ECMO except:

A. AaDo2 greater than 610 for longer than 8 to 12 hours
B. AaDo2 greater than 620 for 6 hours
C. Severe hypotension requiring inotropic support
D. Oxygen index greater than 40

24. Contraindication for ECMO includes all except:

A. Severe prematurity
B. Weight less than 3 kg
C. Nonreversible pulmonary disease
D. Presence of an intracranial bleed

25. Incorrect about congenital diaphragmatic hernia:

A. Incidence of CDH is 1 in 2000 to 5000 live births
B. Occurs more commonly on the left side
C. Bilateral defects occur in 10%
D. Abnormal liver position at 24 weeks of gestation is strong predictor of unfavorable outcomes

26. The lung area to head circumference ratio (LHR) as prognostic of congenital diaphragmatic hernia is determined by:

A. Addition of the longest two perpendicular linear measurements of the lung contralateral to CDH and is divided by head circumference
B. Product of the longest two perpendicular linear measurements of the lung contralateral to CDH and is divided by head circumference
C. Addition of the longest two perpendicular linear measurements of the lung ipsilateral to CDH and is divided by head circumference
D. Product of the longest two perpendicular linear measurements of the lung ipsilateral to CDH and is divided by head circumference

27. The prenatal diagnosis of CDH is made as early as _____ weeks of gestation.

A. 10 weeks B. 15 weeks
C. 24 weeks D. 32 weeks

28. Congenital diaphragmatic hernia through anteromedial location is:

A. Bochdalek hernia B. Morgagni hernia
C. Hiatus hernia D. Serafini hernia

29. Most common type of congenital diaphragmatic hernia occur through:

A. Right anterolateral
B. Left anterolateral
C. Right posterolateral
D. Left posterolateral

30. Infant was well for hours after delivery and then demonstrated worsening of respiratory function with grunting and chest retraction. Decreased breath sounds with bowel sounds were heard on left sided chest auscultation. What is immediate critical step in management of this condition?

A. Oxygen supplementation with bag mask
B. Endotracheal intubation with ventilation
C. Nasogastric tube insertion
D. Endoscopic tracheal occlusion

31. Infant had difficult birth due to shoulder dystocia and then presented with respiratory distress with inability to wean from ventilator. On chest auscultation decreased breath sound were heard on left side with right sided mediastinal shift. What is the probable diagnosis?

A. Congenital diaphragmatic hernia
B. Diaphragmatic eventration
C. Diaphragmatic rupture
D. Pulmonary hypoplasia

32. Diagnosis of diaphragmatic eventration is confirmed by:

A. Upper GI contrast study
B. CT chest
C. Dynamic USG chest
D. Chest radiography

33. Incorrect about diaphragmatic eventration:

A. Results from shoulder dystocia during a difficult birth
B. Diagnosis is confirmed by dynamic visualization of the diaphragm on fluoroscopy
C. Paradoxical movement of the diaphragm on inspiration is diagnostic
D. Repair is done through thoracic approach

34. All are true about bronchogenic cysts except:

A. Most common type of mediastinal cysts
B. They are usually found near the carina and right hilum
C. Cysts within the pulmonary parenchyma typically communicate with a bronchus
D. Asymptomatic cysts are usually managed by observation

35. Classification used for congenital pulmonary airway malformation:

A. Steinberg B. Stocker
C. Stockholm D. Van Praag

36. All are true about congenital pulmonary airway malformation except:

A. Hamartomatous lesions replaces normal lung tissue
B. They are connected to the tracheobronchial tree
C. Blood supply is from aorta
D. A single course of betamethasone has been shown to be effective

37. False about congenital pulmonary airway malformation:

A. Type I is most common type
B. Type I consist of a numerous cysts, usually measuring less than 1 cm in diameter
C. Type III associated with hydrops and poor prognosis
D. Risk of malignant transformation

38. Pleuropulmonary blastoma risk associated with:

A. Type I CPAM
B. Type II CPAM
C. Type III CPAM
D. Type IV CPAM

39. Which of the following is correct about pulmonary sequestration?

A. Connection to the tracheobronchial tree
B. Can be located intralobar or extralobar
C. Vascular connections are to the pulmonary artery and vein
D. Risk of infection is higher

GASTROINTESTINAL TRACT

40. Which of the following is incorrect about TEF?

A. Incidence of this anomaly is 1 in 1500 to 3000 live births
B. There is hereditary association of VATERL anomalies
C. Most common type, a proximal esophageal atresia with distal TEF (C Type)
D. Routine endotracheal intubation is avoided due to risk of inadequate lung inflation

41. Which is most common type of TEF?

A. Isolated esophageal atresia
B. Esophageal atresia with proximal TEF
C. Esophageal atresia with distal TEF
D. TEF without esophageal atresia

42. Which of the following is not included in VATERL anomalies?

A. Vertebral
B. Renal
C. Imperforate anus
D. Eye deformities

43. Newborn infant has mild respiratory distress, excessive drooling and coughing after oral feeds. An abdominal radiograph shows excessive distension of stomach. What is most likely diagnosis?

A. Bilateral choanal atresia
B. Isolated esophageal atresia
C. Esophageal atresia with TEF
D. Duodenal atresia

44. Newborn presented with coughing on oral feeds. NG tube insertion attempted, but it could not be passed in stomach. Which of the following is incorrect about this condition?

A. It has female predominance
B. Associated nonhereditary VACTERL anomalies
C. Maternal history of polyhydramnios is common
D. Echocardiography and renal USG routinely done

45. Cardinal feature of esophageal atresia is:

A. Excessive drooling of saliva
B. Inability to pass NG tube into stomach
C. Absence of gas in stomach
D. Respiratory distress on oral feeds

46. What is the best surgical approach to repair Type C of TEF?

A. Left thoracotomy
B. Right thoracotomy
C. Median thoracotomy
D. Left cervicotomy

47. Following are the complications of TEF repair:

A. Esophageal motility disorder
B. Gastroesophageal reflux
C. Anastomotic leak
D. All of the above

48. Which is the gold standard procedure for GER in children?

A. Dor fundoplication
B. Nissen fundoplication
C. Toupet fundoplication
D. Both B and C

49. Which of the following is incorrect about Hypertrophic pyloric stenosis?

A. Incidence of 1 in 300 to 900 live births
B. Most common between the ages of 2 and 8 weeks
C. First-born male infants being at highest risk
D. Hypertrophy of the longitudinal muscle of the pylorus

50. 1 month old child presented with upper abdominal pain with visible peristalsis and non bilious vomiting. Which of the following electrolyte imbalance is seen with this condition?

A. Hypokalemic, hypochloremic, metabolic acidosis
B. Hyperkalemic, hypochloremic, metabolic acidosis
C. Hypokalemic, hypochloremic, metabolic alkalosis
D. Hyperkalemic, hypochloremic, metabolic alkalosis

51. What is the pathognomonic sign of CHPS?

A. Nonbilious projectile vomiting
B. Visible left to right peristalsis
C. Palpation of the pyloric "olive" tumor in the epigastrium
D. All of the above

52. Following are the diagnostic of CHPS:

A. Palpation of the pyloric "olive" tumor in the epigastrium with visible peristalsis
B. Pyloric muscle thickness of more than 3 to 4 mm on USG with functional obstruction
C. Pyloric length of more than 15 to 18 mm on USG with functional obstruction
D. All of the above

53. What is the gold standard procedure for CHPS?

A. Heller's myotomy
B. Ramstedt procedure
C. Gastroduodenostomy
D. Heineke Mickulicz pyloroplasty

54. What is the most common site of duodenal stenosis?

A. Proximal to ampulla of Vater
B. 3rd part of duodenum
C. Distal to ampulla of Vater
D. At Ligament of Treitz

55. Following is the characteristic of duodenal atresia on plain abdominal radiograph:

A. Single bubble sign
B. Double bubble sign
C. Rat tail appearance
D. Inverted 3 sign

56. Newborn presented with episodes of bilious vomiting. Plain abdominal radiograph shows gaseous distension of stomach with air upto 2nd part of duodenum. What is the probable diagnosis?

A. Congenital pyloric stenosis
B. Duodenal atresia
C. Jejunal atresia
D. Midgut volvulus

57. Newborn presented with bilious emesis with double bubble sign on plain abdominal radiograph. What is best management of this condition?

A. Gastrostomy tube insertion
B. Heineke Mikulicz pylorotomy
C. Duodenoduodenostomy
D. Gastrojejunostomy

58. What is the most common gastrointestinal atresia?

A. Duodenal atresia
B. Jejunoileal atresia
C. Ileocolic atresia
D. Colonic atresia

59. Which of the following is associated with jejunoileal atresia?

A. Down syndrome
B. Anorectal malformation
C. Cystic fibrosis
D. Biliary atresia

60. Apple peel or Christmus tree is which type of ileal atresia?

A. Type II atresia
B. Type IIIa atresia
C. Type IIIb atresia
D. Type IV atresia

61. Which of the following is wrongly matched?

A. Type I – Mucosal web
B. Type II – Blind end with intact mesentery
C. Type IIIa – V shaped mesenteric gap
D. Type IIIb – String of sausage appearance

62. What type of jejunoileal atresia gives "String of sausage" appearance?

A. Type II
B. Type IIIa
C. Type IIIb
D. Type IV

63. During fetal development, intestinal rotation occurs at:

A. Clockwise around axis of SMA by 180 degree
B. Counterclockwise around axis of SMA by 180 degree
C. Clockwise around axis of SMA by 270 degree
D. Counterclockwise around axis of SMA by 270 degree

64. The process of intestinal rotation completes by which gestational age?

A. 10 weeks
B. 12 weeks
C. 14 weeks
D. 16 weeks

65. Which is the most common midgut malrotation?

A. Duodenojejunal nonrotation
B. Complete nonrotation
C. Reversed rotation
D. Incomplete rotation

66. False regarding complete nonrotation anomaly:

A. Duodenojejunal and ileocecal junctions lie close together
B. Midgut is suspended on a narrow SMA stalk, which can twist in a counterclockwise fashion
C. Relationship of the superior mesenteric vessels is reversed or altered
D. Duodenojejunal nor the cecocolic limb undergoes correct rotation

67. Duodenal obstruction by Ladd's band occurs due to:

A. Complete nonrotation
B. Nonrotation of the duodenojejunal limb, followed by normal rotation and fixation of the cecocolic limb
C. Normal rotation of the duodenojejunal limb, followed by nonrotation of the cecocolic limb
D. Nonrotation of the duodenojejunal limb, followed by reverse rotation and fixation of the cecocolic limb

68. Which of the following is incorrect about Ladd's band?

A. Nonrotation of the duodenojejunal limb
B. Normal rotation of the cecocolic limb
C. Relatively broad mesenteric base
D. All of the above

69. Previously well infant presented with sudden onset of bilious emesis and abdominal pain. Plain abdominal X-ray shows gasless abdomen. Which could be most likely diagnosis?

A. Pyloric stenosis
B. Midgut volvulus
C. Intussusceptions
D. Hirchsprung's disease

70. 3 weeks old infant exhibit acute onset bilious vomiting, which would be most appropriate initial diagnostic modality?

A. Abdominal radiograph
B. Abdominal USG
C. Upper GI contrast study
D. CT scan

71. Which of the following is incorrect about midgut volvulus ?

A. It is a true surgical emergency
B. Upper GI contrast study is the diagnostic study of choice in a hemodynamically stable
C. Appearance of a bird's beak in the fourth portion of the duodenum
D. Midgut volvulus is untwisted in a counter-clockwise fashion

72. Ladd's bands extend from:

A. Ascending colon to the anterior aspect of the right upper quadrant
B. Transverse colon to the anterior aspect of the right upper quadrant
C. Ascending colon to the posterior aspect of the right upper quadrant
D. Transverse colon to the posterior aspect of the right upper quadrant

73. 2 months old infant previously normally fed presents with acute bilious vomiting. Upper GI shows bird beak appearance of third part of duodenum. Which of the following is incorrect about management?

A. Ladd procedure is the operation of choice for rotational anomalies of the intestine
B. Midgut volvulus is untwisted in a counter-clockwise fashion
C. Appendectomy is not routinely performed
D. Cecum lies on the left side of the abdomen after the Ladd procedure

74. Cork-screw appearance of duodenum on upper GI contrast is seen in which condition?

A. Duodenal stenosis
B. Midgut volvulus
C. Stammers hernia
D. Periampullary carcinoma

75. Which is the most common GI surgical emergency in neonates?

A. Midgut volvulus
B. Necrotizing enterocolitis
C. Meconium ileus
D. Tracheoesophageal fistula

76. 2 weeks old premature infant presented with abdominal distension and dusky appearance. Patient has abdominal tenderness on examination. What is the most probable diagnosis?

A. Midgut volvulus
B. Meconium peritonitis

C. Necrotizing enterocolitis
D. Ladd's band

77. **What is pathognomonic radiographic sign of necrotizing enterocolitis?**
A. Air fluid levels in distended bowel loops
B. Pneumatosis intestinalis
C. Soap bubble appearance
D. Portal venous gas

78. **2 weeks old premature newborn develops abdominal distension with marked cellulitis. Radiographic finding shows portal venous gas. What is the best step of management for this condition?**
A. Orogastric tube decompression, fluid resuscitation and broad-spectrum antibiotics
B. Bedside peritoneal drain placement
C. Operative laparotomy with stoma creation
D. Laparotomy with resection and anastomosis

79. **Necrotizing enterocolitis is characterized by which of the following?**
A. Term and premature infants affects equally
B. Typically occurs in the first few days of life without the initiation of enteral feeding
C. It almost always require surgical intervention
D. It is associated with premature GI tract which allows translocation of bacterias

80. **Which is the absolute indication for surgery in an infant with NEC?**
A. Pneumatosis intestinalis
B. Portal venous gas
C. Peumoperitoneum
D. All of the above

81. **A premature infant on oral feeds develops abdominal distension with passage of blood streaked stool. What is appropriate management?**
A. Restriction of oral feeds and observation for 48 hours
B. Immediate barium enema to rule out intussusceptions
C. Per anum examination with anoscopy
D. Orogastric tube decompression, fluid resuscitation, IV antibiotics and serial radiographs

82. **Which of the following is most common cause of short bowel syndrome?**
A. Jejunoileal atresia
B. Midgut volvulus
C. Necrotizing enterocolitis
D. Gastroschisis

83. **Which is the most common site of macronutrients and mineral absorption?**
A. Duodenum B. Jejunum
C. Ileum D. Colon

84. **Which procedures are used in short bowel syndrome?**
A. Reversed intestinal segment
B. Colonic interposition
C. Bianchi procedure
D. All of the above

85. **Which of the following is correct about meconium ileus?**
A. It is associated with autosomal dominant CFTR gene mutation
B. It is late clinical manifestation of cystic fibrosis
C. Infants present with cardinal signs after 1 week of birth
D. It presents with bilious vomiting and failure to pass meconium

86. **Which of the following does not suggest meconium ileus?**
A. Dilated small bowel loops with air-fluid levels
B. Soap bubble appearance
C. Contrast enema can both be diagnostic and therapeutic
D. Iontophoresis sweat test is confirmatory of CF

87. **Newborn infant presented with abdominal distension within 24 hours of birth. Radiograph shows dilated small bowel with ground glass appearance and absence of air fluid levels. Patient has not passed meconium. What is appropriate next step of management?**
A. IV fluid resuscitation and observation
B. NG tube, hydration and contrast enema with gastrograffin
C. Sweat chloride test
D. Immediate laparotomy

88. **Pilocarpine iontophoresis sweat is confirmatory of CF if chloride concentration of more than:**
A. 40 mEq/L B. 50 mEq/L
C. 60 mEq/L D. 70 mEq/L

89. **Newborn infant presented with abdominal distension within 24 hours of birth. Patient has not passed meconium. Radiograph shows dilated**

small bowel with calcification and ascites. What is the appropriate next step of management?

A. IV fluid resuscitation and observation
B. NG tube, hydration and contrast enema with gastrograffin
C. Bedside percutaneous drain placement
D. Immediate laparotomy with stoma creation

90. Which of the following is true about meconium plug syndrome?

A. It is clinical manifestation of cystic fibrosis
B. Contrast study shows dilated small bowel with collapsed colon
C. Contrast enema can be diagnostic as well as therapeutic
D. Surgical intervention almost always require

91. Following are the characteristics of Hirschsprung except:

A. It occurs in 1 in 5000 live births
B. Girls being affected four times more frequently than boys
C. It is associated with the RET oncogene
D. An absence of ganglion cells in the myenteric and submucosal plexus of distal colon/rectum

92. Which of the following is correct about Hirschsprung disease?

A. Absent ganglionic cells in both Auerbach and Meissner plexuses
B. Failure to pass meconium in the first 72 hours of birth
C. Best diagnosed with lower GI contrast study
D. Atrophy of submucosal nerve endings in rectal biopsy specimen

93. Most common cause of death in uncorrected Hirschsprung:

A. Enterocolitis
B. Ischemic colitis
C. Meconium peritonitis
D. Meconium aspiration

94. Gold standard for the diagnosis of Hirschsprung:

A. Lower GI contrast study
B. Rectal manometry
C. MRI
D. Full thickness rectal biopsy

95. Which of the following is incorrect about rectal biopsy in Hirschsprung?

A. It is the gold standard for the diagnosis
B. In newborn period, this is performed at bedside using a suction biopsy kit
C. Biopsy specimens obtained at least 2 cm above the dentate line
D. Biopsy shows absent ganglia and atrophic nerve trunks

96. Histopathologic criteria for diagnosis of Hirschsprung does not include:

A. Absent ganglia
B. Hypertrophied nerve trunk
C. Weak staining of acetylcholinesterase
D. Calretitin immunostaining as adjuvant

97. Duhamel procedure is done for:

A. Meconium ileus
B. Hirschsprung disease
C. Midgut volvulus
D. Anorectal malformation

98. Which of the following is not done for Hirschsprung?

A. Soave procedure
B. Swensen procedure
C. Duhamel procedure
D. Ladds procedure

99. Which Hirschsprung disease surgery involves preservation of an aganglionic segment with creation of neorectum?

A. Soave procedure
B. Swensen procedure
C. Duhamel procedure
D. Hartmann procedure

100. Rectal biopsy in older children performed using:

A. Bedside with suction kit
B. Local anesthesia
C. Saddle anesthesia
D. General anesthesia

101. Incorrect about anorectal malformation?

A. Incidence of imperforate anus is 1 in 5000 live births
B. Male predominance
C. Most common defect is an imperforate anus with a fistula
D. By the 8th week of gestation, the urorectal septum moves caudally to divide the cloaca

102. Which is most common anorectal malformation defect?

A. Imperforate anus
B. Imperforate anus with fistula
C. Perineal fistula
D. Cloaca

103. Rectal atresia commonly associated with:

A. Trisomy 15 B. Trisomy 18
C. Trisomy 21 D. Turner's syndrome

104. Most common anorectal malformation in males:

A. Perineal fistula
B. Rectobulbar fistula
C. Imperforate anus without fistula
D. Rectal atresia

105. Most coomon anorectal malformation in females:

A. Rectourethral fistula
B. Rectovestibular fistula
C. Rectal atresia
D. Cloaca

106. Anatomical classification of ARM is done in relationship with:

A. Internal anal sphincter
B. Ischial spine
C. Levator ani muscle
D. Coccyx

107. Regarding anorectal anatomy, false is:

A. Urorectal septum moves caudally to divide the cloaca into the anterior urogenital sinus and posterior anorectal canal
B. Complete or partial failure of the anal membrane to resorb results in an anal membrane or stenosis
C. The perineal body is formed by fusion of the genital tubercles
D. Anatomic classification of anorectal anomalies is based in relationship to the levator ani musculature

108. Which of the following is associated with ARM?

A. Hemivertebrae
B. Spinal cord dysraphism
C. Vesicoureteral reflux
D. All of the above

109. On perineal examination of newborn male shows no anal opening and no perineal fistula. Lateral pelvic film shows rectal gas above coccyx and abnormal sacrum. What is choice of procedure?

A. Anoplasty with serial dilation
B. Single stage repair without colostomy
C. Posterior sagittal anorectopexy with/without colostomy
D. Three stage reconstruction with initial colostomy

110. Initial imaging of choice for ARM:

A. Invertogram
B. Cross table lateral X-ray
C. Lower GI contrast study
D. CT scan

111. Incorrect statement about intussusception is:

A. It is usually idiopathic, without an obvious anatomic lead point
B. It is predominantly ileoileal
C. Meckel diverticulum is found to be the most common identifiable lead point
D. Seen in children from 3 months to 3 years

112. Most common location of intussusception in children:

A. Jejunoileal B. Ileoileal
C. Ileocaecal D. Colocolic

113. 2 years old child came with crampy abdominal pain with history of passing bloody mucus. Examination shows palpable mass. What is the most appropriate diagnostic test?

A. Plain radiograph B. Ultrasound
C. Upper GI scopy D. CT scan

114. Pseudokidney sign is seen in:

A. Midgut volvulus B. Intussusception
C. Pyelonephritis D. Neuroblastoma

115. Red current jelly stools seen in:

A. Intussusception
B. Midgut volvulus
C. Necrotizing enterocolitis
D. Meckel's diverticulum

116. Target sign of intussusception is seen on:

A. Plain X-ray B. Ultrasound
C. CT scan D. Barium enema

117. Correct statement about operative management of intussusceptions:

A. After successful reduction by air enema, exploration needed to rule out lead point

B. After successful reduction by barium enema, delayed laparotomy performed due risk of recurrence
C. Intra-operatively intussuscepted segment is always resected after manual reduction
D. Third recurrence after barium enema is an indication for surgical management

118. Contraindication for reduction of intussusception by barium enema is:

A. Recurrence after prior air enema
B. Age older than 5 years
C. Recurrent symptom in postoperative period
D. Pneumoperitoneum

119. Not an operative indication for intussusceptions:

A. Peritonitis
B. Bowel obstruction at initial presentation
C. Failed hydrostatic enema reduction
D. Second recurrence after air enema

120. Which is most common congenital GI anomaly?

A. Duodenal atresia
B. Intestinal duplication
C. Meckel's diverticulum
D. Hirschsprung disease

121. False regarding Meckel's diverticulum:

A. 2% incidence
B. 2 feet of IC valve
C. 2 inches of base
D. 2 types heterotopic mucosa

122. Meckel's diverticulum is confirmed by:

A. Ultrasound
B. Contrast GI study
C. Balloon endoscopy
D. 99-Tc isotope scan

123. Most common symptom of Meckel's diverticulum:

A. Abdominal pain B. Vomiting
C. Massive bleed D. Diarrhoea

HEPATOBILIARY SYSTEM

124. Extrahepatic biliary atresia is associated with:

A. Asplenia
B. Absence of the IVC
C. Intestinal malformation
D. All of the above

125. Which of the following statement is incorrect about extrahepatic biliary atresia?

A. Associated with anomalies like double spleen, intestinal malformation
B. Immune mediated inflammatory injury is responsible
C. High frequency of HLA B 27
D. Type 3 BA, involving both right and left hepatic ducts, is most common

126. Which of the following HLA type shows high frequency in biliary atresia?

A. HLA B12 B. HLA B 27
C. HLA B 8 D. HLA DQ2

127. Gold standard for the diagnosis of biliary atresia:

A. HIDA scan B. MRCP
C. Liver biopsy D. ERCP

128. Kasai procedure is a procedure of choice for which of the following?

A. Choledochal cyst B. Biliary atresia
C. Caroli's disease D. Biliary dyskinesia

129. Regarding Kasai's procedure which of the following is incorrect?

A. It involves hepatoportoenterostomy, choice for BA
B. Risk of cholangitis is less after successful procedure
C. It does not cure BA, which will inevitably progress
D. If liver transplant is needed, initial Kasai procedure is indicated

130. Which of the following is wrongly matched about choledochal cyst?

A. Type I – Simple CBD cyst
B. Type III – Choledochocoele
C. Type IV – both extra and intrahepatic cysts
D. Type V – Only extrahepatic cysts

131. Most common type of choledochal cyst:

A. Type I B. Type II
C. Type III D. Type IV

132. Caroli's disease is which type of choledochal cyst?

A. Type III B. Type IVa
C. Type IVb D. Type V

133. Which of the following is incorrect about choledochal cyst?

A. Incidence of 1 in 1000 to 5000 live births
B. It has female preponderance
C. Choledochal cysts are considered premalignant lesions
D. It can be associated with duodenal atresia, pancreatic divisum

134. Classical Triad of choledochal cyst includes all except:

A. Abdominal pain
B. Right upper quadrant mass
C. Fever
D. Jaundice

135. Which of the following is appropriate surgical procedure for most common type of choledochal cyst?

A. Observation
B. Choledochojejunostomy
C. Cyst resection only
D. Hepaticojejunostomy

136. Which of the following is incorrect statement describing hereditary pancreatitis?

A. It is an autosomal dominant disorder with high penetrance
B. Representing 10% of chronic pancreatitis
C. Recurrent bouts of pancreatitis usually begin between 5 and 10 years of age
D. Associated with mutation in gene PRSS1 on chromosome 7

137. Biliary dyskinesia is diagnosed with HIDA scan if ejection fraction is less than:

A. 15% B. 20%
C. 25% D. 35%

ABDOMINAL WALL

138. Umbilical cord hernia is defined when central abdominal wall defect is less than:

A. 2 cm B. 3 cm
C. 4 cm D. 5 cm

139. Which of the following is not associated with omphalocoele?

A. Beckwith-Wiedemann syndrome
B. Trisomy 21
C. Anorectal malformation
D. Pentalogy of Cantrell

140. Pentalogy of Cantrell does not include:

A. Omphalocoele B. Sternal cleft
C. Intracardiac defect D. Ectopia vesicae

141. Which of the following is false regarding gastroschisis?

A. Fascial defect is typically 4 cm in diameter
B. Defect is always to the left of an intact umbilical cord
C. Associated with intestinal atresia, however, other major anomalies are rare
D. Risk of late occurrence of NEC

142. Incorrect statement about inguinal hernia:

A. Incidence of inguinal hernia is approximately 3% to 5% in term infants
B. It affects boys six times more often than girls
C. 25% are bilateral
D. 60% occur on the right side, almost all are indirect

143. Silk groove sign is seen in:

A. Undescended testis
B. Inguinal hernia
C. Inguinal lymphadenopathy
D. Torsion testis

144. True about inguinal hernia repair in pediatric population:

A. Transillumination of scrotum differentiate hernia from other swelling
B. Incarceration is higher in the first year of life in premature infants
C. Contralateral inguinal exploration at the time of symptomatic hernia repair is not routinely performed
D. Laproscopic hernia repair is advantageous over open repair

145. Which of the following is incorrect regarding pediatric umbilical hernia?

A. It has a tendency to close on its own in 80% of cases of children
B. Elective repair should be deferred until around 5 years of age
C. Incarceration of an umbilical hernia is common
D. Use of prosthetic patch should never be considered

146. 2 years old child came with swelling at umbilicus without any symptoms. Examination shows 1.5 cm fascial defect. What is most appropriate management?

A. No need to operate
B. Immediate primary closure of defect electively
C. Defect closure using prosthetic mesh
D. Observation and primary repair after 5 years of age

CHEST WALL DEFORMITIES

147. What is the most common congenital chest wall deformity?

A. Pectus carinatum
B. Poland syndrome
C. Pigeon chest
D. Pectus excavatum

148. Which is false about pectus excavatum?

A. Structural deformity where the anterior chest wall is caved-in or sunken
B. More common in males
C. The optimal age for repair is 16 to 20 years of age
D. Nuss procedure is commonly used

149. Haller index is used for which congenital chest wall deformity?

A. Pectus carinatum B. Pectus excavatum
C. Pigeon chest D. Sternal cleft

150. Indications for surgical repair of chest wall deformity:

A. Haller index > 3.2
B. Mitral valve prolapse
C. Presence of murmur
D. All of the above

151. Which of the following is false about Nuss procedure?

A. Nuss procedure has largely replaced the Ravitch (open) procedure
B. The bar is passed through the retrosternal plane
C. The chest wall defect is immediately corrected
D. The bar is removed after 5 years

GENITOURINARY TRACT

152. False about cryptorchidism:

A. It occurs in 25% of full-term infants
B. The undescended testis is associated with histologic and morphologic changes as early as 6 months of age
C. Impaired spermatogenesis can occur by 4 years of age
D. It is most commonly located in the inguinal canal

153. Orchidopexy is performed at the age of:

A. 3 to 6 months B. 6 to 12 months
C. 12 to 15 months D. 15 to 18 months

154. Which of the following is false regarding undescended testis?

A. It is most commonly located in the inguinal canal
B. If both testes are nonpalpable, hCG stimulation test is done to confirm the presence of functioning testes
C. Orchidopexy decreases malignancy risk associated with undescended testes
D. Nonseminomatous germ cell tumors are the most common tumor type with undescended testes

155. About torsion testis, incorrect statement is:

A. Most frequently in early adolescence with a peak incidence at 14 years of age
B. Extravaginal torsion is associated with a bell clapper deformity
C. Radioisotope scanning is the most specific diagnostic test
D. Immediate surgical detorsion through a scrotal medial raphe approach is the standard

PEDIATRIC TUMORS

156. Most common extracranial solid tumor in children:

A. Nephrolastoma
B. Neuroblastoma
C. Hepatoblastoma
D. Rhabdomyosarcoma

157. Most common location of neuroblastoma:

A. Neck B. Chest
C. Abdomen D. Pelvis

158. Blueberry muffin syndrome associated with:

A. Wilms' tumor
B. Neuroblastoma
C. Hepatoblastoma
D. Rhabdomyosarcoma

159. Which of the following is incorrect about neuroblastoma?

A. Most often detected incidentally
B. Associate with MYCN gene amplification
C. Hyperploidy is associated with unfavorable prognosis

D. Infant with stage 4S disease, regress spontaneously

160. Which of the following is associated with good prognosis in neuroblastoma?

A. MYCN amplification
B. Deletion of chromosome 1p
C. Deletion of chromosome 11q
D. Gain of chromosome 17

161. Children's oncology group stratify neuroblastoma based on all except:

A. Age at diagnosis
B. MYCN amplification
C. INSS stage
D. Mitotic index

162. Following syndromes are associated with Wilms' tumor except:

A. Beckwith-Wiedemann syndrome
B. Denys-Drash syndrome
C. Li-Fraumeni syndrome
D. Cowden syndrome

163. Which of the following is incorrect about Wilms' tumor?

A. It is diagnosed in children younger than 5 years of age
B. Bilateral tumors are noted in 30% of patients at diagnosis
C. It is typically discovered incidentally during a physical examination
D. 25% of patients have hypertension

164. Location of WT1 gene:

A. Chromosome 11p13 B. Chromosome 11p15
C. Chromosome 11q13 D. Chromosome 11q15

165. Beckwith-Wiedemann consists of following anomalies except:

A. Macrosomia
B. Abdominal wall defects
C. Neonatal hypoglycemia
D. Gonadal dysgenesis

166. Gene mutation associated with Beckwith-Wiedemann syndrome:

A. p53 B. WT1
C. WT2 D. SDH

167. Denys-Drash syndrome present with which of the following?

A. Macrosomia
B. Gonadal dysgenesis
C. Mental retardation
D. Neuropathy

168. WAGR syndrome presents with all of the following except:

A. Aniridia
B. Hemihypertrophy
C. Mental retardation
D. Abdominal wall defects

169. Which of the following is an unfavorable histology for Wilms' tumor?

A. Blastemal cell tumor
B. Clear cell tumor
C. Stromal cell tumor
D. Epithelial cell tumor

170. Which of the following is favorable histology for Wilm's tumor?

A. Anaplasia
B. Clear cell tumor
C. Rhabdoid cell tumor
D. Epithelial cell tumor

171. Which of the following is false statement regarding Wilms' tumor?

A. SIOP staging system is based on preoperative chemotherapy but is applied after resection
B. NWTSG stratifies patients after resection but before the initiation of chemotherapy
C. Biopsy taken before removal is staged I in NWTSG of Wilms' tumor
D. Residual tumor is confined to the abdomen and of nonhematogenous spread is staged III in NWTSG staging

172. Following is not a type of rhabdomyosarcoma:

A. Embryonal B. Alveolar
C. Pleomorphic D. Fibrous

173. Most common site of rhabdomyosarcoma:

A. Head and neck
B. Chest wall
C. Genitourinary tract
D. Extremities

174. Which of the following is incorrect about rhabdomyosarcoma?

A. There is a bimodal peak in ages at diagnosis

B. Rhabdomyosarcomas involve the proximal limb more commonly
C. Botryoid and spindle cell rhabdomyosarcomas have favorable prognosis
D. At diagnosis, 50% of patients have regional lymph node metastasis

175. Which of the following is correct about hepatoblastoma?

A. Hepatoblastoma represents 80% of all malignant liver tumors
B. Jaundice is common presenting symptom
C. An elevated AFP level is pathognomonic
D. Liver transplant is contraindicated in unresectable hepatoblastoma

176. PRETEXT definition system for hepatoblastoma is classified by:

A. Number of tumor involved segments of liver
B. Number of tumor involved sections of liver
C. Number of tumor free segments of liver
D. Number of tumor free sections of liver

177. Which of the following is false regarding teratoma?

A. More commonly present in females
B. Gonadal teratoma occur primarily in neonates
C. Age at diagnosis is most important prognostic factor
D. Failure to resect coccyx associated with 35% risk of recurrence

178. 'Altman classification' is used for:

A. Neuroblastoma
B. Osteosarcoma
C. Sacrococcygeal teratoma
D. Multiple myeloma

179. Most common ovarian tumor of pediatric population:

A. Serous cystadenoma B. Teratoma
C. Dysgerminoma D. Yolk sac tumor

180. Which of the following is true regarding pediatric trauma?

A. Thoracic injury is the second leading cause of death in pediatric trauma
B. Rib fractures in young toddlers should raise a high index of suspicion for child abuse
C. Thoracotomy is indicated when chest tube blood drainage of 2 mL/kg/hr
D. Traumatic diaphragmatic rupture is more common on the right side

ANSWERS

1. **Ans: B. 23°C**

Ref: Chapter No. 67, Page No. 1845

2. **Ans: B. Closure of ductus arteriosus**

Ref: Chapter No. 67, Page No. 1845

3. **Ans: C. Neonatal lung has higher type II pneumocytes**

Ref: Chapter No. 67, Page No. 1845

4. **Ans: D. 5% Dextrose in 0.45% NS with 20 mEq/L potassium**

Ref: Chapter No. 67, Page No. 1845

5. **Ans: C. Normal saline**

Ref: Chapter No. 67, Page No. 1845

6. **Ans: B. 120 calories/kg/day**

Ref: Chapter No. 67, Page No. 1845

7. **Ans: C. Fat**

Ref: Chapter No. 67, Page No. 1846

8. **Ans: A. 2-3 days**

Ref: Chapter No. 67, Page No. 1846

9. **Ans: B. Restoring enteral nutrition**

Ref: Chapter No. 67, Page No. 1846

10. **Ans: B. Scalp**

Ref: Chapter No. 67, Page No. 1846

11. **Ans: C. They are often osteolytic**

Ref: Chapter No. 67, Page No. 1846

12. **Ans: C. It is characterized by painless regional lymph-adenopathy**

Ref: Chapter No. 67, Page No. 1846

13. **Ans: D. Aggressive and radical resection required**

Ref: Chapter No. 67, Page No. 1846-1847

14. **Ans: C. Just below hyoid bone**

Ref: Chapter No. 67, Page No. 1847

15. **Ans: B. Thyroid diverticulum develops as a lateral ectodermal thickening at the foramen caecum**

Ref: Chapter No. 67, Page No. 1847

16. **Ans: C. Sistrunk procedure**

Ref: Chapter No. 67, Page No. 1847

17. **Ans: D. Thyroid gland**

Ref: Chapter No. 67, Page No. 1847

18. **Ans: D. Third branchial cleft remnants have associated sinuses or fistulas in the suprasternal notch**

Ref: Chapter No. 67, Page No. 1847

19. **Ans: C. Second branchial anomalies located at posterior border of sternocleidomastoid**

Ref: Chapter No. 67, Page No. 1847

20. **Ans: B. Tonsillar fossa or other nasopharyngeal spaces**

Ref: Chapter No. 67, Page No. 1847

21. **Ans: D. All of the above**

Ref: Chapter No. 67, Page No. 1848

22. **Ans: A. Meconium aspiration**

Ref: Chapter No. 67, Page No. 1848

23. **Ans: D. Oxygen index greater than 40**

Ref: Chapter No. 67, Page No. 1848

24. **Ans: B. Weight less than 3 kg**

Ref: Chapter No. 67, Page No. 1848

25. **Ans: C. Bilateral defects occur in 10%**

Ref: Chapter No. 67, Page No. 1848

26. **Ans: B. Product of the longest two perpendicular linear measurements of the lung contralateral to CDH and is divided by head circumference**

Ref: Chapter No. 67, Page No. 1848

27. **Ans: B. 15 weeks**

Ref: Chapter No. 67, Page No. 1848

28. **Ans: B. Morgagni hernia**

Ref: Chapter No. 67, Page No. 1848

29. **Ans: D. Left posterolateral**

Ref: Chapter No. 67, Page No. 1848

30. **Ans: B. Endotracheal intubation with ventilation**

Ref: Chapter No. 67, Page No. 1849

31. **Ans: B. Diaphragmatic eventration**

Ref: Chapter No. 67, Page No. 1850

32. **Ans: C. Dynamic USG chest**

Ref: Chapter No. 67, Page No. 1850

33. **Ans: D. Repair is done through thoracic approach**

Ref: Chapter No. 67, Page No. 1850

34. **Ans: D. Asymptomatic cysts are usually managed by observation**

Ref: Chapter No. 67, Page No. 1850

35. **Ans: B. Stocker**

Ref: Chapter No. 67, Page No. 1850

36. **Ans: C. Blood supply is from aorta**

Ref: Chapter No. 67, Page No. 1850

37. **Ans: B. Type I consist of a numerous cysts, usually measuring less than 1 cm in diameter**

Ref: Chapter No. 67, Page No. 1850

38. **Ans: D. Type IV CPAM**

Ref: Chapter No. 67, Page No. 1850

39. **Ans: B. Can be located intralobar or extralobar**

Ref: Chapter No. 67, Page No. 1850

40. **Ans: B. There is hereditary association of VATERL anomalies**

Ref: Chapter No. 67, Page No. 1852

41. **Ans: C. Esophageal atresia with distal TEF**

Ref: Chapter No. 67, Page No. 1852

42. **Ans: D. Eye deformities**

Ref: Chapter No. 67, Page No. 1852

43. **Ans: C. Esophageal atresia with TEF**

Ref: Chapter No. 67, Page No. 1852

44. **Ans: A. It has female predominance**

Ref: Chapter No. 67, Page No. 1852

45. **Ans: B. Inability to pass NG tube into stomach**

Ref: Chapter No. 67, Page No. 1852

46. **Ans: B. Right thoracotomy**

Ref: Chapter No. 67, Page No. 1852

47. **Ans: D. All of the above**

Ref: Chapter No. 67, Page No. 1854

48. **Ans: B. Nissen fundoplication**

Ref: Chapter No. 67, Page No. 1854

49. **Ans: D. Hypertrophy of the longitudinal muscle of the pylorus**

Ref: Chapter No. 67, Page No. 1854

50. **Ans: C. Hypokalemic, hypochloremic, metabolic alkalosis**

Ref: Chapter No. 67, Page No. 1855

51. **Ans: C. Palpation of the pyloric "olive" tumor in the epigastrium**

Ref: Chapter No. 67, Page No. 1855

52. **Ans: D. All of the above**

Ref: Chapter No. 67, Page No. 1855

53. **Ans: B. Ramstedt procedure**

Ref: Chapter No. 67, Page No. 1855

54. **Ans: C. Distal to ampulla of Vater**

Ref: Chapter No. 67, Page No. 1855

55. **Ans: B. Double bubble sign**

Ref: Chapter No. 67, Page No. 1855

56. **Ans: B. Duodenal atresia**

Ref: Chapter No. 67, Page No. 1855

57. **Ans: C. Duodenoduodenostomy**

Ref: Chapter No. 67, Page No. 1855

58. **Ans: B. Jejunoileal atresia**

Ref: Chapter No. 67, Page No. 1856

59. **Ans: C. Cystic fibrosis**

Ref: Chapter No. 67, Page No. 1856

60. **Ans: C. Type IIIb atresia**

Ref: Chapter No. 67, Page No. 1856

61. **Ans: D. Type IIIb – String of sausage appearance**

Ref: Chapter No. 67, Page No. 1856

62. **Ans: D. Type IV**

Ref: Chapter No. 67, Page No. 1856

63. **Ans: D. Counterclockwise around axis of SMA by 270 degree**

Ref: Chapter No. 67, Page No. 1856

64. **Ans: B. 12 weeks**

Ref: Chapter No. 67, Page No. 1857

65. **Ans: B. Complete nonrotation**

Ref: Chapter No. 67, Page No. 1857

66. **Ans: B. Midgut is suspended on a narrow SMA stalk, which can twist in a counterclockwise fashion**

Ref: Chapter No. 67, Page No. 1857

67. **Ans: B. Nonrotation of the duodenojejunal limb, followed by normal rotation and fixation of the cecocolic limb**

Ref: Chapter No. 67, Page No. 1857

68. **Ans: D. All of the above**

Ref: Chapter No. 67, Page No. 1857

69. **Ans: B. Midgut volvulus**

Ref: Chapter No. 67, Page No. 1857

70. **Ans: C. Upper GI contrast study**

Ref: Chapter No. 67, Page No. 1857

71. **Ans: C. Appearance of a bird's beak in the fourth portion of the duodenum**

Ref: Chapter No. 67, Page No. 1857

72. **Ans: C. Ascending colon to the posterior aspect of the right upper quadrant**

Ref: Chapter No. 67, Page No. 1857

73. **Ans: C. Appendectomy is not routinely performed**

Ref: Chapter No. 67, Page No. 1857

74. **Ans: B. Midgut volvulus**

Ref: Chapter No. 67, Page No. 1857

75. **Ans: B. Necrotizing enterocolitis**

Ref: Chapter No. 67, Page No. 1858

76. **Ans: C. Necrotizing enterocolitis**

Ref: Chapter No. 67, Page No. 1858

77. **Ans: B. Pneumatosis intestinalis**

Ref: Chapter No. 67, Page No. 1858

78. **Ans: C. Operative laparotomy with stoma creation**

Ref: Chapter No. 67, Page No. 1858

79. **Ans: D. It is associated with premature GI tract which allows translocation of bacterias**

Ref: Chapter No. 67, Page No. 1858

80. **Ans: C. Peumoperitoneum**

Ref: Chapter No. 67, Page No. 1858

81. **Ans: D. Orogastric tube decompression, fluid resuscitation, IV antibiotics and serial radiographs**

Ref: Chapter No. 67, Page No. 1858

82. **Ans: C. Necrotizing enterocolitis**

Ref: Chapter No. 67, Page No. 1859

83. **Ans: B. Jejunum**

Ref: Chapter No. 67, Page No. 1859

84. **Ans: D. All of the above**

Ref: Chapter No. 67, Page No. 1859

85. **Ans: D. It presents with bilious vomiting and failure to pass meconium**

Ref: Chapter No. 67, Page No. 1860

86. **Ans: A. Dilated small bowel loops with air-fluid levels**

Ref: Chapter No. 67, Page No. 1860

87. **Ans: B. NG tube, hydration and contrast enema with gastrograffin**

Ref: Chapter No. 67, Page No. 1860

88. **Ans: C. 60 mEq/L**

Ref: Chapter No. 67, Page No. 1860

89. **Ans: D. Immediate laparotomy with stoma creation**

Ref: Chapter No. 67, Page No. 1860

90. **Ans: C. Contrast enema can be diagnostic as well as therapeutic**

Ref: Chapter No. 67, Page No. 1860

91. **Ans: B. Girls being affected four times more frequently than boys**

Ref: Chapter No. 67, Page No. 1860

92. **Ans: A. Absent ganglionic cells in both Auerbach and Meissner plexuses**

Ref: Chapter No. 67, Page No. 1860

93. **Ans: A. Enterocolitis**

Ref: Chapter No. 67, Page No. 1860

94. **Ans: D. Full thickness rectal biopsy**

Ref: Chapter No. 67, Page No. 1860

95. **Ans: D. Biopsy shows absent ganglia and atrophic nerve trunks**

Ref: Chapter No. 67, Page No. 1860-1861

96. **Ans: C. Weak staining of acetylcholinesterase**

Ref: Chapter No. 67, Page No. 1861

97. **Ans: B. Hirschsprung disease**

Ref: Chapter No. 67, Page No. 1861

98. **Ans: D. Ladds procedure**

Ref: Chapter No. 67, Page No. 1861

99. **Ans: C. Duhamel procedure**

Ref: Chapter No. 67, Page No. 1861

100. **Ans: D. General anesthesia**

Ref: Chapter No. 67, Page No. 1861

101. **Ans: D. By the 8th week of gestation, the urorectal septum moves caudally to divide the cloaca**

Ref: Chapter No. 67, Page No. 1861

102. **Ans: B. Imperforate anus with fistula**

Ref: Chapter No. 67, Page No. 1861

103. **Ans: C. Trisomy 21**

Ref: Chapter No. 67, Page No. 1861

104. **Ans: B. Rectobulbar fistula**

Ref: Chapter No. 67, Page No. 1861

105. **Ans: B. Rectovestibular fistula**

Ref: Chapter No. 67, Page No. 1861

106. **Ans: C. Levator ani muscle**

Ref: Chapter No. 67, Page No. 1861

107. **Ans: C. The perineal body is formed by fusion of the genital tubercles**

Ref: Chapter No. 67, Page No. 1861

108. **Ans: D. All of the above**

Ref: Chapter No. 67, Page No. 1862

109. **Ans: D. Three stage reconstruction with initial colostomy**

Ref: Chapter No. 67, Page No. 1862

110. **Ans: B. Cross table lateral X-ray**

Ref: Chapter No. 67, Page No. 1862

111. **Ans: B. It is predominantly ileoileal**

Ref: Chapter No. 67, Page No. 1863

112. **Ans: C. Ileocaecal**

Ref: Chapter No. 67, Page No. 1863

113. Ans: B. Ultrasound

Ref: Chapter No. 67, Page No. 1863

114. Ans: B. Intussusception

Ref: Chapter No. 67, Page No. 1863

115. Ans: A. Intussusception

Ref: Chapter No. 67, Page No. 1863

116. Ans: B. Ultrasound

Ref: Chapter No. 67, Page No. 1863

117. Ans: C. Intra-operatively intussuscepted segment is always resected after manual reduction

Ref: Chapter No. 67, Page No. 1864

118. Ans: D. Pneumoperitoneum

Ref: Chapter No. 67, Page No. 1864

119. Ans: D. Second recurrence after air enema

Ref: Chapter No. 67, Page No. 1864

120. Ans: C. Meckel's diverticulum

Ref: Chapter No. 67, Page No. 1864

121. Ans: C. 2 inches of base

Ref: Chapter No. 67, Page No. 1864

122. Ans: D. 99-Tc isotope scan

Ref: Chapter No. 67, Page No. 1864

123. Ans: C. Massive bleed

Ref: Chapter No. 67, Page No. 1864

124. Ans: D. All of the above

Ref: Chapter No. 67, Page No. 1864

125. Ans: C. High frequency of HLA B 27

Ref: Chapter No. 67, Page No. 1864-1865

126. Ans: A. HLA B_{12}

Ref: Chapter No. 67, Page No. 1865

127. Ans: C. Liver biopsy

Ref: Chapter No. 67, Page No. 1865

128. Ans: B. Biliary atresia

Ref: Chapter No. 67, Page No. 1865

129. Ans: B. Risk of cholangitis is less after successful procedure

Ref: Chapter No. 67, Page No. 1866

130. Ans: D. Type V – Only extrahepatic cysts

Ref: Chapter No. 67, Page No. 1866

131. Ans: A. Type I

Ref: Chapter No. 67, Page No. 1866

132. Ans: D. Type V

Ref: Chapter No. 67, Page No. 1866

133. Ans: A. Incidence of 1 in 1000 to 5000 live births

Ref: Chapter No. 67, Page No. 1866

134. Ans: C. Fever

Ref: Chapter No. 67, Page No. 1866

135. Ans: D. Hepaticojejunostomy

Ref: Chapter No. 67, Page No. 1866

136. Ans: B. Representing 10% of chronic pancreatitis

Ref: Chapter No. 67, Page No. 1866

137. Ans: D. 35%

Ref: Chapter No. 67, Page No. 1867

138. Ans: C. 4 cm

Ref: Chapter No. 67, Page No. 1867

139. Ans: C. Anorectal malformation

Ref: Chapter No. 67, Page No. 1867

140. Ans: D. Ectopia vesicae

Ref: Chapter No. 67, Page No. 1867

141. Ans: B. Defect is always to the left of an intact umbilical cord

Ref: Chapter No. 67, Page No. 1867-1868

142. Ans: C. 25% are bilateral

Ref: Chapter No. 67, Page No. 1868

143. Ans: B. Inguinal hernia

Ref: Chapter No. 67, Page No. 1868

144. Ans: B. Incarceration is higher in the first year of life in premature infants

Ref: Chapter No. 67, Page No. 1869

145. Ans: C. Incarceration of an umbilical hernia is common

Ref: Chapter No. 67, Page No. 1869

146. Ans: D. Observation and primary repair after 5 years of age

Ref: Chapter No. 67, Page No. 1869

147. Ans: D. Pectus excavatum

Ref: Chapter No. 67, Page No. 1869

148. Ans: C. The optimal age for repair is 16 to 20 years of age

Ref: Chapter No. 67, Page No. 1869

149. Ans: B. Pectus excavatum

Ref: Chapter No. 67, Page No. 1869

150. Ans . D. All of the above

Ref: Chapter No. 67, Page No. 1869

151. Ans: D. The bar is removed after 5 years

Ref: Chapter No. 67, Page No. 1869

152. Ans: C. Impaired spermatogenesis can occur by 4 years of age

Ref: Chapter No. 67, Page No. 1870

153. Ans: B. 6 to 12 months

Ref: Chapter No. 67, Page No. 1870

154. Ans: C. Orchidopexy decreases malignancy risk associated with undescended testes

Ref: Chapter No. 67, Page No. 1870

155. Ans: B. Extravaginal torsion is associated with a bell clapper deformity

Ref: Chapter No. 67, Page No. 1870

156. Ans: B. Neuroblastoma

Ref: Chapter No. 67, Page No. 1871

157. Ans: C. Abdomen

Ref: Chapter No. 67, Page No. 1871

158. Ans: B. Neuroblastoma

Ref: Chapter No. 67, Page No. 1871

159. Ans: C. Hyperploidy is associated with unfavorable prognosis

Ref: Chapter No. 67, Page No. 1871

160. Ans: D. Gain of chromosome 17

Ref: Chapter No. 67, Page No. 1871

161. Ans: D. Mitotic index

Ref: Chapter No. 67, Page No. 1871

162. Ans: D. Cowden syndrome

Ref: Chapter No. 67, Page No. 1873

163. Ans: B. Bilateral tumors are noted in 30% of patients at diagnosis

Ref: Chapter No. 67, Page No. 1873

164. Ans: A. Chromosome 11p13

Ref: Chapter No. 67, Page No. 1873

165. Ans: D. Gonadal dysgenesis

Ref: Chapter No. 67, Page No. 1873

166. Ans: C. WT2

Ref: Chapter No. 67, Page No. 1873

167. Ans: B. Gonadal dysgenesis

Ref: Chapter No. 67, Page No. 1873

168. Ans: D. Abdominal wall defects

Ref: Chapter No. 67, Page No. 1873

169. Ans: B. Clear cell tumor

Ref: Chapter No. 67, Page No. 1873

170. Ans: D. Epithelial cell tumor

Ref: Chapter No. 67, Page No. 1873

171. Ans: C. Biopsy taken before removal is staged I in NWTSG of Wilms' tumor

Ref: Chapter No. 67, Page No. 1873

172. Ans: D. Fibrous

Ref: Chapter No. 67, Page No. 1874

173. Ans: A. Head and neck

Ref: Chapter No. 67, Page No. 1874

174. Ans: B. Rhabdomyosarcomas involve the proximal limb more commonly

Ref: Chapter No. 67, Page No. 1874

175. Ans: A. Hepatoblastoma represents 80% of all malignant liver tumors

Ref: Chapter No. 67, Page No. 1875-1876

176. Ans: D. Number of tumor free sections of liver

Ref: Chapter No. 67, Page No. 1876

177. Ans: B. Gonadal teratoma occur primarily in neonates

Ref: Chapter No. 67, Page No. 1876

178. Ans: C. Sacrococcygeal teratoma

Ref: Chapter No. 67, Page No. 1877

179. Ans: B. Teratoma

Ref: Chapter No. 67, Page No. 1878

180. Ans: D. Traumatic diaphragmatic rupture is more common on the right side

Ref: Chapter No. 67, Page No. 1879

68

Neurosurgery

1. **About production of CSF fluid:**
   A. Production at the rate of 20-25 ml/Hr
   B. Production is affected by increased ICP
   C. Ventriculitis causes decreased production
   D. CSF production is not constant

2. **Following is avoided in hyperperfusion state with elevated $PaCO_2$:**
   A. Increased ventilation B. Diuretics
   C. Mannitol D. Barbiturates

3. **Reversible brain ischemia occur with blood flow:**
   A. 0.30 to 0.50 ml/g/min
   B. 0.20 to 0.25 ml/g/min
   C. 0.15 to 0.20 ml/g/min
   D. 0.1 to 0.15 ml/g/min

4. **Duret haemorrhages seen in:**
   A. Ventricle B. Midbrain
   C. Medulla D. Cerebellum

5. **Carotid-cavernous fistula due to acquired (traumatic) cause is:**
   A. Type 1 B. Type 2
   C. Type 3 D. Type 4

6. **Imaging modality of choice for Cavernous hemangioma:**
   A. CT B. MRI
   C. DSA D. PET

7. **False about AVM:**
   A. Congenital lesion of an abnormal collection of blood vessels
   B. Often progress from high-flow lesions at birth to lower flow lesions in adulthood
   C. Risk of hemorrhage rate is up to 4% per year
   D. SRS is usually reserved for lesions less the 2.5 cm in diameter

8. **False about Cavernous Malformations:**
   A. Benign vascular lesion consisting of irregular thin-walled sinusoidal vascular channels
   B. Located in brain with intervening neural parenchyma
   C. Low-pressure, low-flow lesions, hemorrhage is typically not catastrophic
   D. Demonstrates a characteristic dark hemosiderin ring on MRI

9. **Which of the following not treated with surgery:**
   A. Capillary telangiectasia
   B. Venous angioma
   C. Both A and B
   D. None of the above

10. **False about Venous Angioma of brain:**
    A. Abnormally configured venous drainage system
    B. Typical appearance is that of a hydra
    C. Treatment includes SRS or surgical resection of lesion
    D. Characteristic feature is poorly collateralized venous bed

11. **Spetzler-Martin grading used for:**
    A. Aneurysm B. SAH
    C. AVM D. Meningioma

12. **Spetzler-Martin grading includes all except:**
    A. Nidus size
    B. Location in brain
    C. Eloquence
    D. Pattern of drainage

13. **Characteristic of traumatic Carotid-cavernous fistula is:**
    A. Pseudoaneurysm at anterior circulation

B. Dilated superior ophthalmic vein
C. Intra-parenchymal hemorrhage
D. Dilated jugular vein

14. Major cause of death in patients with SAH:

A. Cardiac event
B. Rebleeding
C. Seizures
D. Vasospasm

15. According to Hunt and Hess grading for SAH, patient having focal deficit is of which clinical grade:

A. Grade 1
B. Grade 2
C. Grade 3
D. Grade 4

16. CT based grading used for SAH:

A. Hunt and Hess Grading
B. World Federation of Neurological Surgeons grade (WFNS)
C. Simpson Grading
D. Fischer Grading

17. Following are true about Subarachnoid hemorrhage except:

A. Trauma is most common cause of SAH
B. Most common aneurysms occur at anterior circulation
C. Risk of rupture is greater with posterior circulation aneurysms
D. Charcot-Bouchart aneurismal rupture occurs in internal capsule

18. Which of the following is incorrect about Amyloid angiopathy:

A. Seen in older patients with dementia
B. Multiple episodes of hemorrhages
C. Centrally located intracerebral hematomas
D. All of the above

19. Moyamoya disease characterized by all except:

A. Atherosclerotic narrowing of minor cerebral vessels
B. Bilateral and not necessarily symmetrical
C. Multiple clusters of collateral vessels giving "puff of smoke" appearance
D. Subarachnoid or basal ganglia hemorrhage are most common presentations

20. Surgical bypass for Moyamoya disease typically done between:

A. ECA and ICA
B. ICA and PCA
C. ICA artery and PCA
D. Superficial temporal artery and MCA

21. Most common presenting symptom of brain tumor:

A. Headache
B. Seizure
C. Nausea and vomiting
D. Focal deficit

22. Which is wrongly matched symptom?

A. Frontal lobe – personality change
B. Temporal lobe – Memory change
C. Parietal lobe – Alexia
D. Infratentorial lesion – Cranial nerve deficits

23. Which of the following is incorrect:

A. Gadolinium contrast MRI – Localize small metastases
B. Diffusion weighted MRI – Distinguish between glioma and abscess
C. Functional MRI – Presurgical planning in eloquent areas
D. Diffusion tensor MRI – Predict response to radiotherapy

24. Most common primary brain tumor in adults:

A. Pilocytic astrocytoma
B. Lymphoma
C. Glioblastoma multiforme
D. Meningioma

25. Glioblastoma Multiforme is:

A. WHO grade 1
B. WHO grade 2
C. WHO grade 3
D. WHO grade 4

26. Drug of choice for Glioblastoma multiforme:

A. Dacarbazine
B. Temozolamide
C. Carmustine
D. Bevacizumab

27. MRI characteristic of glioblastoma multiforme:

A. Ring enhancement with edema
B. Target lesion
C. Ring enhancement without edema
D. Both A and B

28. Pilocytic astrocytoma is classified by WHO grade as:

A. Grade 1
B. Grade 2
C. Grade 3
D. Grade 4

29. Anaplastic astrocytoma is:

A. WHO grade I
B. WHO grade II
C. WHO grade III
D. WHO grade IV

30. Oligodendroglioma all are true except:
- A. Tumor presented at 40 years of age
- B. It has male preponderance
- C. Favorable response with gain of Chromosome 1p and 19q
- D. It is aggressive anaplastic

31. Spinal drop metastasis seen with:
- A. Oligodendroglioma
- B. Ependymoma
- C. Meningioma
- D. Midbrain glioma

32. Spinal drop mets of ependymoma seen at:
- A. Subdural
- B. Subarachnoid
- C. Spinal canal
- D. Spinal cord

33. Lhermitte-Duclos disease is:
- A. Glomus jugulare tumor
- B. Multiple sclerosis
- C. Dysplastic cerebellar gangliocytoma
- D. Pineoblastoma

34. Parinaud syndrome is:
- A. Supranuclear vertical gaze palsy by compression of tectal plate
- B. Supranuclear vertical gaze palsy by compression of tegmen
- C. Supranuclear downward gaze palsy by compression of tectal plate
- D. Supranuclear downward gaze palsy by compression of tegmen

35. Spinal drop mets are seen in all except:
- A. Ependymoma
- B. Pineoblastoma
- C. Medulloblastoma
- D. Hemangioblastoma

36. Papillary tumor of pineal region is WHO grade:
- A. Grade I
- B. Grade II
- C. Grade III
- D. Both B and C

37. False about medulloblastoma:
- A. Infratentorial tumor of childhood
- B. Female preponderance
- C. Disseminate through CSF with drop mets
- D. Sensitive to radiotherapy and chemotherapy

38. True about Schwannoma is:
- A. Bilateral tumors may be associated with NF-1
- B. Tumors less than 3 cm are always resected
- C. Nerve resection is always done
- D. It is slow growing tumor

39. Simpson Grading used for:
- A. Meningioma
- B. Schwannoma
- C. Oligodendroglioma
- D. Glioblastoma

40. Hemangioblastoma is seen with:
- A. NF 1
- B. NF 2
- C. VHL
- D. Cowden

41. Which of the following is false about Primary CNS lymphoma:
- A. Observed in 2% to 6% of patients with AIDS
- B. Dramatic short lived response to steroids
- C. Intrathecal methotrexate reserved for young patient
- D. Peak incidence seen at 35 years with immuno-competent

42. Parinaud syndrome is:
- A. Upward gaze palsy
- B. Convergence
- C. Accommodation
- D. All are true

43. All are true about germ cell tumors of brain:
- A. Most present between 10 and 20 years of age
- B. Suprasellar tumors more common in males
- C. Presented with hydrocephalus or Perinaud syndrome
- D. Sensitive to radiotherapy and chemotherapy

44. Embryonal carcinoma of brain is:
- A. It is seen prepubertal age
- B. It is considered malignant and invasive
- C. It is associated with Klinefelter syndrome
- D. All are true

45. About non germ cell tumors of CNS, incorrect is:
- A. Most common in ages 0 to 3 years
- B. They have worse prognosis
- C. Mixed germ cell is variety of non-germ cell tumor
- D. None of the above

46. "Stalk effect" seen with prolactin levels:
- A. Less than 25 ng/ml
- B. 25-150 ng/ml
- C. 150-300 ng/ml
- D. > 300 ng/ml

47. Diagnostic levels of prolactin for prolactinoma:
- A. > 50 ng/ml
- B. > 100 ng/ml
- C. > 150 ng/ml
- D. > 200 ng/ml

48. Parinaud syndrome seen with:

A. Pineocytoma
B. Suprasellar tumor
C. CNS germ cell tumors
D. All of the above

49. All are true about craniopharyngioma except:

A. Peak incidence between 5 and 10 years of age
B. Tumor is histologically benign
C. Most frequent postoperative complications include diabetes insipidus and hypothalamic injury
D. All are true

50. Which of the following is false about brain metastasis?

A. Most common brain tumor in adults
B. Highest incidence of brain metastasis is seen in the fifth to seventh decades of life
C. Equally common among men and women
D. Anticonvulsant recommended for all patients

51. Shortest interval to develop brain metastasis:

A. Breast B. Melanoma
C. Lung D. Adrenal

52. Following can be option for multiple brain metastasis:

A. Excision of symptomatic lesion or multiple lesions
B. Stereotactic radiosurgery
C. Hippocampal sparing whole brain radiotherapy
D. All are feasible

53. False about Diffuse axonal injury:

A. It is rotational injury of white matter pathways
B. Diagnosed with CT brain
C. Causes deterioration of GCS
D. Functional or anatomic disruption of pathways

54. GCS of patient with eye opening to pain, inappropriate words and withdrawal to painful stimuli:

A. 8 B. 9
C. 10 D. 11

55. Any clot or contusion is operated if volume is more than:

A. 20 ml B. 30 ml
C. 40 ml D. 50 ml

56. Wrong about ICP monitoring required with severe brain injury:

A. Age >40 years B. GCS < 10
C. Unilateral posturing D. SBP < 90 mm of Hg

57. Not recommended for traumatic brain injury:

A. CPP between 60-70 mm of Hg
B. $PaCO_2$ 30-35 mm of Hg
C. SBP > 100 mm of Hg
D. ICP > 20 mm of Hg

58. First line therapy to decrease ICP post trauma:

A. Sedation and paralyze
B. Barbiturate coma
C. CSF drainage
D. Craniotomy

59. Recommendation for traumatic brain injury:

A. Early prophylactic hypothermia is required
B. Nutrition initiated at 5 days of injury
C. Seizure prophylaxis prevents late post traumatic seizures
D. Steroids are used to relieve edema

60. Most common Lumbar disc herniation:

A. Anterior B. Posterior
C. Anterolateral D. Posterolateral

61. Reflex lost with C6-C7 disc herniation:

A. Deltoid B. Biceps
C. Brachioradialis D. Triceps

62. Most common cervical disc herniation seen at:

A. C4-C5 B. C5-C6
C. C6-C7 D. C7-T1

63. Spurling sign is seen with:

A. Atlantoaxial subluxation
B. Cervical disc herniation
C. Cervical vertebra fracture
D. Thoracic canal stenosis

64. Gamma knife for SRS uses:

A. Nd:YAG B. Cobalt - 201
C. Yttrium 90 D. Cu – 64

65. Parkinson best treated with stimulation of following:

A. Globus pallidus interna
B. Vim nucleus

C. Globus pallidus externa
D. Subthalamic nuclei

66. Wrong about deep brain stimulation therapy:

A. Parkinson disease is most common movement disorder treated
B. Subthalamic nucleus stimulation most effective for tremors and dystonia
C. Vagus nerve stimulation approved by FDA for intractable seizures
D. Subthalamic nucleus as a target of choice has replaced GPi nucleus for Parkinson

67. Regarding epilepsy treatment wrong is:

A. Wada test used for language dominance
B. Anterior temporal lobectomy is the most commonly performed operation
C. Hemispherectomy reserved for young children with Rasmussen syndrome
D. Corpus callosotomy eliminate epilepsy focus

68. Offending vessel in Trigeminal neuralgia is:

A. Posterior cerebellar artery
B. Superior cerebellar artery
C. Basilar artery
D. Inferior cerebellar artery

69. Triad of Normal pressure hydrocephalus except:

A. Dementia B. Paraparesis
C. Gait ataxia D. Incontinence

70. Dandy-Walker malformation characterized by except:

A. Cystic expansion of forth ventricle
B. Hydrocephalus
C. Descent of cerebellar vermis
D. Abnormally high tentorium

71. Following is not an obstructive hydrocephalus:

A. Chiari type II malformation
B. Vein of Galen aneurysm
C. Arachnoid cysts
D. Intraventricular hemorrhage

72. Most common type of encephalocele in western population:

A. Frontal B. Temporal
C. Occipital D. Basal

73. Occult spinal dysraphism frequently associated with:

A. Hair tufts
B. Dermal sinus tracts
C. Tethered spinal cord
D. All of the above

74. False about Chiari I malformation:

A. Congenital malformation usually diagnosed in adults
B. Downward displacement of medulla
C. Associated syringomyelia of cervical spinal cord
D. May cause cranial nerve palsy or cerebellar syndrome

75. Most common suture involved in craniosynostosis:

A. Coronal B. Sagittal
C. Lambdoid D. Metopic

76. Wrong about subdural empyema:

A. Most common route is hematogenous
B. 60% are associated with frontal and ethmoid sinusitis
C. Cause cortical sinus thrombosis leading to cerebral infarction
D. Anticonvulsant require even in absence of seizures

77. All are true about bacterial meningitis except:

A. Infection of the subarachnoid spaces and meninges
B. Pneumococci and meningococci are the most common causative organisms in both children and adults
C. Associated with obstructive hydrocephalus
D. Neonatal meningitis associated with Group B streptococci or E. coli

78. Brain abscess shows all except:

A. Contiguous spread of infection as the most common route
B. Contrast-enhanced CT and MRI reveal a ring-enhancing lesion with surrounding edema
C. MR spectroscopy shows elevated lactate, high choline peaks
D. Prophylactic anticonvulsant and steroids used for treatment

79. Brain abscess distinguished from brain mets using:

A. MR Spectroscopy
B. DWI MRI
C. MRI STIR sequence
D. Both A and B

80. Ring enhancement seen on MRI except:

A. Brain abscess

B. Brain mets

C. Brain primary lymphoma

D. All of the above

81. Most common cause of ventriculitis:

A. Contiguous spread from paranasal sinusitis

B. Ruptured brain abscess

C. Retrograde spread from dural venous sinus

D. Shunt infection

82. Risk of posttraumatic meningitis increases with persistent CSF leak more than:

A. 5 days B. 7 days

C. 10 days D. 14 days

83. Causative organism for vertebral osteomyelitis:

A. Strep. pneumoniae B. Strep. epidermidis

C. Staph. aureus D. N. meningitides

84. Most common CNS opportunistic infection in AIDS:

A. Toxoplasmosis

B. Cryptosporidiosis

C. Histoplasmosis

D. Pneumocystis jiroveci

85. Target lesions (irregular enhancing mass) seen in CNS lesions of:

A. Toxoplasmosis

B. Primary lymphoma

C. Pneumocystis jiroveci

D. Metastasis

ANSWERS

1. **Ans: C. Ventriculitis causes decreased production**
   Ref: Chapter No. 68, Page No. 1884
2. **Ans: C. Mannitol**
   Ref: Chapter No. 68, Page No. 1884
3. **Ans: C. 0.15 to 0.20 ml/g/min**
   Ref: Chapter No. 68, Page No. 1885
4. **Ans: B. Midbrain**
   Ref: Chapter No. 68, Page No. 1885
5. **Ans: A. Type 1**
   Ref: Chapter No. 68, Page No. 1886
6. **Ans: B. MRI**
   Ref: Chapter No. 68, Page No. 1886
7. **Ans: B. Often progress from high-flow lesions at birth to lower flow lesions in adulthood**
   Ref: Chapter No. 68, Page No. 1886
8. **Ans: B. Located in brain with intervening neural parenchyma**
   Ref: Chapter No. 68, Page No. 1886
9. **Ans: C. Both A and B**
   Ref: Chapter No. 68, Page No. 1886
10. **Ans: C. Treatment includes SRS or surgical resection of lesion**
    Ref: Chapter No. 68, Page No. 1886
11. **Ans: C. AVM**
    Ref: Chapter No. 68, Page No. 1887
12. **Ans: B. Location in brain**
    Ref: Chapter No. 68, Page No. 1887
13. **Ans: B. Dilated superior ophthalmic vein**
    Ref: Chapter No. 68, Page No. 1887
14. **Ans: B. Rebleeding**
    Ref: Chapter No. 68, Page No. 1889
15. **Ans: C. Grade 3**
    Ref: Chapter No. 68, Page No. 1889
16. **Ans: D. Fischer Grading**
    Ref: Chapter No. 68, Page No. 1889
17. **Ans: D. Charcot-Bouchart aneurismal rupture occurs in internal capsule**
    Ref: Chapter No. 68, Page No. 1889
18. **Ans: C. Centrally located intracerebral hematomas**
    Ref: Chapter No. 68, Page No. 1889
19. **Ans: A. Atherosclerotic narrowing of minor cerebral vessels**
    Ref: Chapter No. 68, Page No. 1892
20. **Ans: D. Superficial temporal artery and MCA**
    Ref: Chapter No. 68, Page No. 1892
21. **Ans: A. Headache**
    Ref: Chapter No. 68, Page No. 1892
22. **Ans: C. Parietal lobe – Alexia**
    Ref: Chapter No. 68, Page No. 1892
23. **Ans: D. Diffusion tensor MRI – Predict response to radiotherapy**
    Ref: Chapter No. 68, Page No. 1893
24. **Ans: C. Glioblastoma Multiforme (Grade IV WHO)**
    Ref: Chapter No. 68, Page No. 1893
25. **Ans: D. WHO grade 4**
    Ref: Chapter No. 68, Page No. 1893
26. **Ans: B. Temozolamide**
    Ref: Chapter No. 68, Page No. 1893
27. **Ans: A. Ring enhancement with edema**
    Ref: Chapter No. 68, Page No. 1893
28. **Ans: A. Grade 1**
    Ref: Chapter No. 68, Page No. 1894
29. **Ans: C. WHO grade III**
    Ref: Chapter No. 68, Page No. 1894
30. **Ans: C. Favourable response with gain of Chromosome 1p and 19q**
    Ref: Chapter No. 68, Page No. 1894
31. **Ans: B. Ependymoma**
    Ref: Chapter No. 68, Page No. 1895
32. **Ans: B. Subarachnoid**
    Ref: Chapter No. 68, Page No. 1895
33. **Ans. C. Dysplastic cerebellar gangliocytoma**
    Ref: Chapter No. 68, Page No. 1895
34. **Ans: A. Supranuclear vertical gaze palsy by compression of tectal plate**
    Ref: Chapter No. 68, Page No. 1895
35. **Ans: D. Hemangioblastoma**
    Ref: Chapter No. 68, Page No. 1895
36. **Ans. D. Both B and C**
    Ref: Chapter No. 68, Page No. 1895

37. Ans: B. Female preponderance
Ref: Chapter No. 68, Page No. 1896

38. Ans: D. It is slow growing tumor
Ref: Chapter No. 68, Page No. 1896

39. Ans: A. Meningioma
Ref: Chapter No. 68, Page No. 1896

40. Ans: C. VHL
Ref: Chapter No. 68, Page No. 1896

41. Ans: D. Peak incidence seen at 35 yrs with immunocompetent
Ref: Chapter No. 68, Page No. 1896

42. Ans: D. All are true
Ref: Chapter No. 68, Page No. 1897

43. Ans: B. Suprasellar tumors more common in males
Ref: Chapter No. 68, Page No. 1897

44. Ans: D. All are true
Ref: Chapter No. 68, Page No. 1897

45. Ans: D. None of the above
Ref: Chapter No. 68, Page No. 1897

46. Ans: B. 25 -150 ng/ml
Ref: Chapter No. 68, Page No. 1897

47. Ans: C. > 150 ng/ml
Ref: Chapter No. 68, Page No. 1897

48. Ans: D. All of the above
Ref: Chapter No. 68, Page No. 1895

49. Ans: D. All are true
Ref: Chapter No. 68, Page No. 1898

50. Ans: D. Anticonvulsant recommended for all patients
Ref: Chapter No. 68, Page No. 1898

51. Ans: C. Lung
Ref: Chapter No. 68, Page No. 1898

52. Ans: D. All are feasible
Ref: Chapter No. 68, Page No. 1898

53. Ans: B. Diagnosed with CT brain
Ref: Chapter No. 68, Page No. 1899

54. Ans: B. 9
Ref: Chapter No. 68, Page No. 1900

55. Ans: B. 30 ml
Ref: Chapter No. 68, Page No. 1901

56. Ans: B. GCS < 10
Ref: Chapter No. 68, Page No. 1901

57. Ans: D. ICP > 20 mm of Hg
Ref: Chapter No. 68, Page No. 1901

58. Ans: C. CSF drainage
Ref: Chapter No. 68, Page No. 1901

59. Ans: B. Nutrition initiated at 5 days of injury
Ref: Chapter No. 68, Page No. 1901

60. Ans: D. Posterolateral
Ref: Chapter No. 68, Page No. 1902

61. Ans: D. Triceps (C7 root)
Ref: Chapter No. 68, Page No. 1902

62. Ans: C. C6-C7
Ref: Chapter No. 68, Page No. 1904

63. Ans: B. Cervical disc herniation
Ref: Chapter No. 68, Page No. 1904

64. Ans: B. Cobalt 201
Ref: Chapter No. 68, Page No. 1906

65. Ans: D. Subthalamic nuclei
Ref: Chapter No. 68, Page No. 1906

66. Ans: B. Subthalamic nucleus stimulation most effective for tremors and dystonia
Ref: Chapter No. 68, Page No. 1906

67. Ans: D. Corpus callosotomy eliminate epilepsy focus
Ref: Chapter No. 68, Page No. 1907

68. Ans: B. Superior cerebellar artery
Ref: Chapter No. 68, Page No. 1908

69. Ans: B. Paraparesis
Ref: Chapter No. 68, Page No. 1909

70. Ans: C. Descent of cerebellar vermis
Ref: Chapter No. 68, Page No. 1909

71. Ans: D. Intraventricular hemorrhage
Ref: Chapter No. 68, Page No. 1909

72. Ans: C. Occipital
Ref: Chapter No. 68, Page No. 1910

73. Ans: D. All of the above
Ref: Chapter No. 68, Page No. 1910

74. Ans: B. Downward displacement of medulla
Ref: Chapter No. 68, Page No. 1911

75. Ans: B. Sagittal
Ref: Chapter No. 68, Page No. 1911

76. Ans: A. Most common route is hematogenous
Ref: Chapter No. 68, Page No. 1912

77. Ans: C. Associated with obstructive hydrocephalus
Ref: Chapter No. 68, Page No. 1912

78. **Ans: C. MR spectroscopy shows elevated lactate, high choline peaks**

Ref: Chapter No. 68, Page No. 1912

79. **Ans: D. Both A and B**

Ref: Chapter No. 68, Page No. 1912

80. **Ans: D. All of the above**

Ref: Chapter No. 68, Page No. 1913

81. **Ans: D. Shunt infection**

Ref: Chapter No. 68, Page No. 1912

82. **Ans: B. 7 days**

Ref: Chapter No. 68, Page No. 1913

83. **Ans: C. Staph. aureus**

Ref: Chapter No. 68, Page No. 1913

84. **Ans: A. Toxoplasmosis**

Ref: Chapter No. 68, Page No. 1913

85. **Ans: B. Primary lymphoma**

Ref: Chapter No. 68, Page No. 1914

69

Plastic Surgery

SKIN GRAFT

1. **Triad for setting the reconstructive goals for defect is consist of following except:**
   A. Form
   B. Function
   C. Safety
   D. Sensation

2. **Following are good skin closure techniques except:**
   A. Incision with scalpel at 45 degrees to skin
   B. Careful handling of tissue
   C. Precise approximation of edges with minimal tension
   D. Natural skin line runs at right angle to the long axis of underlying muscles

3. **Which of the following is not a good graftable bed for skin grafts?**
   A. Periosteum
   B. Perichondrium
   C. Perforated bone surface
   D. Tendon

4. **Which of the following is not a poor wound surface for skin grafting?**
   A. Exposed bone B. Cartilage
   C. Paratenon D. Tendon

5. **What is the thickness of split skin graft?**
   A. 0.001-0.005 inch
   B. 0.006-0.025 inch
   C. 0.025-0.05 inch
   D. 0.05-0.1 inch

6. **Which of the following is incorrect about split thickness skin grafting?**
   A. STSG can be taken from anywhere on the body
   B. STSG takes readily on the recipient site
   C. They develop contracture over time
   D. It has more durability than FTSG

7. **Graft taken from same species is known as:**
   A. Autograft B. Allograft
   C. Homograft D. Xenograft

8. **All are disadvantages of split skin grafts except:**
   A. Contracture
   B. Abnormal pigmentation
   C. Less durable when subjected to trauma
   D. Limited area of harvest

9. **All are advantages of full thickness skin graft except:**
   A. More durable
   B. Same texture as adjacent skin
   C. Grows hair and sebum secretion
   D. Graft takes readily on recipient site

10. **Correct sequence of phases in skin graft uptake:**
    A. Imbibition, Inosculation, Neovascularization
    B. Imbibition, Neovascularization, Inosculation
    C. Inosculation, Imbibition, Neovascularization
    D. Inosculation, Neovascularization, Imbibition

11. **Following are the phases of graft uptake:**
    A. Imbibition B. Inosculation
    C. Organization D. All of the above

12. **Which is wrong statement about skin grafting?**
    A. Serum imbibitions occurs during the first 48 hours nourishes the graft
    B. Grafts are securely adherent to the bed by days 10 to 14
    C. Reinnervation begins at approximately 4 to 5 weeks

D. Temperature and light touch sensations return first

13. Which is the first sensation returns after graft uptake?

A. Pain
B. Temperature
C. Light touch
D. Vibration

14. Most common cause of skin graft failure is:

A. Infection
B. Hematoma
C. Poor vascularity of donor site
D. Thickness of graft

15. Duration required for cultivation of human epidermal cells in vitro:

A. 1 to 2 weeks
B. 2 to 3 weeks
C. 3 to 6 weeks
D. 6 to 8 weeks

16. Which is not the characteristic of in vitro culture of epidermal cells?

A. Grown in multilayer
B. Increased fragility
C. Risk of malignancy
D. Sensitive to infection

17. Which histologic change is seen in skin after tissue expansion?

A. Dermal thickening
B. Epidermal thickening
C. Subcutaneous fat hypertrophy
D. Effect on skin appendages

18. Following are the contraindications for tissue expansion except:

A. Malignant neoplasm
B. Hemangioma
C. Open leg wound
D. Prior irradiation

19. What is the most common cause of tissue expansion failure?

A. Inadequate blood supply
B. Inadequate duration for implant
C. Inadequate pocket for implant
D. Inappropriate location

20. Which is false statement regarding tissue expansion?

A. It uses a mechanical stimulus to induce tissue growth
B. Expanders should be placed under tissue that best matches the lost tissue
C. Filling of the expander is initiated after 48 hours of surgery
D. Normal sensibility of the transferred tissue is retained

FLAPS

21. Skin bearing flaps are classified based on all of the following except:

A. Composition
B. Method of movement
C. Blood supply
D. Anatomical region

22. Which of the following is false about local flaps?

A. It usually matches the skin at the recipient site
B. Flaps should be the same size and thickness as the defect
C. Local flaps rely on the inherent elasticity of skin
D. They are raised with known blood supply

23. Which is not the example of random flap?

A. Rotation flap
B. Transposition flap
C. Advancement flap
D. Fasciocutaneous flap

24. Local flaps are based on blood supply from:

A. Dermal plexus
B. Subdermal plexus
C. Subcutaneous vessel
D. Fascial perforator

25. Viability of local flaps depend on which of the following factors?

A. Flap design
B. Extrinsic pressure
C. Undue tension during wound closure
D. All of the above

26. Muscle flaps are classified according to:

A. Location
B. Pattern of vascular anatomy
C. Composition
D. Function

27. Example of dual dominant pedicle muscle flap:

A. Trapezius
B. Latissimus dorsi
C. Serratus anterior
D. Gastrocnemius

28. Example of muscle flap with single dominant pedicle:

A. Tensor fascia lata B. Gracilis
C. Tibialis anterior D. Sartorius

29. Sartorius is classified as which type of muscle flap?

A. Type I B. Type II
C. Type III D. Type IV

30. Latissimus dorsi is which type of muscle flap?

A. Single pedicle
B. Dual dominant pedicle
C. Dominant with minor pedicles
D. Dominant with secondary segmental pedicles

31. Tensor fascia lata is which type of muscle flap?

A. Type I B. Type II
C. Type III D. Type IV

32. Latissimus dorsi is classified as which type of muscle flap?

A. Type I B. Type III
C. Type IV D. Type V

33. Gluteus maximus is classified as which type of muscle flap?

A. Type II B. Type III
C. Type IV D. Type V

34. What is the example of dominant pedicle with secondary segmental pedicles type of muscle flap?

A. Trapezius B. Serratus anterior
C. Sartorius D. Latissimus dorsi

35. Which group of muscle flaps are most useful?

A. Type I, Type II, Type III
B. Type I, Type III, Type IV
C. Type II, Type III, Type V
D. Type I, Type III, Type V

36. Choke vessels are present in:

A. Dermal plexus B. Subcutaneously
C. Fascial plexus D. Muscle

37. False about muscle flaps:

A. Muscle has small-caliber choke vessels with bidirectional flow
B. They have more robust blood supply
C. Useful in wounds compromised by irradiation
D. Vascular anatomy is unpredictable and difficult to identify

38. What is the anatomic features of a fasciocutaneous flap?

A. Angiosome B. Choke vessel
C. Fascial perforator D. Source vessel

39. Following are examples of fasciocutaneous flaps except:

A. ALT flap B. Radial forearm flap
C. TRAM flap D. Lateral arm flap

40. False statement regarding fasciocutaneous flaps:

A. Deep fascial perforators are frequently anomalous in caliber and location
B. It can be distally based
C. Blood flow in the fascial plexus is multi-directional
D. They are effective in the irradiated or infected wound

41. Which type of flap pedicle can be distally based and transposed to cover a defect located at the end of an extremity?

A. Muscle flap
B. Musculocutaneous flap
C. Fasciocutaneous flap
D. Perforator flap

42. Following is true regarding perforating flap:

A. Preservation of functional muscle and fascia at donor site
B. Versatility of flap design
C. Both A and B
D. None of the above

43. Which is incorrect about perforator flap?

A. Difficult dissection needed to isolate the perforator vessels
B. Anatomic variability of position and size of perforator vessels
C. Long pedicle length available
D. Perforators give versatility of flap design

44. Following are the recommendations for harvesting a perforator flap except:

A. Identification of at least one vessel with a diameter of 1 mm or more
B. Inclusion of at least two or more perforators
C. Sufficient pedicle length for the procedure
D. Preservation of a subcutaneous vein to use for venous outflow

45. Minimum diameter of perforator require for perforator flap:

A. 0.3 mm
B. 0.5 mm
C. 0.8 mm
D. 1 mm

46. Muscle tolerate warm ischemia time upto:

A. 1 hour
B. 2 hours
C. 4 hours
D. 6 hours

47. Warm ischemia time tolerated by skin and fasciocutaneous flaps:

A. 1 to 2 hours
B. 2 to 4 hours
C. 4 to 6 hours
D. 6 to 10 hours

48. Which is correct concerning post operative management of free tissue flap?

A. Improved survival rate with anticoagulation regimen
B. Most free flap thromboses occur in the first 24 hours after surgery
C. Thrombosis of arterial anastomosis is the most common finding at reoperation
D. Salvage rates are low

49. Supermicrosurgery involves diameter of vessel:

A. 0.05 to 0.1 mm
B. 0.1 to 0.3 mm
C. 0.3 to 0.8 mm
D. 0.8 to 1.5 mm

HEAD AND NECK PLASTIC SURGERY

50. Which of the following is wrong about craniosynostosis?

A. It occurs approximately 1 in 2500 live births
B. It is usually sporadic
C. Skull grows perpendicular to the affected suture
D. Correction during the first 6 months of life appears to be associated with better neurodevelopmental outcomes

51. Craniofascial microsomia is due to vascular compromise of:

A. Mandibular artery
B. Facial artery
C. Maxillary artery
D. Stapedial artery

52. Which is correct statement about cleft lip and palate?

A. Cleft lip repair at 6 months
B. Cleft palate repair before 24 months
C. Alveolar bone graft when permanent dentition begins
D. Rotation-advancement repair is known as Millard technique

53. What is the primary measure of outcome after cleft palate repair?

A. Facial symmetry
B. Feeding problem
C. Dental occlusion
D. Speech articulation

54. Which of the following incorrect about giant melanocytic naevi?

A. Giant naevi are more than 20 cm in diameter
B. The risk of melanoma development is up to 10%
C. They have increased incidence of leptomeningeal involvement
D. Early excision and reconstruction are always recommended

55. Which is correct management of faciomaxillary trauma?

A. Nasotracheal intubation is contraindicated in skull base fractures
B. Maxillomandibular fixation is an emergent indication for tracheostomy
C. Extraocular muscle entrapment treated within the first 48 hours
D. Fractures are treated after 2 weeks of injury

56. Inappropriate method of hemorrhage control in facial trauma:

A. Applying pressure or packing
B. Bedside clamping and ligation
C. Angiographic embolization
D. Fracture reduction and fixation

57. What is the most effective way of bleeding control in blunt trauma with midfacial fracture?

A. Intranasal packing
B. Fracture reduction and fixation
C. Pressure application
D. Angiographic embolization

58. What is correct concerning management of facial wound?

A. Questionable tissue should be debrided in treating facial lacerations and avulsions
B. Primary repair of facial injury should not be delayed due to risk of infection
C. Even grossly contaminated wounds are irrigated extensively, debrided and left open
D. Parotid duct injuries should be identified and treated immediately over stent

59. All are upper midface fractures except:

A. Malar (zygoma) fractures

B. Nasoorbitoethmoid fractures
C. Orbital fractures
D. Maxilla fracture

60. Angle classification used to describe which of the following?

A. Facial symmetry
B. Maxilllary fractures
C. Relationship of the upper and lower teeth
D. Mandibular fractures

61. What is the appropriate treatment of mandibular fractures?

A. Conservative approach
B. Closed reduction
C. Maxillomandibular fixation
D. Open reduction and internal fixation

62. Which of the following is false regarding management of scalp defects?

A. Skin graft can be placed on intact periosteum
B. Scalp flaps are elevated at the subgaleal level
C. Tissue expansion also can be used for the reconstruction of larger defects with hair-bearing tissue
D. The pedicled muscle flap is preferred for coverage of near-total or total scalp defects

63. All are about nasal repair except:

A. Small nasal defects can be closed with local nasal flaps
B. Large defects of nose repaired with forehead flap
C. The forehead flap is based on the supraorbital vessels
D. Composite grafts from the ear are useful for defects of the nasal ala

64. Abbe flap is which type of flap?

A. Transposition flap B. Rotational flap
C. Pedicled flap D. Free tissue flap

65. Which of the following false about Abbe flap?

A. Used to reconstruct lateral defects of the upper lip
B. Pedicled flap based on the labial artery
C. The flap is transferred in a staged fashion
D. Donor pedicle divided 2 to 3 weeks after flap inset

66. Rhytidectomy referred for:

A. Brow lift
B. Eyelid ptosis correction
C. Nasolabial reconstruction
D. Face and neck wrinkling correction

67. Most common nerve injury involved in facelift:

A. Auriculotemporal nerve
B. Greater auricular nerve
C. Facial nerve
D. Accessory cervical nerve

68. What size of punch biopsies are taken for hair transplant?

A. 0.1 to 0.4 mm B. 0.4 to 0.8 mm
C. 0.8 to 1.2 mm D. 1.2 to 1.5 mm

MAMMOPLASTY AND ABDOMINOPLASTY

69. Most commonly used technique for reduction mammoplasty:

A. Vertical breast reduction
B. Liposuction
C. Wise pattern
D. Inverted T pattern

70. Breast cancer screening before reduction mammoplasty is done:

A. Not required
B. Only if family history is present
C. Above 35 years
D. Above 45 years

71. Regnault classification is used for:

A. Eyelid ptosis B. Breast ptosis
C. Rhinoplasty D. Gynecomastia

72. Which of the following is incorrect about breast implant?

A. Saline implants have flexibility in adjusting size
B. Higher incidence of rippling or wrinkling of the saline implant
C. Smooth implants are more prone to capsular contracture when placed in the subglandular plane
D. Implant deflation is early complication

73. Which of the following is false regarding breast implant?

A. Submuscular placement gives better visualization of the breast by mammography
B. Less chance for development of capsular contracture with submuscular placement

C. Submuscular placement results in longer recovery
D. It is recommended that gel implants be studied by MRI at intervals of 1 year

74. Silicon gel implants are best studied by:

A. Ultrasonography
B. Mammography
C. MRI
D. Physical examination

75. Which type of incision provides excellent access for breast implant placement?

A. Periareolar B. Inframammary
C. Axillary D. Inverted T shape

76. Which cancer is associated with breast implants?

A. Lobular carcinoma
B. Inflammatory carcinoma
C. Anaplastic large cell lymphoma
D. Non-Hodgkin's lymphoma

77. Which type of implants are associated with lymphoma?

A. Round implants
B. Smooth implants
C. Gummy bear implants
D. Surface texture implants

78. About breast implant associated–ALCL, which of the statement is incorrect?

A. It is seen after around 10 years of implant placement
B. It is seen with surface texture silicon implants
C. Sentinel biopsy performed as axillary metastasis can be present
D. Staging is done with positron emission tomography (PET)/CT

79. Breast implant associated anaplastic large cell lymphoma is positive for receptor:

A. CD 3 B. CD 20
C. CD 30 D. CD 45

80. What is the most common clinical presentation of BIA-ALCL?

A. Implant rupture B. Peri implant seroma
C. Implant contracture D. Peri implant fibrosis

81. Which of the following is wrong concerning gynecomastia?

A. Most frequent cause is idiopathic
B. It occurs bilaterally in 50% of cases
C. Most patients with gynecomastia are asymptomatic
D. Symptomatic gynecomastia persisting for more than 6 months in adolescent boy is operative indication

82. Fleur-de-lis abdominoplasty uses what type of abdominal incision?

A. Lower horizontal B. Vertical midline
C. Inverted T shape D. I shaped

83. Abdominoplasty following bariatric surgery is planned if patient maintains weight stability for:

A. 6 months B. 12 months
C. 18 months D. 24 months

84. Panniculectomy is defined as:

A. Upper trunk abdominoplasty
B. Lower abdominal fold resection
C. Abdominoplasty with rectal diastasis repair
D. Abdominoplasty with umbilical preservation

85. Which of the following is false about liposuction technique?

A. Liposuction can be performed in an outpatient setting
B. Liposuction can be performed with tumescent anesthesia
C. Blunt-tip and smaller cannulas are used
D. Superficial fat layers should be suctioned primarily

WOUND MANAGEMENT

86. Which is the most common chronic wound?

A. Ischemic ulcer B. Venous ulcer
C. Pressure sore D. Diabetic foot

87. Which is the most common chronic leg ulcer?

A. Arterial ulcer B. Venous ulcer
C. Pressure ulcer D. Marjolin ulcer

88. Which is the most common chronic foot wound?

A. Arterial ulcer B. Pressure sore
C. Diabetic foot D. Traumatic ulcer

89. What % of diabetic foot infections will lead to amputation?

A. <5% B. 20%
C. 30% D. 50%

90. Most common area to develop pressure sore:

A. Heel B. Ischium
C. Sacrum D. Occiput

91. National Ulcer Advisory Panel classification used for:

A. Arterial ulcer B. Venous ulcer
C. Pressure ulcer D. Diabetic ulcer

92. Loss of the epidermis and a blister or a superficial wound is classified as what stage of pressure ulcer?

A. Stage I B. Stage II
C. Stage III D. Stage IV

93. Full thickness loss of the skin and exposed subcutaneous tissue is classified as what stage of pressure ulcer?

A. Stage I B. Stage II
C. Stage III D. Stage IV

94. Exposed muscle, tendons and bone can be observed through the damaged skin is classified as what stage of pressure ulcer?

A. Stage I B. Stage II
C. Stage III D. Stage IV

95. Which of the following is incorrect about pressure ulcer classification?

A. Blanchable erythema seen in the affected area is stage I ulcer
B. In Stage III ulcers, there is a full thickness loss of the skin
C. Exposed muscle, tendons wound is classified as Stage IV
D. Ulcer covered by an eschar or necrotic tissue is unstageable

96. Which type of flaps are not used for pressure sore?

A. Rotational flap
B. V-Y advancement flap
C. Fasciocutaneous flap
D. Free tissue flap

97. Pressure sore with exposed sacrum is treated with following except:

A. Sharp debridement and serial excision of wound
B. Negative-pressure wound vacuum (NPWV) therapy
C. Flaps of the superior half of the muscle are constructed and moved in to the defect as a rotational flap
D. TRAM free muscle flap as it has robust blood supply

98. Gustilo classification is used for:

A. Osteomyelitis
B. Pelvic fracture
C. Open wound fracture
D. Long bone fracture

99. Open fractures with wound 1 to 10 cm with moderate tissue damage is Gustilo type:

A. Gustilo I B. Gustilo II
C. Gustilo III D. Gustilo IV

100. Inadequate soft tissue with periosteal stripping and bone exposure is included in which Gustilo type?

A. Gustilo II B. Gustilo IIIA
C. Gustilo IIIB D. Gustilo IIIC

101. Vascular injury irrespective of open wound size is which type of Gustilo wound?

A. Gustilo II B. Gustilo IIIA
C. Gustilo IIIB D. Gustilo IIIC

102. Absolute indications for lower limb amputation after trauma except:

A. Older age
B. Multilevel injuries
C. Warm ischemia longer than 6 hours
D. Infection

103. Most commonly used muscle flap for femoral prosthetic vascular graft:

A. Gracilis B. Sartorius
C. Tensor fascia lata D. Adductor longus

104. Correct choice for origin and insertion of Sartorius:

A. Anterior superior iliac spine, Tibial tuberosity
B. Anterior superior iliac spine, Medial condyle of tibia
C. Pubic tubercle, Lateral condyle of tibia
D. Anterior superior iliac spine, Medial condyle of femur

ANSWERS

1. **Ans: D. Sensation**
Ref: Chapter No. 69, Page No. 1916

2. **Ans: A. Incision with scalpel at 45 degrees to skin**
Ref: Chapter No. 69, Page No. 1917

3. **Ans: D. Tendon**
Ref: Chapter No. 69, Page No. 1917

4. **Ans: C. Paratenon**
Ref: Chapter No. 69, Page No. 1917

5. **Ans: B. 0.006-0.025 inch**
Ref: Chapter No. 69, Page No. 1917

6. **Ans: D. It has more durability than FTSG**
Ref: Chapter No. 69, Page No. 1917

7. **Ans: C. Homograft**
Ref: Chapter No. 69, Page No. 1917

8. **Ans: D. Limited area of harvest**
Ref: Chapter No. 69, Page No. 1917

9. **Ans: D. Graft takes readily on recipient site**
Ref: Chapter No. 69, Page No. 1917

10. **Ans: B. Imbibition, Neovascularization, Inosculation**
Ref: Chapter No. 69, Page No. 1917

11. **Ans: D. All of the above**
Ref: Chapter No. 69, Page No. 1917

12. **Ans: D. Temperature and light touch sensations return first**
Ref: Chapter No. 69, Page No. 1917

13. **Ans: A. Pain**
Ref: Chapter No. 69, Page No. 1917

14. **Ans: B. Hematoma**
Ref: Chapter No. 69, Page No. 1917

15. **Ans: C. 3 to 6 weeks**
Ref: Chapter No. 69, Page No. 1917

16. **Ans: A. Grown in multilayer**
Ref: Chapter No. 69, Page No. 1917

17. **Ans: B. Epidermal thickening**
Ref: Chapter No. 69, Page No. 1917

18. **Ans: D. Prior irradiation**
Ref: Chapter No. 69, Page No. 1917

19. **Ans: C. Inadequate pocket for implant**
Ref: Chapter No. 69, Page No. 1918

20. **Ans: C. Filling of the expander is initiated after 48 hours of surgery**
Ref: Chapter No. 69, Page No. 1918

21. **Ans: D. Anatomical region**
Ref: Chapter No. 69, Page No. 1919

22. **Ans: D. They are raised with known blood supply**
Ref: Chapter No. 69, Page No. 1919

23. **Ans: D. Fasciocutaneous flap**
Ref: Chapter No. 69, Page No. 1919

24. **Ans: B. Subdermal plexus**
Ref: Chapter No. 69, Page No. 1919

25. **Ans: D. All of the above**
Ref: Chapter No. 69, Page No. 1919

26. **Ans: B. Pattern of vascular anatomy**
Ref: Chapter No. 69, Page No. 1920

27. **Ans: C. Serratus anterior**
Ref: Chapter No. 69, Page No. 1920

28. **Ans: A. Tensor fascia lata**
Ref: Chapter No. 69, Page No. 1920

29. **Ans: D. Type IV**
Ref: Chapter No. 69, Page No. 1920

30. **Ans: D. Dominant with secondary segmental pedicles**
Ref: Chapter No. 69, Page No. 1920

31. **Ans: A. Type I**
Ref: Chapter No. 69, Page No. 1920

32. **Ans: D. Type V**
Ref: Chapter No. 69, Page No. 1920

33. **Ans: B. Type III**
Ref: Chapter No. 69, Page No. 1920

34. **Ans: D. Latissimus dorsi**
Ref: Chapter No. 69, Page No. 1920

35. **Ans: D. Type I, Type III, Type V**
Ref: Chapter No. 69, Page No. 1920

36. **Ans: D. Muscle**
Ref: Chapter No. 69, Page No. 1920

37. **Ans: D. Vascular anatomy is unpredictable and difficult to identify**

Ref: Chapter No. 69, Page No. 1920

38. **Ans: C. Fascial perforator**

Ref: Chapter No. 69, Page No. 1921

39. **Ans: C. TRAM flap**

Ref: Chapter No. 69, Page No. 1921

40. **Ans: D. They are effective in the irradiated or infected wound**

Ref: Chapter No. 69, Page No. 1921

41. **Ans: C. Fasciocutaneous flap**

Ref: Chapter No. 69, Page No. 1921

42. **Ans: C Both A and B**

Ref: Chapter No. 69, Page No. 1921

43. **Ans: C. Long pedicle length available**

Ref: Chapter No. 69, Page No. 1921

44. **Ans: A. Identification of at least one vessel with a diameter of 1 mm or more**

Ref: Chapter No. 69, Page No. 1921

45. **Ans: B. 0.5 mm**

Ref: Chapter No. 69, Page No. 1921

46. **Ans: B. 2 hours**

Ref: Chapter No. 69, Page No. 1922

47. **Ans: C. 4 to 6 hours**

Ref: Chapter No. 69, Page No. 1922

48. **Ans: C. Thrombosis of arterial anastomosis is the most common finding at reoperation**

Ref: Chapter No. 69, Page No. 1922

49. **Ans: C. 0.3 to 0.8 mm**

Ref: Chapter No. 69, Page No. 1922

50. **Ans: C. Skull grows perpendicular to the affected suture**

Ref: Chapter No. 69, Page No. 1922

51. **Ans: D. Stapedial artery**

Ref: Chapter No. 69, Page No. 1924

52. **Ans: B. Cleft palate repair before 24 months**

Ref: Chapter No. 69, Page No. 1924

53. **Ans: D. Speech articulation**

Ref: Chapter No. 69, Page No. 1924

54. **Ans: A. Giant naevi are more than 20 cm in diameter**

Ref: Chapter No. 69, Page No. 1925

55. **Ans: A. Nasotracheal intubation is contraindicated in skull base fractures**

Ref: Chapter No. 69, Page No. 1925-1926

56. **Ans: B. Bedside clamping and ligation**

Ref: Chapter No. 69, Page No. 1926

57. **Ans: B. Fracture reduction and fixation**

Ref: Chapter No. 69, Page No. 1926

58. **Ans: D. Parotid duct injuries should be identified and treated immediately over stent**

Ref: Chapter No. 69, Page No. 1926

59. **Ans: D. Maxilla fracture**

Ref: Chapter No. 69, Page No. 1927

60. **Ans: C. Relationship of the upper and lower teeth**

Ref: Chapter No. 69, Page No. 1927

61. **Ans: D. Open reduction and internal fixation**

Ref: Chapter No. 69, Page No. 1927

62. **Ans: D. The pedicled muscle flap is preferred for coverage of near-total or total scalp defects**

Ref: Chapter No. 69, Page No. 1927

63. **Ans: C. The forehead flap is based on the supraorbital vessels**

Ref: Chapter No. 69, Page No. 1927

64. **Ans: C. Pedicied flap**

Ref: Chapter No. 69, Page No. 1928

65. **Ans: A. Used to reconstruct lateral defects of the upper lip**

Ref: Chapter No. 69, Page No. 1928

66. **Ans: D. Face and neck wrinkling correction**

Ref: Chapter No. 69, Page No. 1929

67. **Ans: B. Greater auricular nerve**

Ref: Chapter No. 69, Page No. 1930

68. **Ans: C. 0.8 to 1.2 mm**

Ref: Chapter No. 69, Page No. 1930

69. **Ans: C. Wise pattern**

Ref: Chapter No. 69, Page No. 1931

70. **Ans: D. Above 45 years**

Ref: Chapter No. 69, Page No. 1931

71. **Ans: B. Breast ptosis**

Ref: Chapter No. 69, Page No. 1932

72. **Ans: D. Implant deflation is early complication**

Ref: Chapter No. 69, Page No. 1932

73. **Ans: D. It is recommended that gel implants be studied by MRI at intervals of 1 year**

Ref: Chapter No. 69, Page No. 1932

74. **Ans: C. MRI**

Ref: Chapter No. 69, Page No. 1932

75. Ans: B. Inframammary

Ref: Chapter No. 69, Page No. 1932

76. Ans: C. Anaplastic large cell lymphoma

Ref: Chapter No. 69, Page No. 1932

77. Ans: D. Surface texture implants

Ref: Chapter No. 69, Page No. 1932

78. Ans: C. Sentinel biopsy performed as axillary metastasis can be present

Ref: Chapter No. 69, Page No. 1933

79. Ans: C. CD 30

Ref: Chapter No. 69, Page No. 1933

80. Ans: B. Peri implant seroma

Ref: Chapter No. 69, Page No. 1933

81. Ans: D. Symptomatic gynecomastia persisting for more than 6 months in adolescent boy is operative indication

Ref: Chapter No. 69, Page No. 1933

82. Ans: C. Inverted T shape

Ref: Chapter No. 69, Page No. 1933

83. Ans: A. 6 months

Ref: Chapter No. 69, Page No. 1934

84. Ans: B. Lower abdominal fold resection

Ref: Chapter No. 69, Page No. 1934

85. Ans: D. Superficial fat layers should be suctioned primarily

Ref: Chapter No. 69, Page No. 1935

86. Ans: C. Pressure sore

Ref: Chapter No. 69, Page No. 1936

87. Ans: B. Venous ulcer

Ref: Chapter No. 69, Page No. 1936

88. Ans: C. Diabetic foot

Ref: Chapter No. 69, Page No. 1936

89. Ans: B. 20%

Ref: Chapter No. 69, Page No. 1937

90. Ans: C. Sacrum

Ref: Chapter No. 69, Page No. 1938

91. Ans: C. Pressure ulcer

Ref: Chapter No. 69, Page No. 1938

92. Ans: B. Stage II

Ref: Chapter No. 69, Page No. 1938

93. Ans: C. Stage III

Ref: Chapter No. 69, Page No. 1938

94. Ans: D. Stage IV

Ref: Chapter No. 69, Page No. 1938

95. Ans: A. Blanchable erythema seen in the affected area is stage I ulcer

Ref: Chapter No. 69, Page No. 1938

96. Ans: D. Free tissue flap

Ref: Chapter No. 69, Page No. 1938

97. Ans: D. TRAM free muscle flap as it has robust blood supply

Ref: Chapter No. 69, Page No. 1938

98. Ans: C. Open wound fracture

Ref: Chapter No. 69, Page No. 1939

99. Ans: B. Gustilo II

Ref: Chapter No. 69, Page No. 1939

100. Ans: C. Gustilo IIIB

Ref: Chapter No. 69, Page No. 1939

101. Ans: D. Gustilo IIIC

Ref: Chapter No. 69, Page No. 1939

102. Ans: D. Infection

Ref: Chapter No. 69, Page No. 1941-1942

103. Ans: B. Sartorius

Ref: Chapter No. 69, Page No. 1942

104. Ans: B. Anterior superior iliac spine, Medial condyle of tibia

Ref: Chapter No. 69, Page No. 1942

70

Hand Surgery

ANATOMY

1. **Abduction of the thumb is defined as:**
   A. Motion away from the long finger axis
   B. Motion toward the axis of the long finger
   C. Motion that occurs at 90 degrees away from the plane of the palm
   D. Motion that occurs at 90 degrees in the same plane as of the palm

2. **All are intrinsic muscle of thenar eminence except:**
   A. Flexor pollicis brevis
   B. Opponens pollicis
   C. Palmaris brevis
   D. Adductor pollicis

3. **Origin of lumbricals is from:**
   A. Flexor digitorum superficialis tendon
   B. Flexor digitorum profundus tendon
   C. Body of metacarpal bones
   D. Extensor digitorum communis tendon

4. **Which of the following is incorrect about interossei and lumbricals:**
   A. There are three dorsal interossei and four palmar interossei
   B. Action of palmar interossei is adduction of fingers
   C. Action of dorsal interossei is abduction of fingers
   D. Combined action bring about flexion at the MP joints

5. **All are supplied by median nerve except:**
   A. Abductor pollicis brevis
   B. Opponens pollicis
   C. Adductor pollicis
   D. Flexor pollicis brevis

6. **Which nerve supplies dorsal interossei?**
   A. Median nerve
   B. Ulnar nerve
   C. Radial nerve
   D. Posterior interosseous nerve

7. **Mobile wad comprises following muscles except:**
   A. Brachioradialis
   B. Extensor carpi ulnaris (ECU)
   C. Extensor carpi radialis longus (ECRL)
   D. Extensor carpi radialis brevis (ECRB)

8. **How many compartments are present deep to the extensor retinaculum at the dorsum of the wrist?**
   A. 4 B. 5
   C. 6 D. 7

9. **Boundary of anatomical snuff box is formed by following extensor tendons except:**
   A. Abductor pollicis longus (APL)
   B. Extensor pollicis brevis (EPB)
   C. Extensor pollicis longus (EPL)
   D. Extensor carpi radialis longus (ECRL)

10. **Which of the following muscle is not supplied by median nerve?**
    A. Abductor pollicis brevis
    B. Abductor pollicis longus
    C. Flexor pollicis brevis
    D. Flexor pollicis longus

11. **Identify wrong match regarding extensor compartments of extensor retinaculum:**
    A. First compartment - APL and EPB
    B. Second compartment - ECRL and ECRB
    C. Fourth compartment - EDM
    D. Sixth compartment - ECU

12. **Palmaris longus muscle may be absent in:**
    A. 5% B. 10%
    C. 15% D. 25%

13. **Deep layer of flexor compartment consist of following muscles except:**

A. Flexor pollicis longus
B. Flexor digitorum profundus
C. Pronator quadrates
D. Pronator teres

14. **The flexor retinaculum is attached to all of the following carpal bones except:**

A. Scaphoid
B. Hamate
C. Pisiform
D. Trapazoid

15. **Which of the following statement is incorrect?**

A. The median nerve passes through the carpal tunnel
B. The palmar cutaneous branch of the median nerve originates from its radial side 5 to 6 cm distal to cubital fossa
C. The ulnar nerve passes through Guyon canal
D. As an absolute rule, the palmar surfaces of the index and little fingers are always served by the median and ulnar nerves, respectively

16. **Which of the following is composite muscle?**

A. Flexor digitorum superficialis
B. Flexor digitorum profundus
C. Pronator quadrates
D. Adductor pollicis

EXAMINATION AND TREATMENT

17. **Which test is used to detect nerve injury in an unco-operative patient?**

A. Two-point discrimination
B. Tinels test
C. Tactile adherence
D. Pin prick test

18. **Which is the most sensitive method to test sensory loss?**

A. Two-point discrimination
B. Stereognosis
C. Graphesthesia
D. Pin prick test

19. **Motor function test of which muscle gives an absolute diagnosis of median nerve injury?**

A. Opponens pollicis
B. Flexor pollicis longus
C. Abductor pollicis brevis
D. Flexor pollicis brevis

20. **Motor function test of which muscle gives an absolute diagnosis of ulnar nerve injury?**

A. Adductor pollicis
B. Flexor digiti minimi
C. Abductor digiti minimi
D. Flexor carpi ulnaris

21. **Which of the following statement is false?**

A. Clawing of the little and ring fingers is due to distal ulnar nerve palsy
B. The little finger assumes an abducted position and cannot be adducted to the adjacent fingers is a Wartenberg sign
C. Froment sign is loss of thumb opposition
D. Ability to extend the DIP joint when the PIP joint is passively flexed is pathologic, Elson test makes this diagnosis

22. **Following signs are seen with ulnar nerve palsy:**

A. Ulnar claw hand
B. Wartenberg sign
C. Froment sign
D. All of the above

23. **Maximum safe dose of Lidocaine:**

A. 3 mg/kg
B. 4 mg/kg
C. 6 mg/kg
D. 7 mg/kg

24. **What is false regarding tourniquet use?**

A. The cuff selected needs to be as wide as the diameter of the arm
B. Standard pressures used are 100 to 150 mm Hg
C. Cuff is deflated every 2 hours for 15 to 20 minutes
D. 5 minutes of reperfusion for every 30 minutes of tourniquet time

25. **Median nerve block is given at:**

A. At wrist, between Flexor digitorum superficialis and Flexor carpi ulnaris tendons
B. AT wrist, between Flexor pollicis longus and Flexor digitorum superficialis tendons
C. At wrist, between Palmaris longus and Flexor carpi radialis tendons
D. At wrist, between Flexor digitorum superficialis and Flexor carpi radialis tendons

26. **Protected position of wrist for splint application is:**

A. Extension at wrist of 40 to 50 degrees
B. 70 degrees of flexion at MP joint
C. IP joints in a neutral position
D. All of the above

HAND TRAUMA

27. **Which is the inotrope of choice after free flap surgery for hemodynamic support?**

A. Adrenaline
B. Norepinephrine
C. Vasopressin
D. Dobutamine

28. **Flexor tendon injuries are divided into how many zones?**

A. 3
B. 4
C. 5
D. 6

29. **In which flexor tendon zone, tendons are not surrounded by synovial sheath?**

A. Zone 1
B. Zone 2
C. Zone 3
D. Zone 4

30. **Which flexor tendon zones heal well with good blood supply through paratenon?**

A. Zone 1 and 2
B. Zone 1 and 4
C. Zone 3 and 5
D. Zone 2 and 4

31. **Which of the following is false regarding flexor tendon zones?**

A. Flexor tendon injuries are divided into five zones
B. Zones 1 and 2 have a precarious blood supply through the vincula
C. Tendons in the carpal tunnel is zone 5
D. Tendon zones to the thumb are T1 through T3

32. **Following are the contraindications for immediate tendon repair except:**

A. Injuries more than 6 hours old
B. Tendon loss of more than 1 cm
C. Injury at multiple sites along the tendon
D. Destruction of the pulley system

33. **Which flexor tendon zone is called Bunnell no man's land?**

A. Zone 1
B. Zone 2
C. Zone 3
D. Zone 4

34. **Which of the following is wrong about tendon repair?**

A. Tendon injuries greater than 50% are repaired
B. Narrowest part of the flexor tendon sheath is A2 pulley
C. At least a four- or six strand core suture tendon repair is needed
D. The strength of the initial tendon repair decreases by approximately 25% during the first 3 weeks

35. **Which suture material is not used for tendon repair?**

A. Nylon
B. Polyblend
C. Polyester
D. Polydaxone

36. **Which is wrong about forces generated on flexor tendon activity?**

A. 600 g during passive finger flexion
B. 3000 g during active finger flexion
C. 8000 g during strong active finger flexion
D. The work of flexion (resistance) increases by a factor of 50% after tendon repair

37. **Tenodesis brace for postoperative rehabilitation after flexor tendon repair does not allow:**

A. Full wrist flexion
B. Wrist extension of 30 degrees
C. Maintenance of MP joint flexion of at least 60 degrees
D. Maintenance of IP joints in extended position

38. **Extensor tendon injuries have been divided into how many zones?**

A. 5
B. 7
C. 9
D. 11

39. **Volar subluxation of DIP joint is treated with:**

A. Stack splint
B. Relative motion splint
C. K wire fixation
D. Open reduction and internal fixation

40. **Extensor tendon injury at the distal insertion on DIP joint causes:**

A. Mallet finger
B. Boutonnière deformity
C. Drop finger
D. Claw finger

41. **Extensor tendon injury at the central slip over the proximal interphalangeal joint causes:**

A. Mallet finger
B. Boutonnière deformity
C. Drop finger
D. Claw finger

42. **Extensor tendon injury proximal to PIP joint causes:**

A. Mallet finger
B. Boutonnière deformity
C. Drop finger
D. Claw finger

43. 'Sunderland classification' is used for:

A. Tendon injury
B. Nerve injury
C. Vascular injury
D. Ligament injury

44. Axonal regeneration occurs at the rate of:

A. 0.5 mm/day
B. 1 mm/day
C. 2 mm/day
D. 3 mm/day

45. Which of the following is false?

A. Sunderland classification divides nerve injuries in five grades
B. Nerve conduction studies are valuable within 3 weeks after injury
C. Wallerian degeneration occurs in the entire segment distal to the injury and 1 to 2 cm proximal to it
D. Surgical exploration with repair is indicated after 3 months if no clinical recovery is detected

46. Primary nerve repair is done within:

A. 12 hours
B. 24 hours
C. 48 hours
D. 72 hours

47. Which nerve is used for Oberlin transfer?

A. Median
B. Ulnar
C. Radial
D. Musculocutaneous

48. Hypothenar hammer syndrome affects:

A. Median nerve at carpal tunnel
B. Ulnar nerve at Guyon canal
C. Ulnar artery at Guyon canal
D. Radial artery at Styloid artery

49. Which of the following is wrong statement?

A. Axillary or brachial artery injuries are always repaired
B. Isolated radial or ulnar artery injury can be safely ligated
C. Need for arterial reconstruction necessitates assessing the adequacy of collateral circulation
D. Routine fasciotomy after revascularization procedure is not required

50. Replantation is contraindicated under the following circumstances except:

A. Multilevel injury of the amputated part
B. Single-digit amputations in children
C. Patients with severely atherosclerotic arteries
D. Amputation of a single digit proximal to the FDS distal insertion

51. Indications for replantation of amputated parts are as follows except:

A. Single digits that have been amputated proximal to the FDS insertion
B. Multiple injured digits
C. Thumb amputation
D. Guillotine-sharp clean amputations at the hand, wrist, or distal forearm

52. Thumb provides ___ % of hand function.

A. 20%
B. 30%
C. 40%
D. 50%

53. Acceptable warm ischemia time for amputated digits:

A. 4 hours
B. 6 hours
C. 8 hours
D. 12 hours

54. Which is the most unfavorable type of amputation for replantation?

A. Guillotine amputation
B. Crush amputation
C. Avulsion amputation
D. All of the above

55. What is the transportation method of amputated digit for replantation?

A. Directly placed on top of ice at 4 to 10°C in container
B. Wrapped in saline gauze, sealed in plastic bag, placed on top of ice at 4 to 10°C
C. Wrapped in saline gauze, submerged in ice bag at 4 to 10°C
D. Sealed in plastic bag, submerged in ice bag at 4 to 10°C

56. Correct order of repair during replantation:

A. Bone–tendons–muscle–arteries–nerves–veins
B. Bone–tendons–muscle–nerves–arteries–veins
C. Bone–tendons–muscle–veins–nerves–arteries
D. Bone–tendons–muscle–nerves–veins–arteries

57. Which is false regarding fracture fixation?

A. Kirschner wires provide rigid fixation
B. Screws or plates allow early finger mobilization
C. Plates fixation require extensive soft tissue dissection
D. Screws have high stability

58. **An avulsion fracture of the insertion of the FDP tendon into the distal phalanx is called as:**

A. Mallet finger B. Jersey finger
C. Bennett fracture D. Rolando fracture

59. **Dorsally angulated fractures at the neck of the little finger metacarpal is called:**

A. Bennett fracture
B. Rolando fracture
C. Boxer fracture
D. Reverse Bennett fracture

60. **Oblique fractures at the base of the thumb metacarpal is called:**

A. Bennett fracture
B. Rolando fracture
C. Boxer fracture
D. Reverse Bennett fracture

61. **Bennett fracture is produced due to deforming force exerted by:**

A. Extensor pollicis longus tendon
B. Abductor pollicis longus tendon
C. Adductor pollicis tendon
D. Flexor pollicis longus tendon

62. **Comminuted fractures at the base of the thumb metacarpal is called:**

A. Bennett fracture
B. Rolando fracture
C. Boxer fracture
D. Reverse Bennett fracture

63. **Fracture at the base of the little finger metacarpal is called as:**

A. Bennett fracture
B. Rolando fracture
C. Boxer fracture
D. Reverse Bennett fracture

64. **Which is the most common carpal bone fracture?**

A. Scaphoid B. Lunate
C. Trapezium D. Hamate

65. **What is scaphoid view?**

A. Posteroanterior image with the wrist in full ulnar deviation
B. Anterioposterior image with the wrist in full ulnar deviation
C. Lateral image with the wrist in full ulnar deviation
D. Oblique image with the wrist in full ulnar deviation

66. **Thumb spica cast is used in which condition?**

A. Lunate dislocation
B. Displaced scaphoid fracture
C. Non displaced scaphoid fracture
D. Scaphoid dislocation

67. **Which is false concerning scaphoid fracture?**

A. Clinical examination shows tenderness over the anatomic snuffbox
B. Displaced scaphoid fractures require open reduction with internal fixation
C. The blood vessels enter the scaphoid mainly through its proximal half
D. Nonunion needs to be treated with cancellous bone grafting

68. **Salter-Harris classification is used for:**

A. Diaphyseal injury
B. Cancellous bone injury
C. Epiphyseal injury
D. Tendon injury

69. **Stener lesion (Ski-pole injury) is:**

A. Fracture of base of thumb metacarpal
B. Fracture of styloid process of radius
C. Detachment of ulnar collateral ligament of thumb
D. Detachment of radial collateral ligament of thumb

70. **Bone graft and flap depend on following principles except:**

A. Osteoconduction B. Osteoinduction
C. Osteogenesis D. Osteointegration

71. **Vascularised bone graft has properties of:**

A. Osteoconduction B. Osteoinduction
C. Osteogenesis D. All of the above

INFECTION

72. **Which is the most common infection of hand?**

A. Paronychia
B. Felon
C. Palmar space infections
D. Pyogenic tenosynovitis

73. **Space of Parona is present in:**
A. Palm
B. Wrist
C. Proximal forearm
D. Distal forearm

74. **Which of the following is false?**
A. Generous communication is established trough incisions on ventral and dorsal aspects for web space infection
B. An incision is made parallel to the flexor retinaculum for thenar space infection
C. A longitudinal curvilinear incision is the preferred approach for drainage of midpalmar space
D. Kanavel four cardinal sign is seen in Pyogenic flexor tenosynovitis

75. **Kanavel four cardinal signs include all except:**
A. The finger is held in flexed position
B. Symmetrical fusiform swelling of the entire finger
C. The slightest attempt at passive flexion of the affected digit produces exquisite pain
D. Site of maximum tenderness is at the proximal cul-de-sac

76. **Chronic paronychia is caused by:**
A. Staph aureus
B. Atypical mycobacteria
C. Candida albicans
D. Fusobacterium

77. **What is hallmark of muscle and nerve ischemia in compartment syndrome?**
A. Swelling
B. Pain
C. Loss of sensation
D. Decreased range of movement

78. **A stenosing tenosynovitis of the first dorsal compartment of the wrist is known as:**
A. Intersection syndrome
B. de Quervain's disease
C. Trigger thumb
D. Ski pole injury

79. **Finkelstein test—On clasping the thumb and brisk ulnar deviation to the hand elicits extreme pain, seen in:**
A. de Quervain's disease
B. Intersection syndrome
C. Trigger thumb
D. Ski pole injury

80. **Pain and crepitus at the point at which the APL and EPB tendons cross over the tendons of the second dorsal compartment (ECRL and ECRB) seen in:**
A. de Quervain's disease
B. Intersection syndrome
C. Trigger thumb
D. Ski pole injury

81. **Constricting tenosynovitis of the flexor tendons at the level of the MP joint (A1 pulley) is called as:**
A. de Quervain's disease
B. Intersection syndrome
C. Trigger thumb
D. Ski pole injury

NERVE COMPRESSION SYNDROMES

82. **Cubital tunnel syndrome caused by entrapment of:**
A. Median nerve
B. Posterior interosseous nerve
C. Ulnar nerve
D. Radial nerve

83. **Radial tunnel syndrome caused by entrapment of:**
A. Radial nerve at radial groove
B. Posterior interosseous nerve at proximal forearm
C. Posterior interosseous nerve at distal forearm
D. Radial nerve at anatomical snuff box

84. **Pronator syndrome is caused by entrapment of:**
A. Median nerve at proximal forearm
B. Ulnar nerve at proximal forearm
C. Anterior interosseous nerve at distal forearm
D. Posterior interosseous nerve at proximal forearm

85. **What is the most common peripheral nerve entrapment syndrome?**
A. Carpal tunnel syndrome
B. Cubital tunnel syndrome
C. Guyon canal syndrome
D. Radial tunnel syndrome

86. **Which of the following is false regarding carpal tunnel syndrome?**
A. Normal pressures in the tunnel are 20 to 30 mm Hg

B. Earliest symptom is pain characteristically more obvious at night
C. Durkan sign is positive
D. Surgical decompression performed by transversely dividing the flexor retinaculum

87. Pronator syndrome caused by entrapment of the median nerve in proximal forearm between:

A. Two heads of the FDS
B. Two heads of the pronator teres
C. Ligament of struthers
D. All of the above

TUMORS OF HAND

88. Most common tumors of hand:

A. Glomus tumor
B. Squamous cell carcinoma
C. Basal cell carcinoma
D. Melanoma

89. Patient has severe, exquisite pain at the fingertips and a violaceous hue deep to the nail plate. What is probable diagnosis?

A. Basal cell carcinoma
B. Acral lentiginous melanoma
C. Glomus tumor
D. Clear cell sarcoma

90. Most common primary bone tumor of hand:

A. Osteoid osteoma B. Enchondroma
C. Chondroarcoma D. Giant cell tumor

91. Which of the following is false regarding ganglion?

A. An outpouching of the synovial membrane from a joint or tendon sheath
B. Dorsal aspect of the wrist is most common location
C. Ganglions are more common in males
D. Mucous cyst are often associated with osteoarthritis of that DIP joint

92. Which statement is false about giant cell tumor of hand?

A. It is pigmented villonodular synovitis
B. It occurs more common in bones of hand
C. It is usually benign but extends along tendon sheaths and around neurovascular structure
D. Complete surgical excision is the treatment of choice

93. Which is false about pyogenic granuloma of hand?

A. It is highly vascular granulation tissue
B. Occur at the site of previous trivial trauma
C. Histologic confirmation of the diagnosis is necessary
D. They are slow growing

94. Which of the following is wrong about osteoid osteoma?

A. Classically causes pain that is worse in morning
B. Pain is unrelated to use or motion of the hand
C. Symptoms are relieved by nonsteroidal anti-inflammatory drugs (NSAIDs)
D. Radiography shows cortical sclerosis surrounding a radiolucent area of nidus

95. Which of the following is false about osteochondroma?

A. It is also known as exostosis
B. Growth stops after skeletal maturity reached
C. Multiple osteochondromatosis is autosomal dominant
D. It is malignant bone tumor

96. Which is wrong about giant cell tumor of bone?

A. Expansion soap bubble lesion in bone
B. Aneurysmal bone cyst may be derived from Giant cell tumor
C. It may be locally aggressive and even metastasize
D. Irradiation used as treatment option

97. Which of the following is false about enchondroma?

A. Most common bone tumor of hand found incidentally
B. More commonly seen in females
C. Ollier disease is multiple enchondromas
D. Maffucci syndrome has malignant potential

CONGENITAL ANOMALIES

98. Surgical separation of the syndactyly is done at which age?

A. At birth B. 6 months
C. 1 year D. 2 years

99. Duplicated thumb correction is carried out at which age?

A. At birth B. Before 1 year
C. At 5 years D. 10 to 15 years

100. Which is false statement about apert syndrome?

A. It is autosomal dominant disorder
B. It involves craniofacial anomalies
C. Severe form of bilateral polydactyly
D. Surgical treatment involves local flap and the use of full-thickness skin grafts for reconstruction

101. Wassel classification is used for:

A. Syndactyly B. Polydactyly
C. Camptodactyly D. Clinodactyly

102. Most common type of thumb polydactyly:

A. Type I B. Type II
C. Type IV D. Type VII

103. Blauth classification is used for:

A. Thumb polydacytyly
B. Thumb hypoplasia
C. Camptodactyly
D. Clinodactyly

104. Curving of the digits in a radial or ulnar direction is known as:

A. Camptodactyly B. Ectrodactyly
C. Clinodactyly D. Syndactyly

105. Congenital flexion deformity of digit is known as:

A. Camptodactyly B. Ectrodactyly
C. Clinodactyly D. Syndactyly

106. Osteophytes at the DIP joint are called:

A. Heberden nodes B. Osler nodes
C. Bouchard nodes D. Janeway lesion

107. Osteophytes at the DIP joint are called:

A. Heberden nodes B. Osler nodes
C. Bouchard nodes D. Janeway lesion

108. In osteoarthritis, when cartilage weakens and develops cracks is called as:

A. Fragmentation B. Fibrillation
C. Eburnation D. Enchondrosis

109. In osteoarthritis, sclerosis of the subchondral bone is called as:

A. Fragmentation B. Fibrillation
C. Eburnation D. Enchondrosis

110. Which of the following is not seen with rheumatoid arthritis?

A. Swan neck deformity
B. Boutonnière deformity
C. Joint subluxation
D. Sclerosis of subchondral bone

111. Which is false about Dupuytren contracture?

A. Hereditary Mendelian dominant disorder
B. It is six times more frequent in females
C. Predominantly involves the ring and little fingers
D. Occurs in the normal bands of collagen tissue that form the palmar fascia, natatory ligaments and digital sheaths

112. Which of the following is wrong regarding Volkmann contracture?

A. It is most common contracture results from untreated compartment syndrome of the forearm
B. Ulnar nerve and brachial artery are commonly affected
C. Digits are characteristically flexed, with passive extension of the wrist worsening the flexion deformity of digits
D. It is most likely associated with supracondylar fracture of the humerus

ANSWERS

1. **Ans: C. Motion that occurs at 90 degrees away from the plane of the palm**

   Ref: Chapter No. 70, Page No. 1946

2. **Ans: C. Palmaris brevis**

   Ref: Chapter No. 70, Page No. 1946

3. **Ans: B. Flexor digitorum profundus tendon**

   Ref: Chapter No. 70, Page No. 1946

4. **Ans: A. There are three dorsal interossei and four palmar interossei**

   Ref: Chapter No. 70, Page No. 1946

5. **Ans: C. Adductor pollicis**

   Ref: Chapter No. 70, Page No. 1947

6. **Ans: B. Ulnar nerve**

   Ref: Chapter No. 70, Page No. 1947

7. **Ans: B. Extensor carpi ulnaris (ECU)**

   Ref: Chapter No. 70, Page No. 1947

8. **Ans: C. 6**

   Ref: Chapter No. 70, Page No. 1947

9. **Ans: D. Extensor carpi radialis longus (ECRL)**

   Ref: Chapter No. 70, Page No. 1947

10. **Ans: B. Abductor pollicis longus**

    Ref: Chapter No. 70, Page No. 1947

11. **Ans: C. Fourth compartment – EDM**

    Ref: Chapter No. 70, Page No. 1947

12. **Ans: B. 10%**

    Ref: Chapter No. 70, Page No. 1947

13. **Ans: D. Pronator teres**

    Ref: Chapter No. 70, Page No. 1947

14. **Ans: D. Trapazoid**

    Ref: Chapter No. 70, Page No. 1947

15. **Ans: B. The palmar cutaneous branch of the median nerve originates from its radial side 5 to 6 cm distal to cubital fossa**

    Ref: Chapter No. 70, Page No. 1947-1948

16. **Ans: B. Flexor digitorum profundus**

    Ref: Chapter No. 70, Page No. 1948

17. **Ans: C. Tactile adherence**

    Ref: Chapter No. 70, Page No. 1949

18. **Ans: A. Two-point discrimination**

    Ref: Chapter No. 70, Page No. 1949

19. **Ans: C. Abductor pollicis brevis**

    Ref: Chapter No. 70, Page No. 1949

20. **Ans: B. Flexor digiti minimi**

    Ref: Chapter No. 70, Page No. 1949

21. **Ans: C. Froment sign is loss of thumb opposition**

    Ref: Chapter No. 70, Page No. 1949-1951-1954

22. **Ans: D. All of the above**

    Ref: Chapter No. 70, Page No. 1951

23. **Ans: B. 4 mg/kg**

    Ref: Chapter No. 70, Page No. 1951

24. **Ans: B. Standard pressures used are 100 to 150 mm Hg**

    Ref: Chapter No. 70, Page No. 1952

25. **Ans: C. At wrist, between Palmaris longus and Flexor carpi radialis tendons**

    Ref: Chapter No. 70, Page No. 1954

26. **Ans: D. All of the above**

    Ref: Chapter No. 70, Page No. 1955

27. **Ans: B. Norepinephrine**

    Ref: Chapter No. 70, Page No. 1955

28. **Ans: C. 5**

    Ref: Chapter No. 70, Page No. 1956

29. **Ans: C. Zone 3**

    Ref: Chapter No. 70, Page No. 1957

30. **Ans: C. Zone 3 and 5**

    Ref: Chapter No. 70, Page No. 1957

31. **Ans: C. Tendons in the carpal tunnel is zone 5**

    Ref: Chapter No. 70, Page No. 1957

32. **Ans: A. Injuries more than 6 hours old**

    Ref: Chapter No. 70, Page No. 1957

33. **Ans: B. Zone 2**

    Ref: Chapter No. 70, Page No. 1957

34. **Ans: B. Narrowest part of the flexor tendon sheath is A2 pulley**

    Ref: Chapter No. 70, Page No. 1958-1960

35. **Ans: D. Polydaxone**

    Ref: Chapter No. 70, Page No. 1959

36. **Ans: B. 3000 g during active finger flexion**

    Ref: Chapter No. 70, Page No. 1960

37. **Ans: D. Maintenance of IP joints in extended position**

    Ref: Chapter No. 70, Page No. 1960

38. **Ans: C. 9**

Ref: Chapter No. 70, Page No. 1960

39. **Ans: D. Open reduction and internal fixation**

Ref: Chapter No. 70, Page No. 1961

40. **Ans: A. Mallet finger**

Ref: Chapter No. 70, Page No. 1963

41. **Ans: B. Boutonnière deformity**

Ref: Chapter No. 70, Page No. 1963

42. **Ans: C. Drop finger**

Ref: Chapter No. 70, Page No. 1963

43. **Ans: B. Nerve injury**

Ref: Chapter No. 70, Page No. 1963

44. **Ans: B. 1 mm/day**

Ref: Chapter No. 70, Page No. 1963

45. **Ans: B. Nerve conduction studies are valuable within 3 weeks after injury**

Ref: Chapter No. 70, Page No. 1964

46. **Ans: D. 72 hours**

Ref: Chapter No. 70, Page No. 1964

47. **Ans: B. Ulnar**

Ref: Chapter No. 70, Page No. 1965

48. **Ans: C. Ulnar artery at Guyon canal**

Ref: Chapter No. 70, Page No. 1965

49. **Ans: D. Routine fasciotomy after revascularization procedure is not required**

Ref: Chapter No. 70, Page No. 1965

50. **Ans: B. Single-digit amputations in children**

Ref: Chapter No. 70, Page No. 1966

51. **Ans: A. Single digits that have been amputated proximal to the FDS insertion**

Ref: Chapter No. 70, Page No. 1966

52. **Ans: C. 40%**

Ref: Chapter No. 70, Page No. 1966

53. **Ans: D. 12 hours**

Ref: Chapter No. 70, Page No. 1966

54. **Ans: C. Avulsion amputation**

Ref: Chapter No. 70, Page No. 1966

55. **Ans: B. Wrapped in saline gauze, sealed in plastic bag, placed on top of ice at 4 to 10 °C**

Ref: Chapter No. 70, Page No. 1966

56. **Ans: A. Bone – tendons - muscle - arteries - nerves - veins**

Ref: Chapter No. 70, Page No. 1966

57. **Ans: A. Kirschner wires provide rigid fixation**

Ref: Chapter No. 70, Page No. 1967

58. **Ans: B. Jersey finger**

Ref: Chapter No. 70, Page No. 1967

59. **Ans: C. Boxer fracture**

Ref: Chapter No. 70, Page No. 1968

60. **Ans: A. Bennett fracture**

Ref: Chapter No. 70, Page No. 1968

61. **Ans: B. Abductor pollicis longus tendon**

Ref: Chapter No. 70, Page No. 1968

62. **Ans: B. Rolando fracture**

Ref: Chapter No. 70, Page No. 1968

63. **Ans: D. Reverse Bennett fracture**

Ref: Chapter No. 70, Page No. 1968

64. **Ans: A. Scaphoid**

Ref: Chapter No. 70, Page No. 1968

65. **Ans: A. Posteroanterior image with the wrist in full ulnar deviation**

Ref: Chapter No. 70, Page No. 1968

66. **Ans: C. Non displaced scaphoid fracture**

Ref: Chapter No. 70, Page No. 1969

67. **Ans: C. The blood vessels enter the scaphoid mainly through its proximal half**

Ref: Chapter No. 70, Page No. 1969

68. **Ans: C. Epiphyseal injury**

Ref: Chapter No. 70, Page No. 1969

69. **Ans: C. Detachment of ulnar collateral ligament of thumb**

Ref: Chapter No. 70, Page No. 1969

70. **Ans: D. Osteointegration**

Ref: Chapter No. 70, Page No. 1970

71. **Ans: D. All of the above**

Ref: Chapter No. 70, Page No. 1970

72. **Ans: A. Paronychia**

Ref: Chapter No. 70, Page No. 1971

73. **Ans: D. Distal forearm**

Ref: Chapter No. 70, Page No. 1973

74. **Ans: B. An incision is made parallel to the flexor retinaculum for thenar space infection**

Ref: Chapter No. 70, Page No. 1973

75. **Ans: C. The slightest attempt at passive flexion of the affected digit produces exquisite pain**

Ref: Chapter No. 70, Page No. 1973

76. **Ans: C. Candida albicans**

Ref: Chapter No. 70, Page No. 1974

77. **Ans: B. Pain**

Ref: Chapter No. 70, Page No. 1975

78. **Ans: B. de Quervain's disease**

Ref: Chapter No. 70, Page No. 1976

79. **Ans: A. de Quervain's disease**

Ref: Chapter No. 70, Page No. 1976

80. **Ans: B. Intersection syndrome**

Ref: Chapter No. 70, Page No. 1977

81. **Ans: C. Trigger thumb**

Ref: Chapter No. 70, Page No. 1977

82. **Ans: C. Ulnar nerve**

Ref: Chapter No. 70, Page No. 1978

83. **Ans: B. Posterior interosseous nerve at proximal forearm**

Ref: Chapter No. 70, Page No. 1978

84. **Ans: A. Median nerve at proximal forearm**

Ref: Chapter No. 70, Page No. 1978

85. **Ans: A. Carpal tunnel syndrome**

Ref: Chapter No. 70, Page No. 1978

86. **Ans: D. Surgical decompression performed by transversely dividing the flexor retinaculum**

Ref: Chapter No. 70, Page No. 1978

87. **Ans: D. All of the above**

Ref: Chapter No. 70, Page No. 1979

88. **Ans: B. Squamous cell carcinoma**

Ref: Chapter No. 70, Page No. 1980

89. **Ans: C. Glomus tumor**

Ref: Chapter No. 70, Page No. 1980

90. **Ans: B. Enchondroma**

Ref: Chapter No. 70, Page No. 1980

91. **Ans: C. Ganglions are more common in males**

Ref: Chapter No. 70, Page No. 1981

92. **Ans: B. It occurs more common in bones of hand**

Ref: Chapter No. 70, Page No. 1981

93. **Ans: D. They are slow growing**

Ref: Chapter No. 70, Page No. 1982

94. **Ans: A. Classically causes pain that is worse in morning**

Ref: Chapter No. 70, Page No. 1985

95. **Ans: D. It is malignant bone tumor**

Ref: Chapter No. 70, Page No. 1985

96. **Ans: D. Irradiation used as treatment option**

Ref: Chapter No. 70, Page No. 1985

97. **Ans: B. More commonly seen in females**

Ref: Chapter No. 70, Page No. 1985-1986

98. **Ans: B. 6 months**

Ref: Chapter No. 70, Page No. 1987

99. **Ans: B. Before 1 year**

Ref: Chapter No. 70, Page No. 1987

100. **Ans: C. Severe form of bilateral polydactyly**

Ref: Chapter No. 70, Page No. 1987

101. **Ans: B. Polydactyly**

Ref: Chapter No. 70, Page No. 1987

102. **Ans: C. Type IV**

Ref: Chapter No. 70, Page No. 1987

103. **Ans: B. Thumb hypoplasia**

Ref: Chapter No. 70, Page No. 1987

104. **Ans: C. Clinodactyly**

Ref: Chapter No. 70, Page No. 1987

105. **Ans: A. Camptodactyly**

Ref: Chapter No. 70, Page No. 1987

106. **Ans: A. Heberden nodes**

Ref: Chapter No. 70, Page No. 1989

107. **Ans: C. Bouchard nodes**

Ref: Chapter No. 70, Page No. 1989

108. **Ans: B. Fibrillation**

Ref: Chapter No. 70, Page No. 1989

109. **Ans: C. Eburnation**

Ref: Chapter No. 70, Page No. 1989

110. **Ans: D. Sclerosis of subchondral bone**

Ref: Chapter No. 70, Page No. 1989

111. **Ans: B. It is six times more frequent in females**

Ref: Chapter No. 70, Page No. 1990

112. **Ans: B. Ulnar nerve and brachial artery are commonly affected**

Ref: Chapter No. 70, Page No. 1993

71

Gynecologic Surgery

ANATOMY

1. **Hart line is present at:**
   A. Lung
   B. Pelvis
   C. Inguinal region
   D. Vestibule of vulva

2. **Bartholin glands are homologous to which male urogenital structure?**
   A. Prostate
   B. Seminal vesicles
   C. Bulbourethral glands
   D. Skene glands

3. **Skene glands are homologous to which male urogenital structure?**
   A. Prostate
   B. Seminal vesicles
   C. Cowper glands
   D. Bartholin glands

4. **Alcock canal is the fascial tunnel present along:**
   A. Levator ani
   B. Obturator internus
   C. Obturator externus
   D. Pyriformis

5. **Neurovascular bundle present in Alcock canal:**
   A. Internal obturator
   B. Internal pudendal
   C. External pudendal
   D. Inferior gluteal

6. **Nerve root of internal pudendal nerve:**
   A. Anterior rami of S1 S2 S3
   B. Anterior rami of S2 S3 S4
   C. Posterior rami of S1 S2 S3
   D. Posterior rami of S2 S3 S4

7. **Cervical intraepithelial neoplasia occurs at:**
   A. Uterocervical junction
   B. Internal cervix
   C. Transition zone
   D. External os

8. **Peg cells are seen in:**
   A. Cervix
   B. Uterus
   C. Fallopian tube
   D. Ovary

VULVA AND VAGINA

9. **Diethylstilbestrol exposure in utero is a risk factor for development of:**
   A. Vulval cancer
   B. Vaginal cancer
   C. Uterine cancer
   D. Ovarian cancer

10. **Word catheter is used for:**
    A. Penile abscess drainage
    B. Bulbourethral abscess drainage
    C. Bartholin abscess drainage
    D. Perineal abscess drainage

11. **LeFort procedure for vaginal prolapsed is:**
    A. Anterior colporrhaphy
    B. Posterior colporrhaphy
    C. Colpocleisis
    D. Sacrospinous ligament suspension of vagina

CERVIX

12. **Which is false statement regarding CIN?**
    A. CIN is a premalignant condition of the cervix caused by HPV infection
    B. The lifetime cumulative risk of HPV infection is 80%
    C. HPV types 6 and 11 have a high rate of progression to CIN
    D. Average time from HPV infection to invasive disease is generally over 15 years

13. **Which HPV types have high risk of developing cervical cancer?**

A. 6 and 11
B. 16 and 18
C. 31 and 33
D. 45 and 52

14. Current cervical cancer screening guidelines include following recommendations except:

A. Use of cytology alone every 5 years for women 9 to 21 years
B. Use of cytology alone every 3 years for women age 21 to 29 years
C. Contesting with cytology and high-risk HPV testing for women age 30 to 65 years
D. High-risk HPV testing only every 5 years for women age 30 to 65 years

15. Loop electrosurgical excision procedure (LEEP) is used for:

A. Vaginal cancer
B. Penile cancer
C. CIN – Cervical cancer
D. SIN – anal cancer

16. Staging of cervical cancer is based on:

A. Clinical
B. Radiological
C. TNM
D. Pathological

17. Which is false regarding Loop electrosurgical excision procedure (LEEP)?

A. LEEP may be performed in the office setting
B. It uses a wire loop that is heated by electrical current
C. Excision of the transformation zone of the cervix with the involved areas of CIN
D. Figure-of-8 retention sutures are placed at the 3 and 9 o'clock positions

18. Piver-Rutledge-Smith classification is used for:

A. Extent of resection in penile cancer
B. Extent of resection in prostate cancer
C. Extent of resection in cervical cancer
D. Extent of resection in ovarian cancer

19. According to Piver-Rutledge-Smith classification, the modified radical hysterectomy is classified as:

A. Type I
B. Type II
C. Type III
D. Type IV

20. Radical trachelectomy can be considered in following conditions except:

A. Women who desire future fertility with early stage cancer
B. Malignant lesions 2 cm or less in diameter
C. FIGO stage IA1 cancer cervix
D. FIGO stage IB2 cancer cervix

UTERUS

21. Most common cause of postmenopausal bleeding is:

A. Malignancy
B. Vaginal and endometrial atrophy
C. Fibroid
D. Hormone replacement therapy

22. Indications of endometrial biopsy in post menopausal women are:

A. Endometrial thickness greater than 4 mm
B. Difficulty visualizing the endometrium
C. Persistent bleeding despite a normal ultrasound
D. All of the above

23. Cervical fibroids are classified as:

A. Type 2
B. Type 4
C. Type 6
D. Type 8

24. What is false regarding uterine fibroids?

A. They are the most common benign gynecologic tumor
B. Affect up to 30% of women
C. There is a predominance in white women
D. Type 6 and 7 fibroids are subserosal in location

25. Which of the following is not a characteristic sonographic feature of adenomyosis?

A. Heterogeneity in the myometrium
B. Blurring of the junction between the endometrium and myometrium
C. Focal asymmetric thickening of the myometrium
D. Presence of "cysts" within the myometrial layer

26. All are true about adenomyosis except:

A. Found more commonly in nulliparous women
B. Heavy, irregular menstrual bleeding
C. Non-cyclic pelvic pain
D. Simple hysterectomy is the surgical intervention of choice

27. Which is most common gynecologic cancer?

A. Ovarian cancer
B. Endometrial cancer
C. Vaginal cancer
D. Cervical cancer

28. All of the following are risk factors for endometrial cancer except:

A. Age
B. Multiparity
C. Obesity
D. Diabetes

29. Which of the following hereditary syndrome has highest risk of endometrial cancer?

A. Li Fraumeni syndrome
B. Gardner syndrome
C. Lynch syndrome
D. Cowden syndrome

30. Which genetic mutation of lynch syndrome has highest risk of endometrial cancer?

A. MLH1 B. MSH6
C. PSM2 D. MLH3

31. Mayo criteria is used for:

A. Low risk cervical cancer
B. Leiomyosarcoma
C. Low risk endometrial cancer
D. Ovarian cancer

32. What is recommended time interval for post myomectomy conception?

A. 2 months B. 6 months
C. 1 year D. 2 years

FALLOPIAN TUBES/OVARY

33. What is the risk of ovarian cancer in female with BRCA1 mutation?

A. 20% B. 40%
C. 50% D. 60%

34. Sonographic evidence of 'Blob sign' is related to:

A. Subserosal fibroid
B. PCOD
C. Ectopic pregnancy
D. Bartholin abscess

35. Which of the following condition is referred as "Chocolate cyst"?

A. Ectopic pregnancy
B. Endometrioma
C. Ovarian teratoma
D. Mesenteric cyst

36. A 36 years old females presents with pelvic pain and dysmenorrhea. USG pelvis suggestive of a 6 cm right ovarian cyst with low echogenicity and ground glass appearance. Left ovary and uterus are normal in appearance. What is the management for this patient?

A. Medical therapy
B. Right sided cystectomy
C. Bilateral salpingo-oophorectomy
D. Simple hysterectomy with oophorectomy

37. Following procedures are used for tubal sterilization except:

A. Pomeroy procedure
B. Irving procedure
C. Parkland procedure
D. Fothergill procedure

ANSWERS

1. **Ans: D. Vestibule of vulva**
   Ref: Chapter No. 71, Page No. 1999
2. **Ans: C. Bulbourethral glands**
   Ref: Chapter No. 71, Page No. 1999
3. **Ans: A. Prostate**
   Ref: Chapter No. 71, Page No. 1999
4. **Ans: B. Obturator internus**
   Ref: Chapter No. 71, Page No. 1999
5. **Ans: B. Internal pudendal**
   Ref: Chapter No. 71, Page No. 2000
6. **Ans: B. Anterior rami of S2 S3 S4**
   Ref: Chapter No. 71, Page No. 2000
7. **Ans: C. Transition zone**
   Ref: Chapter No. 71, Page No. 2001
8. **Ans: C. Fallopian tube**
   Ref: Chapter No. 71, Page No. 2001
9. **Ans: B. Vaginal cancer**
   Ref: Chapter No. 71, Page No. 2005
10. **Ans: C. Bartholin abscess drainage**
    Ref: Chapter No. 71, Page No. 2005
11. **Ans: C. Colpocleisis**
    Ref: Chapter No. 71, Page No. 2007
12. **Ans: C. HPV types 6 and 11 have a high rate of progression to CIN**
    Ref: Chapter No. 71, Page No. 2008
13. **Ans: B. 16 and 18**
    Ref: Chapter No. 71, Page No. 2008
14. **Ans: A. Use of cytology alone every 5 years for women 9 to 21 years**
    Ref: Chapter No. 71, Page No. 2008
15. **Ans: C. CIN – Cervical cancer**
    Ref: Chapter No. 71, Page No. 2008
16. **Ans: A. Clinical**
    Ref: Chapter No. 71, Page No. 2008
17. **Ans: D. Figure-of-8 retention sutures are placed at the 3 and 9 o'clock positions**
    Ref: Chapter No. 71, Page No. 2009
18. **Ans: C. Extent of resection in cervical cancer**
    Ref: Chapter No. 71, Page No. 2009
19. **Ans: C. Type III**
    Ref: Chapter No. 71, Page No. 2009
20. **Ans: D. FIGO stage IB2 cancer cervix**
    Ref: Chapter No. 71, Page No. 2009
21. **Ans: B. Vaginal and endometrial atrophy**
    Ref: Chapter No. 71, Page No. 2010
22. **Ans: D. All of the above**
    Ref: Chapter No. 71, Page No. 2010
23. **Ans: D. Type 8**
    Ref: Chapter No. 71, Page No. 2011
24. **Ans: C. There is a predominance in white women**
    Ref: Chapter No. 71, Page No. 2011
25. **Ans: C. Focal asymmetric thickening of the myometrium**
    Ref: Chapter No. 71, Page No. 2011
26. **Ans: A. Found more commonly in nulliparous women**
    Ref: Chapter No. 71, Page No. 2011
27. **Ans: B. Endometrial cancer**
    Ref: Chapter No. 71, Page No. 2011
28. **Ans: B. Multiparity**
    Ref: Chapter No. 71, Page No. 2011
29. **Ans: C. Lynch syndrome**
    Ref: Chapter No. 71, Page No. 2011
30. **Ans: A. MLH1**
    Ref: Chapter No. 71, Page No. 2011
31. **Ans. C. Low risk endometrial cancer**
    Ref: Chapter No. 71, Page No. 2012
32. **Ans: B. 6 months**
    Ref: Chapter No. 71, Page No. 2014
33. **Ans: B. 40%**
    Ref: Chapter No. 71, Page No. 2017
34. **Ans: C. Ectopic pregnancy**
    Ref: Chapter No. 71, Page No. 2018
35. **Ans: B. Endometrioma**
    Ref: Chapter No. 71, Page No. 2018
36. **Ans: B. Right sided cystectomy**
    Ref: Chapter No. 71, Page No. 2018
37. **Ans: D. Fothergill procedure**
    Ref: Chapter No. 71, Page No. 2019

72

Surgery in Pregnant Patient

1. **Which of the following statement is false regarding physiological changes during pregnancy?**
   A. The diaphragm can be elevated in pregnancy up to 4 cm and the lower chest wall can widen up to 7 cm
   B. Increase in the incidence of gastroesophageal reflux
   C. The incidence of symptomatic cholelithiasis during pregnancy is more as compared to the incidence in age-related nonpregnant women
   D. Fivefold increase in the risk of venous thromboembolism during pregnancy

2. **What is most common presentation of portal hypertension during pregnancy?**
   A. Esophageal varies
   B. Dilated superficial abdominal veins
   C. Hemorrhoids
   D. Splenomegaly

3. **Which of the following does not increase during pregnancy?**
   A. Tidal volume
   B. Cardiac output
   C. Serum creatinine
   D. Glomerular filtration

4. **What is accepted maximum dose of radiation during pregnancy?**
   A. 0.5 cGy B. 5 cGy
   C. 0.5 Gy D. 5 Gy

5. **Minimum radiation dose associated with congenital malformation:**
   A. 5 cGy B. 10 cGy
   C. 20 cGy D. 50 cGy

6. **Which of the following is incorrect statement?**
   A. The accepted maximum dose of ionizing radiation during the entire pregnancy is 5 cGy
   B. Highest risk from radiation exposure upto 15 weeks' gestation
   C. MRI is useful modality during the first trimester of pregnancy
   D. No effect on the fetus has been observed after the use of gadolinium contrast medium with MRI

7. **Highest radiation exposure is seen with which modality of imaging?**
   A. Abdominal CT B. Barium enema
   C. Upper GI series D. HIDA scan

8. **Teratogenic drugs are included in which category of drugs?**
   A. Category C B. Category D
   C. Category H D. Category X

9. **Which category includes drugs having clear health risk for fetus?**
   A. Category B B. Category C
   C. Category D D. Category X

10. **Which of the following drug use is contraindicated during pregnancy?**
    A. Aminoglycosides B. Cephalosporin
    C. Sulfonamides D. Vancomycin

11. **Which of the following anticoagulant is contraindicated in pregnancy?**
    A. LMWH B. Danaparoid
    C. Warfarin D. Fondaparinux

12. **Which of the following is associated with warfarin use during pregnancy?**

A. Miscarriage
B. Neurodevelopmental problems
C. Birth defect
D. All of the above

13. Which of the following is true concerning drug use during pregnancy?

A. Low dose aspirin (60-100 mg) is safe during pregnancy
B. Clopidogrel is stopped 7 days before an elective delivery
C. NSAIDs are generally used for postoperative pain control
D. Post operative oral narcotic use is contraindicated

14. What is the rate of premature labor induced by nonobstetric surgical intervention?

A. <1% B. <5%
C. 5-10% D. 10-15%

15. What is management of patient with 27 weeks pregnancy undergone laparoscopic appendectomy and presented with uterine contraction?

A. Termination of pregnancy
B. Observation and fetal monitoring
C. Indomethacin
D. Terbutaline

16. What is the tocolytic of choice after 32 weeks of gestation?

A. Indomethacin B. Terbutaline
C. Both of the above D. None of the above

17. Which of the following statement is incorrect regarding laparoscopy use during pregnancy?

A. Laparoscopy is safely performed during any trimester when indicated
B. CO_2 pressure of 10-15 mm Hg can be safely used
C. Laparoscopy has low incidence of preterm labor than open technique
D. If inadvertent entry into uterus occur during trocar access, simple closure of defect and monitoring is adequate

18. Which is not the complication associated with laparoscopic intervention during pregnancy?

A. Decreased uterine blood flow
B. Preterm labor
C. Fetal alkalosis
D. Uterine injury

19. Which of the following is false statement concerning breast masses?

A. Most breast lesions that are diagnosed during pregnancy and lactation are benign
B. Pregnancy-associated breast cancer is defined as breast cancer diagnosed during pregnancy or within one 6 months after pregnancy
C. Mammography has a high false-negative rate
D. Core biopsy remains the standard for tissue diagnosis during pregnancy

20. Which is most common non gynaecological malignancy in pregnancy?

A. Ca breast B. Ca lung
C. Ca colon D. Lymphoma

21. Regarding pregnancy-associated breast cancer, which is correct statement?

A. Most common pathologic type is lobular carcinoma
B. Pregnancy-associated breast cancer have a similar stage-related prognosis compared with non-pregnant
C. High incidence of estrogen receptor–positive cancer
D. MRI is recommended for breast imaging in the pregnant patient

22. 34 years old woman with 12 weeks of gestational age presented with 2 cm biopsy proven DCIS in right breast with clinically node negative. What is the appropriate management for this patient?

A. Continued clinical examination till delivery
B. Modified radical mastectomy followed by chemotherapy after delivery
C. Breast conservation surgery with axillary dissection and chemotherapy
D. Breast conservation surgery with partial breast radiotherapy

23. Chemotherapy can be given for pregnancy associated breast cancer in the following conditions except:

A. During second trimester
B. Node positive breast cancer
C. Size > 1 cm with node negative
D. During breastfeeding

24. 16 weeks pregnant female presented with stage III breast cancer. What is most appropriate treatment?

A. Wait till delivery followed by radiation therapy
B. Elective termination of pregnancy for appropriate therapy

C. Modified radical mastectomy followed by radiation post delivery
D. Systemic chemotherapy

25. Which of the following is false about acute fatty liver of pregnancy?

A. It is more common in female with male fetus
B. It usually occurs during the second trimester
C. Liver function typically returns to normal after delivery
D. It carries a 20% maternal and fetal mortality rate

26. Which of the following is not associated with acute fatty liver of pregnancy?

A. First pregnancy
B. Twin pregnancy
C. Pregnant with male fetus
D. Previous miscarriage

27. What is the diagnostic modality of choice in preeclampsia with upper right quadrant pain?

A. USG B. CT
C. MRI D. Plain radiograph

28. LeBeau and Mandel guidelines used for the treatment of:

A. Pheochromocytoma B. Hyperthyroidism
C. Hypothyroidism D. Gestational diabetes

29. Which of the following statement is incorrect regarding thyrotoxicosis in pregnancy?

A. Gestational thyrotoxicosis is usually self-limited
B. Spontaneously resolves by 28 weeks of gestation
C. Most common cause is Graves' disease
D. Mainstay of treatment is medical treatment with thionamides

30. Thyroidectomy advised for Graves in pregnancy for following situations:

A. Compressive symptoms due to size
B. Allergic to thionamides
C. High dose PTU (> 600 mg/day) or methimazole (> 40 mg/day)
D. All of the above

31. What is the most common non-obstretric abdominal surgical problem in pregnancy?

A. Acute appendicitis
B. Acute cholecystitis
C. Intestinal obstruction
D. Diverticulitis

32. Non operative management for small bowel obstruction can be done upto what period of time during pregnancy?

A. 2 to 4 hours B. 4 to 6 hours
C. 6 to 8 hours D. Upto 12 hours

33. Which statement is false concerning acute appendicitis during pregnancy?

A. It occurs in 1 in 1000 to 1500 pregnancies
B. Treatment of suspected acute appendicitis in the pregnant patient is emergent appendectomy
C. Negative appendectomy rate of 40% to 50% has been accepted during pregnancy
D. MRI is preferred adjust for accurate diagnosis during pregnancy

34. Find incorrect statement of the following:

A. Laparoscopic cholecystectomy can be done safely during 12 to 24 weeks of gestation
B. Surgery for pheochromocytoma should be done before 20 weeks of gestation
C. Thyroid cancer is diagnosed late in gestation, surgery can be performed after delivery
D. In acute iliofemoral thrombosis during pregnancy, caval filter is placed in infrarenal location

35. What is cut off size of splenic artery aneurysms for surgical intervention during pregnancy?

A. 1 cm B. 1.5 cm
C. 2 cm D. 2.5 cm

36. What is the most common cause of fetal death after blunt trauma?

A. Uterine rupture
B. Preterm labor
C. Abruptio placentae
D. Maternal hypovolemia

37. Which is false about use of REBOA in uncontrolled obstetric hemorrhage?

A. It has demonstrated lower transfusion volumes than other occlusion techniques
B. It may put women at a higher risk of arterial thrombosis and ipsilateral limb ischemia
C. Zone 3 (Infrarenal) occlusion is generally tolerated for several hours
D. Sheath should ideally removed within 48 hours of initial placement

38. What is most common cause of massive hemorrhage after delivery?

A. Uterine atony
B. Retained placenta
C. Uterine inversion
D. Coagulopathy

39. What is minimum volume of blood required for cell salvage?

A. 250 ml
B. 500 ml
C. 1000 ml
D. 1500 ml

40. What is current consensus about delaying planned pregnancy after bariatric surgery?

A. 6 months
B. 1 year
C. 2 years
D. 4 years

41. What is best method of fertility preservation for woman with breast cancer?

A. IVF
B. Embryo cryopreservation
C. Surrogacy
D. Ovarian stimulation

42. Which of the following is correct about diagnosed malignancy in pregnancy?

A. There is negative effect of pregnancy on recurrence rate and survival in patients treated for breast cancer
B. Survival is affected by hormonal receptor status
C. Premenopausal women with breast cancer should wait two years before attempting to conceive
D. The occurrence of preterm labor or miscarriage is similar in patients with breast cancer compared with those with no history of breast cancer

ANSWERS

1. **Ans: C. The incidence of symptomatic cholelithiasis during pregnancy is more as compared to the incidence in age-related nonpregnant women**
Ref: Chapter No. 72, Page No. 2026-2027

2. **Ans: C. Hemorrhoids**
Ref: Chapter No. 72, Page No. 2027

3. **Ans: C. Serum creatinine**
Ref: Chapter No. 72, Page No. 2027

4. **Ans: B. 5 cGy**
Ref: Chapter No. 72, Page No. 2028

5. **Ans: B. 10 cGy**
Ref: Chapter No. 72, Page No. 2028

6. **Ans: C. MRI is useful modality during the first trimester of pregnancy**
Ref: Chapter No. 72, Page No. 2028

7. **Ans: B. Barium enema**
Ref: Chapter No. 72, Page No. 2028

8. **Ans: D. Category X**
Ref: Chapter No. 72, Page No. 2029

9. **Ans: C. Category D**
Ref: Chapter No. 72, Page No. 2029

10. **Ans: C. Sulfonamides**
Ref: Chapter No. 72, Page No. 2029

11. **Ans: C. Warfarin**
Ref: Chapter No. 72, Page No. 2031

12. **Ans: D. All of the above**
Ref: Chapter No. 72, Page No. 2031

13. **Ans: A. Low dose aspirin (60-100 mg) is safe during pregnancy**
Ref: Chapter No. 72, Page No. 2032

14. **Ans: B. <5%**
Ref: Chapter No. 72, Page No. 2032

15. **Ans: C. Indomethacin**
Ref: Chapter No. 72, Page No. 2032

16. **Ans: B. Terbutaline**
Ref: Chapter No. 72, Page No. 2032

17. **Ans: C. Laparoscopy has low incidence of preterm labor than open technique**
Ref: Chapter No. 72, Page No. 2032-2034

18. **Ans: C. Fetal alkalosis**
Ref: Chapter No. 72, Page No. 2034

19. **Ans: B. Pregnancy-associated breast cancer is defined as breast cancer diagnosed during pregnancy or within one 6 months after pregnancy**
Ref: Chapter No. 72, Page No. 2034-2035

20. **Ans: A. Ca breast**
Ref: Chapter No. 72, Page No. 2035

21. **Ans: B. Pregnancy-associated breast cancer have a similar stage-related prognosis compared with non-pregnant**
Ref: Chapter No. 72, Page No. 2035

22. **Ans: C. Breast conservation surgery with axillary dissection and chemotherapy**

Ref: Chapter No. 72, Page No. 2035

23. **Ans: D. During breastfeeding**

Ref: Chapter No. 72, Page No. 2035

24. **Ans: D. Systemic chemotherapy**

Ref: Chapter No. 72, Page No. 2036

25. **Ans: B. It usually occurs during the second trimester**

Ref: Chapter No. 72, Page No. 2036-2037

26. **Ans: D. Previous miscarriage**

Ref: Chapter No. 72, Page No. 2036

27. **Ans: B. CT**

Ref: Chapter No. 72, Page No. 2037

28. **Ans: C. Hypothyroidism**

Ref: Chapter No. 72, Page No. 2039

29. **Ans: B. Spontaneously resolves by 28 weeks of gestation**

Ref: Chapter No. 72, Page No. 2039

30. **Ans: D. All of the above**

Ref: Chapter No. 72, Page No. 2039

31. **Ans: A. Acute appendicitis**

Ref: Chapter No. 72, Page No. 2039

32. **Ans: C. 6 to 8 hours**

Ref: Chapter No. 72, Page No. 2039

33. **Ans: C. Negative appendectomy rate of 40% to 50% has been accepted during pregnancy**

Ref: Chapter No. 72, Page No. 2039

34. **Ans: D. In acute iliofemoral thrombosis during pregnancy, caval filter is placed in infrarenal location**

Ref: Chapter No. 72, Page No. 2039-2041

35. **Ans: C. 2 cm**

Ref: Chapter No. 72, Page No. 2041

36. **Ans: C. Abruptio placentae**

Ref: Chapter No. 72, Page No. 2041

37. **Ans: D. Sheath should ideally removed within 48 hours of initial placement**

Ref: Chapter No. 72, Page No. 2043-2044

38. **Ans: A. Uterine atony**

Ref: Chapter No. 72, Page No. 2044

39. **Ans: B. 500 ml**

Ref: Chapter No. 72, Page No. 2044

40. **Ans: C. 2 years**

Ref: Chapter No. 72, Page No. 2044

41. **Ans: B. Embryo cryopreservation**

Ref: Chapter No. 72, Page No. 2045

42. **Ans: D. The occurrence of preterm labor or miscarriage is similar in patients with breast cancer compared with those with no history of breast cancer**

Ref: Chapter No. 72, Page No. 2045

73

Fetal Surgery

1. **The first open fetal surgical intervention was done for:**
   A. Twin-twin transfusion syndrome (TTTS)
   B. Obstructive uropathy
   C. Myelomeningocele
   D. Congenital diaphragmatic hernia

2. **First open fetal surgery performed by:**
   A. Liley
   B. Rodek
   C. Harrison
   D. Warren

3. **All are the maternal risks of fetal surgery except:**
   A. Chorioamnionitis
   B. Placental abruption
   C. Preterm premature rupture of membrane
   D. Polyhydramnios

4. **What is the Achilles heel of fetal surgery?**
   A. Maternal hemorrhage prevention
   B. Preterm labor prevention
   C. Placental abruption prevention
   D. IUFD prevention

5. **Which of the following is incorrect about open fetal repair of meningomyelocele?**
   A. Repair is targeted to mid second trimester
   B. Hysterotomy is done with low transverse uterine incision
   C. Decreased need for ventriculoperitoneal shunting with fetal repair
   D. Improved motor function compared to the postnatal surgery group

6. **MOMS Trial was done for:**
   A. Metastatic melanoma
   B. Maternal hemorrhage control
   C. Meningomyelocele
   D. Medical termination of pregnancy

7. **Non immune fetal hydrops is not seen with which of the following condition?**
   A. Twin-twin transfusion syndrome
   B. Sacrococcygeal teratoma
   C. CPAM
   D. Gastroschisis

8. **Sacrococcygeal teratoma can be managed with following procedures except:**
   A. EXIT-to-resection procedure
   B. Radiofrequency ablation
   C. Open fetal resection
   D. Aspiration

9. **Most common approach used for sacrococcygeal teratoma:**
   A. Aspiration
   B. Radiofrequency ablation
   C. EXIT procedure
   D. Maternal hysterotomy with resection

10. **What is EXIT procedure?**
    A. Extrauterine intraamniotic treatment
    B. Extraamniotic intrauterine treatment
    C. Ex utero intrapartum treatment
    D. Ex utero intervention therapy

11. **EXIT-to-airway procedure is done for:**
    A. Fetoscopic tracheal occlusion
    B. Fetal endotracheal intubation before EXIT procedure
    C. Maternal endotracheal intubation during EXIT procedure
    D. All of the above

12. **Which of the following is correct about EXIT procedure?**
    A. In EXIT-to-resection procedure, mass is resected first and an airway is established later

B. EXIT procedure is done under spinal anaesthesia
C. Contraction of the uterus is ideal because it is hemostatic
D. Fetus undergoes premature transition from fetal to neonatal circulation

13. Symptomatic in utero congenital lung lesion can be managed by:

A. USG guided aspiration
B. Thoracoamniotic shunt placement
C. EXIT procedure
D. All of the above

14. Criteria for fetal intervention regarding congenital lung lesion:

A. Presence of CPAM
B. Bronchopulmonary sequestration with hydrops
C. Large symptomatic macrocyst
D. Placentomegaly with fetal cardiomegaly

15. Thoracoamniotic shunt is done for which of the following conditions?

A. Congenital diaphragmatic hernia
B. Tracheoesophageal fistula
C. Congenital pulmonary airway malformation
D. Cystic hygroma

16. Which of the following is true regarding congenital diaphragmatic hernia (CDH)?

A. Neonatal death commonly due to pulmonary hypoplasia
B. CDH present as isolated defect
C. Estimated survival of fetus with CDH is about 50%
D. Fetal tracheal occlusion shows improved survival

17. Twin-twin transfusion syndrome seen with:

A. Monochorionic monoamniotic twins
B. Monochorionic diamniotic twins
C. Dichorionic monoamniotic twins
D. Dichorionic diamniotic twins

18. Fetal laser ablation can be performed for Twin transfusion syndrome during:

A. 6 to 10 weeks of gestation
B. 12 to 16 weeks of gestation
C. 18 to 24 weeks of gestation
D. 25 to 28 weeks of gestation

19. Application of in utero stem cell transplantation is useful in all of the following except:

A. Sickel cell anemia
B. Osteogenesis imperfecta
C. Gastroschisis
D. Hemophilia B

20. Which of the following is incorrect about "Biobag"?

A. It is extracorporeal placenta aimed at improving outcomes for extreme premature infants of 22 to 23 weeks of gestation
B. A pump assisted arteriovenous circuit where the fetus heart drives blood flow
C. A closed fluid environment with continuous fluid exchange
D. Access through umbilical vessels

ANSWERS

1. **Ans: B. Obstructive uropathy**

   Ref: Chapter No. 73, Page No. 2050

2. **Ans: C. Harrison**

   Ref: Chapter No. 73, Page No. 2050

3. **Ans: D. Polyhydramnios**

   Ref: Chapter No. 73, Page No. 2051

4. **Ans: B. Preterm labor prevention**

   Ref: Chapter No. 73, Page No. 2051

5. **Ans: B. Hysterotomy is done with low transverse uterine incision**

   Ref: Chapter No. 73, Page No. 2052

6. **Ans: C. Meningomyelocele**

   Ref: Chapter No. 73, Page No. 2052

7. **Ans: D. Gastroschisis**

   Ref: Chapter No. 73, Page No. 2052-2053

8. **Ans: D. Aspiration**

   Ref: Chapter No. 73, Page No. 2053

9. **Ans: D. Maternal hysterotomy with resection**

   Ref: Chapter No. 73, Page No. 2053

10. **Ans: C. Ex utero intrapartum treatment**

    Ref: Chapter No. 73, Page No. 2053

11. **Ans: B. Fetal endotracheal intubation before EXIT procedure**

    Ref: Chapter No. 73, Page No. 2053

12. **Ans: A. In EXIT-to-resection procedure, mass is resected first and an airway is established later**

    Ref: Chapter No. 73, Page No. 2053

13. **Ans: D. All of the above**

    Ref: Chapter No. 73, Page No. 2054

14. **Ans: A. Presence of CPAM**

    Ref: Chapter No. 73, Page No. 2054

15. **Ans: C. Congenital pulmonary airway malformation**

    Ref: Chapter No. 73, Page No. 2054

16. **Ans: A. Neonatal death commonly due to pulmonary hypoplasia**

    Ref: Chapter No. 73, Page No. 2054

17. **Ans: B. Monochorionic diamniotic twins**

    Ref: Chapter No. 73, Page No. 2055

18. **Ans: C. 18 to 24 weeks of gestation**

    Ref: Chapter No. 73, Page No. 2055

19. **Ans: D. Hemophilia B**

    Ref: Chapter No. 73, Page No. 2057

20. **Ans: B. A pump assisted arteriovenous circuit where the fetus heart drives blood flow**

    Ref: Chapter No. 73, Page No. 2058

74

Urology

ANATOMY

1. **All are true statements regarding adrenal gland except:**
   A. The cortex of the adrenal gland and is derived from mesoderm
   B. The adrenal medulla is directly innervated by postsynaptic sympathetic fibers
   C. The adrenal glands lie within Gerota fascia
   D. Splenic vein is anterior to the cortical surface of left adrenal gland

2. **Adrenal medulla is derived from:**
   A. Ectoderm B. Mesoderm
   C. Endoderm D. Neural crest cells

3. **Which is false about renal anatomy?**
   A. Gerota fascia forms the renal capsule
   B. The spleen is situated anteromedial to the left kidney
   C. Renal artery originates from aorta at the level of L2
   D. Each segmental artery of kidney is an end artery

4. **Following are the tributaries of left renal vein except:**
   A. Left inferior phrenic vein
   B. Left adrenal vein
   C. Left gonadal vein
   D. Left lumbar vein

5. **All are true about ureteric anatomy except:**
   A. Ureteropelvic junction lies posterior to the renal artery
   B. Each ureter is 22 to 30 cm in length
   C. Ureter has three distinct narrowing point
   D. The lower ureteral segments have a medial vascular supply

6. **Prostatic venous plexus is also known as:**
   A. Batson plexus B. Santorini plexus
   C Burow plexus D. Sappey plexus

7. **Prostate is related to following fascial layers except:**
   A. Lateral pelvic fascia B. Endopelvic fascia
   C. Waldeyer fascia D. Denonvilliers fascia

8. **Fossa navicularis is another name for:**
   A. Prostatic urethra
   B. Membranous urethra
   C. Bulbar urethra
   D. Glandular urethra

9. **External pudendal artery supplies following structures except:**
   A. Penile skin B. Corpora cavernosa
   C. Scrotum D. Labium majora

10. **Internal spermatic fascia is derived from:**
    A. Transversalis fascia
    B. Transversus abdominis
    C. Internal oblique
    D. External oblique

ENDOSCOPIC UROLOGIC SURGERY

11. **What is the size of adult flexible cystoscope?**
    A. 10 Fr B. 14 Fr
    C. 16 Fr D. 20 Fr

12. **Which is false about flexible cystoscope?**
    A. Local anesthesia can be used
    B. Require specific patient positioning
    C. Bedside procedure
    D. It has large deflection radius

13. **False about flexible ureteroscope:**
    A. 6 Fr to 7.5 Fr at the tip
    B. 8.4 Fr to 10.1 Fr at base
    C. Deflection of the tip ranges from 130 to 250 degrees in one direction
    D. Deflection of the tip ranges from 160 to 275 degrees in the opposite direction

14. **What is the size of rigid nephroscope?**
    A. 14 – 16 Fr B. 18 – 20 Fr
    C. 22 – 24 Fr D. 25 – 28 Fr

15. **Identify the instrument used for urologic procedures:**

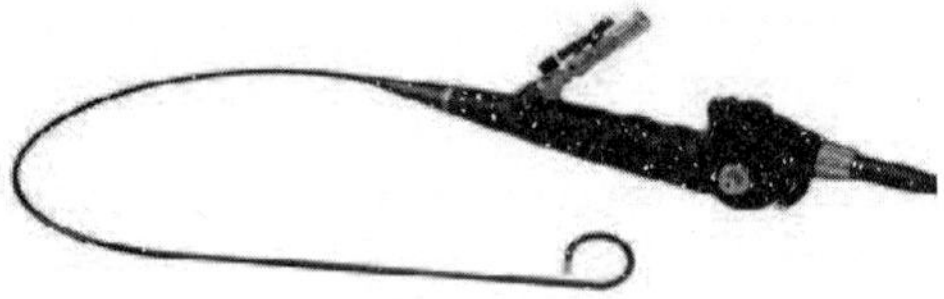

    A. Flexible cystoscope
    B. Flexible ureteroscope
    C. Resectoscope
    D. Semirigid nephroscope

UROLOGIC INFECTIOUS DISEASE

16. **Which is wrong statement about urinary tract infection?**
    A. Females are more commonly affected
    B. UTI in men is generally considered "complicated"
    C. Midstream urine specimen is preferred for diagnosis
    D. Presence of 10^3 CFU on urine culture is diagnostic of UTI

17. **Presence of ___ CFU on urine culture is diagnostic for catheter associated UTI.**
    A. 10^2 B. 10^3
    C. 10^4 D. 10^5

18. **What is the most common cause of UTI?**
    A. Neisseria gonorrhoeae
    B. Staph. saphrophyticus
    C. E. coli
    D. Klebsiella pneumoniae

19. **Which of the following is the example of uncomplicated UTI?**
    A. Immunocompetent female
    B. Current indwelling Foley catheter
    C. Upper urinary tract infection
    D. Infection with resistant organism

20. **Which is the example of uncomplicated UTI in males?**
    A. Immunocompetent male
    B. Prior urologic surgery
    C. Spinal cord injury
    D. None of the above

21. **What is the most common cause of emphysematous pyelonephritis?**
    A. Proteus mirabilis
    B. E. coli
    C. Klebsiella pneumoniae
    D. Enterobacter

22. **46 years old female presented with palpable left sided abdominal mass with symptoms of fever with chills. Patient is known diabetic since 7 years. CT findings as follows. What is the probable diagnosis?**

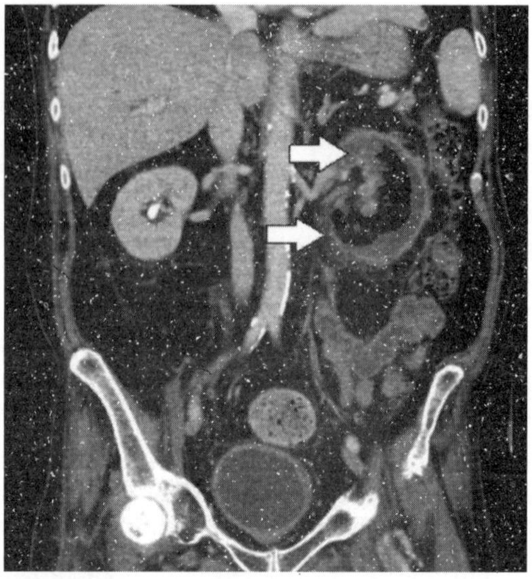

    A. Angiomyolipoma
    B. Emphysematous pyelonephritis
    C. Xanthogranulomatous pyelonephritis
    D. Renal cell carcinoma

23. **Which is false regarding xanthogranulomatous pyelonephritis?**
    A. It is an acute infectious process
    B. Secondary to renal obstruction or renal calculus
    C. Foamy, lipid-laden, macrophage infiltrate in the renal parenchyma with extensive inflammation is characteristic
    D. Involvement of adjacent tissue due to extensive fibrotic reaction

24. Which is false about prostatic abscess?

A. Digital rectal examination should be performed
B. Prolong duration of symptoms
C. Poor antibiotic response
D. Require transurethral de-roofing of abscess

25. Which is the most common sexually transmitted organism causing UTI?

A. Neisseria gonorrhoeae
B. Chlamydia trachomatis
C. Trichomonas vaginalis
D. E. coli

26. Patient presented with following clinical signs. Presence of pain, tenderness, necrotic patches and foul smelling discharge from scrotum. Which is incorrect regarding this condition?

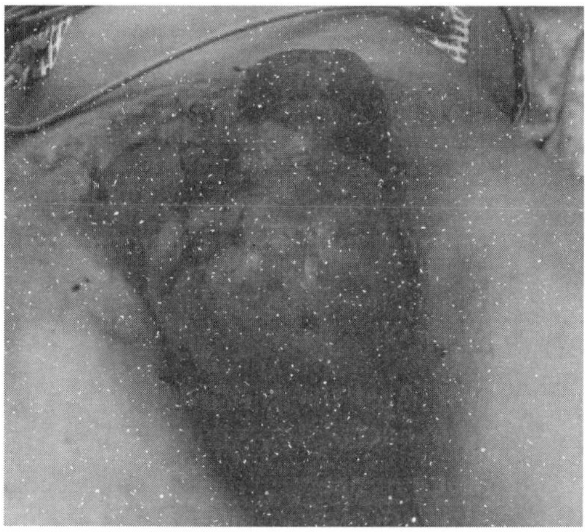

A. It is usually a polymicrobial infection
B. Diabetes mellitus, alcoholism and immunocompromised states are known risk factors
C. Treatment requires emergency aggressive debridement of the necrotic tissue with intravenous broad spectrum antibiotics
D. It commonly involves the testicles or deep tissues of the penis

27. Most commonly affected genitourinary organ in schistosomiasis:

A. Kidney B. Bladder
C. Testes D. Urethra

NEUROGENIC BLADDER

28. Which is false about neurogenic functions of urinary bladder?

A. Bladder storage is driven by the sympathetic nervous system
B. Bladder emptying is driven by the parasympathetic stimulation of cholinergic receptors
C. Voiding is initiated at the level of the pontine micturition center
D. The periaqueductal gray located in the midbrain has stimulatory effect on micturition center

29. All of the following are features of sacral nerve lesion except:

A. Nonfunctional detrusor muscle
B. Abnormal elasticity of the bladder
C. Contracted urinary sphincter
D. Incomplete emptying

30. Following are storage related symptoms of bladder except:

A. Frequency B. Hesitancy
C. Urgency D. Nocturia

31. The sudden, compelling desire to pass urine that is difficult to defer is known as:

A. Strangury B. Urgency
C. Hesitancy D. Frequency

32. Nocturia is defined as:

A. Involuntary urinary leakage during sleep
B. Interruption of sleep due to involuntary urinary leakage
C. Interruption of sleep one or more times due to need for urination
D. Interruption of sleep two or more times due to need for urination

33. What is the first line therapy for overactive bladder?

A. Pharmacotherapy
B. Behavioral therapy
C. Neuromodulation
D. Onabotulinum toxin

34. What is mainstay of treatment for overactive bladder?

A. Pharmacotherapy
B. Bladder training
C. Onabotulinum toxin
D. Augmentation cystoplasty

35. Which is incorrect about urinary incontinence?

A. It is more common in females above 20 years of age
B. In the neurologically normal patient, surgical management is the first step in treatment
C. Patients are counseled to limit fluid intake to around 2 L/day

D. Placement of a midurethral sling in females provides long-term cure and high success rates

BENIGN PROSTATIC HYPERPLASIA (BPH)

36. All are true about BPH except:

A. BPH is most prevalent in men between the ages of 60 and 69 years
B. The degree of bladder outflow obstruction correlates with the severity of LUTS
C. PSA testing is recommended in patients with a life expectancy of more than 10 years
D. The mainstay of treatment for LUTS due to BPH is α1-adrenergic receptor blockers

37. Following are indications for surgical intervention in BPH except:

A. Acute urinary retention
B. Increased PSA
C. Recurrent UTI
D. Bladder calculi

38. 5α-reductase inhibitors alter PSA levels by:

A. Increases by 25% B. Reduces by 25%
C. Increases by 50% D. Reduces by 50%

39. 62 years old male presented with symptoms of LUTS. Cystoscopic findings are as follows. What is the probable diagnosis?

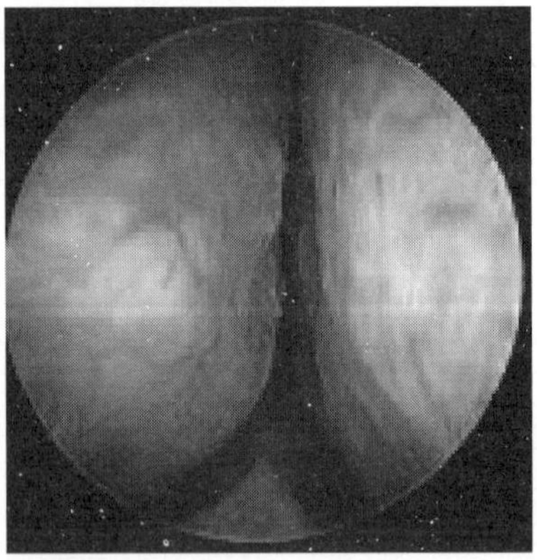

A. Urethral stricture
B. Urethral diverticulum
C. Benign prostatic hyperplasia
D. Bladder carcinoma

40. Following are the complications of TURP procedure except:

A. Persistent bleeding
B. Urethral stricture
C. Retrograde ejaculation
D. Hypernatremia

MALE SEXUAL DYSFUNCTION

41. Which is false regarding male infertility?

A. The male factor is the primary or sole factor in 36% to 75% of infertility cases
B. Infertility is defined as a couple's inability to achieve pregnancy after one year of unprotected intercourse
C. Perineal and rectal examinations are routine assessment
D. The semen analyses should be separated by two month and preceded by 1 week of abstinence

42. Male infertility is divided according to following causes except:

A. Anatomic causes
B. Behavioral and environmental causes
C. Iatrogenic causes
D. Idiopathic causes

43. Correct method of semen analysis:

A. The semen analyses should be separated by one month and preceded by 1 week of abstinence
B. The semen analyses should be separated by one month and preceded by 2 - 3 days of abstinence
C. The semen analyses should be separated by two months and preceded by 1 week of abstinence
D. The semen analyses should be separated by two months and preceded by 2-3 days of abstinence

44. Which is false regarding management of male sexual dysfunction?

A. Erectile dysfunction is considered an early marker for cardiovascular disease
B. The basis of medical therapy for ED is phosphodiesterase type 5 inhibitor
C. Revascularization of the penis is usually achieved using an inferior epigastric artery pedicle flap
D. The goal of therapy is maintenance of testosterone levels between 100 and 400 ng/dL

45. Which is wrong about penile implant surgery?

A. Use of malleable, inflatable silicone implants
B. Implanted bilaterally in the corpora
C. Pumping device is placed in medial thigh region
D. Fluid reservoir positioned in the retropubic space extra-peritoneally

46. Testosterone deficiency is associated with following symptoms except:

A. Lack of energy
B. Decreased cognitive acuity
C. Reduced body fat
D. Irritability

47. Following are adverse effect of testosterone therapy except:

A. Cardiovascular events
B. Polycythemia
C. Gynecomastia
D. Decreased cognitive acuity

48. Target testosterone levels maintained in case of hypogonadism:

A. 100 to 300 ng/dL
B. 400 to 700 ng/dL
C. 700 to 900 ng/dL
D. 1000 to 1200 ng/dL

UROLITHIASIS

49. Which are most common type of urinary stones?

A. Calcium oxalate B. Uric acid stone
C. Struvite stones D. Calcium phosphate

50. Which stones are radiolucent?

A. Calcium oxalate B. Uric acid stones
C. Cystine stones D. Struvite stones

51. Which stones are formed in urinary infection?

A. Calcium phosphate B. Calcium oxalate
C. Uric acid stones D. Struvite stones

52. Following bacterial infections are associated with formation of struvite stones except:

A. Proteus mirabilis
B. Staph. aureus
C. Klebsiella pneumoniae
D. E. coli

53. Which is false statement regarding urinary stones?

A. Calcium stone are formed in urine with low citrate
B. Uric acid stones form in a low pH urine
C. Struvite stones are magnesium ammonium phosphate
D. Indinavir stones are radiopaque

54. What is investigation of choice for renal stones?

A. Plain radiograph
B. Ultrasonography
C. Intravenous urography
D. Non contrast CT abdomen

55. All are true regarding management of renal stones except:

A. Patients who present with upper tract UTI and obstruction should undergo expeditious drainage with either cystoscopic ureteral stent placement or percutaneous nephrostomy tube placement
B. The single most important treatment is increased fluid intake to achieve more than two liters of urine output daily
C. Calcium consumption is reduced in case of calcium stones
D. Alkalinizing agents are used to raise urinary pH in cases of uric acid stones

56. Which is incorrect about shock wave lithotripsy?

A. It is transcutaneous noninvasive method
B. Stone fragmentation monitored with fluoroscopy
C. Non-radiopaque and proximal ureteric stones can be treated
D. Steinstrasse is characteristic complication of SWL

57. ESWL can be safely used for stones upto size of:

A. 1 cm B. 1.5 cm
C. 2 cm D. 2.5 cm

58. Which is false regarding percutaneous nephrolithotomy procedure?

A. Larger working endoscopes
B. Numerous intracorporeal lithotripsy devices are available
C. Postoperative renal drainage required
D. Steinstrasse

59. What is procedure of choice for renal calyceal stones?

A. ESWL
B. Ureteroscopic laser lithotripsy
C. PCNL
D. Laparoscopic nephrolithotomy

UROLOGIC TRAUMA

60. Urologic injury is present in _______% of all abdominal and pelvic trauma patients.

A. 5% B. 15%
C. 25% D. 35%

61. Which is incorrect about traumatic renal injury?

A. The majority of renal injuries are the result of blunt trauma
B. 70% of all patients who sustain renal injury are male
C. In penetrating renal injury, hemodynamically stable patients with gross hematuria should undergo surgical intervention
D. Contrast-enhanced CT scan, is the preferred study to evaluate the renal injuries

62. Following are indications for imaging in case of blunt renal trauma except:

A. Gross hematuria
B. Systolic blood pressure > 90 mm Hg
C. Microscopic hematuria of > 5 RBC/hpf in adults
D. Suspicion of injury on screening radiographs

63. According to AAST renal injury grades, renal laceration with extravasation of urine is:

A. Grade II B. Grade III
C. Grade IV D. Grade V

64. According to AAST renal injury grades, which grade includes non-expanding perirenal hematoma confined to renal retroperitoneum?

A. Grade I B. Grade II
C. Grade III D. Grade IV

65. Wrongly matched AAST renal injury grade of the following:

A. Grade I - Microscopic or gross hematuria urologic studies normal
B. Grade II - Subcapsular, nonexpanding hematoma without parenchymal laceration
C. Grade III - > 1 cm cortical renal laceration without urine extravasation
D. Grade V - Avulsion of renal hilum

66. According to AAST renal injury grades, which grade includes main renal vascular injury?

A. Grade II B. Grade III
C. Grade IV D. Grade V

67. Which is an absolute criteria for operative exploration of renal trauma?

A. Arterial injury
B. Persistent renal bleeding
C. Incomplete renal staging
D. Persistent urinary extravasation

68. According to AAST system, which renal injury grade is shown in the following figure?

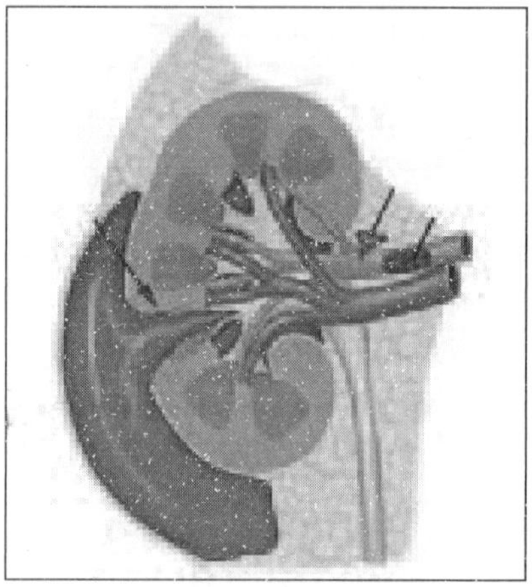

A. Grade II B. Grade III
C. Grade IV D. Grade V

69. Following are the indications for renal angiographic embolization in cases of renal trauma except:

A. Intravascular extravasation of contrast material
B. Perirenal hematoma rim distance of more than 25 mm
C. Medial hematomas
D. Those who have received more than four units of blood transfusion

70. 35 years old male with RTA presented as gross hematuria and severe abdominal pain on left flank region. On examination, P–110/min, Bp–100/70 mm Hg, conscious. CECT abdomen imaging as follows:

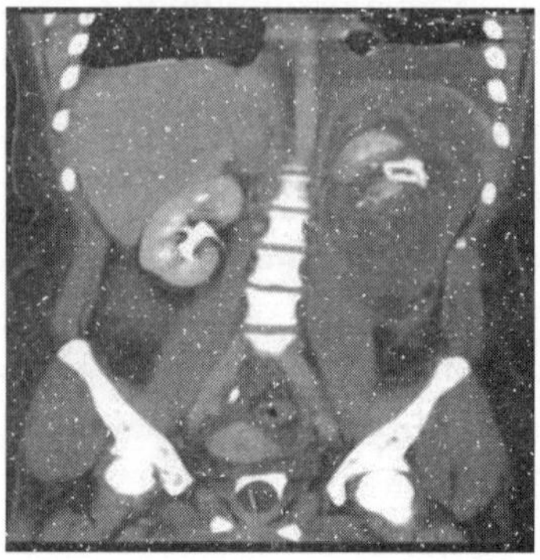

What is best step of management for this patient?

A. Conservative management with serial imaging
B. Percutaneous drain placement
C. Exploratory laparotomy with abdominal packing
D. Exploration with left nephrectomy

71. Which is false about ureteric injuries due to trauma?

A. Up to 5% to 10% of penetrating abdominal or pelvic injuries have ureteral involvement
B. Contrast enhanced CT scan is investigation of choice
C. While repair, ureter is skeletonized along the length
D. Surgical repair of ureter is always preferred when permitted

72. Which is incorrect regarding traumatic bladder injury?

A. Most of the patients with bladder injury will present with pelvic fracture
B. Patients with suspected bladder injury should be evaluated with retrograde cystography
C. Most extra peritoneal bladder injuries can be managed with catheter drainage
D. Defects in the bladder wall are closed with absorbable 2-0 sutures in one layer

73. Patient presented with blunt trauma to abdomen with post traumatic retention of urine. Patient is hemodynamically stable and has suprapubic tenderness. Retrograde cystographic findings are as follows:

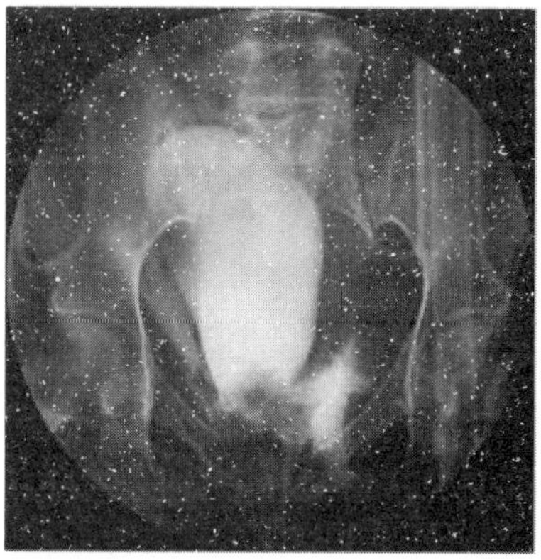

What is the most appropriate management for this patient?

A. Observation with repeat cystogram
B. Non-operative management with catheter drainage
C. Cystoscopy to rule out urethral injury
D. Bladder repair surgery

74. Following are the indications for surgical repair of extra peritoneal bladder rupture except:

A. Penetrating bladder trauma
B. Bone fragment in the bladder
C. Concomitant urethral injury
D. Bladder neck injuries

75. Which is incorrect regarding urethral injury?

A. Most commonly injured segment is the bulbar urethra
B. "Butterfly" hematoma is due to rupture of Buck fascia in case of urethral injury
C. Retrograde urethrography should be performed before attempting the insertion of a Foley catheter
D. Penetrating anterior urethral injury repair is done in delayed fashion

76. Most commonly injured segment in urethral trauma:

A. Prostatic
B. Membranous
C. Bulbar
D. Penile

77. Following are features of urethral injury except:

A. Blood at meatus
B. Ascended prostate
C. Gross hematuria
D. Butterfly hematoma

78. Patient presented with blunt trauma to pelvis. On examination blood was present at meatus and ascended prostate on DRE. Patient is hemodynamically stable. What is immediate next step of management?

A. Gentle urethral catheterization
B. Retrograde urethrogram
C. Suprapubic cystostomy
D. Exploratory laparotomy

79. Pie in the sky bladder on radiography is seen in:

A. Bladder rupture
B. Membranous urethral rupture
C. Bulbar urethral rupture
D. Pelvic fracture

80. Patient presents with blunt lower abdominal trauma. Retrograde urethrogram shows pubic rami fracture with extravasation of contrast below pelvic diaphragm. Patient has complaint

of urinary retention. What is the best step of management?

A. Observation with follow up imaging
B. Gentle per urethral catheterization
C. Suprapubic cystostomy
D. Exploration and urethral reconstruction over catheter

81. **Which is incorrect about genital injuries management?**

A. Ultrasonography is used as an initial imaging modality in genital injuries
B. Blunt testicular injuries should always be explored
C. Penile fracture should be surgically explored and repaired primarily
D. Aggressive debridement of tissue in case of penile injuries should be avoided

82. **Which factor does not constitute "the lethal triad"?**

A. Hypothermia
B. Hypotension
C. Acidosis
D. Coagulopathy

83. **A Renal injuries that are incompletely staged or unstaged without suspicion of active bleed can be managed with delayed reconstruction:**

A. Renal injuries that are incompletely staged or unstaged without suspicion active bleed can be managed with delayed reconstruction
B. Ureteral injuries in unstable patient managed initially with externalized stents
C. The external catheter should be tied to the very end of the injured ureter at the injury site
D. Ligation of the injured distal ureteral limb is recommended

NONTRAUMATIC UROLOGIC EMERGENCIES

84. **Surgical exploration of torsion testis should be done within:**

A. 1 hour
B. 4 hours
C. 8 hours
D. 10 hours

85. **Which is false about management of testicular torsion?**

A. Irreversible damage to testis begins as soon as four hours
B. The most consistent physical examination finding is loss of the cremasteric reflex of the testicle
C. In patients with suspected testicular torsion, Doppler examination is necessary to check viability
D. Contralateral orchiopexy should be done at the same setting

86. **All are true statements about priapism except:**

A. Priapism is a prolonged, painful penile erection that occurs in the absence of sexual arousal or stimulation
B. Intervention is needed, if priapism persists longer than 8 hours
C. Ischemic priapism is managed with initial needle aspiration of the corpora cavernosa and irrigation with saline
D. Non-ischemic priapism is caused by traumatic arteriovenous fistula

87. **Intervention is recommended in case of priapism persisting for:**

A. 2 hours
B. 4 hours
C. 8 hours
D. 12 hours

RENAL CANCER

88. **Which factor does not constitute the classic triad of renal cell carcinoma?**

A. Flank pain
B. Microhematuria
C. Gross hematuria
D. Palpable abdominal mass

89. **Which is incorrect about incidence of renal cell carcinoma?**

A. Renal cell carcinoma typically presents in the sixth to eighth decade of life
B. It is more common in men
C. Majority are diagnosed incidentally by cross-sectional imaging
D. The classic triad of renal cell carcinoma is seen in 50% of patients

90. **The classic triad of renal cell carcinoma is seen in ___% of patients.**

A. < 5%
B. 10%
C. 20%
D. 50%

91. **Which urologic malignancy is associated with the Stauffer syndrome?**

A. Prostate
B. Bladder
C. Kidney
D. Penile

92. **What is Stauffer syndrome?**
    A. Multiple bone metastasis in RCC
    B. Concomitant bladder and urethral carcinoma
    C. Reversible hepatitis without hepatic metastasis
    D. Uremic encephalopathy in case of RCC

93. **Following are risk factors for renal carcinoma except:**
    A. Obesity B. Hypertension
    C. Smoking D. Hyperlipidemia

94. **Following occupational exposures are associated with renal cell carcinoma except:**
    A. Aromatic hydrocarbons
    B. Arsenic
    C. Cadmium
    D. Asbestos

95. **Most common chromosomal aberration associated with clear cell carcinoma:**
    A. Chromosome Y B. Chromosome 3
    C. Chromosome 7 D. Chromosome 11

96. **Most common familial cancer syndrome associated with clear cell carcinoma of kidney:**
    A. Lynch syndrome
    B. Cowden syndrome
    C. von Hippel-Lindau syndrome
    D. Tuberous sclerosis

97. **Fuhrman grading is used for:**
    A. Prostatic cancer B. Testicular cancer
    C. Renal cancer D. Bladder cancer

98. **Fuhrman grading is based on:**
    A. Morphological grade B. Anatomical grade
    C. Nuclear grade D. Clinical grade

99. **Renal cancer extending into the vena cava above diaphragm without involvement of regional nodes and distant metastases is staged according to AJCC as:**
    A. T3a N1 M0 B. T3b N0 M0
    C. T3c N0 M0 D. T4 N0 M0

100. **According to AJCC, contiguous extension into ipsilateral adrenal gland is:**
    A. T3a B. T3b
    C. T3c D. T4

101. **According to AJCC, Tumor grossly extends into the renal vein or invading perirenal fat but not beyond gerota fascia considered T stage:**
    A. T2 B. T3a
    C. T3b D. T4

102. **Renal carcinoma of 8 cm confined to kidney with involvement of regional lymph node but no evidence of distant metastasis is staged as:**
    A. Stage I B. Stage II
    C. Stage III D. Stage IV

103. **Which is false about active surveillance in cases of renal tumors?**
    A. Incidentally diagnosed
    B. Mass < 2 cm in size
    C. Intolerance to ablative therapy or surgery
    D. Yearly imaging follow up

104. **Patient incidentally diagnosed with 4 cm upper pole renal carcinoma confined to left kidney without regional lymph node or distant metastasis on imaging studies. What will be preferred management for this patient?**
    A. Active surveillance
    B. Ablative therapy
    C. Partial nephrectomy
    D. Radical nephrectomy

105. **Which is false regarding radical nephrectomy procedure?**
    A. The entire Gerota fascial envelope, containing the perinephric fat as a margin around the tumor, is excised intact
    B. In comparison to partial nephrectomy, radical nephrectomy has a lower rate of complications
    C. The adrenal gland is removed with radical nephrectomy
    D. Ligation of a renal artery must precede vein ligation during dissection of renal pedicle

106. **Thermal ablation techniques in treating renal carcinoma can be used for tumors of size upto:**
    A. 2 cm B. 3 cm
    C. 5 cm D. 7 cm

107. **Patients with poor risk clear cell renal carcinoma are offered targeted therapy:**
    A. Sunitinib B. Temsirolimus
    C. Pazopanib D. Sorafenib

BLADDER CANCER

108. **Which is false about bladder cancer etiology?**
    A. The urothelium has a variable thickness of three to six cell layers

B. Transitional cell carcinoma arises from the basal cell layer
C. The tumor arises most frequently in the eighth decade of life
D. The most common presenting symptom in bladder cancer is frequency

109. Which is the most common symptom of bladder cancer?

A. Frequency B. Dysuria
C. Urgency D. Hematuria

110. Following are risk factors for bladder cancer except:

A. Tobacco smoke B. Asbestos
C. Schistosomiasis D. Arylamines

111. Following lymph node stations are considered as N1 disease in bladder cancer except:

A. Obturator B. Hypogastric
C. Presacral D. Common iliac

112. Noninvasive papillary carcinoma of bladder is considered T stage:

A. Tis B. Ta
C. T1 D. Tx

113. Bladder carcinoma invading deep muscularis propria with common iliac lymph nodes involvement has stage:

A. T2b N2 B. T2b N3
C. T3a N2 D. T3a N3

114. Bladder tumor invading prostatic stroma or seminal vesicles is staged:

A. T3a B. T3b
C. T4a D. T4b

115. Which is incorrect regarding management of NMIBC?

A. Urine cytology is most sensitive for high-grade tumors
B. Cystoscopic examination is must for all cases of suspected bladder cancer
C. Urine tumor markers have high specificity for bladder cancer detection
D. At the time of TURBT, patients should undergo a bimanual examination of the bladder

116. Palpable mass after TURBT suggest tumor stage of:

A. T2b B. T3a
C. T3b D. T4

117. Patient diagnosed with T1 high grade bladder cancer on initial presentation, has undergone TURBT. Specimen shows absence of muscle. What will be the next step of management?

A. Surveillance with cystoscopy
B. Repeat TURBT within 2 to 6 weeks
C. Immediate mitomycin C instillation
D. Radical cystectomy

118. Immediate intravesical chemotherapy post TURBT reduces the tumor recurrence by:

A. 15% B. 25%
C. 35% D. 45%

119. Which agent is most commonly used for immediate intravesical instillation following TURBT?

A. BCG B. Mitomycin C
C. Epirubicin D. Gemcitabine

120. Which agent is contraindicated in perioperative intravesical instillation?

A. BCG B. Mitomycin C
C. Epirubicin D. Gemcitabine

121. Which is false about management of NMIBC?

A. Immediate intravesical chemotherapy refers to intravesical administration of an antineoplastic agent within 24 hours of TURBT
B. Standard immunotherapy for NMIBC consists of serial BCG intravesical instillations for induction and periodic maintenance therapy
C. Maintenance BCG instillations reduce the risk of recurrence and progression
D. Periodic surveillance is mandatory in patients as 10% to 20% of tumors recur

122. What is ideal treatment for BCG refractory NMIBC?

A. Active surveillance
B. Intravesical mitomycin C instillation
C. Systemic chemotherapy
D. Radical cystectomy

123. What is tumor recurrence rate in BCG refractory NMIBC?

A. 10 – 20% B. 30 – 40%
C. 50 – 60% D. 60 – 80%

124. In higher grade NMIBC, ____% of tumor progress to higher stage or muscle invasive tumors.

A. 5 – 10% B. 10 – 15%
C. 15 – 20% D. 20 – 25%

125. **Which muscle invasive bladder cancer has better prognosis?**
A. Squamous cell carcinoma
B. Urothelial cell carcinoma
C. Adenocarcinoma
D. Small cell carcinoma

126. **Neoadjuvant chemotherapy regime for MIBC involves following agents except:**
A. Mitomycin C B. Vinblastine
C. Doxorubicin D. Cisplatin

127. **Which neoadjuvant chemotherapy regime is commonly used in bladder cancer?**
A. BEP B. MVAC
C. CEF D. VIP

PROSTATE CANCER

128. **Most common cancer in men:**
A. Lung B. Prostate
C. Colon D. Lymphoma

129. **Which is false regarding prostate cancer screening?**
A. Screening for prostate cancer is performed with PSA levels and DRE
B. Current recommendations are for screening in men aged more than 60 years
C. Routine screening interval to occur every 2 years
D. Screening should not be performed in men with a life expectancy of less than 10 to 15 years

130. **Routine screening for prostate cancer is recommended in men aged:**
A. Above 40 years B. 40 to 55 years
C. 55 to 69 years D. Above 70 years

131. **Standard prostate biopsy template involves __ core biopsy:**
A. 6 B. 12
C. 18 D. 36

132. **What is rate of patients suffering from bacteremia following TRUS prostate biopsy?**
A. 3% B. 7%
C. 12% D. 18%

133. **Gleason grading system is used in which cancer diagnosis?**
A. Prostate cancer B. Renal cancer
C. Bladder cancer D. Testicular cancer

134. **According to AJCC, prostate cancer diagnosed after needle biopsy performed due elevated PSA is staged as:**
A. T1a B. T1b
C. T1c D. Tx

135. **According to AJCC, prostate tumor involving seminal vesicles is staged as:**
A. T2c B. T3a
C. T3b D. T4

136. **Following are criteria for active surveillance of prostate cancer except:**
A. Clinical stage < T1c
B. Gleason score ≤ 6
C. PSA < 10 ng/mL
D. Low volume on biopsy

137. **Incorrect about the anatomical landmarks for radical prostatectomy:**
A. Pubic symphysis anteriorly
B. Bladder neck cephalad
C. Prostatic membranous junction distally
D. Rectal wall posteriorly

138. **Which is false regarding radiotherapy treatment for prostate cancer?**
A. The typical treatment dose for IMRT-based prostate cancer therapy is 76 to 86 Gy
B. Most commonly used radionuclides for brachytherapy are iodine-125 or palladium-103
C. Low- and intermediate-risk prostate cancers have outcomes after radiotherapy similar to those of radical prostatectomy
D. Brachytherapy is most useful in high risk prostate cancer

TESTICULAR CANCER

139. **Which is incorrect about testicular cancer?**
A. Spermatocytic seminomas present in men less than 20 years of age
B. The most common presenting symptom is a painless testicular mass
C. Scrotal ultrasonography is the diagnostic study of choice
D. Initial treatment of suspected testicular tumor is radical inguinal orchiectomy

140. **All are true statements about testicular cancer except:**
A. Clinical staging for testicular cancer includes imaging and post-orchiectomy serum tumor markers

B. Embryonal carcinoma is notorious for hematogenous spread early to distant sites
C. From the right testis cancer, primary landing zone is to the infrarenal interaortocaval node
D. Retroperitoneal lymph nodes are the primary metastatic site in more than 70% of patients with metastatic testicular cancer

141. Half life of α-fetoprotein is:

A. 24 – 36 hours
B. 3 – 5 days
C. 5 – 7 days
D. 7 – 10 days

142. Early distant hematogenous metastatic spread is seen in which testicular cancer?

A. Spermatocytic seminoma
B. Endodermal sinus tumor
C. Choriocarcinoma
D. Embryonal carcinoma

143. Which is false regarding management of testicular cancer?

A. For seminoma stage IIA and IIB, radiotherapy of the retroperitoneal lymph nodes is standard therapy
B. For seminoma stage IIC or III, platinum-based chemotherapy is standard therapy
C. For NSGCT stage IIA with normal levels of tumor marker, primary RPLND is recommended
D. For NSGCT stage IIB, RPLND followed by three or four cycles of cisplatin-based chemotherapy is standard

144. According to AJCC, which stage is wrongly matched?

A. Tumor involving the tunica vaginalis is pT2
B. Tumor invading epididymis or tunica albuginea without lymphovascular invasion is pT1
C. Pulmonary metastasis is M1b
D. Nonregional nodal metastasis is M1a

145. According to AJCC, testicular tumor extending to spermatic cord is stage as:

A. pT1b
B. pT2
C. pT3
D. pT4

146. Which testicular tumor markers levels correlate with stage S3?

A. LDH >3× normal
B. hCG >10,000 IU/L
C. AFP >10,000 ng/mL
D. None of the above

147. Which testicular tumor markers levels correlate with stage S1?

A. LDH <3 × normal
B. hCG <5,000 IU/L
C. AFP <100 ng/mL
D. None of the above

148. Testicular tumor of 5 cm invading scrotal wall, presence of retroperitoneal lymph nodes metastasis of < 2 cm, no evidence of any other distant metastases with normal tumor markers is staged as:

A. Stage IB
B. Stage IIA
C. Stage IIB
D. Stage IIIA

149. According to AJCC, testicular NSGCT with hCG levels 20000 IU/L is staged as:

A. Stage IIC
B. Stage IIIA
C. Stage IIIB
D. Stage IIIC

150. According to AJCC, tumor limited to the testis and epididymis with lymphovascular invasion without any lymph nodal and distant metastasis and normal tumor markers are staged as:

A. Stage IA
B. Stage IB
C. Stage IS
D. Stage IIA

ANSWERS

1. **Ans: B. The adrenal medulla is directly innervated by postsynaptic sympathetic fibers**
Ref: Chapter No. 74, Page No. 2061-2062
2. **Ans: D. Neural crest cells**
Ref: Chapter No. 74, Page No. 2061
3. **Ans: A. Gerota fascia forms the renal capsule**
Ref: Chapter No. 74, Page No. 2062
4. **Ans: A. Left inferior phrenic vein**
Ref: Chapter No. 74, Page No. 2062
5. **Ans: D. The lower ureteral segments have a medial vascular supply**
Ref: Chapter No. 74, Page No. 2062
6. **Ans: B. Santorini plexus**
Ref: Chapter No. 74, Page No. 2063
7. **Ans: C. Waldeyer fascia**
Ref: Chapter No. 74, Page No. 2063
8. **Ans: D. Glandular urethra**
Ref: Chapter No. 74, Page No. 2063
9. **Ans: B. Corpora cavernosa**
Ref: Chapter No. 74, Page No. 2063
10. **Ans: A. Tranversalis fascia**
Ref: Chapter No. 74, Page No. 2063
11. **Ans: C. 16 Fr**
Ref: Chapter No. 74, Page No. 2064
12. **Ans: B. Require specific patient positioning**
Ref: Chapter No. 74, Page No. 2064
13. **Ans: A. 6 Fr to 7.5 Fr at the tip**
Ref: Chapter No. 74, Page No. 2064
14. **Ans: D. 25 – 28 Fr**
Ref: Chapter No. 74, Page No. 2064
15. **Ans: B. Flexible ureteroscope**
Ref: Chapter No. 74, Page No. 2064
16. **Ans: D. Presence of 10^3 CFU on urine culture is diagnostic of UTI**
Ref: Chapter No. 74, Page No. 2065
17. **Ans: B. 10^3**
Ref: Chapter No. 74, Page No. 2065
18. **Ans: C. E. coli**
Ref: Chapter No. 74, Page No. 2065
19. **Ans: A. Immunocompetent female**
Ref: Chapter No. 74, Page No. 2065
20. **Ans: D. None of the above**
Ref: Chapter No. 74, Page No. 2065
21. **Ans: B. E. coli**
Ref: Chapter No. 74, Page No. 2066
22. **Ans: B. Emphysematous pyelonephritis**
Ref: Chapter No. 74, Page No. 2066
23. **Ans: A. It is an acute infectious process**
Ref: Chapter No. 74, Page No. 2067
24. **Ans: A. Digital rectal examination should be performed**
Ref: Chapter No. 74, Page No. 2067
25. **Ans: B. Chlamydia trachomatis**
Ref: Chapter No. 74, Page No. 2067
26. **Ans: D. It commonly involves the testicles or deep tissues of the penis**
Ref: Chapter No. 74, Page No. 2068
27. **Ans: B. Bladder**
Ref: Chapter No. 74, Page No. 2068
28. **Ans: D. The periaqueductal gray located in the midbrain has stimulatory effect on micturition center**
Ref: Chapter No. 74, Page No. 2068-2069
29. **Ans: B. Abnormal elasticity of the bladder**
Ref: Chapter No. 74, Page No. 2069
30. **Ans: B. Hesitancy**
Ref: Chapter No. 74, Page No. 2069
31. **Ans: B. Urgency**
Ref: Chapter No. 74, Page No. 2069
32. **Ans: C. Interruption of sleep one or more times due to need for urination**
Ref: Chapter No. 74, Page No. 2069
33. **Ans: B. Behavioral therapy**
Ref: Chapter No. 74, Page No. 2069
34. **Ans: A. Pharmacotherapy**
Ref: Chapter No. 74, Page No. 2069
35. **Ans: B. In the neurologically normal patient, surgical management is the first step in treatment**
Ref: Chapter No. 74, Page No. 2070

36. **Ans: B. The degree of bladder outflow obstruction correlates with the severity of LUTS**

Ref: Chapter No. 74, Page No. 2071

37. **Ans: B. Increased PSA**

Ref: Chapter No. 74, Page No. 2071

38. **Ans: D. Reduces by 50%**

Ref: Chapter No. 74, Page No. 2071

39. **Ans: C. Benign prostatic hyperplasia**

Ref: Chapter No. 74, Page No. 2071

40. **Ans: D. Hypernatremia**

Ref: Chapter No. 74, Page No. 2072

41. **Ans: D. The semen analyses should be separated by two month and preceded by 1 week of abstinence**

Ref: Chapter No. 74, Page No. 2073

42. **Ans: D. Idiopathic causes**

Ref: Chapter No. 74, Page No. 2073

43. **Ans: A. The semen analyses should be separated by one month and preceded by 1 week of abstinence**

Ref: Chapter No. 74, Page No. 2073

44. **Ans: D. The goal of therapy is maintenance of testosterone levels between 100 and 400 ng/dL**

Ref: Chapter No. 74, Page No. 2075-2076

45. **Ans: C. Pumping device is placed in medial thigh region**

Ref: Chapter No. 74, Page No. 2075

46. **Ans: C. Reduced body fat**

Ref: Chapter No. 74, Page No. 2075

47. **Ans: D. Decreased cognitive acuity**

Ref: Chapter No. 74, Page No. 2076

48. **Ans: B. 400 to 700 ng/dL**

Ref: Chapter No. 74, Page No. 2076

49. **Ans: A. Calcium oxalate**

Ref: Chapter No. 74, Page No. 2076

50. **Ans: B. Uric acid stones**

Ref: Chapter No. 74, Page No. 2076

51. **Ans: D. Struvite stones**

Ref: Chapter No. 74, Page No. 2076

52. **Ans: D. E. coli**

Ref: Chapter No. 74, Page No. 2076

53. **Ans: D. Indinavir stones are radiopaque**

Ref: Chapter No. 74, Page No. 2076

54. **Ans: D. Non contrast CT abdomen**

Ref: Chapter No. 74, Page No. 2076

55. **Ans: C. Calcium consumption is reduced in case of calcium stones**

Ref: Chapter No. 74, Page No. 2077

56. **Ans: C. Non-radiopaque and proximal ureteric stones can be treated**

Ref: Chapter No. 74, Page No. 2077

57. **Ans: C. 2 cm**

Ref: Chapter No. 74, Page No. 2077

58. **Ans: D. Steinstrasse**

Ref: Chapter No. 74, Page No. 2077

59. **Ans: C. PCNL**

Ref: Chapter No. 74, Page No. 2077

60. **Ans: B. 15%**

Ref: Chapter No. 74, Page No. 2078

61. **Ans: C. In penetrating renal injury, hemodynamically stable patients with gross hematuria should undergo surgical intervention**

Ref: Chapter No. 74, Page No. 2078

62. **Ans: B. Systolic blood pressure > 90 mm Hg**

Ref: Chapter No. 74, Page No. 2078

63. **Ans: C. Grade IV**

Ref: Chapter No. 74, Page No. 2078

64. **Ans: B. Grade II**

Ref: Chapter No. 74, Page No. 2078

65. **Ans: B. Grade II - Subcapsular, nonexpanding hematoma without parenchymal laceration**

Ref: Chapter No. 74, Page No. 2078

66. **Ans: C. Grade IV**

Ref: Chapter No. 74, Page No. 2078

67. **Ans: B. Persistent renal bleeding**

Ref: Chapter No. 74, Page No. 2079

68. **Ans: C. Grade IV**

Ref: Chapter No. 74, Page No. 2079

69. **Ans: D. Those who have received more than four units of blood transfusion**

Ref: Chapter No. 74, Page No. 2080

70. **Ans: D. Exploration with left nephrectomy**

Ref: Chapter No. 74, Page No. 2081

71. **Ans: C. While repair, ureter is skeletonized along the length**

Ref: Chapter No. 74, Page No. 2082

72. **Ans: D. Defects in the bladder wall are closed with absorbable 2-0 sutures in one layer**

Ref: Chapter No. 74, Page No. 2084

73. Ans: B. Non-operative management with catheter drainage

Ref: Chapter No. 74, Page No. 2084

74. Ans: C. Concomitant urethral injury

Ref: Chapter No. 74, Page No. 2084

75. Ans: D. Penetrating anterior urethral injury repair is done in delayed fashion

Ref: Chapter No. 74, Page No. 2084-2085

76. Ans: C. Bulbar

Ref: Chapter No. 74, Page No. 2084

77. Ans: C. Gross hematuria

Ref: Chapter No. 74, Page No. 2085

78. Ans: B. Retrograde urethrogram

Ref: Chapter No. 74, Page No. 2085

79. Ans: B. Membranous urethral rupture

Ref: Chapter No. 74, Page No. 2086

80. Ans: C. Suprapubic cystostomy

Ref: Chapter No. 74, Page No. 2086

81. Ans: B. Blunt testicular injuries should always be explored

Ref: Chapter No. 74, Page No. 2086-2088

82. Ans: B. Hypotension

Ref: Chapter No. 74, Page No. 2088

83. Ans. D. Ligation of the injured distal ureteral limb is recommended

Ref: Chapter No. 74, Page No. 2088

84. Ans: B. 4 hours

Ref: Chapter No. 74, Page No. 2089

85. Ans: C. In patients with suspected testicular torsion, Doppler examination is necessary to check viability

Ref: Chapter No. 74, Page No. 2089

86. Ans: B. Intervention is needed, if priapism persists longer than 8 hours

Ref: Chapter No. 74, Page No. 2090

87. Ans: B. 4 hours

Ref: Chapter No. 74, Page No. 2090

88. Ans: B. Microhematuria

Ref: Chapter No. 74, Page No. 2090

89. Ans: D. The classic triad of renal cell carcinoma is seen in 50% of patients

Ref: Chapter No. 74, Page No. 2090

90. Ans: A. < 5%

Ref: Chapter No. 74, Page No. 2090

91. Ans: C. Kidney

Ref: Chapter No. 74, Page No. 2090

92. Ans: C. Reversible hepatitis without hepatic metastasis

Ref: Chapter No. 74, Page No. 2090

93. Ans: D. Hyperlipidemia

Ref: Chapter No. 74, Page No. 2090

94. Ans: B. Arsenic

Ref: Chapter No. 74, Page No. 2090

95. Ans: B. Chromosome 3

Ref: Chapter No. 74, Page No. 2090

96. Ans: C. von Hippel-Lindau syndrome

Ref: Chapter No. 74, Page No. 2090

97. Ans: C. Renal cancer

Ref: Chapter No. 74, Page No. 2091

98. Ans: C. Nuclear grade

Ref: Chapter No. 74, Page No. 2091

99. Ans: C. T3c N0 M0

Ref: Chapter No. 74, Page No. 2091

100. Ans: D. T4

Ref: Chapter No. 74, Page No. 2091

101. Ans: B. T3a

Ref: Chapter No. 74, Page No. 2091

102. Ans: C. Stage III

Ref: Chapter No. 74, Page No. 2091

103. Ans: D. Yearly imaging follow up

Ref: Chapter No. 74, Page No. 2091

104. Ans: C. Partial nephrectomy

Ref: Chapter No. 74, Page No. 2091

105. Ans: C. The adrenal gland is removed with radical nephrectomy

Ref: Chapter No. 74, Page No. 2091

106. Ans: B. 3 cm

Ref: Chapter No. 74, Page No. 2092

107. Ans: B. Temsirolimus

Ref: Chapter No. 74, Page No. 2092

108. Ans: D. The most common presenting symptom in bladder cancer is frequency

Ref: Chapter No. 74, Page No. 2092

109. Ans: D. Hematuria

Ref: Chapter No. 74, Page No. 2092

110. Ans: B. Asbestos

Ref: Chapter No. 74, Page No. 2092

111. Ans: D. Common iliac

Ref: Chapter No. 74, Page No. 2092

112. Ans: B. Ta

Ref: Chapter No. 74, Page No. 2092

113. Ans: B. T2b N3

Ref: Chapter No. 74, Page No. 2092

114. Ans: C. T4a

Ref: Chapter No. 74, Page No. 2092

115. Ans: C. Urine tumor markers have high specificity for bladder cancer detection

Ref: Chapter No. 74, Page No. 2093

116. Ans: C. T3b

Ref: Chapter No. 74, Page No. 2093

117. Ans: B. Repeat TURBT within 2 to 6 weeks

Ref: Chapter No. 74, Page No. 2093

118. Ans: C. 35%

Ref: Chapter No. 74, Page No. 2093

119. Ans: B. Mitomycin C

Ref: Chapter No. 74, Page No. 2093

120. Ans: A. BCG

Ref: Chapter No. 74, Page No. 2093

121. Ans: D. Periodic surveillance is mandatory in patients as 10% to 20% of tumors recur

Ref: Chapter No. 74, Page No. 2093

122. Ans: D. Radical cystectomy

Ref: Chapter No. 74, Page No. 2093

123. Ans: D. 60 – 80%

Ref: Chapter No. 74, Page No. 2093

124. Ans: B. 10 – 15%

Ref: Chapter No. 74, Page No. 2093

125. Ans: B. Urothelial cell carcinoma

Ref: Chapter No. 74, Page No. 2093

126. Ans: A. Mitomycin C

Ref: Chapter No. 74, Page No. 2093

127. Ans: B. MVAC

Ref: Chapter No. 74, Page No. 2093

128. Ans: B. Prostate

Ref: Chapter No. 74, Page No. 2094

129. Ans: B. Current recommendations are for screening in men aged more than 60 years

Ref: Chapter No. 74, Page No. 2094

130. Ans: C. 55 to 69 years

Ref: Chapter No. 74, Page No. 2094

131. Ans: B. 12

Ref: Chapter No. 74, Page No. 2094

132. Ans: A. 3%

Ref: Chapter No. 74, Page No. 2094

133. Ans: A. Prostate cancer

Ref: Chapter No. 74, Page No. 2094

134. Ans: C. T1c

Ref: Chapter No. 74, Page No. 2094

135. Ans: C. T3b

Ref: Chapter No. 74, Page No. 2094

136. Ans: A. Clinical stage < T1c

Ref: Chapter No. 74, Page No. 2094

137. Ans: A. Pubic symphysis anteriorly

Ref: Chapter No. 74, Page No. 2095

138. Ans: D. Brachytherapy is most useful in high risk prostate cancer

Ref: Chapter No. 74, Page No. 2095

139. Ans: A. Spermatocytic seminomas present in men less than 20 years of age

Ref: Chapter No. 74, Page No. 2095

140. Ans: B. Embryonal carcinoma is notorious for hematogenous spread early to distant sites

Ref: Chapter No. 74, Page No. 2095

141. Ans: C. 5 – 7 days

Ref: Chapter No. 74, Page No. 2095

142. Ans: C. Choriocarcinoma

Ref: Chapter No. 74, Page No. 2095

143. Ans: D. For NSGCT stage IIB, RPLND followed by three or four cycles of cisplatin-based chemotherapy is standard

Ref: Chapter No. 74, Page No. 2096

144. Ans: C. Pulmonary metastasis is M1b

Ref: Chapter No. 74, Page No. 2097

145. Ans: C. pT3

Ref: Chapter No. 74, Page No. 2097

146. Ans: C. AFP >10,000 ng/mL

Ref: Chapter No. 74, Page No. 2097

147. Ans: B. hCG <5,000 IU/L

Ref: Chapter No. 74, Page No. 2097

148. Ans: B. Stage IIA

Ref: Chapter No. 74, Page No. 2097

149. Ans: C. Stage IIIB

Ref: Chapter No. 74, Page No. 2097

150. Ans: B. Stage IB

Ref: Chapter No. 74, Page No. 2097